The Principles and Practice of
Surgery for Nurses
and Allied Professions

The Principles and Practice of
Surgery for Nurses
and Allied Professions
Sixth edition

D. F. Ellison Nash F.R.C.S.

Senior Surgeon, St. Bartholomew's Hospital (London), Sydenham Children's
Hospital; Surgeon, Chailey Heritage Hospital; Lecturer in Surgery and
formerly Dean, St. Bartholomew's Hospital Medical College, University of
London; past Chairman Court of Examiners, Hunterian Professor, Arris and
Gale Lecturer, Royal College of Surgeons; Examiner in Surgery, Diploma in
Nursing, University of London.

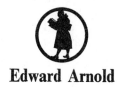

Edward Arnold

© **D. F. Ellison Nash 1976**

First published 1955
by Edward Arnold (Publishers) Ltd.
25 Hill Street, London W1X 8LL

Reprinted 1956, 1957, 1959, 1960
Second edition 1961
Reprinted 1963
Third edition 1965
Reprinted 1967
Fourth edition 1969
Reprinted 1972
Fifth edition 1973
Sixth edition 1976

ISBN: 0 7131 4273 1

Printed in Great Britain by William Clowes & Sons Ltd.
London, Beccles and Colchester

Preface to Sixth Edition

This sixth edition comes at a time when the development of health services in the United Kingdom has been checked by lack of financial provision. The universal introduction of well equipped intensive care units and of ward accommodation which would allow the development of 'progressive nursing care', is unlikely to become a reality during the lifetime of this edition. Although the Report of the Committee of Nursing (Briggs) foreshadowed a two-tier nursing education, economic restraints are certain to frustrate this development. However, the advancement of surgical skill and potential continues and the responsibility of the nurse in the surgical team is heavier than it ever has been. There have been few fundamental changes in surgical management. The chemotherapy of malignant disease has altered the pattern of cancer surgery to the extent of limiting operative treatment, but at the same time involving repeated patient re-admissions for treatment with cytotoxic drugs. Radiotherapy departments are now linked with problems of oncology and in this field of patient management the nurse plays an absolutely vital role. Infection and deep venous thrombosis remain as the two constant hazards of surgery.

One specialist field in which there has been a radical change is that of ophthalmology. The conservative post-operative bed rest regime has been replaced by early ambulation and the introduction of photocoagulation for retinal disease has greatly increased the scope of the specialty. Improved radiological techniques (especially neuro-radiology) and the further development of fibre-optic endoscopy for the alimentary tract have increased the extent of investigation of a patient's condition without his admission to hospital. This in turn has speeded up the turnover in a surgical ward and increased still further the pressure on the nursing staff.

The recent introduction of the Système International d'Unités (SI units) for recording pathological data is a source of bewilderment for those already established in health care professions, and only the essential changes have been made in the text. Hospital staffs are provided with conversion tables. SI units (kilo pascals) for blood pressure and blood gases are not used universally. The calorie value is retained as an energy unit in discussion on nutrition, though the joule may come to be used in due course.

v

ACKNOWLEDGEMENTS

I am grateful to my nursing and medical colleagues for continued assistance in up-dating this book and in particular to Miss Jean Bailey, Miss Elizabeth Capper, Mrs Pamela Curtis, Dr Richard Ellis and Mr John Mercer, and the Department of Medical Illustration, St Bartholomew's Hospital. Acknowledgement is made in the text to those who have assisted in the provision of illustrations. Miss Joy Lee, my personal secretary, continues to shoulder the burden of this revision and the final preparation of the text.

Contents

SECTION VI

SECTION VII

SECTION VIII

SECTION IX

Tables

Introduction

With the sixth edition this publication comes of age. Though the scope of surgery has continued to expand the basic requirements of the surgical patient remain very much the same. An advanced knowledge of surgery is not necessary for nursing but a clear understanding of the scientific basis is essential. In the first edition an attempt was made to explain in each section the fundamental principles involved, and that objective has been retained.

An endeavour has been made to provide in each section sufficient information not only to cover examination requirements, but also to enable the trained nurse to refresh her memory, or with reasonable confidence to face new problems in which she has had little or no experience. The author has been gratified to find over the years that this book has become a reference volume in many surgical wards, and as such it is clear that it must contain advanced and detailed information for those already trained. There has been a great increase in the number of nurses taking post-registration and post-enrolment courses in all specialties. Although many nursing procedures which formed an essential part of the training syllabus 20 years ago have now become obsolete and the role of the nurse has somewhat changed, the correct nursing management is in many cases the key to successful surgery. No textbook can be a substitute for bedside teaching and it is not possible to lay down more than an average routine in nursing treatment and to point out possible errors to be avoided. Personal wishes of individual surgeons vary considerably and extreme views may be adopted over what may appear to the nurse to be a triviality, but individual prejudices are usually based on some unfortunate experience with a particular drug or method. The nurse is a member of her team and her value in that team will depend not only on her ability to work, but also on her power of observation, her curiosity and her intelligence. Surgery is essentially a practical subject. Things happen quickly. Sometimes conditions alter suddenly and the unusual and unexpected have always to be watched for. It is exacting and at the same time both gratifying and frustrating. There are brilliant successes and bitter disappointments in which every member of the team shares.

Provided the nurse understands the basic principles of her method and takes care always to find out *why* a particular practice or routine procedure is adopted, she will not be criticised. The blind following of rules is apt to lead to trouble and it is always wiser to ask than to make mistakes. Intuition may save a situation occasionally, but intuition is extremely dangerous as a basis for nursing in the modern surgical team.

SECTION I

1

Hospital Organisation

The nursing of surgical patients is essentially a practical and very personal affair both for the patient and for the nurse whose individual responsibility is not always clearly defined. The management of any patient's progress through a period in hospital is sometimes more of a pilgrimage by the time various hurdles of consultation, admission, treatment, convalescence and rehabilitation have been negotiated. Only the patient can appreciate fully the significance of any one stage in this journey on which so many personal contacts are made.

Method of introduction of the patient

In British medical practice the general practitioner—family doctor—has the primary care of patients and, except in cases of accident and emergency occurring away from home, access to the hospital services is through the family doctor. He makes arrangements for the attendance at the appropriate consultant out-patient clinic at a hospital of his choice. Alternatively the patient may elect to visit a particular consultant privately in the first instance. If the case is a more urgent one, the doctor may call in a consultant to visit the patient's home. Again this may be a consultant of the patient's or the doctor's choice and the visit may be arranged at the patient's expense, or, in Britain, as part of the National Health Service Domiciliary Visit Scheme. If, on the other hand, the family doctor wishes for immediate admission to hospital, this will probably be arranged either direct with the medical staff on duty at a particular hospital or through the Emergency Bed Service for the area. The EBS is an organisation for 'pooling' vacant beds in the various hospitals in a particular zone and its purpose is to avoid unnecessary delay in obtaining emergency admission.

Whatever approach is made, all these patients who are referred for hospital treatment arrive with a tentative diagnosis and a letter from the family doctor. They are therefore directed to the appropriate department without any further 'sorting'.

There are, however, a large number of patients who attend at hospital without being referred there by their family doctor. Such attendances frequently give rise to difficulty when the patient is dissatisfied with medical advice which has been given elsewhere.

Other patients are brought into the hospital casualty department as the result of accident or illness at work, at school or in the street.

Hospital out-patient organisation

Much depends on the size of the hospital and its particular function in relation to its locality. Specialist hospitals have simple out-patient consultation clinics without a casualty department of any type. In a large general hospital in a busy industrial district where a considerable number of patients arrive without appointment, the out-patient organisation has to be arranged in such a way that there is an initial sorting into medical and surgical cases and a further direction of certain patients to special departments.

Many hospitals follow a general pattern in which there is a casualty department supervised during the daytime by a junior member of the medical staff, sometimes a senior house-officer, sometimes a registrar. Hospitals with a fully developed accident and emergency department have a consultant in charge. A very large proportion of 'emergencies' coming to such departments are medical—e.g. heart attacks, drug overdose, strokes, asthma, and acute chest infections.

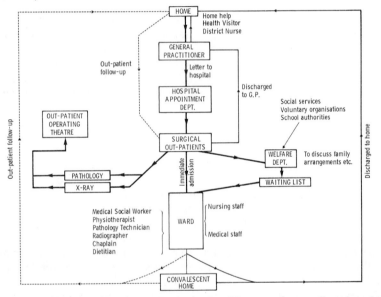

Fig. 1.1 The patient's progress in the hospital organisation. Illustrates the complicated machinery which is set in action by the initial request from the General Practitioner. It will be seen that the patient has contact with many individuals in the various sections of the Hospital Service.

Regular consultant clinics are attended by the senior medical staff who see, by appointment, patients referred with doctors' letters, others referred from the casualty department, and some who have returned for follow-up observation or treatment after a previous admission to hospital.

Owing to the large size of such out-patient clinics, the surgeon or physician is assisted by more junior staff. The larger the hospital, the less likely is the patient to see the same doctor on all subsequent attendances.

Alongside this diagnostic section are the facilities of the x-ray department, the pathology department and the medical social worker. A large number of operations are performed in surgical out-patient clinics under local or general anaesthesia, and there may be a recovery or observation 'day' ward where a patient is permitted to stay before being discharged home or formally 'admitted' to the hospital, as an in-patient. Modern 'short acting' anaesthetic drugs have made it safe to allow patients to go home soon after general anaesthesia.

Accompanying the patient at every move on his course through various departments is his clinical note recording the consultant's opinion and the results of various investigations. It will be readily understood that no matter how small the hospital is, the administrative work connected with the smooth running of an out-patient department is of vital importance and frequently falls upon the shoulders of the nurse. The impression which a patient receives at her first attendance at a hospital out-patient department is a lasting one. A nurse must remember that all patients are apprehensive at this stage; for many it is like embarking on a long journey with an unknown destination. It is remarkably easy for nurses and doctors who are used to the atmosphere of hospital to become indifferent to the patients' ignorance of hospital procedure, but it is at this very 'front door' of the hospital that a nurse should learn the importance of personal attention being given to every patient. An individual's attitude to investigations, treatment and all the subsequent horrors of hospital is often determined by the way in which she is received and cared for on this first day.

Welfare department

Patients whose names are placed on the waiting list are usually interviewed in an admissions office and, if necessary, referred to a trained medical social worker. Advice may be needed to help the patient, particularly the mothers of young children, in connection with the forthcoming admission to hospital. Ambulance and hospital car services and other travelling arrangements usually come under the control of this department. Admission to convalescent homes and arrangements for continued nursing at home are further duties of the department, integrated with the Social Welfare organisation of the local city or county authority, by whom the trained social workers are employed.

Surgical in-patient organisation

The accepted system in large hospitals is that the surgical staff is organised into teams. This 'unit' system has been progressively developed in the British Isles as the hospital service expanded and the field of surgery widened. Each unit consists of one or two consultants and a first assistant of registrar or senior registrar status. This assistant is able to deputise for the consultants who may be working in more than one hospital. The junior staff consists of one or perhaps two house surgeons, and each unit has its own out-patient clinic, follow-up clinic and frequently a particular social worker and physiotherapist.

The consultants in charge of the unit may have a special interest, for instance in surgery of the stomach or of blood vessels; it is therefore common to find that the individual units have a bias towards cases of one particular kind. From the point of view of the nurse's training this is an unsatisfactory tendency, although the standard of nursing in each special field undoubtedly improves. The sister in charge has had an opportunity to develop special techniques. In most large hospitals each general surgical unit is on 'emergency take-in' in rotation and therefore deals with most forms of emergency surgery.

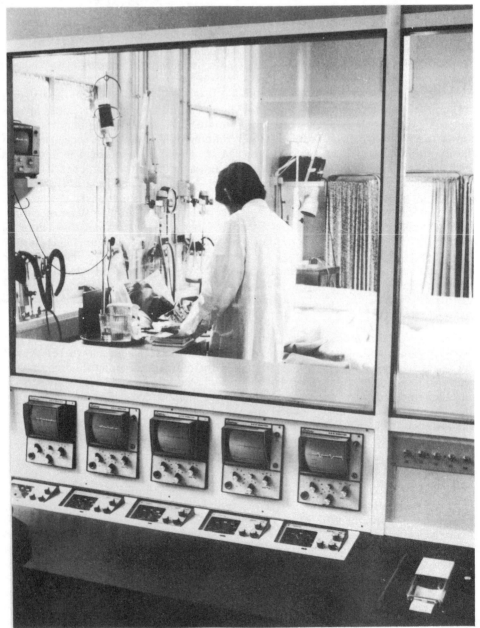

Fig. 1.2 Duty nurse station showing ECG Recorder for each bed. An intensive care unit provides constant electronic monitoring of vital functions, on-the-spot facilities for resuscitation, artificial respiration, infusion, specially trained nursing staff in constant attendance: physiotherapy plays a vital role here. Electrolyte balance is maintained from repeated blood gas analysis: peritoneal renal dialysis may be required. (Cambridge Scientific Instruments Ltd.)

'General' surgery is less inclusive than it was. For instance in a large centre a special gastro-intestinal department may have a combined medical and surgical function. Nephrology and urological patients come together in combined renal units.

Alongside these developments is the evolution of '**progressive nursing care**', in which patients are grouped according to the degree of their disability rather than by the nature of their disorder. 'Minimal care wards' provide hostel-type self-service accommodation for patients undergoing investigations, having radiotherapy, or in a post-operative pre-convalescent stage.

At the other end of the scale is the intensive care unit (ICU) with a small number of beds with medical and surgical patients from any department. There may be patients in the immediate post-operative phase requiring artificial respiration, or dialysis for instance, or a coronary thrombosis patient who requires ventilation (Fig. 1.2). In addition a recovery unit takes all other post-operative patients until consciousness returns. The main wards provide intermediate care. Restructuring hospital organisation in this way changes entirely the nurse training programme. This provision has been made even more necessary in hospitals where there is a great shortage of trained nursing staff. It does, however, take away a great deal of the interest and satisfaction that is derived by a ward nursing team involved in the complete care of the patient during his hospital stay.

Day surgery

Many surgical procedures can be undertaken without the need for a patient to stay overnight. The organisation of 'day surgery' requires certain special provisions.

1. A ward designed and equipped for this specific purpose.
2. A well ordered booking and admission procedure, with blood tests and investigations completed before the patient is called in.
3. Patients must not have to come from so far away as to arrive exhausted from travelling.
4. Operations performed under general anaesthetic must be short and be finished in time to allow *full* recovery before ward closing time, unless an ambulance service is available to take patients home.
5. Facilities for admitting the occasional case unfit to go home.
6. Adequate information service to ensure that the patient's home doctor who might be called out, is fully informed as to what has been done.
7. Clear-cut instructions to patients on discharge, with a supply of analgesics (if needed), urinary antiseptics (after cystoscopy), or other medicines.

Routine endoscopic examinations, special x-ray investigations, minor gynaecological operations, removal of small tumours and biopsy, orthopaedic manipulations and many minor plastic operations can be done under these conditions.

This is a good alternative to admitting day patients as 'lodgers' in general wards, and enables the surgeon to have the use of full operating theatre facilities rarely found in association with out-patient clinics where much of this surgery was done hitherto. There is no lessening of the pre-operative routine care or post-operative vigilance.

In many old hospitals accommodation was arranged so that each unit had its own male and female wards with theatre suite adjoining. However, with the growing complexity of surgery and the need to provide a very wide range of expensive instruments and apparatus to be available in every theatre, modern hospitals are more often built with all their theatres grouped together as one big service. As this theatre suite may be some distance from the wards from which the patients would come, there is either a recovery ward or 'intensive care unit' or both. Where there is adequate space the patient is transferred to the recovery ward on the day before operation so that the immediate pre-operative care is carried out by a specially trained staff who meet the patient at this critical point. After operation, fully trained and experienced nursing is immediately available and such resuscitation and transfusion equipment as may be needed is constantly at hand. This system leads to more efficient after-care for the hours while the patient is still unconscious.

During recent years with the introduction of new methods and new drugs, the rate at which patients recover after operation has been greatly increased. Few patients remain in hospital for more than three weeks unless there has been some complication. Many leave within a week after such operations as those for hernia or appendicitis. There is thus a considerable increase in the number of patients passing through a hospital ward each week.

Table 1   The Surgical Division

GENERAL SURGERY
  Sub-specialties or special clinics
                          Gastro-intestinal
                          Rectal and Colonic
                          Urological
                          Vascular
                          Thyroid or Endocrine
                          Children's
                          Traumatic
        (The accident unit may be under separate control or under the Orthopaedic Department)
  * NEUROSURGERY
  * THORACIC SURGERY
    ORTHOPAEDIC SURGERY
  * PLASTIC SURGERY with BURNS UNIT unless this is a separate Accident Unit
    EAR, NOSE and THROAT SURGERY
    OPHTHALMIC SURGERY
    (GYNAECOLOGY and OBSTETRICS is usually organised as an independent major division)
  * RADIOTHERAPY; closely associated with all other departments

---

   * One Regional Centre may serve several hospital areas.

Ancillary services

In addition to the performance of her nursing duties, the ward nurse has to learn to become one of a team, adaptable, patient and able to work smoothly with the many technical assistants who enter the ward from time to time to deal with various aspects of a patient's illness. Every one of these medical auxiliaries (Fig. 1.1) has a personal task to perform and it is the nurse's duty to help rather than regard their visits as an inconvenience. Frequently we find our patients have been unable to obtain assistance or advice in a particular direction simply through lack of knowledge on the part of those dealing with their discharge from hospital.

On discharge from hospital

Many patients have their treatment completed before discharge, require no follow-up, and are fit to resume their full work within a week of leaving hospital. There are few deaths. On the other hand there are patients of all ages in whom the surgical treatment has been merely the door to recovery and who require prolonged convalescence. For these, arrangements need to be made for their supervision at home under the care of their family doctor, or for their transfer to a convalescent home. After prolonged illness very few patients are able to enjoy this enforced convalescence at their own expense. Special country and seaside homes are provided either under the control of the Hospital Authority or under some voluntary charitable organisation. On return home either directly from the ward or after a stay in a convalescent unit, a patient may still require nursing help at home, or a young invalid mother may require help with the children. In many areas of Great Britain there are special rehabilitation centres to which convalescent patients are sent in order that they may receive active treatment by physiotherapy, occupational therapy and remedial exercises and, in some cases, psychological treatment. This is particularly desirous after severe or prolonged illness in order to speed a man's recovery and fitness to resume his normal occupation. Sometimes, as for instance when a man has had a leg amputated, it is necessary for him to be trained for a different occupation and he may then be sent to a special training centre run by the Department of Health and Social Security.

The ward sister, with the help of the medical social worker, is responsible for seeing that all these arrangements are made and fully understood by the patient before his discharge. Mention has already been made of the impact on a patient of the impressions gained during the first visit to hospital in the out-patient department. It is equally important that when the time comes for the patient to leave hospital he has a very clear idea of what he is permitted to undertake in the way of activity, that he has an adequate supply of dressings and medicines if these are required, and that he has been given instructions about diet. Those who have had hypnotics regularly in hospital find they cannot sleep and, as this is a common experience, such patients need reassurance that the normal sleep pattern may take some weeks to return. Many patients quite unnecessarily believe that they should continue on a restricted diet when they leave hospital simply because no one has discussed the matter with them.

Follow-up departments

Both for the purposes of research, and in order that any recurrence may receive early treatment, all cases of cancer when they leave hospital are brought within an organised scheme which will ensure either their return attendance in the out-patient clinic or the receipt of a report on progress from the family doctor. Such a follow-up arrangement is sometimes criticised on the ground that the patient is repeatedly reminded of the risk of recurrence. On the other hand, most patients who have undergone an operation for this condition are aware of the nature and hazards and are only too willing to return in order to be reassured.

In some hospitals this department also arranges for the follow-up of certain other types of case, for instance, peptic ulcer and thyrotoxicosis, after operation.

Special departments

In large hospital centres, separate units with their own wards and operating suites have been developed for the treatment of particular classes of disease. Table 1 lists such special departments. It will be seen that some branches, instead of being represented in each hospital, are developed as 'regional centres'. This segregation applies particularly to neurosurgery, thoracic surgery and plastic surgery because the organisation of small units scattered in different localities is wasteful both in relation to medical staff and special nursing.

The nurse in the organisation

Most surgical wards admitting acute cases have two trained nurses—the sister and the staff nurse. The other members of the nursing team are in training, and in order to cover the syllabus and obtain all-round experience it is necessary for each nurse to move from unit to unit every few months. It may be necessary for her to spend several months in special hospitals associated with the parent unit. Gradually the student nurse is losing her role as an active participating member of the nursing team with increasing responsibility. Her learning programme is more organised, and she is less involved with the patient and his illness. The classroom instruction over an increasing field of knowledge inevitably leads to less intimate personal 'in service' experience. A nurse may become confused by being taught different methods for carrying out one procedure: a good nurse will learn from personal observation the good points and bad points in each method, for there are very few completely standard procedures in nursing. In the chapters that follow no attempt has been made to enumerate all the methods of carrying out routine procedures, but stress has been laid on the vital points which have to be observed in any one method. Like most medical students, during her training a nurse will almost certainly develop personal likes and dislikes for particular types of work. When her training is complete and examinations are over, she will have an opportunity for further specialisation.

2

The Basic Principles of Treatment

TYPES OF SURGICAL DISORDER AND DISEASE

Almost every disease or disorder falls into one of six great categories, according to the principal cause.

1. Congenital	4. Neoplastic
2. Infective	5. Metabolic
3. Traumatic	6. Degenerative

1. Congenital disorders. This group includes all those diseases which have their origin in the period before birth. Some of these conditions are hereditary, passed on in the 'genes' of the parent, but others result either from infection or damage to the embryo during its development. It is therefore possible to have a disease which is both congenital and infective;

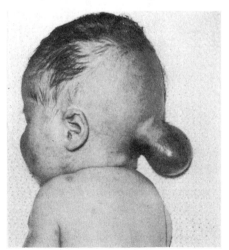 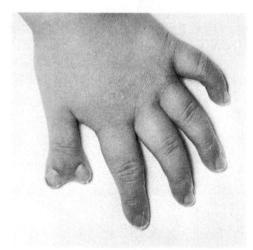

Congenital Disorders
Fig. 2.1 (*left*) Occipital meningocele. This was removed and the child is otherwise normal.
Fig. 2.2 Double thumb; this type of deformity is often familial: surgery is not urgent.

for instance, congenital syphilis. Included under the heading of congenital disorders are all the inborn deformities, such as webbed fingers, club foot and Meckel's intestinal diverticulum. Most inguinal hernias are congenital in origin, although they may not come to light for many years after birth. We know very little about the origin of many congenital lesions, and one of the most difficult things is to comfort the parents of a child who has been born with a serious defect through no fault of theirs.

2. Infective disorders. In this group come the majority of ills that affect the human body at all ages. Although in the healthy individual resistance of the tissues to infection is very great, there are certain periods of life when individuals are more susceptible to attacks of micro-organisms. Fatigue from over-work, exposure to cold, malnutrition and anaemia all lower a patient's resistance to infection. All these things are therefore factors in the production of infective disease, and much of our surgical nursing is directed to removing or lessening such factors. Many surgical conditions are not infective, but bad nursing may allow the complication of infection to arise. Infection is more likely to attack the very young and the very old; healthy age groups between ten and sixty are less liable to such conditions, but there are certain specific infective diseases, such as mumps and glandular fever, which attack young adults, but which are rare in the elderly. The presence or the risk

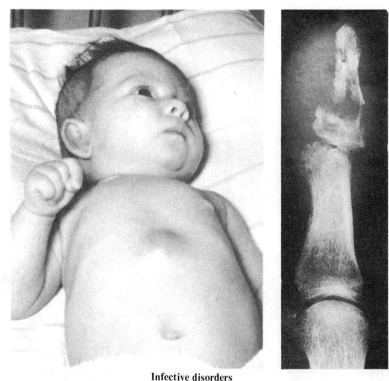

Infective disorders

Fig. 2.3 (*left*) Infection. Abscess in abdominal wall arising in the closed fetal vein between umbilicus and liver, from neonatal umbilical sepsis.

Fig. 2.4 (*right*) Radiograph showing necrosis of phalanx resulting from a pulp whitlow.

of infection plays a big part in determining the surgeon's decision to operate on any particular condition. Since the discovery of the sulphonamide drugs and antibiotics, much of
the terror has departed from the infective complications of surgery. The nurse to-day
rarely sees a case of spreading streptococcal cellulitis or a septic finger which needs to be
amputated. Nursing technique in relation to infective conditions is therefore very greatly
simplified. Nevertheless, the nurse plays a vital part in the recovery of the patient suffering
from infection, since these chemicals and antibiotics merely kill the attacking army of
germs, but do not repair the damage which has been done, neither do they build up the
patient's resistance against succeeding attacks.

   3. Traumatic disorders. Persons of all ages may be injured, but the more active decades
from the age of ten to the age of forty bring the majority of cases of injury. The great bulk of
traumatic surgery is therefore performed on patients who, before the injury, were fit and
active. Similar injuries inflicted on elderly people produce much greater problems of
nursing. Here, again, the technique of nursing the injured has been very greatly simplified

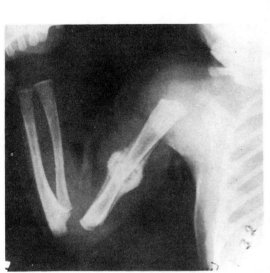 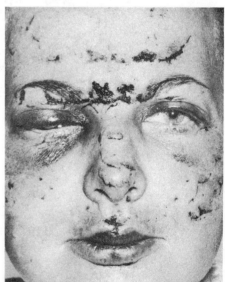

Traumatic disorders

Fig. 2.5   Fracture of humerus due to birth injury. Note the formation of callus. The baby was 2 weeks old
at this stage.
   Fig. 2.6   Typical motor accident. Windscreen glass lacerations: injury to eye: fractured nose.

by the reduction of infection. Rarely now does a nurse see a compound fracture pouring
pus for weeks on end. On the other hand, she has to be prepared for the patient to receive
immediate skin grafts within a few hours of an injury. All injuries produce a certain degree
of shock, and preventive nursing plays a large part both in the stage of first aid and in the
active surgical treatment of injury.

   Poisoning by drugs and other chemicals comes into this category of injury.

   4. Neoplastic disorders. A large proportion of surgery concerns the removal of growths;
some are harmless, but many are malignant (Chapter 23). Many such cases are complicated.

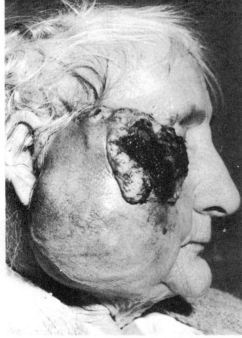

Fig. 2.7 Malignant growth of the parotid, ulcerating through the cheek.

Neoplastic disorders

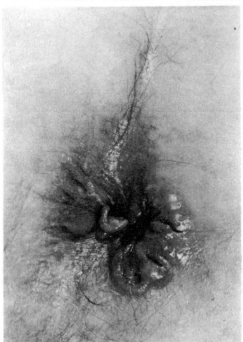

Fig. 2.8 Rodent ulcer of the anus. Note the rolled edges which are typical of malignant ulcers. This is an unusual site for this type of growth. A nurse may recognise this abnormality when washing a patient or giving an enema—the patient may have been unaware of its presence.

The patient may complain of a tumour in the breast or an ulcer on the tongue. The surgeon determines the diagnosis, and operation follows for the removal of the growth. On the other hand, the presenting symptoms may be intestinal obstruction or bleeding, and the primary concern will be to save his life, though the cause of the obstruction or bleeding may not yet be established. Such complications of the primary disease usually present the greatest nursing problems and during the phase of initial (and perhaps urgent) treatment the patient is often, in fact, being prepared for a later major operation to remove the initial cause of the trouble. The surgery of malignant disease frequently becomes a prolonged affair, and the nursing of these patients calls for the greatest degree of tact and cheerfulness and a high standard of skill. Malignant disease affects all ages, though it is most common over the age of forty. The younger the patient the more vicious is the malignancy, and very old patients may have a growth for years with very little disturbance or distress. The surgery for malignant disease in the elderly is, therefore, sometimes less radical and more hopeful than it is in the young individual. Many cases of malignant disease are treated by radiotherapy or chemotherapy with or without surgery, and this adds further to the problems of nursing (Chapter 23). Treatment with cytotoxic drugs (page 434) may continue for several years.

5. Metabolic disorders. Here we have a large group of diseases in which some particular physiological function of the body has gone wrong. Diabetes mellitus is perhaps the best example, but simple obesity is a metabolic disorder and carries with it particular

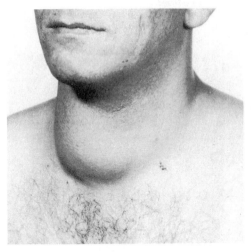

Metabolic disorders

Fig. 2.9 Non-toxic goitre.

complications. Thyrotoxicosis is another metabolic disorder which comes to the surgeon's notice. When a patient's metabolism is disturbed the whole person is affected, not just one particular organ; the problems of diet and nutrition are, of course, particularly important. There are metabolic aspects of diseases of other groups, such as those due to infection. High fever increases tissue activity, and therefore increases the patient's need for nutrition. A metabolic disease such as diabetes mellitus lowers the patient's resistance to infection; if a surgical operation is planned on a diabetic patient, special arrangements have to be made to control the patient's sugar metabolism and every care taken to prevent infection which would be particularly dangerous in such a person.

With rapid advances in biochemistry, more and more hitherto obscure disorders are found to be due to disturbance of endocrine glands or of enzyme production. The clinical investigation of many of these patients takes place in the medical wards and the surgeon is not called in until operation on a gland or tumour is required (page 767).

6. Degenerative disorders. As age advances, or as an infective process affects different parts of the body, the tissues undergo the process of degeneration; this is really 'wear and tear'. Some diseases and disorders occur purely as the result of this degeneration of tissue.

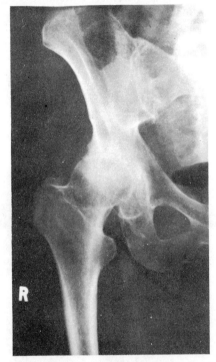

Degenerative disorders

Fig. 2.10 Severe osteoarthritis of the hip joint showing loss of point space and partial destruction of the head.

Arteriosclerosis is one such condition, and complications which arise from the deterioration in the walls of the arteries include such disasters as coronary (artery) thrombosis or the thrombosis of vessels in the brain. The surgery of peripheral vascular disease is devoted largely to the treatment of the circulation in limbs whose arteries have undergone these degenerative processes. Much orthopaedic surgery is concerned with the 'old age' degenerative change in joints, particularly in the hip.

The rate at which different people 'age' is very variable, but modern medicine and surgery, by saving the lives of so many middle-aged people, has created a great problem of a large 'aged' population. This in turn brings new problems of surgery, particularly of the blood vessels.

In any particular nursing problem one should therefore consider whether a disease affecting the patient falls clearly into one of these big groups and then whether, because of the age or type of patient, he may be liable to complications of a particular type. For instance, an elderly man undergoing an operation for appendicectomy is much more liable to cerebral or coronary thrombosis as a complication than would be a younger man undergoing a bigger operation. Though much nursing can be done by rule of thumb, an intelligent consideration of these many factors which cause disease will make a nurse more adaptable in her method and more helpful in the prevention of complications in surgery.

Any particular disease may attack different individuals in various ways. A chronic 'smouldering' condition may suddenly flare up into a grave emergency. The treatment, for instance, of a chronic gastric ulcer presenting as an acute condition (bleeding or perforation) is quite different from the planned treatment of the uncomplicated ulcer. The nurse who has to deal with surgical emergencies needs to act quickly, deliberately and frequently with great resourcefulness. The patient is usually ill-prepared for his disaster, is frequently in a state of shock and has had no time to acclimatise himself to the surroundings of the surgical ward. On the other hand, the planned or 'cold' operation calls for meticulous care in the preparation of the patient and everything possible has to be done to minimise the risk.

In some hospitals it has been possible to segregate all the acute emergency work and further to divide this into acute abdominal emergency work and the surgery of injury. In the majority of hospitals, however, the general surgical ward has to be prepared to deal with all types of surgical illness, whether as an emergency or as part of the planned week's work. Surgical emergencies can arise in patients who are already in hospital for some other condition. A nurse must therefore, very early in her career, become familiar with the treatment and prevention of shock (Chapter 8).

If she once masters both the theoretical and practical principles involved in these aspects of surgery, she will have progressed a long way to becoming an efficient surgical nurse; she will be able to deal well with cases with which she has had no previous experience. The nurse who knows what to do with particular cases, or thinks she does, but has no appreciation of the basic principles of surgical nursing, is a danger to herself, her colleagues and her patients. There is no room for bluff in surgery, nor is there ever an end to learning.

The patient's individuality

With her intimate and daily contact with the patient, the nurse has the privilege of gaining the patient's confidence and gleaning information concerning the social, economic and clinical background of the patient's condition in a way which is not open to a doctor. The nurse should never pry into the patient's affairs but should be ready to pass on to her superior, and to the doctor, any facts which may emerge and which might be relevant.

Patients vary so much both in their anticipation and physical reaction to operation, that after-care is an individual matter and cannot always follow an absolute routine. The management of diet and use of sedatives depends on both the physical stresses and strains imposed by the disease, and to a great extent on the personality of the patient. After an operation on the stomach it may be the surgeon's wish that the nasogastric tube should remain in position with regular aspirations of the stomach contents for several days. Many patients will tolerate this without any distress, but an occasional patient is so disturbed by the presence of the tube that he becomes really distressed, and it may be wise to take an additional risk in order to give him peace of mind. The removal of the tube may itself, by relieving his distress, expedite the restoration of normal intestinal function. We must at all times be adaptable in our methods, and in such circumstances the surgeon will be ready to adjust the 'routine' to which he is accustomed.

The apprehensive patient may lie completely still for fear of pain after operation and will add greatly to his risk of respiratory disorder and even of the occurrence of venous thrombosis and embolus. On the other hand, a particular patient may be very active and difficult to restrain from over-activity after operation. To-day we rarely fear over-activity, but we do fear the lethargic patient who is difficult to get going. It is a great mistake to attempt to make all the occupants of a surgical ward conform to the same standard of activity, appetite and position during sleep and rest. A nurse must observe a patient's particular inclinations in the early stages of the stay in hospital and do her best to conform to the patient's wishes on the more personal aspects of nursing. Particularly is this individuality shown in relation to food. Many people loathe the sight of green jellies or green soups, others dislike pastry, or some may have a life-long obsession about fruit. These desires may be quite unrelated to the disease in question. The study of the individual becomes most important when the nurse is dealing with patients of various nationalities and race. She must realise, also, that a great many patients really need a most sincere form of sympathy during their illness, whilst others who have been used to discipline and being dragooned, continue to need a certain amount of firm treatment and definite instruction during their illness to prevent them drifting into a state of apathy. The highly intelligent patient often requires more sympathetic consideration on this account and the less educated may accept everything as being good for him, without question.

The nurse must remember that each patient has a real right to be an individual and to have individual attention. Nursing as we know it to-day has its foundation in the great Christian institutions of the past. In the Christian faith it is the individual and not the crowd on whom the greatest value is to be placed.

Common clinical types

Textbooks of medicine and surgery are apt to introduce a disease by a long list of symptoms which may or may not be present. A nurse does not, of course, need to know all these symptoms, but it is a great help to know the common groups which are most likely to occur together in a particular age or type of patient. Thus we have certain common 'clinical types' of any particular disease and each of these may have its own particular line of treatment. It is in a young adult that appendicitis most commonly appears with a right-sided pain, early loss of appetite and low-grade fever: this is what we call the acute catarrhal appendicitis. It is uncommon for the young person to develop an appendix abscess (although this may indeed happen even in a baby); in the elderly, however, appendicitis often presents as an abdominal abscess with fever perhaps over several weeks. These clinical types are dealt with later in the various sections on particular diseases and it is important to realise the great variation which occurs in the way in which the same disease affects different people.

PRINCIPLES OF TREATMENT

In spite of this background of individuality—in the origin of diseases, in the types of patient and in the manifestation of the complaint—we may nevertheless outline certain general principles of treatment which can be applied to very nearly every disease, disorder or injury. When treatment is becoming so much more a matter of administering life-saving antibiotics, blood transfusion and dramatic operations, it is very easy to lose sight of the

Table 2   The basic principles of treatment

1. Rest	General
	Local
2. Hygiene	The nurse
	The ward
	The patient
3. Diet	
4. Medicinal treatment	Specific
	Non-specific
5. Special therapy	Surgical operation
	Radiotherapy
	Physiotherapy
	Occupational therapy
	Rehabilitation

general principles, the neglect of which may delay recovery, add to discomfort or even prove fatal. It is around these general principles that the main part of the nurse's training centres. Her experience is measured by the judgement and the skill with which she applies these general principles. These will, therefore, be considered in detail, and in discussing the nursing treatment of particular conditions in later chapters it will be assumed that the nurse is consistently applying these general principles.

Rest

Rest is a vital part of the treatment of disease, to encourage the resolution of inflammation and to permit healing, but too much inactivity is harmful or even dangerous to a patient (page 63). Inflamed or injured limbs need to be kept still by splintage or by sling, perhaps even by extension. In the case of the alimentary tract a restriction of diet is necessary to rest the stomach and intestines (Fig. 2.11). The heart is rested by a restriction of the patient's activity. The mind is rested by the removal of unnecessary stresses and perhaps by the use of sedatives. Rest has therefore to be applied generally in all compartments of the patient's life during the stage of an acute illness. In this great principle of rest (as with the other four principles) we can speak of **general** treatment for the whole patient and **local** treatment—that is, rest for the diseased part or organ. Mumps demands that the unfortunate patient should retire to bed to lessen the general illness by complete rest. It also demands that the diet should consist of bland and uninteresting drinks which will not stimulate the activity of the inflamed saliva-producing glands. A fractured humerus similarly requires that the patient should have complete rest, although this may only be for a day or so, while local rest for the fractured limb is achieved by a plaster cast. Reference will be made later to the danger of too much rest in the case of limb injuries where muscle must be kept in good condition. Care has to be taken to avoid

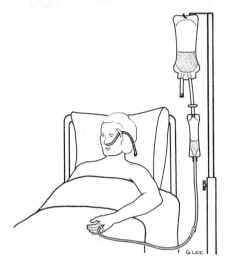

Fig. 2.11   The principle of rest applied to the alimentary tract. No food is given by mouth: the swallowed saliva and gastric secretions are removed periodically through the indwelling gastric tube. Nutrition is maintained by intravenous infusion. Peristalsis is restricted by keeping the stomach empty and by administration of drugs such as pethidine or morphine.

unnecessary inactivity and to realise the complications which can arise from a period of complete bed rest; especially is this so in the elderly patient. For instance, a patient has perhaps spent four weeks in a medical ward being prepared for a thyroidectomy; the operation is complete and she is feeling very much better, but her feet are now so painful and stiff when she walks that her recovery is impeded. This could have been prevented. Routine ward exercises for patients in bed have done a great deal to minimise the risks of prolonged bed rest necessitated by severe illness or injury.

Hygiene

The nurse's personal hygiene

It is part of the nurse's training to be scrupulously careful about her own person. It must never be forgotten that in dealing with surgical conditions the risks of infection are always present. Never must precautions to avoid infection be sacrificed to the desire in the nurse to improve her personal attractiveness. The wearing of caps by nurses on ward duty has as its purpose the prevention of contamination of the nurse's hair by ward dust. Cross-infection in wards takes place largely through the dust and, although short hair is now so much more common and the risk correspondingly less, a real danger exists where nurses persistently leave most of their hair outside their caps, frequently adjusting their forelock with their hands during their ward duties. The next few years may see the disappearance of nurses' caps: they have ceased to contribute to hygiene but are considered by many to be a pleasing feature to distinguish the nurse from the numerous medical auxiliaries and other technicians who take part in the patient's treatment.

Though it may not be fashionable, nails should be kept sufficiently short for them to be kept clean with a nail-brush, as this is the only possible way in which hands may be kept reasonably safe. With very frequent washing a nurse may find in the cold weather that her hands and nail-beds become cracked. A few extra seconds spent in drying the hands thoroughly each time will usually prevent this, but if deep cracks develop they should be treated at once by the application of friar's balsam (pig. benz. co.). In the cold weather the regular application of a 'barrier' hand cream at the end of duty periods and at bedtime may become a necessity.

A word is necessary here on the wearing of masks. Whilst it is very desirable that during the course of a dressing all those present should wear face masks, it is quite unnecessary for the nurse to walk around the ward performing her other duties with the mask in position. It becomes a habit with some people, particularly with midwives, and consequently lack of proper ventilation of the nasal air passages leads to the harbouring of organisms in the nurse's nose and to a rise in the number of streptococcal and staphylococcal carriers among the staff.

The nurse must pay careful attention to her teeth and must not neglect regular dental treatment. Fetor oris in the nurse is distressing to the patient and oral infection is dangerous.

The personal fitness and happiness of the nursing staff plays a very great part in the successful management of a surgical ward. Fatigue and indisposition lead to irritability: the team work becomes frayed and efficiency is soon reduced by tension amongst the staff.

Ward hygiene

Perhaps one of the most important duties of a ward sister is the management, organisation and constant vigilance over everything that takes place in the ward in order to prevent the spread of infection. In any climate the principal problem is one of the control of dust. Infection gains entry to a patient through an unhealed wound when the dressing is inadequate and through the nose, lungs and mouth by dust, food and drink. There are at all times present in the dust, germs which in the normal person or in normal tissues will give rise to very little reaction, but if they gain entrance to a wound or, for instance, to the bladder from contaminated catheters, they may set up serious and even disastrous infection. The gravity of complications by infection has been greatly diminished by the advent of modern chemotherapy. There are some operations and some tissues where the effects of infection are so devastating that it is customary to take extra preventive means, such as special skin preparations of a knee for meniscectomy. This is perhaps an illogical procedure as our precautions should always be of the very best, no matter what the surgical procedure is going to be; there should be no exceptions.

One of the greatest dangers to-day is that an organism, for instance *Staphylococcus aureus,* may be present in a form in which it is resistant to penicillin and other antibiotics, and this resistant strain of germ may travel very rapidly round the ward. This has become such a problem that very large sums of money have been spent on altering the design of hospitals to provide more isolation facilities and better ventilation. Most of the infection arises from patients who bring the germs into hospital as a nose infection. It is almost impossible to avoid the presence of such germs in the air, but an attempt is made to reduce the density of the germs in the surroundings. The strictest discipline is required to achieve this. If a number of staphylococcal wound infections arise in patients whose operations were 'clean' surgical procedures, suspicion is at once aroused as to the source of infection. Ward nursing and medical staff have nasal swabs taken to identify possible carriers.

Dust infection is borne in the atmosphere by the movements of furniture, bedding and curtains. Infection travels from a person's throat by means of droplet spread and becomes deposited on the fibres of blankets. Blankets cannot be sterilised by ordinary methods of laundry, although linen is adequately freed from infection by ironing. Thus the blanket dust becomes a very great danger and many methods have been introduced to prevent or limit this dust spread. Blankets have been impregnated with various forms of oil, but sterilisation by steam autoclaving is the only really effective way of dealing with the problem. Many hospitals have replaced their wool blankets by cotton or polypropylene 'blankets' which can be laundered with the linen.

Hospital wards and furniture have been designed particularly to prevent the accumulation of dust, but for many years to come surgical nursing will still have to take place in both house and hospital under conditions which are structurally far from ideal; under such circumstances the responsibility of the nurse becomes even greater. Such matters as the placing of the ventilators and the proper use of window-opening to provide adequate ventilation without carrying streams of air to and fro across the ward, contribute greatly to safety of a ward. One of the most treacherous sources of dust accumulation is the ordinary central-heating radiator, especially when this is composed of columns of pipes which cannot be adequately cleaned. The stream of warm air which rises from these radiators carries with it a heavy load of infected dust, so that certain positions in the ward may be more dangerous than others.

There are well recognised methods of treating floors to eliminate a great deal of dust. Wax and oil polishing result in the dust accumulating as fluff; this prevents to some extent its circulation in the air. More recently, plastic preparations have been introduced which can be painted on to polished wood floors, rendering them slip-proof and completely impervious to infective material which may be spilt. Such surfaces merely require a damp mop to keep them clean. Most trouble is experienced with concrete or stone floors, and these are similarly treated with a 'plastic' sealer. Suction cleaners, damp sweeping and damp dusting all play their part in the elimination of dust as a source of contamination.

In recent years the old-fashioned wheeled bed screens have been replaced in some of the large and modern hospitals by curtains suspended round each bed on runners. Since the curtains are seldom washed as often as the old-fashioned screen cover, a new source of dust accumulation has been introduced. A nurse should always be conscious of this risk when she draws these curtains in the rush of her routine duties. The disturbance and effort required to draw the curtains is much reduced by the regular application of a smear of ordinary furniture cream to the running rails.

Good surgery and careful nursing can reduce the risk of dust infection to a level at which it becomes almost insignificant, but a relaxation of rigid routine may result in a flare-up of infection which brings disappointment and distress to the patient, the nurse and the surgeon. To avoid wound contamination the dressings are sealed whenever possible and each day the *dressing* (not the wound) is inspected to make certain that the edges have not become lifted, allowing dust particles to be introduced from the bedclothes. The old-fashioned many-tailed bandage with a large layer of cotton wool around the patient with an abdominal wound did much to eliminate this dust contamination, but because of its instability and the desire of nursing and surgical staff alike to look at the wound regularly, the constant adjustment of this bandage led to further contamination. Many surgeons seal gauze along the line of the wound by use of pigmentum iodoformi co. (Whitehead's varnish), or a plastic sprayed on the wound (Nobecutane) or Opsite. Besides excluding dust, the adhesive dressing covered by adhesive strapping makes for greater comfort by preventing friction in the region of the wound. If adhesive strapping is put over a dressing, a small puncture should be made in the centre to allow the wound to 'breathe' to some extent: this prevents an accumulation of moisture from perspiration; the ideal adhesive plaster is the 'porous variety', unless it is deliberately desired to exclude air. Much is to be said for leaving wounds open to the air so that the healing tissue is not injured but becomes protected by a dry natural scab (pages 398, 962).

Beds and bedding. One of the best tests of a nurse's consideration and appreciation of her problems is the way in which she makes a bed. If with great gusto she picks up the pillows and bangs them into shape, clapping them down behind the patient with a great air of satisfaction, she has clearly no appreciation of the dangers of dust. She can do her job with greater efficiency by smooth and gentle movements, although she may not appear to be quite so impressive. The same applies to the way in which she handles the blankets and sheets. It is usual for nurses to wear masks when doing dressings, but the very organisms which they are guarding against may be firmly established in every article of bed-clothing.

The various types of bed and bed-fittings will be dealt with in the section on ward equipment, but from the point of view of hygiene there are certain points worth considering at this stage. Latex-foam mattresses have done a great deal to reduce bed dust. Rubber or plastic foam pillows are safer, more comfortable, dust-free and more easily cleaned.[1] The sterilisation of linen, rubber sheets and air rings which have been contaminated is dealt with in Chapter 17.

Dressings. The frequency with which surgical wounds need to be dressed is now very much reduced by the improved control of infection. A wound discharging pus is a rarity in civilian hospitals in industrial centres, but in isolated districts of the world where patients have come many miles for treatment, sepsis is far more prevalent. The nurse's basic training must include a rigid discipline with regard to dressing technique (page 395). Whether the dressings are changed in a special dressing-room set aside for the purpose as an annex to the ward or whether the dressings are done in the open ward, there should always be on the dressing-trolley a bowl or bucket sufficiently large to accommodate the *whole* dirty dressing. Frequently one has seen a large soiled dressing balanced precariously on the edge of a small bowl; this is dirty and unnecessary. A plastic pail with a lid or, better still, an ordinary domestic bin with a pedal-operated lid is far better. Such a pail or bin should be

[1] Terylene or Nylon pillow slips should never be used in an oxygen tent because of the risk of static electricity.

lined with paper so that when it needs emptying the whole of the contents and the paper may be destroyed without the dirty dressing having to be touched. In the case of small dressings it is sufficient to have an open paper bag in a bowl to receive the soiled swabs. Some hospitals have an incinerator on each ward for the immediate destruction of dirty dressings.

Flowers. The effect of well arranged flowers is clearly good: it has recently been shown that a very virulent organism which attacks plants, *Erwinia*, can cause disease and deaths from septicaemia have been recorded, the infection having come from plants in the ward. Flowers must be banned rigidly from high-risk areas, i.e. intensive care units, labour wards and dressing areas. *Pseudonomas pyocyanea* can readily be spread in flower vases which are rarely 'sterilised'.

Flies. Especially is it necessary in warm climates to pay attention to the menace of flies. Again, it is so much a matter of the nurse becoming conscious of this danger so that care is taken to prevent the exposure of food to which the flies may be attracted. Although it is unlikely that the flies will have an opportunity of settling in a patient's wound, they will be purveyors of germs which lead to attacks of gastro-enteritis. In tropical climates adequate window screening will be essential to protect the ward both from flies and mosquitoes. Fly-papers, although unsightly, are very logical. No dust or insect which settles on a fly-paper will ever escape. The walls of the ward kitchen and storage cupboards which are usually ill-ventilated and rather warm, should be sprayed each spring with a 'persistent insecticide' solution. Flies settle particularly on the edges of partitions and the rounded beadings of window-frames, and in heavily infested areas it is well worth spraying the whole of the ward at the beginning of the warm season. These anti-fly measures may be taken by the hospital authorities as part of the normal routine, but often these things are overlooked unless the ward sister makes a specific request. Similar appropriate measures should be taken in any private house where there is an invalid.

The ward kitchen. Reference has already been made to the protection of food against infection, but perhaps the most vital link in the chain of activity to protect the patient is the attention which is paid to the washing-up of dirty crockery. A disease-causing staphylo-coccus from a patient who is a 'nasal carrier' may very easily find its way from the patient's fingers to a cup, and the infection is spread through lukewarm washing-up water and soiled drying cloths. All ward crockery after use should be washed in really hot water containing either soda or one of the modern detergent solutions. It should be allowed to dry in the air. Drying 'tea towels' are a cause of infection particularly encouraging pseudomonas organisms which like the damp. The new detergents are more effective than soap because they are fat solvents and form no scum, but if used lavishly in washing up by hand the skin is affected by the removal of skin fats. Centralised 'washing-up' for the whole hospital is preferable, for all utensils are then sterilised and heat dried.

The swill bin must not leak and must have a well fitting lid. Other refuse is placed in disposable waterproof containers instead of the old-fashioned rubbish bin. These are destroyed in an incinerator and containers do not have to be washed or returned: there is far less risk of dirt or infection. Sinks, cupboards and refrigerators must be kept scrupulously clean.

The ward bathroom and toilet annex. The nurse will learn in her medical training and elementary nursing the basic principles of hygiene in these departments. It must again be stressed that the risks of infection by gastro-enteritis are still present even in the surgical ward. If there are patients in the ward suffering from septic conditions, clearly the 'bath list' must be organised in such a way that these patients come last, whatever other precautions are taken to prevent the spread of infection.

The patient's personal hygiene

In educated communities perhaps little needs to be said on the subject of personal hygiene in regard to the patient on admission. The nurse, nevertheless, has duties in this connection, no less clear than her other responsibilities. However unpleasant and embarrassing the task may be, both to the patient and the nurse, every individual on admission to hospital should be examined for signs of skin infection and infestation of the head with lice, or more commonly their eggs (i.e. nits). It used to be common practice for there to be a 'head book' in each female ward, and the nurse who examined the patient's head on admission would have to record the fact to make certain the examination had been carried out. In Britain, now that so many women have shorter hair, heavy infestation with lice is uncommon; the regular inspection of children at school had almost eliminated this condition from the children's wards, but there is again an increase of infestation in children and particularly in boys who now cultivate long hair. During the Second World War, women recruits to the three services in the United Kingdom were all examined on entry and a steady twenty per cent were found throughout the period of the war to arrive at their recruiting depot carrying nits in their heads. It is in the interests of the nurse herself, as well as in the interests of the ward as a whole, that these infections should be detected and treated. The application of the appropriate specific lotion or hair oil (Esoderm or Lorexane) containing gamma benzene hexachloride is not distasteful to the patient.

Scabies is another infestation by a minute insect which burrows into the skin. This shows itself mainly by the patient having inflicted scratches on his skin so that there are tiny little scabs, particularly on the arms and legs. Scabies can also attack such areas as the umbilicus and nipple, producing ulcers which acquire secondary infection by other germs: thus the original underlying scabies infection may go unnoticed. The initial examination takes place usually at the first bath before the patient has been put to bed. In the case of emergencies the nurse who helps the patient undress must be held responsible for this initial examination, and she must *always*, without hesitation, report any suspected case of infestation or infection. Scabies is treated by scrubbing the affected areas with benzylbenzoate lotion and applying this over the whole body. Athlete's foot (**tinea pedis**) is another condition which should be looked for specifically and reported so that it may be dealt with This shows itself as sodden patches of peeling skin between the toes, and occasionally a similar infection (**tinea cruris**) is found in the groin and on the inner side of the thighs, where it presents as a bright red, slightly raised and irritant area. The presence of this must *always* be reported (page 720). *Any* septic skin spots should be reported to the ward sister: their presence may be sufficiently important to postpone operation, and the patient may be a 'staphylococcus carrier'—a grave risk to the ward.

The mouth and teeth. During the surgical treatment of any patient, his ability to taste is important, and the presence of unpleasant tastes in his mouth will depress him. The mouths of surgical patients become dry either as the result of their being given atropine or hyoscine before operation, or from post-operative dehydration. The flow of saliva is reduced and the mouth is rendered highly susceptible to infection. The salivary glands also may become infected, and if this happens it is a reflection on the nursing technique. The care of the mouth is of particular importance in patients where dental sepsis is present and cannot be dealt with before a surgical operation is performed. These patients run a risk of the infection spreading to their lungs.

A mouth-wash solution ('collutorium') suitable for general ward use is collutorium thymol co. BPC.[1] This is supplied as a compound thymol solution tablet, solv. thymol co., one tablet being dissolved in 60 ml (2 ounces) of warm water on each occasion of use. Stock solutions are highly dangerous as the antiseptic value is mild and pseudomonas organisms in particular may proliferate in the solution.

In the seriously ill, the nurse must herself attend to the patient's oral hygiene by cleansing the mouth at least every four hours. If the patient is having no fluid by mouth, then the cleansing routine must take place more frequently. A small mop of cotton-wool on a wood probe or sinus forceps, is dipped in an antiseptic solution and the whole of the inside of the mouth, including the tongue, is carefully sponged, the mop being changed several times. A dilute solution of sodium bicarbonate helps to dissolve the sticky mucus in the mouth (Fig. 2.12).

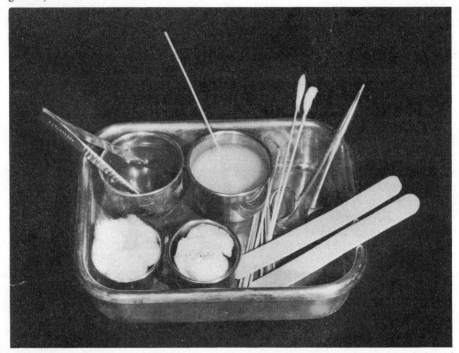

Fig. 2.12 Mouth-cleansing tray. The gallipots contain water, fresh antiseptic mouth-wash solution, pieces of white lint for wiping the mouth or tongue and cotton wool for use on the wood probes. The sinus forceps are for picking up any large particles of food or for retrieving a pledget of wool which may have fallen off the probe. The tray remains on the patient's locker. Used wool and probes are placed in a paper bag and thrown away after each treatment. A good light is essential. These items may be issued as prepacked sets from the CSSD.

[1] British Pharmacopoeia Codex.

Antibiotic drugs, especially those given by mouth, kill many harmless bacteria which keep the mouth healthy and at the right degree of acidity. As a result of this change, fungus infections (moulds) thrive in the mouth and the patient may develop a serious ulcerative condition (**thrush**) such as is found in babies. These fungus infections sometimes spread to the lungs where they do not respond to treatment. As most seriously ill patients nowadays are having some form of antibiotic treatment, the care of the mouth is extremely important. If fungus infection occurs in the mouth it appears as woolly white patches on the gums and palate, eventually covering the whole pharynx. Treatment is urgent. A specific fungicide is nystatin used as a solution or in jelly form, painted or smeared round the mouth. Gentian violet (2 per cent solution in water) is sometimes used but is very messy. Nystatin is also given as tablets to prevent 'thrush' in the intestinal tract when a patient as prolonged antibiotic therapy. Similarly monilial infection attacks the vagina leading to a white discharge, and is commonly found in girls and women who have had antibiotics. If untreated it spreads to the bladder and is difficult to eradicate. The vaginal infection is treated with nystatin pessaries.

Dentures should be washed and lightly brushed. They should never be placed in antiseptic solutions, but preferably kept completely covered with clean water to prevent warping which may occur if they become very dry: all antiseptics in general use may contain substances injurious to the plastic compound of which the dental plate is made, quite apart from the fact that an unpleasant flavour may be imparted to the denture. The nurse must remember that a patient is very often extremely sensitive about his 'plate', and it must be treated as part of his person. Great care must be taken not to confuse dentures and return the wrong ones after cleansing: such a mistake may seem amusing at the time, but the incident will be remembered by the patient as a major event. Again, provided there is no likelihood of a patient vomiting, the wearing of dentures should be left entirely to the patient's discretion. Some people feel undressed without their teeth. Others find them a nuisance, usually because they are a bad fit. The stay in hospital may be an opportunity for the necessary adjustments which have been deferred because the patient was ashamed to be seen without teeth! Dentures and appliances of any type, however small, must be removed from a patient about to undergo operation. The nurse must remember that young people and children sometimes have tiny single-tooth dentures which are very dangerous during anaesthesia and which may easily be overlooked.

The back and pressure points. The development of bed sores is usually considered to indicate bad nursing. They occur from interruption of the nutrition of areas of skin where the blood supply has been impaired by pressure and in some circumstances it is impossible to prevent their development. The very thin, the very heavy, the incontinent and those who through some injury to the spine have lost the sensation of the skin at these points are most likely to develop pressure sores. Common sites for bed sores are the sacral area and the heels. In patients with septic conditions, nutrition is impaired by prolonged fever and there is frequently anaemia. Their toxic condition renders them less likely to move about and the greatest care needs to be taken to prevent the development of these pressure ulcers. Frequent change of position and massage of pressure points with spirit followed by powder is still the best method of prevention. Early post-operative mobilisation of all patients who are fit to get up has done much to prevent this distressing complaint (page 205).

Mention will be made again of this feature as a complication in neurological cases. In unconscious patients or those who have had some injury to the spinal cord, a large pressure sore can develop as soon as twelve hours after the injury or onset of the illness. A bed sore on the sacral area may even develop from the patient's position on the operating table during a long operation and the theatre staff need to be watchful, especially when the patient is particularly thin. Although pressure sores rarely develop over the scapula or the elbows, these points are subject to soreness and require similar preventive treatment when the patient is washed. An ulcer may develop on the shin from the weight of the other leg, if the legs of an unconscious patient are left crossed.

Constipation. Personal hygiene includes attention to the bowel, and much discomfort can be caused by the onset of constipation. An active person confined to hospital by reason of an accident or illness rapidly loses the normal rhythm of his bowel action. As well as his physical discomfort he is mentally disturbed, and the judicious use of laxatives is necessary if there is no reason against this on account of his particular illness. Purging by the use of cascara, Epsom salts or castor oil should never be allowed, unless it has been specifically ordered by the doctor in charge. The *routine* use of liquid paraffin is also fraught with danger, especially in patients with trouble in the alimentary tract. The reason for this is that if an anastomosis of bowel has to be performed the presence of a small amount of liquid paraffin in the bowel may cause a seepage of infection through the stitch holes. Liquid paraffin, preferably as an emulsion, if permissible, is the best aid to restoring normal function in those whose constipation has resulted from the inactivity of being in hospital (page 388). Sometimes constipation is the result of loss of sensation in the rectum, either from ignoring the natural desire to empty the bowel, or from interference with the nerve supply. Habit training of the bowel is then essential, aided by a stimulant laxative.

Many patients have developed a 'laxative habit' over a period of years and a stay in hospital may be a convenient opportunity to break them of this habit: if the facilities are such that the patients are able to have regular abdominal exercises, then with a correctly balanced diet, the patient will need no laxative after the first two or three days. It must, however, be remembered that the patient may know best what suits him, and he should be allowed 'his usual' *if he needs it*. He may require a little assistance after an operation and usually this is given in the form of an initial post-operative enema or stimulant suppository. Much has been done to eliminate the distress of constipation by the early mobilisation of patients after operation and by permitting them to use a bedside commode. The bedpan is uncomfortable and discouraging, and except for the very ill, unnecessary: even after a prostatectomy the average patient may be allowed to sit on a bedside commode on the first day (Fig. 51.5). It is necessary to stress the need for very careful toilet after the patient has had the use of his bowels. The Closomat automatic closet pedestal which cleans the anal area with a warm water spray and dries it with warm air is widely used. Bidets also eliminate a great deal of nursing care both for men and women patients who have undergone perineal surgery.

Barrier nursing

By this we mean the special isolation of a patient with a particularly infective condition who may be still nursed in an open ward. It is not always possible to put such a patient into a single side room or cubicle. Even if accommodation is available it is not always convenient for a very sick patient to be in a room by himself, especially when nursing staff is short. In a surgical ward it is always necessary to 'barrier nurse' any patient who develops **haemolytic streptococcal** infection. Infections due to staphylococci are often very resistant to antibiotics and it is ideal also to isolate and 'barrier nurse' such patients. *Pseudomonas pyocyanea* which forms green pus when in wounds is another rapidly spreading infection often present in the bowel of hospital patients. It thrives in moist areas and particularly attacks the urinary tract. It is spread by contaminated feeding utensils, especially if after washing, such utensils are dried with a cloth. In barrier nursing, feeding utensils must be kept separate from the general supply and sterilised by boiling or steam.

Nurses when dealing with the patient (bed-making or doing dressings) must wear marked gowns which are left by the bedside when not in use: screens should be left between the patient and adjacent beds, and if possible the bed should be at the end of the ward if no cubicle is available: a hand-basin of antiseptic lotion such as chlorhexidine (Hibitane 0·2 per cent) should be left on a table at the foot of the bed, with individual hand towels and a receptacle for used towels: paper hand towels are of value here.[1] There must of course be a special thermometer reserved for the patient who is 'barrier' nursed, if the normal ward routine does not provide for individual thermometers. Unless the ward equipment includes a steriliser for bedpans and urinals, marked ones must be reserved for the patient. Books and magazines must not be used from the hospital library unless they may be burned subsequently.

The effectiveness of barrier nursing depends to a large extent on the ventilation in the ward. If this is inadequate, cross-draughts may spread the infection to neighbouring patients. Cubicle nursing is preferable, but not always possible.

Diet

The intake and digestion of food requires at all times the expenditure of energy. In addition, certain types of food produce a variable increase in activity of particular tissues or organs. Consequently when the body is stricken by injury or disease there has to be a balance between the principle of rest and the principle of nutrition in treatment. This balance is largely a task for the nurse.

Illness accompanied by prolonged fever necessitates a diet with a very high nutritive value. The tissues burn themselves up faster than normal; protein and carbohydrate are therefore necessary in increased amount. In a short febrile illness nutritive diet often has to be withheld and the body's fat reserves are used up. These reserves need to be replaced in the convalescent stage.

The standard 5 per cent dextrose intravenous infusion is totally inadequate for calorie requirements, and without high calorie supplements a patient on parenteral (intravenous) fluids only is living on his reserves. The calorie requirement of a patient in bed without fever is just under 2000 calories per day, but in severe illness the expenditure may go up to 5000 calories per day. (See Preface, page v.)

The 'bricks' for building protein are amino-acids and these are essential in parenteral feeding if the patient cannot be fed normally. A major operation may result in the loss of 500 G of body tissue a day and this requires about 100 G protein. Amino-acids have to be given with extra fuel to enable the body to use them and so additional calories in the form of sorbitol or fructose or fat are added (page 139).

Even if a patient is eating normally a standard hospital diet may be deficient in protein. Injured and diseased tissues call for an extra amount of vitamin C (ascorbic acid) and

[1] Hibitane hand cream applied after drying the hands is a useful safeguard to the nurse and against spread of infection.

many people in all walks of life are deficient in their storage of this vitamin. In treatment not only does there have to be a daily maintenance dose but the 'backlog' may need to be made up. Without vitamin C, wound repair is very defective; wounds burst open and ulcers fail to heal. Similarly, bone repair requires the presence of vitamin D. The application of vitamins in surgery is described in Chapter 7.

In addition to the increased nutritional needs of illness, there is often a real deficiency to be made up. Many surgical patients have been on a reduced diet for weeks. Almost all forms of disease of the alimentary tract lead to loss of appetite and many are accompanied by vomiting or diarrhoea or a failure of absorption of the food from the bowel. These food intake deficiencies lead to a depletion of mineral reserves—calcium and iron especially. Consequently, anaemia develops and if, in addition, the patient is toxic from sepsis or malignant disease (e.g. from stasis and fermentation in the bowel obstructed by growth), the bone marrow becomes poisoned and red blood cell manufacture falls off.

Such are the general dietetic factors to be considered. In addition, we need to take into account the particular condition, disease or injury from which our patient is suffering. These local factors will determine the way in which the necessary diet is prepared and presented—a field in which the nurse has real opportunity for enterprise and skill. She needs to exercise ingenuity, common sense and patience. It is ridiculous to give to a patient with mumps savoury or tasty foods which will stimulate his inflamed salivary glands; it is equally ridiculous to serve a boiled egg in an egg-cup to a man with one arm immobilised in a splint!

Fluid requirements are dealt with in detail in Chapter 8. The fluid balance is a dietetic matter and there are very few occasions on which an increase in fluid intake over normal is not beneficial. Much trouble and discomfort can arise from insufficient fluid. In intestinal cases and burns, 'fluid balance' measurement is not likely to be overlooked, but it is very important in *all* disease, especially where there is fever. Salt depletion (sodium chloride) makes a patient very languid and may lead to a failure of renal function, especially if the patient is anaemic (page 136).

Diet, then, in quantity, quality and presentation, is one of the greatest principles of treatment, and one which needs to be considered from a very practical standpoint. The dietician who knows all the theory but cannot cook usually knows very little about the presentation of food. The cook knows nothing of the patient's illness, capacity or requirements. It is her duty to see that food reaches the patient in an attractive and palatable form, and that any deficiencies in the standard meals are made good by supplemental feeding in some way. It is the nurse who co-ordinates these skills. She will only receive guidance along very broad lines from the medical staff.

Medicinal treatment

Medicinal preparations, whether administered as drugs or applied as dressings, may be grouped according to the purpose for which they are given. Some may be used for the treatment of *symptoms* such as a headache or constipation, irrespective of the nature of the condition which has led to these symptoms. As far as the disease is concerned, these medicines are non-specific. The second group includes those substances which are used for the treatment of a particular disease; for instance, carbimazole in the treatment of thyrotoxicosis, or diphtheria antitoxin in diphtheria.

In her management of the patient, the nurse has at her disposal a considerable number of drugs used generally in the treatment of symptoms. With the constant advance of scientific knowledge, more and more drugs are coming into use with specific actions which strike at the very causes of individual disease processes, for instance use of cytotoxic drugs for cancer (page 434).

The supply, mode of action, and administration of medicinal preparations used in surgical conditions are discussed fully in Chapter 7.

Special therapy

(a) **Surgical operation.** There could be no treatment more specific: each operation, though perhaps following well used methods, presents its own difficulties and requires its own special technique. Even the most experienced surgeon is repeatedly meeting new problems and making fresh decisions. Surgery is being divided into smaller and smaller special fields of work as science makes possible greater extensions of surgical treatment.

It is, of course, the 'operation' which forms the climax of treatment in many surgical cases, but it is the skilful and conscientious application of the other great principles of treatment which makes operative surgery possible and successful. Perhaps the greatest argument in favour of the development of specialised surgical units is not so much the greater experience of the surgeon, but the very much more efficient nursing which can be developed in such units. The establishment of special centres for the treatment of burns proved the truth of this claim beyond doubt.

(b) **Radiotherapy.** This is a specialised field of surgical treatment used alone or in conjunction with operation, mainly in the treatment of malignant growths. Certain rays, similar to wireless or light waves but with a very much smaller wave-length (higher frequency), have a damaging or lethal effect on rapidly growing tissues. Special high-voltage x-ray plants and radium emit these waves. Radium is a solid substance which produces a gas—radon— which itself emits these rays. Many other radioactive substances, as these 'emitting' chemicals are called, are becoming available for special treatment and research, and the nurse needs to be familiar with the principles and management of these treatments (Chapter 23).

(c) **Physiotherapy.** The trained physiotherapist is called upon to help in surgical treatment in many ways. Routine exercises designed to maintain the strength of limb and abdominal muscles during periods of enforced confinement to bed, lessen the risk of venous thrombosis and hasten convalescence. Special exercises are used to restore the function of damaged joints and muscles after fractures and soft-tissue injuries. Lung expansion is encouraged in the prevention and treatment of thoracic disease.

By the use of various methods of applying artificial heat, the blood and lymphatic circulation may be improved and muscular spasm and pain relieved. The physiotherapist is an invaluable member of the surgical team. From time to time her activities may interfere with ward 'routine', but co-operation from the nursing staff is essential. Physiotherapy is prescribed by the surgeon just as he orders other treatments and a patient must not miss her treatment merely because it is inconvenient.

(d) **Occupational therapy.** This seeks to aid recovery in two ways. First, by providing a hobby during prolonged illness, occupational therapy helps the patient's mind, by relieving boredom and giving purpose to what may seem otherwise wasted days. Second, by selected handicrafts the patient may be encouraged to do repetitive exercises for joints—perhaps fingers—which have been injured. A third and increasingly vital role is in guiding the handicapped patient—with arthritis, or paralysed after a stroke or injury—in aspects of daily living. This includes, for instance, the supply of gadgets for turning taps, modification of domestic equipment and toilets, supply of bathseats, 'tongs' for picking things up from the floor, and specially designed cutlery. Social, welfare and educational services are all brought into action.

Convalescence

Recreation, occupational therapy and remedial exercise constitute what is termed collectively 'rehabilitation'. This phase of recovery starts in hospital. After minor accidents or operation patients need very little active help, but after severe and multiple injuries, major orthopaedic procedures, vascular and lung surgery, gradual return to normal needs special help and encouragement. Rehabilitation centres which provide all these services accept patients direct from hospital wards or from, for instance, a fracture clinic at a suitable stage after injury. These may be day or residential centres. Convalescent homes, providing a little nursing care, special diet and usually a country or seaside atmosphere of peace are needed for patients whose home conditions are not ideal for recovery after illness.

The role of the surgical nurse

In many small hospitals, in rural areas and countries where social services are not so advanced, the nurse may have to combine with her duties the function of a social worker and physiotherapist; she may also need to instruct her patients in occupational therapy. In the past she spent much time changing dressings, applying poultices and packs. Today she helps the post-operative patient to cough, moves his joints systematically when bed making, and plays an active role in this recovery phase. In her training she must be eager to watch and to learn as much as possible of these 'ancillary services'; her career may well lead her to areas where surgery is practised under the most difficult and primitive conditions. A thorough appreciation during training of the basic principles of treatment will enable her to make the best use of all available resources and, where facilities and amenities are poor, to improvise.

Common sense has been described as the amount of sense possessed by the average individual. A nurse needs more than this—a sense of sympathy, a sense of humour, a sense of urgency and a sense of thrill in her work. Drudgery comes from lack of inspiration and purpose. Let any who feel that nursing is drudgery, consider again the tremendous scope of these great outlines of treatment. The nurse, especially at the beginning of her career, may feel that she is a small cog in a large machine; but if a small cog is broken or bent, the whole machinery may stop.

3

Tissue Repair and Replacement

When any portion of body tissue has been destroyed by disease or violence, the adjacent tissues at once set to work to repair the gap. Clearly their task will depend on the extent of the gap and the presence of any factors which hinder normal tissue activity. When a clean surgical incision has been made and the edges sewn closely together, the gap to be bridged is very thin. On the other hand, if there has been an abscess and a large area of tissue has been dissolved away, the problem is very much greater. There are many factors which influence the rate of the body's power of healing, and it is necessary to understand the process of tissue repair in order that we may see where the various factors of nursing have their effect.

Where a gap has been left in the tissue, the 'raw' surfaces are covered with blood clot and any intervening cavity may in fact be filled with blood. From the ends of the capillaries which have been cut on either side, cells grow rapidly into this **haematoma** (a collection of blood in the tissues) and form **granulation tissue**, which is thus a mass of tiny little capillary buds with fibrous tissue cells (Fig. 3.1). As the days go by, the very rich blood supply enables fibrous tissue to grow rapidly and become more dense, and finally to cement the gap. Weeks later the blood vessels die off and firm fibrous **scar tissue** remains. This becomes slowly tighter and tighter. This process we know as contraction, so that what may appear to be quite a large scar shrinks down over a period of months to become sometimes invisible. Perhaps the best example of this is the cavity left by the removal of the slough from a large carbuncle; in a very few months there is a small white, irregular scar marking the centre of the great cavity where the carbuncle existed.

If the wound has involved other tissues than connective tissue—for instance, the mucous membrane of the cheek, or the skin—then the very specialised epithelial lining also grows across as a sheet of cells and covers up the granulation tissue. The same process occurs in the intestinal tract; when an **anastomosis** (artificial opening between two hollow organs or vessels) has been performed, the cut edges of the mucous membrane are stuck together temporarily by fibrin, and over a period of days the cells lining the stomach or intestine grow rapidly across the gap. When a bone is broken, repair takes place in a similar way: calcium substances from the blood are deposited in the granulation tissue forming **callus**. Into this callus the specialised cells which form true bone migrate from the surrounding damaged bone: over a period of weeks or even months the minute structure is rebuilt to join up exactly with the bone on either side of the break (Fig. 3.2).

The healing power of the body is influenced by many factors. An adequate supply of oxygen is necessary for these tissue repairs, and, as oxygen is carried to the tissues by the blood, anaemia results in a very poor healing rate. Vitamins, especially vitamin C, are necessary for the repair of tissues, so that patients whose reserve of vitamin C has been depleted heal more slowly and may in fact not heal at all. Patients who are ill use more

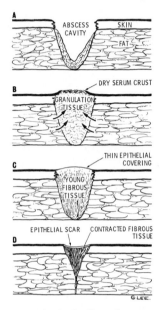

Fig. 3.1   Stages in the healing of an open wound.

vitamin C than the normal healthy individuals and sometimes, unless their requirement is met, a wound may come apart even a week or more after operation, showing no sign of healing whatever. Infection always delays healing as it interferes with the activities of the cells at the edges of the wound. Similarly, if the patient's general health has been impaired by long-standing disease or bad nourishment his powers of healing are poor, as the substances required for the repair are in short supply. The presence of foreign bodies or a poor blood supply (such as occurs in arteriosclerosis, or if the stitches have been tied too tight) will also delay sound healing. In addition, there are many personal and undetermined factors which must be responsible for the fact that some people heal quickly and others heal very poorly. Age is important; babies and children repair their tissues very much more rapidly than old people. This is because the growing child has much more vitality in all his cells. A fracture of the humerus in a new-born baby may be soundly united in ten days: in an adult the same fracture would require eight weeks.

From the point of view of nursing, we have learnt, therefore, that if a patient has the task of repairing a large area of injured tissue, for instance after a major operation, he has for a variable time before and after operation the following requirements:

(a) **A really nutritious diet,** preferably with a high protein content (page 27).

(b) An adequate supply of vitamin C. In the case of an operation like a gastrectomy we are particularly careful to see that the patient has had perhaps 1000 mg a day for five days before operation. The normal hospital patient requires a maintenance dose of 100 mg daily, but if he is feverish or has a septic condition, this requirement may go up to as much as 500 mg a day. Few hospital diets are rich in vitamin C as the prolonged cooking necessary in a large institution destroys the vitamin C content, both of potatoes and green

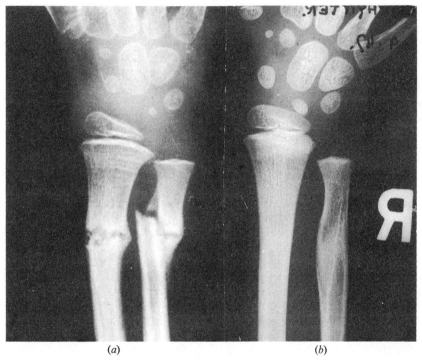

(a)   (b)

Fig. 3.2 Fracture of radius and ulna in a boy aged six years. (a) Three weeks after the fracture, showing callus formation in the healing. (b) Six months later. The site of the fracture has been completely remodelled by the periosteum and the normal minute structure has been restored.

vegetables which form a very important source of the vitamin in the ordinary small household. Many bottled fruit juices—lime, orange and lemon—contain little or no vitamin C and therefore reliance must not be placed on these drinks as a source of the vitamin, which is normally administered as synthetic **ascorbic acid**.

(c) An adequate intake of iron. If anaemia is present or likely to occur as a result of prolonged sepsis, iron is given by mouth in the form of ferrous sulphate. If the patient's haemoglobin is found to be under 10 g/100 ml before operation, many surgeons would prefer to transfuse the patient rather than delay treatment until the haemoglobin level rose naturally.

(d) Adequate rest for the diseased part, such as splintage for an injured or diseased limb, a carefully arranged diet for disorders of the alimentary tract, or protection of an injured eye to prevent its use and movement.

(e) **Avoidance of infection** at every stage in the nursing of the patient by the highest standards of personal and ward hygiene, and particularly by the avoidance of frequent dressings.

Delayed healing of wounds

Even when all these factors have received adequate attention there remain a number of patients whose healing will be slow, a number of sites in the body which always heal more slowly than others, and certain diseases which by their very nature resist every effort of the body to repair their damage. Patients with malignant disease, although it is not quite clear why, tend to heal badly. Patients with kidney disease and a raised blood-urea level do not heal well. Patients with jaundice tend to suffer from delayed healing because there is frequently an interference with the formation of proper blood clot: bleeding into the tissues prevents the proper closure of the wound: vitamin K (page 583) is given to lessen this tendency. Certain fractures, because of poor blood supply to the fragments, are subject to delayed union.

The skin of an ordinary surgical incision should be soundly bridged across in five or six days, but in some areas of the body it is even quicker. In the neck, skin stitches need not be left in a thyroid wound for more than two days: this is largely because the skin is very loose and therefore it is not put under tension by the movement of the head. Occasionally, for instance on the abdominal wall, if an incision has been made across the line of pull of the normal abdominal muscles and skin, the scar will 'stretch' and several months after the operation it will be found to be a broad white scar. This stretching occurs particularly where there has been infection in the wound which has led to delayed healing or a 'bursting' of the tissues beneath the skin, so that a greater pull than normal has come on the skin itself. The surgeon aims at sewing up the tissues under the skin in such a way that there is very little pull on the skin: consequently he needs to tie the skin sutures only loosely, and so avoid as far as possible any mark which a tight skin stitch will otherwise produce.

There are then certain diseases, certain types of patient, and certain local conditions in which delayed healing is to be anticipated. The underlying causes are summarised in Table 3.

It is known that adrenalin (which is released especially in conditions of stress) inhibits the normal division (mitosis) of skin cells, and severe or prolonged stress may have a profound effect upon the repair processes. More important is the knowledge that the multiplication of skin cells is much faster during sleep than at other times. Lack of sleep may therefore actually delay wound healing.

It will be seen that some of these factors depend on the patient, some on the surgeon, and some on the nursing and general care of the patient.

Gangrene

The term **necrosis** means death of cells. This may be brought about by poisoning of or by direct injury to the cell. If, however, a piece of tissue dies because its blood supply has been cut off, this type of necrosis is spoken of as **gangrene**. The blood conveys not only oxygen but other substances vital to the life of the cells. The branch of a tree withers and dies when it is broken from the trunk because its supply of vital sap has been cut off. Gangrene is a similar process.

Table 3   Causes of delayed wound healing

In infected wounds	drug-resistant organisms
	inadequate drainage of abscess
	fistula from internal organ
	foreign body or sequestrum
In surgical wounds	sutured under tension
	edges of skin turned in
	edges burnt by diathermy
	neoplasm present in wound
	haematoma formation
	irritant ligatures (e.g. chromic catgut too near the skin)
In accidental wounds	bruising of skin edges
	skin loss
	exposed tendon or aponeurosis
	burnt tissue
General condition of patient	anaemia
	cardiac insufficiency
	pulmonary disease
	stress
	uraemia
	jaundice
	malnutrition (protein or vitamin shortage)
	cortisone therapy

There are four main causes of gangrene.

1. Arterial obstruction. An artery may become blocked by the clotting of the blood within it or from the entry of a clot which has been formed in the heart or at another point on the arterial tree. Arteriosclerosis, injury and inflammation of the arterial wall and syphilis produce 'arteritis' which may lead to thrombosis. Heart disease, especially if there has been atrial fibrillation, may allow the formation of clots within the heart. If these become detached, they pass out to lodge usually in the arteries of the limbs (page 67).

2. Infection. When infection is established in the tissues, the cells may be killed by the bacteria and their poisons. Infection also attacks the artery walls, especially of the very tiny vessels, and tissue necrosis occurs as the result of these two processes. This condition is **infective gangrene**. A particular form of this is **gas gangrene**, which is produced by organisms which form gas from the decomposing tissues (page 300).

3. Injury. Direct violence to tissues tears the blood vessels as well as damaging the cells. Burning coagulates the blood vessels. Thus, as with infective gangrene, the tissues die from a double assault on their own protoplasm and on their blood supply.

4. Diabetes. Diabetic patients develop degenerative changes in their small arteries and are thus more liable to gangrene from the resultant **'ischaemia'** (lack of blood). If the diabetes is not adequately controlled by diet or insulin, the tissues themselves are devital-ised and much more susceptible to infection. The gangrene of diabetes is a combination of tissue damage from infection and blood vessel damage from degeneration.

The aim in treatment of gangrene

Since gangrene is the result of lack of blood, and therefore of oxygen, in the tissues, it might seem that the obvious way to improve the oxygen supply would be to dilate the blood vessels by applying local heat. However, heat increases tissue activity and therefore increases oxygen consumption. In order to make the best of a bad blood supply, one needs to cool the tissues which are threatened with gangrene, rather than to heat them. The threatened limb is therefore left exposed to the air, or under certain circumstances actually cooled with ice-packs. In many cases, however, as we have seen, the blood vessels

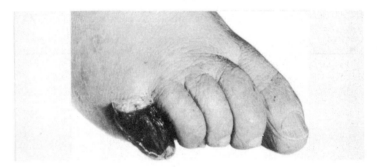

Fig. 3.3   Arteriosclerotic gangrene of toe with superimposed infection

themselves are diseased and rigid: thus they are incapable of dilating to allow a better flow of blood. The body is so constructed that there is a tremendous network of small arteries, and most tissues have what is known as a 'collateral' circulation—that is, a by-pass or alternative route—which opens if the principal artery should become blocked. Thus a piece of tissue which is threatened with gangrene is in the same position as a free graft from another part of the body, in that it has to survive on a reduced oxygen supply until the by-pass is adequately opened up. This development of the collateral circulation is partly dependent on the nerve supply to blood vessels and partly on local chemical changes.

If the devitalised tissue does not become infected one of two things happens. If the dead area is very small it gradually becomes converted into fibrous tissue and is in effect a scar. This applies particularly to small infarcts (page 62) in solid organs such as the liver or kidney. When skin or mucous membrane is affected by gangrene the epithelium has to be shed along with any portion of deep tissue that has also died: the gap is filled up by granulation tissue and new epithelium as already described (page 31). When large areas of tissue die they have to be removed surgically—a toe, a leg, or an area of skin which has been killed by a burn.

If, however, infection supervenes the dead tissue is gradually rotted by infection and is separated from healthy tissue by enzyme action. Healing is greatly delayed until this

slough is removed surgically or by natural processes. In the deeper tissues of the body an abscess forms and has to be dealt with by operation (e.g. in the lung).

Treatment of gangrene of limbs and of gas gangrene has led to the use of hyperbaric oxygen to limit the extent of tissue death. The patient is nursed for periods in a closed cabinet in an atmosphere of high pressure oxygen (Fig. 23.7).

Ulceration

An ulcer is a gap in the skin or epithelial surface of an internal organ. It may arise from a simple injury or from chronic irritation—a dental ulcer on the tongue produced by a jagged tooth. Gangrene of the skin results in ulceration. Malignant disease of the skin produces a non-healing ulcer, **epithelioma**; a tumour beneath the skin may break through leading to secondary ulceration. Ulcers in internal organs—stomach, bowel, bladder— may be inflammatory, infective or malignant. Whatever the cause of an ulcer, symptoms are produced by seepage of serum, bleeding from erosion of blood vessels, and pain from exposure of nerves with inflammation of surrounding tissue. Because of the uncertainty of the cause of ulcers, biopsy is often required.

Tissue restoration by grafting

The great risk and difficulty in tissue grafting is that the cells of the graft are called upon to live on a very low supply of oxygen during the period required for new blood vessels to grow into the graft from the tissues round about. During that interval of lowered vitality, the graft is very liable to infection. Since the introduction of antibiotics and other means of controlling infection, many new forms of tissue grafting have been made possible, while the well established techniques of skin grafting have become much more extensive (Chapter 49).

The various forms of grafting are described in the appropriate chapters.

The introduction of chemically stable metals (e.g. vitallium), and 'plastics' opened a new field of 'replacement surgery'. Metallic and plastic joints are now a practical proposition to replace joints wrecked by arthritis, and diseased arteries are replaced by woven Terylene and Dacron tubes.

The replacement of damaged or lost skin by healthy skin removed from other parts of the body is commonplace and a procedure which forms part of the routine treatment in accident units. Skin grafting is by no means confined to plastic surgical centres and the general surgeon may be called upon at any time to cut skin grafts to bridge the gaps left in the treatment of malignant or other disease. Bone is similarly grafted from one part of the body to another in the repair of fractures or to fix joints which have become painful or unstable. Damaged sections of nerves are sometimes replaced by using healthy sections of less-important nerves. Tendons may be transplanted to alter the function of muscles.

In all these instances the grafted tissue is an **'autograft'** (*auto* = self). Autografting of blood vessels is undertaken occasionally, a vein being used to replace a vital diseased or damaged artery, but more commonly the arterial grafts are obtained from other human beings who have died as a result of accidents or from some non-communicable disease. The cornea obtained from the healthy eye of a person recently dead is used to restore the sight of patients blinded by corneal scarring. When the transplanted tissue comes from another human being—in other words there is a donor—it is described as **homogenous** (*homo* = same, *genus* = species). **Heterogenous** grafting is a process by which tissues of one species are planted successfully in an animal of a different species (*heteros* = other). Although this is sometimes successful in research experiments there is yet very little application to human surgery. Valves from a pig's heart have been used to replace human heart valves. This can be successful because the valves are made of fibrous tissue which produces very little rejection reaction. The dead tissues of animals are of course used in the form of catgut (from sheep's intestines).

In some instances the living tissue from the donor's homograft becomes part of the living tissue of the recipient. This is so in the case of the cornea which is nourished by tissue fluid and has no direct blood supply.

Table 4   Common examples of tissues used for grafting are:

Tissue	Donor site	When used
Skin (p. 952)	Any area of matching colour	Following burns or skin loss from injury
Bone (p. 928)	Tibia; iliac crest	Un-united fractures; arthrodesis in arthritis (e.g. tuberculous)
Tendon (p. 927)	Palmaris in forearm; plantaris in leg	Tendon injury; paralysis (e.g. leprosy)
Cornea (p. 844)	From the recently dead	To replace scarred cornea
Arteries (p. 941)	From the recently dead (or synthetic tubes)	To replace blocked arteries or to by-pass obstruction or aneurysm
Intestine (pp. 500, 685)	Small bowel or colon	To replace oesophagus, ureter, or bladder

Other tissues which are transplanted, such as arteries, never become part of the living structure of the recipient patient but merely act as temporary scaffolding which serves the function of the replaced tissue. This scaffolding is gradually invaded by the tissues of the host and surrounded by fibrous tissue.

Live sections of endocrine glands including the ovary and adrenal have been transplanted from one human being to another and the grafted tissue has continued its normal function of producing a hormone. In recent years many attempts have been made to establish the grafting of whole organs from one person to another. Each individual has specific chemicals in his cells which clash with those of every other individual. The exception to this is a pair of identical twins and successful kidney transplantation has been achieved from one twin to the other.

Organ transplantation

The transfer of living tissue from one individual to another (**homograft**) depends not only upon an adequate blood supply being picked up from the recipient body, but is affected by what is known as the **graft** *versus* **host reaction**. Just as an individual develops immunity to particular infections so he becomes immune to different proteins introduced to his body from outside. The donor tissue acts as an **antigen** and the natural immunological mechanism which the body of the host possesses rejects the grafted tissue just as it deals with bacterial infection. The leucocytes in the blood are probably the main agents responsible for the immunity reaction and the cornea survives as a homograft because in its new site it is not in contact with blood vessels but is nourished by the fluid in the eye.

Various methods of controlling this immune response have been introduced with considerable success. It is possible to suppress the body's response by total body irradiation, or by the use of cytotoxic drugs (page 434) which depress the activity and multiplication of the body's leucocytes. These methods necessarily lower the patient's resistance to infection. In the early days of renal transplantation the patient had to be nursed under very special bacteria-free conditions. Many of these problems have now been overcome through a better understanding of what is known as tissue specificity. As individuals have blood groups so they have tissue types. The success of heart-transplant operations has been due to the effective tissue typing of host and donor so that the two can be matched as far as possible and tissue-type reference centres are being established to enable donor and recipient to be matched. The particulars of patients awaiting kidney transplants are filed in a computer bank. When a donor kidney becomes available, the 'bank' is notified and the patient with the most compatible tissues is called. In Europe, matching is now international and donor organs are transported by air if necessary to the transplant centre.

Nevertheless in spite of all the advances in homografting, particularly in kidney transplantation, there is no universally successful method of preventing the rejection of a grafted organ. With improvements in vascular surgery the actual technique of coupling up the arteries and veins of donor organs to the recipient's blood vessels is now not a major problem, but there is no method of reconnecting the sympathetic or other nerve supply of transplanted organs.

Prosthesis

This term is applied to a structure or material used as a substitute for human tissue or organ. A prosthesis may be composed of synthetic material such as stainless steel, vitallium, Teflon or Dacron. In recent years silicone rubber has been used extensively because it produces no tissue reaction, and is therefore tolerated by the body. Modelled portions of this material are used to build up the contour of a nose, or chin which has been damaged by disease or accident. In cosmetic surgery silicone is injected into the area of the breast to build up the bust contour. Artificial fallopian tubes, parts of the external ear and finger joints are also being made of this material. As all these substances are in fact dead they have no natural ability to kill bacteria and any organisms circulating in the blood stream may therefore be attracted to such a buried substance in the body and set up a nidus of infection. This happens from time to time in the little valves used for the management of hydrocephalus (page 854). Artificial limbs, eyes and wigs are prostheses, but as these are not implanted in the tissue there is no rejection problem. Sometimes, however, there is an allergic reaction by the skin to a particular synthetic material.

4

Inflammation

The process by which tissues respond to injury or infection is known as **inflammation**. The term arose of course as a graphic description of the 'fieriness' of the tissues in this condition. Everyone is familiar with classical symptoms and signs of inflammation. It is important to realise that the tissues respond both to injury and infection in a similar manner, although the response to infection is usually more dramatic and accompanied by a greater general effect on the patient. Infection and inflammation are not synonymous. Inflammation arising from injury alone, repeated over a long period of time, is illustrated by the condition 'housemaid's knee' (Fig. 4.1): this can be secondarily infected.

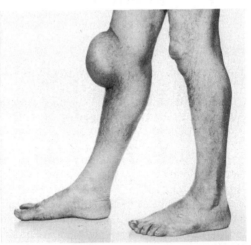

Fig. 4.1 Chronic trauma—pre-patella bursitis. 'Housemaid's knee', an occupational disorder in carpet and floor fitters; also in miners who wear special knee protectors. Constant minor injury and friction enlarge the natural bursa. A bunion and an olecranon bursa arise similarly from friction and pressure.

The underlying change in inflamed tissue is the great increase in the amount of blood flowing into the area involved. The chemicals released by the damaged tissues produce dilatation of the arteries, veins and capillaries to such an extent that serum exudes from the capillaries into the tissues, producing **oedema**. This distension of the tissues with fluid—the inflammatory exudate—is the main factor producing pain in inflammation. Pain and swelling together result in loss of function. This local inflammatory reaction is the beginning of the healing process and is at the same time a means of defence against infection. White blood cells appear at the site of inflammation in great numbers and are responsible for the local control of bacteria which may have gained entrance. The invading organisms or the poisons which they have produced are carried away from the site of inflammation, partly by the veins and partly by the lymphatic system. As infection travels up the lymphatic vessels, these too become involved in the inflammatory process (**lymphangitis**). The lymph glands to which these lymphatics drain will become similarly inflamed, large and tender (**lymphadenitis**).

Where there has been injury without infection, in addition to the local reaction (inflammation), poisonous substances are released from the damaged tissues and these circulate in the blood stream, producing a general effect on the whole body which may become a state of shock (pages 43 and 114). A collection of blood in the tissues following an injury is a **haematoma**. This undergoes a clotting process making a solid lump unless the blood is withdrawn through a needle before clotting takes place.

The nurse needs to know the early symptoms and signs of inflammation so that the process may be detected and 'arrested' if it is occurring as a complication of surgery. The development of pain, or a change in the character of pain already present, especially if throbbing develops, is almost always the first symptom of which the patient complains. This pain may only be present when the tissues are touched—that is 'tenderness'. At this stage in the superficial tissues, inflammation will produce reddening of the overlying skin. As the process advances, the skin itself becomes thickened by oedema; pressure with a finger on the reddened area will produce temporary blanching and will leave a little depression where the oedema fluid has been squeezed from the tissues (**pitting**).

The course of inflammation

Aseptic inflammation—that is resulting from injury without infection—usually subsides within a few days, and if there has been destruction of tissue the processes of repair proceed without interruption. If a haematoma has formed and clotted, a digestive enzyme in the tissues, **fibrinolysin**, works on the clot and makes it fluid again; a small amount of blood is absorbed into the tissues but a larger collection will need evacuating by excision or aspiration, and forms a very ready focus for infection with a subsequent formation of an abscess (Figs. 2.3 and 4.2). If on the other hand there is infection, much depends on the general resistance of the body, and the precise nature of the organism which has gained entry. Chemical irritation of the tissues (as, for instance, by urine leakage, or injection of an irritant drug) produces prolonged inflammation; infection may gain entry to the tissues thus devitalised.

The word-ending '**-itis**' indicates inflammation which is usually, but not always, infective in origin. Thus cellu**litis** merely means inflammation of the connective tissue of the body. The term is incorrectly assumed by some to mean a specific condition of streptococcal infection of the subcutaneous tissue, akin to **erysipelas**.

Erysipelas is in fact an infection of the skin due to a highly contagious haemolytic streptococcus. It may occur as a specific condition or as a complication of infection in a wound. The area affected is bright red and very painful; it often occurs on the face.

Severe inflammation is already established in many conditions by the time the patient first seeks advice. The inflammatory process, and the complications which may result as it progresses, need to be fully understood.

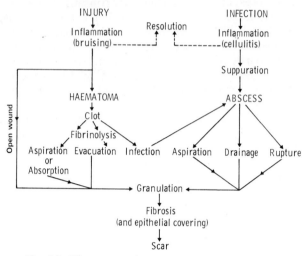

Fig. 4.2   The process of repair of injury and infection.

Resolution. If the power of the infecting germs is low, the natural resistance of the patient high, and the degree of local injury is slight, then the infection may be rapidly controlled by the body's own resources without any treatment: the inflammatory process is reversed, the swelling subsides, the redness disappears and function returns. This recovery process is '**resolution**' (Fig. 4.2). Our aim from the medical and nursing point of view is that all inflammatory processes should end in this way. If the cause of the inflammation is non-infective and infection does not gain access through an open wound, resolution follows as soon as the cause is removed. Extravasation of urine is a good example of this (page 632).

Suppuration. If the invading organisms are more virulent they grow in the inflammatory exudate and some of the surrounding tissue dies. The collection of fluid which results is heavily laden with bacteria, dead white cells, and the remains of tissue cells digested by the infection. This infected fluid is 'pus' and a collection of **pus** in the tissues, frequently walled off by a firm layer of the inflammation, is an '**abscess**'.

Infective gangrene. All tissues depend upon oxygen carried in the blood for their survival. If the blood supply is cut off the cells will die. When inflammation reaches the small arteries, these vessels undergo thrombosis (Chapter 5). Thus as the process of inflammation spreads, areas of the tissue involved may die from lack of oxygen before the infection actually reaches them. This process is known as 'gangrene' and has been referred to already (page 34). The area of dead tissue is described as 'slough' (pronounced 'sluff').

When suppuration or gangrene has occurred, the pus and dead tissue need to be removed. This may happen spontaneously by an abscess bursting on the surface of the body or a surgical operation may be necessary for the removal of the dead tissue or for the drainage of an abscess. Then follows the formation of granulation tissue and the normal process of repair (Fig. 3.1 and page 31).

Sinus and fistula. These terms are used to describe a track leading from a deep area of the body on to the surface. A 'sinus' is usually the result of some deep persistent infection. The presence of a foreign body, such as a metallic particle, may prevent an abscess from healing and the track which leads from the foreign particle to the surface is a sinus. 'Fistula' is used to describe a track leading from a hollow organ on to the surface of the body or into another organ (Fig. 4.3). A fistula is also frequently infected.

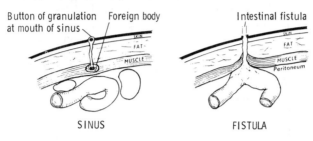

Button of granulation   Foreign body   Intestinal fistula
at mouth of sinus

SINUS   FISTULA

Fig. 4.3   Sinus and fistula.

An example of a common internal fistula is that which arises from '**diverticulitis**' of the large bowel. The inflamed pocket in the bowel wall becomes adherent to the bladder cavity. This is a 'vesico-colic' fistula and of course the urine becomes grossly infected. Such a fistula will not heal without surgical intervention to separate the two organs and overcome the infection.

Allergy

Sensitivity of an individual to substances foreign to his body produces an inflammatory reaction and in many cases the development of antibodies (page 38). Allergy to certain antiseptics, drugs and dressings (such as adhesive strapping) produces a local inflammation similar to injury or infection. Sometimes a local reaction may lead to blister formation and secondary infection and a general reaction may occur as well (see below). Treatment is with antihistamine drugs and local antihistamine creams.

The general reaction of the body to inflammation

After a severe **injury**, substances arising from damaged tissues are absorbed into the blood stream and have a general effect on the patient. This contributes to the development of oligaemic shock (page 110) and will not be further discussed here.

The general response of the body to inflammation arising from **infection** is of course entirely different. The degree of general disturbance depends more on the potency of the infecting germ, than on the size or severity of the local reaction. A very large abscess due to a 'weak' infection may produce far less constitutional disturbance than a very small streptococcal whitlow. If infection occurs in the deep-seated areas of the body, such as in the liver or kidney, the diagnosis is made principally upon the general reaction of the body rather than on the local examination of the inflamed area.

Malaise ('not feeling very well'), headache, loss of appetite and perhaps shivering are the early symptoms of infection. The observant nurse, by recognising these, may be able to avert the development of serious infection following surgical operation. Pyrexia and increase of pulse rate are the early signs, together with sweating and restlessness. Sweating is often severe and the patient rapidly becomes dehydrated. The urine becomes concentrated and the patient thirsty.

Suppuration is usually detected by the onset of a swinging temperature—the so-called 'hectic chart'—in which the temperature is sub-normal in the morning and rises to a variable degree in the evening.

Fig. 4.4 is the temperature record of a woman with acute mastitis following childbirth. In the first few days of acute inflammation, the temperature had risen to 39 °C (102 °F) and the breast was swollen and extremely painful. In spite of the use of penicillin,

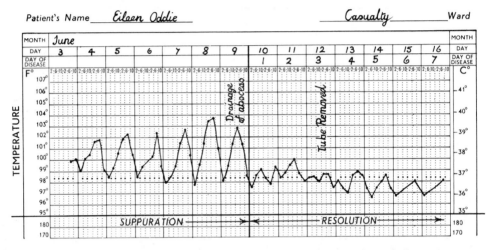

Patient's Name __Eileen Oddie__   __Casualty__   Ward

Fig. 4.4 Acute infective mastitis with abscess formation. The swinging temperature indicates the presence of pus under pressure (see text).

the infection was not controlled and pus formation occurred with the development of a large breast abscess. The onset of this suppuration was indicated by the gradual increase in the swing of the morning/evening temperature. The examination of the breast to detect 'fluctuation'—the sign of a collection of fluid—was prevented by extreme pain, so that the change in the temperature chart was the main indication that an abscess had formed. Drainage of the abscess relieved the condition and the temperature rapidly subsided.

The nursing management of inflammation

Because of the dramatic response of many infective conditions to modern drug treatment, the traditional special nursing methods have been largely eliminated. Before the introduction of the sulpha drugs and penicillin, the management of acute infections, such as cellulitis of the arm or a septic finger, was a highly skilled and exacting task involving the general care of a very ill patient and the local treatment of his inflamed tissues. Such grave conditions still arise occasionally when an infection does not respond to specific drug therapy. The principles involved in the management of inflammation follow the general pattern outlined in Chapter 2 and should be applied to a greater or less extent in every case until the response to specific drug treatment is known.

Rest. Inflamed tissues require rest and this can only be achieved by immobilisation. Infective conditions of the arm and hand require a sling if the patient is ambulant. In the more severe conditions when he is confined to bed (Fig. 4.5), the arm may be suspended from an overhead bar or may be propped up by pillows; the purpose is to support the hand and forearm higher than the upper arm and axilla, thus promoting adequate lymphatic

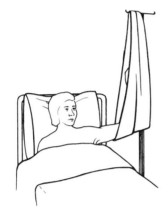

Rest is essential in the treatment of inflammation—the arm is elevated in a folded towel or sheet,

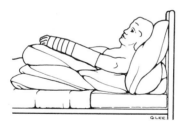

or on pillows so that the wrist is above the elbow and above the axilla.

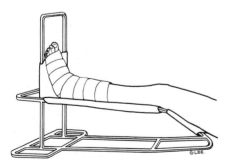

The leg is elevated on a Bohler frame to relax both calf and thigh muscles.

Fig. 4.5

drainage and preventing venous congestion. Similarly an inflamed or infected leg is protected from the weight of the bedclothes by means of a cradle from which the leg can be slung. This, or a splint, is usually more comfortable for the patient than having the leg elevated on pillows[1] (Fig. 4.5). Cellulitis and other infective conditions in the neck should similarly be splinted by placing the patient's head between sand-bags which anchor a folded towel across his forehead. An ambulant patient may be treated in a plaster-of-Paris cast to rest the soft tissues, even if there is no fracture.

Pyrexia—its effect and control. Both acute and chronic infective conditions produce some degree of pyrexia. This is part of the body's defence mechanism and is associated with a speeding-up of the general metabolism. The increase of tissue activity is shown by increased need of oxygen which in turn leads to a rise in pulse rate. There is an abnormal consumption of calories and a need for an increased energy value in the diet. During a fever of short duration, the body draws on its food reserves and the calorie value of the diet is of little or no importance. If, however, fever is prolonged more than three or four days, the administration of food with sufficient nutrient value, or of intravenous glucose, is essential. On general principles, therefore, illnesses accompanied by fever create a need for a high-calorie diet.

A 'rigor' is an attempt by the body to generate heat from muscle action to counteract the sudden fall in temperature that sometimes occurs in severe infections. A patient with a rigor therefore needs to be kept warm to lessen the violent muscle activity which is attempting to raise the body temperature.

The fever and increased metabolism due to infection produce, in turn, an abnormal loss of fluid by sweating. This is the natural attempt of the body to reduce its temperature to a normal level, but sometimes in severe infections the temperature control mechanism is damaged and the patient's skin remains quite dry. If the temperature rises above 39·5°C (103°F), tepid sponging frequently makes the patient more comfortable and in fact may be essential to prevent death from heat-stroke. It depends for its effectiveness upon the evaporation of water from the body surface. It cannot therefore be done in a hurry and its effect is completely lost if the patient is covered with blankets.

Excessive sweating, produced partly by the toxaemia and partly by the body's attempt to reduce its temperature, aided by the use of too many bedclothes is dangerous in that it produces dehydration. The correct state to achieve is that the patient's skin should be moist, but the sweating should never be sufficient for 'beads of perspiration' to appear on the patient's face. Sweating also results in excessive chloride (salt) loss, and this needs to be made good in the diet or in some cases by infusion. Dehydration in severe infections increases the risk of a patient going into a state of shock.

Diet. It has already been mentioned that the increased metabolism due to fever results in an increased calorie requirement which must be made good by additions to the food. The diet of a febrile patient should be easily digested and yet have a high calorie content. Vitamin supplement is necessary, including vitamins A, B, C, and D. Particular attention must be paid to the fluid balance. Many surgical patients in whom infection has occurred will already be on measured fluid intake and output because of the intrinsic nature of their condition or recent operation. If, however, infection supervenes in a case not on 'fluid balance', the necessary records must immediately be initiated. In cases of prolonged fever

---

[1] A small table or stool placed on the bed will serve the same purpose in the patient's home.

such as occur with deep-seated infection (e.g. subphrenic abscess, pyelonephritis), not only should there be a fluid balance chart, but there should be a calorie record chart on which is recorded the amount of food and other nourishment such as intravenous glucose actually *consumed* by the patient each day. It is of course completely useless to record the amount of food which has been taken to the patient's bedside if some of it is not eaten. The protein value of the diet must also be high to replace the tissue protein which is being destroyed.

Sedation. Inflammation produces pain. Fever produces restlessness. Sweating produces discomfort. Rest and satisfactory sleep is of supreme importance both psychologically and physically and there should be no hesitation in the use of drugs to aid sleep. If the simple mixtures containing aspirin or phenacetin are used it must be remembered that these drugs also reduce temperature. Their use brings great benefit but will produce a misleading temperature record and it is an advantage if the administration of such drugs is indicated on the temperature chart. In carrying out the other treatments for an infective condition—local drugs, etc.—the nurse must bear in mind that the treatment should be so organised that the patient may have the longest possible periods of rest.

Local treatment of inflamed area. Distinction must again be made between the inflammation due to injury and that due to infection. In the former, the reaction is due to chemicals released by the injury; these are not increasing in amount but tend to be absorbed: all that is required is to encourage this absorption and relieve discomfort: cold compresses or simple immobilisation are alone sufficient. In infective inflammation the bacteria are constantly increasing the amount of local tissue poison and the objective of treatment is to increase the blood supply and therefore the defensive cells and antibodies, and to increase the lymphatic drainage to aid absorption of oedema. In other words, to imitate nature's reaction.

For centuries heat has been regarded as essential in the relief of inflammation. Time-honoured methods include poultices and radiant heat lamps. It is very doubtful whether the local application of heat does anything to help the tissues overcome infection. Whatever arguments there may be against the use of heat, there is no doubt that the patient is usually comforted. It has to be remembered that the inflamed tissues already have an increased blood supply and are therefore hotter than the surrounding tissues. Very little can be achieved by the application of *hot* poultices, though one has occasionally been convinced of the benefit of the classic hot fomentation. From the point of view of the patient's comfort, all that is required may be achieved by enclosing the inflamed area in an insulating material which will prevent the loss of natural heat from the body. This is much simpler and just as effective as adding heat in the form of a poultice, which must in any case cool to body temperature within a very few minutes. Cold kaolin is therefore as effective as hot kaolin and it is also common experience that cold compresses do perhaps just as much to relieve the pain of inflammation as hot applications. The use of deep heat derived from electrical apparatus such as infra-red lamps and ultra short-wave diathermy, is prescribed for specific purposes, and such treatment should never be administered by a nurse.

Counter-irritation is another method of producing an increase in the 'local heat'. A chemical is applied to the surface of the body and by its irritation produces dilatation of the skin vessels and thus an increase in blood supply. Embrocations, liniments, and certain of the substances, such as oil of wintergreen which are included in kaolin poultice, act in this way when applied to the skin; counter-irritants are also thought to increase the blood supply to the deep tissues by a nerve reflex. Probably the massage employed in rubbing in the liniment is in fact the main benefit.

Historically the process known as 'wet cupping' was used to produce counter-irritation in the hope of 'drawing out' the inflammation. Tiny cuts were made in the skin with a spring-loaded brass instrument with multiple blades. A heated glass cup was then placed over the cut area, and as it cooled it sucked out tissue fluid and blood (Fig. 4.6). Without scarification of the skin the procedure was 'dry cupping'.

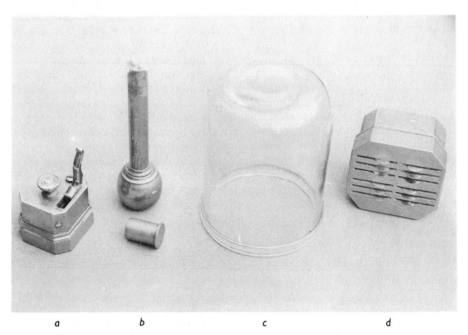

| a | b | c | d |

Fig. 4.6 'Cupping' set. (*a*) Small cutter, with spring setting lever. (*b*) Spirit lamp for heating glass cup. (*c*) Large cup. (*d*) Large cutter—twelve blades which spring out and across the slots very fast when the release button on the side is pressed.

The use of antiseptics. The spread of infection in the tissues cannot be controlled by the local application of any form of antiseptic. On the other hand, bacteria on the surface of the body, in an ulcer or in an abscess cavity, can be killed by the application of a suitable antiseptic. Antibiotics (particularly penicillin) and sulpha drugs are used for injection into the tissues, instillation into abscess cavities or for application to ulcers. Other antiseptic substances are of little use for this purpose because they are too destructive and damage the delicate granulation tissue or healthy young epithelium. Mild antiseptic substances such as noxytiolin (Noxyflex) and dilute povidone iodine are used in the urethra, bladder and vagina. Dettol (chloroxylenol) and chlorhexidine (Hibitane) are used also for their surface effect. Stronger antiseptics such as a liquor iodi mitis BP, povidone iodine, or spirit are used to clean the skin around a discharging sinus, abscess or boil. Here, however, the antiseptic is used both to prevent the entry of other organisms from the surrounding skin into the open wound and partly to prevent the discharge infecting the surrounding skin.

The local surface application of an antiseptic forms the major treatment in a number of skin conditions such as impetigo and tinea pedis (athlete's foot). Antibiotic powders (neomycin, polymyxin) are used in aerosol form (Fig. 7.6).

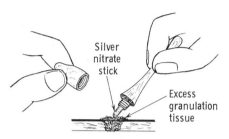

Silver
nitrate
stick

Excess
granulation
tissue

Fig. 4.7   Cauterising excessive granulation tissue in an ulcer or at the mouth of a sinus.

The management of suppuration. The pus which forms in an open infected wound will discharge freely on the surface. The cavity of a wound should never be 'packed' but gauze should only be laid lightly in the cavity to prevent the edges joining together before sufficient healing has taken place in the base of the wound. Pus must be allowed to escape and must not be kept in by plugging. Similarly, gauze applied over a discharging wound should be fluffed up so that its absorbing power is increased. It must never be applied in its folded flat state. When the dressing is changed, the surrounding skin should be cleaned with an antiseptic which will not damage the tissue and for this purpose cetrimide 2 per cent with chlorhexidine 1 : 1000 (Savlon or Cetrex) is perhaps the best. The cleansing should be done with small balls of cotton wool held in a pair of non-toothed dressing forceps.

An abscess may form from infection of fluid already present (e.g. haematoma, cyst), or cellulitis may proceed to tissue necrosis and pus formation.

When pus has accumulated in the tissues and formed an abscess, drainage by surgical incision through the overlying tissues is the usual treatment. Under certain circumstances the contents of an abscess may be aspirated through a wide-bore needle by means of an ordinary 20-ml syringe. A large collection of pus such as occurs in empyema thoracis (page 613) is more conveniently aspirated with a special syringe using a three-way adaptor: this eliminates the need for repeated disconnection of the syringe from the needle. Very thick pus, such as occurs in tuberculous abscesses, requires a specially powerful syringe and wide-bore needle or trocar. The Gauvain syringe was designed for this purpose in treating psoas abscesses arising from tuberculous spinal disease.

When a surgical incision has been made into an abscess cavity and the pus evacuated, it is usually necessary to take steps to prevent the skin edges (probably healthy tissue) from healing together before the cavity of the abscess has been filled with granulation tissue. If surface healing takes place too rapidly, pus will again accumulate and further drainage will be necessary. The surgeon, therefore, after evacuating the abscess, passes into the cavity a strip of corrugated plastic or rubber, a length of rubber tubing, or sometimes a strip of disused rubber glove material. He may be content to leave a strip of ribbon gauze in the wound as a wick. Tube drains are invariably stitched to the skin edge by one suture and a sterile safety-pin is sometimes inserted into the projecting end to minimise the risk of the drain disappearing into the abscess cavity. It is the nurse's duty to know exactly what has happened to a drainage tube, or to drainage gauze. There is no absolute rule about how long a drainage tube should be left in an abscess cavity and the surgeon will normally give instructions about its removal. The usual procedure with an abscess, occurring for instance in the breast, is for the 'tube' to be left undisturbed for two days; if there is then only a slight discharge, its anchoring suture is removed and the tube shortened by withdrawing it, cutting off the outside 1 inch (2·5 cm) and replacing the safety-pin. The shortening process is repeated every two days if the amount of discharge is decreasing and if the patient's temperature has settled. If a drainage tube is left in position too long, healing will be delayed. If it is removed too soon, the infection will persist and a sinus will result; the wound may close over too rapidly and produce a recurrence of the abscess.

After suppuration, the repairing granulation tissue may be excessive and protrude from the former site of the drainage tube as a button of moist flesh. This excessive granulation tissue is cauterised by a silver nitrate stick (Fig. 4.7) so that the epithelium from the surrounding edge may grow over to complete the healing. If the abscess has been a deep one, the sinus may persist for several weeks while the cavity and drainage tract are being obliterated. Usually the persistence of a sinus means that there is dead tissue or perhaps a retained foreign body in the depth of the wound (Fig. 4.3). For instance a knot of chromic catgut or silk will keep an infected abdominal wound discharging for weeks. This complication is seen when a discharging sinus forms over an area of unhealed osteomyelitis in which there is a sequestrum (page 925).

Recovery of function after inflammation

Whether the site of inflammation has been in a limb or in an internal organ, the recovery of function may often be delayed for weeks or months. When the acute phase of the inflammation has passed, whether it has been due to infection or injury, active movement of the infected limb must be encouraged as soon as possible. This applies particularly to affections of the fingers and feet. There is very little that can be done towards restoring the function of inflamed internal organs except to realise that the process may be slow, and therefore an appropriate limitation must be placed on the patient's diet and general activity. Food must be tasty and attractive.

Patients who have been ill with infections, especially if they have had severe pain, may have lost their morale and self-confidence. Encouragement is an essential part of the nurse's daily duty, but this must always be accompanied by sympathy.

The anti-inflammatory action of cortisone

This hormone is one of the 'steroid' group of chemicals produced naturally by the suprarenal glands. In severe infections and in shock there is over-activity of the suprarenal with sometimes excess cortisone production which masks inflammatory response and lowers resistance to infection. The patient's metabolism and blood chemistry go wrong and collapse may follow. As the synthetic hormone is used extensively in the treatment of rheumatism, advanced carcinoma of the breast, ulcerative colitis and other diseases, patients being so treated do not show the normal response to infection: the inflammatory response is suppressed and an overwhelming spread of infection may occur. Any patient undergoing treatment with cortisone and allied drugs must be warned to report any feeling of illness such as colds or abdominal pain, and must be warned always to report his previous treatment to any doctor under whose care he comes. If prolonged treatment is stopped abruptly sudden collapse may ensue.

For instance, a patient receiving cortisone for arthritis developed gangrenous appendicitis and peritonitis with practically no pain. Operation was undertaken, and cortisone was not given because in the emergency she did not tell the hospital that she was having treatment; she collapsed in a state of extreme shock after operation under general anaesthetic. Patients receiving steroid treatment must be given an 'identity' card to hand to any doctor or hospital in case of urgent treatment being needed so as to avoid such a calamity.

Boil and carbuncle

A boil (**furuncle**) is an abscess of a hair follicle, produced by infection with a staphylococcus. The abscess and central core usually discharge through a hole at the site of extrusion of the hair. Healing is by granulation tissue.

A **carbuncle** is a similar but more severe infection usually by staphylococcus or streptococcus or both together, involving a group of hair follicles. The tissue between the infected

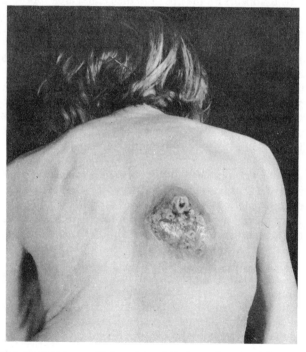

Fig. 4.8   Large carbuncle showing multiple points of discharge in a necrotic area over the lower ribs. There was a loss of full thickness of skin and fat from an area 6 × 6 cm. A split-skin graft was necessary.

follicles dies because of interference with its blood supply. This area of gangrene gradually separates as the 'core' or slough. A carbuncle, if it is not treated with penicillin or some equally effective anti-bacterial agent, may be several centimetres in diameter and the tissue loss involves the whole thickness of the skin. A carbuncle, before the introduction of the antibiotics and sulpha drugs, was an extremely painful and sometimes fatal condition. The management of such a lesion now consists of the general management of inflammation, local cleanliness and antiseptic application to the skin together with the administration of the anti-bacterial drug.

Boils should never be squeezed and considerable relief from pain is usually achieved by placing over the boil a disc of Elastoplast to extend at least one inch (2·5 cm) beyond the edge of the infected area. No dressing is placed underneath this adhesive which is changed when it becomes contaminated by discharge. Cleanliness is vital to prevent the infection entering other hair follicles. The axilla is a common area for such recurrent boils and antiseptic ointment is advisable to prevent re-infection.

Syphilis and gonorrhoea

Infection by the **spirochaeta pallida** (syphilis) or by the **Neisserian gonococcus** (gonorrhoea), occur as the result of sex contact with infected persons: these conditions are normally treated in special centres. The initial stage of syphilis is a **'chancre'** which resembles a large infected wart. It appears on the lips or in the genital area, but frequently this stage of the disease is overlooked and heals spontaneously. **Primary syphilis,** as this stage is called, may then pass unnoticed. The **secondary** stage lasts for several weeks and is characterised by rashes and ulcerative lesions in the mouth. This stage also may be overlooked and if treatment is not instituted the patient will develop **tertiary syphilis** of which there are various manifestations. One is the development of a syphilitic tumour or **gumma** which breaks down and produces an ulcer—gummatous ulcer. Tertiary syphilis also affects the nervous system, producing **tabes dorsalis** (locomotor ataxia). In this condition the victim develops degenerative changes in the joints (Charcot's joints)[1] and perforating ulcers in the feet. The presence of latent syphilitic infection is of great importance in surgery because it prevents the healing of wounds and the infection so often simulates other diseases such as carcinoma.

The child of an infected mother may be born with **congenital syphilis** which shows itself during the first two or three years of life in special changes which affect the child's bones, liver and eyes.

Gonorrhoea affects mainly the urinary tract producing urethritis, cystitis and infections of the uterine tube (**salpingitis**) in the woman and of the epididymis (**epididymitis**) in the man. Sometimes these initial infections also are overlooked and chronic inflammation occurring in the female genital tract, or producing stricture in the male urethra, is frequently the result of untreated gonorrhoea. Urethral or vaginal discharge is almost always examined bacteriologically for gonococcal infection.

Syphilis and gonorrhoea can both be contracted by doctors or nursing staff treating such patients since the lesions produced by these infections are extremely contagious. A cut or a prick on the finger sustained during an operation on a patient who has syphilis

---

[1] Charcot's joints also develop in other diseases of the nervous system when the sensory side in particular is affected. Gross painless arthritis and dislocation results.

may produce the disease in the surgeon. The eyes are particularly sensitive to the gono-coccus, and gonorrhoeal conjunctivitis may be contracted if the attendant's hands are not adequately washed after dealing with catheters or other things which may have been contaminated. Both these organisms are very sensitive to exposure to air and the risk of the infection being passed from one person to another by the use of toilets or bathrooms is almost negligible.

Gout

This is a metabolic disorder in which the amount of uric acid in the body is much higher than normal. The chemical becomes deposited in soft tissues as a chalky substance. It is an example of inflammation without infection. The ears, the fingers and the elbows are typical sites for these **tophi**. In the chronic form bones and joints become involved, pro-ducing gouty arthritis. Renal colic due to uric acid stones is common.

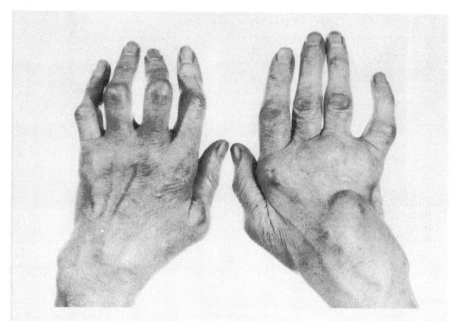

Fig. 4.9   These hands are severely affected by gout around the joints and in the soft tissues of the wrist.

The disease also occurs in an acute form frequently attacking the big toe joints. There is intense pain and the foot becomes bright red, swollen and very tender. Gout can also affect soft tissues of the limbs, bringing about a condition which is in fact chemical cellulitis often confused with phlebitis or infective cellulitis. Acute gout is treated with colchicum 0·5 mg given hourly until the patient is nauseated or develops diarrhoea; up to twelve tablets may be used but relief is dramatic. Phenylbutazone is also effective. The presence of gout appearing as a first attack is confusing if the patient is in hospital for some other condition. Chronic gout is treated with probenecid which greatly aids the elimination of uric acid in the urine. Gout sufferers are usually advised to adopt a milk and vegetarian diet.

Immunisation and antitoxins in surgery

Many organisms when they gain entry into the body provoke a response of the defence mechanisms which results in the production of antibodies. These substances are either antitoxic or antibacterial. Certain organisms liberate a poison (exo-toxin) which is directly neutralised by the antitoxin in the patient's serum. Other organisms are attacked directly by anti-bacterial substances constantly being manufactured in the body. There are many diseases against which the body gains a prolonged protection as the result of a single attack of that particular infection. Poliomyelitis is an example of this process of **acquired natural active immunity**. In some conditions the active immunity is lifelong as in the case of polio-myelitis, and in others it only lasts for a few weeks. For instance, erysipelas may result in

Table 5. Immunisation

Disease	Preparation used for passive immunisation	Preparation used for active artificial immunisation
Smallpox		Calf lymph vaccine (virus of cowpox)
Diphtheria	Horse serum antitoxin	Toxoid (toxin from bacteria)
Poliomyelitis		Vaccine (virus)
Tetanus	Horse or human serum antitoxin	Toxoid
Pertussis (whooping cough)		Vaccine (bacteria)
Typhoid and paratyphoid		Vaccine (bacteria)
Tuberculosis		Vaccine (bacteria) (BCG)
Gas gangrene	Horse serum antitoxin	
Measles	Gamma globulin (or serum from convalescent measles patient)	Vaccine (virus)
Influenza		Vaccine (virus)
Yellow fever		Vaccine (virus)
Cholera		Vaccine (bacteria)
Rabies	Serum	Vaccine (virus)

the development of antibodies in the patient's blood which will prevent him developing another lesion from infection by that particular streptococcus during several succeeding months. Immunity may not, however, be lasting.

Tetanus and gas gangrene

Two of the most dreaded infections are **tetanus** and **gas gangrene**, both of which are particularly liable to develop as the result of contamination of accidental wounds, especially those contaminated with soil. The 'anaerobic' organisms causing these infections produce spores which are particularly resistant to the usual forms of sterilisation by antiseptics, and they thrive in injured or dead tissue. Both these organisms can to some extent be controlled by artificially induced immunity. By an injection of a regulated amount of toxin derived from tetanus organisms, the body's defence mechanism can be stimulated so that the patient develops an acquired **active immunity** without having had the infection himself. Injections of tetanus 'toxoid' are used for this purpose to protect those particularly liable to injury—members of the armed forces, firemen and farm workers. If an individual who has not received such protection is injured in a road accident, he may be given artificial protection against the infection for a period of several weeks. This **passive immunity** is achieved by the use of antitoxic serum from a horse which has been immunised by receiving injections of toxoid. If he has been previously immunised he is given a 'boost' dose of toxoid after injury to stimulate his natural defences, but he does not require anti-tetanus serum (ATS) (Table 6).

Table 6 Anti-tetanus measures

ACCIDENTAL WOUND
|
Surgical Toilet
Removal of dead tissue

If the wound is clean with very little tissue damage	Severe wounds (all soil contaminated wounds; road and agricultural injuries; gunshot wounds)
Toxoid unless booster dose has been given within one year	If immunised previously by toxoid, booster dose and penicillin, or tetracycline for two weeks
If never immunised, further **toxoid** at six weeks	If **no** previous immunisation, **toxoid** plus antibiotic for four weeks and further toxoid at six weeks

Tetanus Antitoxin (i.e., passive immunity) is given only to high risk cases: contaminated wounds more than six hours old; war casualties; if injured tissues have poor blood supply (e.g. complicated by burns or arteriosclerosis). The dose is ATS 1500 international units by subcutaneous injection irrespective of age.
ATS must not be given if the patient has had it previously, or has asthma or other allergic disorders.

In the case of gas gangrene there is no known means of producing active immunity in the human being. The infection is due to a group of organisms and antitoxic horse serum is available to produce passive immunity in cases of injury. This serum is given in larger doses in the treatment of a case of established gas gangrene. The organisms are present in the bowel and any operation on the intestinal tract may be followed by gas gangrene of the abdominal wall.

Certain fractions of blood are known to contain defensive substances, or **antibodies**. Gamma globulin is one such fraction and this substance or serum from a patient who has already had measles, is sometimes used in a surgical ward to produce passive immunity in children if one of them has developed measles.

The spores of tetanus and gas-gangrene organisms are found from time to time in substances such as catgut (which is manufactured from sheep's intestines) and in packing materials such as cardboard. Particular care has to be taken, therefore, in the sterilisation of these items (Chapter 17).

Active immunity is acquired either by suffering from the disease or by being given an inoculation of the disease by injection of killed organisms or prepared toxin. Individuals can now be protected from poliomyelitis by injection of vaccine (dead organisms). To maintain a high level of immunity boost doses are given at long intervals.

Administration of serum. Antitoxic serum prepared from the blood of horses provokes in the human circulation the production of antibodies against the horse serum. Injection of the serum sometimes produces an allergic reaction, particularly in patients who have had serum on a previous occasion. It may be a mild reaction, or it may be dramatic and fatal in a matter of seconds. There is no certain way of avoiding reaction. Skin tests are unreliable. The usual safety measure is to inject 0·05 ml of the serum subcutaneously as a test dose and wait for thirty minutes. If this produces a marked swelling or shivering, or a rise of pulse rate, the rest of the serum should not be given. An injection of adrenaline and a syringe must always be immediately at hand. If there is an unexpected reaction 0·5 ml of adrenaline injection (1 in 1000 solution) is given to an adult immediately and repeated in five minutes. If a doctor is present a larger dose may be ordered. Sometimes an intravenous injection of 100 mg of hydrocortisone may be life-saving and this should be available wherever serum is used. The necessity for giving tetanus antitoxin to injured people can be avoided completely by protective immunisation of the whole population by means of toxoid, and ATS is in fact now only given to very few accident patients, reliance being placed on active immunity, thorough surgical toilet of wounds, and antibiotics to prevent the development of tetanus. Abnormal reaction to serum is 'serum sickness' or **anaphylactic shock**.

Septicaemia

In many bacterial infections living organisms circulate in the blood stream and are carried to other parts of the body where they produce local abscesses. This state of 'bacteraemia' is one of the causes of the general reaction to infection. If the circulating organisms multiply faster than the body defences can deal with them a clinical state of **septicaemia** is present. The patient has a high hectic fever (page 46) and is very ill. Abscesses may arise in the brain, lungs, liver and kidney (as shown by albumen or blood in the urine). Sometimes fragments of dead tissue and pus cells get into the blood vessels and make matters worse (pyaemia). If septicaemia is suspected a blood sample is taken for direct culture. Chronic septicaemia is sometimes seen, with little general reaction. This occurs usually when there is some persistent focus of infection in the body such as osteomyelitis or a chronic brain abscess. The patient becomes very anaemic with an abnormally high white blood count, evening temperature and chronic weight loss (page 115, bacteraemic shock).

Rabies

This virus infection attacks the nervous system and is transmitted to man by animals of the canine species—dogs, foxes or wolves. The virus is most frequently implanted in human tissues by a bite. Infection, however, may arise from a dog licking either a scratch or abrasion, or the lips of a child. Rabies is virtually non-existent in Great Britain having been stamped out by rigorous quarantine regulations, but in India for instance 150,000 persons bitten by infected animals seek treatment every year. At the time of the bite the dog may not necessarily be showing any symptoms of rabies (hydrophobia) and if the dog remains healthy for 10 days it is extremely unlikely that it will have been infected. The incubation period of the disease may be anything from 2 to 10 weeks depending on which part of the body has been bitten. The nearer the laceration is to the brain the sooner the disease starts, as the virus travels up the nerve trunks.

As with other injuries of this type, treatment is directed to local toilet of the wound, and if it is known that the animal that has inflicted the injury has rabies, the wound may be cauterised with nitric acid or an electric cautery. Such severe treatment is justified by the fact that the mortality even in treated cases may be as high as 25 per cent. It is this fear of rabies that has led to the traditional scare of all dog bites, but in fact in Great Britain a dog bite is no more serious an injury than a wound inflicted in other ways where soil may be a contaminant. The chief risk is tetanus.

In countries where rabies is endemic all dog bites are regarded as being potentially infected with rabies and an intensive system of treatment combining anti-rabies serum and vaccine giving both passive and active immunity is now the standard practice. Serum is also injected at the time of original wound toilet into the area of the bite. Vaccine injections have to be given daily and this automatically means the retention of the patient in hospital, or in a special centre in the underdeveloped countries where the disease is prevalent.

Perhaps the importance of the condition in Great Britain to-day lies in the fact that the incubation period is a long one and a great many people go for holidays abroad, travelling widely in areas where the disease may well be endemic

Veterinary surgeons and animal attendants who are at risk should have prophylactic inoculation with vaccine.

Symptoms. The clinical picture of rabies is characterised by high fever and violent pharyngeal spasms in which the patient is dyspnoeic, grips his throat and is unable to swallow. Drooling and grave distress, with staring eyes, accompany each spasm and the attacks are brought on by the slightest external stimulus such as noise or a draught. In contrast, the muscle spasm in tetanus is continuous and sustained and does not occur in attacks. Apart from the specific treatment with serum, tracheostomy is often required with full antibiotic treatment and heavy sedation.

5

The Principles of Blood Clotting and

Anticoagulant Therapy

In order to understand some of the complications of medical and surgical disease it is necessary to review the factors which lead to the formation of a blood clot. **Thrombosis** is the term which is used when clotting takes place inside a blood vessel, as distinct from the formation of a clot on the surface of the body, within a body cavity, or in blood which has been shed. During surgical operation or injury, when small blood vessels are cut across, bleeding is stopped partly by contraction of the muscular wall of the artery or vein, and finally by the blocking up of the tiny hole by formation of a clot. Only the larger vessels are tied with a ligature. Very deep anaesthesia, relaxant drugs (page 219) and certain poisons prevent this contraction of the blood vessels, and oozing in consequence may be very severe.

Mechanism of clot formation (Fig. 5.1)

The trigger which sets off the clotting of blood is a chemical substance which comes from damaged tissues or from blood platelets; this part of the process takes place only in the presence of calcium. Sufficient calcium is normally present in the blood to enable clotting to occur when the trigger substance (**thromboplastin**) is released from damaged tissues, or when the blood is shed. When we remove blood from a patient for a blood transfusion, sodium citrate is added to the blood collecting bottle and is thus mixed with the blood as it leaves the vein; this combines with the calcium in the blood and turns it into a compound which cannot take part in the clotting process. Thus we can store blood for long periods without clotting taking place. Similarly when blood is removed from the patient for certain chemical investigations the calcium is rendered inactive by the addition of oxalic acid contained in the tiny tubes used for the collection of specimens.

If we go further back in the process of blood clotting, we find that normally there are two substances (Fig. 5.1), **prothrombin** and **heparin,** both of which are manufactured by the liver and which exist side by side in the blood in such quantities that they cancel out one another's effects. The granules in the basophil white blood cells are probably heparin.

We can therefore prevent the clotting of blood by increasing the amount of heparin present or by decreasing the amount of prothrombin. Heparin is given intravenously and produces an immediate effect which is only transient: it needs to be given continuously or every six hours. Injected subcutaneously it is absorbed very slowly and is sometimes given twenty-four hours before operation to reduce the risk of thrombosis, and yet not impair the coagulability of the blood sufficiently to make haemostasis difficult. Daily injections may be repeated for the first post-operative week.

Prothrombin is formed by the liver from vitamin K absorbed from the bowel: vitamin K itself can be given by mouth but is probably manufactured normally in the intestine. When phenindione, or alternatively dicoumarol, is given by mouth it prevents the liver

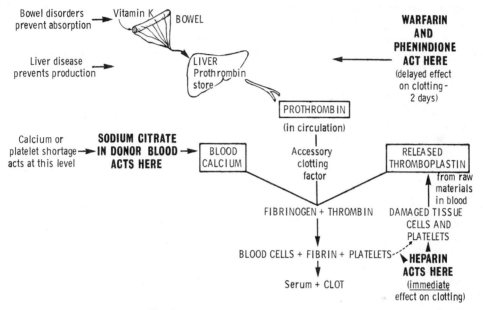

Fig. 5.1 Stages in the clotting of blood.

Table 7 Blood-clotting factors

Factor I	(Fibrinogen)
Factor II	(Prothrombin)
Factor III	(Thromboplastin)—tissue extract
Factor IV	(Calcium)
Factor V	(Proaccelerin)
Factor VII	(Proconvertin, SPCA)
Factor VIII	(Antihaemophilic factor) Cryoglobulin—isolated by freezing methods
Factor IX	(Plasma thromboplastin component—PTC)
Factor X	(Stuart-Prower factor)
Factor XI	(Plasma thromboplastin antecedent—PTA)
Factor XII	(Hageman factor)

Due to misinterpretation of certain experimental findings a factor number VI was given to a substance which subsequently was found not to exist as a special entity.

using vitamin K; it thus interferes with the manufacture of prothrombin, and its effect becomes apparent when the circulating prothrombin has been used up. Warfarin is therefore used as a slow and prolonged method of reducing the clotting power of the blood, while heparin is used for an immediate effect. The two are frequently used in conjunction, in the management of arterial and, more commonly, venous thrombosis.

Obviously there are very great disadvantages in reducing the clotting power: excessive reduction leads to severe bleeding from the kidneys, bowel or elsewhere. The use of anticoagulant therapy in the prevention and management of post-operative thrombosis has to be very carefully controlled by frequent testing of the clotting time of the blood (page 66). The effect of heparin can be neutralised by intravenous injection of another substance called protamine sulphate. An overdose of phenindione (or dicoumarol) can be remedied to some extent by intravenous phytomenadione (vitamin K), but usually a blood transfusion is required to restore to the circulation the missing factors.

The clotting mechanism is a very complicated one and there are at least twelve different chemicals involved in the various stages. For scientific clarity these have been given numbers—Factors I–XII. Certain rare bleeding disorders such as haemophilia are known to be due to the absence of one or more of the Factors (page 117, 'Bleeding Diseases'). A nurse does not need to know the details but may like to refer to a chart for a 'bleeder'.

Fibrinolysis

The word *lysis* is derived from a Greek word meaning to free, or loosen. The body contains certain enzymes which dissolve solid protein. The particular lysin which will dissolve fibrin is **fibrinolysin**; it is present in blood and body tissues and is named plasmin. Just as in the clotting mechanism, **fibrin** comes from a precursor substance, **fibrinogen**, plasmin comes from **plasminogen** and is released by a substance called an **activator**, or **kinase**. Depending on the situation in the body where the clot has formed, a variable amount of fibrinolysin may collect and dissolve the clot so that it can be more easily absorbed, or aspirated through a needle. This liquefaction of clot, or prevention of clot formation, is therefore a natural process. Fibrin also forms as a result of inflammatory processes affecting for instance joints, pleura and peritoneum. Normal tissue contains an inactive substance which under certain conditions changes to the **activator**. Stress, electric shock and violent exercise set this reaction going and therefore increase the liability for bleeding to continue. Sudden death liberates the activator which inhibits the clotting of blood after death. Plasmin also destroys the fibrin precursor fibrinogen, and thus further reduces coagulability of the blood. Normal blood contains in addition a plasmin inhibitor.

Urine contains a plasminogen activator, **urokinase**, and this by retarding the normal clotting mechanism may prolong bleeding from injury or disease in the kidney. In other diseases such as acute pancreatitis (page 599) a similar fibrinolysis may occur, adding to the haemorrhage and severity of the disease. Activator substances, as well as being present in the body, particularly in the walls of the veins, may be derived from bacteria such as haemolytic streptococcus—streptokinase. A patient who has had an infection with haemolytic streptococci develops antibodies to this **streptolysin**: the amount of this antibody in the blood may be measured to give some indication of the severity of the infection—the antistreptolysin titre.[1]

[1] titre = chemical measure of quantity or strength.

Urokinase and **streptokinase** are used in a purified form in treatment. They may be injected into the cerebral ventricles to prevent fibrin formation, or to dissolve fibrin which is formed in meningitis, and sometimes this is very effective in clearing the particles of fibrin which block the catheters of a Spitz Holter valve (page 854). **Streptokinase** has been used in arterial and venous blockage in order to diminish clot formation and prevent extension of clot. In fact there is evidence that these substances will dissolve the clot and allow circulation in vessels which have previously been blocked. Plasmin with an additional enzyme is used to break up blood clots in the bladder or haematoma areas (Elase, page 635)

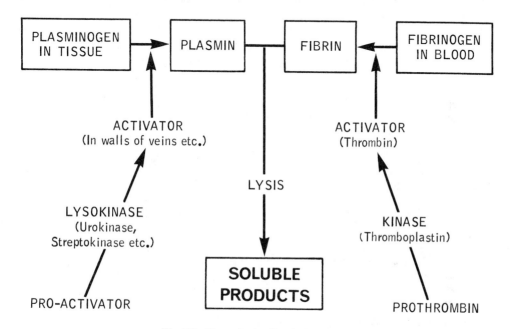

Fig. 5.2   Stages in the dissolution of clot.

A further substance, **aminocaproic acid,** prevents the action of the activator substance and therefore inhibits fibrinolysis. Thus, where there is a bleeding tendency due to excess of these lysins, aminocaproic acid (Epsikapron) may be given over a course of several days.

Thrombosis

There are thus many chemical mechanisms involved in the clotting process. The normal fluidity of the blood is maintained by a balance of enzymes which induce clot formation and those which either prevent it, or increase the solubility of the fibrin as it forms. Whether from chemical damage or from chemical changes in the blood, injury to the walls of the blood vessels upsets this delicate balance and intravascular clotting occurs. Likewise, thrombosis is induced by inflammation of the walls of the veins and arteries and by the spread of infection from surrounding tissues or arterial disease such as the thickening which occurs with arteriosclerosis. Circulating platelets become attached to the wall of the blood vessel and very soon the clot becomes piled up so that the lumen is completely blocked. Once this clotting process has started it spreads rapidly up and down the vessel, blocking the mouths of the little branches, and consequently the blood flow to or from the part affected becomes completely obstructed. If it is an artery which is blocked by this process, gangrene may supervene very rapidly. Arterial thrombosis occurs frequently in the coronary arteries of the heart: the heart muscle is deprived of oxygen and the patient collapses: if the clotting extends to one of the bigger vessels of the coronary circulation, the patient dies. If a vein becomes affected and arterial blood is still being pumped into the part, the tissues become greatly swollen and painful. Venous thrombosis occurs perhaps most commonly in the veins of the leg following operation, leading to the formation of an oedematous leg which is called 'white-leg'.

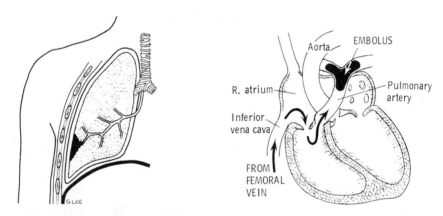

Fig. 5.3 (*left*) A small pulmonary embolus has blocked a branch of the pulmonary artery.
Fig. 5.4 (*right*) The main pulmonary artery is blocked by a large clot which has travelled from the leg.

If part of the clot within the vessel becomes detached and carried on into the circulation, it is known as an 'embolus', and will be carried to distant parts, blocking smaller vessels. Blood emboli travelling in the venous circulation pass through the right side of the heart into the pulmonary artery and thence into the smaller arterioles of the lungs (Fig. 5.3). If a large pulmonary artery is blocked (Fig. 5.4) this condition of **pulmonary embolism** produces sudden death (page 392).

The area of the lung which has been deprived of its blood supply is an **infarct.** A small infarct is compatible with life. The surrounding area of lung becomes inflamed and an area of pleurisy develops. Healing may take place without trouble or, if infection occurs in the dead area, a lung abscess results.

Venous thrombosis

While there are many factors which lead to the formation of thrombosis, the principal ones are damage to the vessel wall and the slowing of the circulation. Much of our nursing is directed to the prevention of the fundamental causes of thrombosis.

Blood is returned to the heart from the legs partly by the pumping action of the muscles which surround the veins, the veins themselves being fitted with non-return valves. The blood is transmitted through the vena cava in the abdomen by the changes in abdominal pressure brought about in turn by diaphragm movement. If the patient is confined to bed by illness or has, because of old age, been reduced to sitting in a chair for long periods of the day, this venous return is slowed down considerably; spontaneous clotting may occur in the veins, particularly in the calf. The stagnation of blood in the veins may be further increased by back pressure from the heart when there is a mild or severe degree of cardiac failure. Similarly this back-pressure effect will be brought about by a tumour in the pelvis pressing on the iliac vein: the weight and size of the pregnant uterus contributes in this way to the development of venous thrombosis and 'white-leg' of pregnancy. When an elderly person is admitted to hospital for a surgical operation, or indeed is in a medical ward undergoing prolonged treatment or investigation, particular care **must** be taken to encourage muscular activity in the legs. In former times, the use of a pillow across the bed, underneath the knees—the 'donkey'—was almost universal in hospital wards as it helped to prevent the patient from sliding down the bed. The resultant partial flexion of the knees, together with the pressure of the pillow in the popliteal fossa and on the calves, continued to add further to the venous stagnation. The use of such a 'donkey' is now regarded as dangerous.

The nurse must repeatedly encourage the patient to move his toes and ankles and bend his knees up and down whenever the bed is made, and at frequent intervals during the day. If he is unconscious it is even more important for his limbs to be exercised. The ideal arrangement is that routine ward exercises should be organised for all patients. Where this is possible bedclothes are turned back, leaving the legs free below the knees. It is a mistake to limit such exercises to the convalescent patient: the ill and lethargic person is the one who is most in need of such gentle preventive exercises. Virtually no strain is placed on the patient's physical (cardiac) resources by this routine. Every time even a small pulmonary embolus occurs, the event must be regarded as an alarm; the medical and nursing staff must ask themselves whether they are being sufficiently thorough in their preventive measures.

Pre-operative use of heparin in patients who may be particularly at risk for thrombosis has been described on page 58. This group includes those over forty years old, women 'on the pill' and patients undergoing pelvic surgery. While awaiting operation, patients must be encouraged to be up and about as much as possible. They should not be allowed to sit around the fire all day, if they are fit to do something more active. Similarly after operation, patients must be got out of bed and encouraged to move about as soon as possible. Some surgeons insist that patients should leave their beds on the first day after operation. The nurse must of course carry out the medical officers' instructions, but everyone needs to remember that it serves no useful purpose to get a patient on his feet at the expense of producing severe pain and discomfort. There are, however, very few surgical operations which require the patient to remain in bed for more than a week.

Venous thrombosis in the arms, or in fact in the superficial veins of the legs, occurs after the administration of drugs intravenously and particularly from the site of infusions or transfusions. Certain substances, such as glucose and thiopentone, tend to produce thrombosis more readily than others. Infection at the site of introduction of the needle is another very common source of thrombosis, and it is negligent to place an ordinary piece of zinc oxide strapping directly over the needle at the point at which it enters the skin and vein. This is apt to happen in an operating theatre when transfusions are put up in a hurry. A patient after a major operation may say quite sincerely that his greatest discomfort was from a thrombosed vein in the arm where his life-saving transfusion was administered. In spite of every precaution, however, a certain number of transfusions and simple infusions will be followed by a venous thrombosis which is sufficiently severe to give rise to pain and swelling. This will be dealt with in the section on transfusion (page 153). Dehydration is a factor which tends to produce thrombosis, and this is yet another reason why the nurse must take care to see that fluid intake is always adequate.

Compression of calf veins by the weight of the leg on the operating table should be prevented by the use of a small sponge rubber block under the Achilles' tendons to keep the calves clear of the table, even though the table itself is covered with sponge rubber (Fig. 5.5).

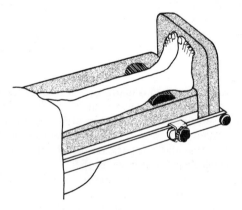

Fig. 5.5 Compression of the calf muscles and their enclosed venous plexus is prevented by elevating the Achilles' tendon on a pad when a patient is on the operating table. This provides some degree of protection against venous thrombosis.

Spontaneous thrombosis occurs sometimes in varicose veins. Intravenous clotting is produced deliberately in the treatment of varicose veins either by ligature or by the injection of sclerosing fluids. As the blood flow in varicose veins has already been reduced or reversed, embolism is extremely unlikely: there is no flowing stream from incoming tributaries to carry the embolus upwards.

Diagnosis of venous thrombosis. Venous thrombosis in the calves or in the veins of the pelvis may go completely unnoticed, and the first sign that anything untoward has occurred is the occurrence of a pulmonary embolus. Thrombosis may be painless, and when pain occurs, it is usually either due to infection or to spasm of the blood vessels irritated by the presence of clot. This spasm further narrows the channel within the vein and encourages the spread of the clot. We have therefore to take very seriously any complaint by the patient of pain in the calf, when he has been confined to bed for medical or surgical treatment. A great deal of risk and inconvenience can be avoided by the early diagnosis of a venous thrombosis, and the nurse in her daily round must always be ready to take note of such complaints of leg pain. When she makes the bed she must look particularly for the slightest swelling of the ankles or of the skin over the shins. There is usually a slight rise in temperature, perhaps up to 37·8 °C (100 °F) when on the preceding days it has been normal. Thrombosis may start at any time after operation, but it is generally noticed about the fifth day. The first and only symptom may be an otherwise unexplained pyrexia. Haemoptysis may be the first indication that thrombosis is present somewhere (page 62). Ultrasonic testing, post-operatively, is used to detect rate of flow in main leg veins. The apparatus sends out ultrasonic vibrations which bounce back from the blood vessel: changes in the rate of flow show up on the meter. Venous return to the heart varies with respiration: inspiration which increases intra-abdominal pressure as the diaphragm descends, slows the venous flow in the legs. The ultrasound detector over the vein indicates whether the flow is varying with respiration. Absence of variation or difference between the two legs confirms the probable thrombosis and is an indication for anticoagulant therapy. The presence of thrombosis may be detected by giving an intravenous injection of radioactive fibrinogen and 'scanning' the legs daily in the post-operative period. If clot forms the radioactivity is concentrated. The fibrinogen is labelled with radioactive [125]iodine and to prevent this being taken up by the thyroid, the patient's thyroid is saturated with iodine by being given daily sodium iodide.

Complications of thrombosis of veins. When a clot becomes detached and begins to travel the patient usually complains of intense pain in the vein where the clot has parted: if this embolus is a large one and passes through the heart into the pulmonary artery, it will be accompanied by pain in the region of the heart. If the main pulmonary artery is blocked, the patient will collapse at once and will become pulseless for a while. The traditional story is that the patient sits up in bed suddenly and asks for a bed pan. This request is brought about by the passage of clot through the abdominal vena cava producing intense abdominal pain. Death may be instantaneous or the patient may survive for a few hours.

On the other hand, if the clot is a small one, it will pass into some very small branch of the pulmonary artery and the first symptom will be in the chest, the pain of pleurisy. Haemoptysis occurs during the next day or so and there is a rise in temperature, which is not due to thrombosis but due to the presence of an infarct in the lung (Fig. 5.3).

When superficial veins undergo thrombosis—such as the antecubital vein in the arm following a transfusion—there is no residual disability, except a hard cord-like structure under the skin. The vein may at some later day regain its lumen. If, however, the deep veins of the leg are affected, the valves are destroyed, and when the patient becomes ambulant again the swelling is persistent. The amount of swelling will depend upon the length of the main vein which has been involved. Unfortunately, if the pelvic veins have been affected, and clot has formed in the whole length of the femoral vein, even though the main veins regain their lumen, the absence of valves makes them relatively ineffective in returning blood to the heart. Thus the 'white-leg' which occurs following child-birth, is frequently a permanent disability.

A similar deep thrombosis affecting a main vein occurs in the axilla, occasionally after such operations as a radical mastectomy. The vein itself has been exposed, and perhaps pressed with the retractors in the axilla. The swelling of the arm is often permanent.

Management of venous thrombosis

Conservative treatment. If venous thrombosis in the legs is suspected, very close observation is kept and the circumference of the thigh and calf measured daily. An indelible ink mark to indicate the level of measurement, should be made 10 cm above and 10 cm below each patella. In the absence of embolism, and if the leg swelling is slight, a surgeon may decide that the only treatment is bed rest, elevation of the leg, and a crêpe bandage.

Anticoagulant therapy. When, however, there is no longer a risk of post-operative haemorrhage—and this is usually the case at the end of the first week, when thrombosis appears—it is now common practice to administer drugs which reduce the coagulability of the blood. There are two types of drugs which can be used. The first is **heparin** which has to be given intravenously. This acts directly on the clotting mechanism and inhibits it. It is usual to continue an infusion of heparin for 48 hours, and the result on the pain in the limb is sometimes quite dramatic. At the same time the second type of drug, either **dicoumarol** or **phenindione**, is given by mouth; these drugs act by stopping the production of prothrombin in the liver. After the drug has been administered by mouth, all prothrombin which is circulating in the blood already has to be used up before the clotting time of the

Table 8   Chart for anticoagulant therapy in an adult patient

---

1st day
> Heparin* by intravenous injection. 10,000 to 15,000 international units every 4 hr or the equivalent by continuous infusion.
>> *Antidote to heparin.* 1% protamine sulphate. 5–10 ml by intravenous injection. (1 ml of 1% protamine sulphate is equivalent to 1000 international units of heparin.)
>> *Note.* Although heparin is dispensed in amounts measured in milligrams, the strength of different makes varies, and dosage must be in standard units.
> (Warfarin) by mouth in tablet form (one tablet = 50 mg), 50 mg every 4 hr for 6 doses (i.e. 300 mg).

2nd day
> Prothrombin estimation carried out by laboratory.
> (Warfarin) 50 mg every 6 hr (i.e. 200 mg).

3rd and subsequent days
> Prothrombin estimation carried out by laboratory.
> (Warfarin) 50 mg every 12 hr.

Note. Phenindione (Dindevan) is more rapid in its action but less prolonged. The risk of over-dose is therefore less serious and treatment is easier to control.

1st day
> Phenindione by mouth, 100 mg every 12 hr.

2nd day
> Phenindione by mouth, 50 mg every 12 hr.

Maintenance dose, 50 mg by mouth (or less) every 12 hr.

---

    * Dextran sulphate (Dexulate) is a synthetic heparin substitute.

blood is reduced. This takes more than twenty-four hours, and phenindione is therefore used to continue the work of heparin. In addition to the risk of haemorrhage from un-healed wounds spontaneous bleeding may occur from the gastro-intestinal or urinary tract, if the clotting power of the blood is reduced too far. The administration of these drugs has therefore to be controlled by laboratory tests, and the result is expressed as **prothrombin time**. An average scheme of treatment is given in full in Table 8, but this will be varied by the doctor in accordance with results of blood tests which have to be made daily.

Surgical measures. If, however, repeated pulmonary embolus has occurred in spite of anticoagulant therapy treatment, certain surgical procedures are available. The first of these is to tie the vein from which the emboli are believed to be coming. This is possible if one leg is affected and the femoral vein can be explored and tied. If, however, the emboli are coming from the iliac veins which frequently become involved in post-operative thrombosis, the inferior vena cava can be pleated (plication). That is, its lumen is reduced in size with stitches or a small plastic clamp, folding it up to prevent the passage of large clots.

The third method is to remove the clots by opening the vein and sucking out the con-tents. The modern method of doing this is to clamp the vein above the site of incision and then to pass a **Fogarty** catheter downwards through the soft clot as far as it will go (Fig. 5.6). The balloon is then inflated and the catheter is withdrawn clearing all the clot from the vein. An advantage of this method is that circulation can be resumed through the vein which would otherwise become solid and permanently obstructed, or if it recanalised would do so with its valve damaged.

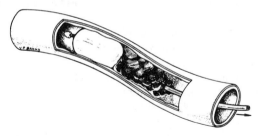

Fig. 5.6   Fogarty balloon catheter. The artery or vein is clamped on the cardiac side of an incision into its wall into which the catheter is threaded through thrombotic clot, inflated and withdrawn bringing the clot out of the vessel. The incision is repaired and the clamps released.

Unfortunately these operative methods are only applicable to thrombosis occurring in the veins of the pelvis and lower limbs, and to a lesser extent in the arms.

In spite of these great advances in the treatment of thrombosis, nothing is better than prevention, and the nurse has a constant and all-important part to play in this.

Arterial thrombosis

The arteries most commonly affected are the coronary arteries in the heart and the arteries in the brain. The condition occurs when previous disease in the arteries (arteritis, arteriosclerosis, atheroma) has already led to a restricted blood flow. Arterial thrombosis sometimes follows bruising of a previously healthy artery; a 'strangulation' type of neck injury, or a bullet wound, may produce spasm of a carotid artery and subsequent thrombosis.

Shock following an operation or injury results in lowered blood pressure and this in turn may lead to thrombosis in brain, heart or limb. Prevention lies mainly with the surgeon and anaesthetist, but the nurse needs to be watchful for marked post-operative fall in blood pressure sometimes brought about by the excessive use of sedative drugs.

The symptoms of arterial thrombosis depend of course on the site. Coronary thrombosis may present as a dramatic incident in which the patient collapses and becomes unconscious, and the condition can only with difficulty be distinguished from pulmonary embolism: it may however be detected only when the nurse notices that the pulse is irregular. Cerebral artery thrombosis is sometimes much more elusive. If a large vessel is affected the patient may develop hemiplegia and become unconscious: this is fortunately rare as a post-operative complication. More commonly a small vessel is involved and the changes may be so slight as to go unnoticed for a time. An alteration in the behaviour, or personality, of an old person after an operation is sometimes due to the occurrence of a cerebral thrombosis. Speech which has been perfectly normal before operation becomes slurred and perhaps incoherent. The nurse must always be on the alert to notice such signs and symptoms when she has the care of old people.

Arterial embolism. When clotting commences on the wall of a major artery a portion of the clot may become detached, travel down the limb and block important branches around which there is no alternative route for the blood. Gangrene supervenes, unless the clot can be extracted by operation. Similarly, flakes become detached from the thickened lining of diseased arteries and result in sudden obstruction of limb arteries. Because the patient's vessels are thick and inelastic, thrombosis spreads rapidly down the branches arising beyond the point of obstruction (page 940).

Another source of arterial embolism is the left auricular appendage of the heart, when the patient has suffered from auricular fibrillation. In this condition, clots sometimes form on the inside of the heart, and become detached if the rhythm returns to normal. Such an event may occur after thyroidectomy for severe thyrotoxicosis (page 771). The patient complains of sudden pain at the site of the arterial block and the limb beyond this point is blanched.

Management of arterial obstruction. Injury, use of the limb and heating of the limb must be avoided. Anticoagulant drug treatment is used in arterial thrombosis. Sympathectomy (page 943) is performed when the arterial block has jeopardised the blood supply of a limb. After operations for arterial grafting a patient's prothrombin blood concentration is maintained at a low level by anticoagulant drugs for an indefinite period to diminish the possibility of the graft becoming blocked by clots.

Surgical procedures for dealing with chronic arterial obstruction are discussed on page 943. For acute arterial embolism operation may be performed as an emergency. The artery is opened and the clot removed, sometimes by means of a Fogarty catheter (page 67).

The care of the limb which is ischaemic (short of blood) is described on page 944.

Recovery after arterial thrombosis. Blockage of an artery may arise from embolism or from thrombosis which in turn has followed compression of an artery by haematoma or growth. Damage to one of the main blood vessels frequently occurs from fractures and the artery itself may be kinked. Whatever the cause or the degree of mechanical obstruction within the vessel, there is always some spasm of musculature in the artery wall, though in the very hardened arteries of old people this is a minor factor. Relief of pain and general improvement in the patient's circulation as shock passes off lessen the spasm and render ischaemia less likely. With the vast network of junctions between small arteries there is usually an alternative path through which blood may reach a portion of a limb whose main artery has been obstructed. The same state of affairs exists in the organs. There is, however, a time lag between the onset of obstruction and the development of an adequate collateral circulation. If thrombosis occurs in one of the arteries of the heart, sudden ischaemia of the heart muscle stops the beat and consequently there is no time for the alternative pathways to develop. Even in severe cases of coronary thrombosis recovery can be complete as far as function is concerned, although a small scar forms in the heart muscle which has been deprived of its blood supply. Improvement in collateral circulation in limbs or viscera or in the brain may continue for two or three months after the original incident provided there is no further thrombosis. It is absolutely vital therefore that everything possible is done during this convalescent period to lessen strain, risk of injury or infection. Patients who have arterial disease such as arteriosclerosis or an aneurysm are liable to repeated attacks of thrombosis even after grafting operations have been undertaken. This necessarily limits their activity and demands that they should live within easy access of skilled medical assistance. If such patients develop other unconnected disorders their vascular disease becomes of paramount importance.

6

Pain

The nature of pain

Pain is the most common symptom of disease. It is due to chemical changes in nerve cells brought about by direct injury to the nerve cell from physical violence—e.g. heat and cold, or cutting—or by poisons derived from other cells which in turn have been damaged by infection, or injury. For this reason the famous physiologist Sherrington defined pain as the psychical adjunct of the protective reflex. The importance of pain to the sufferer is that it tells him that something is wrong. It is a minute-by-minute experience of daily living in all of us. As a result of physical sensation we learn to live in a normal environment and to protect ourselves from all ordinary hazards. Most of these sensations which we experience along pain pathways in the nervous system are of such a low intensity that our body automatically takes protective action without the mind being aware of what has happened. When an area of the body loses its sensation, for instance with paralysis due to a spinal cord injury, the tissues which have lost the power of sensation are very easily damaged, ulcers develop and infection supervenes. Similarly, gastric or intestinal discomfort prevents us from taking more food until the alimentary tract has recovered. To this extent pain is a psychological experience. The intensity of physical suffering in any individual depends not only on the severity of the stimulus, but on the mental state of the sufferer. The person who is unconscious from injury, or who is mentally defective or drugged, cannot experience pain to the same extent as someone who is fully conscious. Conversely, the more alert a patient's mind the more acutely he is aware of injurious processes taking place in his body.

The effect of pain on the individual is very much worse if he does not understand why that pain has arisen. For instance if a man develops a septic thumb which swells and throbs he becomes anxious because he does not understand what is going on, neither can he forecast the outcome of his disease. On the other hand if that same man hits the same thumb with a hammer while mending his fence, even though the swelling is just as great, the pain will not be nearly as serious because he knows that after a certain number of days the whole thing will settle. It is very important for all those who have to do with the sick to appreciate how anxiety intensifies pain. Confidence, reassurance and kindness go a long way to alleviating pain, and **sedative** drugs, by diminishing fear, can act as pain killers.

Even when we have made allowance for fear and anxiety, we are often baffled by the fact that individuals vary so widely in their reaction to incidents of disease which we know to be painful. Pain is an experience, and it is wrong to say that people react differently to pain; they act differently to the stimulus which produces pain. It is important to recognise that people cannot help their reactions to those nervous stimuli any more than they can stop vomiting if they feel sick. The skill of an experienced nurse is to be found in her ability to decide in a patient who is apparently in pain, whether his pain indicates something severe or significant in his body, or whether he is 'over-acting' to an unimportant stimulus because of some anxiety. The patient with poor morale tolerates pain badly, but the brave man may suffer severely though he complains little.

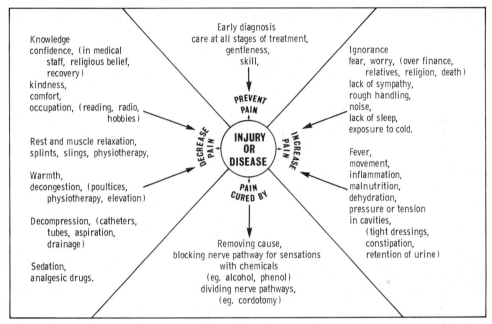

Fig. 6.1   The relationships of pain.

In the later years of life many people suffer from 'involutional depression'. In this condition the patient has 'pains' in various parts of his body, and will describe all sorts of symptoms, some of which are misleading. They may imitate severe organic disease. The doctor has to decide the importance of the symptom of pain in such an individual, and without x-ray and other investigations he may be unable to come to a certain conclusion that the patient's pain has its origin in his mind, and has no organic basis.

Types of pain

The recognition of various types of pain is an aid to diagnosis. Pain produced by inflammation is constant; it is often described as 'aching', and is due to engorgement of the tissues affected by the inflammatory process. This increase of blood supply to the inflamed area is so great that each beat of the heart can be felt—the throbbing feeling. In fact, when infection produces an abscess the pressure of pus in the cavity is often so great that the patient describes the sensation as 'bursting'.

Muscle spasm produces one of the most severe types of pain. In ordinary life it is experienced in the form of cramp arising from exercise. In the voluntary muscles of the limb this spasm is due to the accumulation of tissue breakdown products, particularly when the muscles are overactive. The violent crippling contraction of muscle fibre is so severe that the sufferer cannot move the limb in any way. Similar violent contraction of involuntary muscle in viscera and blood vessels can be brought about by inflammation or injury. When it occurs in the abdomen it is called colic. This type of pain can arise in any organ where there is 'smooth' (non-striped) muscle such as the kidney or ureter, any part of the intestinal tract, bile or pancreatic ducts. The passage of some stone or abnormal particle through the ducts is the usual cause of such colic. 'Labour pains' are due to contraction of the smooth muscles of the uterus.

The third type of pain is produced by stretching of nerves and is most common in abdominal conditions due to the **distension** of an organ such as the stomach, the bowel or the bladder. This is a constant aching pain varying in intensity from time to time as the organ tries to empty itself; thus in some ways it resembles colic. In fact the two forms of pain frequently occur together; spasm of the muscle is an effort to move the obstruction, and distension of the organ follows if the colic has failed to move the blockage. This combination is most common in intestinal obstruction.

Recognition of pain

Pain is an indicator of disease. When a patient complains, or shows signs of being in pain even without complaining, our first duty is to determine why a particular pain has arisen. A nurse must never be so busy as to overlook a patient's complaint of pain, nor to be weary of his complaining. We must never assume that because a patient has had an operation he will necessarily have pain and therefore his complaint may be ignored. This is very important in the nursing of patients in the post-operative phase because the intensity, type and site of pain are usually the earliest clues to any complication which may develop. Unless the nurse pays attention to the patient's complaints which may seem trivial the success of an operation may well be jeopardised. Reassurance that all is well may turn out to be a deception, and all trust in the staff will be lost. Nursing skill and knowledge is at its highest in the recognition of pain and in its prevention and relief.

Measures for the relief of pain

When we know that a patient is likely to experience pain, as indeed is most probable after any major operation, we must take steps beforehand to see that he is prepared for this but relieved of anxiety, otherwise after operation he may develop the idea that everything is going wrong because of his pain. We must never frighten patients before operation. Mention has already been made of the use of sedative rather than pain-killing drugs in the post-operative period, and if we find that a drug given for the relief of pain has proved ineffective we may frequently produce an immediate response by giving in addition a drug which relieves anxiety, e.g. intramuscular phenobarbitone, *with* morphine.

By a pleasant atmosphere of kindness and sympathy much can be done to reduce a patient's sensitivity to pain. It is important to remove the unnecessary annoyance of noise from banging doors, metal bedpans and the washing-up of crockery. Music, daily newspapers, flowers and colour schemes in decoration all play their part in providing a calm and soothing environment. Careless bedmaking, tucking in the clothes too tightly, or leaving breadcrumbs under the patient all contribute to the severity of pain, and are avoidable.

Almost at every stage of surgical treatment measures are taken to prevent or relieve pain. Skilful surgery with very gentle technique, the avoidance of large retractors and gentle swabbing on the part of the assistant, all contribute to a patient's freedom from pain, because the tissues are less bruised. After injury or operation to an arm or leg the limb is elevated on pillows or in a sling, to reduce congestion and thus reduce the pain. The intestinal tract is rested after surgery and a naso-gastric tube is used in the stomach to prevent the accumulation of secretions. After operations on the urinary tract steps are taken to make sure that there is no accumulation of blood or urine which will distend the organs and produce profound shock from pain (pages 635, 671). Long-acting local anaesthetic agents (bupivacaine) injected along the line of the main nerve supply to an operation area may be a great help (e.g. in operations for hernia or undescended testis).

The use of drugs

Medicines used in the relief of pain are described in the next chapter. It must, however, be realized that the use of a drug to relieve pain is a provisional or palliative measure, and is not aimed at curing the disease which produced the pain. It is far better to prevent pain, or to take steps to strike at the underlying cause. It is for this reason that a nurse must be instructed repeatedly in bedside methods designed to make a patient comfortable. Care in the giving of injections, in the administration of enemas, washing and in many other nursing procedures will eliminate much discomfort, and may reduce the demand for drugs. Nevertheless, the nurse must be familiar with the drugs most commonly used, she must be acquainted with their dosage, the methods of administration and particularly with the choice of a drug whose action is most appropriate to the type of pain from which a patient is suffering. For instance a surface pain from abrasions or bruises is adequately relieved by aspirin or phenacetin. To give the stock mixture of these two drugs containing caffeine would only help to keep the patient awake and it should not be given late in the day. Again, pain arising from a laceration which has been sutured will not be adequately relieved by pethidine whose main function is to relax muscle; morphine or methadone (amidone) should be used for this purpose. Renal colic on the other hand has no better treatment than pethidine, combined with atropine.

Intractable pain

If a main nerve trunk becomes involved in injury, or more commonly in malignant disease, the resultant pain is one of the most serious with which we have to deal. This state of affairs arises particularly in cancer of the pelvic organs such as the bladder, the uterus or the rectum when surgical removal has not been possible. When the pain becomes too severe for it to be controlled by drugs such as morphine (unless given in such quantity that the patient would be unconscious) operations are performed to 'block' the sensory nerves which carry the pain sensations up the spinal cord to the brain. Epidural anaesthesia may be tried and if it relieves the pain temporarily the effect may be made more permanent by injecting phenol (page 238). Alcohol or phenol can be injected into the spinal theca (the fluid 'bath' in which the spinal cord and nerves rest) in a manner similar to that used for the production of spinal anaesthesia. The spread of the drug around the spinal cord is controlled by the position of the patient. Alternatively the surgeon may decide to expose the spinal cord by cutting away part of the vertebrae (laminectomy); he then makes a small cut into the spinal cord at the exact point through which run the nerve fibres carrying the pain-producing sensations from the pelvis to the brain. This operation (cordotomy) is sometimes very dramatic and precise in its effect, but it involves a major operation. Injection of phenol or alcohol is a minor procedure, and almost always damages some other nerves as well as those carrying the painful sensations, but when faced with severe and intractable pain desperate measures are sometimes called for.

When malignant disease spreads to other parts of the body from an organ such as the breast, or prostate, the secondary deposits are sometimes extremely painful. Although we cannot expect to cure the patient we may be able to relieve the pain from this secondary growth by x-ray treatment, by the injection of chemicals, or by the use of hormones. For instance, in advanced cancer of the breast the ovaries may be removed; subsequently the adrenal glands may be removed and sometimes the pituitary gland is excised or destroyed by radiation, not with the intent of curing the patient, but for the sole purpose of relieving suffering and making life more tolerable.

The relief of pain which has failed to respond to ordinary measures remains one of the major problems in the management of patients with advanced disease. Some hospitals have established 'pain clinics' for the treatment of such intractable pain by nerve block and nerve section, and by the planned prescription of drugs.

For the surgeon, for the nurse, and indeed in all forms of medical practice the aim should be to produce conditions in which pain is largely eliminated. It is vital to maintain a constant vigil in order that where pain is inevitable, the surroundings, the handling of the patient and every aspect of the care of that individual shall make it easier for him to bear the pain. This is better in every way than numbing his senses by drugs. A skilled physio-therapist will succeed in building a patient's confidence to overcome pain in breathing: she will by experience be able to judge the extent to which exercise can be permitted. Confidence in those who care for him, and surroundings as congenial and comfortable as possible, contribute so much to the relief of pain and suffering that these abstract possessions should be sought and treasured as the secrets of success in any hospital team work.

7

Action and Administration of Drugs

In hospital practice it is usual for all patients in the surgical ward to be 'signed up', 'written up' or 'boarded' for certain groups of medicines such as sedatives, vitamins, laxatives and enemata. These are given at the discretion of the ward sister as and when they may be required. They are substances needed for the relief of symptoms rather than for the treatment of some specific condition. A nurse must however always remember that there may be very good reasons for withholding the most simple drugs which would seem quite harmless. For instance, aspirin must be withheld from a patient whose temperature record is of particular importance, since the drug lowers the temperature artificially: liquid paraffin should never be given to a patient who is about to have, or has already had, a resection of intestine as the oil may seep through the sutures and produce peritonitis.

No sharp distinction can be made between non-specific (symptomatic) and specific drugs, but it is convenient to group together as specific those drugs which are reserved for treatment of individual diseases rather than for the relief of symptoms alone. Specific treatment is always prescribed in detail for each particular case and is to be regarded as a 'must be given' in contrast to some of the non-specific 'may be given' treatments. The effect of drugs depends upon their rate of absorption and the rate of breakdown in the body and the excretion usually by the kidneys.

Poison Law

In Great Britain the prescription of a large range of drugs which are potentially dangerous is regulated by the Misuse of Drugs Act 1971, which supersedes all previous legislation. Amplification of the Act came in the Misuse of Drugs Regulations 1973. There are severe penalties for infringement of these regulations. Hospitals have their own internal rules concerning the use and storage of drugs controlled by the poison laws and orders. Official ward record books are issued in the National Health Service for the registration of the issue and administration of these controlled drugs.

Schedule I of the Poisons Act is an official list of poisonous substances, not necessarily used in medicine. This list includes such substances as arsenical weed-killer, certain antiseptics, and sodium nitroprusside (used in certain chemical tests). The chemist is only permitted to sell such substances to persons who are known to him personally and the purchaser is required to sign his poison register.

Schedule IV of the Poisons Act includes many drugs used in medical and veterinary science, and these substances may only be supplied on the prescription of a medical or veterinary registered practitioner. Each prescription has to comply with the regulations, bearing the patient's name and address and the qualifications of the doctor. The prescription also has to state whether and how often it may be repeated. Schedule IV drugs include barbiturates and the list of scheduled substances is added to from time to time as new drugs are discovered.

Origin and supply of drugs

The majority of substances used now in medical and surgical treatment are pure chemicals. Many have been synthesised artificially, and some have been extracted from a naturally occurring source and purified. Crude solutions of plant extracts are rarely used now, though occasionally the nurse will come across such medicines as dried extract of belladonna or infusion of quassia or senna. The sulphonamide drugs are synthesised as pure chemicals while many of the hormone preparations are extracted from animal glands. Whatever the source of the drug, all medicinal preparations in Britain have to conform to certain standards set out in the British Pharmacopoeia (BP) and the British Pharmacopoeia Codex (BPC). The manufacture, purity, method of supply, and safe dosage are all specified. For the convenience of individual doctors and of hospital dispensing there is also a National Formulary in which are set out the details of a wide selection of compounds or mixtures in general use. Some hospitals also have their own local pharmacopoeia to cover the usual requirements of the medical staff.

Many substances in common use are supplied under trade names, and credit for the discovery of most modern drugs has to go to the research laboratories of the great manufacturing chemists. Where possible, drugs should always be described with their BP or BPC name as the pharmacist is then able to supply a brand of the drug which is probably considerably cheaper than that with the proprietary name. There is a great deal of confusion over these multiple names for the same substance, and often difficulty arises because the name of a new drug is well established in the minds of the public and of the medical profession before it receives an official name for inclusion in the Pharmacopoeia.

All hospitals have a 'pharmacy' in the charge of a qualified pharmacist. It is worth noting that there is a distinction between 'pharmacist' and 'dispenser'. The former is a member of the Pharmaceutical Society (MPS), is more fully trained and able to accept a greater degree of responsibility, particularly in the preparation of substances used in medical and surgical treatment, while the dispenser has had a much shorter and less comprehensive training and is working under the supervision of a pharmacist. These persons are responsible for maintaining hospital stocks and controlling their distribution. The nurse, during the course of her training, will be taught the methods in use in her particular hospital. It is usual for each ward to have its 'dispensary book' in which is placed the daily order for medicinal preparations in common use. Because of the deterioration of most drugs in storage, it is wasteful and even dangerous to keep large supplies of drugs in the ward medicine cupboard. Certain mixtures such as those containing aspirin deteriorate.

Storage

In addition to the general storage space of the ward where bottles of lotions, ointments, antiseptics and other preparations are kept, there is always a poison cupboard in which is placed every drug subject to the poison regulations (page 75). In some hospitals there is also a special cupboard for the safe storage under lock and key of the preparations subject to the more stringent control of the Misuse of Drugs Act. In a small hospital it is unlikely that controlled drugs will be kept in every ward and each dose has to be collected from the dispensary. There may be a night drug box in charge of the night sister. The key to the poison cupboard and controlled drug box or cupboard should only be in the possession of a trained nurse or doctor; no unregistered person is allowed access to such drugs. The same arrangements apply to the operation theatre, out-patient and other departments, and each has to make special provision for the storage of poisons. Every dose of a controlled drug given to a patient has to be recorded in the central ward register, and the record witnessed by another person.

Labelling

There are detailed statutory regulations controlling the dispensing and labelling of all medicinal preparations, and under no circumstances must the nurse transfer a tablet, capsule, or liquid from one container to another. Serious accidents have occurred in the use of multiple pill boxes for the storage of medicines, where the patient's name or the name of the drug has been written on the lid of the pill box alone. The lids of more than one box may be removed simultaneously and the wrong lids replaced. However, if drugs are supplied in pill boxes, the patient's name or the name of the drug, or both, must be written on the bottom of the pill box. Fluids should always be poured from the bottle on the side away from the label so that the drips do not run down the side and damage the label. All fluids are dispensed in bottles with caps: corks are not used as they harbour infection.

All poisonous lotions and antiseptics should have distinctive colours, and it is common practice for a hospital dispensary to add a dye to white or colourless fluids so that they will not be confused. Diluted Dettol resembles milk in appearance and fatal accidents have occurred to babies by their being fed with a bottle of Dettol instead of milk. Most hospitals now therefore tint their Dettol solutions with a red dye.

Many drugs are supplied in more than one form—tablets or solutions for use by mouth, and powder or solution for injection. Great care has to be exercised so that oral preparations are not used for injection and the nurse should **never assume that any powder or solution is safe, unless it is labelled clearly as suitable for injection**. Glass ampoules should be labelled by etching in the glass since adhesive labels are readily detached when the ampoule becomes wet. Any such ampoule separated from its label should be returned to the hospital pharmacy at once.

To the nurse who has been trained in a large hospital, many of these simple observations may seem redundant, but in the small hospital, where the turnover of drugs is less rapid, there may still be preparations bearing out-of-date names or packed and labelled in a manner quite unfamiliar to her.

PHARMACOLOGY

The action of drugs

Drugs are used extensively in the management of surgical cases and may be grouped according to their action on the human body. Many drugs have more than one action, and while they may be used because of their principal effect, they may have side-effects which in any particular individual can be sufficiently severe to preclude their use.

Personal sensitivity

There is a very wide individual variation in response to particular drugs: some patients are severely disturbed by certain mild sedative drugs, while others may develop an allergic reaction including 'drug fever' and an urticarial rash. If at any time a patient mentions having had any such reaction following a particular drug, the nurse must always report this fact so that alternative treatment may be given and the necessary measures taken to relieve the allergic symptoms (see below). Drugs, like microbes, lead to the production of specific antibodies which may persist in the body indefinitely.

Pregnancy and drugs

In the early weeks of pregnancy a patient may fail to call the doctor's attention to her belief that she has conceived and there is inherent danger in the use of many drugs at this stage of pregnancy. The 'thalidomide tragedy' in 1961 resulted in the birth of many deformed children because their mothers were given this drug as a sedative (Fig. 7.1). Great care must therefore be taken in the selection of drugs to be given to women in early pregnancy.

Sedatives, hypnotics, analgesics and narcotics

Drugs which affect the nervous system may do so in various ways, the intensity of each action depending on the dose.

Sedatives and **hypnotics** are drugs which quieten the patient or produce sleep. Such drugs are ineffective in the presence of pain unless they are given in amounts which are dangerous. Chloral, phenobarbitone, diazepam (Valium) and nitrazepam (Mogadon) are ones in common use. Phenobarbitone given twice in the day is most suitable if it is desired to sedate the patient for the whole of the 24-hour period.

Analgesics are drugs which relieve pain whether given by mouth (thereby affecting the whole body) or applied locally to the painful area. Aspirin, phenacetin, and codeine are used for this purpose, separately or in mixtures. Aspirin has the disadvantage of producing gastritis and the patient may be sensitive to the extent of developing haematemesis. Phenacetin rarely produces any side-effects but prolonged use damages the kidneys. Codeine has a constipating effect. A patient who is repeatedly taking codeine (in the usual form of compound tablet of codeine, Veganin) requires also a gentle laxative. Paracetamol is a derivative of phenacetin, and has less side-effects.

Narcotics are drugs which act on the higher centres of the brain and usually have a depressive effect also on the vital centres, slowing respiration and the pulse. They produce

Table 9 Drugs of the barbiturate group in common use

BP name	Trade name	Mode of supply	Adult dose Metric	Approximate duration of effect	Remarks
Phenobarbitone	Luminal, Gardinal	Tablet	30–120 mg	12–16 hr	Long-term sedative
Phenobarbitone sodium	Soluble Luminal	Tablet: ampoule for injection	30–200 mg	12–16 hr	Use as single dose intramuscular or intravenous injection
Barbitonum soluble	Medinal	Tablet	300–600 mg	8–16 hr	Less 'hangover', more rapid effect
Butobarbitone	Soneryl	Tablet	90–200 mg	4–8 hr	
	Sonalgin	One tablet contains: Butobarbitone 60 mg Codeine 10 mg Phenacetin 225 mg Dose: 1–2 tablets			Analgesic and hypnotic combination
Amylobarbitone	Amytal	Tablets or capsule	100–300 mg	3–6 hr	Use by intramuscular or intravenous injection for rapid action
Amylobarbitone sodium	Sodium amytal	Tablet: ampoule	200–600 mg		
Pentobarbitone	Nembutal	Capsule or tablet	100–200 mg		
Hexobarbitone	Evipan Cyclonal	Tablets	250–500 mg	4–8 hr	Can be used to produce a short sleep (e.g. early hours of the morning)
Quinalbarbitone	Seconal	Tablet: capsule	50–200 mg		
Thiopentone	Pentothal Intraval sodium	Ampoule of powder	Dose according to anaesthetic requirement, intravenously		Dissolved in water immediately before use
			0·5–1 G in water, by rectum		Basal anaesthetic

Note. These drugs are all Schedule IV poisons (page 76).

sleep in the presence of pain. Morphine, in its various forms and combinations, is the commonest narcotic. Diamorphine hydrochloride (heroin) has certain advantages over morphine but is now rarely used because of its habit-forming properties. Some patients are extremely sensitive to morphine, which produces in them intense and distressing vomiting.

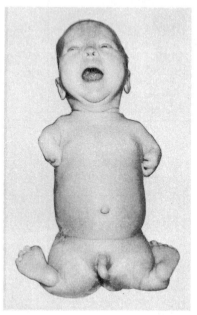

Fig. 7.1 Phocomelia (short limbs) occurring as a congenital defect produced by the administration of thalidomide to the mother in the early weeks of pregnancy. Note also the 'birthmark' affecting the nose and forehead.

Patients who are likely to be in need of morphine or its modern counterpart—papaveretum (Omnopon)—should be asked if they have ever had this drug before. Pethidine is used extensively as a narcotic because it has practically no unpleasant side-effects, is less constipating, and has the additional advantage of relaxing smooth muscle and therefore relieving colics of all types. Pethidine inhibits bladder activity and may produce retention of urine. Drugs of the morphine group which all have the disadvantage of depressing respiration should be used as sparingly as possible, in the post-operative phase.

   Morphine is sometimes given by mouth, but an effective substitute is dipipanone (Pipadone). Given by mouth it acts rapidly and is equal in effect to that of morphine by injection. It was found that certain drugs which counteract morphine themselves have a pain relieving effect. Nalorphine is used to neutralise morphine but not for its own analgesic effect. **Pentazocine** (Fortral) either by mouth or injection is as powerful as morphine and without the same side-effects of habit formation and respiratory depression. It has however no sedative effect and can be combined with intramuscular phenobarbitone or diazepam by mouth, or by injection. Some patients are severely disturbed by pentazocine which may produce severe hallucinations—bad dreams.

To reduce the risk of nausea or vomiting, **anti-emetic** drugs (as used to prevent sea-sickness) are frequently given with morphine preparations and Pipadone, e.g. Pipadone compound tablets (25 mg dipipanone) with 50 mg **cyclizine hydrochloride.**

Other anti-emetic drugs used pre- and post-operatively are promethazine (Avomine, Phenergan). The action of these drugs is mainly anti-allergic (anti-histamine). They are used also in the treatment of drug sensitivity rashes (page 244).

For the relief of mild pain, the safe and usual combination is an aspirin mixture with one of the barbiturate drugs (e.g. Sonalgin—butobarbitone, codeine and phenacetin). In a surgical ward many patients, particularly during the first few nights of their stay in hospital, are unable to sleep merely because of the strange surroundings and the constant movement of nursing staff and other patients. Short-acting hypnotic drugs of the barbiturate group or nitrazepam (Mogadon) should be given without hesitation to such patients, and these are usually prescribed as routine 'discretionary' drugs to be given as the nursing staff feel necessary. Table 9 shows drugs of the barbiturate group most commonly used and the approximate duration of their action. The dose required depends on the size of the patient, the age and the general state of activity. Old persons should always be given the minimum quantity of barbiturates as they readily become mentally deranged. Welldorm (dichloral-phenazone) is a safe non-barbiturate hypnotic widely used and not habit-forming, but produces 'heart-burn'.

Drugs for the treatment of constipation

Reference has already been made to the management of the patient's bowel action (page 26). Only mild laxatives are called for in surgical wards; magnesium hydroxide (cream of magnesia) is the most commonly used but occasionally a more irritant drug such as senna is called for. Liquid paraffin in **emulsion form** is an ideal laxative for routine administration.[1] It is often prescribed in combination with magnesium hydroxide (Mil-Par).

Neostigmine (Prostigmin) is given by subcutaneous or intramuscular injection to stimulate peristalsis in the management of post-operative distension. The injection is usually followed by an enema twenty minutes later. Neostigmine is never used when there is any risk of peritonitis or organic intestinal obstruction. It must never be given without a specific prescription on each occasion (see page 480 for its use in paralytic ileus).

Neostigmine is also used specifically in the treatment of myasthenia gravis for its effect on the junctions of nerve fibres with muscle.

Bowel stimulant suppositories such as glycerine or Dulcolax (bisacodyl BP) are safe and dramatic in action without undue disturbance of the small bowel. Bisacodyl is also given by mouth in very severe constipation. It acts as a wetting agent and softens the faecal masses.

Enema (plural 'enemas', enemata)

Except for the period immediately before defaecation, the rectum is normally empty. Various forms of fluid may be introduced into the rectum and colon. The very slow in-

---

[1] No preparation containing liquid paraffin is permitted before or immediately after surgery involving the alimentary tract as the oil may interfere with healing at the site of the anastomosis.

jection of water or saline is used as a means of counteracting dehydration as the rectal and colonic mucous membrane readily absorbs water. Certain drugs are also absorbed in this way. Thiopentone and paraldehyde are given rectally either as a pre-operative sedative or in cases of extreme restlessness such as occurs in cerebral concussion. Prednisolone retention enemas are used in ulcerative colitis (Table 10). Evacuant enemas are used in the treatment of constipation or in the preparation of the bowel for barium enema examination by x-ray, or for operation. Antiseptic enemas (using an emulsion of insoluble phthalyl-sulpha-thiazole or succinyl-sulphathiazole) are used to prepare the bowel for colonic surgery.

Occasionally, constipation is so extreme that a mass of hard faeces becomes impacted in the rectum and has to be removed under anaesthesia. There are certain conditions in which such extreme constipation is common (megacolon, and conditions in which there has been interference with the pelvic nerves) and the introduction of concentrated ox-bile into the bowel softens these hard masses of faeces and allows them to be evacuated more readily.

There are of course certain risks in the administration of an enema. Extreme shock may be produced especially if the fluid is too cold or too hot. In evacuant enemas, the patient is placed on the left side during the introduction of the fluid and is then turned on his back with the foot of the bed elevated. Gravity is thus used to assist the passage of the fluid into the descending colon. The 'rolling enema' aims at taking the fluid across the transverse colon to the right by turning the patient over on to his right side. Peristalsis is thus more effectively stimulated and evacuation more complete. The technique of enema administration is important and will be learnt in ordinary ward routine work. A summary

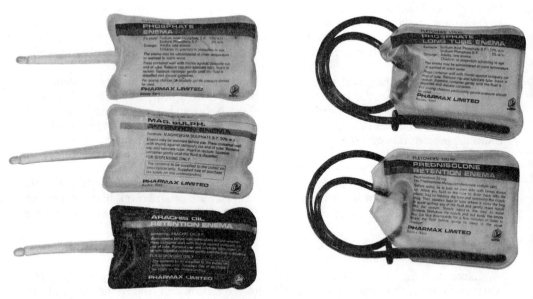

Fig. 7.2 Fletcher's 'disposable' enemas. Great care must be taken that the semi-rigid nozzle does not damage the rectum. The volume in a single pack is inadequate for a high colonic evacuation. When an enema has to be retained, the foot of the bed must be elevated. (Pharmax Ltd.)

Table 10   Composition of enemas

Quantity—as an evacuant enema, 500–600 ml (20 ounces) (up to 1000 can be given safely if the colon has not been operated upon).

Total enema volume for children depends on the size of child: a condition in childhood requiring repeated enemas is megacolon, and 'adult' quantities can then be used. Otherwise an approximate guide is 30 ml (1 ounce) for each year of age.

Temperature—40°C (105°F) in the container.

Pressure—30 cm (12 inches) above the anus, with patient in lateral position.

Method—Funnel and soft rubber catheter (Jaques) with aseptic eye, Size 42 Benique (12 E).

Note: a Higginson syringe should not be used, as there is a very real danger of injury to the rectum. A metal or vulcanite nozzle must never be used.

Lubricant—Soft paraffin should be smeared over and around the anus to protect the sensitive skin from the irritant action of the enema solution. Especially is this important with turpentine enemas.

SIMPLE ENEMA—600 ml tap water.

SOAP ENEMA—30 G soft soap 600 ml water.

OX-BILE ENEMA—15 ml ox bile solution
          15 G soft soap
          300 ml water

VERIPAQUE ENEMA (Oxyphenisatin)—Veripaque is a substance which stimulates contraction of the large bowel. It has been used in radiography mixed with barium to outline the colon. It is, however, used without the barium as a cleansing enema to ensure complete evacuation of the whole colon prior to a barium enema examination. One vial of Veripaque (3 G) is dissolved in a litre of warm water and administered as a rolling enema. Half the fluid is given slowly with the patient in the left lateral position and the foot of the bed raised. The patient then rolls on to his face and slowly over to the right lateral position in which the rest of the fluid is run in. The enema should be retained for at least fifteen minutes if possible. The enema is given $1\frac{1}{2}$ hours before a barium enema and is followed by 15 mg of propantheline given 30 minutes before the x-ray examination.

MOLASSES ENEMA—60 G molasses-black treacle
          200 ml milk

GLYCERINE ENEMA—Up to 16 ml pure glycerine, with syringe and catheter.

(If the patient is severely constipated, and the bowel contains hard faecal masses, these may be softened by inserting into the rectum at night, and evacuating with a soap enema in the morning, either:
olive oil, 150 ml or ox-bile solution, 150 ml)

RECTAL WASH-OUT

The purpose of this is to cleanse the rectum without stimulating the colon higher up. Normal saline is used and 100 ml is run in and allowed to return by lowering the funnel over the receiving pail. The process is repeated until the returning fluid is clean.

Occasionally hot rectal wash-out is prescribed in the treatment of pelvic cellulitis, or to encourage a pelvic abscess to discharge into the rectum (page 481) 3000 ml of water at 45°C 112°F) is run in and out as above. Useless if water is allowed to cool to blood temperature.

RETENTION ENEMA

Prednisolone (steroid) 20 mg in water, administered daily for local steroid treatment of ulcerative colitis or proctitis.

---

of the main types of enema, their use and composition, is given in Table 10. Instead of nurses having to assemble a funnel, tubing and catheter, most hospitals now use commercially packed disposable apparatus. Some of these are administered by gravity using a long tube and some merely by squeezing a plastic pack.

With the introduction of wetting agents and harmless bowel stimulants has come the 'micro-enema'. A small quantity of fluid (5 ml only) is supplied commercially prepared (Microlax) in a plastic tube fitted with a pliable nozzle. It contains sodium citrate, sorbitol and a wetting agent. These small stimulant enemas are more effective than suppositories and yet eliminate the need for ordinary enema apparatus. To avoid the cost of commercial preparations the hospital pharmacy can provide single enema bottles containing bisacodyl 5 mg with glycerine 0·5 ml in water to 2 ml. This is injected with a discarded 2-ml plastic syringe through a 5-cm length of soft polyvinyl (transfusion) tubing. Both syringes and tubing can be sterilised by washing in a chlorhexidine solution.[1]

Nutritional medicines

Resistance to disease and healing after injury or operation are influenced by nutrition.

Iron, calcium, and other essential elements are administered either by mouth or by injection when there is likely to be insufficiency of these substances in the diet. Extracts of liver and stomach are used in the treatment for certain forms of anaemia (page 123).

Many severe surgical conditions are associated with prolonged malnutrition and the patient suffers from a gross shortage of protein. In conditions such as extensive burning, this shortage can be made up by feeding a high protein diet. Unfortunately many of these conditions of protein deficiency are associated with disease of the alimentary tract. Special, easily absorbed, protein preparations can be given by mouth (Casilan) or protein hydrolysate can be given as an intravenous infusion (Aminosol, Casydrol). Glucose is of course the simplest nutritional substance given intravenously and it is used at some stage in most major surgical cases but fructose is used as a high calorie source. Preparations of fat are also available for intravenous use and this is given in the form of cottonseed oil (page 139).

Vitamins in surgery

The role of these essential chemicals has an important part in the management of both medical and surgical illness. Gross deficiencies of any particular vitamin as the result of diet insufficiently are almost unknown in the Western world and a diet which is adequate for calorie requirements is almost always adequate in vitamin content. Occasionally, as the result of some disease, both the intake and the utilisation of a particular vitamin may be interfered with and a clinical condition may arise which is due to this vitamin shortage alone. Prolonged use of oral contraceptives is thought to aggravate vitamin shortage, particularly the B vitamins.

Nevertheless, there is evidence that if certain vitamins are in moderately short supply, normal tissue activity is interfered with and the repair of disease processes or injury is slowed down.

---

[1] The re-use for any purpose of disposable syringes is generally to be discouraged, but for this purpose it is safe.

Vitamin A—retinol—is fat-soluble substance which occurs naturally in fish-liver oils and some other meats. A similar pure chemical substance, carotin, is found in certain vegetables. Gross deficiency of vitamin A leads to night blindness and a severe destructive condition of the conjunctiva. It is thought that vitamin A protects epithelial surfaces (such as the mucous membrane lining to the urinary and alimentary tract) against infection or degeneration. This vitamin rarely needs to be given in the treatment of surgical conditions.

Vitamin B. The 'B complex'is not one pure chemical substance but a group of chemicals which in their natural sources are found together and have similar physical properties. The early attempts to isolate vitamin B as a chemical failed to distinguish these various separate fractions. Thiamine (aneurine) (vitamin B_1) deficiency leads to the clinical condition of beri-beri which is characterised by neuritis, general weakness and oedema. It was seen in World War II in prison and internment camps in the Far East where the diet was grossly defective. Riboflavine (vitamin B_2) deficiency is one of the earliest indications of a defective diet and it is seen in this country in patients with disease of the alimentary tract. The tongue becomes beefy-red, swollen and sore. Cracks develop at the angles of the mouth and the lips become fissured. Deficiency is common in the elderly (Fig. 7.3). Nicotinic acid (niacin) (pellagra-preventing factor) is used in medicine as a pure substance for its effect in dilating peripheral blood vessels. If there is a gross deficiency of nicotinic acid in the diet, the clinical condition of pellagra arises, with mental disorder, dermatitis, and diarrhoea. Pyridoxine is another member of the B group. It is used in patients with severe tissue breakdown, for instance during radiotherapy; it also counteracts the nerve weaknesses which may develop during treatment with isoniazid. Cyanocobalamin (vitamin B_{12}) is essential for the prevention of anaemia and it is the shortage of this substance which leads to the development of macrocytic anaemia (which resembles pernicious anaemia) after such operations as partial gastrectomy.

Vitamin C—ascorbic acid. Severe shortage of this vitamin leads to scurvy, a condition in which spontaneous haemorrhage occurs into the tissues, especially when the disease affects children. The joints, epiphyses, and periosteal covering of the long bones are sites where bleeding occurs. Vitamin C is essential for the proper formation of fibrous tissue

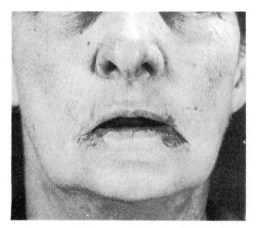

Fig. 7.3   Shortage of vitamin B (riboflavine); ulceration at angle of mouth (cheilosis; rhagades).

Table 11

Vitamin	Food source	Diseases produced by gross deficiency	Importance in surgery	BP or BPC preparations	Approx. daily requirement in health
A	Fish oils Margarine (supplemented in United Kingdom) Eggs, milk, cheese	Xerophthalmia Night blindness	Protective against epithelial infection	Capsules Vit. A, 4500 units each Concentrated Vit. A, solution 50,000 units per G	2500 units
B					
B_1 Thiamine (Aneurine)	Yeast Marmite Eggs Meat Milk	Beri-beri	Shortage may cause certain forms of neuritis Deficiency from failure of absorption occurs after gastric or intestinal operations in pancreatic or biliary disease and other forms of steatorrhoea	Aneurine hydrochloride tablets 3, 10, 50 mg	1–2mg
B_2 Riboflavine	Cereals	Stomatitis		Ampoules, riboflavine 10 mg Tablets 1, 3, 10 mg	1–2 mg
Nicotinic acid (amide)		Pellagra	during radiotherapy	Tablets, nicotinamide 50 mg	10–20 mg
B_6 Pyridoxine		Dermatitis Nerve lesions	during treatment with isoniazid	Tablets, pyridoxine 25 mg	
B_{12} Cyanocobalamin		Macrocytic (pernicious) anaemia	from prolonged antibiotic therapy	Inj. cyanocobalamin. ampoules 20, 50, 100, 1000 mcg	
C Ascorbic acid	Fresh fruits Vegetables (esp. potato)	Scurvy	Essential for wound healing, especially in intestinal tract	Tablets, ascorbic acid 50 mg Ampoules 500 or 1000 mg for intramuscular or intravenous use	30 mg

D Calciferol	Fish oils Margarine (UK) Eggs, milk	Rickets	Essential for bone development and healing Used in treatment of tuberculous conditions	Capsules, 3000 units Concentrated solution (oral), 500,000 units per ml Tablets, 50,000 units	150 units
E Tocopherol	Wheat germ Green leaves	Sterility	Prevention of threatened abortion Fibrous tissue diseases	Tocopheryl acetate, ampoules 30 mg Tablets 3, 10, 50 mg	
K	Certain vegetables and probably manufactured in bowel	Haemorrhagic disease	Antidote for dicoumarol and phenindione Prevention of bleeding in patients with liver damage (i.e. jaundice)	Tablets—by mouth 10 mg Ampoules 10 mg. by injection (not in BP) Vit. K substitutes are acetomenaphthone BP—oral, tablets, 10 mg Menaphthone injection BP ampoules, 10 mg Phytomenadione	

Note. The normal requirement of vitamins A and D is raised in childhood and pregnancy. The daily requirement of vitamins A, B, C, D, otherwise is supplied in full by 3 compound vitamin capsules BPC. In those surgical cases in which vitamin deficiency is expected to be present, or which show frank symptoms, mass dosage is achieved with Parentrovite supplied in paired ampoules to be mixed for intravenous or intramuscular injection, usually put into an infusion. This supplies ascorbic acid (in glucose) and the 'B complex'.

in the healing of wounds. Where the deficiency is not great enough to cause scurvy it may be sufficient to lead to delayed healing and so to the breakdown of surgical wounds. In patients who have been on a deficient diet, or have been vomiting and feverish, ascorbic acid is sometimes given intravenously (1000 mg daily for 3–5 days).

Vitamin D—calciferol. Rickets, a disease in which the bones are soft and bend under stress, results from severe shortage of vitamin D. In certain tuberculous conditions where during treatment it is desired to encourage calcification of a lesion, vitamin D is administered in large doses. In tuberculous conditions of the skin (lupus vulgaris), the administration of vitamin D seems to aid the healing process without the addition of calcium.

Vitamin E—tocopherol. Certain cases of sterility are thought to be due to the shortage of vitamin E and it is used in the treatment of repeated threatened abortion.

Vitamin K (page 59). This is allied to prothrombin and a shortage of this vitamin leads to hypoprothrombinaemia, which in turn leads to haemorrhagic disease. This condition is particularly seen in new-born babies and is cured immediately by the injection of vitamin K or synthetic substances allied to it (acetomenaphthone).

Cause of vitamin deficiency

An individual may be short of one or several vitamins for the following reasons.

(*a*) His diet in its natural state may have contained insufficient vitamin.

(*b*) His food may have been over-cooked or have been exposed to the air for too long a period. Vitamin C is decomposed by oxygen in the air, and vitamin A similarly loses its effectiveness. The action of light on fish oils also destroys their vitamin A content. All the water-soluble vitamins (the various factors of the B complex, and vitamin C) are destroyed by heating or by alkalis. Thus if food is cooked with the addition of soda, it will have no vitamin value. If as the result of disease (for instance, gastritis or carcinoma of the stomach), or gastrectomy, the acid-producing power of the stomach has been reduced (**achlorhydria**), these water-soluble vitamins will pass through the stomach into the duodenum and be destroyed there by the alkaline digestive juices.

(*c*) If any condition exists which causes intestinal hurry, there will be insufficient time for the vitamins to be absorbed from the bowel. Any condition of chronic diarrhoea may thus produce a vitamin shortage.

(*d*) There are certain disorders of fat absorption which result in the fatty elements of the diet being passed with the faeces. This condition is **steatorrhoea**, and occurs in certain recognised conditions such as sprue and coeliac disease, but is also present if there has been an obstruction to the outflow of pancreatic juice into the duodenum or if there is insufficient bile to aid fat digestion. It has now been shown that if as the result of surgical operation on the intestinal tract there is a cul-de-sac or blind loop, the presence of this loop may lead to abnormal digestive processes and interference with vitamin absorption (leading especially to macrocytic anaemia).

Newly discovered vitamins have been used in the treatment of disease often without sufficient information. If a hospital diet is properly prepared only patients with severe debilitating disease, or receiving antibiotic therapy, require vitamin supplements. The routine distribution of multiple vitamin pills is wasteful and expensive.

(*e*) It is thought that certain parts of the vitamin B complex are actually manufactured in the intestinal tract by the action of bacteria. The prolonged use of antibiotics, particularly of aureomycin, interferes with this normal bowel function and the defective production of vitamin B has to be made good by the administration of the vitamin by injection. The bowel is sterilised deliberately before intestinal surgery by insoluble sulphonamide drugs, or neomycin by mouth.

Table 11 shows the names of the vitamins, their uses in surgery, the natural source of supply and the preparations which are used in clinical practice.

Anti-infective drugs

Strictly speaking, **chemotherapy** describes treatment with synthetic chemical compounds: **antibiotic** drugs are derived from 'natural' living sources such as fungus and bacterial growth and having a distinctive action on other organisms. For general purposes now the term 'antibiotic' is used for any anti-infective drug and *chemotherapy* is used mainly in connection with cancer treatment. The division is artificial, since many antibiotics are synthesised chemically.

Sulphonamides. Drugs of the sulphonamide group are used extensively in both medicine and surgery but have been largely replaced by antibiotics. They are supplied in tablet form or as a fluid suspension suitably flavoured, and some are suitable for intramuscular or intravenous injection. Sulphadimidine is the most commonly used, especially in the treatment of urinary infection: it diffuses readily into the cerebrospinal fluid (CSF) and is used to prevent or treat meningitis (e.g. fractured skull with CSF leak from ear or nose). Sulphamethoxazole combined with trimethoprim (Septrin, Bactrim) is a widely used combination with a prolonged action: it is given every 12 hours. If the patient is dehydrated or the dose is excessive, these drugs, as they are excreted by the kidney, form crystals in the urinary tract so that haematuria or suppression of urine may result. Patients receiving sulphonamide therapy must therefore have a positive fluid balance. A daily intake of at least 2500 ml is to be aimed at and the urinary specific gravity should be kept below 1020.

Sulphaguanidine, succinylsulphathiazole (Sulfasuxidine) and phthalylsulphathiazole (Sulfathalidine) are drugs of this group which are practically insoluble. They are therefore not absorbed when given by mouth, but destroy organisms in the bowel. Large doses are given in the preparation of the large intestine for operation, and a suspension of the drug is used for injection into the rectum or perhaps into a colostomy opening.

Sulphathiazole may be used as a powder for local application or applied with an insufflator (Fig. 7.6) as an antiseptic in abdominal and other wounds.

Sensitivity to sulphonamide drugs is shown by the development of various forms of urticarial rash and there is sometimes an otherwise unexplained fever. A development of any such rash must be reported immediately to the surgeon. Sulphonamide powder should not be applied to any area of the skin which is exposed to light, especially to direct sunlight, as sensitisation occurs very readily.

Antibiotics

Penicillin, the first of the antibiotic substances, and its various derivatives (Table 13) are used in the treatment of many surgical conditions, particularly streptococcal and

Table 12   Sulphonamide drugs in common use

FOR GENERAL USE IN PYOGENIC AND OTHER INFECTIONS

Oral Tablets or Suspension		*Parental Injection Ampoules*
BP, BPC Name	*Trade Name*	
sulphadimidine	Sulphamezathine	sodium sulphadimidine
sulphadiazine	—	sodium sulphadiazine

FOR INTESTINAL STERILISATION

BP Name	*Trade Name*
succinylsulphathiazole	Sulfasuxidine
phthalylsulphathiazole	Thalazole, Sulfathalidine
sulphaguanidine	

FOR URINARY INFECTIONS (easily excreted: very little use in other infections)

BP Name	*Trade Name*	*BP Name*	*Trade Name*
sulphafurazole	Gantrisin	sulphamethoxydiazine	Durenate
sulphacetamide sodium	Albucid	sulphamethoxypyridazine	Lederkyn
sulphamethizole	Urolucosil	sulphadimethoxine	Madribon
		These are long acting, requiring one dose daily.	

FOR TOPICAL APPLICATION AND IRRIGATION
    Eye Drops—sulphacetamide sodium (Albucid) 10% or 30%
    Bladder irrigation—sulphacetamide 1 in 500

---

staphylococcal infections. It is also given prophylactically, especially in the prevention of post-operative lung complications. Penicillin is administered by intramuscular injection and there are many types of preparation. Crystalline (soluble) penicillin (benzylpenicillin when given) by intramuscular injection or used in intravenous infusion achieves an effective blood level very quickly. It is used in the initial treatment of severe infections such as osteomyelitis. It can be given by mouth but is not reliable by this route. The range of penicillin preparations with their characteristics is set out in Table 13.

Penicillin is also used in solution for instillation into abscess cavities, joints, the eye and the ear. When used as a local application in powder form it is diluted by mixing with sulphathiazole powder (see above).

Many common infecting organisms are killed by penicillin but certain strains become resistant and a surgeon may therefore prescribe a combined course of, for instance, sulphadimidine and penicillin. It may, on the other hand, be supplemented with another antibiotic.

Quite a number of persons are sensitive to penicillins and very severe reactions have occurred with high fever, sometimes severe dermatitis, and intestinal disturbance. A common symptom, even when the drug has not been given by mouth at all, is for the patient to complain of a sore tongue. The soreness spreads through the pharynx and oesophagus, resulting in loss of appetite and dysphagia. It is always wise to enquire from a patient whether he has received penicillin on any previous occasion. Nurses become sensitised easily.

Particularly when penicillin has been given by mouth (as lozenges or chewing gum), the patient is liable to develop a 'black hairy tongue'. This is a fungus infection, like thrush,

Table 13   Widely used penicillin derivatives

Type		Route	Notes
Benzylpenicillin—soluble, crystalline		I-M or I-V	Rapid action
Phenoxymethylpenicillin—resists digestive acid (**Penicillin V**)		Oral	4-hourly dosage (allied proprietary preparations—Broxil, Penspek, Ultrapen)
Procaine penicillin		I-M	Long acting—once daily injection
Cloxacillin (**Orbenin**)	Effective against strains of organism which have become resistant to other penicillins	I-M or oral	Used for penicillin-resistant strains—e.g. hospital cross-infections
Methicillin (**Celbenin**)		I-M only	
Ampicillin (**Penbritin**)	Wide range activity but resistance develops easily	Oral	Used only after bacteriological tests for sensitivity: urinary tract infections 8-hourly dosage
Carbenicillin (**Pyopen**)		I-M	Especially effective against **pseudomonas pyocyanea**
Amoxycillin (**Amoxil**)		Oral	Especially for the urinary tract; 8 hourly dosage

which has been allowed to thrive since the normal protecting organisms in the mouth and saliva have been killed.

Those who administer antibiotics frequently may themselves become sensitised. A dermatitis develops which interferes with nursing duties. Sensitization dermatitis is avoidable and it is the nurse's duty to take this elementary precaution by avoiding spillage and any personal contact with the solution. If a nurse becomes allergic to an antibiotic she is then unable to be treated with it herself if the occasion should arise. Now that a wide range of penicillin derivatives are available for longer periods of activity treatment is required less often.

Streptomycin is not absorbed from the alimentary tract unless there is severe ulceration (e.g. colitis); it is therefore used in the same way as the insoluble sulpha drugs to reduce the bacteria in the intestine before operation: it is given by mouth 0·5 G a day for three days. Streptomycin in excess damages the 8th cranial nerve producing vertigo and deafness. It was the first antibiotic to be found effective against tuberculosis and revolutionised the management, thus ultimately eliminating the large 'sanatorium' hospitals built to treat tuberculosis. Now, with **rifampicin,** it is usually combined with other anti-tubercular chemicals, the principal ones being **sodium amino salicylic acid (PAS), isoniazid (INAH), ethambutol** and **ethionamide.** Ethambutol may damage the 2nd (optic) nerve and patients are instructed to report any visual disturbance. PAS causes thyroid enlargement and may also lead to toxic hepatitis; isoniazid sometimes induces psychotic disorder.

Tetracycline and its derivatives chlor- and oxytetracycline are very powerful antibiotics used when penicillin and streptomycin are not effective. They are given in capsules or tablets by mouth, and occasionally injected intravenously. All these drugs affect the bowel, sometimes producing diarrhoea, but invariably resulting in the passage of bulky soft stools for 2–3 weeks after treatment. Very severe itching of the anal area is a common complication at this time and local treatment with nystatin lotions or ointment destroys the candida or monilial fungus infection which causes the symptoms. Tetracycline given to infants may produce yellow staining of the first teeth with severe damage.

Chloramphenicol (Chloromycetin) is not used extensively in surgery, but is of some value in certain cases of urinary infection. Prolonged use of chloramphenicol or repeated use carries with it a risk of damage to the bone marrow and fatal anaemia.

Neomycin is not absorbed from the bowel unless there is ulceration (e.g. it should never be used in ulcerative colitis as a bowel sterilising agent) and is used to sterilise it before intestinal operation. It is also used on the skin in ointments and powders.

Polymyxin is used particularly for certain urinary infections. It may produce renal damage and sometime severe neuritis of the limb nerves, with paralysis.

Novobiocin (oral), **erythromycin** (oral; i-m), **kanamycin** (i-m; i-v), **gentamicin** (i-m; i-v), and **cephaloridine** (i-m; **cephalexin**—oral) are used in the treatment of penicillin-resistant and other organisms.

Fucidin (sodium fusidate—oral; i-v) a chemical allied to penicillin is used as a surface application and by injection for staphylococcal infections, such as osteitis.

Side effects of anti-infective drugs. Prolonged administration of sulpha drugs or antibiotics leads to an interference of normal bacterial activity in the large bowel and subsequently to a shortage of vitamin B—sore tongue, oesophagitis (dysphagia), pruritis ani. The vitamin B complex is therefore administered to all patients undergoing this form of treatment. Sulphonamide and antibiotic treatment should be recorded on the patient's temperature chart so that the responsible medical officer observes each day that the treatment is continuing. It is not necessary to record on this chart each dose, but merely the fact that the drug is still being given. Treatment usually extends over a few days only, and prolonged intensive treatment is dangerous. All these substances come within the poisons regulations, and signed prescriptions are necessary.

It cannot be stressed too strongly that antibiotics or chemotherapy can be fatal and, short of that, often produce many unpleasant side-effects.

Hormones

Treatment by various endocrine gland extracts or synthetic hormones is not uncommon in surgery. **Thyroid extract** (thyroxine) is used in the treatment of myxoedema accompanied by colloid goitre or following total thyroidectomy for malignant disease of the thyroid gland. It is occasionally required after thyroidectomy for toxic goitre. **Parathormone** is very occasionally needed if all parathyroid tissue has been removed as for instance in a very wide resection of thyroid carcinoma. **Calcitonin** is a calcium retaining hormone also produced by part of the thyroid gland and is used in treating Paget's disease of bone.

Pituitrin, the secretion of the posterior portion of the pituitary gland, is sometimes given by injection as an intestinal stimulant. It is also used in obstetrics to promote contraction of the uterus after the child has been born. It may be injected into the wall of the uterus at the end of the operation for caesarean section.

Oxytocin, another hormone produced by the posterior lobe of the pituary, also stimulates the uterus and is used in obstetrics.

A secretion of the anterior lobe of the pituitary gland, **ACTH** (**adrenocorticotrophic** hormone), is used in the treatment of certain collagen (connective tissue) diseases, and acts by its stimulation of the adrenal gland cortex. It is used for a variety of other conditions, especially where there has been a gross disturbance of body chemistry. It causes water to be retained in the tissues, thereby producing a gain in weight and oedema. It is an extremely powerful drug, sometimes dramatic in its action, but it is also dangerous and is not generally available.

Other anterior pituitary hormones are not used often in surgery (the body-growth and gonad-stimulating secretions), but the cells which produce these hormones may also give rise to neoplasms which themselves then produce an excess of the secretion, leading to excessive skeletal growth (gigantism, or acromegaly), or to alteration in secondary sex characteristics.

Corticosteroids are produced by the adrenal cortex (page 697) and have two main effects. Aldosterone controls water and electrolyte balance, and hydrocortisone also controls carbohydrate and protein metabolism. (Excess male hormone arises from the adrenal tumour or from adrenal hyperplasia.) Cortisone, hydrocortisone and their derivatives when given therapeutically have a water- and salt-retaining effect which produces oedema and gives the patient a 'bloated' appearance. Commonly used preparations are **betamethasone, dexamethasone, fludrocortisone** and **prednisolone** which is also injected into injured ligaments (e.g. tennis elbow) and arthritic joints.

Cortisone is required daily for patients who have had both adrenal glands removed or excision of a pituitary tumour or of the normal pituitary in the treatment of advanced breast carcinomas.

A further disadvantage of corticosteroid therapy is that the natural adrenal function wanes, and if treatment is stopped suddenly the patient may collapse and die. For this reason all patients receiving steroid therapy are given a card indicating the treatment they are having, so that this information is available to any doctor treating the patient for some infection or other illness which may require an added dose.

The dangers of steroid therapy are referred to on pages 35 and 51.

Adrenaline, the secretion of the adrenal medulla, is used for its effect in causing the contraction of the walls of blood vessels. When combined with local anaesthetic solution or saline infiltration, it diminishes the bleeding in the field of operation (page 128) and is sometimes used on a gauze swab in the nose or tonsillar fossa for the same purpose. It is given in emergency by injection to raise the blood pressure in cases of collapse and is sometimes injected directly into the heart. It is also used in severe allergic conditions such as asthma or collapse due to drug sensitivity or for serum rash (anaphylactic shock). Adrenaline must be available in every surgical ward and department and is always at hand when an anaesthetic is being administered. It is provided for injection in ampoules of 0·5 or 1 ml solution of adrenaline tartrate. Noradrenaline, a more powerful adrenal hormone, is also used in the treatment of shock (page 111).

Oestrogens (female sex hormones), **stilboestrol, ethinyloestradiol** and **dienoestrol** are used extensively in gynaecology, but they have a peculiar additional property. Carcinoma of the prostate is particularly liable to spread to the bones and this form of growth can be largely controlled by these hormones. They also produce water retention in the tissues, and the patient on intensive stilboestrol treatment may become oedematous and suffer from heart-failure unless the drug is stopped.

Androgens (male hormones—testosterone and derivatives) are used where there is a deficiency of natural secretion, for instance from bilateral testicular absence or atrophy. Other synthetic male-type hormones are used to promote protein 'body-building' in rachitic state, and to diminish the bone softening (osteoporosis) which occurs in old age or prolonged cortisone treatment. These drugs are used illicitly to increase the stamina of athletes in important competitive sports. The most commonly used is nandrolone (Deca-Durabolin) given as an injection at three-week intervals.

Both male and female hormones are used in the management of breast cancer (page 885) and dramatic improvement is seen in some cases from norethisterone.[1] If prolonged action is required hormones may be administered as small pellets introduced through a special trocar which punctures the skin and 'implants' the pellet in the subcutaneous tissues where it is absorbed very slowly, the effect lasting for several weeks.

Prostaglandins are a group of hormones discovered first in seminal fluid from the prostate. These substances are in fact found widely distributed in body tissues. Prostaglandins cause contraction of uterine muscle and are now used to induce labour when a baby's birth has to be accelerated.

Insulin, the endocrine secretion of the pancreas used normally in the treatment of diabetes mellitus, is sometimes given in non-diabetic conditions to increase glycogen storage in the liver when there has been liver damage.

Antitoxic sera and vaccines (page 54)

There is very little use for these substances in surgery except for the routine use of tetanus antitoxin and anti-gas gangrene serum in cases of road or other open-air accidental injuries. Tetanus toxoid is used to promote active immunity against tetanus infection as a preventive in people particularly liable to injury.

Antiseptics

There are scores of antiseptic substances in common use. Each hospital seems to have its own particular fads.

The practical use of various antiseptics is further described in Chapter 17 on sterilisation.

Sulphonamide drugs and antibiotics are of course antiseptic in their action but are not used outside the body, except in the preservation of tissues for grafting.

The nurse needs to be familiar with the main groups of antiseptic chemicals in common use.

Phenol (carbolic acid) was used for many years as a general-purpose antiseptic for ward utensils which cannot be boiled. It is an unnecessary and dangerous antiseptic. It does not destroy viruses (e.g. poliomyelitis) and is thus unreliable for thermometers in preventing cross-infection. **Cresol** is similar in its action, and with soap solution it was used for many years as a general disinfectant.

Sudol is also a coal tar derivative with similar action but is less caustic and destructive to material and tissues. For ward and theatre use Sudol is now used generally and all carbolic acid and lysol preparations may be excluded. For other purposes such as thermometer sterilisation **chlorine** is regarded as the most satisfactory and safe antiseptic. It is used as 'hypochlorite solution', Eusol, Milton, Dakin's solution, Domestos and other commercial bleach preparations.

[1] Norethisterone, acetate is SH 420.

Chloroxylenol solution. This substance, supplied with the trade name of Dettol, is an extremely powerful antiseptic. It is used in a special concentrated clear yellow preparation for sterilising instruments and equipment. The Cheatle's forceps are often kept in a jar of this solution. It is also used as a vaginal or rectal douche. When mixed with water it has the appearance of milk, and is therefore tinted in hospitals with a dye to prevent accidents (page 77).

Iodine compounds in spirit are used for sterilising the skin, but iodine is extremely expensive and severe burns of the skin may occur if a patient happens to be sensitive. **Povidone-iodine** is a safe preparation used with a detergent as a 'scrub-up' soap and for local application to treat fungus (monilial and tinea) infection.

Dyes—crystal violet, brilliant green, proflavine— are used in the sterilisation of the skin. Proflavine is used occasionally in wounds.

Detergent solutions such as ether soap, spirit soap and cetrimide, are used mainly for cleaning the skin; Stergene or other liquid domestic detergent should be used for ward equipment before sterilisation. Alcohol in 70 per cent solution (methanol, spirit) is a most powerful and safe skin antiseptic.

Formalin as a gas (derived from heated tablets or powder) or as formaldehyde solution is used for instrument and catheter sterilisation and for the preservation of pathological specimens and pieces of tissue removed for biopsy (page 261). Formalin and phenol are used together in embalming the dead and for this purpose they are injected into the femoral artery under high pressure.

Ethylene oxide gas is used in hospitals and commercial practice for bulk sterilisation of materials and apparatus.

Chlorhexidine[1] (Hibitane) is the most versatile non-injurious antiseptic in common use now for skin sterilising, apparatus and most instruments which cannot be autoclaved. It is also used for cavity and wound irrigation and as a nasal cream in the treatment of staphylococcal 'carriers' (page 19). One per cent chlorhexidine in spirit is a standard pre-injection skin antiseptic.

Anti-fungal agents

Particularly after treatment with antibiotics patients develop troublesome infections in the mouth, body creases (groins, buttocks) and around the anus due to infection by monilia or candida.

Nystatin is given orally for mouth, intestinal or anal infection and it is not absorbed. It may be applied to the skin as a lotion or ointment.

Noxytiolin (Noxyflex) is used as an irrigation for bladder or vagina, and a derivative, **polynoxylin** (Anaflex), as a cream.

Griseofulvin taken by mouth is used for chronic fungal infection of nail beds in particular, or tinea.

Iodine in spirit or as povidone-iodine is an effective fungicide for local application.

---

[1] Prolonged use of chlorhexidine or hexachlorophane, where it can be absorbed from the skin or wounds, is thought to be inadvisable and for this reason hexachlorophane soaps are no longer used for bathing newborn babies.

Table 14 Antiseptics

BP name	Trade or alternative name	Recommended strength	Common use
Chloroxylenol	Dettol	5% aqueous soapy solution 1 in 40 1 in 300 Spirituous	Glassware, china, etc., instead of phenol For vaginal douche As mouthwash Sharp instruments: needles and 'non-boilable' items
	Instrument Dettol		
	Sudol	1%	Ward utensils, trolleys, etc.
Cetrimide—plain with chlorhexidine	Cetavlon Savlon	1% aqueous 1% in alcohol	For skin sterilisation and wound cleaning For skin sterilisation
Chlorinated soda	Milton (Eusol, Dakin's solution) Domestos	1 in 20 to 1 in 40 Dilution to produce 1% available chlorine	Irrigation of wounds, cavities and ulcers Feeding utensils Clinical thermometers
	(Concentration of 'bleach' solution varies with the brand)		
Iodine in spirit	Tincture of iodine	Liq. iod. mitis 2½% in spirit	Skin preparation: may cause burning of skin
Povidone-iodine	Betadine	Cream, solution, pessaries	Skin preparation, and 'scrub-up' Vaginal infection
Crystal violet	Gentian violet Bonney's blue	1% aqueous 1% in spirit	Aqueous solutions for irrigation of mouth, vagina and wounds or bladder
Proflavine	Flavine	1:1000 aqueous 1:1000 in spirit	Spirit solutions for skin sterilisation
Formalin	Liquor formaldehyde Liquor boracis et formaldehyde (p. 307)	10% in water	Instrument antiseptic for needles, scalpel blades, etc.: borax is included as a rust preventive
Paraformaldehyde	Paraform	Tablets for vaporisation	For dry vapour sterilisation of catheters, cystoscopes
Glutaraldehyde	Cidex	2%	Cystoscope, glassware, etc.
Chlorcresol with sodium benzoate	Liquor Sodi Benzoate BPC surgical instrument preservative	It will only *maintain* the sterility of instruments which must therefore be boiled or autoclaved first: rust preventive, but unsatisfactory	
Chlorhexidine	Hibitane	0·5 or 1%	In soaps for scrubbing up
Hexachlorophane	Active agent in Ster-Zac powder and in Cidal soap	0·33%	In cream for treatment of skin or nasal staphylococcal 'carriers': in solution for instruments and glassware In spirit for skin cleaning

Barrier creams

These are substances which are applied to the skin around a fistulous opening to protect it from the digestive effect of the discharge which probably contains enzymes. Many of these have a complicated formula but the most effective ones contain silicones which have a water-repelling effect and are unaffected by the chemical action of the ferments (page 469). Plastic spray-on substances are equally effective but cannot be applied to moist skin.

Coagulants and anticoagulants

Special preparations are available to encourage the clotting of blood at an operation site or to prevent the oozing of blood from a raw area. **Silver nitrate** is perhaps the simplest. The 'styptic pencil' as used by the barber to staunch the bleeding from accidental razor cuts. is a stick of silver nitrate used to destroy granulation tissue (Fig. 4.7). A solution of silver nitrate (1 part in 500) is sometimes used in bladder irrigation in persistent haematuria.

Tissue extracts and derivatives of blood plasma essential for the clotting mechanism are also available in purified form.

Anticoagulant drugs for the prevention and treatment of thrombosis are fully discussed in Chapter 5.

Stimulants

Alcohol has very little place in surgery but is nevertheless useful as a source of energy (calories) in a patient whose appetite is small, quite apart from its effect in stimulating the desire for food. The patient already severely addicted to alcohol is liable to develop delirium tremens after a day or so in hospital where he is deprived of his usual quota of alcoholic drinks. The management of delirium tremens as a complication of a surgical operation is by no means easy.

Nikethamide (Coramine) is a respiratory stimulant, very rarely used.

Chlorpromazine (Largactil) produces a feeling of well-being and restores confidence after operation or in advanced disease. It reduces worry without producing drowsiness.

Diazepam (Valium) is often used to allay anxiety but several of these tranquilliser drugs necessitate careful control. Diazepam is given orally. It has a muscle relaxant effect. It is not water soluble and for injection it is dissolved in glycerol; it must be given by *deep* intramuscular injection. If it is placed superficially in the fat or the buttock it is not absorbed and may produce necrosis. It is used intravenously in anaesthesia.

Tranquilliser drugs known as 'monamine oxidase inhibitors' can produce serious and even fatal hypertension if given with certain other drugs or foods. Patients who have taken these drugs within three weeks, or are currently being given them, must under no circumstances be allowed cheese, Bovril, Oxo, Marmite, or alcohol or broad beans if eaten with pods. Liver, yoghurt, cream, bananas and coffee **are** permitted, though there have been deaths in the past. The MAOI group includes isocarboxazid (Marplan) and tranylcypromine (Parnate).[1] The presenting symptom is often one of intense headache and collapse resembling subarachnoid haemorrhage. A similar reaction may occur after **perphenazine** (Fentazin) (page 387). Patients do not always reveal what drugs they have had prior to admission.

[1] Emergency treatment of this reaction is intravenous 5 mg phentolamine mesylate (Rogitine).

Diuretics

Drugs may be given to increase renal output in the treatment of heart failure, over-transfusion or oedema. Bendrofluazide, frusemide (Lasix) and chlorothiazide are most commonly used. Patients who have been taking diuretics for long periods without added potassium may be hypokalaemic. This adds to the danger of surgery unless corrected.

Special solutions for intravenous infusion

There are various standard preparations used for infusion. The essential feature of all these solutions is that they must be made with specially distilled water free from any dissolved matter which would cause an untoward reaction in the patient. Sterile, pyrogen-free water, as it is called, should also be used for the dilution of any drugs given intravenously, or by intramuscular and subcutaneous injection. The composition and use of intravenous infusions is described in Chapter 9.

Drugs used in anaesthesia

The action and application of these drugs is described in Chapter 12.

ROUTE AND TECHNIQUE OF ADMINISTRATION OF DRUGS

Oral

Drugs for administration by mouth may be supplied as tablet, dry powder, powder in watery suspension, emulsions (of oily substance), syrup, and simple water mixtures.

In the majority of cases a drug will be administered in the form in which it has been supplied by the pharmacist. Many patients find difficulty in swallowing tablets or capsules and a drink should always be at hand. Post-operatively, if a patient has a naso-gastric tube in place drugs supplied by the oral route may be given through the tube: tablets may be crushed, suspended in water and injected into the tube with a syringe. When gelatine capsules (usually containing hypnotic drugs) are administered pre-operatively, each end of the tube should be pricked with a needle to ensure rapid dispersal of the contents and therefore rapid action of the drug.

Oily substances are particularly difficult to swallow as their presence in the pharynx does not stimulate the normal reflex. It is preferable for such substances as liquid paraffin to be given in an emulsion form flavoured with peppermint and thickened with mucilage.

Rectal

Paraldehyde is administered in saline. Quinalbarbitone and pentobarbitone are particularly useful in children when given by this route; the capsules are pierced at each end with a stout needle and are readily inserted into the rectum. Thiopentone dissolved in water may also be given rectally as a basal anaesthetic agent. Morphine is used frequently in general practice in the form of a suppository; the drug is released slowly from the cocoa-butter base which forms the bulk of the suppository and the action is thereby prolonged. There is of course a difference between drugs introduced into the rectum to be *absorbed* for their general effect on the body, and those which are applied for their local effect on the rectum, colon or anal canal.

Whatever the precise form in which the drug is introduced, the manoeuvre must be extremely gentle to avoid stimulation of peristalsis in the rectum and consequent ejection of the fluid.

Retention enemas of prednisolone are used in ulcerative colitis (page 548).

Parenteral—subcutaneous, intramuscular and intravenous injections

Drugs given otherwise than by the alimentary (enteric) canal are introduced into the circulation either directly by intravenous injection or by rapid absorption from the very vascular muscle tissue or by more gradual absorption from the less vascular tissue immediately beneath the skin. The speed with which an injection acts depends on the site of injection and the blood supply to that site. Certain drugs because of their chemical effects on the tissues must **never** be given subcutaneously or necrosis of the tissues will occur and an abscess is almost certain to form. Similarly there are certain drugs which should not be given intramuscularly. Conversely the nature and dose of the drug may be such that it needs to be absorbed slowly from the subcutaneous area: if such an injection is given in error into the muscles or intravenously, the full dose will at once take effect with sometimes fatal results. These two hazards may be illustrated by two common examples. Morphine is normally injected subcutaneously. If, however, the injection is given to a patient severely shocked as the result of operation or accident, the blood supply to the skin and surface tissues (as shown by pallor) is for the time being extremely poor and the morphine is not absorbed with sufficient rapidity. The patient may therefore appear to require a further dose which may again in error be given subcutaneously. As the shock passes off the blood supply returns to the subcutaneous tissues and both injections are rapidly absorbed, the patient being subsequently poisoned by overdose. In cases of shock, morphine should be given intravenously, or if this is not possible, at least intramuscularly. On the other hand, if certain preparations, such as sulphonamides, are injected into the subcutaneous tissues by mistake or by movement of the needle, instead of into the vein, severe inflammation may develop at the injection site. Thiopentone also has a destructive effect if it is not injected into the vein, and paraldehyde for intramuscular injection will produce necrosis of fat and skin if given too superficially.

Injection Technique. The nurse must observe certain basic precautions in giving injections of drugs. She will be shown the correct technique in each case during her training, but this simple and oft-repeated act is too often performed in a slovenly and slip-shod manner; the complications and difficulties that arise from incorrectly placed injections are manifold.

The nurse will not normally be expected to give intravenous injections, except into an already established infusion line. A 'flash ball' or rubber section in the delivery tube provides a site for injections of the required dose directed into the infusion line. If a 'Buretrol' type drip set is used (page 146) the drug may be injected into the graduated reservoir so that it is delivered more slowly. Drugs are not now normally put into the infusion flask. The correct location for intramuscular injections is shown in Fig. 7.4.

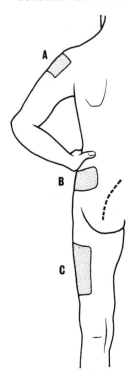

(A) Injections of 2 ml or less may be placed in the deltoid muscle. Clothes must be removed; the temptation to push up the sleeve instead will result in the injection being given too low. A short needle should be used and it should be directed downwards through the muscle toward the axilla in order to avoid the subdeltoid bursa and the shoulder joint.

(B) Larger volumes should be placed in the gluteal muscle mass, using the upper outer quadrant of the buttock above the top of the great trochanter. The sciatic nerve will be damaged if the injection is given near the midline.

(C) A convenient site for *small* volumes is the lateral muscle mass of the thigh.
(Particular care is needed in paraplegic patients whose leg muscles are very wasted: the main bulk is fat and if drugs are injected into the fat necrosis and ulcers will result.)

Fig. 7.4   Intramuscular injection sites.

The following points of procedure should be noted for intramuscular or subcutaneous injections:

(*i*) All apparatus for injections must of course be absolutely sterile and completely free of antiseptic. The sterilisation and preparation of syringes is described in Chapter 16, though most hospitals now use commercially sterilised apparatus.

(*ii*) From the patient's point of view, the sharpness matters far more than the thickness of the needle. When withdrawing solution from a glass ampoule, care must be taken not to injure the point of the needle on the bottom of the ampoule. (Unless the needle is a new disposable one, the nurse should develop the habit of testing the point by drawing the needle across a sterile swab which she is going to apply to the skin at the site of injection. If there is a hook on the end of the needle, it must on no account be used.)

(*iii*) The needle must be a really tight fit on the nozzle of the syringe. Many injections are lost in part or in entirety by this joint being blown apart as the fluid is compressed in the syringe.

(*iv*) All air must be expressed from the syringe and needle **through the needle which is actually to be used for the injection.**

(*v*) A spare needle of the right size should always be at hand, especially when giving penicillin injections as the needle is apt to get blocked.

(*vi*) The hand which is holding the syringe should **always** be in such a position that it is resting against the patient's skin while the injection is being given. This is the only way of making certain that the needle remains stationary and of guarding against its breakage should the patient move. Particularly is this true of intramuscular injections given into the thigh or buttock: the syringe should be held like a pen between the thumb and first two fingers so that the ulnar side of the hand

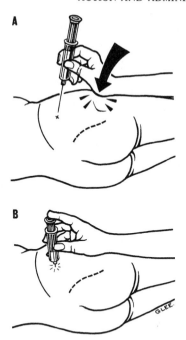

Fig. 7.5   Gluteal intramuscular injection technique. The syringe is held like a dart, or pen, and plunged into the muscles as the inner side of the hand strikes the great trochanter: if the arm is kept behind the patient's upper leg, this ensures that the injection is made far forward away from the sciatic nerve. It is better to penetrate down to bone and withdraw than to inject superficially into the fat where an abscess may be produced.

strikes the patient's arm or leg (the great trochanter of the femur) as the needle pierces the skin (Fig. 7.5).

(*vii*) Subcutaneous injections are often given by inserting the needle into the base of a fold of skin which has been pinched up by the opposite hand. The purpose of this is to ensure that the injection is not placed deeper than the subcutaneous tissue, but it can be a very painful method: if the skin is put under tension instead, a fine needle is inserted rapidly through the skin and it can be felt to slide through the fat. The syringe should be kept as nearly parallel to the skin as possible but a weal should not be raised as the fluid is injected.

(*viii*) If subcutaneous injections are given in the orthodox sites—the outer side of the upper arm or the outer side of the thigh—the risk of penetrating a vessel, and thus giving the injection intravenously in error, is extremely slight. If, however, an intramuscular injection is being given, the piston must always be withdrawn after insertion of the needle, and if blood appears in the syringe, the needle must be moved to a different site. Occasionally one sees a haematoma at an injection site from damage to a major vessel, usually by the needle having passed right through it.

(*ix*) When the injection is completed, an antiseptic swab should be placed on the point of entry and the needle withdrawn rapidly. The site of injection should be massaged very gently to seal the needle track in order to avoid leakage, and to prevent pooling of the fluid which has been injected. If more than 2 ml of any substance is injected intramuscularly or subcutaneously, the needle should be advanced during the course of the injection or withdrawn a little and advanced to a different site, the plunger again being pulled back momentarily to guard against the needle having entered a vessel.

(*x*) Glass ampoules should always be filed at the neck and broken cleanly. It is quite easy to inject small fragments of glass inadvertently.

(*xi*) Multidose containers of drugs for injection always contain in addition an antiseptic preservative fluid. This is principally to prevent the growth of moulds, but it is not an absolute guarantee that any infection introduced carelessly through the rubber cap will be killed. The cap must therefore be adequately sterilised and probably iodine in spirit, or methylated ether, is the best rapid antiseptic for this purpose. A cursory wipe with a swab dipped in cetrimide is quite insufficient. If several patients are to receive injections within a few minutes, the needle (its size depending on the consistency of the fluid) is inserted into the container and left in position until the last injection has been given. The smaller the needle for this purpose, the less likely will there be contamination of the fluid within, but the needle must always be adequate in size for easy filling. Air must always be injected into the container in the same quantity as the fluid it is desired to withdraw. If an excessive amount of air is injected, the drug will continue to squirt through the needle after the syringe has been removed. When the needle has been withdrawn from the container, the cap should be wiped with an antiseptic and the metal cap (if there is one) should be replaced.

(*xii*) If the multidose container or ampoule contains powder to be dissolved in water, only sterile pyrogen-free water provided for the purpose may be used: the exact quantity to be injected into the ampoule or container is indicated on its label. Sometimes of course the whole of the powder content of an ampoule is to be given in one dose and the exact quantity of water does not then matter.[1]

A haematoma or bruising discovered later at an injection site should be reported. It may be the first sign of a bleeding tendency.

A very heavy responsibility rests on anyone who uses a syringe to administer drugs; once the injection has been given, the process cannot be reversed. Each hospital has its own rules for checking and double-checking the nature and quantity of drugs before injections are given. Different drugs should not be mixed in the syringe before injection and a separate syringe should be used for each drug on account of interaction of the drugs in their concentrated form.

Topical application

Instead of the drug being carried to the site of action by the blood stream, it is applied to the lesion direct. This is the action of some substances given by mouth, for their local effect on the gastro-intestinal tract.

Ointments containing antiseptics, sedatives or hormones are used for **inunction**.

Pine, menthol and friar's balsam are used for **vapour inhalation** while penicillin and other drugs may be given by an 'atomiser' as a very fine spray (page 284). Anaesthetic gases and oxygen are in a different category since they are given not for their topical effect but for their general effect, when absorbed through the lungs.

Instillation is the introduction of 'drops' or larger quantities of solution—into the eye, ear, nose or joint cavities. Penicillin may be injected into an abscess cavity or, for instance, into an infected maxillary air sinus, after aspiration of the pus: this is **replacement** therapy.

Insufflation of antiseptic powder (usually neomycin or bacitracin) is achieved with a

---

[1] Drugs supplied in multidose containers have an added preservative such as chlorocresol or chlorbutol. The amount is harmless unless injected into the spinal canal and any substance provided for injection **via lumbar puncture** must be taken from a single-dose sealed glass ampoule.

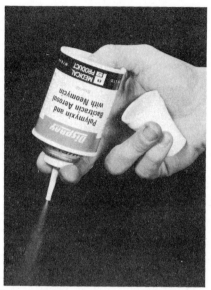

Fig. 7.6 Anti-bacterial powders are supplied in pressurised cannisters: except when in use the spout must be covered to prevent contamination: the outlet must be held at least 25 cm from the wound to prevent the propellent gas from freezing the tissues.

special spray or pressurised container; wounds, burnt areas, or the vagina may be treated in this way (Fig. 7.6).

WEIGHTS, MEASURES AND DOSAGE

The 'Imperial' system (pints, ounces, drachms and minims) has been replaced by the metric system. For some years to come, nurses will need to be familiar with both systems, but it behoves doctors and nurses alike in hospitals to attempt to conform with the new standards.

Prescription

For any drug, the amount to be prescribed will depend on the patient's weight, age and state of activity. For instance, a child of 6 stones weight (38 kilograms) will require a larger dose of papaveretum or morphine than an elderly lady of the same weight. It is not uncommon for old folk to be overdrugged by being given the dose for a healthy adult without reference to age and weight.

The dose of drug to be given on a particular occasion is, in the majority of cases, specifically written down by a medical officer. There will, however, remain those drugs to be used at the discretion of the nursing staff.

Pain-relieving drugs such as morphine and its allied substance pethidine are often prescribed in limited quantity to be given at the discretion of the nursing staff;[1] the prescription has to be signed in the doctor's handwriting and may be marked 'as required'

[1] The old signs p.r.n. = *pro re nata*, as the occasion demands and s.o.s. = *sic opus sit*, if necessary, are no longer used and the instructions are written in full.

and may be repeated; or 'if necessary'—a single dose only. For instance, a patient about to undergo appendicectomy may be 'written up' or prescribed:

    (1) Pre-operative Inj. Morphine sulphate 10 mg.
                   Inj. Atrophine sulphate 0·6 mg.
    (2) Post-operative Inj. Morphine sulphate 10 mg as required.

    Item 1 **must** be given; item 2 **may** be given if required.

Strictly, the doctor should limit the total dose by writing 'not to be repeated' or 'repeat if necessary in 4 hours'. A great deal of authority in the administration of such drugs as morphine is delegated to responsible nursing staff; all nurses must show great care in the use of these 'non-specific' and 'discretionary' treatments. Drug-recording sheets are now being introduced widely so that each dose prescribed is signed for by the nurse administering it.

The effect of drugs depends upon accurate administration: the nurse needs to make specific enquiry from the doctor as to whether he wishes a patient wakened to be given medicine which has been prescribed, or whether a dose may be omitted or delayed. The night nurse must obtain her instruction on such matters from the ward day sister. If a dose has been omitted by nursing error, by the patient's sleep or refusal, or if an oral medicine has been returned by vomit, the fact must be reported to the doctor in charge.

Poisoning from overdosage or sensitivity

All patients suffering from poisoning should be treated for shock which is partly the result of pain, partly from the poisoning of the vital centres and heart, and from consequent anoxia (Chapter 10).

Morphine or pethidine. In surgical practice poisoning from these narcotics arises from time to time. A small elderly adult may have been given a dose appropriate for a healthy young person of average build. To avoid such accidents, all patients are weighed on admission and the weight should be recorded on the temperature chart. A dose of morphine in excess of 10 mg prescribed for a patient of small stature (under 8 stone, 50 kilos) and over sixty years of age should be queried with the medical officer. On the other hand, a second dose may have been given before the first injection has been completely absorbed, in a case of shock (page 99).

Slow respiration (less than 10 breaths per minute), small pupils and pallor are evidence of excessive morphine. If the patient has also had atropine, the pupils may not be constricted.

The specific antidote for morphine, papaveretum (Omnopon), pethidine and amidone (methadone, Physeptone), is **nalorphine** (Lethidrone). It is given intravenously and should be at hand in all wards.

If this drug is not available, nikethamide (Coramine) should be given (5 ml initially), preferably into a vein, as a respiratory stimulant. Oxygen should be administered if respiration is very slow, although the patient's oxygen requirement is greatly reduced by the general effect of morphine in depressing tissue activity.

As this eventuality arises usually in the post-operative period, it is vital to pay particular attention to chest-expansion exercises when the effect of the drug has passed off.

Procaine and allied drugs. Certain patients are extremely sensitive to these local anaesthetic agents: it seems that the fact of the patient having had a previous injection without reaction is no safeguard. Pallor and collapse is very frightening for all concerned. This reaction has been thought to be due to the adrenaline which is sometimes given with procaine. The patient is treated as for shock. Nalorphine (the specific antidote for morphine) is effective and can be given by intramuscular or intravenous injection. Barbiturate drugs act to some extent as an antidote to the cocaine group.

Barbiturate hypnotics. Intentional (suicidal) or accidental poisoning with barbiturates results in deep coma which may be prolonged, if not fatal. The time available to prevent death depends on the nature of the particular drug, its rate of destruction or elimination from the body, and the amount taken. The drug has usually been taken by mouth and the stomach should be washed out with sodium bicarbonate or magnesium sulphate solution. If the patient survives the immediate crisis there is still the additional risk of pulmonary collapse or pneumonia. Special treatment centres are maintained for the management of drug addition and cases of acute drug poisoning. Renal dialysis is frequently required.

Mercurial compounds. The accidental administration of mercurial antiseptics occurs occasionally. The initial effect is upon the lining of the oesophagus and stomach. The immediate administration of egg white or blood plasma by mouth is of value as the protein combines with the mercury salts which may still be unabsorbed. The later effect is upon the kidneys, and anuria may result, necessitating renal dialysis (page 674).

Mercuric perchloride is occasionally used as a surface application to areas upon which malignant cells may have been spilled, for instance in the removal of a pelvic growth. There is a very serious risk that the drug may be absorbed from the peritoneum or other raw areas and produce severe renal damage. Such treatment has to be used with great caution.

Phenol and Lysol. If either of these has been swallowed, the stomach should be immediately washed out with strong magnesium sulphate solution—1 teaspoonful to a pint (4 G to 600 ml)—or the patient should be given a drink of strong magnesium sulphate and made to vomit by tickling the pharynx with a spatula or tube. Sixty millilitres of liquid paraffin should be given and removed by lavage after ten minutes: this should be repeated several times, and a further quantity left in the stomach. The oil absorbs the phenol or cresol but is not itself digested or absorbed from the bowel.

The golden rule about poisons is that they should be kept locked up when not in use. Prevention of poisoning is always better than treatment. Not only should the nurse be extremely careful about the administration of drugs, but she should remember that in any hospital ward, especially where patients are waiting for operation, there may be those who are depressed, worried and easily tempted to seize an apparent opportunity to escape from their problems by suicide.

Artificial respiration, probably prolonged and with tracheostomy, is sometimes required, and the artificial kidney is used to eliminate drugs which should normally be excreted by the healthy kidney (page 677).

Poison bureaux. In the United Kingdom there is a network of Hospital Poison Information Centres to which doctors can refer by telephone for information on antidotes for less well-known poisons such as weedkillers and industrial preparations.

SECTION II

8

Haemorrhage, Shock and Fluid Balance

Bleeding is usually the result of injury or operation, but it may occur spontaneously without either accident or apparent injury. Shock accompanies almost all injuries and surgical operations; even procedures which appear trifling, may produce fatal collapse. Both haemorrhage and shock have a similar effect on the well-being of the victim. Each lowers the pressure in the arterial side of the circulation; this is turn leads to oxygen shortage in the tissues. The anoxia has its first and most important effect on the brain, leading to a rapid series of nervous reactions designed to protect the body and to restore the pressure in the circulation. If this compensatory mechanism is inadequate, loss of consciousness occurs and the heart itself may fail. If the patient has already been rendered unconscious by head injury or anaesthesia, the onset of this 'collapse', whether from haemorrhage or shock, will not be so apparent and may be overlooked in the early stage at which treatment can be most effective.

To avert disaster and even more commonly to allay anxiety, a nurse needs to be very well informed about the management of haemorrhage and shock. As with many other aspects of surgical nursing, it is far better to have a clear understanding of the simple fundamentals which guide our actions than to attempt nursing management by rule of thumb.

Although for descriptive purposes haemorrhage is to be dealt with as a distinct subject in its various aspects, it must be emphasised at this point that—

(a) **Haemorrhage** (i.e. loss of blood from the circulation) if at all severe is always accompanied by shock.

(b) **Shock,** though it can be produced by haemorrhage, frequently occurs without any blood loss.

Body fluid distribution

Fluid in the body is distributed mainly in three ways:
(1) The plasma in the circulating blood (consisting of water, dissolved protein and dissolved salts): 5 per cent of the body weight.
(2) The tissue fluid and lymph (with a similar composition to that of plasma): 15 per cent of body weight. This fluid is distributed throughout the tissues of the body and has to be distinguished from:

(3) The intracellular fluid which is in fact part of the living protoplasm within each cell: 50 per cent of body weight. Thus water may form between 60 and 70 per cent of total body weight (Figs. 8.1, 22.3) in relation to total body size.

The blood plasma might be described as the wholesaler of the chemicals and foodstuffs which the tissues require; the tissue fluid acts as the retailer or 'shop' and, without using the chemicals and foodstuffs itself, supplies the needs of the cells in its district. The blood plasma draws its supplies from many factories such as the liver and the intestinal tract. If at any time there is a crisis, the water and salts which are in the tissue fluid may be recalled back into the blood plasma, and in extreme crises the tissue fluid may withdraw chemicals and water from the cells. This distribution of fluid in the three 'compartments' of the body is regulated largely by osmotic pressure, which depends mainly on the protein content of the fluid and on the concentration of the various chemical salts called electrolytes. The cells need an exact amount of such chemicals as calcium, potassium, sodium and chloride. If any one of these chemicals is present in excess it may act as a poison, or if it is in short supply, tissues may die (Tables 15, 16).

It will thus be seen that when fluid has been lost from the body in excessive quantity, it needs to be replaced by a fluid with the right composition and the right osmotic pressure.

The distribution of fluid in the body is shown in Fig. 8.1.

DISTRIBUTION OF BODY FLUID

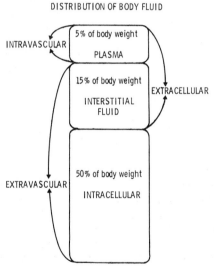

Fig. 8.1   Half the body weight consists of water which is actually within the cells. It is held there by the electrolyte balance, mainly potassium; clearly if dehydration is prolonged the time of recovery of the tissues to their full content of water is also prolonged and cannot be achieved very rapidly without overloading the circulation. This is why the treatment of dehydration due to vomiting or diarrhoea or any other cause, must be managed very carefully with regular electrolyte estimations.

Electrolyte balance

Certain chemicals when dissolved in water break down into component ions; thus sodium chloride breaks down into sodium (Na^+) and chloride (Cl^-) ions.

The principal alkaline (base) ions in the blood are calcium, potassium and sodium; the acid ions are chlorine and carbonic acid (HCO_3—from carbon dioxide dissolved in water and protein compounds). The balance of cations (positive, alkaline or base) to anions (negative, acid) determines the acidity of the blood and tissues at any given time. The amount of any chemical dissolved in water can be given as milligrams per 100 ml but this tells us nothing of the combining power of the dissolved substance. The concentration of electrolytes can be expressed in terms of their molecular weight (milli-mol per litre) and with the introduction of the new international (SI) units this term has replaced the former mEq/l which was more expressive. (See Preface, page v). Except for calcium and magnesium mEq/l and mmol are numerically the same. Compound substances such as protein and organic acids cannot be expressed as mmol in the same way. The Term mEq/l has been retained in Tables 15 and 16 for the sake of comparing the anion and cation equivalent content of the blood which is approximately 154 of each. In reports

Table 15   Anions

Anions	Plasma concentration mEq/l	
HCO_3	24	
Cl (Chloride)	105	Normal base/acid balance is mainly
P (Phosphate)	2	due to base bicarbonate excess over
Proteinate (protein compounds)		carbonic acid: carbonic acid is
Organic acids		'blown off' by breathing; base bi-
(pyruvic, citric, lactic)	Approx. 23	carbonate is regulated largely by
Sulphate		kidney function. Acidosis may
		therefore be **metabolic** (renal) or
		respiratory in origin.

For simplicity mEq/l is retained in this chart. See text.

on electrolyte estimations it will be seen that there is an excess of base ions over acid ions because HCO_3, the carbonic acid part, is not shown. This excess is the 'alkali reserve' or 'carbon dioxide combining power' of the plasma. The carbon dioxide in the body is adjusted through the lungs by respiration and thus the individual has a very rapid means of balancing the acidity of the blood. Over-breathing 'blows off' too much CO_2 and alkalosis occurs. In normal plasma there are 140 parts of sodium to 100 parts of chlorine; if normal saline (sodium chloride) with 154 mmol of sodium and 154 mmol of chlorine is given in large quantity the patient will have an excess of chlorine: this acidity is more than he can correct by getting rid of carbon dioxide through his lungs. Therefore, in order to keep the balance right in prolonged infusion we use sodium lactate one part, to two parts of sodium chloride. The lactic acid portion decomposes and goes off from the lungs as carbon dioxide, leaving the sodium in excess (page 138).

Other disturbances of electrolyte balance occur in certain renal diseases, with the use of cortisone, and after diuretics like chlorothiazide. Excessive potassium may be lost from the kidney under these conditions. Vomiting produces a heavy loss of chloride resulting in

Table 16 Cations

Cation	Specific actions	Plasma concentration mEq/l	Effects of variation	
			Excess	Deficiency
Na$^+$ Sodium	Maintenance of extra cellular (tissue) fluid	142	Thirst Oedema Oliguria Restlessness Overbreathing	Fatigue Anxiety Oliguria Convulsions
K$^+$ (Potassium)	Maintenance of intra cellular fluid	5	Renal failure Diarrhoea Cramp Paraesthesia ECG elevation of T wave	Ileus Muscular weakness (paralysis) Bradycardia and coupled beats ECG depression of T wave
Ca^{++} (Calcium)	Bone metabolism neuromuscular activity	2·25–2·60	Coagulation defect Renal stones	**Acute** Paraesthesia Twitching Tetany **Chronic** Rickets Osteomalacia
Mg^{++} (Magnesium)	Essential for enzyme activity (hence effect on neuro-muscular mechan-ism)	0·7–1		Confusion Tremor Convulsions Tetany

alkalosis whilst diarrhoea causes the loss of sodium and potassium from the bowel and results in acidosis.

If we use potassium chloride to give a patient potassium, he receives equal quantities of potassium and chloride. If we use potassium bicarbonate, he gets rid of the HCO_3 (the bicarbonate) through his lungs and is less likely to be acidotic.

Magnesium is essential for enzyme action and because clinical symptoms arising from shortage of this element are uncommon and are similar to symptoms arising from other causes, shortage of magnesium is easily overlooked. It occurs principally when there has been prolonged starvation, and is often precipitated by severe diarrhoea. Twitching and convulsions occur, and the clinical picture is a little like calcium depletion, but it is not relieved by giving calcium nor are the symptoms of calcium shortage relieved by giving magnesium. The remedy lies in intravenous magnesium sulphate. A 50 per cent sterile solution is used and the initial dose is 10 ml given slowly in not less than 500 ml of dextrose solution over a period of at least three hours. It can be given intramuscularly; no more than 3 ml of this solution should be injected at any one muscle site.

All these complicated matters become vitally important in any patient who is severely ill from injury or major surgery, and skilful management of electrolyte balance may save an otherwise 'hopeless' patient. The nurse cannot be expected to remember details and the only way of becoming familiar with the complexity of blood chemistry is to study individual patients in relation to the facts outlined here. The important principle is never to give a bottle of intravenous fluid unless it has been prescribed specifically: guesswork may be fatal (page 134).

The nature of shock

What is shock? No one really knows the answer to this question, but for all practical purposes it may be regarded as a state of abnormally low blood pressure. This fall in the blood pressure may be brought about in various ways:

(a) **By diminished heart action.** The heart is under nervous control and severe pain may, by nervous reflex, slow the heart and reduce its output. Pain may stop the heart (page 191). Under-perfusion (anoxia) of certain tissues, the pancreas in particular, leads to the production of a substance known as myocardial depressant factor (MDF) which has a direct effect on the heart.

(b) **By a leak in the circulation,** if a main blood vessel bursts and blood pours out into a body cavity (such as bleeding into the peritoneum from a ruptured spleen) or into a hollow organ (for instance into the stomach from a bleeding ulcer).

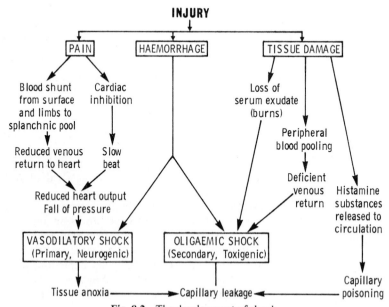

Fig. 8.2   The development of shock.

(c) **By a sudden shunting of the blood to a different part of the circulation**. There are certain areas of the body which normally contain vessels of small calibre. Nervous stimulation of various types may bring about a sudden 'opening-up' of these blood vessels so that they contain much more blood than normal. There is then insufficient pressure in the main circulation for the brain to receive its full supply of oxygen. This is the basis of what is known as **primary** or **neurogenic shock.** Some people refer to this as **vasovagal** shock because it is brought about through the pathways of the vagus nerve, but the most rational descriptive name is **vasodilatory shock,** and the 'pooling' is in the splanchnic (abdominal) vessels. However, the shock stimulus releases the hormones **noradrenaline** and **adrenaline** from the adrenal glands. These affect the heart directly and the peripheral vessels. Noradrenaline constricts the peripheral vessels causing pallor and raising the blood pressure; adrenaline accelerates the heart and dilates the coronary vessels. There is peripheral vasoconstriction at first, but the mixed effect of these hormones is not clear cut. Shock may be present without pallor if the adrenaline 'beta' effect on the peripheral vessels dominates the 'alpha' noradrenaline (page 697). The contraction of small arteries all over the body reduces blood flow and insufficient blood returns to the heart to maintain pressure. The term **stagnant shock** is now applied to this phase and if rapid infusion is not given, the anoxic state of the peripheral tissues leads to vasodilation and pooling of blood with capillary leakage and an irreversible condition.

(d) **By a gradual seepage of fluid from the circulation over a very wide area.** In the normal state of affairs, the millions of blood capillaries have walls which are capable of retaining water except for the small amount which the tissues deliberately withdraw to meet their needs. If these capillary walls become damaged and 'porous' it is obvious that water will ooze from the capillary network all over the body. The capillaries are in fact damaged by a substance called histamine which is a toxin coming from injured cells. A bruise or a scratch is followed by production of histamine which produces local swelling (oedema). If a large quantity of this toxin is absorbed from a damaged area and circulates in the blood, then the capillaries all over the body are affected. Such a condition occurs particularly with extensive burns. Severe lack of oxygen has a similar effect on the capillaries and makes them porous. This type of shock is therefore described as **secondary** or **toxigenic** (generated by toxin), and the water seeps out into the tissue spaces.

The shock produced by severe blood loss (i.e. haemorrhage into an organ or body cavity or from a wound) has an effect similar to that arising from toxigenic shock and we speak of both these conditions as being **oligaemic** shock (in Greek ὀλίγος, 'oligos', means little or few).

Tissue respiration and tissue perfusion

To acquire a clear understanding of many of the procedures in the care of the very ill, in the management of shock, of lung disease and of post-operative complications, it is essential to grasp the basic principles of the physiology of respiration and circulation. Strictly, respiration is the physiological process by which each cell obtains oxygen and discharges carbon dioxide—**tissue respiration.** Clearly, this depends on the integrity of the blood supply to the part. The flow of blood through the capillary bed depends basically on the pumping action of the heart, but is regulated by the contractile power of the small arteries. The outflow of blood from the capillary bed depends largely on the pressure exerted by the veins or by tissues surrounding the veins thus preventing free drainage. This process of blood moving through the tissues is referred to as **tissue perfusion**, a term now widely used in discussion on shock. The peripheral circulation—that is the small arteries, the capillary bed and the veins—is capable of great variation in size. Large volumes of blood may pool in the periphery in certain circumstances so that the return of blood to the central circulation is inadequate to keep up the pressure required for satisfactory tissue perfusion.

Thus, tissue respiration depends on the mechanical act of breathing which we refer to as respiration in the gross sense, and upon the related blood flow through the lungs. Inadequate lung perfusion leads to anoxia even if ventilation is normal (Fig. 8.3b).

Cyanosis (Greek 'kyanos'—dark blue)

This is the description applied to tissues which are purple or dusky instead of being of normal pink oxygenated hue (derived from the blueness of copper salts).

Central cyanosis is usually due to respiratory obstruction, and there is then likely to be hypercapnia (excess CO_2 in blood) as well and thus a struggle to breathe.

However, a patient breathing with a clear airway may become cyanosed if part of the lung bed is unaerated and 'blue' blood passes through unchanged (Fig. 8.3d). This vascular 'shunt' is the most common cause of central cyanosis in the fully conscious post-operative patient. Other causes of central cyanosis are defects in the septa of the heart or abnormal communications between the great vessels.

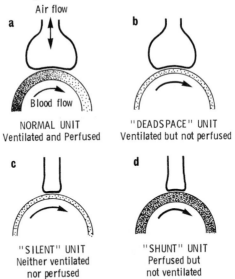

Fig. 8.3   The effectiveness of breathing depends both upon the airflow into lung units and upon the related blood flow. Decreased expansion or decreased perfusion have the same effect in producing anoxia. Cyanosis may be due to deficient aeration or to deficient perfusion. **a.** Normal respiration. **b.** Breathing normal: shock or other cause of low cardiac output: anaemia has the same effect. **c.** Shock with respiratory depression: collapsed area of lung: capillary shut down. **d.** Consolidation or bronchial or broncheolar obstruction.

Peripheral cyanosis is due to venous stagnation in the surface tissues. In such a state if the 'blue' lips or 'blue' ears are rubbed they may become pink: but will not do so if the cyanosis is due to some central cause, or if the arterioles are in spasm, as in certain phases of surgical shock where blood is pooled in the periphery, or in Raynaud's disease and other forms of acrocyanosis (page 944).

Respiration

We now return to the mechanics of respiration and to consider exactly what happens in the lungs. We have to understand first that the air which we breathe contains oxygen at a certain pressure, nitrogen at a lesser pressure and carbon dioxide in negligible amount. It is general knowledge that at high altitudes the air is 'thinner'—that is, that the oxygen pressure is less than at sea level. It is the pressure of oxygen in the atmosphere that enables us to maintain normal oxygen exchange in health. If there is any degree of obstruction to respiration, for instance by narrowing of the bronchioles, the oxygen tension (pressure) that reaches the tiny air cells of the lungs is diminished. Also if the lining membrane of the pulmonary alveoli is inflamed or congested (by oedema from cardiac failure or over-infusion), normal atmospheric oxygen tension is insufficient to drive the oxygen through into the blood. In abnormal conditions such as bronchitis or patchy pneumonia, parts

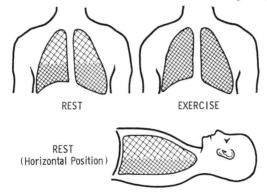

REST   EXERCISE

REST
(Horizontal Position)

Fig. 8.4   Maximum perfusion and aeration occur in the densely shaded areas.

of the lung may be functioning normally while other parts are only receiving an inadequate amount of oxygen. The blood flow through the lungs continues both to the healthy and unhealthy parts: that which goes through the unhealthy or unaerated portions of the lung returns to the left atrium unoxygenated, but mixed with the oxygenated blood from the rest of the lung (Fig. 8.3c,d). The state of oxygenation of the *arterial* blood is described in terms of this oxygen pressure and is known as Pa_{O_2}: this is simply written as P_{O_2}. Pressure of oxygen in the *alveoli* themselves is described as PA_{O_2} but this term is not used generally in clinical work. The normal Pa_{O_2} is 95–100 mm mercury (Hg) pressure. [1]

In health the amount of lung being fully aerated depends on the oxygen demand and on the posture of the individual. Figure 8.4 illustrates the relationship of expansion of the lungs to perfusion by the blood stream. At rest the flow of blood through the lungs is

[1] In SI units this pressure is expressed in pascals (11–15 kPa) but the change is not applying to blood and gas pressures.

greater to the lower portions. In exercise more oxygen is obtained by increasing the perfusion of the whole lung field as well as by more expansion. In the supine position blood flow to the posterior part of the lungs is greater.

Similarly, if we look at the carbon dioxide exchange there is the normal Pa_{CO_2} and the normal PA_{CO_2}. As the body loses carbon dioxide through the lungs during the mechanical process of respiration the P_{CO_2} is reduced and is normally at about 40 mm Hg. When Pa_{CO_2} is raised the clinical state is called **hypercapnia** (Greek 'kapnos'—smoke)—and there is **respiratory acidosis.**

Tissue perfusion

Moving now into the circulation itself, the transport of oxygen and carbon dioxide depends on there being sufficient red blood cells and each red blood cell having sufficient haemoglobin. Thus we can see that a failure of the central pump, a pooling of blood in the peripheral circulation, loss of blood from haemorrhage or the poor quality of blood—acute or chronic anaemia—may all lead to a condition in which the oxygen saturation of the tissues and the elimination of carbon dioxide is inadequate though the pulmonary function may be good. One of the most important changes which occurs is the poisoning of the tissues by carbon dioxide. If tissue perfusion is inadequate the peripheral blood vessels become incapable of contracting: the blood pools so that it is not available for the central circulation. One of the body's early responses to injury is the production of adrenalin which in turn produces constriction of the small arterioles all over the body (except in the heart and lungs) as a defence mechanism to raise the blood pressure to maintain adequate perfusion to the brain and to the heart itself. If this constriction persists, in order to maintain an adequate central circulation, the peripheral tissues become deprived of oxygen for such a long period that they then are permanently impaired. When eventually circulation is restored, the blood stagnates at the periphery and the state of shock becomes irreversible. There is an apparent paradox here because a 'shocked' person may for a short time have a high pressure and give the appearance of being safe.

It will be seen that it is really impossible to separate the circulatory aspects of shock from those of respiration. When shock in its various forms is discussed, we have constantly to bear in mind that there must be adequate return of blood to the right side of the heart.

Shock treatment

In primary or neurogenic shock, the blood fluid is still in the body, still in the blood vessels but in the wrong blood vessels: the treatment must therefore be to return the blood to the normal vessels of the main circulation. This happens spontaneously if the nervous stimulation passes off or pain is relieved, but if primary shock persists, lack of oxygen (from lowered blood pressure) may damage the capillaries and oligaemic shock will ensue.

The treatment of secondary or oligaemic shock is different. Either we have to pour fluid into the circulation from outside, or to draw it back from the tissues into which it has leaked through the porous capillaries.

Unfortunately we cannot repair the capillaries and this damage is sometimes so severe that the patient dies, no matter what temporary improvement is obtained from transfusion. We know that it is almost useless to give saline or glucose saline solutions in the presence of such capillary damage. Simple saline solutions are of real value only in the treatment of oligaemic shock which has arisen from dehydration—that is from an external loss of the water and salt components of blood, but not of the plasma and cells. In order to raise the blood pressure and the power of the blood to draw water back from the tissues into the circulation, it is necessary to give some solution which behaves more like plasma. Plasma obtained from 'blood donors' can be dried, stored for long periods and reconstituted by the addition of distilled water; this method was employed with dramatic success for several years. Plasma infusions are still very useful, but there is a risk of passing on to the patient the virus of infective jaundice which survives the drying process. The risk of this infection is much greater than with a simple blood transfusion since the plasma comes from 'pooled' blood, so that one bottle may represent blood from a considerable number of donors.

From extensive researches in organic chemistry, there have arisen several synthetic plasma substitutes. Dextran is now in general use instead of plasma for this 'supportive' therapy. Dextran is lost only slowly from the circulation; at least 60 per cent of the amount given intravenously remains in the circulation for 24 hours.

Dextran is supplied in standard transfusion bottles of 540 ml in 6 per cent solution, with normal saline, glucose, or both. It is far the best solution for emergency use in severe shock due to blood loss, pending the grouping and necessary arrangements for the transfusion of whole blood. **Blood for grouping must be taken before dextran or its substitutes are given as some of these substances interfere with the grouping procedure.**

In practice, the management of shock cannot really be considered in isolation from that of haemorrhage, and dehydration. Nursing measures to be adopted in the prevention and treatment of shock and haemorrhage are outlined on page 129. The management of fluid balance generally in relation to dehydration, water intoxication and salt balance is described on page 133.

Haemorrhagic shock

This is sometimes described as though it were a special condition. It is a form of oligaemic shock which can be completely corrected by transfusion if this is sufficiently early and adequate in amount (page 120).

Septicaemic (bacteraemic) shock

One of the most dramatic conditions is what we call bacteraemic (or endotoxic) shock, because the toxins are derived from bacteria. This occurs sometimes following major abdominal surgery where the bowel or urinary tract has been involved: it can occur from burns or injury, or even from catheterisation. The organisms involved are usually the so-called 'gram-negative' bacteria of the coliform type, perhaps *Pseudomonas pyocyanea*, which are not controlled by the antibiotics used most commonly. The condition might for instance occur a few hours after a transurethral resection of the prostate in a patient who has been previously in a good condition. Sudden collapse, with a shivering attack, a blood pressure falling to 70 with an imperceptible pulse, is the usual onset picture. Death will supervene in a very few hours unless immediate action is taken. The endotoxins which have circulated paralyse the peripheral blood vessels and there is a sudden pooling of blood. The initial treatment is, therefore, the rapid transfusion of dextran in particular, followed by saline in order to keep up the blood pressure, and the immediate intravenous injection of a suitable antibiotic—for instance gentamicin or cephaloridine. If the condition is treated quickly it is completely reversible and in a very few hours the patient returns to normality.

Anaphylactic shock

This is a particular type of primary shock or collapse which sometimes follows the injection of serum (page 56) given in the prevention or treatment of tetanus or some other disease. It also occurs after the administration of certain drugs to which a patient may be sensitive; the exact physiological mechanism is not known. It is dramatic in its onset and may prove fatal. Adrenaline is usually injected as a counter-measure and 100 mg of hydrocortisone is given intravenously. Artificial respiration and external cardiac massage will of course be required if the heart stops. This is an extremely rare accident but one for which we have to be constantly prepared in casualty departments and wards.

The heart in shock

The amount of blood pumped out by the heart depends obviously upon the rate of beat and upon the strength of each contraction of the heart. It also depends upon the size of the heart. The muscle of the heart requires a particularly rich supply of oxygen and in any condition in which there is a reduction in the oxygen capacity of the blood (whether from lung disease or from anaemia) the heart is the first organ to notice this oxygen shortage. It responds usually by an increase in rate. Injured patients or others who have suffered from severe haemorrhage show what is called 'air hunger'. They breathe rapidly with gasps. If the chest has been damaged or the patient has been so severely injured that the brain is not responding to the normal stimulus to respiration, lung function is inadequate and the heart at once is working under greater difficulty. We have already referred to the effect of the vagus nerve in primary neurogenic shock. Stimulation of this nerve puts a brake on the heart's action and may bring it to complete standstill. We now know that we can massage the heart by vigorous repeated compression of the sternum towards the spine and this external cardiac massage is sometimes sufficient to start the heart by pumping blood artificially for a few seconds until an oxygen supply returns to the muscle of the heart itself. In thinking of primary shock we must therefore always give very urgent consideration to the heart's action. The term **angina** (strictly meaning pain) is used to describe the pain of cramp of the heart muscle when it is deprived of oxygen. This occurs if the coronary arteries are diseased and the heart is called upon to do more work than it is capable of with a reduced blood supply to its own muscles. When thrombosis occurs in a coronary artery this intense angina is sufficient to produce a degree of shock which stops the heart. Consequently an individual may die with a coronary thrombosis which is only affecting a very small part of the heart muscle. If coronary thrombosis occurs and an individual is at hand who can perform external cardiac massage life may be saved but of course the time interval available when such a measure can be effective may only amount to a few seconds. Nevertheless, this is sufficient in an operating theatre in a case of cardiac arrest which occurs reflexly from surgery or from injury.

The action of the heart is greatly helped by the administration of oxygen but no amount of oxygen is any use unless the chest is rising and falling with respiration naturally or as a result of artificial respiration.

When we come to deal with secondary or oligaemic shock which comes on at a later stage after operation or severe injury, the heart is just as important and careful and continuous observation of its action as shown by repeated blood pressure recordings and continuous record of the pulse rate will indicate the onset of shock in time for corrective measure to be taken. The heart's action can be monitored by electrocardiograph displayed on an oscilloscope screen.

'Circulatory failure' occurs when the heart output becomes inadequate to maintain blood flow to vital organs. This may occur as a result of primary cardiac disease, blood loss or shock. The detection of its onset is vital in the management of emergency transfusion and long term fluid balance maintenance (page 133).

HAEMORRHAGE

The cause of bleeding

Blood may escape from the blood vessels as a result of injury. Capillaries are fractured by simple abrasion, veins with their very fragile walls are easily torn, while arteries are usually injured by a cut, either accidental or intentional. Infective or malignant disease, as it eats its way through tissues, may invade the wall of a blood vessel which subsequently gives way allowing free escape of blood. In the case of capillaries and veins, the inflammatory process involving the vessel usually sets up thrombosis so that haemorrhage does not occur. With arteries, while thrombosis may sometimes occur as the result of the inflammation, severe haemorrhage frequently follows erosion. Perhaps the most common site of such arterial haemorrhage is in the base of a gastric ulcer. Because of the inflammation in the walls of the artery which may be coursing through the base of the ulcer, the vessel is prevented from contracting, and when it bursts the hole is held rigidly open with resultant severe and sometimes fatal haematemesis (vomiting of blood).

High blood pressure is frequently associated with disease of the walls of the arteries, which lose their elasticity. In most parts of the body, the arteries are surrounded by fairly firm tissues which tend to support them, but this is not the case in the brain, which is the most common site for the rupture of small arteries. Such cerebral haemorrhage is responsible for one form of apoplexy.

The wall of an artery may be weak from injury, from congenital defect or from disease, and instead of it bursting it develops a large bulge which continues to increase in size as the years go by. The surrounding tissues become eroded by the continuous beating of the artery and eventually the stretched-out thin-walled sac bursts. This arterial bulge is known as **aneurysm.** A congenital form occurs near the base of the brain. Aneurysm follows gunshot wounds in the region of arteries and the aorta undergoes a similar change as the result of arteriosclerosis or syphilis.

Bleeding diseases

Many patients believe that they are particularly liable to prolonged bleeding after injury or operation. Commonly their fear is based on an experience of a single dental extraction—an injury from which tiresome and prolonged bleeding is by no means uncommon. Shock and certain types of injury raise the fibrinolysin content of the blood and reduce the normal clotting power of the blood (page 59).

Normal wear and tear of the body tissues is not followed by haemorrhage because of the very efficient processes of repair involving platelets and the normal clotting mechanism (page 59).

There are however some well recognised disorders of blood vessels and the blood-clotting mechanism, and the existence of these conditions has a direct bearing on surgery.

Haemophilia is one well known form of bleeding disease. It is an hereditary condition passed on by the mother who is not herself affected although all her male children are afflicted, and her daughters carry the same latent fault which they pass on to their own children. It used to be thought that no female could be affected but this is not so. Girls may in fact suffer from haemophilia. Trivial injuries produce gross haemorrhage and even the normal wear and tear on the joints is sometimes accompanied by tremendous **haem-arthrosis** (blood in the joint).

Haemophilia is known to be due to an absence of certain clotting factors and is incurable. 'Closed' haemorrhage—that is haemorrhage under the skin or into an internal organ or joint—is usually self-limiting. A large haematoma results and in the case of a joint the haemarthrosis leads to stiffening and deformity. Surgical operation for any condition in a haemophiliac is extremely hazardous but transfusion with fresh (not stored) blood improves the clotting power of the blood for a few hours. Sooner or later almost every sufferer from haemophilia requires blood transfusion which has the dual effect of replacing lost blood and adding factors which produce clotting at the site of bleeding.

In haemophilia, the usual methods of blood control by pressure, heat or chemicals are completely ineffective and the only local application of value has been the venom from a particular species of adder, Russell's viper. This substance is supplied as a dry powder in glass ampoules and is useful for controlling the bleeding from small areas such as a tooth socket. A solution is made with water and applied on a small cotton wool swab. The management of incidents of bleeding in haemophilia has, however, been revolutionised by the isolation of clotting factor VIII (page 59) from human serum. This is done by freezing methods and the resulting preparation is known as **cryoprecipitate**[1] or **cryoglobulin**. Immediately a haemophilia sufferer has an injury, as shown for instance by a sudden swelling of a knee, he is taken with all possible speed to one of the special centres in Great Britain where treatment has been organised for this condition. An immediate infusion is started to administer cryoprecipitate and the necessary physiotherapy is given. Joints can then be kept mobile and the very serious deformities which used to develop are prevented. A purer preparation of anti-haemophilia factor (AFH) is available in some centres. This is more stable and the volume of injection is small so that treatment can be given at home and may be self-administered.

Thrombocytopenic purpura. In this condition there is a shortage of platelets due to excessive destruction. It is treated by removing the spleen (splenectomy). Occasionally blood transfusion is required at such an operation, but there is very little risk of bleeding being excessive since the number of platelets in the blood rises rapidly once the spleen, which has been destroying them, is removed. In fact, the number of platelets circulating in the

[1] cryo- is a Greek word meaning cold. Cryo-surgery includes procedures carried out by intensely cold instruments in which liquid nitrogen is used as the freezing agent (page 844).

blood for the few days following the operation may become so excessive that spontaneous thrombosis may occur in veins (page 594).

Marrow replacement. The red corpuscles, platelets and granular white cells are manufactured in the bone marrow. Leukaemia in its varied forms results in overcrowding of the red cell and platelet forming tissue by deposits of the white cell growth. Persistent anaemia and a tendency to bleed (purpura) arise as the disease progresses. A similar marrow replacement occurs in advanced cancer where metastatic deposits have arisen in the bones.

In the prevention and treatment of post-operative thrombosis, drugs are given which interfere with the clotting mechanism, and in excess such drugs may lead to severe spontaneous haemorrhage.

Time of haemorrhage (primary, reactionary, secondary)

Bleeding which occurs at the time of injury or operation from the severance of a blood vessel, is referred to as **primary haemorrhage**. This is normally controlled by the contraction of the cut end of the blood vessel, by immediate formation of clot, or in the case of an operation wound, by ligature, by pressure or by surgical diathermy (page 128) which is used to produce artificial clot and seal the cut ends of blood vessels.

Reactionary haemorrhage is bleeding which occurs a few hours after an injury or after operation, and is due to the return of blood pressure to its normal level after a period of hypotension (low blood pressure) resulting either from primary shock, or from the particular method of anaesthesia which has been employed: intravenous thiopentone almost always lowers the blood pressure. As the pressure rises and shock passes off, the muscle in the cut vessel tends to relax and release any clot which has been blocking its open end. With good anaesthesia and careful surgery, reactionary haemorrhage should not occur, but it is particularly liable to happen in areas such as an anastomosis between the stomach and intestine (page 526), when clamps have been used at the site of anastomosis and when the stitches have not been put close enough to constrict the many vessels in the cut ends of stomach and intestine. From the nurse's point of view, continued primary haemorrhage or reactionary haemorrhage must never be forgotten as a possibility in the first twenty-four hours. Many a child has died following the removal of tonsils because the post-operative bleeding was either not detected or not controlled. Not only does the loss of blood itself constitute a risk to life, but the presence of blood in the tissues, in the throat or perhaps in the intestinal canal is an additional danger.

Secondary haemorrhage occurs usually during the second week after injury or operation and is due to infection which erodes the clot in the end of a major vessel. The clot becomes soft from sepsis and is dislodged. When haemorrhage occurs from the invasion of the wall of a blood vessel by infection or malignant disease, as mentioned above, it is also described as secondary. In surgical practice today, post-operative secondary haemorrhage is a rarity and perhaps the most common site for its occurrence is from the prostatic bed after a prostatectomy. The almost complete elimination of secondary haemorrhage is due to the fact that infection after operation or injury is now so readily controlled. Before the antibiotic era, infection in the stumps of limbs amputated following severe injury was extremely common. Secondary haemorrhage was feared from one of the major vessels in the stump. It is because of this risk that all cases of amputation are nursed in such a way that the bandaged stump is visible outside the bedclothes (page 916) and a rubber tourniquet is attached to the end of the bed so that it is immediately available should haemorrhage occur.

Sites of haemorrhage

From a wound open to the surface of the body, the blood will escape and apart from making a mess it will do no harm. Bleeding occurring from the nose (**epistaxis**), mouth or throat, may be swallowed or may trickle down the trachea into the lungs if the patient is unconscious. Blood aspirated into the lungs may be sufficient to drown the victim or in smaller quantities will produce an aspiration broncho-pneumonia. Blood which is swallowed ferments and invariably produces vomiting, the vomiting in turn being liable to produce broncho-pneumonia by aspiration.

Bleeding from the stomach and duodenum is frequently an indication for surgical operation. Bleeding from gastric ulcers (page 520) usually produces **haematemesis**, some of the blood passing into the intestinal tract and being evacuated from the bowel as 'melaena'. Bleeding from a duodenal ulcer, though it may be just as severe, less commonly leads to the vomiting of blood but produces massive melaena. The presence of blood in the intestinal tract leads to abnormal fermentation, distension, the passage of large quantities of flatus and produces considerable distress to the patient, quite apart from the loss of blood and its immediate effect.

Bleeding may occur from any part of the alimentary tract, particularly from growth or from ulceration; the passage of blood from the rectum is often the earliest sign of serious disease. In the thorax, disease of the lung tissue produces **haemoptysis** (spitting of blood) and bleeding into the pleural space, following injury or operation, produces haemothorax (page 608), which constitutes a danger to life by compressing the lung.

In the urinary tract, bleeding from the kidney is frequently the first warning of the presence of disease. Bleeding into the bladder from growth or following operation leads to 'clot' retention of urine, and is a surgical emergency.

In the field of gynaecology, grave and frequently fatal haemorrhage occurs into the peritoneal cavity from the rupture of an ectopic pregnancy where the fetus has become lodged in the uterine tube. Excessive loss of blood from the uterus, either from growth or from endocrine disorder, is the principal reason for which hysterectomy (removal of the uterus) is performed.

Thus it will be seen that the detection of the source of the bleeding, the prevention and control of bleeding, and the treatment of the patient who has lost blood, constitute another major portion of surgical nursing.

Effects of haemorrhage

Acute blood loss. The rapid loss of 500 ml or more of blood from the circulation is likely to produce collapse (fainting) and a picture which at first strikingly resembles neurogenic shock. The patient is cold and pale, shivering, restless and frightened. He may be unconscious. If the loss has occurred very suddenly the pulse is at first slow but later rises rapidly. If however the accumulation of blood within the body is producing pain, the pulse may remain slow for a longer period. For all practical purposes a person must be presumed to be bleeding seriously if he has had an operation or injury and is cold, pale and restless, with a feeble pulse which is rising in rate.

On the other hand a smaller but nevertheless significant quantity of blood may be lost on several successive occasions, but on none of the occasions is the amount sufficient to produce collapse. Such bleeding occurs from growths or ulcers in the intestinal canal. The patient feels ill, rapidly becomes pale, complains of fatigue and has a fast pulse.

If severe visible bleeding takes place, the amount of blood lost is very difficult to assess. Haematemesis, haematuria, or the passage of altered blood (melaena) or bright, fresh blood from the bowel, demands immediate measures to prevent collapse. The principle of treatment must be to maintain an adequate blood supply to the brain and an adequate oxygen intake through the lungs. The pulse volume is not a very reliable guide as it is impossible to detect the gradual fall of blood pressure from the alteration of the pulse beat felt at the wrist. The blood pressure must be measured at the earliest possible opportunity, and at intervals of fifteen minutes during the first hour of observation at least. The nurse must acquaint herself with the use of the sphygmomanometer and come to regard this measurement of blood pressure as part of nursing routine.

Any fluid lost from the body and suspected to contain blood must be saved for inspection by the surgeon who will be able to form a very rough estimate of the volume of blood lost.

The management of a patient who is bleeding severely is the same as for the management of the shocked patient, and will be described later (page 129). The important difference between acute blood loss and severe oligaemic shock, from the nurse's point of view, is that by the careful observation of early symptoms and signs, a nurse may be able to report the occurrence of bleeding in time for transfusion to take place, before the onset of oligaemic shock. In acute haemorrhage, the initial blood loss is made good by contraction of the spleen and by the diversion of blood from the skin and peripheral vessels to the more vital parts of the circulation, in the brain and coronary vessels. The resultant pallor from this defensive reaction, and pain from the accumulation of blood in tissues or body cavity, may sound the alarm before there is any detectable change in the pulse or blood pressure. The body temperature falls and will almost certainly be below normal even in a patient who has previously been feverish. Table 17 shows the effect of reduction in the haemoglobin on oxygen transport by the blood. With a haemoglobin down to 10 grams the work done by the heart is very materially increased and it will be seen that the effect of giving pure oxygen is relatively slight.

Table 17   Oxygen transport—effect of anaemia

Cardiac output (litres/min)	15 grams haemoglobin		10 grams haemoglobin	
	In Room air	In Pure O_2	In Room air	In Pure O_2
10	2000 ml	2200 ml	1330 ml	1555 ml
5	1000 ml	1100 ml	665 ml	770 ml

Severe haemorrhage results in damage to the kidneys from oxygen deprivation. Anuria may occur, followed by uraemia. Unfortunately the changes in the kidney are often irreversible and the patient dies, in spite of the blood loss being replaced by transfusion (Fig. 8.6).

Table 18   Common sources of severe haemorrhage

EXTERNAL

Nose (epistaxis)

   Usually from a small vessel on the septum near the front (there is no purpose in the patient lying flat unless the amount of blood loss has already been great: even and continuous pressure along the upper lip from one cheek to the other for a minute or two is frequently sufficient to allow the vessel to block. This simple manoeuvre is effective but the temptation to move the finger in order to mop the nose must be resisted).

Lung (haemoptysis)

   Brisk haemorrhage usually indicates growth or tuberculosis: the patient should be put at complete rest, flat.

Oesophagus and stomach (haematemesis)

   Swallowed blood from mouth or nose.

   Oesophagel varices (in cirrhosis of liver and other forms of portal hypertension, page 483).

   Gastric ulcer or neoplasm.

   Occasionally in severe gastritis (e.g. aspirin sensitivity).

Duodenum and small intestine (melaena = black stools)

   Ulceration, Meckel's diverticulum, bleeding disease. (Often remains concealed and internal for several hours, but blood speeds up peristalsis.)

   Melaena may arise from swallowed blood, or gastric bleeding.

Colon and rectum (usually red blood in stools; sometimes melaena from digestion of blood pigment)

   Intussusception.

   Neoplasm—polyp, adenoma, carcinoma.

   Diverticulitis. Ulcerative colitis. Haemorrhoids.

Renal tract (haematuria)

   Neoplasm, cystitis, nephritis, stone, prostatic enlargement.

Uterus and vagina

   Excessive menstruation (metrorrhagia).

   Neoplasm.

   Abortion (and other mishaps of pregnancy).

Wounds

   Primary, reactionary, or secondary.

INTERNAL

Intraperitoneal

   Injured viscus—liver or spleen.

   Ruptured ectopic gestation (tubal pregnancy).

Retroperitoneal

   Ruptured kidney, aneurysm of aorta; fractured pelvis.

Intra-thoracic (haemothorax)

   After injury (especially fractured rib).

Interstitial (into tissues)

   Fractures.

Intracranial

   Rupture of congenital aneurysm of basilar artery.

   Injury.

   Arteriosclerosis.

(**N.B.**—The blood loss in cerebral haemorrhage is insignificant compared with the neurological damage done to the brain.)

Table 18 shows some common causes of severe bleeding in various sites, with the local symptoms which may be produced.

Chronic blood loss. At the other extreme is the patient who is losing blood continuously—the steady ooze from ulcerative colitis, or the daily but small loss from bleeding haemorrhoids. This patient over a period of weeks will become tired and languid. He will develop pallor but may be completely free from other symptoms which might help the surgeon to locate the disease. Particularly is this true of the patient who is bleeding from piles, and who has become accustomed to passing a little blood with each motion. He regards this as normal for himself and may not even tell his doctor, as he does not consider the amount of blood lost on each occasion is significant.

The blood manufacturing process of the body (haemopoiesis) breaks down in the face of continued or repeated blood loss and the symptoms are due to severe anaemia. Since many of the patients who are suffering from such blood loss have diseases which themselves are producing toxins, the bone marrow which is responsible for haemopoiesis is poisoned and blood replacement is impaired.

Recovery

Anaemia, therefore, either from acute blood loss, repeated severe loss, or chronic loss, is a matter which demands attention in a great many surgical cases, before or after operation.

Acute severe loss may be made good by a rise in blood pressure brought about by dilution with body fluid from other compartments. The haemoglobin will be low for several days, but if the patient's general health is satisfactory and the bone marrow is normal, a pint of blood may be replaced naturally in a week. (A blood donor may give 500 ml of blood every two weeks if he is in good health.) If however the bone marrow is unhealthy from toxaemia or is partly replaced by malignant deposits (Hodgkin's disease, leukaemias, metastasis from carcinoma of the prostate), this acute blood loss will not be made good. The patient's haemoglobin will remain low with consequent impairment of healing, lethargy, depression and prolonged hospitalisation.

Repeated loss of lesser degree or chronic loss has the same effect on the patient, and if haemorrhage continues over several weeks the bone marrow becomes exhausted, the supply of new red cells fails and the haemoglobin falls rapidly. Indications for blood transfusion in anaemia are discussed in Chapter 9, but many surgeons feel that if a patient's haemoglobin is under 60 per cent transfusion is called for in order that the necessary surgery (if any is needed) can be undertaken early, and that recovery of full activity may be accelerated. Although blood transfusion carries a very slight risk, to wait for a natural rise of haemoglobin and blood replacement is not justified. If the haemoglobin is over 60 per cent, the surgeon will be guided by whether he expects there to be further blood loss, whether there is sepsis present and whether the patient is free from any other debilitating disease which impairs his nutrition.

Persistent anaemia in surgical cases

Severe and persistent anaemia can occur without bleeding or may accompany and therefore intensify the effects of bleeding. Toxaemia from the presence of sepsis inhibits the normal replacement of red blood cells and platelets. This kind of toxaemia arises in patients with extensive burns (page 958) and particularly in patients with kidney infection (chronic pyelonephritis), arising perhaps from long-standing urinary obstruction. Persistent anaemia also occurs if the bone marrow is replaced by leukaemic or neoplastic deposits. Carcinoma of the prostate is particularly liable to spread to the bones but the disease is also to some extent controlled in its development by hormone treatment; the anaemia which results may be the most troublesome problem in treatment. The hormone stilboestrol also may cause fluid retention in the tissues. This puts further strain on the heart, and in the presence of severe anaemia may lead to cardiac failure.

Table 19   Common sources of persistent (chronic) anaemia

Aplasia—bone marrow replacement by metastatic neoplasm
　　　　bone marrow repression by uraemia, or toxins from sepsis
　　　　wide skeletal irradiation
　　　　chronic renal disease (erythropoietin deficiency)
Iron deficiency
　(microcytic anaemia)—dietetic
　　　　　　　　　　　non-absorption, achlorhydria and after gastrectomy (acid is necessary
　　　　　　　　　　　　for iron absorption)
Folic acid deficiency
　(pernicious macrocytic anaemia)—post-gastrectomy (absent intrinsic factor)
　　　　　　　　　　　　　　steatorrhoea
Haemolysis—burns, infection
　　　　　　spherocytosis
Blood loss—usually from alimentary tract, hiatus hernia, peptic ulcer, colitis, haemorrhoids

---

Anaemia of a different type arises if there is deficient absorption of iron from the alimentary tract. Conditions such as chronic gastric ulcer or gastritis in which there is a low digestive acid or none at all (achlorhydria) are often accompanied by severe anaemia. After removal of part of the stomach there may likewise be a deficiency of the 'intrinsic' factor, produced in the stomach wall, and essential for the production of red blood cells. Thus gastrectomy is sometimes followed by a 'pernicious' type of anaemia, sometimes by an 'iron deficiency' type.

The control of haemorrhage

When bleeding occurs through accidental or surgical injury or from disease, the physiological defence mechanisms of the body at once come into play. The contraction of the muscle wall of the divided vessel, and the formation of clot in and around its mouth, limit the blood loss. If the loss is severe the whole cardiovascular system is automatically adjusted in such a way that the flow in the limbs and superficial areas of the body is reduced to maintain the essential oxygenation of the brain. **Haemostasis**—the stemming of the flow of blood—occurs naturally in most minor injuries.

First aid

In the first-aid treatment of accidental external haemorrhage, pressure at the site of bleeding must be achieved by the application of a pressure dressing held firmly in place with a bandage, or by the hand until a bandage is available. Very rarely is it necessary to use a tourniquet on the limb, and even arterial haemorrhage occurring in wounds below the elbow or below the knee, can usually be controlled by a tight bandage and a pressure dressing applied at the site of the wound.

It is common in first-aid instruction to speak distinctively of capillary, venous and arterial bleeding, but such distinction is unnecessary and misleading.

Pressure points

It is essential to have an accurate knowledge of the points at which the main artery to each limb may be compressed against the bone as an emergency measure while a tourniquet or compression dressing is being applied.

The particular pressure points are:

(**a**) **Upper limb:** subclavian artery: two fingers pressed firmly back against the first rib above the mid-point of the clavicle. This manoeuvre should be practised on oneself. Some pain is produced at the same time due to compression of the brachial plexus. If in your test you have located the correct spot, you will notice that when you clench your fist tightly maintaining the pressure above the clavicle, the palm of your hand will remain blanched when you open the hand again. On releasing your digital pressure, the hand will be seen and felt to become engorged with blood.

(**b**) **Upper limb:** brachial artery: compressed against the inner side of the upper end of the humerus. This may be tested in a similar manner.

(**c**) **Lower limb:** femoral artery: very firm pressure requiring at least three fingers in the hollow of the groin immediately below the inguinal ligament. The femoral artery is thus compressed against the front of the hip joint.

(**d**) **Carotid artery:** deep wounds in the upper neck may occasionally involve carotid vessels but the bleeding from 'cut throat' injuries is usually from veins. The common carotid artery may be compressed by a thumb with its tip against the side of the larynx, the pulp pushing firmly backwards against the transverse processes of the cervical vertebrae. Carotid vessel pressure is useless and dangerous in bleeding from lacerations of the scalp as there are so many pathways by which blood reaches this area. Attempts to compress the neck merely result in obstruction to the veins, and so to increased bleeding.

Tourniquets

Owing to the fact that the main arteries for the limbs are for the most part surrounded by muscle, any attempt to compress them with a tourniquet must involve:

(*a*) A very tight constricting force.
(*b*) Simultaneous compression of muscles and nerves.
(*c*) Complete ischaemia (bloodlessness) of all the tissues beyond the point of application of the tourniquet.

Risks of applying a tourniquet are therefore:

1. Insufficient compression of the artery but occlusion of the vein only, leading to congestion and increased bleeding from the ends of the cut veins.
2. Peripheral nerve injury and subsequent paralysis.
3. If the tourniquet remains in position too long, ischaemia and damage to muscles resulting in their contracture.
4. Damage to the artery wall, especially if it is already affected by arteriosclerosis. Subsequent arterial thrombosis may occur.

In severe injuries where there has been considerable muscle damage, there is one distinct advantage in the application of a tourniquet. It prevents the return to the circulation of the histamine products of tissue damage, and as long as a tourniquet is in position there is less likelihood of severe surgical (secondary) oligaemic shock. Immediately the tourniquet is removed, however, these substances reach the general circulation and the onset of oligaemic shock may be very rapid.

In operations upon the limbs, the surgeon is able to work in a bloodless field by means of a suitably applied tourniquet. For the lower limb the rubber 'Esmarch' bandage tourniquet is used. The application of this tourniquet involves stretching the rubber almost to its limit and applying a continuous compression force by bandaging from the toes to the upper thigh. Several turns of the tourniquet are taken at the top, or a separate bandage is used at this point. The rubber bandage is then unwound from the toes upwards so that the limb is left with its veins empty and its arterial supply temporarily closed. If the tourniquet has been applied correctly, it may be left in place with safety for an hour or even more during operation, because the limb has been exsanguinated before the artery was occluded.

In the upper limb because of the greater risk of damage to nerves, a pneumatic tourniquet or blood pressure cuff is used. This may be applied as a first-aid measure in casualty departments when it is desired to inspect a wound of the hand or forearm, in order to assess the extent of the damage. After the cuff has been evenly applied the pressure must be raised rapidly to 200 mm Hg, or higher if the patient is known to be hypertensive. It should never be left in position for more than half an hour without deflation, though this period can be exceeded at operation if the limb has been emptied of blood by means of an Esmarch bandage.

Various types of tourniquet are in supply for first-aid purposes. A simple piece of stout rubber tubing tied as tightly as possible round the upper thigh, can be made effective in persons of moderate build. It can then be tightened by a stick or pencil (windlass fashion) if necessary. The standard emergency tourniquet available in most hospitals is the 'Samway' anchor tourniquet in which the rubber is held in position round a steel hook. The more complicated the pattern of tourniquet, the less effective it is likely to be. For operations upon a finger or toe, a thin piece of rubber drainage tube is used, pulled tight and clipped round the base of the digit, by a pair of pressure forceps.

Simple rules for the use of tourniquets are:

1. **Don't use them unless pressure at the site of bleeding has failed.**
2. **Always note the time of application.**
3. **Never apply a tourniquet to the bare skin; there must always be a pad of lint or clothing beneath to spread the pressure (except in case of a toe or finger).**

4. If you hand the patient on to someone else's care, always repeat, and preferably record, the time of application. In operation cases or after first-aid treatment, if the tourniquet has already been removed, the theatre or casualty nurse must always report to the ward the fact that a tourniquet has been used.

5. A limb which has had a tourniquet applied is liable to develop oedema after the tourniquet is removed. The limb should therefore be elevated for at least twenty-four hours.

6. Never cover a tourniquet with dressings, clothing, or bedclothes. Its presence may be forgotten.

Complications may arise from the use of tourniquets for surgical operations. They are fortunately rare and usually the result of ignorance in the technique of application. In the upper limb, wrist drop is sometimes seen from injury to the radial nerve and subsequent paralysis of the extensor muscles of the wrist. In the lower limb, foot drop occurs from paralysis of the anterior tibial and peroneal muscles resulting from compression of the lateral popliteal nerve against the back of the head of the fibula. Particular care must be taken as the Esmarch bandage is wound round this area, to avoid excessive pressure near the head of the fibula where the nerve can easily be felt. Frequently the lower limb is placed in plaster-of-Paris after operation and the foot drop may not be discovered until several weeks later (page 899).

Serious accidents have occurred from a tourniquet being left in position too long. It is difficult to believe how the surgical team and the nursing staff can overlook the presence of a tourniquet, but there are numerous cases on record where the patients have been returned to the ward and the tourniquet has been discovered several hours later. Such an accident does not necessarily lead to loss of the limb, but is extremely likely to lead to permanent muscle damage and crippling.

First aid in internal haemorrhage

There is no practical measure that can be taken to speed the arrest of haemorrhage occurring internally from accident or disease. All that can be done is to keep the patient absolutely still and quiet, and institute anti-shock measures. If he is vomiting blood or has a severe haemoptysis, he should be nursed on his side or on his face, so that he may more readily clear the blood from his throat.

Severe bleeding may occur following the injection of haemorrhoids and if medical assistance is not available, a swab of cotton wool soaked in adrenaline solution should be placed inside the anal canal.

Surgical haemostasis

There are several methods of controlling bleeding during surgical operations:

1. When an incision is made, much of the bleeding comes from the skin edges and from subcutaneous tissue: small towels are often used, clipped to the edges of the wound to protect the cut surface, and prevent the repeated rubbing away of clot which would otherwise occur. These are called variously 'side towels', 'skin towels' or 'tetra towels'. The last-named term arose as these towels are commonly attached with four-pronged forceps ('tetra forceps', Greek τετρα 'tetra' = four). Self-adhesive transparent plastic drapes are sometimes used instead.

2. By pressure. As the surgeon makes his incision, he or his assistant applies a gauze swab to the raw area. Capillary and most venous bleeding stops almost immediately, and does not re-start unless the surface is rubbed.

3. Pressure forceps (artery forceps) are applied to the cut ends of arteries, as little of the surrounding tissue as possible being included in the jaws of the forceps. These bleeding points are dealt with at some later stage in the operation in one of four ways.

(*i*) The artery forceps are simply removed. Bleeding does not recur as the crushed end of the vessel has sealed itself off.

(*ii*) Surgical diathermy current is applied to the pressure forceps, thus coagulating the end of the blood vessel.

(*iii*) A surgical ligature is tied round the tissue included in the forceps which are then removed.

(*iv*) A stitch is inserted and tied round the tissue held in the forceps in order to secure more firmly the end of the cut vessel.

4. Surgical diathermy is used to make the incision through the muscle and deep tissue layers. This technique is used especially in the treatment of cancer and particularly in the removal of vascular structures such as the breast. Small blood vessels are thus sealed as the tissue is divided.

5. The application of gauze soaked in adrenaline solution. This drug constricts the ends of the vessels and is particularly useful in the nose. Where extensive bleeding may be expected—such as in plastic operations on the face—the operation area is sometimes infiltrated with a saline solution of adrenaline. By the time the effect of the adrenaline has passed off, the divided vessels have become blocked by clots.

6. The application of hot packs. The combination of pressure and heat speeds the clotting process and the retraction of the cut ends of vessels.

7. Reference to the chart on page 59 will recall that thromboplastin released by enzymes from damaged tissue is essential to start the clotting process. There is very little damage in a clean surgical incision and thromboplastin formation can be brought about by the surgeon taking a small piece of muscle, and pulping it by repeated crushing with pressure forceps. This 'muscle graft' is applied to the bleeding area. Purified thrombin is supplied in powder in sterile ampoules ready to mix with sterile water: the solution is then applied with a swab or a spray and is particularly useful under skin grafts, where it acts as a kind of glue. Fibrin foam is another preparation used extensively in neurosurgery, where even a small amount of bleeding into the brain or nerve may do irreparable damage.

Gelatin 'sponge' supplied in small biscuit-like strips, can be used in bleeding cavities or tied to the surface of a bleeding organ. The sponge acts as an artificial network in which clotting occurs and the substance is itself absorbed. Oxycel (oxidised cellulose) acts in a similar way and promotes rapid clotting. It is used in such sites as the prostatic cavity and can be tied around the catheter which is left in place at the end of operation.

Calcium alginate is a similar preparation and is manufactured from sea-weed. The raw oozing surface is moistened with one solution which is then activated by spraying with a second solution containing calcium.

All these artificial coagulants are only of use for 'low pressure' bleeding—that is from capillaries or small veins.

The nursing management of shock and haemorrhage

The history of the treatment of shock has been interesting in that it is clear that we have in the past sometimes done entirely the wrong thing in treating severe shock due to blood loss or toxaemia. Noradrenaline, a substance allied to adrenaline and producing constriction of peripheral blood vessels, raises the blood pressure dramatically and for some years was used as a means of keeping the blood pressure up in cases of extreme shock. It was not realised, however, that by doing this the peripheral tissues were being deprived of blood and consequently became anoxic and permanently damaged, with the result that the maintenance of blood pressure was only transient and the shock state then became irreversible. Today the principle in the treatment of shock is to transfuse large volumes, safeguarding the patient against over-transfusion by watching the pressure on the venous side of the heart—the management of the **central venous pressure** (page 134).

Factors which combine to affect the maintenance of normal blood pressure and normal tissue respiration may be summarised as follows:

1. The oxygen tension in the air which is being breathed. In the normal atmosphere this is 150 mg (20 kPa) Hg but may be raised to over 300 (40 kPa) by supplementary oxygen.

2. The ease with which this air is transmitted to the alveoli of the lung. Respiratory obstruction, bronchial and alveolar inflammation affect this phase. Physiotherapy plays a vital part here.

3. Adequate perfusion of the lung tissues—this depends on the amount of venous return to the heart so that the pressure produced by the right ventricle may be sufficient. In chronic lung disease where the right side of the heart has been working for years against a high resistance in the lungs, right-sided heart failure may develop. This might arise also from a coronary occlusion affecting the right ventricle or irregularities of the heart rate or rhythm. Distension of the external jugular vein in the neck, when the patient is sitting up, suggests right-sided heart failure. This central venous pressure is monitored to regulate transfusion volumes (page 134).

4. Anaemia from blood loss, or from inadequate haemoglobin in each red cell.

5. Left-sided heart failure, for instance when the patient has had a high blood pressure for a long period of time and the musculature of the left side of the heart has become fatigued, back-pressure produces pulmonary oedema.

6. Peripheral arteriolar vasoconstriction, or arterial obstruction from disease of the arteries.

7. Tissue oedema. This is part of a vicious circle because the oedema interferes with tissue perfusion. Right-sided heart failure leads to obstruction to the venous return and to oedema in the more dependent parts of the body, as left-sided heart failure leads to oedema of the lungs. Fortunately, diuretics such as bendrofluazide and frusemide have the effect of dehydrating the tissues very quickly, and thus of improving the circulation.

8. Hypercapnia (CO_2 retention) producing acidosis. Excess carbon dioxide in the blood is hypercapnia (Greek 'kapnos'—smoke). If we breathe pure oxygen instead of atmospheric oxygen with nitrogen, our oxygen requirement may be met with less respiratory movement; ventilation is reduced and then becomes insufficient to get rid of carbon dioxide (carbonic acid). This accumulates for a while in the blood and is neutralised chemically until all available base is used up, and the patient becomes acidotic. Thus oxygen intake must be adequate to prevent tissue **hypoxia** but the total ventilation must be sufficient to get rid of

CO_2. In all the nursing problems connected with the unconscious patient with shock, lung disease or artificial respiration, we have constantly to consider this gas exchange going on in the lungs and the effect of its inadequacy on other tissues. In such conditions in which heart and lung function may become defective, blood gas analysis carried out at regular intervals by means of the Astrup apparatus reveals at any time the concentration of oxygen and carbon dioxide in the blood.

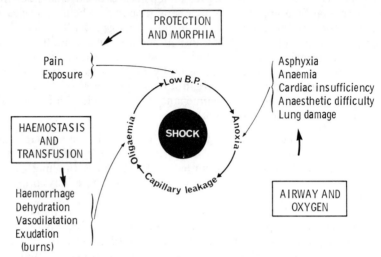

Fig. 8.5 Factors in the management of shock. The so-called 'cycle of death' is reversed by appropriate protective measures directed to the various causative factors.

We have now considered the physiological factors which affect the distribution of fluid in the body under various abnormal conditions. We have seen that the effects of shock must be considered in relation to blood loss and dehydration, and that dehydration and haemorrhage are similar in that they tend to promote shock. We have also seen the vital role of adequate pulmonary ventilation.

Nursing management must therefore be directed first to prevention. Attention is drawn again to the importance of the heart's action (page 116). Figure 8.2 shows the factors which encourage the development of **vasodilatory** (primary or neurogenic) shock. The diagram also shows other factors which particularly encourage the onset of **oligaemic** shock. Preventive measures are directed against each of these factors. When an operation is planned, the constitution of the patient, his state of nutrition, and fluid balance have to be estimated in relation to the magnitude of the operation which he is to undergo. The degree of shock to be expected after injury can also to some extent be estimated and forestalled. Particularly is this true in the case of burns (page 958).

With a correct understanding of the fundamental nature of shock, treatment is along simple lines directed to maintain or restore circulation of adequately oxygenated blood to the brain. Whether in prevention of shock or in treatment of the fully developed condition, the management is similar.

In routine surgical practice, neurogenic shock is very common in the immediate postoperative stage. The adequate and efficient treatment of this—mainly by pain-relieving drugs, correct positioning and perhaps oxygen—will avoid the development of tissue anoxia and lessen the risk of true oligaemic shock.

Shock is a condition which rarely occurs by itself. Perhaps this is over-stating the obvious. Shock, though of vital importance, is but one of the main features needing attention in an injured person or in one who has undergone a major surgical operation. There may be gastric tubes, catheters, wounds or splints requiring attention. The nurse's main function is to observe and report progress in relation to shock, and to undertake other nursing attention which the patient may require, in such a way that there will be as little pain and disturbance as possible.

The management of shock in the post-operative period is referred to particularly in Chapter 20.

First aid

The treatment of shock after injury is in effect very little different from the simple measures used in the routine care of the patient returning from the theatre, after operation. Remembering that shock and haemorrhage are frequently associated, the first major principle is that haemorrhage must be stopped, by pressure with the finger, by tightly applied bandage, or by tourniquet in extreme cases. Apart from this the general principles involved are:

(*a*) Avoidance of all unnecessary movement: in limb injuries, the minimum amount of disturbance in the application of first-aid dressings and splints.

(*b*) Reassurance of the victim and protection from unnecessary questioning, fussing, and 'flap' on the part of those around.

(*c*) Protection from cold: the application of artificial heat is unnecessary and dangerous since it reverses the natural defence mechanism, which has withdrawn blood from the surface of the body to maintain the more vital circulation to the brain.

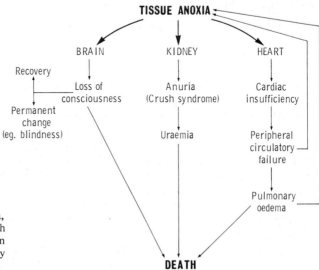

Fig. 8.6 The triple path of anoxia, showing the three main targets each of which has a profound effect in addition to the general capillary leakage.

(d) The administration of hot sweet drinks if it is certain that there is no abdominal injury and the patient is conscious.

(e) The administration of morphine if this is available. Ships, ambulances and aircraft carry a supply of morphine for use by nursing personnel or by the crew in cases of emergency. This use outside the ordinary provisions of the poisons regulations is covered by special Home Office Orders in Great Britain.

These first-aid measures may suffice to reverse the progress of the shock mechanism.

Initial hospital treatment

On arrival in hospital, an injured patient with shock is received into a warm room and the same principles of treatment are applied initially. Pulse and blood pressure recordings must be taken immediately and repeated at quarter of an hour intervals. This may be the duty of the nursing staff. If the injuries are severe, intravenous infusion will be essential at once. Time is very easily wasted at this stage and it is the duty of the nursing staff to be certain that all necessary emergency apparatus is at hand and in a serviceable condition. If a bleeding wound is easily accessible, a small quantity of blood should be taken in a test tube so that the serum may be used for grouping as a preliminary to blood transfusion.

Oxygen equipment must be available and oxygen should be administered without hesitation if the shock is severe.

There must be provision for elevating the foot of the bed, stretcher, or trolley.

An oral anaesthetic airway, mouth-gag and tongue forceps with the necessary swabs and bowl must also be placed by the patient's side.

The resuscitation of shocked patients has been the subject of much thought, extensive research and many changes of fashion. There is in surgical practice frequently no clear line of distinction between the two types of shock. The one fades into the other. The importance lies in the fact that this change must never be missed. In broad outline the hospital treatment of shock may be said to lie basically in:

1. Protection—from movement, pain and anxiety.
2. The maintenance of respiration—a clear airway, an unrestricted thorax, and an active respiratory mechanism. In the absence of the latter, artificial respiration is necessary.
3. The use of oxygen—this can do no harm if correctly administered. It may be life-saving. It can do no good if administered with a funnel.
4. The prompt infusion of blood, dextran or plasma.

Primary infusion. If there has been marked blood loss or more than one major fracture (i.e. thigh and arm) whole blood must be given as soon as possible. Until blood is available, and for all other cases where blood pressure is low or likely to be low from the nature of the injuries, dextran is given intravenously—one unit (600 ml) rapidly and then at fast drip rate (60 drops/min). Dextran is a synthetic commercial preparation which acts like plasma in holding water in the blood vessels; it has a high osmotic pressure and does not leak from the capillaries (Rheomacrodex is a form of dextran which is thought to be more effective in maintaining a good flow as it prevents 'sludging' of the blood and keeps it more fluid).

If plasma is available it is to be preferred to the synthetic dextran, especially in burns.

When a shocked patient is being moved from a casualty or reception department to a surgical ward, particular care must be taken during the journey. It is quite wrong for such a patient to be accompanied only by one nurse and a porter. Sudden collapse, vomiting with subsequent obstruction of the airway, the onset of haemorrhage, or the sudden excitement of a patient with a mild head injury, are all incidents which may cause disaster if not correctly handled by the nurse. There should always be three attendants.

The successful management of severe shock calls for prompt action, constant observation, and a personality that can organise the necessary help from other members of the team without creating panic and confusion.

FLUID AND ELECTROLYTE ('SALT') BALANCE

Dehydration[1]

This means quite simply that the body is short of water. This water depletion is probably associated with a loss of salts, especially of sodium, potassium and chloride. The kidneys require a certain volume of water passing through their vessels to flush out the waste products of metabolism. The blood requires a certain volume of water in which to carry the glucose, sodium, chloride, potassium and other salts to meet the constant requirements of the body's tissues. Every cell needs water in order to live. In certain types of oligaemic (toxigenic) shock, though there is plenty of water in the body, it is in the wrong place. The tissues are flooded with water but there is insufficient passing through the kidneys and renal failure, with uraemia, develops very rapidly. On the other hand, in cases of severe vomiting, so much fluid is lost from the body that every cell is called upon to give up some of its water and the patient becomes extremely ill. Fluid may be lost in large quantities from a burnt surface of the body so that dehydration and oligaemic shock will be present together.

Fluid replacement and 'water intoxication'

From all these considerations of haemorrhage, shock and dehydration, it is obvious that one of the most vital functions of the nurse is to see that the patient receives sufficient fluid one way or another. There are many ways in which fluid can be given—by mouth, by rectum, by subcutaneous infusion, by intramuscular or intravenous infusion. There are also many ways in which fluid can be lost from the body—by vomiting, by the removal of fluid from the stomach or intestine through an aspirating tube, by diarrhoea, and of course by the passage of urine. There is a constant 'insensible' loss of fluid from the body by respiration and by sweating and this cannot be measured. We know that an individual both in health and in disease must receive more fluid than his measured loss. It is possible without detriment to have a deficient fluid intake for several days in normal health, but in illness and especially after surgical operation, water deficiency may well lead to the development of oligaemic shock.

The accurate measurement and recording of all fluid received by the patient and all fluid known to be lost is called the *fluid balance*.

The function of the kidney tubules is not only to get rid of waste products but to conserve such chemicals as are needed to maintain normal tissue activity. The tubules

---

[1] The section on renal failure (page 674) should be read in this relation to this subject.

also have the specific property of being able to withdraw water back into the circulation from the fluid that has altered through the glomerulus of each kidney excretory unit (nephron). In certain diseases the glomerular filtration continues but the tubules are unable to concentrate the urine and, in order to get rid of the waste products of metabolism, large quantities of very dilute urine are manufactured. This excessive urinary water loss leads to thirst and so we have a well recognised association of 'polydipsia' (excessive drinking) and 'polyuria' (excessive urine formation).

If in the treatment of shock or dehydration, more fluid is administered (perhaps intravenously) than is required in the body, the excess is eliminated by the kidneys. Sometimes however, under such circumstances, the kidneys themselves may be impaired in function by disease or physiological control (page 674) and they may be unable to eliminate this excessive fluid. This happens particularly if the infusion is given too fast. Excessive infusion, excessive drinking, or deficient elimination by the kidneys leads to generalised oedema which is noticed first in the lower portions of the body, that is in the legs and sacral area when the patient is in bed. This tissue oedema may spread very rapidly and fluid begins to pour into the lower portions of the lung producing 'pulmonary oedema'. Clearly even a slight impairment of the function of the lungs by oedema may have a very serious effect in a patient who is already ill and suffering from anoxia (page 113). Particularly is this likely to happen if large quantities of saline are given intravenously instead of substances such as plasma or dextran, which hold the water in the circulation and prevent its seepage into the tissues. If the kidney is unable to excrete salts then it must hold back sufficient water in the body for their solution; 'water intoxication' and oedema again occurs.

The earliest clinical evidence of excessive hydration is a rise in the respiration rate with the patient perhaps developing a 'bubbly' cough. The pulse rate will also rise since a decrease in efficiency of the lungs has to be compensated by the heart pumping blood through them at greater speed. If this pulmonary oedema occurs it is sometimes treated by an intravenous infusion of concentrated plasma, but will usually clear if fluid intake is stopped, provided there is not additional renal damage. A rational way of eliminating excessive fluid would be by purging, but the patient may well be one with peritonitis or some other gastro-intestinal disorder.

A confused state of mind may be produced by oedema of the brain caused in turn by excessive hydration. There are of course many possible causes of mental confusion following injury or operation, and this is only one of the things which needs to be borne in mind when a patient's behaviour seems irrational.

Central venous pressure (CVP). This is the pressure in the right atrium measured in centimetres of water and the normal range is 4–6 cm.[1] In heart failure when there is a greater return of blood to the right side of the heart than can be pumped away by the ventricle, pressure rises in the superior vena cava and the external jugular veins are visibly distended. If there has been a great loss of fluid from the body from whatever cause, the return of blood to the right side of the heart is diminished and there is insufficient to fill the ventricle with each beat. In shock conditions it is often necessary to give blood or dextran in large quantities and there is clearly a danger that this might be overdone. For this reason the central venous pressure is monitored to make sure that an adequate volume of fluid is given but that this does not go on to be excessive. A catheter is inserted through an intravenous trochar into the internal jugular vein and passed down into the atrium. Alter-

[1] The SI units of pressure are not being used in connection with CVP.

natively it is placed in an ante-cubital vein in the forearm at a normal infusion site and advanced into the superior vena cava; its position is checked by x-ray. Either a 'drum' catheter or flexible 60-cm plastic one is used (Fig. 9.2). The catheter may pierce the wall of the heart causing the pericardium to fill with blood. 'Tamponade' occurs (page 606). Blood pressure falls very rapidly and the heart sounds are muffled. Death occurs unless the pericardial space can be emptied rapidly by aspiration with a needle.

The pressure is measured on a manometer coupled to the infusion line. The zero mark on the manometer should be at the level of the right atrium, but this is difficult to locate and various 'points of reference' for the zero are taken. The manubrium of the sternum is approximately 5 cm above the point of entry of the superior vena cava into the atrium and if this sternum is taken as zero level the pressures registered on the manometer are about 5 cm above the true atrial pressure. This does not matter because the main purpose is to record changes in pressure. The correct height is obtained by using a spirit level on a bar or arm hinged to the drip stand or a telescopic gun sight. A third method is a length of catheter tubing filled with water to within a hand's breadth of each end. One end is attached to the stand with adhesive tape, and the other is held on the sternum: when not in use, the ends of this levelling tube can be stoppered with plastic covers from disposable needles.

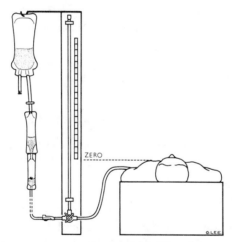

Fig. 8.7 Central venous pressure measurement. When the CVP is to be measured the zero is levelled with the sternum. When the zero of the manometer is level with the sternum, the infusion line is opened so that the manometer fills through the 3-way tap (Fig. 9.4(c)). The tap is then turned to cut off the line from the flask and to put the manometer column in continuity with the intravenous catheter. There will be an initial fall of saline in the manometer tube and a reading is taken when the level becomes static. There is a variation of level of 1–2 cm with respiratory movements or if the patient coughs. A CVP registering under 5 cm with the patient flat indicates under-infusion: over 12 cm is dangerous and input must be restricted.

A condition in which CVP measurement is extremely useful is internal haemorrhage from peptic ulceration. In the absence of repeated haematemesis it is difficult to detect continued bleeding and this may be recognised by CVP fall before there is a marked rise in pulse or fall in BP.

Post-operative fluid balance

If there has been pre-operative vomiting, the patient will receive intravenous infusion in adequate amount, for the 24-hour period preceding operation. If he has been admitted to hospital as an emergency, there will have been no time for such measures.

In cases of limb surgery, hernia, skin grafting not involving the face, and similar procedures, there need be no special provision of extra fluid intake for the 24-hour period in which the operation takes place. The deficiency will be made good very rapidly.

If, however, there has been pre-operative shock or the thorax or abdomen have been opened, then there must in every case be special provision for increased fluid intake. In the adult a major operation involves the loss of about 3000 ml of body fluid by respiration, bleeding, serum loss and urine, over the 24-hour period. The aim in nursing must therefore be a positive fluid balance before and immediately after operation, sufficient to cover this expected loss. If the patient is to undergo an operation which will necessarily prohibit or restrict oral fluid intake for more than 12 hours, steps will be taken to supplement this through other routes (i.e. parenteral). Rectal tap-water infusion is the simplest method which can be adopted without the assistance of medical staff, and for one or two days this may be adequate.

Table 20   Potential loss of digestive juices containing water and electrolytes from the gastro-intestinal organs in 24 hours

	ml
Saliva—swallowed but lost if naso-gastric suction used	1500
Gastric secretions—aspiration or fistula	2500
Bile—biliary fistula	500
Pancreatic juice—small bowel or pancreatic fistula	700
Intestinal secretions—small bowel fistula or diarrhoea	3000
Total	8200
In normal conditions all is reabsorbed except about 100 ml lost in faeces.	

The average daily 'insensible' loss—the unmeasurable fluid loss from respiration and sweating—is 800 ml, in health. This is decreased by bed rest but increased by fever. The daily balance must therefore show a gain of at least 800 ml (30 oz).

Figure 13.3 shows a simple chart for recording the fluid intake and output, arranged so that the staff can see at a glance whether the balance is positive over each 24-hour period. For the convenience of nursing staff it is usual to have the day and night balance shown separately. There are many varieties of chart, some far too complicated. It is helpful to have the time intervals printed. If any item of output cannot be measured through unattended vomiting, or incontinence, it is assessed and entered as the customary +, ++, or +++; the amount which is lost in this way is relatively small and is unlikely to be more than 100 ml. In cases where the measurement is important, there will usually be a gastric aspiration tube in position and so vomiting does not occur. Post-operative urinary incontinence is rare. The nurse has to remember that the contents of every drainage bottle, every urinal and every sputum mug must be measured and recorded.

The total 24-hour intake and output is entered on the temperature chart also: in this way the daily progress can be more readily assessed in relation to pulse and temperature records. Figure 13.1 shows the application of these records in the pre- and post-operative course of a patient who underwent resection of her colon.

The disturbance of a major operation leads to the production of excess anti-diuretic hormone, by the pituitary. This hormone prevents the kidneys from eliminating water so that for one or two days after operation, the urinary output is low no matter how much water has been administered. It is also known that after operation, the kidneys are unable to excrete sodium for a variable time and the administration of saline (sodium chloride) may act as a poison and produce oedema. Though this oedema may be insufficient to be seen in the surface tissues, it may occur at the operation site, in the wound or anastomosis and prevent healing.

The management of fluid and electrolyte administration is therefore a very complicated process. It is considered that not more than 4·5 G of sodium chloride (500 ml of normal saline) should be given in any 24-hour period, unless there is an excessive loss of sodium from the intestinal tract, as for instance by diarrhoea. In addition, it is now considered necessary for patients undergoing major surgical operations to receive extra potassium which is given in the infusions at the rate of 6 G potassium chloride in 24 hours, if there has been a period of dehydration or starvation. Refer again to page 107, the chemical principles of electrolyte balance.

From the nursing point of view, the essentials of fluid administration are therefore summarised as follows:

(a) Adequate pre-operative fluid intake is vital at a time when the kidneys can adjust the body's chemistry.

(b) A diminished urinary output is usual for the first 24-hours after operation, no matter how great the fluid intake has been.

(c) Because of the inability of the kidneys to excrete electrolytes in the immediate post-operative period, the estimation of chloride in the urine is not a reliable guide.

(d) Excessive sodium chloride administration is dangerous and the intake should not normally exceed 500 ml of normal saline, or its equivalent (4·5 G NaCl).

(e) The remaining fluid, if administered intravenously, should be in the form of glucose 5 per cent solution.

(f) 6 G of potassium chloride should be included in the total intravenous fluid in a 24-hour period, in patients who have been severely dehydrated, especially those with intestinal obstruction.

(g) The total intake of fluid should not exceed 3 litres (3000 ml) in the 24-hour period of the operation.

The accurate measurement of a patient's fluid balance is thus of paramount importance. It must be done accurately and conscientiously. In spite of all precautions, excessive dehydration or excessive hydration still occurs occasionally in the course of treatment.

NUTRITION BY INTRAVENOUS INFUSION

An adult at rest in bed, apart from fever or making up for malnutrition, requires a minimum of 2000 calories of energy a day (see Preface, page v): 5 per cent glucose (4 calories per G) can only give 200 calories per litre; 10 litres infusion a day is about 3 times the average need and much glucose would be lost in the urine. It is therefore impossible to meet nutritional requirement completely without protein and fat or some other source of energy. To provide for tissue replacement protein is required and amino-acid (protein components) solution is used. Alcohol can be given intravenously and so can fat in special emulsion form, devised from cotton-seed or soya-bean oil (Table 23). Plasma and whole blood given intravenously have no nutritional value, and a form of nitrogen which can escape from the blood into the tissues to be assimilated is essential. Amino-acid solutions meet this need (Table 23), but require additional calories to provide energy for metabolism of protein.

In providing for the patient's metabolic needs we must supply between 2000 and 3000 calories, 10–14 G of nitrogen (for protein replacement) in approximately 3 litres of fluid. This would require for example a combination of fat emulsion (intralipid 20%, 2000

Table 21   Fluids for intravenous infusion

All solutions must be prepared with special 'pyrogen-free' water, sterilised by autoclave.

Sodium chloride   'normal saline'
                   0·9%, i.e. approx. 1 G in 100 ml. 5 G per standard 540-ml transfusion bottle.

Dextrose   strong
                   50% in small quantities for treating insulin overdosage: occasionally for coma due to head injury.

Dextrose   5% for treatment of dehydration or shock without chloride loss.

Dextrose   4·3%   ⎱ This is 'isotonic' and is the most commonly
Sodium chloride   0·18% (⅕ normal saline)   ⎰ used solution for post-operative replacement of water and salt loss: it avoids excess salt.

Blood substitutes
  Plasma   natural
  Plasma   reconstituted from dry powder; also used double or quadruple strength.
  PPF   plasma protein factor in saline; free from fibrinogen. Must not be used unless it is crystal clear.

Dextran 110   6% (Intradex, Dextraven 110, Macrodex)
Dextran 40   10% Low molecular weight special: increases rate of blood flow (Intraflodex, Lomodex, Rheomacrodex). Dextrans are supplied in normal saline or in 5% dextrose.

                   N.B.   *Blood for grouping should be taken before these solutions are given.*

Sodium lactate compound solution
    (Hartmann's or Ringer–Lactate solution) i.e.:
        sodium lactate   0·26%
        sodium chloride   0·6%
        potassium chloride 0·04%
    Each 1000 ml contains approx. 0·4 G potassium.

This is insufficient to make up potassium *deficiency* and special potassium chloride solution is needed, or potassium citrate by mouth to give 6 G a day (page 137). Sterile potassium is supplied in ampoules 1 G to 20 ml of water: 1 ampoule may then be added to each litre of infusion solution.

In severe acidosis 2% sodium lactate solution is used (i.e. to give *sodium* ions (base) without *chloride* ions (acid)).

Mannitol 5%, 10%, 20% for acute anuria following shock, but not if there is known renal impairment. This is an alcohol which is not metabolised but is excreted rapidly and acts as a diuretic.

See Table 23 for additional substances used in parenteral nutrition.

---

calories per litre) and aminosol 10% (320 calories + 12 G nitrogen per litre). The remaining litre would contain sugar in the form of glucose (or fructose—see below) and the necessary electrolytes and vitamins.

The requirements where there is acute renal failure have to be modified to reduce the intake of nitrogen. Patients having renal dialysis must have their caloric needs met by the addition of fat (Table 23).

Table 22   Milli-mol strengths of common infusion fluids (p. 108)

			Milli-mol per litre		
	Ca^{++}	K^+	Na^+	HCO_3^- equivalent	Cl^-
Normal plasma	5	4·5	142	26	103
Potassium chloride injection (0·3 per cent)*		40			40
Sodium chloride injection (normal)			154		154
Sodium lactate injection			167	167	

* This strength is prepared by diluting sterile potassium chloride solution to 50 times its volume.

Fructose has been extensively used instead of glucose, since it does not require insulin for its metabolism, but is broken down directly by the liver to provide an energy source. It is for this reason thought to be of value in diabetic crises and in shock states. It is now known that if fructose is used in the presence of liver damage, renal function impairment or severe shock, a rapid build up of lactic acid occurs in the bloodstream and acidosis follows which is usually fatal. The liver cannot dispose of the lactic acid sufficiently fast. It is probably therefore unwise for fructose to be used in acute conditions though if administered very slowly to a patient who is undernourished, but has a good liver, it may be a satisfactory substitute for glucose. Fructose also produces a high uric acid state, and may thus precipitate an attack of gout. In severe malnutrition, as for instance if the patient has an intestinal fistula, the route usually selected for intravenous feeding is through the internal jugular vein or femoral vein with a flexible catheter passed well into the superior or inferior vena cava. An ever present danger of extended intravenous medication is fungal infection with candida albicans which may prove fatal. Extreme care must be taken. The patient is usually on wide spectrum antibiotics which encourage fungus infection.

Table 23   Fluids for parenteral nutrition

Fructose and sorbitol 30% (12 calories per litre) are used as alternatives to dextrose as a source of calories. They have the advantage of not requiring insulin for their metabolism.

Amino-acid (protein replacement solutions—Trophysan (Servier) in various forms. Aminosol vitrum is a proprietary combination of Aminosol, fructose and ethanol (alcohol).

Aminoplex 5 (5 G nitrogen/litre) with Sorbitol and alcohol is similar. Aminoplex 14 is a concentrated solution of amino-acids only, 14 G/litre.

Fat emulsion compound*—Lipiphysan (10% or 15% cotton oil seed with 5% Sorbitol at 1780 and 1240 calories per litre respectively). Intralipid (soya-bean oil, glycerol) 20% 125 ml (2000 calories but is given in 500 ml water) 10% 500 (1100 calories).

* The giving set must be changed before and after infusion of fat emulsions.

9
Infusion and Transfusion

The maintenance of body fluid is a primary requirement in the treatment of disease (page 133). Under normal conditions the alimentary tract is capable of handling an adequate food and water intake. When kidney function is unimpaired and the digestive system intact, these mechanisms adjust themselves to abnormal requirements of the tissues in disease or injury. Unfortunately, in some medical and in many surgical conditions, the normal mechanism has to be replaced or supplemented by parenteral feeding. Not only water but protein and electrolyte balance has to be adjusted artificially.

Such conditions of depletion arise:

(a) In disorders of the alimentary tract—congenital obstruction, inflammation, injury or neoplasms. Obstruction and infection are the chief lesions.

(b) In disorders of renal function. The chemical control of the body is thus disturbed and there is an upheaval in the distribution of body fluid in the various 'compartments' (page 106).

(c) In injury or overwhelming disease where the natural mechanisms, though still efficient, are inadequate to meet the abnormal demands (e.g. oligaemic shock).

Parenteral feeding is achieved by one of several routes:

(a) intravenous,
(b) subcutaneous,
(c) rectal or colonic.

By **infusion**[1] is meant the introduction of significant amounts of water (with dissolved chemicals) into the body so that it enters the general circulation.

Transfusion refers to the infusion of blood in some form, transferred from another individual. Whole fresh blood, stored blood, concentrated blood or plasma, may be administered by the intravenous route.

The choice of method, composition of the fluid or the necessity for transfusion of blood is a matter of very great importance and may be considered outside the realm of nursing. However, the nurse manages the patient during these procedures and it is on her observations and records that the programme of fluid administration is based. She must be aware of the hazards and of the importance of the procedures employed.

[1] Infusion, in another sense, means a concoction of a drug, e.g. infusion of senna.

This section is concerned with techniques, management, and complications of these procedures, rather than with the indications for treatment by these methods.

The choice of route

The majority of infusions are by the **intravenous route**. This makes it possible for blood to be administered without an alteration of technique. The intravenous route makes rapid administration possible but requires the presence of a medical officer to set it up initially. Large quantities of fluid may be given and the infusion continued for many days. Unfortunately venous thrombosis is a common complication at the site of infusion, and it follows that many of the available superficial veins become unserviceable if prolonged treatment is necessary. Infusion thrombosis is a very painful complication and many patients declare that this is worse than the discomfort at the operation site. Drugs may be administered at the same time by injection into the tube and perhaps one of the chief merits of the intravenous method is that the drug produces its effect almost immediately, in contrast to the delay in other methods.

Subcutaneous infusion was largely abandoned in favour of the intravenous route. There was, before the era of chemotherapy, the great risk of uncontrolled spreading of infection in the water-logged area of subcutaneous tissue and the greater rapidity of the intravenous method was an advantage. The subcutaneous route is however very convenient and rapid for babies and small children where the layer of fat is not great. The amount of infusion that can be introduced in a given time by the subcutaneous route depends upon the rate of absorption: a visible swelling must never be produced. The introduction of the spreading agent **Hyalase** completely reinstated the subcutaneous route as a vital treatment, and has made it possible to extend the use of subcutaneous infusion. There is a great increase in the rapidity with which the water is absorbed, and plasma, and other substances can now be given in this way. In practice the subcutaneous route has the distinct advantage that it can be set up by a nurse, and is less likely to 'block' or go wrong in a child than an infusion given by the intravenous method.

The **rectum** provides an area of mucous membrane which absorbs water very readily and 500 ml can be administered by this route in 4 hours. Tap-water is the least irritant substance. The addition of sugar (glucose) and other chemicals tends to produce inflammation of the rectum and very few patients are able to tolerate rectal infusion for more than 24 hours. A convenient and trouble-free method is by means of a long ureteric catheter introduced into the sigmoid colon through a sigmoidoscope. The level of entry of infusion is then much higher than the rectum and is in fact in the area of bowel designed for the absorption of fluid. This is a very practical way of administering as much as 3000 ml in 2 hours for several days. It is tolerated extremely well and has become standard practice in some surgical units for use in cases of gastric resection and other major abdominal operations.

Excessive infusion by the intravenous route occurs very easily. The subcutaneous route having a slower rate of absorption is to some extent a safeguard against overhydration provided no visible swelling is allowed to form. The risk of overhydration is extremely small if the rectal or colonic route is used, since the bowel will only absorb the amount the body requires.

With the increasing magnitude of surgical procedures, many more patients at some time during their treatment receive an infusion by one of these routes. The choice of route will depend on the expected time for which parenteral feeding will be required, upon the condition and accessibility of the patient's veins, and upon the urgency with which it is desired to raise the patient's circulating blood volume.

Time of infusion

Modern anaesthesia frequently calls for the use of intravenous injection of drugs. Observation of the patient's pulse and blood pressure during operation is the responsibility of the anaesthetist. Consequently the setting up and maintenance of infusion or transfusion during operation is frequently undertaken by the anaesthetist. Preparation for this procedure will then be the responsibility of the operating theatre staff. The infusion may or may not be continued after return to the ward.

Parenteral feeding may be necessary for varying periods, perhaps even two or three weeks.

Apart from operative and immediately post-operative periods there are many occasions on which dehydration or shock requires treatment by infusion before the time arrives for operative surgery.

INTRAVENOUS INFUSION

Technique

There are two distinctive methods—the 'stick-in' (injection) and the 'cut-down'. These colloquial terms indicate that in the first method a sharp needle is inserted through the skin into the vein. In the second method the vein is exposed through a skin incision, opened deliberately, and a blunt tube (cannula) inserted into it under direct vision. The preparation for the stick-in technique is of course simpler, nothing more being required than for an intravenous injection. Sometimes it is impossible for the medical officer to see or feel a surface vein: even if one can be felt it is sometimes preferable to cut-down and be absolutely certain that the cannula is tied into the vein. After repeated infusions and in babies, venepuncture without a cut-down may be difficult or quite impossible.

Needles and cannulae. In the stick-in technique, a short bevel serum type needle is used, but to simplify the procedure various special needles have been devised with an inside rod or stilette which is itself bevelled or pointed. Once the needle is in the vein the inner sharp stilette is withdrawn, leaving the cannula in the vein. There is then less likely to be damage to the lining of the blood vessel than if a sharp needle remains in position during the whole of the infusion period.

A cannula is really a point-less needle. Metal cannulae which have to be resterilised are now rarely used. When a cut-down infusion is initiated, the vein is exposed through a small transverse incision and a ligature is passed underneath the vein distal to the point at which the needle or cannula is going to be inserted. Sometimes this ligature is tied, but more often it is only left there temporarily to put traction on the vein while the needle is being inserted. The saphenous vein immediately in front of the medial malleolus at the ankle is a constant vein and is sometimes used in emergencies when no other veins can be found, particularly in babies. When this cut-down procedure is used, it is now standard practice to insert a fine Nylon or plastic catheter for several centimetres into the vein tying it there with a piece of fine plain catgut before stitching up the wound.

The **butterfly needle** is used very widely now. This was originally designed for scalp vein infusion in babies. It is short with a short bevel and two plastic wings with which it is held during insertion. The wings can then be strapped to the skin to keep it in place. The fine plastic tube which is attached to the needle carries a mount at the inlet end to which a syringe or drip-set can be attached, or a sterile plug can be applied into which intermittent injections can be given. The butterfly needle is particularly useful for intermittent intra-venous infusion when drugs such as heparin are being used by intermittent rather than continuous administration.

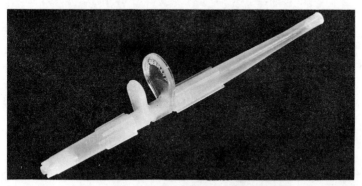

Fig. 9.1   Disposable Braunula intravenous cannula (half size). A rigid plastic cannula with an inner steel needle is seen on the right within a protective plastic cover. The Luer fitting input end is seen on the left within a further plastic case. The steel-introducing needle on which is mounted the smaller wing is removable and the infusion tubing is plugged into the second Luer opening at the base of a large wing. After insertion, the cannula is fixed in place by a piece of strapping with a slot placed over the wing. (Armour Pharmaceutical Co.)

For the measurement of central venous pressure a long catheter is required which will reach from the forearm vein into the right atrium. A suitable catheter for this purpose is the drum catheter (Fig. 9.2).

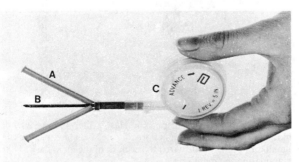

Fig. 9.2   Intravenous drum catheter. Plastic wings A protect the introducing needle B. When this is in the vein, the fine plastic cannula is advanced by rotating the drum C, the distance being measured by the number of turns. When the desired length is in, the needle is withdrawn from the vein and the wings A are closed to prevent fracture of the catheter over the point of the needle. This long cannula (or catheter) is passed into the superior vena cava for central venous pressure measurement, or through a leg vein to the inferior vena cava for prolonged intravenous feeding with amino-acids and lipid (page 139).

Flasks and fluid packs. Figure 9.3 shows the type of 'blood bottle' which has become standardised in Great Britain with its sampling bottle for cross-matching the blood. There is a groove near the base into which fits a metal clip for suspension. Each bottle has a screw-cap with a rubber washer. The bottles are never filled completely. Space has to be

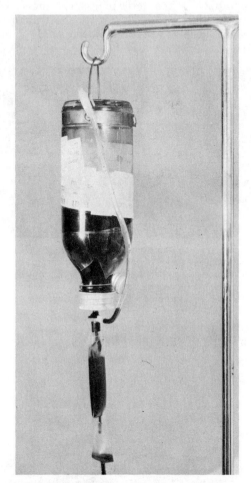

Fig. 9.3   Standard transfusion bottle. The disposable plastic filter with an air inlet tube (the bottom of which is filled with blood in the illustration) has a trochar needle which pierces the rubber diaphragm on the bottle. Note the small 'sampling' bottle wired to the neck of the main flask. This makes cross-matching possible without contaminating the main unit.

allowed for expansion of the fluid during autoclaving of solutions, and for the insertion of the delivery tubes and filter. Sterilised solutions for infusion are available commercially and one of the widely used types is the Baxter Vacoliter.

Flasks are litre or half-litre capacity. Some bottles are graduated so that the amount which has been administered may be measured accurately. This is of particular importance when an infusion is being given to children and, if the bottles are not supplied with complete graduations, a slip of paper with printed graduations is attached to the outside of the bottle in the hospital pharmacy. Adhesive tape is fixed around the neck of the cap when the apparatus is sterilised.

Plastic containers are now being used widely for intravenous fluids. These have the advantage that they are easily destroyed after use and they require no air inlet as the bag collapses as the fluid is withdrawn. Fluid from glass containers, however they have been prepared, has been shown to contain minute particles of silica (from the glass); this risk is eliminated with plastic packs.

Plastic packs (Fenwal) are now used in some regional blood transfusion depots. Each pack contains considerably less blood than the standard 540 ml bottle and the total volume of blood is usually about 340 ml. Thus, if two standard units of blood (540 ml each) are needed, the equivalent in plastic packs will be three units to produce just under a litre of blood. One of the principal disadvantages is the difficulty in inserting the giving-set.

There are certain rigid rules in relation to flasks and their usage.

1. If the seal around the cap is broken, the bottle should not be used.
2. If the label showing the composition of the solution is missing or is indistinct, the bottle must be discarded.
3. If the volume of fluid indicated on the label is not present in the bottle this suggests that there has been a crack or the bottle has been opened previously. It should not be used.
4. If there is any solid matter floating in the solution, the particular bottle must be discarded; if saline and electrolyte solutions are not crystal clear they must be discarded.
5. The suspension clip must be inspected to make quite certain it will not come loose or fall off.
6. The patient's name should be written on the flask so that if there is any untoward reaction the discarded flask can be traced. If the flask has a serial number, this number should be stated on the patient's fluid balance chart.
7. If it is necessary to mix the contents of two bottles, special care must be taken not to contaminate the solution as it is poured. The cap is removed from each bottle and the outside of the neck must not be touched. The rubber washers are lifted away **with sterile forceps** and the edge of one bottle rested firmly on the edge of the other. If solutions are to be mixed, a proportion of one bottle will have to be discarded. Care must be taken that any solution which drips down the side of the bottle, does not run back towards the sterile lip when the bottle is inverted. In many hospitals mixing of intravenous fluids on the ward is prohibited.

Giving-sets. The apparatus which connects the infusion flask to the patient is described as the 'giving-set' (Fig. 9.4). Plastic packs may have the giving-set sealed to the outlet so that no separate apparatus is required. Glass bottles, however, require an administration set which consists of a sharp plastic tube with bevelled end, through which protrudes a second tube as an air inlet; alternatively a separate long pointed tube may be inserted through the diaphragm stopper. The short tube is the outlet, the second tube allows air to run into the bottle and is connected to the loose plastic side tube which carries a wool filter (Fig. 9.3). The trochar of the giving-set is pushed through the rubber diaphragm top

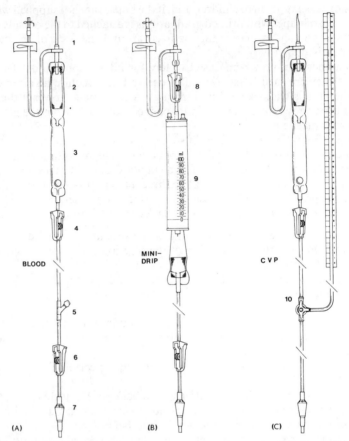

Fig. 9.4 Types of infusion administration units. (A) Standard set for blood or saline solutions. (B) 'Buretrol' with fine drip needle giving 60 drops per ml. (C) Central venous pressure disposable manometer set incorporating 3-way tap **10**. (Travenol Laboratories.)

Key: 1. Fluid outlet with integral air inlet (inlet kept closed when used with plastic reservoir). **2.** Filter. **3.** Drip chamber with safety floating ball (to prevent accidental run-through). This reservoir also acts as a pressure pump: the air is ejected; the chamber fills when released; the ball floats in the full chamber; when pumped again the ball blocks the inlet and so prevents reflux. **4.** Flow control. **5.** Side port with rubber cap. This can be used to inject drugs or to connect a second infusion set. **6.** Final flow control. **7.** Flexible connection: rubber flash-ball for injection of drug through the thin dimples on the cone. **8.** Control unit to shut off supply when metered amount has been run into the burette. **9.** Burette with air vent and rubber cap for injection of drugs. Fine mini-drip delivers into filter. **10.** Three-way stopcock.

of the infusion bottle when the foil seal has been torn away. When inverting the bottle to start the infusion, care must be taken that the air tube is not allowed to hang down at any time or it may fill with blood during the inversion process. The drip chamber contains a filter, sealed to a length of plastic tube at the distal end of which is a syringe type fitting (male Luer nozzle). Some sets have a short length of rubber tube interposed between the needle mount and the end of the plastic tube. This 'flash-ball' is used for injecting drugs in the vein without disconnecting the infusion. When drugs known to irritate the vein are given, the infusion rate is speeded up for a few seconds to wash the drug through.[1]

Additional equipment. Occasionally a medical officer will wish to inject a bleb of local anaesthetic (procaine) before inserting the needle. Syringe and needles must always be available.

The stand on which to hang the blood bottle may be an independent unit or a simple metal rod which clamps to the bed.

In the cut-down method the surgeon requires, in addition to the usual towels, dressings and bandages, the following:

1. A scalpel blade (with or without handle), No. 10 or 15.
2. Very fine, sharp pointed ophthalmic scissors.
3. Very small dissecting forceps.
4. A small aneurysm needle or curved suture-passer with which to thread the ligature deep to the vein.
5. Ampoule of local anesthetic solution (2 per cent procaine with adrenaline).
6. Pair of artery pressure forceps (small, mosquito).
7. A curved cutting-edge needle (30 mm).
8. The appropriate cannula (probably contained in the giving-set).
9. One sachet of '00' plain catgut or fine silk.

Insertion and connection

A blood-pressure cuff, a length of bandage, or a length of rubber tubing is applied above the intended site of injection in order that the veins may be made more prominent for the stick-in method. If a cut-down is being used, the surgeon locates the vein by palpation and a tourniquet is not necessary. The needle or cannula is then inserted. The exact location is checked by allowing a drop of blood to flow backwards out of the needle and the giving-set is then connected. The position of the needle in the vein is adjusted so that its axis is the same as that of the vein. Care is taken that the point does not press outwards towards the skin: a small pad is sometimes placed under the needle mount to prevent this. In any case the butt of the needle and its point of junction with the tubing must be firmly fixed by adhesive strapping to prevent lateral movement.

The flow is allowed to be rapid for the first few seconds, and the control clip is then adjusted to the necessary flow-rate which will probably be between 20 and 40 drops a minute, depending on the particular circumstances.

[1] Baxter giving-sets are widely used. Some contain a separate air inlet trochar which is used with the infusion bottles. If blood is to be given from a plastic pack the air inlet tube is not required. When the blood transfusion is over, if the saline bottle with the inlet tube has been discarded a new giving-set will have to be opened to provide an additional inlet tube for the next bottle of saline. It is wise, in any case, to use a complete new giving-set when switching from blood back to saline, disconnecting at the I-V needle or cannula.

In countries where labour is plentiful and apparatus is in short supply, transfusion sets may be made up in the hospital, autoclaved, and returned to the department to be cleaned and reissued, but this practice has now almost disappeared because of the risk of conveying virus infections on the sets. Certainly, in hospital practice in Great Britain, the nurse will be called upon only to use disposable equipment with a variety of needles and needle fittings, each individually packed and usually sterilised by gamma radiation.

A sterile dressing is strapped over the point of entry and the end of the delivery tube is anchored with adhesive strapping. In the upper limb, the tube can then rest between the thumb and index finger and be reversed back up the forearm where it is incorporated in a bandage. In the leg, the tube is taken between the first and second toes, looped back onto the dorsum of the foot where it is bandaged. This large loop is essential to allow for accidental pulling on the tube, and if the patient is particularly restless, it is wise to strap this loop independently beneath the bandages. An arm or leg into which an intravenous infusion is running should if possible be elevated above the level of the heart to assist venous return and thus lessen the risk of thrombosis (Fig. 2.11). The occurrence of 'drip' arm—painful thrombo-phlebitis—is more likely if the hand and forearm are unsplinted, or if the same giving-set is used for more than 24 hours.

Control and maintenance

Infusion rate. The rate at which fluid should be infused clearly depends upon the volume prescribed for a given period of time. In order to initiate treatment of shock, fluid is administered as a continuous stream and probably as much as 1 litre may be given. Other than in an acute crisis the amount to be infused will be prescribed for a 24-hour period. The type of fluid to be given over each section of the 24 hours will also be recorded by the medical staff. The nurse has to regulate the drip accordingly. Most infusions are given at approximately 30 drops a minute but there needs to be an hourly check to prevent over- or under-infusion. The best method is for an adhesive strip to be inscribed in ink and attached vertically to each infusion bottle. This will show the time at which a particular bottle has to start and end with the intervening hours marked at the appropriate levels. This is known as the 'water clock' system and has the merit that the correctness of the rate can be checked by anyone at any time without reference to books or charts.

The drip rate may vary from hour to hour, depending on the rate of spasm of the vein and on the exact position of the needle, but for ordinary purposes or post-operative hydration the aim is approximately one bottle (540 ml) every 4 hours. In children the amounts are considerably less.

If the infusion or transfusion is to be given very slowly or in small volumes, for instance, for children, or for drugs such as heparin, the best accurate control is by the use of an intermediate 'burette'; the volume to be given over a set time (e.g. 30 ml in 2 hours) is run into this and the main supply clipped off (Fig. 9.4B). For intravenous chemotherapy even more accurate control is achieved by the use of a very fine 'drip' tube. The standard apparatus allows approximately 20 drops to 1 ml. The buretrol illustrated gives 60 drops to 1 ml.

The ideal is achieved by the use of an electronic controlled regulator (Fig. 9.5). Here the drip tube passes through an 'electric eye' which counts the drops and feeds the information

---

Fig. 9.5 Decca automatic infusion control unit. The drips are counted in the drip chamber by the photo-electric eye **E**. The flow tube passes through the regulator **R** at which the compression is varied by the control unit, to comply with the drip rate selected. Each drip flicks the meter up to the selected number. The 'over-drip' selector rings the alarm **S** if more than the maximum permitted variation occurs over a minute. With fixed settings infusion rate is affected by the patient's position, venous pressure and state of the vein. The alarm **S** has a buzzer and a light. The outlet tube **V** is the standard infusion line, with the flow control open. (Decca Radar Ltd.)

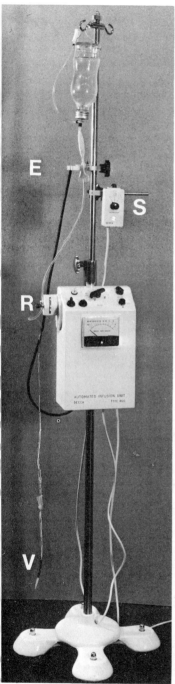

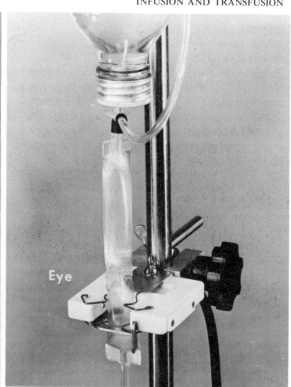

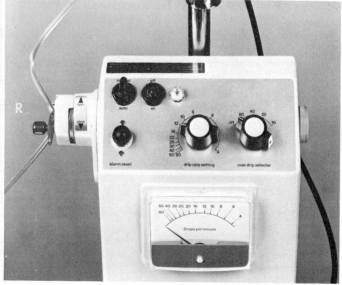

into the control box which in turn compresses or releases the tube to correct the flow rate to the 'drops per minute' which has been set on the dial. If the drops are too slow or too fast the alarm rings.

The apparatus shown in Fig. 9.5 depends upon gravity for the flow. An alternative is an infusion pump (e.g. Ivac 501) which forces fluid through the tube at a regulated rate. It stops if the resistance to flow is excessive but because it is absolutely constant there is less liability to blockage.

When rapid infusion is required this is usually supervised by a medical officer and the rate at which the infusion is given is, if possible, controlled by a reference to the central venous pressure (page 134). Occasions on which rapid infusion or transfusion are required are:

(a) Severe injury and loss of blood. In the casualty reception area the infusion is started with saline; blood is taken for cross-matching and, only after blood has been taken, dextran is given until blood is available. Two drips may be put up simultaneously in order to administer sufficient fluid while blood is being obtained.

(b) Sudden torrential haemorrhage during operation.

(c) Bacteraemic shock. In the circumstances of both (b) and (c), the patient's blood group will already be known. Dextran can be used and the infusion can be increased by connecting a pressure bulb to the air inlet of the transfusion bottle, but this must only be done under the direct supervision of the medical officer.

A special pump is required for intra-arterial transfusion or infusion (page 435, neoplasia).

Interruption of flow. There is an old saying 'the show must go on', the inference being that incidents or accidents may occur on the best-ordered stage. Intravenous infusion is capricious. It stops when everything appears to be in order and it starts again when hope of this has been abandoned! The reason for this variation and uncertainty is that the vein is muscular. It goes into spasm, and while it is in spasm, clotting may occur in some tributary and later spread into the main vein. Cold saline, glucose, and certain drugs are particularly liable to set the vein into spasm and positive pressure is sometimes needed in the initial few minutes of an infusion. This can be achieved by 'milking' the tube of the giving-set. An effective way of relieving venous spasm is the injection of 1 per cent procaine (1 ml) into the tubing at the flash-ball or into the cannula direct with a needle. (Such a course is only to be undertaken if it has been prescribed by the medical officer.) Once the 'drip' has started satisfactorily, the causes of unexpected stoppage are:

(a) *Alteration of needle position brought about by limb movement, a slipping splint, or dragging on the tube.*

REMEDY—very gentle alteration of needle position either by rotation or lifting the mount so that the point is depressed. Under no circumstances must an attempt be made to advance or withdraw the needle. Such action will tear the vein or produce a haematoma.

(b) *The needle has punctured the vein wall opposite the point of insertion and caused a leak, shown by swelling at the site of injection.*

REMEDY—the infusion must be transferred to a different site.

(c) *The needle or cannula has become blocked. Blood may have flowed back into the needle mount and a small clot formed there at the beginning of the infusion.*

REMEDY—the lumen must be tested by disconnecting the tube and passing a stilette (in the case of a cannula) through the needle. Blood or infusion fluid should flow back if the needle is clear. If there is no flow a syringe should be attached and some saline injected.

(*d*) *Kinked delivery tube.*

REMEDY—inspect and rearrange.

(*e*) *Bandages or clothes too tight above the injection site.*

REMEDY—release.

(*f*) *Air locks. (If the delivery tubing has been correctly filled as described above, there can be no air lock.)*

REMEDY—disconnect the giving-set from the needle and flush through.

(*g*) *Air inlet to bottle blocked. This may occur if the air inlet carries a short tube and filter which has become kinked, or filled with blood (in transfusion).*

REMEDY—cut the air inlet tube with **sterile** scissors near the filter end or change the giving-set.

(*h*) *Venous thrombosis.*

REMEDY—none. The infusion is transferred to a different site.

Most of these causes are obvious, but venous spasm is probably the most irritating and yet most common. Stroking with fingers along the line of the vein above the injection site sometimes starts the infusion again. The spasm may relax spontaneously as the limb warms up inside the bandages.

The nurse's main duty is to take simple steps as outlined above if the drip ceases, but she should not disconnect the giving-set tubing from the needle unless instructed to do so. Correct splintage, elevation of the limb, and constant observation are essential if the drip is to be maintained for any reasonable length of time, and if complications are to be avoided.

Changing the bottle. The infusion bottle should be changed before the level of the fluid reaches the bottle neck. The control clip is closed, the bottle taken down and stood on the table or locker. A fresh bottle is uncapped and the giving-set trochar inserted through the rubber diaphragm. The air inlet tube is attached at the suspension point of the bottle.

The drip chamber may become too full at any stage during an infusion and the rate of drip cannot then be observed. This may be remedied in one of two ways. The control clip is closed and air injected with a sterile needle and syringe into the tubing immediately above the drip chamber. The surface of the tube is of course sterilised with an antiseptic first. It is not really necessary to *inject* air because if a sterile needle is inserted into the tube, air will be drawn in as the drip continues. The needle is removed and the control clip readjusted. Alternatively, when the bottles are to be changed, the drip may be allowed to continue after the old bottle is empty, until sufficient air has entered the drip chamber. The principal cause of the chamber filling with fluid is the vigorous milking of the delivery tube, a procedure sometimes adopted to overcome a resistant vein: air is in this way driven from the chamber upwards through the filter into the bottle. Double chamber giving-sets have a side air inlet with a plug, which may be removed, after closing the bottle outlet, to allow air into the chamber, or for injection of drugs (Fig. 9.4B).

The giving-set should be changed after blood, plasma or fat emulsion infusions.

Drug administration via infusion line

When there is intravenous infusion it is convenient to use this for the administration of any drugs which are required. If the action of the drug is required immediately it may be injected into the 'flash-ball', or rubber connector adjacent to the needle or cannula and the infusion accelerated for a few moments to wash the drug out of the vein (bolus technique). Certain antibiotics can be given similarly. Some drugs are given more conveniently over a prolonged period by mixing with infusion fluid in the flask. This latter procedure carries a serious risk of reaction occurring between the drugs and the infusion fluid. Antibiotics lose their potency when diluted and left mixed for prolonged periods before injection and the general rule is that drugs should not be mixed with the injection fluid, but only mixed by the 'bolus' technique described above.

Observation during infusion

Temperature and pulse should be taken at the commencement of any infusion or transfusion, and recorded hourly during the first 4 hours. The pulse record may need to be more frequent if shock is present. Reference has already been made to the complete graduations necessary on the bottle if the infusion is for a child, and the level in the bottle must be recorded on the patient's chart every hour. It is possible by over-infusion to produce cardiac and lung failure in less than half an hour.

The programme of infusion is planned by the medical officer. It is usual if the drip is to be continued for long periods to alternate glucose infusions with simple glucose-free saline, as glucose solutions are liable to cause thrombosis by their acidity.

Discontinuing the infusion

If the vein has blocked or the time has come to discontinue the 'drip', the control clip is closed and a small sterile bandage and dressing prepared. Splints, all other dressings and strapping are removed from the limb. The fresh dressing pad is then pressed on the site of injection and the needle or cannula withdrawn smartly from the vein. Even if the cannula has been tied into a vein, a jerk is sufficient to remove it, but pressure must be kept on the vein while this takes place. The pad is then firmly bandaged in place to prevent the formation of a haematoma. Elevation of the limb should continue for 24 hours.

If the 'drip' is blocked or has been deliberately stopped, under no circumstances must there be unnecessary delay before withdrawing the needle or cannula. Any such delay is calculated to induce thrombosis, or infection.

Complications of intravenous infusion

These may be described as general and local. The patient may react abnormally to something contained in the infusion. Such a reaction is now extremely rare because the water used in the preparation of infusion solution is freed completely from 'pyrogenic'[1] material. Plasma or other 'blood expanding' solutions may occasionally produce an untoward reaction which will be shown by rigor or rapid rise of temperature.

A rise of pulse rate of more than ten beats a minute during the first 15 minutes of an infusion should be regarded as abnormal, and a constant watch kept for generalised reaction.

Over-infusion. A bubbly cough, a rising pulse, or a rising respiration rate are early indications of excessive fluid intake. The patient may however become oedematous about the face, lumbosacral region or legs without any signs of cardiac failure or pulmonary

---

[1] Pyrogenic = fever or heat producing: foreign protein matter is mainly responsible (e.g. dead bacteria or moulds).

congestion, if the electrolyte balance is disturbed and water retention is occurring (page 133). If there is the slightest suspicion in the nurse's mind that any of these signs are present, she must report her observations (CVP, page 134).

Thrombosis. This is by far the most common complication of infusions and is probably the end result of more than half of all infusions given into a vein. Frequently the clotting process is limited to a few centimetres above the injection site, but sometimes the thrombosis spreads up the full length of the surface vein of the limb, and is extremely painful. It is shown by a red line and extreme tenderness along the course of the vein. It is usually accompanied by slight fever. Apart from stopping the infusion, there is very little treatment for such thrombosis. Kaolin poultices, cold saline compresses and other local applications may have their place. The main treatment is preventive: the type of needle, efficacy of splintage and the exact degree of acidity of the solution play a considerable part in the production of infusion thrombosis. Infection due to inadequate dressing at the site of injection is another likely cause of thrombosis, but since patients undergoing this treatment are very often receiving large quantities of antibiotics in addition, infection probably plays only a small part. The thrombosis is superficial and the risk of clot becoming dislodged and forming an embolus is extremely remote.

Air embolus. The entry of air into an infusion may be fatal, but nothing very serious is likely to occur unless several millilitres of air have entered. Air entry may occur in several ways.

1. Sufficient time may elapse between the introduction of the needle and the connection of the drip-set for air to enter the vein if the limb is already elevated, and the veins empty.
2. The air may not have been entirely expelled from the giving-set.
3. The infusion bottle may be allowed to run dry: if ever this happens the entire giving-set must be discarded as no one can be certain to what level the fluid has fallen.
4. If positive pressure is used on an infusion bottle, a nurse or doctor must watch continuously to avoid rapid emptying of the bottle and escape of air under pressure into the giving-set.
5. The common practice of 'flicking' or tapping the plastic delivery tube sometimes produces a series of air gaps: the set then needs disconnecting at the I-V needle and the air locks running through.

Sepsis. Infection may gain entry to the blood and cause dramatic and sometimes fatal septicaemia. Sources of infection are many.

1. The infusion solution or blood may be already infected when supplied, through faulty manufacture.
2. Bottles or packs may have been damaged and bottle caps broken.
3. Careless insertion of the giving-set without adequate cleansing of the top before removing the seal.
4. Infections in the giving-set.
5. Inadequate protection of the venepuncture site.
6. Prolonged infusion, especially with glucose.
7. Failure to change the giving-set with sufficient frequency (i.e. every 24 hours). It is a mistake to keep a drip running just to maintain a patent line in case it is needed *unless* the patient has already had several veins used.

8. Patient tampering with the injection site—prevent by using a sealed dressing.

Non-absorbable ligatures used to tie in an intravenous cannula may cause inflammation and leave a tender nodule. Stitches inserted at the site of a cut-down must be removed a week later. It is very easy for such sutures to be forgotten as they are far away from the main site of the patient's operation.

Haematoma and oedema. Extravasation of the infusion around the vein or the formation of a haematoma may be extremely distressing, and if the infusion has been given into the area in front of the elbow, the pressure may be sufficient to restrict the blood flow to the forearm. If haematoma or extravasation has occurred, infusion must be stopped immediately and an injection given of 1000 units Hyalase distributed in several points in the swollen area.

A firm bandage should then be applied and the circulation of the limb examined repeatedly: elevation must continue.

Intravenous infusion is a life-saving measure. It is a procedure in everyday use and therefore one with which all nurses become familiar. It is nevertheless a procedure which calls for skill and care. It is a source of great discomfort to the patient if anything goes wrong. Familiarity with this seemingly simple operation must not lead to lack of attention to detail.

SUBCUTANEOUS INFUSION
(Hypodermoclysis)

When this procedure was first introduced, special multiple-eyed needles were used, but these are quite unnecessary. The size of needle required depends on the size of the patient. This method is hardly ever used on adults but a No. 1 or 2 hypodermic needle is necessary. A No. 14 hypodermic is suitable for most children, while a No. 12 or smaller may be used for infants. The importance is that the needle must be long enough to lie comfortably beneath the subcutaneous fat. Sometimes by means of a Y-connector, a double infusion is maintained from a common reservoir. This method is of value in that it can be initiated by a nurse in emergency or isolated conditions when no medical help for intravenous infusion is available.

Site and technique

Suitable regions for subcutaneous saline infusion are:

(a) The lateral chest wall. The needle is inserted behind the lower border of the pectoralis major muscle, and clear of the breast area. This allows the fluid to go into the loose tissue on the medial wall of the axilla.

(b) The abdominal wall. The needle is inserted lateral to the umbilicus approximately over and parallel to the outer border of the rectus muscle, pointing upwards and outwards. This site is of course unsuitable for patients undergoing an abdominal operation.

(c) Outer sides of thighs. The needle is inserted mid-way between the great trochanter and the knee, pointing to the hip.

In all these instances the needle is pointing upwards so that the infusion tube can be taken down towards the foot of the bed where it interferes least with nursing. The fluid spread is also thus directed upwards along the normal lymphatic stream.

A standard infusion bottle, drip chamber, control clip, and needle mount are required (Fig. 9.3). If two needles are used a Y-connector and twin tubes with needle mounts and individual control clips are necessary. The reservoir and giving-set is prepared as for intravenous infusion.

To aid absorption, hyaluronidase (Hyalase) is injected at the commencement of the infusion. Each ampoule of powder contains 1000 units which has to be dissolved in 1 ml of sterile distilled water or saline. This can be injected directly through the needle before the infusion tube is connected or it can be injected through the rubber tubing as soon as the connection has been made: the tubing must be sterilised with an antiseptic on its outer surface before this injection. A wide area of skin around the site chosen for the infusion should be cleaned with cetrimide or some other innocuous antiseptic. Once the infusion has started, a small sterile dressing must be strapped lightly across the puncture site. This strapping must be arranged with a pad under the butt of the needle in such a way that the point of the needle is prevented from pressing outwards against the skin. A bandage must not be applied over the site of the infusion although the tubing may be anchored to the limb or trunk below the point of injection.

The rate of administration must never exceed the rate of absorption. This means that the injection site must be inspected frequently to make quite certain that no swelling develops. The flow rate depends on the calibre of the needle, the screw-clamp, and the height of the reservoir. The latter should never exceed 1 metre (3 feet) as a safeguard against excessive pressure.

Normal saline or sodium lactate can be administered in this way up to 600 ml an hour, using two needles. Such a rate of flow is never required in a child, and with the aid of Hyalase the continuous drip method can be avoided in many cases. 50 ml of the infusion fluid are injected with a syringe directly into each site which has previously been prepared by the injection of Hyalase. Alternatively the Hyalase may be mixed with the saline. Further injections of 50 ml may be given as required, the approximate maximum rate for a baby being 50 ml per hour, by either method.

It is not necessary to warm the fluid to be given by the subcutaneous route but, if desired, the tube may pass over a hot water bottle when the drip method is used.

Dextrose solution can be given but causes pain unless given very slowly, with Hyalase.

Plasma can be given in this way, but only with the Hyalase technique.

Drugs should not be administered by way of the subcutaneous infusion.

Blood has also been given but such a practice is very unusual.

SUMMARY OF RULES FOR SUBCUTANEOUS INFUSION
1. Use Hyalase.
2. No bandage over injection site.
3. Strict asepsis.
4. Repeated inspection.
5. No drugs by the same needle.
6. Stop and wait if pain occurs.

Risks
1. Local pooling (pain and inflammation).
2. Infection.
3. Over-hydration.

If a visible swelling appears during the course of a continuous infusion, the flow should be interrupted until the swelling has subsided. The site of injection should be changed every 24 hours if prolonged administration is necessary. The injection area should not be tender and if pain develops with redness it is a suggestion that infection has entered, and the infusion should be stopped.

RECTAL AND COLONIC INFUSION

This route of fluid administration is extremely valuable in domiciliary nursing and in conditions of isolation away from hospital facilities no special apparatus is needed. In routine ward work as a pre- or post-operative supplement, it can entirely replace the intravenous therapy in many cases. It is essentially a nursing procedure and requires no special aseptic technique. It can nevertheless be dangerous unless certain simple precautions are taken.

The rectal mucous membrane readily absorbs water and the colon does so with even greater rapidity. Glucose and certain drugs may be administered by this route (page 98), but the presence of glucose in the rectum for more than a few hours causes irritation and proctitis which then makes continuous infusion impossible: glucose and saline solution should be given diluted to less than the normal (isotonic) strength.

Tap-water or saline is normally used, administered by slow drip (40 drops a minute); 540 ml in 4 hours, followed by a rest period of 2 hours and then repeated, is most likely to be tolerated. Patients vary enormously in their tolerance of an indwelling rectal catheter. Absolute contra-indications to the use of the rectal or colonic route are bowel disorders, anal lesions, paralytic ileus or intestinal obstruction of uncertain origin. Peritonitis and pelvic cellulitis also makes this route inadvisable.

The principal requirement is slow administration with the patient in the best position to prevent fluid pooling in the lower rectum. It is therefore ideal for an unconscious patient, who is flat or tilted in the 'head-down' position.

Technique of rectal infusion

The apparatus required consists of a simple Jaques type urethral catheter (Fig. 35.6), preferably with an aseptic eye. The size is immaterial; the smaller catheter is better tolerated but may be too soft to insert. No. 24 Beniqué is a suitable size. A standard (not necessarily sterile) blood bottle with giving-set may be used with the addition of a glass connector for the catheter if the latter is of the funnel-end variety. With a straight-ended catheter an infusion record or Luer tubing mount may be inserted directly into the end of the catheter to receive the drip set. Alternatively, a simple glass reservoir may be used, with a length of rubber tube incorporating a drip chamber.

Before the insertion of a catheter, a digital examination of the rectum must be made to confirm that it is empty. If the rectum and colon is loaded, an enema will be necessary except, of course, if the infusion is being used in the immediate post-operative period. In the latter case a loaded rectum indicates that there was insufficient pre-operative preparation: rectal infusion cannot then be used.

The catheter is lubricated with mucilage jelly and inserted slowly for approximately one-third of its length. Any attempt to push it further than this is almost certain to result in the catheter curling up in the rectum and perhaps irritating it. The catheter is then strapped to the side of the leg. The giving-set is freed from air and connected so that the reservoir is approximately one metre above the patient. The initial drip-rate should not exceed 40 drops a minute. An excessive flow may stimulate the rectum to contract. Without unduly bothering the patient observation should be kept for leakage and the quantity administered must be recorded on the fluid balance chart.

Rectal infusion can be given rather more rapidly in small quantities with a tube and funnel instead of by the continuous method. There is very little advantage in this except the even greater simplicity of apparatus, which makes it particularly suitable for use by the District Nurse, away from hospital organisation. Again the tolerance of the patient may vary a great deal, but 200–300 ml may be administered in 20 minutes. The catheter may be reinserted 2 hours later, and if there is no fluid in the rectum, the infusion may be repeated. By this intermittent method, glucose may be administered satisfactorily.

Technique of colonic infusion

To permit the infusion of larger quantities with less irritation to the rectum and therefore extending over a longer period, a ureteric catheter is inserted into the sigmoid colon through a sigmoidoscope. This procedure has to be undertaken by a surgeon, but if the patient has been adequately prepared this should not add more than five minutes to the preparation of the patient. It is usually carried out after the induction of the anaesthetic before the patient is placed on the operating table. The ureteric catheter is then connected to a standard giving-set and the flow regulated as for a rectal infusion. Glucose is well tolerated when the administration is into the colon rather than the rectum. As much as the full requirement of 3 litres in 24 hours may be administered by this route, and continued at this rate if necessary for several days. It is of particular value in gastric surgery where the patient is having repeated gastric aspiration.

BLOOD TRANSFUSION

The transfer of blood from one individual to another first became a practical proposition during World War I. The recognition of four major blood groups indicated that there were limitations on blood transfusion which necessitated very careful examination of the blood of the two individuals concerned. In the early days of transfusion after preliminary grouping, the blood was transferred from the donor to the recipient by the 'direct' method, using a two-way tap and syringe, so that the blood was not exposed to the air and had no opportunity for clotting.

The 'indirect' method was later introduced in which the donor's blood was received into a solution of sodium citrate which prevented it from clotting by inactivating the calcium (page 59). Within an hour or so the blood was then injected into the veins of the recipient.

Prior to World War II, most large hospital centres in Great Britain maintained a panel of blood donors who were willing to come to the hospital at any hour of the day or night for emergency transfusion. The relatives of patients also were called upon, if with the right blood group, to give their blood.

The necessities of war, and the greater demands of surgery for blood transfusion have led to the establishment of 'blood banks', in which are stored large quantities of blood taken at a convenient time from thousands of volunteers.

With suitable refrigeration, blood may be stored for three weeks with safety and such blood is quite suitable for the treatment of shock and conditions of blood loss. Certain other disorders, mainly medical conditions affecting the formation of red cells in the bone marrow, are preferably treated with the transfusion of fresh blood: this seems to possess properties which become lost in storage.

Blood transfusion performs a double purpose. It replaces the oxygen-carrying red cells and its fluid fraction, the plasma, contributes protein which maintains the circulating blood volume, thus preventing the escape of water into the tissues.

Blood products. Whole blood can be separated into its various constituents. When the cells have been separated by centrifuge, the plasma or serum can be used fresh or stored or it may be dried. In this form it was used extensively during World War II because it could be stored indefinitely and reconstituted by the addition of distilled water when infusion was needed in the treatment of shock.

By the extraction of the fluid portion of the whole blood, the cell content may be concentrated. Such a preparation is known as 'packed cells'. This has become of particular value if it is necessary to raise the haemoglobin rapidly without raising the blood volume unduly. Such a procedure may be required in the treatment of severe anaemia arising from toxaemia.

Blood group incompatibility (concerned with what is known as the rhesus factor) is of great importance in obstetrics. A baby born to parents who are, from the blood group point of view, incompatible, suffers from a particular form of anaemia which is frequently fatal. In the treatment of this condition the new-born baby's blood is replaced entirely by fresh blood from specially suitable donors. This procedure is known as 'exsanguination-transfusion' (page 169).

In the United Kingdom, **plasma protein factor** (PPF) solution is supplied as an alternative to plasma. Other fractions of blood plasma are separated for specific use. **Cryoprecipitate** (obtained by freezing) contains anti-haemophilic factor and **anti-haemophilic globulin** is also available. **Fibrinogen** is another separated blood product. Concentrated suspension of **platelets** is used in platelet-deficiency states.

Occasions for transfusion in surgery

The circumstances which call for blood transfusion vary considerably in their urgency. In fact, they may be grouped for convenience into urgent and non-urgent.

In the management of injuries transfusion of blood is frequently the initial life-saving measure. Occasionally during surgical operations, blood transfusion may be required unexpectedly because the surgeon has met with an unforeseen hazard. Severe haemorrhage occurs spontaneously without either injury or operation, particularly from gastric and duodenal ulcers or from an ectopic pregnancy, and these require most urgent transfusion.

Most other occasions allow for a deliberate planning of blood transfusions for which adequate preparation can be made and the time of the transfusion selected for everyone's convenience. Under such circumstances it is often possible to call upon relatives as blood donors and so avoid drawing from the national blood bank. No matter what degree of skill, or standard of success of a major surgical procedure, blood transfusion may be called for and preparation should be made for such eventuality before the operation commences.

Blood transfusion is in itself occasionally fatal, and such fatalities are usually the result of errors of grouping. Blood transfusion, as any other form of infusion into a vein, should not be undertaken lightheartedly.

Blood groups

Normal red blood cells are of four main groups in relation to their behaviour when mixed with blood plasma (or serum) of another individual. Similarly the plasma (and serum) of each individual belongs to one of four groups. If cells of one group meet plasma of an 'incompatible' group, the cells stick together in blocks. These clumps obstruct blood vessels and may cause death. The interaction of the incompatible cells and plasma is called 'agglutination'. The provocative substance in the cells is called the **agglutinogen**, while the defensive substance in the plasma is the **agglutinin**. A similar mechanism develops in relation to our immunity to infections by certain bacteria and viruses.

Table 24 International (ABO) classification of groups showing associated serum factor and the Moss group used formerly

International group or cell factor	Serum factor (plasma)	Moss group
AB	None	I universal recipient
A	Anti-B	II
B	Anti-A	III
O	Anti-A and anti-B	IV universal donor

In blood transfusion, the amount of plasma administered is small in relation to the large amount of plasma in the recipient's circulation. On the other hand, even a small quantity of cells given to a patient whose plasma will not tolerate that particular type of cell, will lead to clumping of the donor's cells in the recipient's blood vessels. The importance therefore lies in the **cells of the donor** and the **plasma of the recipient**.[1]

Plasma and serum for this purpose are identical and the serum obtained when a small quantity of blood is allowed to clot is used for testing against the donor's red cells. In order to determine a patient's blood group, a small quantity of blood is obtained from a finger or ear prick and immediately mixed with citrate to prevent clotting; the cells are then tested against special serum of known groups. To obtain the patient's serum for cross-matching, 5 ml of blood is taken, by vein puncture, and allowed to clot.

The four common groups have been numbered variously. The **Moss classification** I, II, III, and IV was used extensively until the adoption of the **International A, B, O classification**, which describes the groups according to the presence or absence of the specific cell factors, which are of two types, A and B. Thus we have four blood groups in the inter-

[1] For easy memory, C of D (cells of donor) and S of R (serum of recipient)—these pairs of letters are closest in the alphabet.

national system. In the first of these, both cell factors are present but no serum factors. The serum factors are called anti-A and anti-B, and obviously the cell factor A and the serum factor anti-A could not exist in the same patient. The second group contains cell factor A and serum factor anti-B. The third group contains cell factor B with serum factor anti-A, and the fourth group contains neither cell factor but both serum factors. The fourth group could therefore be given to any of the other groups and the cells, having no clumping factors, would be tolerated in any recipient. On the other hand, the first group with both cell factors could not be given to any other group. The terms **universal donor**, Group O (Moss IV), and **universal recipient**, Group AB (Moss I), were used to amplify the earlier grouping system. Transfusion with the wrong group of blood is usually fatal so that very great care has to be taken in the determination of the blood group, both of donor and recipient.

Table 25   Blood group chart. The agglutination or clumping of the cells which occurs when standard group A (anti-B) and group B (anti-A) serum is used for testing.

Blood group of cells under test	Typing serum	
	anti-B	anti-A
AB	+	+
A	−	+
B	+	−
O	−	−

+ indicates clumping or agglutination.

Unexplained incompatibility was found to be due to the presence of other factors than the A, B, O, agglutinogens. The most important of these is the **rhesus cell factor**. Certain monkeys (Rhesus species) have this factor naturally, but it is present in only 85 per cent of white people in England and America. The other 15 per cent—Rh negative—may become sensitised to Rh positive cells by repeated transfusion of Rh positive blood. A rhesus negative mother whose husband is Rh positive may produce an Rh positive baby. A battle occurs between the unborn baby's cells and the mother's plasma. The baby may die before birth (miscarriage) or be born with very severe anaemia and jaundice. If born alive, the baby is treated by complete replacement of its blood to get rid of the mother's sensitised Rh negative plasma. This is 'exsanguination-transfusion' (page 169).

Blood grouping in preparation for transfusion has become a complex and very responsible task. In most hospitals this is undertaken by specialists—perhaps a pathologist or transfusion officer. A specimen of the patient's blood is taken into sodium citrate and the cell group determined with known anti-A and anti-B sera. From the cell-factor finding, the patient's serum factor is known as well, and the donor of the correct group is selected. As an additional safeguard 'cross-matching' of the two bloods is undertaken (**with every bottle**) using the patient's serum this time with red cells from the bottle of blood which has been provided for infusion.

The nurse's responsibility in relation to blood transfusion is a heavy one. An error is usually fatal. The grouping and cross-matching of blood is a medical officer's responsibility entirely. The nurse may be responsible however for labelling and retaining a sample of the patient's serum for cross-matching. Matched bottles of blood must always be labelled with the patient's name *and* initials *and* some other identity such as bed or ward number.[1] The nurse is frequently responsible for changing the blood bottles during a long-term infusion. Before a further bottle of blood is installed there must be a check, by at least two persons, that it has been correctly cross-matched and labelled. In Great Britain the National Transfusion Service has adopted a colour code for the four main groups with additional easily recognised identification marks. Where a patient has already had a blood transfusion there may be an extra risk of incompatibility with sub-groups and particular care has to be taken over the rhesus factor. The numbered tag from the bottle label is detached and fastened to the patient's notes as a cross-check in case there is any untoward reaction.

Partly because of the rhesus factor and partly because of the occurrence of many other minor factors which influence blood grouping, it is now considered advisable for all blood grouping and cross-matching to be done with special techniques only possible in the pathology laboratory. In dire emergency only should the quicker and less reliable method be adopted in which a drop of the patient's blood is mixed with each of the two test sera on a white tile, the result being deduced from the clumping which occurs with incompatible serum. Direct cross-matching is then undertaken.

Untoward effects of blood transfusion

The reaction of a patient to infusion of blood from another individual may be immediate or delayed.

1. Pyrexial reaction. A slight rise of temperature following blood transfusion is by no means uncommon and in itself is of little significance. A rise of temperature to 38 °C is regarded as significant and its cause must be sought.

Improperly cleaned infusion apparatus, the use of infected blood, or stale blood, and infection at the site of infusion, all lead to pyrexial reactions. Rigor and headache occurring during transfusion must be regarded seriously. It is usual then to reduce the rate to the lowest possible, and if the symptoms continue or become intensified, the transfusion is stopped.

A severe 'anaphylactic' shock may possibly occur with rigors and collapse. It is treated with adrenaline injection.

For the purpose of official records, it is usual to describe febrile transfusion reaction in these grades:

Grade I—associated with a rise of temperature to 38 °C but not other objective features.
Grade II—associated with a similar or greater rise of temperature, the patient complains of feeling cold and shivery, but without the occurrence of a true rigor.
Grade III—associated with a definite rigor.

2. Haemolytic reactions. Haemolysis means the breaking up of red cells. In normal stored blood, the plasma in the upper half of the bottle should be absolutely clear. If it is pink or turbid it is likely that some change has occurred and some of the cells have broken up. The use of such blood may produce severe reaction in the recipient. The over-warming of blood before administration may also produce haemolysis.

[1] There may be more than one patient having the same name in a ward, or beds may be moved during the course of a day's operating, or to make room for an emergency admission. Such incidents have led to fatalities when labelling was incomplete.

The use of incompatible blood will produce severe haemolytic reaction with immediate symptoms. These are usually pain in the back, shivering and collapse. Renal failure with complete suppression of urine or with severe haematuria may follow and is usually fatal though haemodialysis may avert this outcome. Lesser degrees of incompatibility will produce delayed reaction, and when large quantities of blood are transfused the natural breakdown of the red cells may produce jaundice within a few days.

3. Heart-failure. The rapid increase in the circulating blood produced by transfusion of too large a quantity in too short a time, strains the heart. Death may occur from heart-failure and pulmonary oedema.

4. Transfusion lung. When large quantities of blood are required—5 units or more, a Dacron micro-filter must be used in the transfusion line to prevent the entry of minute clumps of red cells. This hazard in which thousands of tiny 'micro-emboli' pass into the lung results in a large number of alveoli being under-perfused with resultant hypoxia (page 112). In the past this condition went unrecognised and the pulmonary complication was thought to be pneumonia.

5. Infective hepatitis is a later complication due to transmission of the hepatitis virus from the donor. To eliminate this risk all donors are now screened for the presence of a specific antigen, 'Australia antigen', found in patients who are known to have had jaundice or may have had a minor attack of hepatitis which has not been sufficiently severe to be recognised. Hepatitis in the past was much more likely to follow infusion of plasma or serum as a single unit of this would have been drawn from pooled blood, i.e. from several donors.

The nursing management of these reactions depends clearly on the cause. The simple rules for prevention are:

(a) Prevent reactions by using only properly prepared apparatus.
(b) Prevent reactions by absolute certainty about grouping, cross-matching and labelling.
(c) Prevent reactions by avoiding rapid infusion, particularly in elderly patients or those with known heart disease.
(d) Headache, rigor, pain in the back, rise of temperature over 38 °C should be reported immediately if these symptoms occur during blood transfusion.

Other complications which may occur from blood transfusion are the same as those which may occur from other forms of intravenous infusion already described. Air embolus, thrombosis, haematoma, and sepsis are all to be guarded against.

If a severe transfusion reaction occurs there is a full investigation by the medical authorities. Empty bottles from which blood has been administered should not be washed out or sent away from the ward for at least twenty-four hours after use, in case the small residue is needed for examination.

Many hospitals have a special card on which the details of each transfusion have to be entered so that there is a permanent record, and untoward reactions can be traced in relation to the source of the blood.

Alternative routes for transfusion of blood

The normal method of giving blood is by a simple intravenous infusion. As with the infusion of saline it may not be possible, particularly in babies, to find a vein suitable for the introduction of a large enough needle for blood transfusion.

Sometimes scalp veins (Fig. 22.7) or the external jugular vein are used, but even these may not be accessible. Blood may be administered into the bone marrow (**intramedullary transfusion**) which has large sinuses, acting somewhat like veins in conveying the blood away rapidly. The marrow of the sternum or the tibia is preferable.

By the use of Hyalase, **intramuscular transfusion** is possible, the blood being absorbed into the circulation. Such a method is by no means reliable.

In some operations, especially in vascular surgery, very large quantities of blood need to be given rapidly and the transfusion is then given by a positive pressure pump into an artery—**intra-arterial transfusion** (page 435).

BLOOD DONATION

Donors

In Great Britain the National Blood Transfusion Centres located in each region are supplied by blood from volunteer donors recruited by local advertising campaigns. The medical and nursing team may visit factories and institutions where there are numbers of willing donors and blood is collected by this mobile team. Other donors may be asked to visit the depot itself. Before World War II, in large cities, the British Red Cross Society maintained panels of volunteer donors, but there was no 'bank' or 'store'.

In hospital, fresh blood is collected from donors who are frequently relatives of the patient needing the blood, or whose names have been obtained from the list maintained by a local voluntary organisation. Whatever the circumstances it must always be remembered that the donor is doing a public service for which he is not being paid. It must also be remembered that many donors have served on several occasions and are therefore familiar with the correct—and perhaps incorrect—method of conducting this operation.

Most healthy individuals can part with 500 ml of blood without any physical disturbance. It is not usual to take more than this quantity from one donor on any particular occasion.

Apparatus for collection of blood

Because of the complexity of blood grouping and cross matching, the taking of blood from donors is now a rare event in hospital. The need may arise if fresh blood is required urgently or if a donor for a very rare group has been located. A special plastic pack (Fenwal) is provided with a long plastic tube to which is sealed a wide-bore intravenous needle. The bag is allowed to hang well below the donor's arm and blood flows by gravity without the need for suction. The bag has no air outlet but expands as the blood fills it. An appropriate volume of anti-coagulant fluid is supplied in the bag and this is mixed by gentle agitation as the blood flows into it. Alternatively, a glass bottle with an air outlet may be used.

In cases of polycythaemia, 'blood letting' (venesection) is sometimes needed and a taking-set may be used in order that the blood may not be wasted but used for some other purpose.

The apparatus required will include:

(a) Taking-set and blood bottle or pack as described above.
(b) A sterile 1- or 2-ml syringe with fine hypodermic needle.
(c) Local anaesthetic solution—sterile (it is customary to insert a tiny drop of anaesthetic over the point of venepuncture).
(d) Sterile swabs and skin antiseptic.

(e) A 5-ml stoppered tube or bijou bottle into which is taken a sample of the donor's blood for subsequent laboratory examination.

(f) Sterile dressing packet and bandage for application to the site of venepuncture when the blood has been taken.

(g) Sphygmomanometer.

In addition, apparatus must be at hand to deal with possible collapse in the donor and this must include:

(a) Vomit bowl, tongue forceps, and mouth gag.

(b) Sterile resuscitation outfit—syringe, needles, adrenaline injection and methylamphetamine ampoules.

Grouping and cross-matching

If the patient has been grouped previously and holds a card which certifies his blood group, the medical officer will proceed to direct cross-matching of the donor's blood with the patient's serum. A small amount of donor's citrated blood may be sent to the laboratory before anything further is done. If the blood is being collected for a blood bank, no further grouping is performed at the time but the sample tube of blood accompanies the original bottle and is clipped to its side. A Wassermann reaction (for syphilis) is performed on all blood taken for the blood banks. Syphilis cannot however be handed on by stored blood as the spirochaetes die as soon as the blood is refrigerated.

Collection technique

The donor must not be kept waiting in a cold corridor but must be received amicably in a warm, well-lit room. His name and address must be checked and recorded on the card which is to accompany the bottle of blood. The medical officer will enquire about the donor's medical history—whether he has had jaundice or any other relevant infective disease. The donor then discards his shoes and sufficient clothing to expose the arms well above the elbows. He is made comfortable on an examination couch and the pneumatic sphygmomanometer cuff applied as high as possible on the arm which has been chosen. The skin of the forearm should be cleaned with soap and water or a detergent solution such as cetrimide, and dried.

When the taking-set and bottle (or pack) is assembled and the medical officer seated, the sphygmomanometer is connected to the cuff and the pressure raised to 80 ml. The skin is cleaned and the needle inserted into the vein. The blood flows immediately but may be slowed down by spasm of the vein or slight alterations of the needle position. Collection of 440 ml of blood may require fifteen to twenty minutes; the rate of flow is variable. During the whole of the collection period, the bottle is agitated gently to mix the fresh blood with the citrate solution and prevent clotting. To encourage the rate of flow, the patient is often asked to clench and open his fist repeatedly. This compresses the blood into the veins of the forearm.

As soon as the bottle has been filled to the 540-ml mark, the cuff is deflated. The sterile dressing is then placed firmly at the site of needle puncture and the needle smartly withdrawn. The donor's arm is lifted in the air and a bandage applied firmly round the elbow. He remains lying down for at least fifteen minutes and should not be allowed to leave for half an hour. During this time he is given a hot drink, usually coffee. The site of venepuncture is inspected before he leaves and he is advised to keep the firm dressing in place for a few hours to prevent the formation of haematoma.

Very occasionally, the rapid withdrawal of blood produces collapse in the donor. The early evidence of this is a desire to vomit and the development of pallor and a feeble pulse. Spontaneous recovery occurs without treatment, but sometimes adrenaline is given by injection. The donor must be asked to return and report any sign of inflammation or persistent discomfort in the arm, if such should occur during the following few days.

The taking-set is removed from the bottle by the medical officer and the screw-cap applied, care being taken not to touch the top of the bottle with the fingers or with the outside of the metal cap. Such contact may lead to infection of the blood. When plastic packs are used the receiving tube is disconnected and the pack sealed.

The donor's name must be written on the bottle or on a label attached thereto, and if the blood is being taken for immediate use and has been cross-matched already, the patient's name must also be written on the bottle.

Care of the blood

Blood taken for transfusion is precious and must be treated with respect. If it is to be used within a few hours it should not be refrigerated. It is not considered necessary to warm stored blood before use if a slow-drip method is to be used, but if rapid infusion is to be given for severe shock or haemorrhage it is preferable for the blood bottle to stand in water at 37 °C for at least 30 minutes before transfusion, if there is time.

When blood is stored in the blood bank, special refrigeration at constant temperature is necessary and the ordinary domestic refrigerator is quite unsuitable and in fact danger-ous.[1] Blood stored for more than three weeks is unsuitable for transfusion. If storage for more than a week is required a special citrate solution is used.

A blood bottle must never be shaken. After storage there should be a clearly dis-tinguished line of separation of the lower red cellular layer, from the upper plasma which should be uniform yellow but not necessarily clear. If the plasma is deep orange or red, haemolysis has occurred and the blood should not be used.

Reference has already been made to concentrated or 'packed cells'. In the preparation of this blood there has been a mechanical separation and additional handling. The blood should therefore be used within three days of preparation. If it is likely that such blood will be required, the blood bank must be notified well in advance.

Some blood depots collecting blood into plastic packs are recommending that unless whole blood is needed (i.e. to increase blood volume in oligaemia), the pack should not be agitated but the cell layer administered through the plastic outlet tube and the plasma returned to the blood depot so that it may be used for the preparation of special fractions such as cryoprecipitate.

Blood which has been drawn from storage and allowed to warm up to room tem-perature must not be returned to the blood store and then used on some subsequent occasion. Special arrangements are made for the use of such unused blood for other purposes.

[1] Refrigerators used for food storage may become too cold. If a blood bottle is placed near the ice cabinet its temperature may fall to freezing point: haemolysis will occur.

BLOOD ADMINISTRATION

The urgency of the occasion will determine both the route and the rate of administration. Severe injury involving considerable blood loss, as for instance from a cut-throat wound, may require the immediate introduction of a 'stick-in' infusion into each arm. On such an occasion plasma or dextran will probably be used to start the infusion while blood is obtained and the patient grouped. Positive pressure may be used on the blood bottle to ensure the introduction of perhaps a litre of blood in 10 minutes. In extreme life-saving urgency the surgeon may use group O (IV) blood without grouping the patient.

These occasions of great urgency are extremely rare. The majority of blood transfusions can be planned and need to take place in an atmosphere freed from drama and excitement. If massive transfusion is required a special filter must be inserted in the giving-set to avoid the risk of transfusion lung (page 162).

If a patient is to undergo a blood transfusion, the procedure should be explained if possible so that his full co-operation may be sought. Very few patients today are upset by the thought of blood transfusion, though its necessity may cause some apprehension, and it may in such patients be unwise to mention the word. Whenever possible, blood transfusion bottles should be suspended in a position where the patient will not be continuously staring at the bottle, bearing in mind of course that the bottle must not be covered or hidden within the bedside curtain: it needs to be watched continuously by the nursing staff.

Non-urgent planned blood transfusion should when possible be arranged to start in the morning, so that the reduced night staff avoid the added burden. Unfortunately in a busy surgical ward the majority of transfusions are started later in the day and continued through the night, since they follow major operations.

In an effort to reduce recurrence of post-infusion thrombosis some surgeons prefer intermittent infusion to the continuous 24-hour drip. It is thus possible to give the necessary volume of blood or other infusion fluid at a faster rate without risk, and consequently the patient and the nursing staff are freed from the worry of night-time infusion.

Administration of blood by the intravenous route requires the same procedure as simple intravenous saline infusion. Even greater care should be taken to avoid contamination of the blood or apparatus, to avoid haematoma, and kinking.

Blood transfusion initiated during surgical operation almost always follows a preliminary infusion of saline: the procedure merely consists of changing the bottle of saline for one of cross-matched blood. The blood bottle must be agitated gently before being inverted, but it must never be shaken. Similarly, care must be taken not to shake the drip chamber as frothing will make it impossible to see whether the drip is running or not.

It is impossible to over-emphasise the importance of ensuring correct cross-matching and labelling of blood.

The method of changing the bottle must follow the same procedure as outlined on page 151 for saline and other solutions. If blood becomes spilt through the air inlet tube, it must be washed off the outside of the bottle and tubing with an antiseptic such as cetrimide. If this is not done, the whole affair looks dirty and becomes an attraction for flies.

Rate of transfusion

Non-urgent transfusions are started slowly as a precaution, so that if a pyrexial reaction occurs the infusion may be stopped. If however there is no reaction in the first two or three minutes, there is no particular reason why the $\frac{1}{2}$-litre bottle should not be administered in twenty minutes if it is being given to make good the loss of blood which has occurred during an operation, or has followed injury. Otherwise, the common practice is to permit a drip-rate of 40 to 60 drops per minute in the adult.

A very anaemic patient, probably also with a weak heart, may require more than 4 units of blood to raise the haemoglobin to 10 G before operation is considered safe. Rapid infusion in such a case might produce immediate heart-failure. To produce the concentration required, 'packed cells' may be used, that is whole blood from which a very large proportion of the plasma has been withdrawn.

The determination of the flow rate is a matter for the medical officer, but the nurse may be called upon to vary this from time to time, in order to ensure that the prescribed quantity is given in the prescribed time. It must be remembered that the rate of flow does not depend solely on the control clip but may be slowed down by spasm of the vein. After such a period of reduced flow the control clip may need to be opened a little to make up for lost time. A 'time schedule' is an essential record for safe transfusion in children and a special metering burette should always be used.

Observation during infusion of blood

Attention has already been drawn to the untoward effects of blood transfusion. The most important initial observation is the reaction of the patient to the first few millilitres of blood. Twitching or shivering or any suggestion of a rigor sounds the alarm. The transfusion must be stopped and the medical officer called at once. Such an initial reaction does not necessarily mean that blood is incompatible or that the transfusion cannot be continued, but this will be decided by the medical officer.

Temperature, pulse and respiration records must be taken at least every quarter of an hour during the first hour of the transfusion, and hourly if the procedure continues. When blood is being given in the treatment of shock, frequently repeated blood-pressure readings must also be taken, and the sphygmomanometer cuff must be left in place (deflated and unconnected) on an arm which is not being used for the infusion: this avoids constant disturbance of the patient.

Vomiting or development of an irregular pulse during blood transfusion must be reported at once.

The urine must be tested for albumen on the morning following blood transfusion, and every specimen must be saved for inspection if there has been any suggestion of untoward pyrexial reaction.

Intramedullary transfusion

This is a rare procedure but sometimes of great use in cases of extensive burns when all four limbs are involved, and no veins are readily accessible. A sternum puncture needle with a sliding guide is used and slow infusion is carried out in the normal way. Alternatively a similar needle is inserted through the subcutaneous surface of the tibia which is relatively soft. The chief risk of intramedullary transfusions is that of sepsis. As far as nursing preparation is concerned, the same giving-set and other apparatus is required as for 'cut-down', with the addition of the special needles (page 147). The greatest possible care is necessary with full aseptic technique.

Autotransfusion

Blood lost during an operation is removed by constant suction. The blood may be passed through a filtration system which removes bubbles and minute clots and is then re-infused. An automatic apparatus is now available and, in selected cases such as severe internal bleeding from a ruptured spleen, provides a readily available method of restoring blood volume. Many years ago this method was used, with a crude filtration technique before 'blood banks' were available.

Transfusion of infants

Blood transfusion in babies is a highly skilled procedure. The amount of blood given is approximately 20 ml for each kilogram body-weight (10 ml per pound). If the quantity is under 100 ml it may be given with a syringe as a slow intravenous injection, perhaps into

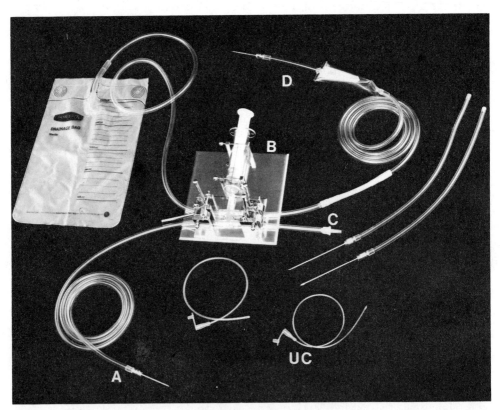

Fig. 9.6 Exchange (exsanguination) transfusion set. Blood is withdrawn from the baby's umbilical vein through a catheter UC attached to tube A; through the 4-way control valves at B the blood is expelled into the waste drainage bag; Rh negative donor blood is taken by catheter and filter D and injected back through A. The process is repeated until the baby's blood has been 'changed'—perhaps 1,000 ml to ensure adequate removal of the Rh antibodies. Heparin solution is taken in through tube C to wash the syringe and valves during the procedure. (Portex Ltd.)

a scalp vein. Sometimes a two-way tap is used to facilitate this transfer from the bottle to the vein. Intravenous Nylon catheters are used for 'cut-down' infusions, and special butterfly scalp vein-needles, with the short bevel and plastic tubing fused to the shank to reduce bulk and weight. In an emergency when intravenous transfusion is impossible blood may be given into the peritoneal cavity from which it is absorbed.

Exsanguination transfusion

The **exchange transfusion** is performed on certain new-born babies for the complete replacement of the baby's blood which has been affected by the anti-rhesus factor from the mother.

A length of polythene tubing is introduced through the umbilical vein stump **immediately** after birth; this acts as a cannula and is passed into the vena cava. (There is in the baby at this time a vein which by-passes the liver but which undergoes thrombosis very soon after birth.) By means of a three-way tap and syringe, 10 ml of blood is aspirated from the vena cava and replaced by a similar quantity of special rhesus negative blood: this process of exchange is repeated until a litre of the donor's Rh negative blood has been given. The new-born baby's total blood is approximately 300 ml and by this means almost all the damaged Rh positive red cells are replaced by cells insensitive to the mother's antibodies. This blood is sufficient to meet the baby's needs until its own blood-forming tissue has produced new Rh positive cells. By this time, the Rh antibodies from the mother will have disappeared from the baby's circulation. During the procedure heparin solution (1000 units to 100 ml normal saline) is used to wash out the tubing and thus prevent clotting. This is necessary as the baby's blood has no anticoagulant in it. The apparatus required is shown in Fig. 9.6.

It is not necessary for the nurse to be familiar with the details of this technique, unless she is a member of a special team which is necessary to undertake this task. Blood tests

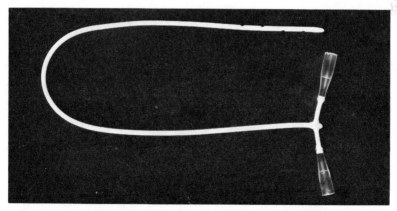

Fig. 9.7   A simple Portex cannula for umbilical vein transfusion. An artery forceps is applied to each cross-limb of the 'T' alternately while blood is withdrawn from one and injected into the other. This eliminates the complications of taps. (Portland Plastics Ltd.)

performed on the mother before the baby is due to be born may indicate the likely necessity for the exchange transfusion and there is then adequate time for preparation.

Conscientious and careful nursing is essential to successful and trouble-free transfusion. The procedure need not, and should in fact never, be an ordeal for the patient, nor a source of great trouble to the nursing and medical staff.

Summary

The whole subject of shock, fluid and electrolyte balance, blood loss and lung function is a very complicated one which involves meticulous attention to detail in all cases of severe illness or injury. These facets of treatment form the real basis of intensive care units. Relevant cross references are:

Body fluid distribution and the physiology of electrolyte balance, page 106
Acute blood loss, page 120
Central venous pressure, page 134
Basic post-operative requirements, page 136
Infusion solutions in common use, page 138
Effect of artificial respiration, page 197

10

Asphyxia, Anoxia and Cardiac Arrest

Pulmonary function and its relationship to tissue respiration and circulation have been described in Chapter 8. If the basic principles of respiratory physiology are understood, the causes and management of asphyxia are easy to follow.

In any organism, respiration is the process of gas exchange between the tissue and its environment. Basically the process is the same whether the environment is air or water and whether the organism has a blood-lung system, a gill system, or merely surface respiration like certain insects and plants. Interference with this process of gas exchange is **asphyxia**. It is just as vital for the organism to get rid of the products of metabolism (e.g. carbon dioxide) as it is for oxygen to be absorbed. In organisms with a lung system, the accumulation of CO_2 (**hypercapnia**) in the blood stimulates breathing rhythm; shortage of air provokes a violent struggle for survival.

Asphyxia thus involves both oxygen shortage and carbon dioxide poisoning. There is a consequent tremendous struggle on the part of the heart, breathing system and muscular system (which thus produces even more CO_2). The effect of asphyxia is not the same as that of anoxia. The result of simple oxygen shortage is shown at high altitudes in flying or mountaineering and can be produced artificially in a 'decompression chamber'. The effects of this anoxia are confused action, mental impairment, lethargy, weakness, and finally collapse without a struggle: carbon dioxide is being removed adequately from the blood until the circulation fails from oxygen shortage.

Causes

Asphyxia in man is most often produced by blockage of the large air passages—'the obstructed airway'. This stoppage may be due to a foreign body or to spasm of the larynx or bronchial muscles (as in asthma, page 374). Approximately a litre of saliva and nasal secretion is produced daily and if this is not removed by natural swallowing or suction, the fluid is inhaled and causes drowning. An unconscious patient very rapidly drowns in his own secretion.

Asphyxia may also arise from disease of the lung epithelium: it may be caused by the tiny air alveoli being filled by inhaled water or exudate from pneumonia or oedema. Over-infusion and congestive heart-failure produce a similar flooding of the lungs with water, and consequently a condition which resembles drowning.

Inhaled vapour or gas, by replacing air, similarly produces asphyxia. The victim 'drowns' in vapour instead of in water. Nitrous oxide anaesthesia (dental gas) acts partly in this way and the accompanying asphyxia then produces violent muscle contraction and struggling. Irritant gases such as ammonia (used in refrigeration), smoke, and chemical warfare agents have a double effect by replacing air and by producing a profuse bronchial secretion which aids the 'drowning'. In fires, carbon monoxide (CO) poisoning renders much of the circulating haemoglobin ineffective for oxygen transport.

Anoxia (occurring for instance in shock) leads to pulmonary oedema from damage to the lung capillaries and this oedema increases the anoxia as well as interfering with the escape of CO_2. A state of asphyxia therefore supervenes.

Thoracic injury, which interferes with the piston action of the diaphragm or the negative pressure in the pleural space, prevents adequate respiration. Entry of air into the pleural space (**pneumothorax**), collection of blood (**haemothorax**), or the presence of a tumour, produces collapse of the lung by compression. The lung resembles a sponge which is being squeezed and the collapsed condition is **atelectasis** (Chapter 34). Atelectasis may also result from blockage of a bronchus (by tumour or by inhaled foreign body): the air in the part of the lung beyond the block becomes absorbed, and as the natural tendency of the elastic lung is to contract, it collapses. A lung has properties alike and yet opposite to those of a sponge. The sponge is air-containing but naturally expands, while the lung is air-containing but naturally contracts. If for any reason a large area of lung ceases to contain air, asphyxia results.

The more common causes of asphyxia are shown in Table 26. It will be seen that there are four main groups:

1. The obstructed airway.
2. Air replacement by 'drowning'.
3. Atelectasis (from compression of the lung or pneumothorax).
4. Respiratory paralysis (originating in the nervous system centrally or at the neuro-muscular junctions).

Apart from these causes there is a condition of congenital or **neonatal asphyxia** arising from an association of various obstructive and paralytic factors. The lungs fail to expand when the baby is born. Positive pressure inflation may be necessary to save the baby's life.

Newborn babies sometimes have a disorder of the pulmonary epithelium which hinders the transfer of gas—this is the neonatal respiratory distress syndrome.

Diagnosis

Asphyxia is a rapidly progressive cycle of events which will probably result in death if it cannot be relieved in less than one minute. The endurance time will depend on the degree to which respiratory movement is impeded, and on the strength of the heart. Frequently there are several factors present together in causing the condition. For instance, poor respiratory effort may be accompanied by vomit, inhalation of foreign matter and spasm.

Relief of asphyxia is by no means simple. In any particular case the reason for asphyxia will usually be apparent from the circumstances under which it has occurred.

Breath-holding, blueness, congestion, or movements of the jaw suggestive of choking, all indicate the likely presence of impending asphyxia and demand **urgent** action.

The obstructed airway is an ever-present risk of general anaesthesia or of unconsciousness from any other cause.

Partial obstruction may be present in the conscious patient due to the presence of tumours in the pharynx or larynx. Goitre or other swelling at the root of the neck may cause tracheal compression. Risk of this obstruction becoming complete during unconsciousness from injury or anaesthesia in such patients is much increased.

Apart from such pathological conditions, obstruction is usually in the unconscious patient and is due to

(*a*) The tongue falling back into the pharynx.
(*b*) The inhalation of mucus, vomit, a tooth or other foreign body which produces intense laryngeal spasm.

This spasm may pass off spontaneously and the obstruction will therefore be relieved, but such spasm alone can be fatal.

Prevention and management

The prevention and recognition of asphyxia is one of the most important tasks in nursing routine. Practical experience in the management of patients in the immediate post-operative phase is essential.

There are five main principles in treatment, both in prevention and in the management of the condition if prevention has been impossible or has failed.

(*a*) Control of the tongue.
(*b*) Position of the patient.
(*c*) Suction or aspiration of foreign matter or secretion from the air passages.
(*d*) Artificial respiration.
(*e*) Tracheostomy if the throat cannot be kept clear.

The application of these principles and other methods are indicated in Table 26 as appropriate to the various disorders producing asphyxia.

Control of the tongue. The tongue is composed of muscles arranged in layers which run in different directions. The 'intrinsic' muscles in the body of the tongue are responsible for alterations in its shape whereas the 'extrinsic' muscles pull the tongue forward from the pharynx and protrude it. The principal extrinsic muscle is the genioglossus (Fig. 10.1), which fans out into the substance of the tongue from a fixed attachment to the mandible at the chin. It is the tone of this and other muscles in the floor of the mouth which prevent the tongue dropping back and choking the unconscious individual. In normal sleep there is sufficient tone remaining in the extrinsic muscles of the tongue to prevent obstruction of the airway at the inlet to the larynx. In deep coma and during anaesthesia, this tone is lost; gravity allows the bulky mass of the tongue to fall back into the pharynx where it acts as a valve and is drawn down over the glottis during inspiration. If the mandible is fractured so severely that the front portion is mobile, this fixed attachment of the tongue drops backwards and asphyxia occurs: a patient with a severe fracture of the mandible must therefore be turned on the face with the head supported so that the fractured jaw and relaxed tongue falls forward.

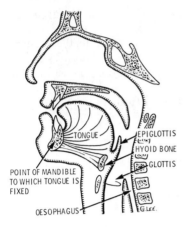

TONGUE

EPIGLOTTIS

HYOID BONE

GLOTTIS

POINT OF MANDIBLE
TO WHICH TONGUE IS
FIXED

OESOPHAGUS

Fig. 10.1 Note the relation of the laryngeal opening (glottis) to the back of the tongue and the oesophagus.

To re-establish the airway, the tongue needs to be pulled forwards. The way in which this is achieved is illustrated in Fig. 10.2. The simplest method and the most commonly applicable is to *lift the mandible forward*, so that the lower teeth are in front of the upper. Pressure behind the angle of the jaw is useless unless it is directed *forward* (pressure inward in this region can produce facial palsy, as the facial nerve lies just below the ear). If no apparatus is available, some solid object is hooked over the back of the tongue to hold it forward into the floor of the mouth. Alternatively tongue forceps may be applied at least 2·5 cm (1 inch) from the tip on the upper surface of the tongue. The further back the forceps are placed, the more effective will be the manoeuvre. The forceps should never pierce the tongue from its upper to its lower surface.

The normal post-operative practice is to insert a rubber or metal shaped airway which extends beyond the back of the tongue and prevents it falling backward; this is left in position until the pharyngeal reflexes return. The likelihood is that the patient will then push it out. When the risk of asphyxia is prolonged as in cases of respiratory paralysis, intubation through the nose or through the mouth is used to maintain the airway. A cuffed tube (Fig. 12.6), carrying a small balloon, will probably be used so that the trachea can be blocked around the tube by inflation of this cuff, to prevent secretions from the mouth trickling down into the lungs. Intubation is however only a very temporary method. If paralysis of respiration is complete it is usually accompanied by paralysis of the muscles of the mouth and pharynx and a tracheostomy may then be necessary.

Position of the patient. Unless mechanical suction apparatus is available to clear the pharynx, the only permissible position is one which places the lips lower than the diaphragm. This can only be achieved by the patient being fully prone (face downwards) or semi-prone with the head turned towards the floor and the body tilted into the head-down position. The main purpose of such positioning is to ensure that no fluid can collect in the pharynx or be aspirated into the trachea. Furthermore, any fluid which has already entered the lung is more likely to escape when the patient begins to recover bronchial reflexes and coughing. The neck must be extended (i.e., 'chin-up' position).

Suction. It is traditional to have a swab holder and swabs when accompanying an unconscious patient who may become asphyxiated, but it is incredibly difficult to clear the pharynx effectively with the aid of a swab. It can only be done if the jaw is widely open

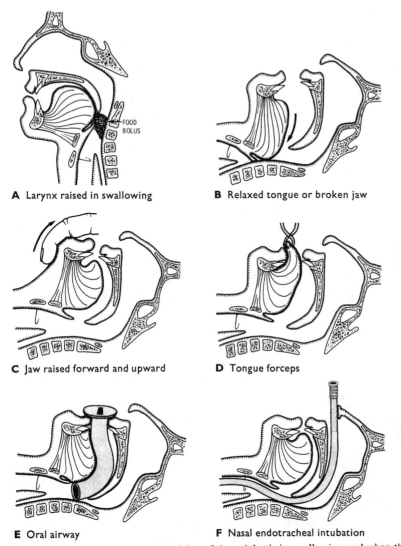

A Larynx raised in swallowing

B Relaxed tongue or broken jaw

C Jaw raised forward and upward

D Tongue forceps

E Oral airway

F Nasal endotracheal intubation

Fig. 10.2 **A** and **B** show alterations in the position of the epiglottis in swallowing and when the tongue falls back into the pharynx. The obstruction may be relieved as shown in **C, D, E** and **F**.

and the tongue pulled far forward: otherwise the swab can do no more than clean the mouth. Many types of mechanical suction device have been introduced (Fig. 16.13). The intake end of a Higginson's syringe with a piece of rubber tubing attached is quite effective for ward use. Special 'mucus catheters' are used in obstetric units for new-born babies, suction being produced by the midwife's mouth. An infusion drip-chamber with a catheter each end is an easily assembled substitute, the chamber acting as a trap to prevent the nurse contaminating her mouth with the secretions aspirated from the baby.

The use of suction in the operating theatre at the end of an operation is essentially preventive: by removing any mucus, blood or other material which has accumulated in the throat, the anaesthetist very greatly diminishes the risk of aspiration pneumonia or

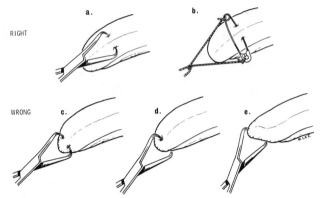

Fig. 10.3 Application of tongue forceps. It is the back of the tongue which causes respiratory obstruction. Traction on the tip does not dislodge the main body of the tongue.   **a.** Correct position, 3 cm from the tip.   **b.** Satisfactory first-aid manoeuvre. The string can be held by anyone. This may be life saving in cases of fractured mandible.   **c.** Ineffective position; too near tip.   **d.** Dangerous; through the tip. **e.** Dangerous; producing haemorrhage from the veins under the tip.

atelectasis. Also, the presence of blood clots or particles of vomited matter in the pharynx is very liable to produce reflex laryngeal spasm or to provoke further vomiting. If such material has in fact been drawn into the trachea or the anaesthetist suspects that mucus has accumulated in the lower air passages, a laryngoscope is used to clear the trachea by catheter suction.

Artificial respiration. In first aid, artificial respiration may be required if there has been a sudden arrest of respiration by interference with the vital centres in the brain stem. Electric shock and cerebral concussion are examples of such conditions. In drowned persons respiratory arrest has occurred from asphyxia, and is complicated by the fact that the lungs are waterlogged. Asphyxia from inhaled poisonous gases occurs in coal mines. In all forms of artificial respiration, blood circulation is also helped by the rise and fall of pressure in the thorax.

If the heart has stopped it is unlikely that artificial respiration will be successful. On the other hand instances are on record of the heart-beat being restored. It is also very difficult to be certain that the heart *has* stopped, and the absence of a pulse at the wrist is unreliable. It is therefore always worth instituting artificial respiration in what may seem to be a hopeless emergency.

In medical and surgical practice, artificial respiration is required in four conditions.
 1. Sudden unexpected respiratory arrest during or after anaesthesia.
 2. Artificially induced respiratory paralysis in controlled anaesthesia where curare-type drugs have been used (Chapter 12).
 3. Thoracic surgery or thoracic injury where the pleural space has been opened.
 4. Respiratory paralysis in poliomyelitis, myasthenia gravis, or from poisoning.

Table 26 Causes of asphyxia

Mechanism	Cause	Treatment
Obstructed airway	Intrinsic obstruction:	
	Tongue	Posture and pull
	Tumour in mouth or pharynx or air passage	Tracheostomy
	Spasm	Avoidance, intubation, removal of irritant factors, antispasmodics
	Inhaled foreign body	Remove
	Oedema of glottis (from infection or injury)	Intubation, tracheostomy
	Diphtheritic membrane	Intubation, tracheostomy
	Extrinsic obstruction:	
	Tumour in neck	Removal of tumour
	Goitre	Thyroidectomy
	Post-operative haematoma	Release by drainage
	Malignant glands	Probably untreatable
	Strangulation (accidental or criminal)	If found before death, tracheostomy may be necessary
	[In criminal cases the hyoid bone is frequently broken]	owing to oedema and damage to larynx
Air replacement, 'drowning'	Inhaled water—submersion	
	Inhaled vomitus	
	Excessive bronchial secretions from irritation	} Aspiration, artificial respiration
	Oedema from over-infusion	
	Heart-failure	} Diuretic
	Flash burns	
	Scalds by inhaled steam	} Intubation, tracheostomy
	Inhaled gases—nitrous oxide	
	ammonia	
	chemical warfare	} Oxygen, artificial respiration
Respiratory paralysis	Poliomyelitis	
	Head injury (vital centres in medulla affected)	
	Cervical spinal cord injury (dislocated neck)	Artificial respiration and preservation of airway
	Operations on the spine	
	Spinal anaesthesia	
	Myasthenia gravis	} Neostigmine and artificial respiration
	Relaxant drugs in anaesthesia	
Atelectasis	Compression of lung, haemothorax, effusion, pneumothorax	Measures to decompress pleural cavity, positive pressure artificial respiration
	Crushing injuries of chest	
	Congenital non-expansion at birth	Positive pressure inflation after clearing airway

Methods of artificial respiration

First-aid methods—physiological principles

There is no one method of artificial respiration which can be applied universally in all circumstances. The nurse will receive practical instruction in the use of several methods and only brief reference will be made to the use of each.

These procedures depend upon the fact that the lungs and thorax possess a natural springiness or power of recoil to a balanced neutral position. The tendency in the lungs is towards complete collapse. The chest wall and diaphragm may be compressed beyond the 'neutral' point, and when released the thoracic cage will expand again, drawing air into the lungs. On the other hand, the thorax can be expanded artificially by pulling the ribs up via the shoulder girdle muscles, or by sucking the abdominal wall and thorax outwards with a mechanical respirator. When released the chest recoils to the neutral position, and this time, by the lung elasticity, air is driven from the lungs. Artificial respiration which depends on the suction effect of chest expansion for inspiration either side of neutral point—i.e. by arm muscle movement, or by recoil after compression—is **negative pressure respiration**.

These simple physiological points may be demonstrated on oneself by passing a tape measure around the lower thorax and noting the respiratory movement. In normal respiration the excursion is 2 cm, by deep breathing one can expand at least 2 cm beyond this normal measurement, and by forced expiration, by lowering the ribs, one can force out air and decrease the circumference to 2 cm less than the normal relaxed position of expiration. The total excursion demonstrates the 'vital capacity', but in normal life we use only a small proportion of this (Fig. 10.4).

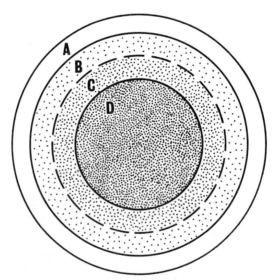

Fig. 10.4 Lung capacity. Zone **A**. The outer reserve range; over-expansion; emphysema. Zone **B**. The normal excursion; 'tidal air'. Zone **C**. The inner reserve range; compression; forced expiration. Zone **D**. The airless lung; atelectasis.

Positive pressure techniques

The 'kiss of life'. This depends on the inflation of the victim's lungs with the exhaled breath of the rescuer. Any revulsion which may be felt against this mouth-to-mouth, or mouth-to-nose, method is overcome by placing a thin handkerchief over the patient's nose and mouth, but in a dire emergency no one should be concerned unduly with finesse. It is clearly no use inflating, or endeavouring to inflate, the lungs when air passages are partly blocked, and therefore, as with other methods of artificial respiration, the first duty is to extend the head and neck and lift the jaw forward to clear the airway. Most emergency resuscitation kits contain a special shaped 'anaesthetic' airway which is double ended so that one end can be placed in the mouth of the operator; e.g. the 'Brook' (Fig. 10.5) or 'Safar' airway. The patient's nose in pinched during the inflation. If no such airway is available the rescuer's mouth is placed over the patient's lips and the rescuer's head can be tilted in such a way that the cheek obstructs the patient's nose: this leaves the two hands free to hold the jaw and the head. Dummies on which nurses may practise are now available in most training schools. This method is now often combined with external cardiac massage (page 191). It is found in practice that when an individual is practising mouth-to-mouth artificial respiration she automatically breathes more deeply herself and therefore the exhaled air contains a higher proportion of oxygen than would normally be the case. Even though the breath has a lower oxygen content and a higher carbon dioxide content than normal air, there is sufficient oxygen to meet the patient's needs and insufficient carbon dioxide to cause damage, but clearly the method cannot be as efficient as artificial respiration performed with an Ambu bag or some other mechanical contrivance using fresh air.

Negative pressure techniques

The alternative to mouth-to-mouth or mouth-to-nose artificial respiration is to use a method which creates a negative pressure in the thorax to induce lung expansion. At the end of this suction movement the elastic recoil of the chest wall expels the air.

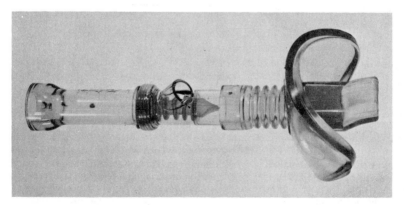

Fig. 10.5   The Brook Airway, which contains a one-way valve enabling the operator to inflate the patient's lungs, the expired air escaping through the side tube. The airway holds the victim's tongue forward out of the pharynx and the nose is pinched to prevent the escape of air during inflation. (British Oxygen Co. Medishield.)

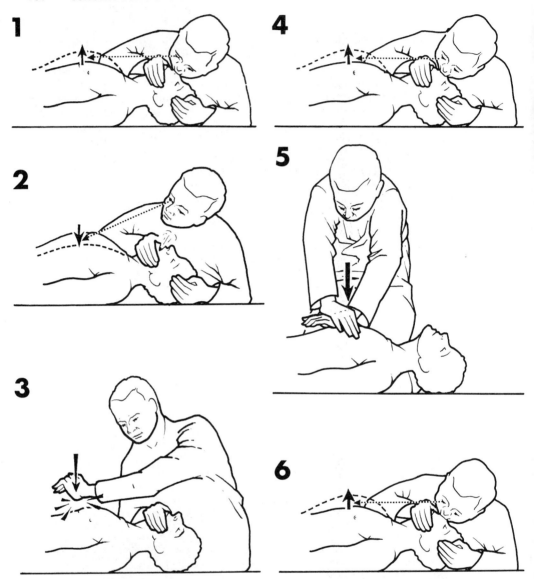

Fig. 10.6 Emergency resuscitation. 1. Mouth-to-nose inflation; watch for rise of chest and feel carotid pulse. **2.** At the end of expiration repeat inflation (approximately every 3 seconds) and continue for 1 minute. **3.** If no pulse or improvement of colour, thump the lower third of the sternum 3 times. **4.** Continue mouth-to-nose respiration for a further minute. **5.** If still no pulse, external cardiac massage 60–80 times for 1 minute, then **6.** Resume artificial respiration.

If single-handed, 2 breaths and 15 chest compressions is approximately the best rhythm. If assistance is available the same rhythm can be maintained and the operators should change places when the one doing cardiac massage begins to tire (page 191 and Fig. 10.19).

Artificial respiration can therefore be achieved in either range—above or below normal inflation. The ideal method clearly is to work both sides of the normal relaxed or neutral position.

The **Schafer** method depends on recoil for inspiration, and compression for expiration (by increasing abdominal pressure, thus raising the diaphragm).

The **Silvester** method depends on recoil (with some added pressure) for expiration, and muscle traction for inspiration.

The **Holgar Neilsen** method combines both principles fully.

The **Eve's rocking stretcher** uses diaphragm movement by means of gravity for both inspiration and expiration. The weight of liver attached to the under surface of the diaphragm acts as a piston. This method has been extensively used in injuries sustained in mining where the chest wall may have been crushed in addition.

In Figs. 10.7, 10.8, 10.10, and 10.11, the normal relaxed expiratory position is indicated by the dotted line and the diagrams illustrate whether the outer range or inner range of lung movement is being used.

Schafer method. The patient is placed on his face with his shoulders raised a little so that the mouth is unobstructed. Pressure is exerted on the patient's loins and lower ribs, thus compressing the abdominal contents and forcing the diaphragm upwards. As the weight is taken off the patient's loins, the abdomen and thorax re-expand and inspiration occurs (Fig. 10.7). This is the simplest method of artificial respiration as it can be performed without assistance and encourages the removal of fluid from the air passages by gravity.

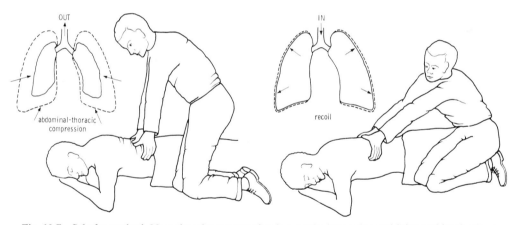

Fig. 10.7 Schafer method. Note that the compression is over the lower ribs and loins and inspiration is entirely by natural recoil. As the patient is face down, fluid can escape freely from the mouth. This method can be used in the presence of arm injuries.

Eve's rocking stretcher method (Fig. 10.8). The apparatus consists of a stretcher pivoted at its centre and of such height that it can be tilted down to an angle of at least 45° either way. The patient is fastened to the stretcher by arm and leg straps, and is placed on his face. As the stretcher is tilted into the full head-down position, expiration is produced by the weight of abdominal

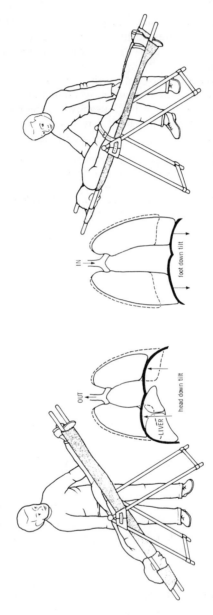

Fig. 10.8 Eve's method. The great merit of this method is its simplicity, lack of fatigue on the part of the operator, and the assistance which is given to circulation by the repeated change in posture.

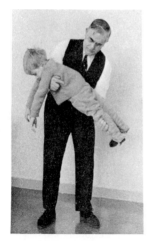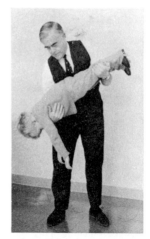

Fig. 10.9 The 'rocking stretcher' principle used as a first-aid measure with a child. It circumstances such as fire, smoke or flooding prevent the use of mouth-to-mouth ventilation this simple method may save life while the rescued child is carried to safety. The act of rocking may sometimes start an arrested heart. *Left.* Inspiration, *Right.* Expiration.

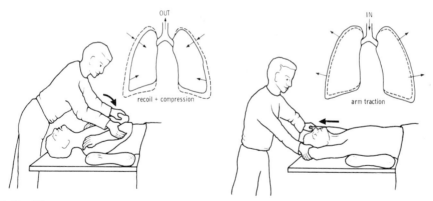

Fig. 10.10 Silvester method. This method is particularly suitable for use on the operating table or with the patient in bed, until the inflation apparatus is available. Note that a cushion is necessary to lift the shoulders off the bed. The respiratory excursion is produced actively by the operator in both phases; the patient is lying on his back. An assistant will probably be needed to hold the tongue forward. This method cannot be used if the arms are injured.

contents pressing the diaphragm upwards. In the foot-down position the diaphragm is pulled downwards and inspiration occurs. The Riley (patent) portable rocking stretcher is one of the most simple and yet effective appliances for unskilled artificial respiration. The application of the method of resuscitation of a child is illustrated in Fig. 10.9 and Eve's 'discovery' of the rocking stretcher method originated in this way in a case of diphtheritic paralysis.

The same principle is the basis of the rocking bed, for constant use by respiratory cripples, for instance in poliomyelitis residual damage. Such patients may be able to maintain adequate

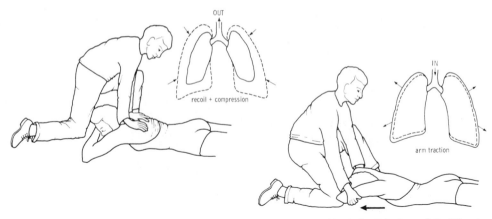

Fig. 10.11 Holgar Neilsen method. This combines the advantages of both the Schafer and the Silvester methods. The patient is face down and the operator is active in both inspiration and expiration. The respiratory excursion is greater than with the other methods. This is not suitable for patients with severe upper limb injuries.

ventilation whilst awake but become hypoxic in sleep. The bed is rocked by an electric motor at the appropriate frequency.

Silvester method. (Fig. 10.10). The patient lies on his back with a folded coat or blanket under the upper part of the thorax. The patient's arms, flexed at the elbow, are abducted and taken above his head so that the pectoral muscles elevate the ribs and expand the chest. As the arms are brought down, with pressure against the sides of the chest, forced expiration is produced. This method really requires an assistant to hold the tongue forward, in order to preserve the airway: a safety pin can be put through the dorsum of the tongue and attached to a string held by the assistant (Fig. 10.3).

Holgar Neilsen method. This method, introduced by the Danish Red Cross Society, is similar in principle to the Silvester method except that the patient lies face downwards. Inspiration (chest expansion) is produced by lifting the arms upwards over the head, and expiration is produced by the operator compressing the chest with hands placed over the patient's scapulae (Fig. 10.11).

The Holgar Neilsen method is the most suitable and most effective for uninjured patients (e.g. after drowning); it cannot be combined with external cardiac massage.

If there is any doubt about the possibility of abdominal injuries, the Schafer and Eve's methods should not be used; if there is a thoracic cage injury, the chest compression methods should not be used. Fractured ribs are a common accompaniment of drowning and the Eve's rocking stretcher method is undoubtedly a very satisfactory way of dealing with persons who have been drowned in shipwreck or have fractured ribs.

In all methods the aim is to produce approximately twelve respirations per minute. All movements must be slow and progressive without violence. Quick jerky movements followed by pauses, are useless. 'Over-breathing' washes out carbon dioxide from the blood so that there is then even less stimulus to the breathing centre in the brain.

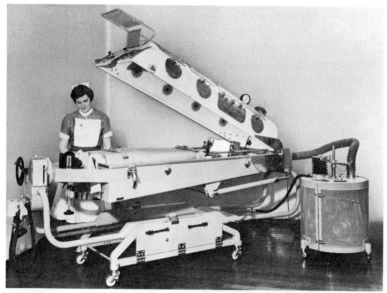

Fig. 10.12   The Cape 'Alligator' rotary tank respirator (Kelleher). Open, showing fibre-glass cuirass placed over patient to hold her in position when the tank is inverted for nursing attention to the back and to relieve pressure points. It thus incorporates the principles of the Stryker bed (page 897). (Cape Engineering Co. Ltd.)

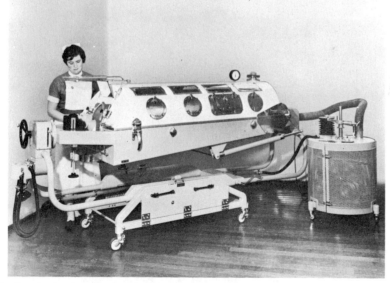

Fig. 10.13   Respiration is maintained by intermittent negative pressure in the tank, causing expansion of the chest and inspiration as there is no other air leak. This tank may be easily rotated by one nurse: toilet attention and other procedures are carried out through the port-holes which fit round the attendant's arms so that respiration continues. (Cape Engineering Co. Ltd.)

Mechanical appliances for artificial respiration

The term respirator[1] is used to describe various forms of appliance which perform artificial respiration.

Apart from the apparatus used in the course of general anaesthesia these appliances may be divided into **negative pressure** and **positive pressure** machines.

Negative pressure appliances

These are of two main types:

(*a*) Cabinet respirators,
(*b*) Cuirass respirators.

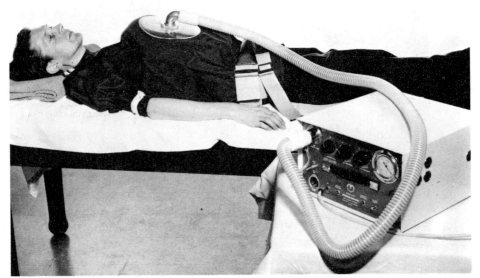

Fig. 10.14 Tunnicliffe breathing jacket. Inspiratory phase; negative pressure in the jacket causes chest expansion. (Department of Medical Photography, St Thomas's Hospital, London.)

Cabinet respirators. The 'iron lung' or **Drinker respirator** was the first successful cabinet machine. This consists of a steel cabinet in which the patient is enclosed completely except for his head and neck. A rubber airtight collar fits round the neck and the cabinet has windows through which inspection and nursing can take place. The pressure in the cabinet is intermittently reduced below the atmospheric pressure by a large electric pump. The principle is an imitation of the natural method by which chest expansion leads to lung

---

[1] The use of the word respirator to denote a gas-mask for protection against chemical warfare was an unfortunate mis-application of the word, since such an appliance interferes with, rather than aids, the movements of respiration.

expansion through the negative pressure in the pleura. This type of respirator is complex and it is very difficult to nurse a patient who cannot be moved from the respirator for more than a few seconds at a time. Nevertheless, the 'cabinet' is the best-known type of respirator for complete respiratory paralysis.

The original cabinet type has been considerably modified and the 'Both' mechanical respirator was widely distributed throughout the British Commonwealth during World War II. This was made possible by the generosity of Lord Nuffield. Further advances in design have been made but the principles remain the same.

Cuirass respirators. The second negative pressure apparatus is the cuirass respirator. The Tunnicliffe jacket (Fig. 10.14) has a rigid plastic shell which forms a bridge over the

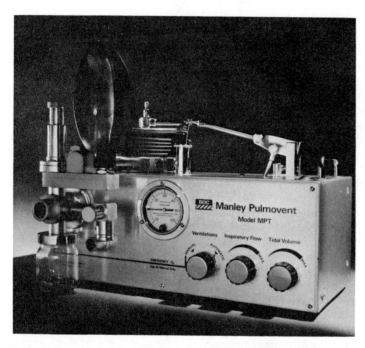

Fig. 10.15 Manley **Pulmovent** ventilator which is independent of electricity supply and is operated by pressure from the oxygen or compressed air cylinder. This apparatus is often incorporated in the theatre anaesthetic apparatus. (British Oxygen Co.)

patient's chest. The airtight seal around the neck and arms ensures that when air is withdrawn from the jacket the chest expands to produce effective inspiration. Expiration occurs from the normal elastic recoil of the chest but may be assisted by positive pressure within the jacket. This appliance is of particular value to poliomyelitis patients with permanent respiratory paralysis who require additional ventilation whilst sleeping though they can manage when conscious and vertical.

Positive pressure appliances

If the lungs are to be inflated by **positive** pressure, certain safeguards are essential to prevent rupture of the tiny alveoli by over-distension. The positive pressure method is essential if the chest wall is open or has been severely injured; it is the best method for prolonged use in respiratory arrest. It is used in the conduct of 'controlled respiration' anaesthesia (Chapter 12). The essential features of an appliance for this purpose are:

1. Regulation of pressure, rate of inflation and volume.
2. Low resistance to expiration, which depends on the natural elastic recoil of the lung.
3. The delivery tube must be capable of attachment to an endotracheal tube, tracheostomy tube or airway, or to a simple face-piece.
4. If the apparatus is electrically driven, it must also be capable of manual operation in the event of electricity failure.

The simplest possible appliance is an anaesthetic mask, wide-bore corrugated delivery tube and rebreathing bag, into which oxygen is delivered in a steady stream controlled by a reducing valve. Rhythmic inflation is performed by squeezing the bag with one hand. (See below, also Fig. 16.13.)

The Ambu bag. This is a simple positive pressure artificial respiration apparatus which consists of a rubber bag the walls of which are reinforced with a resilient plastic foam material making it fully self-expanding. There is a face-piece with a non-return valve which also acts as a safety device to prevent over-inflation of the lung. The face-piece can be held over the patient's mouth, the jaw held forward and the bag compressed intermittently with the same forearm, leaving the other arm free. Oxygen can be fed into the bag if desired. With this simple apparatus artificial respiration can be maintained by relatively untrained persons for prolonged periods. As when any method of artificial respiration is used, so here the bag must be removed from time to time and the pharynx cleared of accumulation of mucus, or blood if the face has been injured.

Mechanical inflators. There are now many designs of automatic mechanical inflation apparatus and no one machine has been standardised throughout the hospitals of Great Britain. Positive pressure is applied initially through a mask or an endotracheal tube as a first-aid measure, but if artificial respiration has to be continued on a conscious patient, or for more than a day or so on an unconscious patient, a tracheostomy is essential. If it appears unlikely that natural respiration and swallowing will return quickly, early tracheostomy is preferable. Positive pressure respiration through a tracheostomy necessitates the introduction of a humidifier in the circuit to avoid the drying action of the air on the lining of the trachea and bronchial tubes.

The automatic respirator, whatever its pattern, must have the following controls:

1. A frequency regulator which determines the number of respirations per minute.
2. A depth regulator which determines the 'tidal air'—that is the amount of air going in and out of the lungs with each respiration. Most machines have a meter attached to this regulator so that the amount of air exchange per minute can be measured readily. This total volume is of course a combination of the depth and frequency of the stroke. Some machines depend upon the natural recoil of the chest to produce the expiratory stroke and others exert a negative pressure to aid expiration. There is a danger when negative pressure is used that the small bronchial tubes may collapse; the negative pressure phase has to be used with great caution if at all.

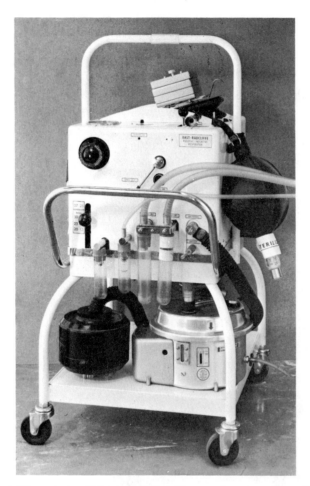

Fig. 10.16 East-Radcliffe respirator. This is a typical positive-negative automatic ventilator. The machine can be used as an anaesthetic apparatus with open or closed circuit. The negative pressure expiration can be varied from 0–15 cm water pressure and the positive pressure inspiration from 5–40 cm water pressure. (East & Co. Ltd.)

All this apparatus is supplied with detailed instructions on its maintenance and any nurse left in charge of a mechanical respirator must be completely familiar with its mode of operation. The majority of machines are electrically driven, but some depend on compressed air or oxygen pressure for their motive power. Electrically driven machines must have an alternative manual method of operation should the electrical supply fail. There is in addition an alarm bell which rings in the event of a power or mechanical failure.

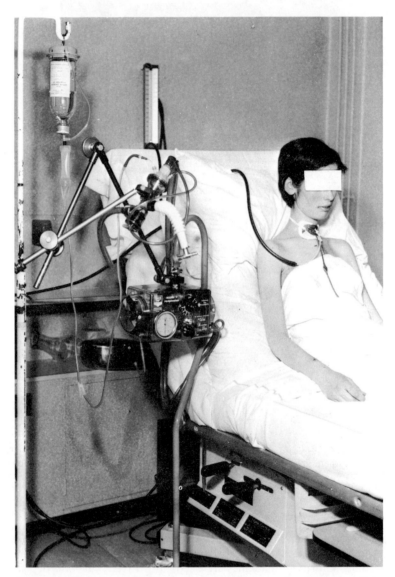

Fig. 10.17   Bird automatic respirator for IPPR. Note that this is operating through a cuffed tracheostomy tube. The motive power of this respirator is compressed air or oxygen. The apparatus is independent of electric current supply. (d'Abreu, *A Practice of Thoracic Surgery*).

Cardiac massage

Asphyxia very rapidly leads to cessation of the heart-beat and sometimes the very act of artificial respiration by altering the pressures in the thorax starts the heart again. If, however, no pulse can be felt and artificial respiration after several breaths has failed to produce any change of colour, the first immediate step is to thump the sternum at its lower end, and sometimes a single shock of this type will start the heart. Should this fail then external cardiac massage must be applied without delay. If the nurse is faced with this situation and has no help she will have to perform both the artificial respiration and the external cardiac massage herself. Although ideally the patient should be on a hard surface (and it is sometimes suggested that the patient should be dragged off the bed on to the floor) it is not always easy to ensure this: provided adequate force is used, massage may be performed on the patient's bed. The operator's two hands are placed on the lower part of the sternum as shown in Fig. 10.19 and really forcible compression made to pinch the heart between the sternum and the vertebral column. Short sharp compressions at the rate of approximately 60 per minute must be interspersed by inflation of the lungs—about 12 heart compressions to one double inflation. It is difficult to assess the rate of massage and perhaps the simplest way is to count, *one-one-thousand-two-one-thousand-three-one-thousand*. The average person speaking at normal rates takes approximately one second over each thousand. If of course there are two operators then the position is much more readily controlled, but they should change position if the person doing the cardiac massage shows any signs of fatigue.

If during the procedure it is possible to raise the foot of the bed or trolley or table on which the patient is lying, this helps the return of blood to the heart and maintains the circulatory pressure. External cardiac massage should produce a pulse which can be felt in the carotids or at the wrist.

When medical assistance has been obtained and if normal rhythm has not be restored, massage must be continued until an electrical appliance known as a '**defibrillator**' can be obtained (Fig. 10.18). The external defibrillator has two electrodes which are applied to the chest wall and a powerful electric shock is delivered over the heart (see figures). This converts ventricular fibrillation into regular rhythm but the method is only applicable under hospital conditions (page 629 for internal defibrillation).

If external cardiac massage fails to restore the heart-beat the doctor may decide that open massage of the heart through an incision in the chest wall is essential. Such a procedure should only be carried out under hospital conditions and in the operating theatre, as it is now generally agreed that simple external cardiac massage can in many cases be just as effective. It does not run the risk of damage to the left pleural cavity which would impair respiratory function.

When occurring as a result of injury or surgical conditions, asphyxia and cardiac arrest are commonly associated, with asphyxia as the primary cause. Severe pain may produce cardiac arrest (shock, page 110) and if the heart stops while there seems to be no obvious cause for asphyxia the initial treatment must be directed to starting the heart. For instance with coronary thrombosis cardiac arrest is primary, not due to asphyxia. External cardiac massage, if applied promptly after the cessation of the heart-beat, may quickly restore the circulation with spontaneous resumption of breathing. Obviously an artificially produced heart-beat will do no good unless the lungs are being inflated.

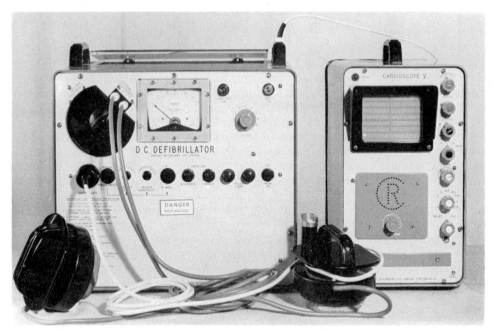

Fig. 10.18(a)   Direct current cardiac defibrillator for external use, with electrocardiograph monitor on which the heart response is watched after each shock.

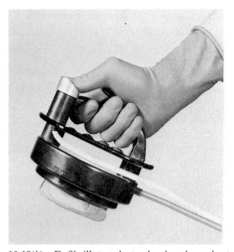

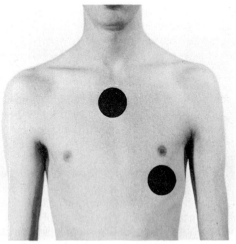

10.18(b)   Defibrillator electrode placed on chest wall: note rubber glove to insulate the operator (see Fig. 10.18(c) for position).

10.18(c)   For external defibrillation the electrodes are placed in the positions shown.

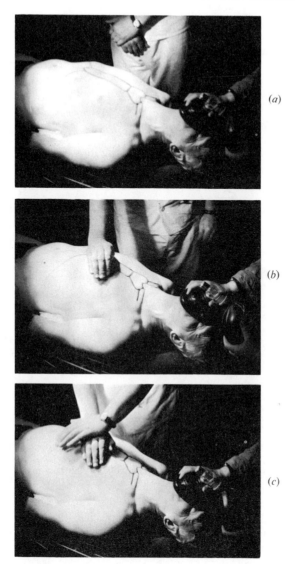

(a)

(b)

(c)

Fig. 10.19 External cardiac massage. (a) The outline of the sternum and costal margin is shown. Artificial respiration is being given with an Ambu bag. (b) and (c) show the position of the hands. Pressure is exerted with the heel of the hands with the fingers lifted clear.

Open cardiac massage—operating room procedure

The anaesthetist maintains artificial positive pressure respiration and must have suction available to remove bronchial secretions. The scrub nurse must have an assistant to fetch urgently needed drugs, but every theatre should have a resuscitation tray with the necessary ampoules on it.

A pre-sterilised set of thoracotomy instruments must always be available.

The surgeon opens the chest through the fifth left intercostal space to the left of the sternum. A rib spreader (or, if this is not available, a pair of retractors or even a mouth gag) is inserted: the sternal ends of the ribs are cut or broken to provide space for the surgeon to open the pericardium and insert his hand. He continues rhythmic pumping to restore adequate circulation and when the patient's colour indicates adequate oxygenation,

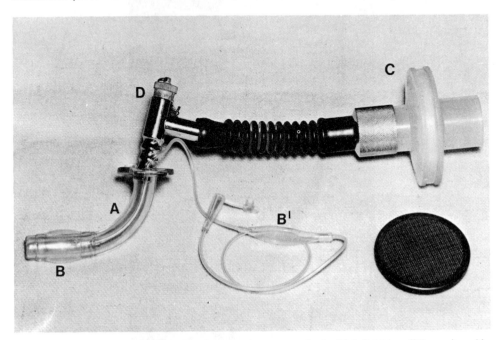

Fig. 10.20   Vitalograph humidifier. The plastic tracheostomy tube **A** with inflatable cuff **B**, monitored by bulb **B¹** is joined through an anaesthetic connector T-piece **D**, to the condenser-humidifier **C**. This contains a gauze disk which traps expired moisture and thus maintains humidity in the inspired air. Intermittent suction is performed by catheters inserted at **D** when the plug is removed.

he may pause to see if the heart beats spontaneously. He may wish to inject 10 ml of 1 per cent calcium chloride into the ventricle. Often the patient is in a state of ventricular fibrillation—the muscle is shimmering. This irregular contraction can be converted to a rhythmic beat by the application of an electric shock. Sterile electrodes soaked in saline are applied direct to the heart and a special electric difibrillator is connected to provide the correct current, initially at 150 volts; 1 in 10,000 adrenaline solution (i.e. 1 ml of liq. adrenaline diluted in 10 ml water = 1 : 10,000) is sometimes used to stimulate a heart which is inert.

When regular rhythm has been restored, the pericardium is closed with a continuous stitch and the pleura closed (if it has been opened) after full inflation of the lung: the chest wall is closed calmly and carefully, and the patient must of course receive continuous nursing supervision until consciousness returns.

(These procedures are summarised in Appendix II).

Intermittent positive pressure respiration (IPPR)

Following resuscitation for respiratory or cardiac arrest, mechanical respiration may be continued through a cuffed endotracheal tube. The patient may resist both the tube and the ventilation phase as consciousness is regained. Sedation with diazepam, or **phenoperidine** (Operidine) depresses this resistance. Elective **IPPR**—that is, instituted for a conscious patient who is not ventilating adequately—may be through an endotracheal tube inserted under local anaesthesia, or may require tracheostomy.

Reference is made to the creation of an artificial opening into the respiratory tract on page 803. In the days when diphtheria was very common in Great Britain, laryngeal obstruction was a frequent complication; an emergency opening into the trachea was a life-saving measure with which every doctor was familiar. When immunisation almost eliminated diphtheria the occasions on which a tracheostomy was performed became extremely rare. During recent years and with an increased knowledge of the physiology of respiration, it has been realised more and more that the elimination of the dead space between the vocal cords and the lips, and likewise the avoidance of any possible obstruction here, adds enormously to the freedom of respiration and thus to the efficiency of gaseous exchange in the lungs, particularly if the lung tissue itself is inflamed, or the circulation feeble.

The reasons for which tracheostomy is performed, other than for the emergency relief of mechanical obstruction to breathing, are therefore grouped according to the underlying disease:

A. In respiratory failure, i.e. failure of the respiration centre in the brain to maintain the necessary stimulus. This may occur as a result of head injury, a stroke or poisoning (from drugs), or in myasthenia gravis or poliomyelitis. The natural impulses from the brain to the respiratory muscles are missing and artificial respiration has to be maintained. For a short period a cuffed endotracheal tube (Fig. 12.6) may be placed between the vocal cords and positive pressure respiration continued through the tube, by hand with a bag or by automatic mechanical respirator (page 186).

B. In cases of head injury in which the face is involved and the jaw is fractured even though the respiratory centre is intact. The purpose here is to prevent the inhalation of secretions from the mouth and to make the nursing of the mouth condition easier. Tracheostomy may be necessary as a preliminary to severe operations on the throat.

C. When there has been infection of the lung or damage to the chest wall and it is desired to give the best possible inflation-expansion.

When artificial respiration is going to be administered through a tracheostomy, a cuffed tube is used (Fig. 12.6) and the pump connected to the opening of the tube. It is obvious that the machine used for this form of pulmonary inflation must be very accurate and contain safety devices to prevent over-inflation and damage to the lungs. Modern machines contain regulators by which the doctor can adjust the amount of air entering the lung with each respiration and can vary the rate of respiration as well. To prevent the trachea and air passages becoming dried a humidifier is also used.

Nursing Management

The following basic rules have to be observed in the routine care of a patient with a tracheostomy and of course these rules have to be greatly amplified where positive pressure respiration is being used.

1. A nurse must check personally that essential ancillary equipment is immediately at hand within arm's reach of the patient, or nurse looking after the patient.

    (*a*) An alarm bell or telephone with which she can call for assistance, a hand lamp which can stand by itself and remain switched on, a note-pad and pencil on which the patient can write if he is conscious.

    (*b*) A supply of sterile rubber or plastic catheters, preferably disposable, for suction; catheter-holding forceps with which to handle the suction catheters, together with a small bowl and a supply of sterile water in which the catheter may be washed and its lumen cleared. A catheter once used must be discarded and not reinserted.

    (*c*) A spare tracheostomy tube and introducing forceps for immediate insertion if the cuffed tube or the other tube should be expelled by coughing.

2. The surgeon will give instructions as to how often the tracheostomy tube and bronchial tree must be aspirated and these instructions must be written down. The frequency will clearly depend on the amount of secretion present. The pharynx will also require repeated aspiration to remove saliva or blood that may have trickled in from facial injury. Each occasion when the suction routine is carried out a fresh sterile catheter must be used and must be handled only with sterile forceps. Suction must be cut off as the catheter is inserted into the tracheostomy tube and this can be achieved by kinking the suction tube or using a connector with a side hole which is closed by a finger when suction is required. Suction to clear mucus and secretion from the trachea or bronchi must be intermittent and never continued for more than 30 seconds at a time. When a patient is on positive pressure respiration it is usual to interrupt the respiration not more than once a minute for the aspiration of secretions. Suction is continued each time during the complete withdrawal of the catheter to avoid any lump of secretion being left in the trachea at the bottom of the tube.

3. Sedation will be needed if the patient becomes agitated or 'fights the respirator'.

4. Pulse and blood pressure records must be made at frequent intervals and when positive pressure pumps are in use, airflow and pressure must also be recorded.

5. If there is any doubt whatever that the tube may be blocked the nurse in charge must sound the alarm without hesitation to summon assistance. Every second is precious. The tube may become displaced or blocked and in the case of cuffed endotracheal tubes a defect may develop either in the cuff itself or in the lumen of the tube allowing the cuff to become blocked. If this is suspected the cuff must be deflated to see if the lumen becomes unblocked. A faulty tube must be replaced. The unconscious patient undergoing artificial respiration this way must receive all the usual nursing treatment given to any unconscious patient. The respiratory problem must not lead to neglect in other directions. Turning every 2 hours is essential to protect pressure areas; passive movements of the legs at all joints and gentle massage of the calves with several forced dorsi-flexion movements of the feet empties the deep calf veins and will help to prevent venous thrombosis.

Feeding is carried out by gastric tube and antibiotics are given by injection.

Patients undergoing artificial respiration may develop severe biochemical disturbances owing to the absence of natural control of the amount of carbon dioxide eliminated by respiration. Electrolyte balance must therefore be watched very carefully and every specimen of urine that is passed must be tested for pH and specific gravity and its volume recorded.

Further information on tracheostomy and its complications is on page 803.

Special respiratory care unit

The regulation of the volume of air used to expand the lungs—the tidal air—the respiration rate and in fact the pressure, is absolutely critical and in cases of severe shock, particularly if there has been some degree of renal failure, the difference between failure and survival may be entirely dependent on the critical management of the artificial respiration. Inadequate tidal air leads to accumulation of carbon dioxide in the blood hypercapnia (page 129): **respiratory acidosis** ensues. Conversely, over-ventilation leads to alkalosis and muscle spasms sometimes amounting to tetany.

In severe shock changes take place in the peripheral circulation which may lead to stasis of blood in the tissues and the accumulation of metabolic products such as lactic acid. As these products find their way back into the circulation the acidity of the blood may be further changed, and this in turn puts an increased load on the kidneys adding to the likelihood of renal failure.

With all these considerations in mind many hospitals have developed special units for the care of patients requiring artificial respiration, or likely to develop cardiac arrest, or indeed all patients with severe shock. Such units are staffed by fully trained nurses who have learned the special techniques required, and usually such a unit is under the immediate control of a consultant anaesthetist.

Frequent blood chemistry investigations have to be undertaken and a special blood gas analysis apparatus known as the Astrup is used for this purpose.

Reference has already been made to the importance of exact control of intravenous fluids in both quantity and type. Measures to prevent the introduction of infection through endotracheal tubes or tracheostomies have already been described and the chapter which follows deals with other aspects of the care of the unconscious patient. In no section of nursing is devotion to detail, a full understanding of the underlying principles, and absolute co-operation between medical and nursing staff more vital than in such intensive care units where the patients have been severely injured, or have undergone some major surgical procedure producing the same complications.

Epilogue

In the course of a full and busy life of surgery or nursing, the occasions when the action of one individual saves a life are extremely rare. The relief of the obstructed airway of an unconscious road casualty is far more important than the major surgery which may be required when the patient reaches hospital. All who are associated with medical practice in any form must be familiar with the necessary procedures and must be ready to act. Death from asphyxia is very common. It is frequently the result of criminal action: sometimes it is the result of negligence or ignorance, when a mother allows a tiny baby to rest its head on a soft pillow in which it buries its face. Sometimes death from asphyxia occurs in the presence of medical and nursing staff who have failed to appreciate its onset or have lacked the resources for its treatment.

It must be repeated again and again that a patient, unconscious from any cause except natural sleep, should never be left out of sight of trained staff. Screens and bed curtains are known to be a wall of death when the nurse is unwary.

11

Care of the Unconscious Patient

Consciousness depends upon the full function of the cerebral cortex. This in turn depends not only upon the presence of normal undamaged brain tissue but upon an adequate supply of oxygen to the brain cells. There are thus two distinct causes of loss of consciousness: direct damage to the brain cells and cerebral anoxia.

Depth

Consciousness implies an awareness of one's environment and an ability to respond to an outside stimulus by speech or by purposeful movement, even if this is merely a change of facial expression. Loss of consciousness is described in terms of 'depth', in the same way that natural sleep can be light or deep.

The nervous activity of the body, both sensory and motor, may be conscious or unconscious. Voluntary movements in response to sensations of touch or temperature are under control of the mind. In the first stage of interference with consciousness, control by the mind is lost and movements in response to stimulus become automatic or 'reflex' but may nevertheless be purposeful: for instance when an attempt is made by the doctor to separate the eyelids to examine the pupil, the patient raises his hand to fight off the interference. The greater the disturbance of the brain, the more widespread is the loss of reflex activity. The last reflex to be lost before death is the automatic rhythm of the respiratory muscles and reflex control of the heart.

In assessing the depth of unconsciousness, various reflexes are used. Inability to answer questions coherently is a feature of the first stage, frequently referred to as a 'state of confusion'. This is found in persons mildly intoxicated with alcohol, but an exactly similar state occurs following a mild degree of concussion. Short nitrous oxide anaesthesia gives the same effect during the brief recovery period.

In the next stage, which corresponds to light anaesthesia, there is complete loss of awareness but the 'primitive' or life-preserving reflexes are still present. Incision of the skin, or the insertion of a towel clip, into the skin, will provoke movement. When he recovers the patient will have no memory of pain produced by such a stimulus and for minor operations such as dental extractions or incision of an abscess, loss of consciousness does not go beyond this stage.

The third stage or plane of unconsciousness corresponds to full surgical anaesthesia in which there is complete paralysis of all voluntary muscles, and no obvious or visible response to stimulus. Deep reflexes may however still be present, and although the pain stimuli do not reach consciousness they affect the nervous system and may produce shock. A patient with multiple injuries, although unconscious perhaps from brain damage, may die from shock produced by unnecessary handling of fractured limbs.

The fourth stage is one of deep coma where the centres controlling heart and respiration are themselves partly affected. Interference with these 'vital centres' in the medulla of the brain is an indication that the patient's condition is extremely grave.

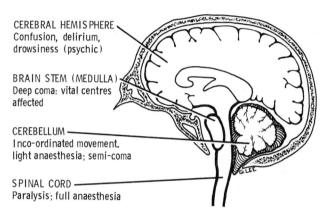

Fig. 11.1   The levels of unconsciousness. Showing the effects of involvement of the main brain areas by anaesthesia or injury.

In describing the depth of unconsciousness, the term 'coma' is used to denote a state in which there is no sign that the patient perceives (in his mind) any external stimulus. There is no alteration in facial expression and no attempt at speech. For convenience these four stages may be defined rather broadly as:

Confusion ('delirium')—speech present, but the replies to questions are irrational; movement usually purposeless: resentful of treatment and handling.
Semi-coma—no coherent speech; movement only in response to painful stimulus; swallowing and pupil light reflexes present.
Coma—paralysis; no speech or response to pain stimulus; swallowing reflex probably still present. Eye reflexes lost or very sluggish.
Deep coma—no reflexes whatever. Breathing automatic and probably irregular in depth.

It is, however, more important to note and record from time to time what reflexes and responses are present, than to rely upon a descriptive term to indicate the depth of unconsciousness. Recognition of and ability to describe and record the patient's depth of unconsciousness is very important in nursing, to ensure a continuity of observations.

Causes of unconsciousness

Loss of consciousness may be brought about by direct violence to brain tissue, arising from skull fractures, bullet wounds, or the bursting of a cerebral artery (page 861). Other causative conditions are shown in Table 27.

Table 27   Causes of loss of consciousness

Congenital—defects of the brain.
Infective—meningitis, cerebral abscess (from infection of middle ear, skull fractures, or septi-
     caemia).
Traumatic—concussion, skull fractures, operation on the brain.
Neoplastic—innocent or malignant growths (arising from brain, meningeal coverings or metastatic
     deposits from other organs).
Metabolic—poisoning of the brain in uraemia, diabetes, or insulin overdose, or drugs.
Degenerative—cerebral arteriosclerosis causing thrombosis or haemorrhage.
Poisoning—by anaesthesia or drugs.
Cerebral anoxia—due to shock, haemorrhage or embolus (including air and fat embolus):
     persistent anoxia due to respiratory depression.
     In general surgical practice there are three common causes of unconsciousness.
     (1) General anaesthesia.
     (2) Cerebral anoxia in shock, haemorrhage or heart-failure.
     (3) Head injury.

Compression of the brain produces temporary interference with its function and if the pressure can be relieved, permanent damage may be avoided. The intracranial pressure may be raised in several ways.

(*a*) By increase of the cerebral spinal fluid (hydrocephalus).
(*b*) By the presence of a growing tumour or abscess in the skull.
(*c*) By the formation of a haematoma between the skull and brain.

(*b*) and (*c*) are called space-occupying lesions in the skull (page 850). Neurosurgery is largely concerned with the investigation and treatment of raised intracranial pressure.

The term **cerebral vascular accident** is applied to thrombosis of one of the brain arteries or from intracranial haemorrhage which is usually due to a ruptured artery or aneurysm. The 'stroke' which results need not necessarily be associated with coma.

Duration of unconsciousness

When loss of consciousness is due to anaesthesia we know approximately how long a patient will take to recover. When it is due to other causes there is no such certainty and there are many aspects of management to be considered. The depth of unconsciousness may vary from hour to hour in response to treatment or progress of the disease. The nurse has therefore to become familiar with the signs and symptoms which indicate the different stages of unconsciousness.

Complications and nursing management

A brief survey of the abnormal conditions which arise as the result of loss of consciousness is essential. No matter what the cause, the risks are similar in nature and only vary in degree according to the depth and duration of the unconscious state. The conditions are described in Table 28 in order of their importance if the patient is to survive: the necessary corrective or preventive nursing measures, to be adopted in each case, are briefly defined.[1]

Complications arise from loss of sensation, from paralysis, and from the general lowering of metabolic activity.

Sensory loss. Anaesthesia of the skin leads very rapidly to pressure sores. The sacral area and the heels are most liable to this trophic ulceration. If the legs of an unconscious patient are crossed, skin may ulcerate on the shin, compressed by the calf of the overlying leg. Hot-water bottles are dangerous and more often than not quite unnecessary: their use is traditional but burns occur very easily from exposed parts of the bottle. Warmth is maintained by blankets: if the temperature rises above 38 °C, the coverings must be reduced.

The loss of corneal and conjunctival reflex with associated muscle weakness prevents blinking, and the eye very easily becomes dry: corneal ulceration occurs from this exposure.

Lack of bladder sensation leads to retention.

In the respiratory tract, with lesser degrees of unconsciousness, the cough reflex may be more excitable than usual and the inhalation of foreign matter such as a small particle of vomit may produce a fatal bronchial spasm. In deep coma any attempt to feed the patient by mouth, or excessive zeal in oral hygiene, will almost certainly result in fluid entering the trachea, since the protective reflex has been completely abolished. Very small and weak babies are particularly liable to 'drown' if they vomit when in coma or in deep natural sleep. Quite apart from vomit or from administered fluid, if the swallowing reflex is affected the natural secretion of saliva (amounting to nearly a litre a day) causes respiratory embarrassment and inhalation pneumonia.

Motor loss. Paralysis of voluntary muscles results in poor heat production in the body so that the temperature of an unconscious patient is subnormal unless infection or some other complication has arisen. Absence of limb movement predisposes to thrombosis, the development of pressure sores, and poor chest expansion.

Respiration. This is affected in various ways. The respiratory centre in the medulla may be intact or affected by oedema or pressure. The absence of normal tracheal reflexes renders the patient liable to inhalation pneumonia. Weakness of respiratory muscles limits chest expansion. The general depression of tissue activity (lowered metabolic rate) results in less demand for oxygen and adds to the respiratory depression. For all these reasons pulmonary atelectasis with infection is an ever-present risk in the unconscious patient.

Metabolism. Nutrition is not a serious matter unless the state of unconsciousness lasts for more than three or four days: metabolic activity has been depressed and the patient's calorie requirement is therefore very low. On the other hand the loss of consciousness may be associated with injuries or other disorders which may themselves require administration of glucose, electrolytes, water, plasma or even blood. 'Gavage' feeding by means of a stomach tube is possible except in deep coma when the sphincter of the upper end of the stomach relaxes and allows the contents to run back into the pharynx. This would be dangerous and might lead to drowning.

Constant attention. In the light stages of unconsciousness when the cough and swallowing reflexes are still present, it is unlikely that a patient will choke. If there is the slightest

[1] Poliomyelitis in its most severe form affects the brain stem and vital centres, and produces almost all the conditions of deep coma except that the patient is still aware of his environment. The nursing measures to be adopted are therefore similar to those used in dealing with the deeply comatose patient.

Table 28   Complications of unconsciousness

Site or nature of complications	Effect	Preventive nursing	Nursing treatment
Pressure necrosis: shoulder blades, sacral area, iliac crests, heels	Blistering: gangrene, ulceration, infection	Very frequent change of position: Avoidance of wet Massage	Relief from pressure and friction. Exposure to air. Antiseptic powder. (Dead tissue may need surgical excision)
Obstructed airway (Chapter 10) Respiratory arrest (apnoea)	Asphyxia	**Watchfulness** intubation: tracheostomy: avoid morphine: stimulants (niketh-amide) (depends on cause)	Withdrawal of tongue: insertion of airway. Oxygen: artificial respiration
Vomiting (cerebral origin or due to ileus)	Laryngeal or bronchial spasm: obstruction, death, atelectasis, or lung abscess	Keep stomach empty, especially if blood has been swallowed Nurse semi-prone	Suction to pharynx. Tilt to head-down position
Eyes—drying	Conjunctivitis Corneal ulceration	Keep covered if lids retract Twice a day irrigation: chloramphenicol drops Swabbing of eyelids	Irrigation and drops For ulcer, homatropine and keep covered
Nose	Infection and ulceration	Frequent cleansing: ointment to nostrils	
Mouth	Infection and ulceration (monilia, 'thrush'). (White patches appear on gums and palate)	Very frequent toilet	Nystatin or crystal violet application
Ears (may be blood or cerebrospinal fluid leak in skull fracture)	Infection	Mopping and cleansing with cetrimide 1%, or spirit. **Do not plug with wool. Never syringe**	Local cleansing with antiseptic

Table 28   Complications of unconsciousness   *continued*

Site or nature of complications	Effect	Preventive nursing	Nursing treatment
Bladder	*a.* Incontinence	No preventive measure	May be automatic micturition: bed must be kept dry. Catheterisation may be ordered to avoid wet bed and to monitor urinary output
	b. Retention *c.* Overflow incontinence (page 633)	No preventive measure ⎫ Early diagnosis ⎬ of retention ⎭ (Prophylactic urinary antiseptic is given)	1. Manual expression may be possible at set intervals 2. 12-hour catheterisation 3. Self-retaining plastic catheter drainage with antiseptic seal 4. Tidal drainage
Genitalia	Vulvitis or balanitis	Very thorough toilet	Antiseptic irrigation
Bowel	Constipation and/or incontinence	Daily enema to avoid soiling which occurs if automatic evacuation is awaited	Regulation of bowel action by laxatives and use of suppositories
Heart	Strain and failure from anoxia	Timely oxygen therapy	Oxygen
Venous stagnation	Thrombosis: Embolism	Avoid pressure on calves: frequent passive movement of legs: elevation of legs above hips.	(Anticoagulant therapy unlikely in unconscious patient)
Nutrition	Malnutrition: vitamin shortage, dehydration	Early assessment of need: (in head injury fluid may be withheld)	Tube feeding. Intravenous infusion
Limbs—muscle paralysis or imbalance	Contractures	Correct posturing: regular movement, stretching, use of bed cradle and foot support	Physiotherapy (surgical operation may be required if severe deformity has developed from neglect)
Joints	Stiffness: Delayed recovery	Regular passive movements of all joints by nursing staff or physiotherapist	

doubt about this, a nurse must remain by the patient's side continuously, and always if an airway or endotracheal tube is still in place.

Far the most important objectives are the maintenance of a free airway, the maintenance of a correct but frequently changed position, and the most scrupulous attention to all aspects of hygiene. These are the three main threads running through all other treatment which may be required for the patient's underlying condition. The preservation of life is always the primary consideration, but this must not be made an excuse for overlooking routine nursing procedures, the omission of which may lead to prolonged disability or even to subsequent loss of the life which has been preserved. The development of bed-sores or infection in the mouth (thrush), or cystitis and pyelitis, is an indication that the nursing has failed.

Position and transportation of the unconscious patient

The unconscious patient must be nursed on one side—semi-prone—to avoid any tendency of the tongue to fall into the back of the throat, and to encourage secretions from the mouth, respiratory tract and oesophagus to drain outwards by gravity.

There are of course exceptions to this rule, but each exception carries with it additional safeguards. In the immediate post-operative stage an unconscious patient is usually nursed on his side unless such a position is impossible or inadvisable because of the nature of the operation. If the patient has to be kept flat initially he should be sat up as soon as possible to improve lung ventilation. A nurse must be constantly present at the bedside in case obstruction to respiration develops. An airway should remain in the mouth until the cough reflex returns. Even after abdominal operations, it is safer for the patient to be nursed semi-prone unless it is known that the stomach is completely empty and vomiting is very unlikely (i.e. a Ryle's naso-gastric tube is in place).

After operations on the nose, mouth, jaws or throat, the patient *must* be kept semi-prone until full return of consciousness. There can be no exception in such cases.

In prolonged unconsciousness, the patient's position will again depend partly on the depth of coma. Every nurse is familiar with the desperate efforts which are made to prevent pressure sores, by massaging the skin with soap, with powder, or with spirit. Though this is a necessary part of nursing technique, it is totally inadequate to prevent the development of skin necrosis in unconscious patients. The only effective method is to change the area of pressure every two hours throughout the day and night. If the patient is not encumbered by splints or extension apparatus, these changes may be from right semi-prone, to recumbent, to left semi-prone, to prone (with the head turned to one side), and so on. If this turning can be carried out reliably, and if there is adequate attention to prevent soiling of the bed by faeces or by urine, additional treatment of pressure areas is unnecessary. This repeated change of position has the additional advantage of decreasing the likelihood of pulmonary stasis (with hypostatic pneumonia) and of stagnation in the urinary tract with subsequent infection. There is less likelihood that contractures of paralysed limbs will develop if the change of position is frequent (Fig. 11.2). If unconsciousness is deep, it is wise to nurse the patient on a foam 'over mattress' without a sheet or draw sheet. Rapid movements of the legs, drawing them up quickly and then extending them again is a feature of restlessness; blisters on the heels may then develop very quickly from friction

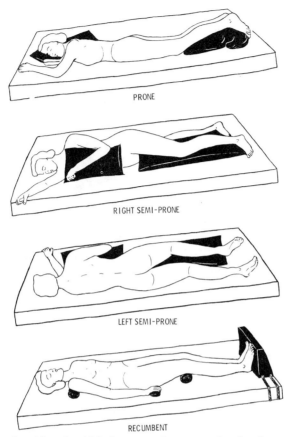

PRONE

RIGHT SEMI-PRONE

LEFT SEMI-PRONE

RECUMBENT

Fig. 11.2   The cycle of positions in which the unconscious or paralysed patient must be placed to avoid pressure sores. Support by pillows is essential to avoid stretching joints, ligaments, or muscles. The bed has a head-down tilt.

on a hard sheet. Foam-lined heel pads, held on with Tubigrip, or Tubipads (Fig. 11.3) are an invaluable nursing aid. If there is sensory loss with or without paralysis, the use of a Ripple mattress is the ideal method of preventing sores and thrombosis (page 875, Fig. 45.16).

Transport of an unconscious patient involves the same strict rules for the maintenance of an airway. If there is any doubt about the presence of adequate cough and swallowing reflexes, the patient must remain in the semi-prone position. If a journey is to be made by ambulance a soft mattress or pillows must be placed underneath the patient on the stretcher, and the position should be changed every hour. Such problems arise in cases of head injury if they are to be transferred to a special neurosurgical centre. To those unaccustomed to this procedure, it may seem at first unwise to send a patient with a brain injury on such a journey. The chances of recovery are however so much improved by the special provisions of a trained neurosurgical nursing and operating team, that the advantages usually more than balance the very slight additional hazard of the journey itself. During such a journey the patient must be accompanied by at least two fully trained nurses. Suction apparatus must be at hand for clearing the pharynx. Oxygen equipment must also be carried and a pulse record made every 15 minutes.

Tracheostomy is performed with increasing frequency in patients with severe head injuries. It greatly simplifies nursing and improves breathing. The chemical, mechanical and nursing problems which arise are described in Chapter 8 and page 803.

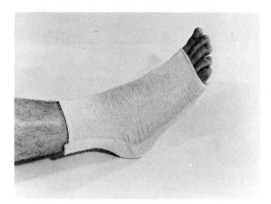

Fig. 11.3   Disposable foam heel protective pad with attached cling-sock. (Tubipad, Seton Products Ltd.)

Return of consciousness

Both in the short post-operative phase and after a period of prolonged unconsciousness from head injury, recovery proceeds through the same planes of depth in reverse sequence. It must be realised that the patient may 'awake' in entirely new surroundings without the presence of a familiar voice or face. In addition to the confusion produced by so many new experiences, there is the added factor of loss of memory, since unconsciousness from any cause may produce a gap in the memory going back several minutes, hours, or days, before the injury or onset of unconsciousness. The patient when fully conscious may be unable at first to appreciate what has happened and where he is.

A patient recovering from operation passes through similar experiences usually of very short duration. **Amnesia** (loss of memory) is increased by the use of hyoscine as a preoperative drug.

Return to the conscious state is accompanied by a resumption of all other normal activities, such as voluntary micturition and normal bowel action. Limbs may be weak or stiff and other treatments such as intravenous infusion may have to be continued. The nurse is responsible for readjusting the patient to these fresh circumstances. Physiotherapy is essential if unconsciousness lasts for more than twenty-four hours. All limb joints must be put through their full range of movement passively at least once a day, and the limbs must be supported in such a way that gravity does not stretch one particular group of muscles. Plantar flexion of the foot and hyper-extension of the knee are the two main errors to guard against.

Warning. It is difficult to be certain during the recovery stage, as to whether the patient is in a state of natural deep sleep from which he can be roused. It is common for patients who have been unconscious to recall something they have heard said by those around. Great care must be taken to avoid conversation that is not essential to the task in hand. Never should there be any critical or personal remarks about the patient or the relatives. Most of all is this important on the journey to the theatre and in the anaesthetic room during induction. The patient may appear to be unconscious, but in the drowsy phase sounds are greatly amplified and whispers may easily be heard.

It must be repeated again and again that a patient, unconscious from any cause except natural sleep, should never be left out of sight of trained staff. Screens and bed curtains are known to be a wall of death when the nurse is unwary.

SECTION III

12

Anaesthesia

Successful surgery depends not only upon surgical and nursing skill, but very largely on satisfactory anaesthesia. The science of anaesthesia has developed through two main channels—advances in our understanding of the physiology of respiration and circulation on the one hand, and the development of many new drugs on the other. Modern 'miracles' of surgery have been made possible largely by these great developments in anaesthetic techniques. This is a specialty for which training has to be very comprehensive and anaesthetists in the modern hospital organisation have taken on the responsibility for 'intensive care' (page 5). In some hospitals they also conduct 'pain' clinics (page 74).

The nurse's duties in relation to anaesthesia fall naturally into three groups.

(*a*) In the ward, before operation.
(*b*) In the operating theatre.
(*c*) In the ward, after operation.

When possible, in order to lessen the tension that exists in a patient's mind it is usual for the patient to have a fairly strong sedative (such as **nitrazepam, dichloralphenazone, butobarbitone** for an adult) the night before operation. The nurse is responsible for the restriction of intake of fluid and food by mouth and the collection of a specimen of urine. The patient is dressed in special garments and other pre-operative treatment is required which is not directly concerned with the administration of the anaesthetic. In addition to the preliminary sedative, even in emergency cases, certain drugs are essential before the administration of a general anaesthetic.

In the operating theatre the nurse needs to be familiar with the pieces of anaesthetic apparatus commonly in use, with their maintenance, and with the cleaning and preparation of the various instruments and accessories which the anaesthetist may require. In many busy operating theatres a special nurse is detailed to assist the anaesthetist. In some large hospitals a trained technician is made responsible for the mechanical maintenance of the anaesthetic equipment. The nurse must be properly trained to assist the anaesthetist during the induction of general anaesthesia and she must be completely competent to take charge of a patient at the end of the operation when the anaesthetic is no longer being administered but the patient is still unconscious.

The journey from the operating table back to bed may occupy perhaps a minute or five minutes, depending on the lay-out of the hospital. At this most critical time, the nurse is in complete command and must be conversant with the emergency drill which may be required.

Special types of anaesthesia such as the spinal block require special after-care and observation.

Principles of anaesthesia

In the choice of an anaesthetic suitable for any particular patient, certain requirements have to be met.

1. Pain. There must be complete relief from pain. This does not necessarily involve complete unconsciousness or the loss of all the sensations of every type. Most nurses will have experienced the removal of a tooth under local anaesthesia only. Though there is no pain one can perceive the movement of the tooth and the pressure of the dental forceps. Similarly during child-birth a woman may be freed from pain without becoming completely unconscious; she may still be able to hear what is being said. Loss of sensation of pain without loss of consciousness is **analgesia. Neuroleptanalgesia** is the technique of producing a 'trance' state in which pain perception and reaction is abolished. The drugs **ketamine** (Ketalar) and **droperidol** (Droleptan) are given for this purpose, and are particularly useful in children and for patients undergoing radiotherapy (page 218), or extensive dressings.

2. Relaxation of muscles. Muscles must be adequately relaxed, if for instance the abdomen is to be opened, and there must be no straining at any stage. This relaxation can be brought about as part of the complete paralysis achieved in deep general anaesthesia; this is, in effect, an extreme degree of the relaxation which occurs in normal sleep. All the voluntary muscles, except those used in respiration are put out of action. In recent years special drugs have been discovered which produce muscular paralysis without affecting the other functions of the body or diminishing consciousness.

3. The circulation. Whatever anaesthetic agent is used nothing must be allowed to embarrass the action of the heart, and at all times the blood pressure must be sufficient to maintain an adequate oxygen supply to the vital centres in the brain. In order to diminish the bleeding which occurs from the field of operation, certain drugs may be used to lower the blood pressure (page 243).

4. Respiration. The fourth essential is that adequate ventilation of the lungs must take place so that the vital centres and the heart muscle receive an adequate oxygen supply. Carbon dioxide must be properly eliminated. The lower the blood pressure and the more anaemic the patient, the more necessary is it that pulmonary ventilation (oxygen intake) shall not be diminished. Most drugs which are used in anaesthesia are in themselves poisonous to some tissues and have undesirable side effects, and any agent which diminishes respiratory muscle movement or lowers the blood pressure will at the same time increase the risk of oxygen lack in the heart and vital centres. Morphine and its derivatives depress respiratory activity.

The choice of anaesthetic, in relation to a particular patient's health and to the type of operation, is therefore made on a basis of safety in relation to these first principles. The administration of the anaesthetic calls for skill and constant vigilance again in respect of these four basic principles. In practice, a common way in which a difficulty arises during anaesthesia is in the development of some obstruction in the air passages. This will be dealt with later. Upon a correct understanding of this problem rests the nurse's ability to deal with emergencies which may arise in the unconscious patient—whether he is un-conscious from anaesthesia or from some brain injury or disease (page 202).

Methods of anaesthesia

When we speak of general anaesthesia we mean that during the operation the patient is unconscious: this is achieved by the administration of a drug which acts on the brain, and the degree of unconsciousness is varied according to the depth required for that particular operation. Just as unconsciousness from any cause may vary in depth so general anaesthesia may be varied. As pain makes the conscious individual 'catch' and hold his breath for a few seconds, so the lightly anaesthetised person will show a change in respira-tion rate when pain is produced.

If we take our 'level' of anaesthesia lower in the nervous system, below the vital centres in the medulla, we can prevent the brain receiving pain impulses from the skin or viscera (or, in fact, from any part of the body) by interrupting the nerve pathway. This is done by injecting certain drugs which poison the nerves, and put them out of action for varying periods of time. The spinal cord can be bathed in such a drug solution, which is injected into the spinal canal and mixes with the cerebrospinal fluid; this produces '**spinal anaes-thesia**' (more correctly 'analgesia'). If on the other hand the anaesthetic drug is injected around the concentration of nerve roots going to the limbs—for instance around the bra-chial plexus at the root of the neck—then only one limb is rendered analgesic. Thus the whole of one arm can be rendered painless and paralysed while the rest of the patient is completely normal. If we proceed further toward the nerve endings, one single nerve, such as that going to a finger, can be blocked with the anaesthetic solution: thus just part of the limb becomes insensitive. If an even smaller area of analgesia is needed then the solution is injected at the operation site. The plexus or nerve block injection is known as **regional analgesia.** Analgesia produced by injection at the site of operation is **local analgesia.**

In addition to these methods, there is **surface analgesia.** This is achieved on mucous membrane surfaces such as the mouth and the nose, by applying a strong anaesthetic solution with swabs or with a spray or, in the case of the urethra, a sterile solution in a small syringe.

Nerves can also be rendered incapable of passing impulses by freezing them: the refrigeration method of producing analgesia in the limb is used occasionally, if, for instance, a leg has to be amputated from a patient who is considered too ill for a general anaesthetic and in whom the injection of a toxic drug as a local anaesthetic might be considered dangerous.

It is essential that the nurse should understand the basic principles of anaesthesia. She needs to know the peculiarities of the various methods employed and to be aware of the particular complications which may arise so that she may watch for them.

During a major operation several methods of anaesthesia may be employed, each carrying its own particular risks. The individual methods will now be considered in detail.

General anaesthesia

As we have already seen, this implies that the patient is unconscious during the opera-tion and the depth of his unconsciousness may be varied according to the needs of the operation.

Pre-medication

The usual method of obtaining general anaesthesia is to employ first a substance administered by mouth or by rectum as a basal anaesthetic. This removes the patient's immediate pre-operative tension. Morphine type drugs such as papaveretum (Omnopon) combined with atropine or hyoscine (scopolamine) to reduce salivary and bronchial secretions is given at least one hour before operation. Trimeprazine (Vallergan) syrup is commonly given to children. The small amount required by mouth is insufficient in volume to be hazardous: no other drink is allowed. This ensures that the child falls into a deep sleep before going to the operating theatre, or the adult is so sleepy that he loses his sense of apprehension but can be roused. The use of these basal anaesthetic drugs means that during the rest of the operation the patient requires far less of the more potent drugs necessary to produce muscular relaxation and relief of pain.

Routes of administration

Substances used to produce general anaesthesia may be given in various ways.

(a) **Through the lungs.** The inhalation of gases is by far the most common method of producing general anaesthesia. Broadly speaking these drugs may be divided into:

(i) those which are supplied as compressed gas and are used direct from cylinders;

(ii) those which are supplied in liquid form and need to be evaporated through some form of chamber.

(b) **Intravenous/intramuscular.** It is possible for major operations to be performed under general anaesthesia produced solely by the injection of drugs such as thiopentone with other drugs such as tubocurarine or Scoline to help relax the muscles. Ketamine by intramuscular or intravenous injection is used increasingly: this produces a trance state, usually without loss of pharyngeal and laryngeal reflexes, though these may be diminished.

(c) **By mouth.** Alcohol, morphine, barbiturate drugs (such as Nembutal) and paraldehyde can be used by mouth to produce a loss of consciousness. The depth of sleep, however, is not great and if an operation were to be performed without the addition of some other substance, the dose necessary would probably be dangerous. Reference will be made later to the use of some of these substances to render the child patient completely unconscious before the journey to the operating theatre.

(d) **By rectum.** Thiopentone and paraldehyde may be used by rectal administration but are not usually employed as the sole means of anaesthesia.

Inhalation anaesthesia

When a drug is administered as a vapour through the lungs, it has to be mixed with sufficient oxygen for the patient's requirements: the rate and depth of breathing has to be sufficient to get rid of the carbon dioxide which would otherwise accumulate in the blood stream. The anaesthetist is then concerned with maintaining adequate respiration as well as with the giving of the drug to produce anaesthesia. The simplest method of administering a gas is to allow the patient to breathe the air naturally in and out through a piece of gauze or cloth which has been soaked in a volatile anaesthetic drug. A substance such as ether will evaporate and be carried into the lungs with the inspired air; the patient's respiration continues automatically even though he is completely unconscious. This is known as the 'open' method of anaesthesia. Chloroform is also used in this way, particularly in hot climates where ether would evaporate too quickly. Trichlorethylene (Trilene), a blue liquid, can similarly be used on a cloth mask: it is an excellent emergency anaesthetic agent and is usually given through a simple inhaler for pain relief in obstetrics or for dressings. Ethyl chloride is another very powerful anaesthetic agent, and because of its rapid rate of evaporation it is supplied in glass tubes with a valve stopper. The drug is squirted on to the mask where it evaporates very rapidly and is inhaled with the air.

The 'open' method of anaesthesia has many advantages. It is simple, it requires no expensive apparatus, and the patient's oxygen requirement is supplied from the air. No cylinders of gas or oxygen are necessary and it remains the ideal method of administering a general anaesthetic in situations where equipment and supplies are short. The method is used very little in general surgery except for children. The 'open' method of anaesthesia was used exclusively from the discovery of chloroform by Simpson (1811–70) in 1847 until the introduction of the anaesthetic vaporising machines of which Magill and Boyle of London were pioneers.

There are many varieties of anaesthetic apparatus, the main functions of which are:

1. to deliver a regulated volume of nitrous oxide, oxygen or cyclopropane.

2. to vaporise into the oxygen/nitrous oxide mixture, volatile drugs such as ether, halothane or Trilene.

3. to 'take over' respiration at a controlled rate when the patient has been given curare or other relaxant.

Very sophisticated machines include pulse, blood pressure and electro-cardiographic monitoring instruments.

Gases used in anaesthesia

To be useful as an anaesthetic gas, the substance must be capable of producing a loss of consciousness, without any significant risk to the heart, brain or any other organ. Many substances which occur as a gas will produce unconsciousness but are at the same time intense poisons. It is well known that carbon monoxide which occurs for instance in motor car exhaust fumes produces drowsiness which is very peaceful and it is not in any way unpleasant as it is inhaled. Carbon monoxide, however, combines with the haemoglobin of the blood so that the red cells become useless for carrying oxygen: this change is permanent and unconsciousness is therefore due to lack of oxygen in the brain and death occurs from relatively low concentration of carbon monoxide. The effect of a gas used in anaesthesia must pass off fairly quickly and completely, and must not interfere with the oxygen carrying capacity of the blood.

Nitrous oxide. This is an odourless gas which is non-explosive; it produces no irritation of the lungs during inhalation, and has a wide safety margin. It is very quick in its action and is therefore used extensively in anaesthetic practice for short operations such as the removal of teeth. It is not possible to produce good muscular relaxation with nitrous oxide. By itself it is not therefore suitable for prolonged operations, but it is an excellent 'vehicle' for administering other drugs such as ether. It can be inhaled in limited quantity so as to produce analgesia without complete loss of consciousness. It is used thus in midwifery.

Nitrous oxide is supplied as a 50 per cent mixture with oxygen under the trade name **Entonox** and may be administered for an 'on demand' inhalation device for intermittent relief of pain such as is required for large dressings (Fig. 12.1). This 50 per cent oxygen-gas mixture may be 'piped' to strategic points such as dressing station, casualty department or obstetric delivery room, and intensive care units.

This mixture has also proved to be invaluable to relieve pain in casualties awaiting rescue, and it can safely be administered by ambulance or nursing staff.

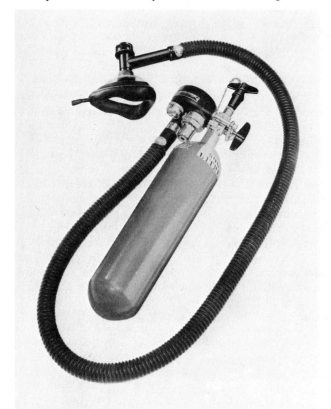

Fig. 12.1 Nitrous oxide-oxygen (Entonox) self-administered analgesic appliance; simple and safer than vaporising machines (Figs. 18.20, 18.21).

Cyclopropane. This is the only other anaesthetic gas commonly used. It is very explosive is extremely powerful and rapid in its action, has no smell and is expensive. Only very small quantities of it need to be used and a special apparatus is necessary to regulate and measure the exact quantity being given to avoid the risk of overdose. The great advantage of cyclopropane is that it will produce muscular relaxation. It is very useful therefore combined with nitrous oxide to give a greater depth of anaesthesia without using an irritant gas, such as ether. Cyclopropane has largely lost its usefulness since the introduction of special relaxing drugs such as tubocurarine and Scoline.

Mention must be made here of other gases used in anaesthesia which are, however, not in themselves anaesthetic drugs.

Oxygen. With the introduction of machines for the administration and mixing of anaesthetic gases and vapours, a constantly regulated supply of oxygen became essential. If the patient is relying on oxygen in inhaled air, the amount of oxygen which reaches his lungs depends entirely on the depth and rate of his respiration. If, however, the anaesthetic is being administered through a machine the anaesthetist can vary the amount of oxygen given. The patient's blood can then be fully oxygenated as it passes through the lungs even though the respiration may be shallow and slow. Oxygen also has to be available for emergencies for the same reason. The presence of oxygen makes the risk of fire very much greater; a tiny electric spark, or the spark produced by the contact of two metals, may be sufficient to start a fire. Particularly is this true when very small quantities of oil or grease are present and it is extremely dangerous for oil to be used on the connections of anaesthetic apparatus even if the valve screws seem to be stiff. **Under no circumstances whatever must oil or grease be applied to the connections of gas cylinders or anaesthetic apparatus.** Occasionally when this warning has been ignored the pressure-reducing valves on the cylinders have caught fire and explosions have occurred.

Carbon dioxide. The respiration of living cells consists of the utilisation of oxygen and the production of carbon dioxide. The accumulation of carbon dioxide in solution in the blood acts as a stimulus to the centre of the brain which controls respiration. Thus after exercise it is not only the demand for oxygen but the accumulation of carbon dioxide which leads to increased breathing. Anaesthesia must provide for an escape of the carbon dioxide. In any open-circuit anaesthetic apparatus, valves must be arranged so that the last air to leave the lungs in expiration is blown off into the atmosphere and not back into the apparatus. In certain types of anaesthetic apparatus using the closed-circuit principle, the carbon dioxide, instead of being blown off into the atmosphere, is absorbed by soda-lime in a special container through which all the expired gases are passed: the purified gases are re-inhaled with added oxygen. During deep anaesthesia, the respiration rate tends to fall because of the depressant effect of drugs on the special brain centres. Morphine, for example, has a particular effect on the respiratory centre and patients who have received large doses of such drugs breathe so slowly and shallowly that they become cyanosed from lack of oxygen. This inadequate respiration may prevent the patient from absorbing sufficient anaesthetic vapour to give the required depth of unconsciousness. The anaesthetist sometimes uses carbon dioxide which is supplied in a special cylinder attached to the anaesthetic apparatus. A small proportion of carbon dioxide is allowed to trickle into the anaesthetic inspired air; this is absorbed through the lungs—the reverse of the physiological procedure—and acts as a stimulus to breathing. The patient is thus compelled to breathe more deeply, and so to inhale the anaesthetic agent, such as ether, which is being used to make him completely unconscious. Similarly, towards the end of the operation when the anaesthetist wishes to expand the patient's lungs to the full, he may produce deep breathing artificially, by using carbon dioxide. Its use in the administration of anaesthesia has largely been eliminated by the adoption of controlled respiration techniques (page 220).

Helium. In America more commonly than in Great Britain, helium is used as a medium in which to convey other anaesthetic agents instead of using additional oxygen or nitrous oxide, especially for patients with obstructive airway disease (e.g. emphysema).

BRITISH STANDARD COLOURS FOR MEDICAL GAS CYLINDERS

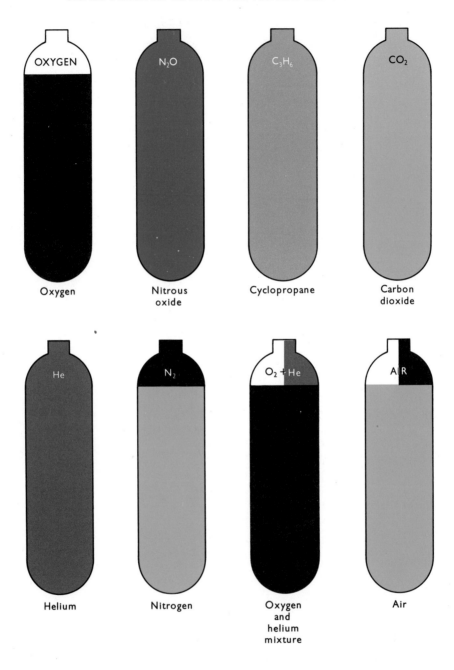

The British Standard colours from BS 1319: 1955, Medical gas cylinders and anesthetic apparatus, are reproduced by permission of the British Standards Institution, 2 Park Street, London W1A 2BS. Entonox (page 213) is supplied in a blue cylinder with a white sector at the top indicating the oxygen content.

Identification of cylinders

On the opposite page are shown the colours employed by international agreement to distinguish the various types of gas cylinder. Many serious accidents have occurred from cylinders being incorrectly connected to the anaesthetic apparatus, or from some individual painting the cylinders all the same colour. **The nurse must be completely familiar with the colours used on the cylinders, so that in a moment of crisis there can be no mistake.** Cylinder connections are designed to fit only in the correct positions on anaesthetic machines.

Volatile liquids used in anaesthesia

These substances are supplied in liquid form, but are evaporated in a suitable apparatus or on a mask made of lint, so that their vapours can be inhaled with air or oxygen and perhaps nitrous oxide.

Chloroform. This was introduced as the first inhalation anaesthetic agent in 1847 by Sir James Simpson, a Scottish obstetrician. It is extremely powerful in its action, has a rather sweet smell and taste, and does not evaporate at ordinary temperatures nearly as fast as ether. It is therefore sometimes used in very hot climates where ether boils too rapidly; although the development of modern vaporisers has largely eliminated the inconvenience of the hot climate. Chloroform has a somewhat dangerous effect on heart muscles and renders the heart very sensitive to nerve impulses. It can be used in an anaesthetic apparatus, but more commonly as a simple method of producing deep anaesthesia, by dripping from a bottle on to a lint mask held over the patient's face. Chloroform becomes easily decomposed by direct sunlight and it is therefore stored in a cool place in dark brown glass bottles. Old chloroform which has been exposed to the light must never be used. It may burn the skin of the face if the liquid form comes in contact. It is not used in normal hospital practice.

Ether. Ether is very much safer for the patient than chloroform, but it is highly inflammable, and it has been the presence of ether in the operating theatre that has been mainly responsible for serious fires and explosions. Ether may be used by dropping it from a bottle as with chloroform on to a lint mask, the patient inhaling it with ordinary air. It is, however, most commonly used in a special machine in which the gases oxygen and nitrous oxide are passed through a vaporiser containing ether, the evaporated chemical thus being carried to the lungs intimately mixed with the gases. Ether has an unpleasant smell which lingers for a long time after an operation is over. During the induction stage of the anaesthetic, it is so irritant that it may send the vocal cords (glottis) into spasm, and make breathing impossible. It also has an irritant effect on the lungs, rendering them more liable to complications from infection. The presence of ether in the body fluids and tissues acts to some extent as a poison. The taste and smell may upset a patient considerably for some days following a major operation. It is an extremely safe anaesthetic agent for use in children, but it is rarely used: halothane has taken its place.

Trichlorethylene (Trilene). This substance is perhaps the most generally used volatile agent. It is supplied coloured blue to distinguish it from chloroform as the smell is somewhat similar. It is used commercially as a dry-cleaning agent. Such cleaning substances are dangerous if the fumes are inhaled. Trilene, like chloroform, is very rapid in its action,

Table 29   Evaporating (volatile) liquid anaesthetic drugs

Drug	Method of use	Comments
Trichlorethylene (Trilene)	In special 'self-administra- tion' inhalers for dressing and obstetrics. In anaes- thetic machines in the 'chloroform' unit. Can be used on open mask	Clear blue liquid. Sweet smell. Rapid action. Does not give muscle relaxation. Non-irritant and does not produce vomiting Non-explosive and safe with diathermy *Forms poisonous gas with soda-lime and must never be used in closed-circuit apparatus.*
Halothane (Fluothane)	Vaporising machines	Extremely powerful and produces rapid loss of consciousness; very short recovery period; non-irritant
Ether	On open mask from drop- bottle or in evaporating unit on anaesthetic machine.	Irritant vapour. Safe anaesthesia. Good muscle relaxation. Bad for pulmonary conditions. Highly explosive. Supplied in glass bottles or cans with screw stoppers. Must not be left in warm cupboards
Vinyl ether (Vinesthene)	Vaporising machines	As for halothane: smells of garlic; may be used on open mask for children
Ethyl chloride	Sprayed on to open mask or into rubber bag. Some- times used for local 'freezing'	Supplied in 50-ml tubes with spray-valve nozzle, plain or eau-de-Cologne scented. Highly inflammable. Often produces vomiting
Chloroform	On open mask or in evapora- ting unit. From small glass ampoules in obstetrics	Sweet smell. Rapid action. Bad effect on heart and adrenaline must be avoided for infiltra- tion. Non-inflammable and therefore can be used with surgical diathermy. Gives deep anaesthesia and full muscle relaxation

but it does not produce the same depth of anaesthesia unless used in amounts which are dangerous. As has been mentioned, some anaesthetic machines contain soda-lime for taking the carbon dioxide out of the gases which are exhaled. Unfortunately, Trilene combines with soda-lime to produce a poison, so that Trilene must not, under any circum- stances, ever be used in a 'closed-circuit' apparatus containing soda-lime. There are special inhalers for using Trilene safely in limited measured quantities; these are used extensively in obstetrics as the patient can administer the vapour to herself when she feels it necessary. Trilene is also extremely useful when administered in a similar way to patients having to undergo painful dressing after operation; surface pain is relieved very quickly without the patient becoming completely unconscious. Trilene is non-explosive but has an action on the heart which may produce irregular rhythm.

Halothane (Fluothane) is now very widely used owing to its power of rapid induction and rapid elimination, so that the recovery period is short. It is very powerful and may easily make the anaesthetist or surgeon drowsy unless care is taken to avoid the exhaled gas. It is now common practice for the exhaled gases to be led away from the operating table to a special exhaust outlet. Specially calibrated vaporisers are used. Patients given Fluothane as their main anaesthetic require post-operative sedation to relieve pain and anxiety sooner than those who have had Trilene or ether.

Methoxyflurane (Penthrane) is a powerful inhalation agent with a smell like paraldehyde.

Ethyl chloride. This substance is one of the earliest used for inhalation anaesthesia and evaporates very rapidly when exposed to the air. Its rapid evaporation produces cooling of the surface to which it has been applied and in addition to its use as an anaesthetic it has therefore been employed extensively for 'freezing' tissues which need to be cut. It is provided in glass tubes with a special valve and lever fitted at one end. The warmth of the hand causes the liquid to expand and evaporate and the pressure that it produces in the glass tube squirts the fluid through a tiny opening when the lever is depressed.

Intravenous anaesthesia

The principal intravenous anaesthetic is thiopentone (Pentothal). This is used to complete the work of the pre-medication drug, such as morphine, producing a much greater depth of unconsciousness in what is called the induction stage. A further dose of the drug may be given during inhalation anaesthesia to increase the depth. Many operations can be performed entirely under intravenous anaesthesia with thiopentone. The original intravenous anaesthetic agent, hexobarbitone (Evipan), is still sometimes used.

Thiopentone is supplied in a powder in sealed glass ampoules containing 0·5 G. The solution is mixed with sterile distilled water immediately before use (20 ml to 0·5 G). The anaesthetist must perform this mixing himself and unused solutions must not be left lying about. Deaths have occurred from the injection of liquid such as spirit which has been mistaken for thiopentone. An eccentric nozzle 20-ml syringe is used with a large-bore needle or cannula for the mixing, but the anaesthetist will usually wish to use a short hypodermic needle for the intravenous injection. The amount of drug required varies with the individual patient but a healthy adult is usually given approximately 0·5 G rapidly; this produces complete loss of consciousness in about ten seconds. As soon as the patient goes off to sleep and while the anaesthetist is still injecting the solution, the nurse is required to hold up the patient's chin to facilitate his breathing. Respiration is reduced by thiopentone and may cease completely for a while (**apnoea**).

One disadvantage of intravenous anaesthesia with thiopentone is that its effect does not wear off very rapidly; therefore it is not suitable for the performance of minor operations where the patient is expected to walk out of the operating theatre and go home shortly afterwards. It is in other respects ideal for such minor operations as the opening of an abscess and for manipulations.

Thiopentone is sometimes used as a continuous intravenous anaesthetic, the anaesthetist mixing the solution into an infusion bottle of intravenous dextrose saline. Though thiopentone produces a loss of consciousness, it does not abolish completely all reflexes, nor does it produce complete muscular relaxation. Although a patient who has had intra-venous thiopentone may then appear to be quite unconscious an attempted passage of an endotracheal tube or a surgical incision may produce a violent response and muscle spasm unless a relaxant has been given as well. Frequently the anaesthetist is able to pass an endo-tracheal tube under intravenous thiopentone anaesthesia by first spraying the pharynx and larynx with a local anaesthetic solution. We now begin to see the advantage of a combina-tion of the various methods of anaesthesia. **Methohexitone** sodium (Brietal) is a short-acting thiopentone substitute increasingly used for out-patient surgery and 'day-cases': **propanidid** (Epontol) is used similarly.

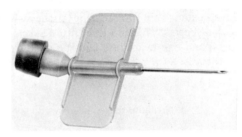

Fig. 12.2   Armoven Gordh type intravenous needle for intermittent injection of drugs during anaesthesia, or long-term heparin administration (Table 8). The backing plate is strapped to the hand to prevent dis-placement of the needle. (Armour Pharmaceutical Co.)

Pethidine is sometimes used intravenously during general inhalation anaesthesia: it is repeated at intervals of perhaps 30 minutes as necessary. It also slows the respiration rate.

Ketamine (Ketalar). This drug, given by intramuscular or intravenous injection, has a rapid action and the patient goes into an hypnotic trance. It produces loss of memory for the immediate part so that a child has no dread of a repetition. It may be followed by inhalation anaesthesia. Ketamine is particularly useful for children who require daily radiotherapy, or for instance extensive burns dressings. The most important rule is that patients under the influence of ketamine must not be disturbed or deliberately awakened, but must be allowed to recover consciousness fully. Unpleasant hallucinations may occur during recovery and this complication is avoided by giving diazepam before the recovery phase.

Althesin (CT 1341) is a steroid, allied to adrenal cortical and sex hormones, which has anaesthetic properties. It is used for brief surgical procedures or supplemented with nitrous oxide for full general anaesthesia.

Rectal anaesthetic administration

Certain drugs are absorbed very readily through the lining of the rectum, and this route can be used to advantage. **Paraldehyde** which is extremely unpleasant to take by mouth is one such drug. Its administration takes at least five minutes and the appropriate dose is mixed with saline. It is administered through a small rubber catheter inserted as high into the rectum as possible at least half an hour before the operation is due. The depth of anaesthesia produced is not great, but it enables a child to be taken to the operating theatre and an inhalation anaesthetic commenced without the patient even being aware that he has left his bed. Used in this way, paraldehyde is described as a 'basal' anaesthetic agent, and by the elimination of fear it has contributed greatly to the care and management of the sick child who needed an operation. The usual dosage, based on body weight, is 2·5 ml per kilo.

Thiopentone is also used rectally. It takes 20 minutes to have its effect, and as in other drugs the dosage has to be calculated according to body weight.

Other barbiturates such as quinalbarbitone (Seconal) and pentobarbitone (Nembutal) are also used by the rectal route, particularly in children when difficulty is experienced in persuading the child to swallow a capsule or when the capsule has been vomited. The gelatine capsule containing the appropriate dose is opened by cutting one end off. The capsule is inserted into the rectum half to one hour before operation.

Fluids given rectally for narcosis should be administered with the patient turned well over on to the left side: this position is maintained until the patient goes to the operating theatre: the fluid then passes up into the colon and absorption is more certain.

The disadvantage of rectal administration of anaesthetic agents is that the rate of absorption varies in different patients, so that the effect may vary; the advantage is that the patient experiences nothing unpleasant: there is no needle prick, no feeling of being stifled, and in fact the patient need not have any knowledge that an operation is going to take place in the immediate future. Because of these advantages this method is particularly suitable for children, but because of the irritant local effect, bowel incontinence may occur during operation.

Drugs used to produce muscular relaxation

For many years **curare** has been used by the natives of South America as a poison tip to their arrows. Its effect is to produce muscular paralysis in the whole body, including of course the muscles of respiration. A purified derivative **tubocurarine** is now used extensively in anaesthesia. Many drugs diminish perception of pain, but deep anaesthesia is necessary in order to obtain the relaxation of muscles required in abdominal surgery. It was discovered that when small quantities of tubocurarine were injected intravenously, all muscles of the body were relaxed, especially those of the abdominal wall. Unfortunately the muscles of respiration are affected so that breathing becomes impossible if an excessive quantity of the drug is used. With a modern anaesthetic apparatus, however, it is possible to inflate the lungs rhythmically in artificial respiration. With the introduction of tubocurarine, relaxation can be obtained for major abdominal operations without the deleterious effect of large doses of noxious anaesthetic agents. Other substances similar to curare have been introduced, some of which affect the abdominal muscles in particular and are therefore most suitable. Further, it has been found that the use of a relaxing drug abolishes the spasm of the vocal cords, which sometimes occurs when a tube is passed down into the trachea. The presence of this laryngeal spasm prevents the anaesthetist from passing an endotracheal tube unless he has previously rendered the pharynx and larynx insensitive by spraying them with a local analgesic solution. A relaxant drug, by paralysing the muscles, has the same effect at the other end of the reflex—that is, in preventing the laryngeal muscles contracting. Relaxant drugs (especially tubocurarine) can however in certain patients produce bronchial muscle spasm and asphyxia.

The nurse needs to know little about the various relaxant drugs except that certain precautions are necessary whenever they have been used. Table 30 shows the drugs in

Table 30   Muscle relaxant drugs

Chemical	Trade Name	Properties
Tubocurarine	Tubarine	Prolonged action: reversible by neostigmine
Pancuronium	Pavulon	Prolonged action: less depression of BP than tubocurarine
Suxamethonium	Scoline Anectine	Short acting: rapid destruction, not reversible. Action time prolonged by tacrine (I-V).
Gallamine	Flaxedil	Short acting: dangerous for patients with kidney disease
Alcuronium	Alloferin	Short acting: 20–30 minutes

These are administered intravenously, often in repeated doses during anaesthesia. The injection is made into the tube of an intravenous infusion or through the rubber cap of a special needle usually placed on the back of the hand at the beginning of the operation (Fig. 12.2).

common use. They are given intravenously with a 1- or 2-ml syringe and small hypodermic needle (No. 14). Respiration frequently remains shallow, and oxygen may therefore be required after operation. The effect produced by the drugs is rather like that which occurs spontaneously in the disease known as myasthenia gravis. This condition exists undetected in some people, and if a relaxant drug is given to such a patient, the result may well be fatal. Just as neostigmine is effective in the treatment of myasthenia, so is it a complete antidote to some relaxant drugs, and at the end of the operation the patient may be given an injection of neostigmine in order to restore normal respiration and muscle activity. Neostigmine is supplied in ampoules of 2·5 mg in 1 ml and in glass bottles containing larger quantities.

Apart from anaesthesia, relaxant drugs are used to control convulsions in such conditions as tetanus, and to limit the violent muscle spasms which accompany the electroconvulsive treatment of mental disorders.

Control of respiration

The natural automatic respiration which takes place in an unconscious patient, depends upon (a) the vital nerve centres in the base of the brain, (b) the ability of the muscles of respiration to respond to stimulus of these nerve centres, and (c) the fact that the thorax is a closed airtight compartment so that any increase in its size leads to expansion of the lungs.

Poisoning of the vital nerve centres by drugs (e.g. morphine or thiopentone), reduction of their vitality by lack of oxygen, muscular paralysis, or an open wound of the pleural cavity either accidental or surgical, would each have the same effect—asphyxia. Obstruction to the airway in the throat, larynx or trachea similarly produces asphyxia.

The art of anaesthesia has been to regulate this automatic breathing so that sufficient oxygen is inhaled together with sufficient anaesthetic vapour to produce the required degree of muscular relaxation. With advances in thoracic surgery, when it became commonplace for the pleural cavity to be opened, the anaesthetist had to be armed with an apparatus for inflating the lungs since the natural mechanism for expanding them had been interfered with. With the development of relaxant drugs it then became possible to override the patient's own respiratory rhythm and to continue artificial ventilation with anaesthetic apparatus. This technique of 'controlled respiration' has been applied to the management of respiratory insufficiency quite apart from anaesthetics (page 188).

From the nurse's point of view, when this method of anaesthesia has been used, the patient may be less inclined to breathe spontaneously and fully to expand his lungs, after operation. On the other hand, if the technique has been carried out well it is likely that the whole course of the operation will be smoother and the patient less disturbed.

Airways

These are short sections of rubber or metal tubes especially shaped to be held between the incisor teeth and to fit against the upper surface of the tongue, reaching into the pharynx, but are not long enough to touch the opening of the larynx itself. The more modern rubber airways are flattened from side to side and their shape enables them to fit snugly in the mouth, so that their presence may be tolerated even by a conscious person. Many of these rubber airways have metal connecting pieces which may become detached during use, and as with endotracheal tubes, faulty airways must be discarded. The principal types are shown in Fig. 12.3. Airways must be sterilised by boiling or autoclave. The purpose of an airway is to keep the tongue forward so as to enable the patient to breathe freely through the mouth. During general anaesthesia an airway is used sometimes in the early stage if intubation is to be performed, and throughout the operation if the patient is anaesthetised through a face mask; in almost all cases the airway is left in place when the patient returns to the ward, where it is removed when he shows signs of intolerance. As the insertion of an airway may be an emergency measure the nurse must know how to do it. When in position the curve of the airway is such that the point is directed down the throat. It is very difficult to put it in position this way up, unless the tongue can be held forward with tongue forceps. The airway is therefore moistened or lubricated and inserted upside down so that the tip rides along the palate. When the airway is in to its full length, it is turned round to direct the point downwards. It may be necessary to use a gag to open the mouth sufficiently for this to be done. Once the airway is in position and the jaw lifted forward, respiration will continue without difficulty unless there is also spasm of the glottis produced by mucus or vomitus in the pharynx (page 173).

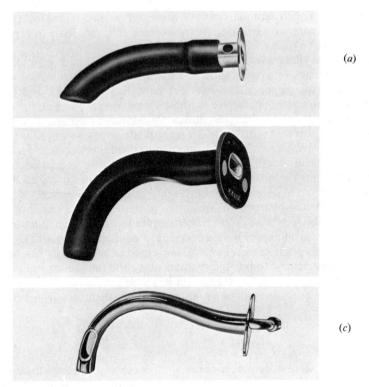

(a)

(c)

Fig. 12.3 Airways. (*a*) Phillips rubber airway, metal inserted, which can be connected with anaesthetic machine. (*b*) Guedel airway. Moulded rubber with metal inserted. (*c*) Waters airway. All metal, with side oxygen tube. (British Oxygen Company.)

Intubation

During operations on the nose, mouth and throat there is a great risk that blood may trickle into the trachea and thus find its way into the lungs. If the quantity is great, the patient will drown, and even with small amounts there will be collapse of areas of the lungs with consequent infection. Many ways have therefore been devised for preventing the inhalation of blood, and the simplest is that in common use for tonsillectomy. Here the patient's head is kept fully extended so that the blood will accumulate in the mouth and in the back of the nose but will not run down the throat. It may be removed continuously by suction apparatus. An alternative method for extensive operations on the mouth and tongue was to perform a tracheostomy and to administer the anaesthetic through the tracheostomy tube. This difficulty is overcome by endotracheal intubation.

Tubes are made of rubber or plastic and are of three main types. First, the rubber tube may be passed through the nose. The natural curve of the pharynx directs the tip of the tube towards the glottis and the anaesthetist may be able to pass the tube into the trachea between the cords 'blind', or may use a laryngoscope to hold the tongue and the epiglottis forward. Nasal intubation is used infrequently but is necessary for extensive surgery

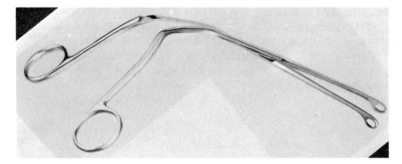

Fig. 12.4 Magill's introducing forceps, for passing endotracheal tubes under direct vision through the laryngoscope (26 cm long). (British Oxygen Co.)

in the mouth. There are two types of oral tube: the plain tube which is similar in structure to the nasal tube has, however, a different curve and a different length and these two are not interchangeable. Great care should be taken to avoid mixing the tubes up: the nasal type, which is also softer, is very easily kinked and its use through the mouth may result in respiratory obstruction and asphyxia. The most commonly used type is the cuffed oral tube which carries an inflatable section around the main tube connected to a pilot bulb

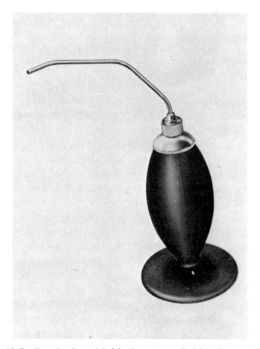

Fig. 12.5 Rowbotham Multicaine spray. (British Oxygen Co.)

which indicates the state of distension of the cuff. The purpose of the cuff is to occlude the airway around the tube to enable the anaesthetist to apply positive pressure, and this type of tube is always used for intermittent positive pressure respiration.

To allow the passage of an endotracheal tube the patient must be unconscious, or have had his larynx made insensitive by spraying with an analgesic solution. Newborn babies may be intubated without preliminary anaesthesia.

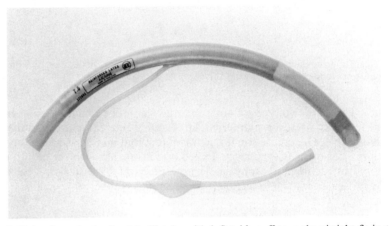

Fig. 12.6 Cuffed endotracheal tube. Magill tube with inflatable cuff to make airtight fit in trachea or bronchus. A 10-ml syringe or small plastic pump is used to inflate the cuff, the degree of inflation being shown by the pilot bulb: a spigot or pressure clip is used to close the end. This is the most commonly used type of tube as positive pressure artificial respiration can then be maintained. (British Oxygen Co.)

Once the tube is in place a gauze pack can be placed in the back of the throat around the tube, eliminating the risk of any blood or foreign matter running down into the trachea. The use of a cuffed tube lessens the need for a pack.

Endotracheal tubes must be treated with care and thrown away if they are even slightly damaged. A metal or plastic adaptor is used to connect the tube to the corrugated delivery tube from the anaesthetic machine and it is essential that these pieces of apparatus fit correctly. If the endotracheal tube is damaged the metal adaptor will almost certainly not fit. After use endotracheal tubes must be carefully cleaned in soap and water and sterilised according to the routine being used in the particular hospital. If chemical sterilisation is to be used glutaraldehyde (Cidex) is the best solution and under no circumstances must carbolic solution be used. Boiling after the tubes have been properly cleaned inside with a brush is satisfactory, but repeated treatment softens the rubber. Undoubtedly the best method of storage is in individual Nylon sleeves, the tubes being autoclaved and stored sterile in the anaesthetic room. Endotracheal tubes need to be lubricated immediately before use, but **oily lubricants such as paraffin or petroleum jelly should not be used.**

The laryngoscope is an absolutely vital instrument and must be available in various sizes. Some units have fibre-light direct vision laryngoscopes, the illumination being through a fibre-glass cable from a separate light source. The majority of units still use

(a)

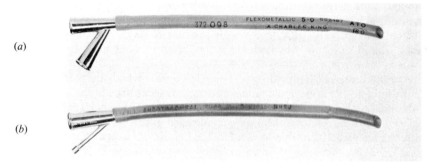

(b)

Fig. 12.7 (a) 'Armoured' tube in which the latex is reinforced by a metal spiral to prevent kinking. (b) Simple standard endotracheal rubber tubes. Both these have a shoulder near the lower end. Only the narrow portion lies below the vocal cords. (British Oxygen Co.)

battery operated laryngoscopes and clearly one of the most important maintenance operations is to check the reliability of the battery and bulbs. Spare batteries and bulbs must always be available. Most laryngoscopes have detachable blades which may be auto-claved. Different sized blades are required for children and babies.

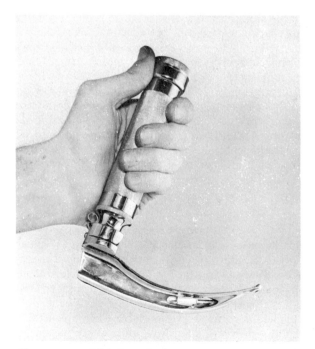

Fig. 12.8 Illuminated laryngoscope. With the patient's head extended the blade is slipped over the tongue so that the rounded tip is positioned in the pit in front of the epiglottis. When the laryngoscope is lifted the epiglottis is thus pulled forward, exposing the glottis through which the endotracheal tube is passed.

'Armoured' tubes have a flexible wire spiral embedded in the upper half to prevent kinking. This addition is used particularly in the small tubes for children (Fig. 12.7a).

The Magill forceps (Fig. 12.4) is a simple instrument angled in such a way that the anaesthetist's hand does not obstruct his vision when he is using it to guide the tube between the vocal cords.

Reference has already been made to the metal adaptors which are used to connect the endotracheal tube to the apparatus: some are straight, some are angled and commonly a connector is used with a side arm which carries a plug; when the plug is removed a catheter may be placed down the endotracheal tube to suck out excessive secretions.

Usually the anaesthetist is able to regulate the depths of anaesthesia so that when the surgeon has finished, the patient will regain consciousness quickly. The aim is that when the endotracheal tube is removed the patient's laryngeal reflexes will be present and the risk of obstruction is greatly reduced. If reflexes have not returned adequately then an airway may be left in place, but occasionally the patient is returned to the ward with the endotracheal tube still present. Under such circumstances the nurse must never remove the tube until told to do so unless the patient is coughing. Removal of the tube may be followed immediately by some laryngeal spasm.

Throat packs

In operations in the mouth and throat when there is likelihood of blood running into the pharynx, a gauze pack is placed well down at the back of the tongue to protect the opening to the glottis. It is usual to use a 5-cm gauze roll which has been wrung out in saline. Some anaesthetists prefer the roll to be soaked in liquid paraffin. It must never be used dry and at the same time it must never be really wet. Once the pack has been placed in position by the anaesthetist or surgeon it is left undisturbed. If it becomes soaked with blood and any attempt is made to remove it, it will result in blood being squeezed into the larynx. Under no circumstances must independent gauze swabs be used for this purpose as they may well be lost or forgotten. It is the duty of the theatre nurse to see that all packs are accounted for before the patient leaves the operating theatre. When a throat pack has been introduced the anaesthetist may write on the patient's forehead or attach an adhesive tag as a safeguard against the pack being left in.

Gags

The partially anaesthetised patient clenches his jaws and if his airway becomes obstructed it is necessary to use force to open the mouth. It is sometimes possible to insert the rubber-covered jaws of a gag towards the back of the mandible, if there is a gap left by the removal of teeth on previous occasions. If the metal gag cannot be inserted then a wooden wedge is used, and it is almost always possible to insert this between the **molar** teeth. The nurse must see that there is always a gag available when a general anaesthetic is being administered; a gag, together with an airway, must always accompany an unconscious patient on his return to the ward. The Mason gag and the Doyen gag (Fig. 12.9) are two common varieties, and both of these have small pieces of rubber tube slipped over the jaws. **This rubber must be a really tight fit and must be renewed if it shows the slightest sign**

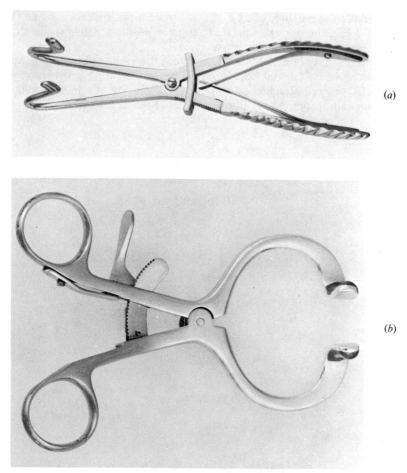

(a)

(b)

Fig. 12.9 Gags. (a) Ferguson gag (ratchet lock). The Mason gag is similar but has a screw lock. The jaws are usually covered with a piece of rubber tubing which must be a very tight fit. This is the only suitable type for use by nurses. (b) Doyen's gag with rubber-covered jaws. (Seward Surgical Instruments.)

of deterioration. A special type of gag is used for tonsil operations—the Boyle-Davis; this consists of an upper section the jaws of which are protected with rubber and fit against the upper incisor teeth. The tongue blade is attached to the frame with a ratchet which regulates the amount of opening. There is a metal tube incorporated in the blade and this is connected to the anaesthetic machine so that oxygen and ether or other gas may be administered through it. The nurse must ensure that this anaesthetic tube in the gag is thoroughly cleaned with a pipe-cleaner immediately after use. The pieces of rubber tubing on a Boyle-Davis gag are actually sewn in position with thread. Various sizes of blade are provided and the complete set must be available so that the surgeon can select one of suitable width and length. The Boyle-Davis gag is also provided with a breast plate which is strapped across the patient's chest and this carries a rod or 'jack'. When the 'jack' is attached to the gag, the gag and jaw are held up in position. This may be done equally well by an assistant or by the anaesthetist.

Short flanged rubber or metal tubes 2–4 cm long are used to prop the jaws apart during minor operations such as dental extractions. These 'props' must always have a length of fine metal chain or cord attached to prevent the possibility of one becoming dislodged into the mouth and dropping back into the throat (Fig. 12.10).

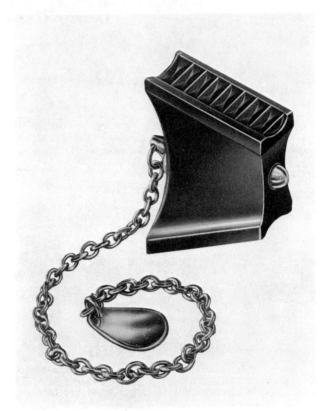

Fig. 12.10   Hard rubber dental prop. (British Oxygen Co.)

Syringes and needles for use by the anaesthetist

The standard range of disposable syringes and needles meets most of the anaesthetist's requirements. Intravenous cannulae of various types also have to be provided (page 142). Special long needles used for brachial plexus block and other forms of regional anaesthesia may be of the non-disposable type which have to be re-sterilised.

'Gordh' needles are angled large intravenous needles with a screw-on head containing a rubber diaphragm to prevent back leakage. (Fig. 12.2). This needle is placed into a vein at the beginning of an operation and strapped in position. There are many variations of this needle. The anaesthetist injects with a very fine needle, through the rubber cap, relaxant and other drugs at appropriate times during the course of operation. Gordh needles must be taken apart, cleaned and dried immediately after use: a faulty diaphragm must be replaced and the needles are sterilised either by boiling or by autoclave. Immersion in antiseptic solution is unsatisfactory; the needle is not adequately filled as it is closed by the cap at one end. Disposable single-use substitutes are now used for these needles.

Many intravenous infusion giving-sets have a 'flash-ball' rubber section near the needle into which drugs may be injected.

An infiltration syringe is illustrated on page 236 and lumbar puncture needles are described in Chapter 16.

For further information on anaesthetic equipment and its maintenance see Chapter 18.

Untoward effects of general anaesthesia

Apart from the most urgent trouble of respiratory obstruction (page 172) the complications of general anaesthesia are many. As far as the nurse is concerned, she needs to know of the occurrence of these so that she may detect them from the early signs which she may observe in the ward. Many of the complications arise from an overdose of the drug in relation to the size of the patient, or from the sensitivity of a particular patient to a normal amount of the drug which has been used. Morphine sometimes has an abnormally great effect on particular individuals. The effect of a morphine overdose is a very slow respiration rate, perhaps four a minute, and consequent cyanosis. The pupils are also constricted by morphine though this finding is not necessarily a sign of overdose. Morphine, when injected subcutaneously into a shocked patient whose skin circulation is poor, will not be absorbed until the circulation returns to the skin when the blood pressure rises. Sometimes a second subcutaneous dose has been given to a shocked patient when the first has had no effect and in consequence both doses are absorbed at the same time; when the circulation begins to recover an 'overdose' occurs. Morphine in shock should be given intravenously (or if this is not possible, intramuscularly) so that its effect is immediate.

Cardiac arrest may occur any time during the operation, but it can be entirely due to the anaesthetic. Trichlorethylene and cyclopropane, chloroform and ethyl chloride may produce primary heart failure. This catastrophe has to be dealt with urgently by artificial respiration, oxygen administration and cardiac massage (page 191). The procedure to be adopted in the event of heart failure is described in Appendix II. One of the main difficulties is knowing when in fact the heart has stopped. Relaxant drugs may produce a very slow heart beat, and so may neostigmine given at the end of an operation to reverse the effect of curare.

Apart from the sudden fatality of asphyxia or heart failure there are some other serious conditions which may occur from the administration of a general anaesthetic. Lack of oxygen either from obstruction or the excessive use of nitrous oxide may lead to permanent brain damage. This may be shown by prolonged stupor following an operation, or by blindness. Fortunately the blindness is very rare and recovery is to be expected. Permanent mental defects have been recorded following the use of nitrous oxide, but if used with 50 per cent oxygen (Entonox, page 213) it is perfectly safe. Paralysis of cranial nerves such as the facial has also been attributed to trichlorethylene.

The pulmonary complications which may ensue after an operation performed under general anaesthesia are discussed in Chapter 20.

A patient's abnormal behaviour after general anaesthetic should always be reported, however slight or odd it may seem. Cerebral haemorrhage, cerebral arterial thrombosis or embolus may show first as abnormal behaviour or speech.

Some drugs used in anaesthesia, particularly the barbiturates, may produce dermatitis in sensitive patients. Liver damage may be caused by chloroform.

Ether convulsions

Convulsions sometimes occur during the administration of a general anaesthetic, especially when ether is being used. The cause is not known but it is certain that excessive heat in the operating theatre is a major factor. It must be remembered that the temperature under the operating towels and other coverings is considerably higher than on the wall of the theatre where the thermometer may be fixed.

Heavy rubber mackintoshes should never be used to cover the patient. Light-weight waterproofed paper or foil should be used, sterile, under the operating towels. A clinical thermometer should always be on the anaesthetic trolley. The convulsions are treated by thiopentone and relaxant drugs but the condition is sometimes fatal. In prolonged major operations, the patient's temperature is monitored throughout with an electronic thermometer.

'Halothane shakes'

Patients recovering after halothane (Fluothane) anaesthesia frequently develop a marked tremor like severe shivering; this passes quickly without any treatment but may worry an unwarned nurse. It is severe especially in the elderly; the added muscle activity requires more oxygen and hypoxia may result: oxygen should be administered until the condition subsides.

Post-operative care after anaesthesia

The principles of nursing the unconscious patient are the same no matter what the cause of the coma. There are, however, certain duties which the nurse must undertake post-operatively which are directly related to the anaesthesia. With very few exceptions patients are turned onto one side at the end of anaesthesia so that any fluid regurgitated into the pharynx will run out and not flood the trachea. The lateral position is routine but clearly the type of operation performed may prevent this. After operations on the nose, mouth or throat the patient is usually kept semi-prone, without a pillow, so that any blood which may accumulate in the mouth will not trickle down into the larynx.

Collection of the patient from the operating theatre

The journey back to the ward may be only a few yards or it may involve a long walk, the use of a lift or even a staircase. However short or long the journey, the nurse must never take her eyes off the patient or relax her attention in any way.

Equipment

The nurse must be armed with:

Kidney dish.

Hand towel.

Known number of small swabs of a type or colour which will not be confused with those used in the theatre.

'Sponge holder.'

Tongue forceps.

Mouth gag of the Mason or Ferguson type with very secure rubbers on the jaws.

Airway (even if the patient is leaving the theatre with an endotracheal tube in place, he may become light enough on the journey to need this removed and replaced by an airway).

Torch if the journey involves more than a few yards.

Instructions. The surgeon or one of his team should write post-operative instructions clearly. The ward nurse is responsible for speaking personally to the anaesthetist, surgeon or house officer. It is her duty to ask and remember what anaesthetic has been used, the nature of the operation, the presence or absence of drainage tubes, and the general condition of the patient at the end of the operation. In addition, she may be required to supervise an intravenous infusion which has been set up and is to continue. She must receive definite instructions as to what the 'next bottle' of infusion is to be and it is customary for a tie-on luggage label to be attached to the 'drip' tube with a record of the intended infusion programme: alternative methods of keeping a record may be used but 'notes' tend to stray!

Examination of the patient. Before leaving the theatre suite the nurse must satisfy herself that the patient has a clear airway and is breathing adequately. There should be no cyanosis and if this is present, the patient should remain in the theatre until the colour is satisfactory.

Similarly if vomiting is imminent, it is best to wait and have a sucker available. If this should occur just outside the theatre, the nurse must not be afraid to return the patient to the theatre where the light and equipment is more adequate and the skilled assistance of the anaesthetist is available.

The pulse must be felt and its rate, rhythm and volume carefully observed. If any irregularity is present, the nurse must inform the anaesthetist and determine its importance. If the nurse is uncertain whether she can feel the pulse she must call for help. Occasionally collapse occurs from shock or internal haemorrhage in the short interval which elapses between the patient being placed on the trolley and the start of the journey to the ward.

Injuries occur from time to time when an arm falls down off the stretcher (page 392). This should not be possible if the blankets have been adequately tucked in. If a journey involves moving to another floor or going into the open, stretcher straps should be used on all cases. The nurse will learn any particular wishes of the medical staff with regard to position on the stretcher.

On the journey

Obstructed airway. The respiration may be obstructed by spasm of the glottis. This in turn is caused by vomit, or by an airway or nasopharyngeal tube being pushed in too far. Apart from removal of the cause, there is nothing that can be done at this stage, and the spasm passes off spontaneously. Obstruction may be due to the tongue dropping back and it is wise to have an airway in position for the journey in all cases. Even those patients who are only lightly anaesthetised, will often tolerate a moulded rubber airway. If this is not tolerated, the patient is light enough to have regained his cough reflex and is unlikely to have difficulty. If the head is flexed by a pillow the jaw falls back and the tongue blocks the airway more easily. The remedy is to turn the head to one side, extend the neck, and lift the mandible forwards (page 173, Fig. 10.2). If this fails, the gag must be inserted between the molar teeth (in the absence of teeth, as far back between the jaws as possible) and opened carefully; the airway is inserted after the tongue has been drawn forwards.

Tongue forceps are of two types:

(a) Those which pierce the tongue, with two spikes. This pattern must be applied to the upper surface of the tongue about 3 cm (1 in.) from its tip. The spikes must never be used under or through the tongue as severe haemorrhage may be produced from the large veins on its under surface (Figs. 10.3 and 12.11).

(b) Those which have a serrated pair of jaws, like a sponge forceps. These are applied with one jaw above and one below the tongue. They squeeze the tongue, are less satisfactory and do more damage than the first pattern.

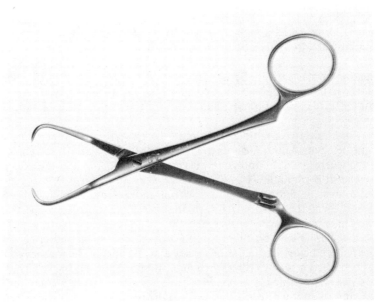

Fig. 12.11   Moynihan tongue forceps. (British Oxygen Co.)

If there has been vomiting or there is excessive saliva, the mouth and pharynx must be cleared with a swab firmly secured to a holder. If the patient is flat on his back the nurse must not hesitate to turn the patient into the semi-prone position if she cannot get the pharynx clear.

If a crisis occurs on the journey to the ward, it is much better to turn into the nearest ward where skilled help may be obtained, than to complete the journey with a cyanosed obstructed patient.

In the ward

The nurse must remain with her patient until transfer to the bed has been completed. She must not cease her watch on the patient's breathing in order to prepare the bed. Someone else must do that. The unconscious patient must never be left alone. It is very easy for a nurse to slip outside the room to fetch bed blocks, or more blankets, thinking she will be only a few seconds. It is in such brief moments that troubles occur and apart from respiratory obstruction an unrestrained 'fling' of an arm or leg may displace a transfusion needle, sweep all the articles off the locker or tear off the dressing.

Only when the patient appears to have his cough reflex again and is swallowing normally, can he be regarded as safe to be left from the point of view of the anaesthetic. The airway or endotracheal tube will have been removed and there will be no risk of tongue swallowing. He will be in a 'sleep' state from which he can be roused. If vomiting occurs, the patient who is semiconscious may inhale the vomitus. The risk of inattention at this stage is greatest if the patient is in a cubicle or single room.

It must be repeated again and again that a patient, unconscious from any cause except natural sleep, should never be left out of sight of trained staff. Screens and bed curtains are known to be a wall of death when the nurse is unwary.

Unconsciousness after operation is not normally prolonged. Many anaesthetists aim at the ideal of having the patient return to consciousness sufficiently to be able to 'cough and clear the throat' before starting the journey back to the ward. With modern anaesthesia, there is very rarely any violent restlessness after operation. With the more rapid return of consciousness, it is then safe to administer morphine, papaveretum or pethidine but these drugs should be withheld if the rate and depth of respiration is small. At the earliest possible opportunity, the patient must be made to take several slow, deliberate and full breaths. Attention to chest expansion before the narcotic is given is essential if pulmonary complications are to be avoided (page 389).

Regional analgesia[1]

By applying to the nerve tissues drugs which in themselves are poisons we can prevent these tissues from performing their normal functions. As we have seen already, this may be done by introducing the drugs into the blood where it circulates to all tissues, and by using a drug which particularly affects the nerve cells. In contrast to this general or circulation anaesthesia, we can limit the effect of the drug to one particular area by applying it in such a way that only a limited number of nerves are affected. Brief mention has already been made of the different ways in which this method of regional analgesia may be applied. It is not necessary for the nurse to be familiar with all the various techniques that are used by surgeons and anaesthetists, but she must be familiar with the drugs which are in common use for this purpose, their method of administration, and the complications which may arise from any particular method.

[1] *Anaesthesia* implies that the patient is unable to perceive any sensation, whereas *analgesia* means the abolition of pain.

Drugs used in regional analgesia

These are almost all related in some way to cocaine which itself is extremely toxic. When a drug is applied for analgesic purposes to the surface of the body or injected into the tissues, the duration of its action depends upon the rapidity with which it is absorbed into the blood stream. Cocaine has the additional property of making the blood vessels constrict, thereby preventing oozing from the cut surface which has been anaesthetised and to some extent preventing its own rapid absorption into the blood stream where it would act as a general poison. Other analgesic drugs have the opposite effect—dilating blood vessels; they need therefore to be used in combination with drugs which constrict the blood vessels, such as adrenaline or ephedrine. The main difference between the various drugs which are used, lies in their rates of absorption in the tissues, and in the degree to which they act as general poisons. Table 31 shows the common substances in use, with some of the trade names which the nurse may come across in her daily work.

Sterilisation and supply

In very large hospitals many of these drugs are obtained by the hospital in powder form, bottled and sterilised in various strengths in the hospital dispensary and supplied to the ward in sterile containers. The smaller hospitals and individual surgeons are more likely to obtain their supplies from one of the large manufacturers and it is usual for the drugs to be presented in small sterile ampoules or rubber-capped bottles for injection in strengths suitable for immediate use without further dilution. To reduce the risk of contamination from the repeated use of one rubber-capped bottle, the lid of which becomes punctured by a needle on several occasions, certain preparations are provided containing an antiseptic which it is claimed makes the solution self-sterilising. All multi-dose containers of substances used for injection contain antiseptic (chlorocresol, phenol or chlorbutol) to prevent the growth of moulds and organisms in the bottle. **Never under any circumstances may substances from such containers (e.g. rubber-capped bottles) be injected into the spinal theca.** The greatest possible precaution must be taken in the preparation of syringes and all apparatus used in connection with local or regional analgesia, since the presence of the drug in the tissues lowers their resistance to infection. Sepsis in the wound is therefore more likely to follow than after general anaesthesia.

It is now convenient to consider briefly the various applications of regional analgesia, the apparatus required for use and the nursing points in connection with each.

Surface analgesia

This is the simplest method of all. The drug is applied direct to the skin or more usually to a mucous membrane. The chemical rapidly penetrates the moist surface such as the lining of the nose, and for the removal of nasal polyps or the insertion of a cannula into the maxillary antrum, cocaine (usually 5 per cent) is applied on pledgets of cotton wool firmly attached to special nasal probes. The nasopharynx may be completely anaesthetised by applying the drug with a fine spray. In the mouth, if only a small area is to be involved, the anaesthetic may be applied on a small pad of wool held in contact with the site of operation. If, however, it is desired to pass an instrument such as a gastroscope, complete anaesthesia of the mouth and oesophagus can be obtained with 2 ml of

2 per cent amethocaine or lignocaine (Xylocaine). Cocaine is not used for the oesophagus as it may be rapidly absorbed from the stomach and act as a poison. The solution of amethocaine is merely dripped into the mouth from a syringe. The patient moves the solution all round the mouth and finally swallows it if anaesthesia of the oesophagus is desired. The larynx and trachea may be anaesthetised by a special angled spray introduced over the back of the tongue and operated as the patient breathes in. Lubricant jellies containing amethocaine are applied to endotracheal tubes so that they cause less irritation to the air passages.

For urethral instrumentation such as cystoscopy, 0·5–2 per cent amethocaine or 2 per cent lignocaine (Xylocaine) are commonly used. Sterile lignocaine gel can be introduced direct from the tube through the special nozzle with which it is supplied.

The solution is inserted into the urethra with a small urethral syringe (Canny Ryall) and is gently massaged backwards into the posterior urethra. Sufficient time has to be allowed for the mucous membrane to become anaesthetised before the instrument is passed.

Local analgesia

Strictly, this means that the analgesic agent is injected merely at the site of operation and no attempt is made to affect any particular nerve. Cocaine must never be used for injection; procaine in the usual strength of 1 or 2 per cent is used for both major and minor operations. The maximum amount of drug which can safely be given to the healthy adult of average size, is one gram of procaine (i.e. 100 ml of 1 per cent solution, or 50 ml of 2 per cent solution). If a large area of tissue is to be infiltrated with the anaesthetic solution (for instance in operating upon a hernia under a local anaesthetic) then a solution of 0·5 per cent is used. Procaine must always contain adrenaline in the solution to prevent its rapid absorption so that the patient is not poisoned and so that effect of the anaesthetic is prolonged. Liq. adrenaline hydrochlor. BP 0·5 ml of 1 : 1000 solution added to 250 ml of anaesthetic solution gives a final strength of 1 : 500,000 adrenaline. The total amount of adrenaline injected should never exceed 0·5 ml of 1 : 1000 solution, and in certain cases must be considerably less (page 242). A strength of 1 : 250,000 is sufficient for most purposes. For minor operations, such as the removal of a wart, a simple 1- or 2-ml record syringe may be used, with the finest possible hypodermic needle. A larger (No. 1) needle should be available with which the surgeon can fill the syringe from the rubber-capped bottle or ampoule. For major operations a 20-ml syringe with special long flexible needles should be prepared. If no such needles are available, a fine lumbar puncture needle forms a useful substitute for this purpose. Special syringes (Fig. 12.12) are in common use with a continuous-flow valve which serves two purposes. When injecting anaesthetic solution, the surgeon has to take care that he does not put the drug directly into a vein. The 'continuous-flow' syringe is filled with a valve so arranged that should the needle enter a vein as the surgeon is withdrawing the plunger, blood will come up the needle into the syringe more readily than it will come down the rubber tube from the receptacle containing the drug solution. In using this syringe the surgeon advances the needle into the tissues as he withdraws the plunger with his thumb. The injection is made as the needle is moved back through the tissues. In order that the solution may be put in the right tissue layers the surgeon feels his way with the needle: for this reason, the piston should be working very freely and the needles should be sharp, fine, with lock fitting, and slightly flexible: an 8-cm needle is commonly employed.

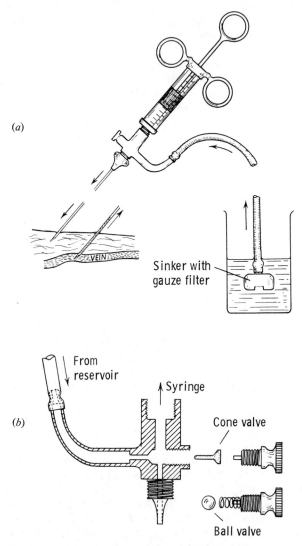

(a)

Sinker with
gauze filter

(b)

From
reservoir

↑ Syringe

Cone valve

Ball valve

Fig. 12.12   (a) Continuous-flow syringe with Dunn valve. As the piston is withdrawn, the barrel fills from a reservoir through the rubber tube. If, however, the needle has entered a vein, blood will be drawn into the barrel at the same time and the surgeon will thus avoid injecting anaesthetic solution into the vein. Long flexible needles are used with this type of syringe. (b) Details of Dunn valve with two types of fitting. Great care must be taken not to lose the cone or ball and spring.

Table 31 Drugs used in regional and local analgesia

BP Name	Supply	Strength	Uses
Cocaine	Powder made up by hospital dispenser	5, 10 or 20%	Surface application to mucous surfaces by swab or spray
		Must not be used for injection	
Procaine	Ampoules or rubber-capped bottles. With and without adrenaline mixed	1 or 2% 0·5%	Regional or local block For extensive infiltration
		Up to 1 G is given by long-period intravenous infusion	
	Ampoules of powder	Mixed with cerebrospinal fluid for spinal anaesthesia.	
Bupivacaine	Ampoules 10 ml with or without 1 : 200,000 adrenaline	0·5% 0·25%	Long-action local or epidural analgesia
Etidocaine	Ampoules	1% solution	Long-action local or epidural analgesia
Amethocaine	Powder made up by hospital dispenser. Also in ampoules	1 or 2%	Surface application or spray for pharynx, oesophagus, trachea
	Sterile bottles	0·5%	For urethral instillation or eyes
	Mucilage jelly	2%	Catheter lubricant
	Sterile solution 1 in 1000 for injection block		
Lignocaine	As for procaine, but more effective and less toxic		
Cinchocaine	Ointment	1%	'Nupercainal' for irritant surfaces
		10%	Cream lubricant
Cinchocaine hydrochloride	Ampoules 3 ml	0·5% (1 in 200) 6% dextrose	'Heavy' spinal
	Ampoules 20 ml	1 in 1500	'Light' spinal
Amylocaine hydrochloride	Sterile ampoules 2 ml	5% in 5% dextrose	'Heavy' spinal

(**Note.** Amylocaine is destroyed by the slightest trace of alkali in a syringe or needle. These must be rinsed in sterile distilled water.)

Five minutes should be allowed to elapse after injection before the operation is commenced and although the patient may be conscious of pressure in the wound, there should be no pain whatever. The tissues, when they are cut, appear relatively bloodless and oedematous from the presence of the solution. Most of the anaesthetic fluid will escape during the progress of the operation except of course in very short minor procedures.

There is a reaction of the tissues to this injection and for several hours after the anaesthetic effect has worn off, the patient will be conscious of a feeling of tension and inflammation in the tissues which have been injected, quite apart from the pain of the incision.

Nerve block analgesia

The interruption of nerve pathways at various levels outside the spinal cord is performed by the injection of 2 per cent procaine with adrenaline, 2 per cent lignocaine or 0·5 per cent bupivacaine.

(a) **Brachial plexus block.** The whole arm may be anaesthetised by the injection of one of these solutions into the area at the root of the neck immediately above the collar bone. Two special 8-cm long flexible needles must be available (or again, fine Howard Jones lumbar puncture needles will do) in addition to smaller needles for raising the initial wheal in the skin. There is a danger in performing this injection that the pleura over the apex of the lung will be penetrated, and the lung itself may be damaged resulting in pneumothorax on the affected side. The technique of producing a brachial plexus block is difficult but this method of analgesia is very suitable for operations on the arm, such as manipulation of fractures. The patient is fully conscious and may walk from the plaster room to the x-ray department, wait for his wet films and then undergo a second manipulation if necessary without further analgesia.

(b) **Paravertebral block.** The principle here is the same as with a brachial plexus block, but the injection is made just at the point where the spinal nerves leave the vertebral column. By a series of injections on one side of the spine, the whole of the chest wall on that side, or the abdominal wall if the injections are lower down, may be rendered anaesthetic. The paravertebral block is used in thoracic surgery for operations such as thoracoplasty, and repeated injection may be used to ease the pain from fractured ribs (see below).

(c) **Epidural block.** In this procedure the local anaesthetic (0·5 per cent bupivacaine) is injected inside the spinal canal, but outside the dura mater which lines it. The solution spreads up and down on the side of the injection and blocks the adjacent spinal roots. A special needle with a stilette is used (Fig. 12.14). It has a blunt tip which pushes the dura away, and allows a polythene cannula to be threaded through the side-eye of the needle to lie in the epidural space. The needle is then removed. Anaesthetic solution may be injected repeatedly to maintain anaesthesia over several days. It is of particular use to relieve the pain of broken ribs and enable the injured patient to breathe fully without pain. By injecting phenol, permanent anaesthesia can be attained to relieve the pain of infiltrating malignant growths.

(d) **Caudal block.** This is a form of epidural block but here the analgesic solution is injected into the small aperture at the base of the spine and it tracks up inside the spinal canal within the sacrum, which the last of the spinal nerves are traversing. The roots of these nerves are then bathed in analgesic solution and the tissues of the perineum are made insensitive. This method is used in childbirth and for operations on the perineum. The

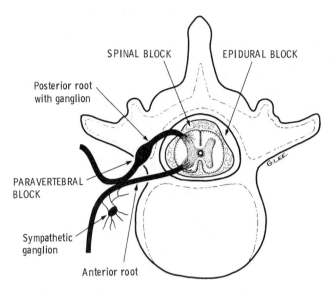

SPINAL BLOCK   EPIDURAL BLOCK

Posterior root
with ganglion

PARAVERTEBRAL
BLOCK

Sympathetic
ganglion

Anterior root

Fig. 12.13   Spinal anaesthesia is achieved by injection into the spinal theca; the anaesthetic agent diffuses up and down with the spinal fluid, bathing both the anterior and posterior nerve roots according to the position of the patient. An **epidural block** is outside the dura mater; the extent of its spread depends entirely on the pressure, which in turn is dependent on the volume injected. A **paravertebral block** is outside the spinal canal entirely; this is sometimes used as a trial sympathectomy.

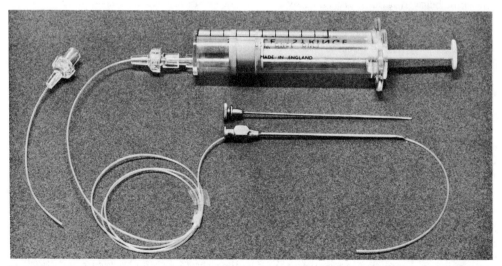

Fig. 12.14   Epidural anaesthesia. Trocar needle introducer with plastic cannula threaded through and directed sideways by the angle of the bevel.

solution is not injected into the spinal theca, and therefore cannot rise to a dangerous high level of the spinal cord.

(e) **Digital block.** This is the simplest form of regional block in which 2 per cent procaine is injected into the skin around the base of a finger or toe. The main digital nerves are thereby affected, and the whole finger becomes insensitive.

(f) **Abdominal field block.** This term is applied to the method in which the abdominal wall is made analgesic by several smaller injections at strategic points where the nerves course round to the front. It is used sometimes for operations on the gall-bladder or for hernia.

(g) **Splanchnic block.** This is a more specialised method in which a more dilute drug is injected into the area of the splanchnic (solar) plexus around the aorta. The injection may be made after the abdomen has been opened, and is sometimes used to reduce the shock from such operations as partial gastrectomy. Alternatively the solution may be injected from behind using special long needles.

(h) **Intravenous field block.** A tourniquet is placed on the upper arm or leg after exsanguination with an Esmarch bandage. An anaesthetic solution (0·5 per cent ligno-caine) is injected into one of the distal veins under pressure. The anaesthetic agent is forced backward down the vein producing complete anaesthesia of the limb.

Spinal analgesia

If an anaesthetic drug in solution is mixed with the cerebrospinal fluid, it percolates into the tissues of the spinal cord and for the time being cuts off all impulses passing up from below the affected point and similarly prevents all movement of muscles whose nerve supply comes from below this same point. The sympathetic nerves connected with the spine below this point are similarly affected and the blood vessels dilate, thereby lower-ing the blood pressure. All forms of spinal anaesthesia therefore have this one great disadvantage, namely that of lowering the blood pressure and thus sometimes producing collapse. Ephedrine is injected into the buttock muscles at the same time as the spinal injection to counteract this effect.

The apparatus required for spinal anaesthesia is the same as that required for an ordinary lumbar puncture. At least two lumbar puncture needles must be available together with an adequate supply of sterile towels and the anaesthetist should always wear sterilised rubber gloves.

Many substances have been used for injecting into the spinal theca. Just as oil will rise to the surface of water, so any solution which has a specific gravity lower than cerebro-spinal fluid will rise towards the brain if injected at the base of the spinal theca. Conversely if the solution is heavier than cerebrospinal fluid, it will settle to the bottom, if the patient is sitting up or is tilted with the head as the highest point. Thus by varying the specific gravity of the solution (heavy = hyperbaric, light = hypobaric) and similarly by varying the position of the patient after the injection of the fluid, the anaesthetist can control the level of the spinal cord at which the drug will work. We therefore refer to 'high spinal' and 'low spinal' anaesthesia. The higher the level the greater will be the degree of blood vessel paralysis and the greater, subsequently, will be the risk of low blood pressure and shock.

Retention of urine may be troublesome after spinal block. Hyperpyrexia occasionally complicates spinal anaesthesia: tepid sponging and elimination of excessive blankets is required.

Although spinal analgesia has largely been replaced by improved methods of general anaesthesia, it is still used in many places where highly trained anaesthetists are not available and where the surgeon has to act as his own anaesthetist. From the nurse's point of view, there are certain salient points which she must remember in connection with spinal anaesthesia.

(a) Blood pressure raising (vaso-pressor) drugs must always be available when spinal analgesia is used.

(b) Owing to the lowering of the blood pressure, patients who receive spinal analgesia are more liable to collapse on return to the ward unless adequate precautions have been taken.

(c) The effects of spinal analgesia are prolonged for several hours and therefore very great care needs to be taken to avoid pressure on the legs or buttocks, and under no circumstances should hot-water bottles be allowed to come in contact with the skin. The risk of burning insensitive skin is very great and the benefits from the use of hot-water bottles in shocked patients are very doubtful. A bed should be warmed but it is far safer to *remove* the hot-water bottles as soon as the patient returns to the bed. The legs must not be left crossed over one another as a pressure sore may develop on the skin of the leg which is beneath.

(d) By the time the patient has returned to bed, the anaesthetic drug which has been injected into the spinal canal will be 'fixed'. This means that it will have been used up or so mixed with the cerebrospinal fluid that its effects will extend no further; therefore a change of position of the patient on his return to the ward is unlikely to bring about any increase in anaesthesia. The surgeon however must always be asked deliberately whether he wishes the patient tilted with the head down or the head up. It is usual for all patients who have had a lumbar puncture performed to be kept for at least two hours with the foot of the bed raised, and not allowed to sit up until 24 hours have passed.

(e) The paralysis of the abdominal muscles or even of the lower (intercostal) muscles which accompanies spinal analgesia, leads to diminished respiratory movement; therefore patients who undergo this form of analgesia are particularly liable to post-operative chest troubles. The nurse must take particular care to see that deep-breathing exercises are performed as soon as possible, and repeatedly.

(f) Post-operative headache is common and may be very troublesome. They are less likely if a very fine lumbar puncture needle has been used as there will be less cerebrospinal fluid leakage.

(g) Care must be taken to avoid bladder distension. If retention occurs, carbachol injection is tried but catheterisation may be necessary.

Although the utmost precautions are taken in the preparation of drugs for spinal anaesthesia, occasionally contamination results when infection occurs during the actual injection process. Meningitis is therefore a complication which unfortunately arises sometimes, and severe post-operative headache accompanied by fever must always give rise to suspicion. Lumbar puncture is performed and the cerebrospinal fluid examined by the pathologist.

Other uses for local anaesthetic drugs

Sometimes a solution of butacaine in oil is injected into the tissues around the anus or into areas of fibrositis. The presence of the oil makes the absorption of the drug extremely slow, and the effect of the anaesthesia is thereby greatly prolonged. There is however an increased risk of infection with these substances, but they are used occasionally for pruritus ani. Bupivacaine with adrenaline has an effect lasting several hours and will effectively reduce post-operative wound pain for this time: etidocaine (Duranest) has an even longer action time.

Cocaine, benzocaine or amethocaine and other drugs are sometimes used in lozenges, particularly to diminish the pain of a malignant ulcer in the mouth or pharynx when other methods have failed. Occasionally these substances are used in ointments for application to particularly troublesome forms of dermatitis, but since the drugs are in themselves irritants, they have to be used with extreme caution.

The anaesthetist is often called upon to administer local or regional block analgesia for patients with pain which is not satisfactorily controlled by other drugs. For instance, multiple rib fractures produce so much pain that respiration is inhibited. Drugs to decrease the pain further depress respiration and pneumonia may follow. If an epidural block (i.e. nerve roots as they leave the spinal cord) is produced, pain-free improved respiration occurs. A tiny tube may be left in position so that continuous or repeated local anaesthetic injection may be given.

Supplementary drugs

Vasoconstrictor (pressor) drugs

Adrenaline (epinephrine), and noradrenaline (Levophed).

Ephedrine.

Methylamphetamine.

By their action in constricting the muscular walls of the small blood vessels, these substances stop bleeding if applied to an oozing surface. When injected hypodermically, subcutaneously, intramuscularly or intravenously they raise the blood pressure artificially. The site of injection is chosen to determine the rate of action required. To prevent the fall of blood pressure which may accompany spinal analgesia, ephedrine is used intramuscularly.

Adrenaline (1:10,000) is injected directly into the heart if 'cardiac arrest' occurs during operation. (Appendix II.)

All these drugs must therefore be available on the anaesthetist's trolley, in ampoule form, sterile and clearly marked.

Adrenaline is also used in dilute solution (made up to 1 part of adrenaline in 500,000 parts of solution down to 1:70,000) mixed with local analgesic procaine solutions to prevent rapid absorption of the procaine and diminish bleeding. Sometimes it is used purely for the latter purpose mixed only with saline.

Occasionally the surgeon requires a swab of gauze or wool soaked in 1:1000 liquor adrenaline (from sterile bottle solution) as a pack to apply to a bleeding raw surface for a few minutes. The anal margin after haemorrhoidectomy and the tonsil bed are sites where adrenaline is used for this purpose.

Drugs used to lower the blood pressure

Hexamethonium iodide (C.6 Hexathide).

Pentamethonium iodide (C.5 Antilusin).

Trimetaphan camphorsulphonate (Arfonad).

Phentolamine (Rogitine)

Guanethidine (Ismelin).

Shock is a state of lowered blood pressure and the prevention of shock is one of the main concerns of all who are connected with the case of the injured or ill. It may seem odd therefore to lower the blood pressure artificially (i.e. to produce **hypotensive anaesthesia).**

The low blood pressure which follows injury is to some extent a protective mechanism of nature which automatically reduces the amount of blood lost from a wound. The danger in shock lies in the fact that it may get out of control and permanent damage may result from the pressure being too low for too long. From experiments with drugs used in the treatment of hypertension (high blood pressure) it has been found that the blood pressure can be safely brought down to levels which have been previously thought to be dangerous. Certain of these drugs are used during operations in order to lower the blood pressure and enable the surgeon to operate in a bloodless field, as he does on a limb to which a tourniquet has been applied for the same purpose. Thus, the prostate gland or the thyroid can be removed almost bloodlessly: tedious and otherwise very bloodsome extensive plastic operations are simplified in this way. Reactionary haemorrhage does not occur as one would expect when blood vessels have been cut across and not tied, since the drug is given in a quantity sufficient to maintain the effect for about four hours after the operation is over. During this time the vessels contract on the small clot which has formed in their cut ends and this prevents reactionary haemorrhage (page 119).

Serious complications have arisen from the use of these drugs; blindness occurs occasionally from thrombosis of the retinal artery; cerebral thrombosis and its sequelae, and cardiac damage have also occurred. If one of these hypotensive drugs has been used the nurse must therefore be on the look-out particularly for untoward symptoms such as abnormal behaviour or visual disturbances which might indicate brain or retinal damage.

Hypotensive anaesthesia is more often induced with a combination of curare and Fluothane. A patient for whom this technique has been used must not be left unattended until the blood pressure has returned to normal.

In certain conditions, blood pressure may rise dangerously high during operation, and phentolamine is used to lower the pressure.

Hyaluronidase (Hyalase)

This is a chemical which has a dispersive effect on other substances when injected into the tissues. This effect is utilised to aid rapid absorption of subcutaneous infusions (page 154). It has been used to help the diffusion of local analgesic solutions, to which a vaso-constrictor has always to be added to prevent rapid absorption of the analgesic drug.

Chlorpromazine (Largactil), **Promethazine**

These drugs, given by mouth or by injection, depress tissue metabolism and reduce oxygen requirements. If used in adequate dosages, a state of **artificial hibernation** is produced. Operations can then be performed on the heart and great vessels, when the circulation has to be curtailed or temporarily suspended (page 626).

Chlorpromazine is also used to relieve depression and post-operative vomiting.

Anti-histamine drugs

To reduce sensitivity to other drugs (such as morphine), and in prevention or treatment of post-anaesthetic vomiting, it is common practice to combine pre-operative atrophine-action drugs with one of the anti-histamine drugs such as **mepyramine** (Anthisan) or **promethazine** (Phenergan). These also have a mild sedative effect and diminish apprehension. When drug sensitivity reactions have occurred the most widely used antihistamine substance is **Piriton (chlorpheniramine** 4 mg tab. orally: up to 10 mg I-M).

Other anti-nausea drugs (such as are used to prevent travel sickness) are **cyclizine** (Marzine) and **prochlorperazine** (Stemetil) (page 387).

Drugs used in resuscitation and cardiac abnormality

Occasionally drugs are needed which stimulate respiration or otherwise counteract the depressive effect of an overdose of anaesthetic agent. The following drugs must therefore be available on the anaesthetic trolley. It is best to arrange them in a small rack which can be improvised from an ampoule box.

Nikethamide (Coramine), a respiratory stimulant—2 ml and 5 ml ampoules for intravenous or subcutaneous injection.

Lobeline, a respiratory stimulant—1 ml ampoules containing 3 mg (1/20 grain).

Picrotoxin is an antidote for the barbiturate drugs such as thiopentone—1 ml ampoules each containing 3 mg.

Bemegride (Megimide) is used particularly for barbiturate poisoning and is given intravenously (50 mg every 5 minutes to a total of 1 G).

Amiphenazole (Daptazole) is another stimulant used with bemegride in barbiturate poisoning (15 mg every 5 minutes up to 300 mg).

Nalorphine (Lethidrone), a direct antidote for drugs of the morphine group—morphine, heroin, papaveretum, pethidine, methadone (Physeptone)—1-ml ampoules containing 10 mg.

Neostigmine (Prostigmin), antimyasthenic and antidote for relaxant drugs such as tubocurarine (ampoules 2·5 mg in 1 ml). Atropine (0·5 mg in 1 ml) must be available in ampoules for injection at the same time to prevent the effect of neostigmine on the bowel. Side-effects are sweating and bradycardia (slow pulse).

Doxapram (Dopram) is a stimulant used to rouse a patient to normal breathing level after controlled respiration with relaxant drugs.

Calcium gluconate, for treatment of tetany from alkalosis sometimes precipitated by overbreathing—10 ml ampoules for intravenous or intramuscular injection (10 per cent solution).

Naloxone (Narcan) is an antidote for morphine: it reverses both the respiratory depression and analgesic effect of the morphine groups.

Digoxin, for use in auricular fibrillation if the pulse rate becomes excessive—0·5 mg in 1 ml as an alcoholic solution. NOTE. This should be diluted with 10 ml normal saline for intravenous injection, unless it is injected into an intravenous infusion tube.

Propranolol (Inderal) is used to control cardiac arrhythmias, or excessive heart rate.

Practolol (Eraldin) is similar in action, but if used for prolonged periods reduces the production of tears and leads to corneal ulceration.

Salbutamol is a cardiac stimulant: it produces some degree of vasodilatation and this reduces the resistance against which the heart pumps. The blood flow and perfusion of tissues increases though the blood pressure is not raised.

SECTION IV

13

Ward Records and Patients' Notes

Each hospital has its own particular system for the collation and recording of the enormous amount of information which is gathered together about each patient. The junior nurse may have little idea of the importance of the many facts which she is observing and reporting. The accuracy and efficiency with which the 'paper work' is handled in a ward is a criterion upon which may be judged the standard of treatment. The basic records in a surgical ward do not differ greatly from those elsewhere, but the general tempo of activity is faster than in a medical ward and the admission of both planned and emergency operating lists, contributes to the difficulty of maintaining ward routine. Treatment may change from hour to hour and it is not possible always for the medical staff to prescribe far ahead. Accurate records are essential.

The nursing records fall in two distinct categories. First there are those for the general use of the nursing staff: second, there are the individual patient's notes and charts.

The repeated observations of temperature, pulse and respiration rates are recorded at the time on the patient's temperature chart by the nurse who makes the observation. Other data such as 'operation', x-ray examination and total fluid balance figures will be entered once in 24 hours by the sister or staff nurse (page 248).

Ward record books

There is a multiplicity of central records in each ward, to cover the many matters of nursing routine. Many hospitals now have a loose-leaf individual patient record system (Kardex) which provides a continuous treatment record for each patient: this system eliminates the tedious rewriting of nursing instructions each day in the treatment book and saves hours of nursing time.

In relation to the patient's treatment, the following items are essential. Where a unified system is not in operation separate books are kept.

(1) **Temperature, pulse and respiration record book.**

(2) **Treatment book.** This contains standing instructions for the nurses in relation to each patient. Serious errors sometimes arise if this book and the temperature record book refer to patients by the numbers of the beds alone, instead of by name. If a patient's bed is for any reason moved to a different place in the ward, trouble may occur because

the necessary alterations in the records have been forgotten. This mistake is apt to happen in the night if a serious emergency case is admitted.

(3) **Report Book.** This contains a summary of salient features of each person's progress during the previous twelve-hour period. This book forms the continuity record between the day and night staff and in a surgical ward needs to refer to any requirements and pre-operative treatment ordered in readiness for the forthcoming day's operations. The Report Book should always contain specific instructions with regard to the management of intravenous infusions which are in progress. It is also usual to include in this book the administration of any dangerous drugs during the previous twelve-hour period. The Report Book whether in hospital or private practice summarises the situation in relation to each patient and is of particular value to the resident medical staff on the night rounds and to the night superintendent sister who may have the responsibility of several wards.

(4) There is usually a book of standing instructions for the routine **pre- and post-operative treatment** preferred by the individual surgeons. Standard preparations for patients about to undergo x-ray and pathological investigations must also be available.

(5) **Admission and discharge records** are also the duty of the nursing staff.

(6) **Diet instructions** are frequently kept in a separate book and the junior nurse needs to be particularly careful over the distribution of food and drinks. Patients are very apt to take all that is offered, even if it is done in error, and many a patient being starved before operation has obtained a meal from an unsuspecting ward orderly!

PATIENTS' PERSONAL RECORDS

1. The temperature chart and essential entries

There are two main types. The three-line chart and the single-line chart. The three-line chart records as three graphs, temperature, pulse and respiration. The single-line chart records as a graph only the temperature, the pulse and respiration rates being inserted in figures on the appropriate line at the foot of the chart. The single-line chart is most unsatisfactory in surgical work and does not give a readily interpreted picture of the patient's condition. Both these types of chart are used in four-hourly and twelve-hourly varieties. During the initial period after admission to hospital and for at least one week after any operation, surgical patients must have a four-hourly record. During the latter part of their convalescence, though it is usual to make the observations four-hourly, twelve-hourly charting is all that is needed. In long-stay cases such as occur most commonly in orthopaedic and plastic surgical units, the twelve-hour record is sufficient.

In cases of injury or where a special post-operative record is needed, a standard chart is modified to show half-hourly pulse rates and blood pressure records.

The three-line chart has the additional advantage of providing adequate space for the supplementary information which should be entered. The routine record of daily urine volume, bowel action, weight (entered weekly if possible), and the results of urine testing must always be included.

Certain other important information is added to individual charts (Fig. 13.1) in such a way that vital day-to-day changes are seen at a glance.

Operation. The name of the operation should be inserted on the appropriate day and

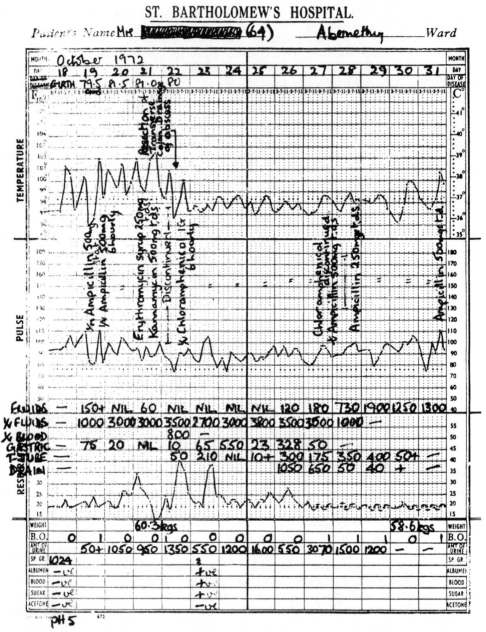

Fig. 13.1 Typical three-line chart. The amount of data, other than temperature, pulse and respiration, which is entered on the chart varies from unit to unit. All landmarks in management such as x-rays, operation, removal of drains or stitches are important when reviewing a case. Very often it is the total pattern of the record over several days which gives more information than any single recording. The start and duration of an antibiotic course is thus related to the temperature response. Adequate entry of data on this chart saves a great deal of time and searching through other notes during a ward round, but clearly more detailed records of fluid balance and drug administration have to be kept separately.

the subsequent days numbered in the 'day of disease' space if this is provided. Such information is helpful both to the medical staff and to the ward sister who has to set out each day the necessary instructions for her staff concerning, for instance, the removal of stitches.

Antibiotic and chemotherapy record. Courses of specific treatment such as the use of sulphonamides, antibiotics or antitoxic sera may be entered on this record by inserting the name of the drug and initial dose from the date of commencement and later inserting any change of dose and the cessation of that particular treatment.

Fluid intake and output. It is not necessary to insert all the details of fluid balance, but the total daily intake and output can be shown. Many important daily items such as gastric aspiration following partial gastrectomy, suprapubic drainage of urine, or the drainage of bile from a 'T' tube in the common bile duct, should be shown as specific amounts, again to give an accurate picture of the daily progress.

Other important incidents. The occurrence of x-ray examination, removal of drainage tube, removal of stitches, or change of plaster cast, are also added.

On first consideration, it would seem that the temperature chart would become a mass of figures and writing which would be quite unintelligible. To the surgeon, however, whether house-officer, registrar, or consultant, if it is neatly compiled, the temperature chart will be fully informative and will enable him to assess progress and vary treatment more speedily and more reliably than if he has to depend upon the memory of the nursing staff or reference to a host of books. Another side of this record which is not readily appreciated by nursing staff, is that many hospital records have to be studied later by doctors investigating the results of any particular form of treatment. Clinical research can be badly hampered by careless omissions from these nursing records.

2. Operation and anaesthetic consent form

For the protection of the hospital, the surgeon and the anaesthetist, all patients are required to sign a form which states their willingness to undergo the performance of an operation and the administration of an anaesthetic. The form of consent in common use in hospitals of the National Health Service is shown in Fig. 13.2. It is the duty of the medical staff to explain in very broad terms the nature of the operation. This has usually been done at an initial consultation in the out-patient department in the case of patients admitted from the waiting list, but it is surprising how many patients reach the morning of operation without having been told what they are about to undergo and even without having enquired. Such is their confidence, but because of claims by patients that they have not been told what is to be done, the form has recently been altered to include the signature of a doctor. In order that the surgeon should not be embarrassed by finding that he needs to perform an operation the nature of which has not been explained to the patient before-hand, there is an escape clause in this form of consent allowing him to extend the operation as necessary. In the case of a child, the form has to be signed by the parent or legal guardian. Since no operation is 'legal' in the strict sense of the word—that is, every operation is technically an assault—there is no official age of consent. It is usual to accept personal consent of young people over eighteen if their parents are not immediately available. In the case of an emergency operation such as may be required on a child injured in a road

Anaesthetic and Operation Consent Form

Unit Registry Number................

CONSENT BY PATIENT

....Hospital.
I.............................. of ....
hereby consent to undergo the operation of ....
the nature and effect of which have been explained to me by
Dr./Mr....................................

I also consent to such further or alternative operative measures as may be found to
be necessary during the course of the operation and to the administration of general,
local or other anaesthetic for any of these purposes.

No assurance has been given to me that the operation will be performed by any
particular surgeon.

Date.............................. (Signed) ....

Patient

_____

I confirm that I have explained to the patient the nature and effect of this operation.
Date.................................. (Signed) ....

(Physician/Surgeon)

CONSENT BY PARENT OR GUARDIAN

....Hospital.
I.............................. of ....
hereby consent to the submission of...
to the operation of...the nature
and effect of which have been explained to me by Dr./Mr...........................
....

I also consent to such further or alternative operative measures as may be found to be
necessary during the course of the operation and to the administration of a general, local
or other anaesthetic for any of these purposes.

No assurance has been given to me that the operation will be performed by any
particular surgeon.

Date.............................. (Signed) ....

(Parent/Guardian)

_____

I confirm that I have explained the nature of this operation to the child's parent/
guardian.
Date.............................. (Signed) ....

(Physician/Surgeon)

Fig. 13.2 Specimen anaesthetic and operation consent forms. Special forms are used prior to electro-
convulsive therapy and for gynaecological operations involving hysterectomy or sterilisation.

accident, if the parent cannot be reached in time, the surgeon proceeds on his own responsibility. In some hospitals, an administrative officer is authorised to give the necessary consent.

Before certain operations it is thought wise to obtain the consent of another relative in addition to the patient's own consent. For instance, before a hysterectomy or sterilisation operation, the patient's husband is usually asked to give his consent.

The consent form must be attached to the patient's notes so that it cannot be lost. It must accompany the patient to the theatre.

3. Prescription sheet

On this individual document is written by the medical officer in charge, all the drug treatment which the patient is to receive. It will show such treatments as may be given at the discretion of the nursing staff—for instance, enemas, inhalations, laxatives and certain sedatives. All drugs covered by the poison regulations will be specified, with the amount, the method of administration, and whether it is to be repeated. Dietary supplements such as vitamins or basic alterations in the diet (e.g. high calorie requirements) will also be specified. If a prescription is written for continuous or repeated treatment, it should be cancelled when the treatment is suspended. If any doubt arises as to whether some drug treatment which has been written down is in fact to be stopped, the prescription sheet must be brought to the medical officer's notice so that clear instructions may be left.

Many hospitals now have a complete drug administration record chart for each patient. This shows the time each dose is given and the initials of the nurse who gave it. Thus the complete treatment is 'programmed' on a time schedule.

In the case of drugs under the poison regulations (Chapter 7) where individual prescriptions are dispensed by the hospital pharmacist, the patient's prescription sheet must be sent to the dispensary. The usual procedure is for the pharmacist to initial the prescription showing that the drug has been issued. In the event of accidents in treatment from errors of dosage or administration, the records on this drug sheet are of vital significance.

The individual's prescription sheet must not be used for obtaining ward stocks. One patient's sheet must not be used for obtaining a drug to be given to another patient. This may be a very convenient procedure if the chart of a patient needing treatment is missing or is perhaps already in the dispensary. It is an easily acquired but dangerous habit.

4. Fluid balance chart

Reference has already been made to the recording of the patient's fluid intake and output and the specimen chart is shown in Fig. 13.3: the daily totals from this detailed record are incorporated in the temperature chart. For babies there will be an additional feeding schedule. As it is common practice to administer certain drugs to patients receiving an intravenous infusion by injecting the drug into the tubing, it is wise to record on the fluid balance chart the time at which each such injection is given.

CH. 18/49   INTAKE AND
                                                                             OUTPUT CHART

Surname	First Names	UNIT No.

DATE................................ **INTAKE**   **OUTPUT**

Time	Mouth	Rectal	Subcu-taneous	Intra-venous	Total	Gastric Content	Vomit	Urine	Faeces	Total	Balance + or −
0800											
0900											
1000											
1100											
1200											
1300											
1400											
1500											
1600											
1700											
1800											
1900											
2000											
2100											
2200											
2300											
2400											
0100											
0200											
0300											
0400											
0500											
0600											
0700											
TOTAL											

DAY (rows 0800–1900)

NIGHT (rows 2000–0700)

Fig. 13.3   Specimen intake/output chart. There are many variations and space may be left for drugs. Antibiotics and other substances administered with an intravenous infusion should be recorded in the appropriate intake column.

5. Diabetic chart

Any patients suffering from diabetes will have a special record showing the result of the daily urine test for sugar, related to the insulin dosage.

6. Pre-operative treatment note

When a patient is taken to the operating theatre, there should be attached to the front of the notes, on a separate form, the details of the drugs which have been given as 'pre-medication'. This should also indicate clearly whether the injection has been given intra-muscularly, subcutaneously or intravenously so that the anaesthetist will not be misled. The form must also show when the patient last passed urine, the quantity and, in the case of a diabetic subject, whether it contained sugar.

This pre-operative record is sometimes incorporated in an anaesthetic report form upon which the anaesthetist enters details of drugs given in the operating theatre. Such drugs will not otherwise appear recorded in the patient's notes or on his prescription sheet.

7. Pathological reports

The careful routine insertion, in the notes, of all pathological reports contributes greatly to the ease of interpretation in complicated cases. It is usual to group these reports so that all blood examinations appear consecutively in the notes with the most recent one uppermost. When a report arrives in the ward from the pathology laboratory, it must be attached immediately to the patient's notes. Any observation of particular significance from the nursing point of view such as a high blood urea figure, or the presence of a haemolytic streptococcus in a throat swab, will be recorded by the sister or staff nurse in the ward Report Book.

8. X-ray reports and films

These reports must be grouped similarly in the patient's notes, the most recent one being uppermost. The procedure varies in different hospitals concerning the storage of patient's x-rays. As these form so often a vital and permanent record of the patient's condition, care must be taken to preserve them from damage. If films are brought to a ward from the x-ray department before they have been adequately washed and dried, they must be returned as soon as possible after inspection by the medical officer. Great care must be taken that the emulsion is not scratched and a special rack for such 'wet films' is a necessary part of every ward equipment. When the films are dry, they may be very easily damaged by splashing water on them or by putting an individual film down on a locker where water has been spilled perhaps from a flower vase. If several films have been removed from the envelope and these represent examinations on different dates, the films should be grouped together with paper clips or in separate paper sheaths and replaced in the envelope in their correct serial order. When the patient has been discharged from hospital, the x-rays should not be retained in the ward but returned to the x-ray department. A patient's x-rays must always accompany him to the operating theatre.

9. Wound infection record

In order to have a constant check on the occurrence of cross-infection it has become standard practice to have a wound infection record book in each ward. The 'clean' surgical wound which at any stage is found to be infected is examined bacteriologically. The date of the operation, the post-operative day on which there was any evidence of infection, the nature of the organism and its sensitivity to antibiotics are included in this record. If there is an 'outbreak' of hospital staphylococcal cross-infection it is very often possible to discover at once the carrier, or the source of the infection, by referring to this book. This record also makes it possible for the hospital authority to assess the efficiency of ward routine and structural design, particularly in relation to ventilation. Many hospitals have a 'control of infection' nursing officer whose duty it is to monitor cross-infection and advise on its control.

14

Pathological Investigation

Many out-patients and all in-patients in a surgical ward undergo some form of pathological investigation—at least an estimation of haemoglobin before an anaesthetic is administered. With the complexity of modern medicine, pathological investigation has become almost an industry and much of it is conducted on factory production principles. Practically all chemical investigations of blood, urine and other fluids are carried out by automatic machines which use a very small amount of blood and simultaneously estimate a number of constituents, printing out the result without the intervention of a human operator. With this sophistication of methods it has been necessary to centralise expensive apparatus so that each well equipped laboratory serves a large number of hospitals. A selection of routine tests may well be done in a local hospital laboratory; routine urine examinations are conducted on the ward or in the out-patient department. The nurse's role in relation to pathology is in the correct collection of specimens and in acquainting the patient with the purpose of the investigation. Some procedures such as gastric test meal analysis involve nursing procedures and the collection of specimens for bacteriology is also usually the duty of the nurse.

A simple hospital laboratory is usually divided into four main sections. Though the work of these overlaps there is an arbitrary division of labour between them and each section is in the charge of a consultant who has specialised in this branch of pathology.

These four sections or sub-departments usually cover the investigations set out below, and the forms on which a medical officer makes his request for an investigation may be distinctive for each department. The usual practice is for all request forms to be sent to a special office or placed in a collecting box. They are then apportioned to the various sections of the pathological department by a pathologist.

1. **Clinical pathology and haematology**
   Bleeding and clotting times
   Blood counts and haemoglobin
   Blood grouping for transfusion
   Erythrocyte sedimentation and fragility
   Examination of sputum, faeces and cerebrospinal fluid, etc.
   Urine testing
2. **Chemical pathology**
   Blood—electrolytes (sodium, potassium, calcium, chloride, bicarbonate), urea, sugar, cholesterol, phosphatase, protein, etc.
   Gastric test meal analysis
   Faeces—percentage of fats, etc.
   Urine—special tests of renal function (page 643).

3. Bacteriology

Throat swabs and swabs of pus from the ear, nose, wound or fistula.

Bacteriological examination of the urine ('clean specimen', page 638).

Faeces for special disease-producing organisms.

Sensitivity tests to determine what chemotherapy or antibiotic is likely to be most effective. This is necessary for the reason that many bacteria become resistant to common forms of treatment.

4. Morbid anatomy and histology

Microscopic examination of pieces of tumour tissue removed for 'biopsy'.

Complete examination of specimens removed at operation, particularly of tumours, to determine their nature and extent of spread.

Post-mortem examinations.

Collection of specimens

This may be considered under four main headings:

(*i*) Specimens collected by special technique by laboratory technician or pathologist. If the patient is ambulant and the laboratory conveniently situated, he will be sent there for the test. All specimens of blood for counts of cells, haemoglobin, sedimentation rate and clotting times will be collected by the technician.

(*ii*) Blood specimens obtained from venous puncture for chemical tests or grouping. These specimens may be taken by the technician or the nurse may be required to obtain the blood. The rules vary in different hospitals, but in many places all specimens requiring venepuncture have to be collected by a medical officer, to minimise the risk of damage to the vein and consequent formation of haematoma. Some large hospitals appoint a trained nurse as a 'bleeder'.

(*iii*) Specimens collected by the nursing staff in the course of normal routine. Urine specimens (ordinary or catheter), stools, sputum, vomit, or discharge from a sinus are placed in special clean containers provided by the laboratory. If bacteriological examination has been requested there will be a sterile container or a 'throat' swab will be used. In domiciliary practice the patient provides a boiled medicine bottle, the cork of which has also been boiled.

(*iv*) Specimens obtained as the result of some surgical procedure. This includes all specimens of tissue removed at operation, pus obtained from an abscess when it is incised or aspirated, swabs of discharge from urethra, vagina or rectum obtained through an endoscopic instrument. The nurses' motto here must always be:

'What has been removed, must be preserved.'

General rules

The nurse has special duties in relation to these four groups.

(1) When a test has been requested, care must be taken to see that the patient is not

allowed to go to another special department or be absent from the ward until the specimen has been collected.

(2) When blood specimens are to be collected by venepuncture, the nurse must provide a tray containing swabs, a dry sterile 10-ml syringe with at least two disposable needles, a piece of rubber tubing to act as a tourniquet, and some skin antiseptic (methylated ether is preferable as it dries quickly and does not contaminate the specimen). Venepuncture sometimes produces a haematoma unless pressure is *maintained* for a minute or so after the removal of the needle. Some tests are performed on plasma or whole blood which is prevented from clotting by a small quantity of oxalic acid, citrate or sequestrene provided in the container. The majority of blood tests are performed on serum and the blood for these must not therefore be received into a container in which there is some anti-clotting chemical. All blood specimens must be dispatched to the laboratory at the earliest possible moment. If they are left in the warm ward atmosphere for more than a few minutes changes may take place which completely invalidate the pathological test.

(3) All specimens of excreta or discharge (urine, faeces, sputum, vomit, etc.) must be sent to the laboratory immediately after collection. The same urgency applies to all forms of throat swabs in order that the specimen may not become dry by evaporation. Delay leads to death of delicate bacteria or parasites and to chemical changes in the specimen from bacterial decomposition.

(4) If at any time during her normal duties the nurse notices something abnormal, such as blood in a sputum mug, urinal, or bedpan, the specimen must be saved so that part of it may be sent to the laboratory for examination if the medical officer so desires.

(5) All containers should be clearly labelled with the patient's name and the name of the ward. To send an unlabelled container to the laboratory, even if it is accompanied by a completed request form and sent by hand, is courting disaster. The nurse sometimes forgets that the pathology laboratory is frequently overburdened by urgent requests from all wards. Many tests take several hours to complete and it is therefore imperative that specimens should be sent as early as possible each day.

(6) When the investigations have been completed, the pathologist's report will be sent to the ward and it is the duty of the nursing staff to see that this report is attached to the patient's notes.

Owing to the danger of infective hepatitis and its easy transmission, there will be special rules for the collection and delivery of blood specimens from patients suspected of having infective hepatitis, or of being carriers. There are very rigid rules for handling such specimens in laboratories (page 162).

Preparation for investigation, and special methods

Many tests require no preliminary preparations on the part of the nursing staff. Others require several hours' or even several days' preparation and standing instructions will usually be available in every ward for the direction of the nursing staff. The technique for some pathological investigations varies from centre to centre, and the exact preparation depends upon the technique adopted by the pathologist concerned. The usual preparation and procedure so far as the ward is concerned is given in relation to some of the more common tests undertaken on surgical patients.

Sputum

If a specimen is to be sent to the laboratory for bacteriological examination, it must be specially collected and the patient must be instructed to spit into the special carton or container only material which he feels he has coughed up. He therefore needs to be provided with an ordinary sputum mug or second carton into which he may eject saliva from time to time. Needless to say, no antiseptic must be added to this specimen. Such an apparrently obvious instruction needs to be given to any out-patient who is asked to produce a specimen. If the examination is specifically for tubercle bacilli, and no suitable sputum is obtained, a Ryle's gastric aspiration tube is passed before any food or drink is taken in the morning: 20 ml of saline are injected into the stomach and re-aspirated. Swallowed tubercle bacilli are often recovered in this way.

Tubeless analysis

The 'Diagnex' test is dependent on the absorption of azuresin taken by mouth and affected by hydrochloric acid in the stomach. The by-product appears in the urine and colours it blue. Detailed instructions will be given for each test. The nurse's duty is to be accurate with the recording of the time at which the granules are given, and urine passed. All urine specimens must be saved. If no blue dye is passed the patient has achlorhydria.

Urinary tract tests (see Chapter 35)

Renal and bladder function tests involve accurate collection and measurement of urinary output and this is a ward responsibility.

Tests for gastric secretion

In the study of digestive disorders, especially if peptic ulcer is suspected, the acid-producing function of the stomach is determined by passing a naso-gastric tube and aspirating the secretion of the stomach at regular intervals and after various stimulants have been applied. Previously 'gruel' and alcohol were used to provoke the flow of secretion.

Two tests are in common use to assess the volume and strength of hydrochloric acid. When the tube is first inserted 50 cm from the front teeth (to a point between the single and double rings on the tube), the resting juice is withdrawn and its volume measured.

In the **histamine test**, after a further 4×15 minute samples have been withdrawn, a subcutaneous injection of histamine is given (0·04 mg per kg body weight), preceded by 50 mg intramuscular injection of mepyramine maleate to stop the unpleasant side-effects of histamine). Further samples are taken at 15-minute intervals for an hour.

In the **pentagastrin test**, using a synthetic hormone stimulant, sample aspirations are taken before and after injection of 6 micrograms per kg. Pentagastrin may itself induce nausea even when the patient has settled after swallowing the tube, which may be rejected. The patient may faint, from lowered blood pressure.

The **insulin test** is used after vagotomy has been performed to stop gastric acid production. After the resting juice has been withdrawn, blood is taken for a blood sugar estimation: 0·2 units insulin per kg body weight is given intravenously and aspiration of gastric juice taken half-hourly for 2 hours. A second blood sugar test is taken 45 minutes after the injection. The blood sugar must fall to 2·5 mmol per litre and there should be no acid. The test is based on 'hunger response'—i.e. a low blood sugar producing acid flow.

Blood sugar and glucose tolerance tests

These tests are performed on patients suspected of suffering from diabetes or certain other endocrine conditions. The test is performed in the morning; prior to this the patient must have no breakfast, biscuit, or chocolate, but may be allowed a cup of unsweetened tea.

After the initial blood sample has been taken to determine the fasting blood sugar, a drink is given containing 50 G of dextrose in 100 ml of water. The quantity is appropriately reduced for children. Blood samples are collected at intervals following this drink and the nursing staff will be required to obtain specimens of urine at the end of the first and second hours after the dextrose drink. These specimens must be clearly labelled with the time. The patient is not permitted to smoke during this test and should remain at rest in bed.

Examination of faeces

If blood escapes into the alimentary tract from an ulcer or growth, the evidence in the stools will depend on the site and amount of the haemorrhage. Blood escaping from the stomach or duodenum is digested in the small intestine and blood cells cannot therefore be found in the faeces. A large amount of altered blood makes the stool tarry black. If only a small quantity of blood has been shed, its presence can be detected by special chemical tests. If on the other hand blood is coming from the large bowel or rectum, it may be visible on the stool; cells may be detected microscopically since digestion will not take place. If there is visible blood on the stool, no laboratory test is necessary, but if the blood is associated with the presence of mucus, a piece of faeces 'the size of a walnut' must be sent to the laboratory, care being taken to include the mucus.

If the test is for **occult blood**—that is blood coming from high in the alimentary tract— the patient needs to have a restricted diet for three days before the specimen is sent. No meat may be eaten and soups or meat extracts must be excluded from the diet.

Another common examination is for the presence of amoeba histolytica, a cause of chronic and acute diarrhoea. These amoebae can only be detected if the stool is fresh, and the specimen must therefore be kept warm and sent to the laboratory as soon as possible.

Chemical examination of faeces is carried out in the assessment of digestive function, particularly in suspected pancreatic disease, and the laboratory will indicate how much is required.

Bacteriological examinations are carried out on an ordinary sample dispatched in a sterile jar, or swabs may be taken by the medical officer through a proctoscope or a sigmoidoscope.

A special Cellophane swab is used to take smears from the anus when the presence of thread worms is suspected. The Cellophane is moistened and rubbed over the anal skin and the swab replaced in its glass tube.

Cytology

Malignant disease can sometimes be diagnosed by microscopic examination of cells found in exudates from body surfaces or secretions from organs. Gastric 'washout' fluid, sputum, discharge from the nipple and smears taken from the uterine cervix are all subjected to this examination, but specimens have to be taken for this specific purpose and pathologists provide the necessary apparatus and instructions.

Special 'well women' clinics are now held by local health authorities and in hospitals for routine examination of the cervix to detect pre-cancerous changes in the epithelium. A scraping is taken from the opening of the cervix using a special wooden spatula (Ayre's scraper). The cell films are examined by expert cytologists.

Regular examination of the urine for malignant cells is undertaken in patients who have had bladder growths, or may have been exposed to industrial toxins known to produce such growths (page 707).

Scrapings of buccal mucosa, the lining of the cheek, are taken from babies of doubtful sex. True female cells have a densely staining 'chromatin' in the cell nucleus.

Vaginal smears

Vaginal discharge may be taken by 'throat' swab for bacteriological examination but the findings are then unreliable. Specimens of discharge from the vagina or cervix uteri should be taken by a medical officer using a speculum. Certain protozoa (*Trichomonas vaginalis*) are found in the vagina as a cause of inflammation and the only reliable method of taking a specimen in a suspected case is for a long sterile pipette (Pasteur pipette) to be used through a vaginal speculum. The vulva is cleaned with soap and water, care being taken that no antiseptic enters the vagina; 2 ml of sterile saline are injected into the vault of the vagina with the pipette and aspirated again. The fluid is sent immediately to the laboratory, and if the organisms are present they are seen spinning around in the fluid.

Urethral discharge

If a male or a female has urethral discharge, the main purpose of bacteriological examination is to exclude the presence of gonococcal infection. Specimens taken with a small swab are quite unreliable as the organism is very delicate and difficult to grow on any culture medium. The usual procedure therefore is to make a smear on a glass microscope slide. This may be done by direct contact of the slide with the urethral orifice or by using a probe or moistened throat swab. The film on the glass slide is then dried in the air and sent to the laboratory in a sterile jar. The dead organisms can be seen inside the pus cells.

Pus

If pus from a wound or aspirated from a cavity is to be sent for examination, care must be taken not to contaminate the specimen with antiseptic. A swab is taken from the wound or ulcer immediately the dressing is removed and before any cleaning up is performed. If the pus is collected from an abscess at the time of incision, it should be transferred to the test tube with a Volkmann's spoon (a form of curette), with a syringe or with a scalpel handle. Care must be taken not to contaminate the outside of the tube as this will constitute a danger to persons handling it.

Biopsy specimens

For microscopic examination, small pieces of superficial tumour are sometimes removed under local anaesthetic from the lip, tongue, mouth or perhaps from the edges of an ulcer on the skin. Pieces of tissue may similarly be removed by the surgeon through a proctoscope or sigmoidoscope, from the rectum and colon. These pieces of tissue must be immediately placed in a hardening solution. This is usually a mixture of formalin and saline—formol-saline. Specimens removed in the operating theatre are usually placed in a screw-cap jar with formol-saline or sent direct to the laboratory without the addition of this preservative fluid. The hardening, cutting and staining processes necessary for full microscopic examination normally take 5–7 days. Biopsy specimens are sometimes sent for immediate examination by a special technique; by freezing the tissue with carbon dioxide snow or liquid nitrogen, microscopic sections may be cut at once. This frozen section examination may be used during the course of an operation to enable the surgeon to decide whether a tumour is malignant or not. The whole examination need not take more than 5 minutes.

Great care must be taken of all biopsy specimens as the patient's life may depend on the findings of this examination. During a search for the notes of a patient who underwent an operation for a rare tumour thirty years ago, the author found the cryptic remark entered against the histological examination, 'Specimen lost by porter'!!

15

Radiological Investigation, Procedure and Preparation

The great discovery of x-rays was made by Wilhelm Röntgen in 1895. He was an experimental physicist working in Germany, and he came upon the remarkable properties of penetration possessed by mysterious rays which escaped from a vacuum tube, in which was being studied the passage of high-voltage electric currents. The application of x-rays to medicine was at the beginning quite fortuitous in that Röntgen used his own hand as a test of penetration by the rays and found that he had a picture of the skeleton of the hand. He was awarded a Nobel prize in 1905, and since then the science of x-rays or radiology has entered into almost every walk of life. There are few men and women in civilised countries who have not at some time had an x-ray photograph taken and many of the machines and metals which make up our environment have been inspected by a special x-ray apparatus.

In the early days x-ray examination consisted of a simple photograph which showed up bony structures, areas of the body in which calcium had been deposited and, as clear spaces, those parts of the body which contained air.

As well as affecting a photographic plate, x-rays can be made to illuminate a specially prepared surface so that it emits a visible image of the structure being examined. This fluorescent screen used in a dark room makes it possible to watch the movements of various parts of the body and to study the function as well as the shape and structure of the various components.

Soft tissues such as the stomach and intestine are not visible on x-ray photographs or on the screen except in so far as their outline may be shown by gas contained within them. Certain chemicals, especially those containing barium, bismuth, iodine, bromine or calcium, prevent the passage of x-rays. If a drink containing any of these substances is swallowed by a patient undergoing x-ray examination, the course of the fluid may be studied all the way through the alimentary tract. It is of course necessary to use a compound which when taken by mouth is not absorbed from the intestine. Barium sulphate is the substance commonly used for examination of the alimentary tract.

This technique of examination of organs and body spaces by contrast media has been greatly extended and it is now possible to inject substances containing iodine, which are harmless to the body and yet are passed rapidly by the kidney, in such concentration that the outline of the kidney pelvis and the rest of the urinary tract can be seen by x-rays. This procedure is **pyelography** or **urography**. Similarly it is possible to give either by injection or by mouth another preparation which is selectively excreted by the liver and concentrated by the gall-bladder so that the shape and function of the gall-bladder may also be studied. By introducing iodine-containing oily substances into the trachea in such small amounts that there will be no harm to the lungs, the whole of the bronchial tree can be outlined and studied. Various radio-opaque dyes are injected into sinuses and body cavities to determine their extent.

Injection of large amounts of contrast media into the arteries and veins enables a block by arteriosclerosis or thrombosis to be identified, and the vascular pattern of tumours can be outlined: this for instance distinguishes between a cyst and a growth in the kidney. The heart is examined by this means and defects of the valves are detected. The scope of radiological examination is indicated in Table 32 with the special contrast medium used in each procedure.

Air is harmless to tissues unless it enters the blood stream, and as it produces clear areas on x-ray photographs it is injected into the ventricular system of the brain in the search for abnormalities inside the skull. It is used as a contrast medium.

The full and adequate x-ray examination of the patient may be prolonged and tedious. The average patient expects just a simple photograph and whenever possible some indication should be given to the patient concerning the extent of the examination in order that his fullest co-operation may be given.

Organisation

Radio-diagnostic departments, so called to distinguish them from radio-therapeutic departments, are in the charge of radiologists. A **radiologist** is a doctor who has undergone a special training in this science and who usually holds specialist qualifications. He is responsible for the organisation of the department, the examination of patients by the fluorescent screen, for the supervision of special techniques and for making reports on the interpretation of all films taken in his department. The x-ray pictures are taken by technical assistants who are not doctors. These **radiographers** have undergone an extensive training which includes, in addition to their technical subjects, the study of anatomy, physiology, surgery and medicine. The radiographer is also responsible for processing the films.

The majority of patients undergoing x-ray examination as out-patients or in-patients, attend in the radiology department, but patients who are unfit to be moved, such as those who have recently undergone operation, are examined in the ward by a mobile x-ray apparatus. Such an examination is rarely as satisfactory as one carried out in the department, mainly because of the difficulty experienced in putting the patient in the correct position on an ordinary bed. Also, because of their portability, these x-ray sets are not as powerful as those in the department. Occasionally a patient who may seem too ill to leave the ward, will in fact need to be transferred to the x-ray department in order that the examination may be adequate.

Many x-ray examinations are now undertaken during the course of certain surgical operations. The radiographer is then required to attend with a mobile set in the operating theatre, or the operation may be carried out in a special x-ray operating theatre where the more powerful equipment is available.

Although all modern x-ray apparatus has to be shock-proof, care is still needed when x-ray examination is carried out in an operating theatre so that there may be no risk of

Table 32 Radiological investigations

	Procedure	Contrast medium	Route	Part examined
	Plain film (skiagram)	Nil		Anywhere
Cardio-vascular	Arteriography (arteriogram) Phlebography (phlebogram)	Diodone 70% Conray (280) 60%	Sterile injection	Arteries and veins
	Angiocardiography (angio-cardiogram)	Diodone 70% Sodium diatrizoate (Hypaque)	Cardiac catheter through arm vein	Heart and great vessels
Pulmonary	Bronchography (broncho-gram)	Iodised oil (Lipiodol) or Dionosil non-oily	Catheter through nose or mouth; injection into trachea	Lungs
Alimentary	Sialography (sialogram)	Dionosil : iodised oil	Sterile injection into duct openings	Salivary gland ducts
	Barium swallow	Barium sulphate suspension	Drink	Oesophagus
	Barium meal Barium follow-through Barium enema	Barium sulphate suspension Barium sulphate suspension Barium sulphate suspension (probably with tannic acid added, but never if liver damage is suspected)	Drink Drink Enema—tube and funnel	Stomach and duodenum Intestine Rectum and colon
	Gastrografin examination Gastro-conray	An iodine compound Gastrografin Gastro-conray	By mouth or tube	Alimentary tract if ob-struction or haemor-rhage suspected.
	Cholecystography (cholecystogram)	Bioptin, Biliodyl Telepaque (iopanoic acid) Osbil (iobenzamic acid) Biligrafin (iodipamide) Biligram (ioglycamate)	By mouth Intravenous	Gall-bladder Biliary tract if oral has failed
	Cholangiography (cholangiogram)	Diodone, Dionosil	By direct sterile injection at operation through biliary fistula	Bile ducts (after oper-ation)

	Procedure	Contrast medium	Method	Region/Notes
Urinary	Excretory pyelography (pyelogram) (Intravenous—commonly called IVP)	Diodone 30 or 50% Sodium diatrizoate (Hypaque) Sodium acetrizoate (Diaginol) Iothalamate (Conray)	Intravenous sterile injection (intramuscular or subcutaneous with Hyalase)	Kidneys and ureters
	Retrograde pyelography	Diodone 20% Retro-Conray	Ureteric catheter; sterile injection (by cystoscopy)	Kidneys when not adequately outlined by IVP
	Cystography	Conray (280) 60% diluted × 3 diodone 10%	Urethral catheter	Bladder
	Urethrography (urethrogram)	Iodised oil	Injection with Ryall urethral syringe	Male urethra
Central nervous system	Ventriculography (ventriculogram)	Air	Ventricular puncture via skull burr holes or as introduced via lumbar puncture	Brain ventricles
	Myelogram (spinal radiculography)	Iodised oil, Myodil, Dionosil	Lumbar puncture	Spinal canal
Miscellaneous	Salpingography (salpingogram)	Iodised oil, Myodil, Dionosil	Sterile injection into cervix via special catheter	Uterine tubes
	Gynaecogram	CO_2	Sterile injection into peritoneal cavity through abdominal wall	To outline pelvic organs for ovarian cysts etc.
	Sinography (sinogram)	Iodised oil, diodone and Dionosil	Direct sterile injection	Any sinus or fistula
	Arthrography (arthrogram)	Air: diodone or iodised oil	Sterile injection	Joints
	Tomography (tomogram)	Nil		Especially the thorax: technique to determine the depth of a shadow in a thick part of the body
	Stereoscopic films	Depending on part to be examined		Twin pictures viewed in special projector to give three-dimensional perception

explosion: inflammable anaesthetic agents should be avoided. Ideally all persons who might be exposed to irradiation should move away from the operating table or be protected by a radio-resistant apron.

Complications of x-ray examination

There are fortunately very few hazards. Most of these are due to sensitivity of the patient (allergy) to one of the contrast media, especially those which contain iodine. Such compounds are used for bronchography, pyelography, sialography, and blood vessel investigations.

Any patient liable to asthma, hay-fever, urticaria, or any other clearly allergic disorder, may be particularly liable to such a reaction and the facts must be brought to the notice of the x-ray department. Injection of an anti-histamine drug may then be prescribed.

When any such investigations are taking place, equipment for resuscitation must always be at hand. Oxygen, adrenaline, hydrocortisone, Piriton injection and two sterile syringes with the necessary needles and antiseptic must be available. The reaction is shown by sudden collapse, sometimes with a preliminary warning of twitching or sneezing. Fortunately this complication is rare, but it has often been fatal. If the patient shows any sign of reaction, intravenous Piriton (10 mg) is given immediately if no previous anti-histamine was used. Intravenous hydrocortisone (100 mg) is held ready and given if the condition deteriorates.

Barium investigation of the alimentary tract sometimes leads to gross constipation, due to impaction of the barium substances in the large bowel. If a barium enema has not been satisfactorily evacuated before the patient is returned to the ward (this is determined by x-ray screening), an enema should be given on the same day.

It is widely known that x-rays have a damaging effect on tissues if used in excess and repeated radiographic examination of one part of the body may have very serious effects. X-rays affect the ovary and testis and produce sterility. They damage the bone marrow and produce anaemia. They damage the skin and produce burns and cancer of the skin which does not develop for many years. The effect of repeated exposure to x-rays accumulates and so may not become apparent for a long time after the exposures have finished. Radiographers and others working in the department, where they may be exposed to repeated doses of x-ray, undergo regular routine blood examinations to guard against the risk of anaemia. X-ray departments and examination rooms are specially screened to prevent the scatter of rays through the walls or doors. Such insulation is of course much more necessary with radio-therapy plant where the output of rays is very much greater. The radiologist or surgeon who is repeatedly examining patients with a fluorescent screen, wears special gloves impregnated with chemicals which will prevent the passage of x-rays on to his hands: he wears also a protective apron.

A single x-ray exposure may damage a very early fetus and a 'ten day rule' is now applied to all female patients of reproductive age to reduce the risk of irradiating a pregnancy. The clinician who requests the x-ray examination has to be certain of the date of the first day of the patient's last menstrual period and this is recorded. Abdominal x-rays will only be undertaken in the first 10 days. The clinician may indicate that the rule does not apply, e.g. children, post-menopausal patients, x-rays of skull or chest. As the rhythm of menstruation is sometimes disturbed by illness or operation, co-operation of nursing staff in noting the onset of a period is vital. Patients who have been on oral contraceptives for more than three months or who have an intra-uterine device in position are regarded as 'safe', but all patients must be questioned closely about this.

The occasion of an x-ray examination should always be noted in the ward record so that it is recalled if any fever or untoward reaction should occur.

In some hospitals an additional precaution is taken in asking the patients to sign a form of consent to special x-ray examination. Although this may seem to be a wise precaution, it is not universally adopted. The disadvantage is that it adds to the patient's anxieties by putting the idea into his head that something may go wrong.

Preparation for x-ray examination

It is the nurse's duty to ensure that the patient is ready for examination at the appropriate place and time. The part to be x-rayed must be completely freed from clothing. In-patients for examination of the chest or abdomen are usually sent to the x-ray department wearing nothing at all except a special full-length gown which ties up behind and has no buttons. The necessity for this divestment should be explained to the patient by the nurse. If it is not carried out, difficulty is almost certain to arise in the x-ray department and delay will occur while the patient is being undressed.

For radiological examination in cases of emergency, there can be no long-term preparation of the patient. **All adhesive strapping (or traces of it on the skin) must be cleaned off and safety pins removed from any bandages or dressings.** Blood-soaked dressings should be changed immediately before the examination. A nurse should be in attendance during the examination in order to attend to the patient's needs and to help in the movement of any injured part.

Apart from these routine items which must be attended to in all cases, special preparations are necessary in certain x-ray investigations, particularly in those of the alimentary tract. These are given below, though they may vary in detail in different hospitals.

Barium examinations of the alimentary tract

Before a **barium meal** the patient must be starved and allowed *nothing* to drink for 6 hours. If there is to be a 'follow-through' examination of the intestine the patient must take no food for 12 hours prior to the x-ray, in order to reduce the bulk of intestinal contents.

Before a **barium enema** the patient is usually given a Veripaque enema (Table 10) or a high colonic washout before the examination. If this is not done and the patient is sent to the department with a loaded colon, the introduction of the barium enema will not be tolerated. Bisacodyl (Dulcolax) suppositories may provide an adequate evacuation and avoid the dangers of colonic washouts, but the radiologist's wishes must be sought in the preparation.

Cholecystography. The usual routine is a normal early supper. Only water may be taken subsequently and the Telepaque dye tablets are given at 9.00 p.m. Nothing further is given by mouth except a cup of black coffee or tea without milk for breakfast. If food *is*, it is likely that the gall-bladder will contract if it is normal, and the dye will be expelled before the x-ray examination has taken place. A mistaken diagnosis of non-functioning inflamed gall-bladder may then be made.

A fatty meal is required during the examination and the patient is therefore asked to take with him a drink of milk and some thickly buttered bread and cheese. A synthetic meal is sometimes supplied by the x-ray department, but by this time the patient is usually very hungry and a meal must be reserved for him in the ward.

If inadequate information is given by oral cholecystography because the gall-bladder fails to concentrate, **cholangiography** follows, using intravenous injection of iodipamide (Biligrafin), which shows the bile ducts.

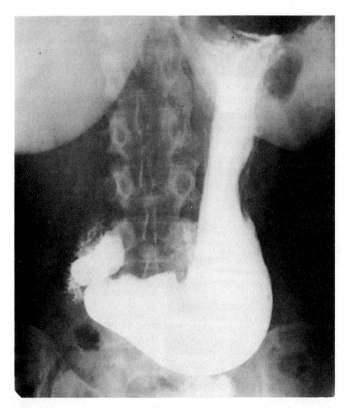

Fig. 15.1   Barium meal. The contrast medium outlines the stomach, pylorus and duodenum.

At operation Conray, diodone or diatrizoate is injected by fine catheter into the bile duct to reveal obstruction or prove that the duct is clear. This is an **operative cholangiogram.**

Excretion (intravenous) pyelography. Two main principles govern the patient's preparation. First the accumulation of gas in the intestine may obscure the kidney shadows. The patient therefore takes a laxative (2 cascara tablets) on the second night before the examination. He is kept up and about as much as possible. Pyelograms on bed-patients are rarely satisfactory because of the accumulation of gas. Some radiologists use an injection of pitressin or pituitrin before the examination to help expel the flatus.

Second, in order to obtain a good concentration of dye, the patient must be producing a concentrated urine. He must therefore drink nothing for at least six hours before the examination. His bladder must be emptied before he is sent to the x-ray department. Conray (meglumine iothalamate) or other iodine containing compound solution (Table 32) is injected intravenously in the x-ray department.

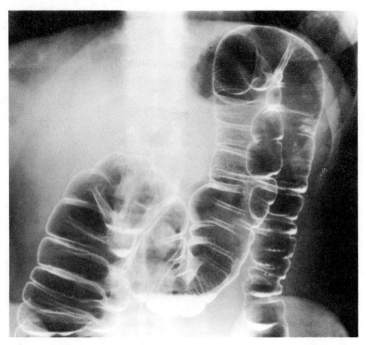

Fig. 15.2   Air contrast barium enema. The barium suspension has been run into the colon and after full screen examination the patient evacuates the enema: the colon is then inflated with air, the adherent barium thus outlining the mucosal folds to reveal ulceration or growth. This film shows the transverse colon with hepatic and splenic flexure.

An additional technique where renal function is poor is to give an intravenous infusion of approximately 100 ml 50 per cent diatrizoate in 100 ml 5 per cent dextrose or normal saline. By induced diuresis this large volume speeds up the excretion of dye.

Angiography. The introduction of dye into an artery, a vein or a lymphatic vessel is a surgical procedure and has to be performed under full operating theatre conditions.

Arteriography is used in the investigation of arteriosclerosis or suspected aneurysm, for instance in the brain or abdominal aorta. By **phlebography** the venous system can be outlined to detect thrombosis, or in the leg deep communication of varicose veins. By

lymphangiography the lymphatic vessels and glands into which they drain can be outlined and this may be helpful in the detection of secondary deposits from malignant disease.

Arthrography. Skin preparation may be requested to reduce the risk of infection.

Cystography. A Foley urethral catheter with 5-ml balloon is passed and the bladder filled with radiopaque solution: catheterisation may be undertaken in the ward and the catheter strapped in position. The bladder is examined by 'image-intensifier' apparatus and perhaps a ciné record taken to show bladder function.

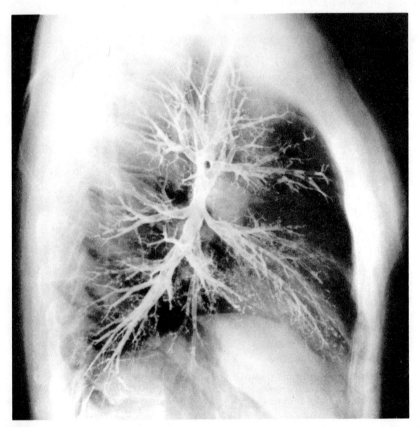

Fig. 15.3 Bronchogram. Iodised oil has outlined the trachea and the right bronchial tree (lateral view).

Myelography. Full preparation as for lumbar puncture is required (page 863). The opaque dye shows the roots of spinal nerves and whether there is a block in the fluid pathway.

Salpingography is a special gynaecological procedure requiring operating room facilities.

Sialography to reveal the salivary ducts in parotid and submandibular glands involves injection of viscous dye into the duct orifice.

Ventriculography (page 865). Preliminary burr holes in the skull are made as an operative procedure.

If these examinations take place in a ward or operating theatre, the nursing staff will be responsible for providing the contrast medium for injection and for the necessary sterile syringes and apparatus.

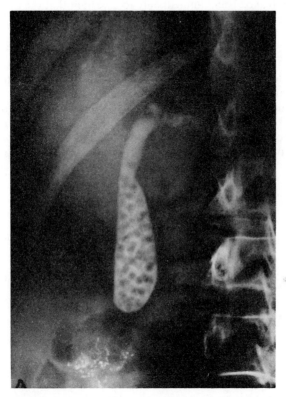

Fig. 15.4 Cholecystogram. The contrast medium, taken by mouth, has been absorbed and excreted by the liver: the dye has concentrated in the healthy gall-bladder in which can be seen clear areas representing stones, two of which are in the cystic duct at the top.

It must be remembered that x-ray examination is expensive; it is an additional item of worry to the patient; it occupies time and may necessarily delay treatment. Inattention to pre-x-ray preparation on the part of the nurse will therefore waste time, money and effort, as well as causing disappointment to the patient and dismay to the x-ray department. On the other hand, in spite of all preparations some investigations are a failure or may have to be repeated in order to obtain satisfactory results.

Ciné radiography and video-recording

During such x-ray investigations as barium meal examination of the stomach or pyelography, observation of the movement of organs is very important. In cardiac catheterisation procedures, the passage of dye through the chambers of the heart is too rapid for recording single pictures. A ciné record of the screen examination can be taken and examined repeatedly and in slow motion. Modern image-intensifier x-ray apparatus records the image on video tape at the same time as the observer watches the 'television' screen. The picture can be 'played back' immediately to ascertain that the examination has been adequate, and the tape forms a permanent record for comparison with later examinations.

Advanced techniques

A new technique of examination has been devised using x-rays to produce a three-dimensional 'shadow' type picture of the body which shows not only the bony structure but details of size and shape of the soft tissue organs. Initially this method has been applied to the skull and provides accurate localisation of brain disorders. A total body EMI scanner utilising this technique has now been manufactured but has not come into general use owing to its extreme cost.

16

Ward Equipment

The care and maintenance of the furnishings and equipment of a ward is essentially a nursing duty. Hospital equipment of all types is invariably of high class and very expensive to replace. Much of it is metal and therefore noisy in use: much of it is easily damaged by thoughtless or ignorant handling.

The nurse must understand thoroughly the purpose of all special apparatus: she must know where to find it, how to fix it up, how to sterilise it (if necessary) and how to clean it. She must return it to the correct place after use, and if it is unserviceable it must be replaced.

The design of all types of equipment is directed to produce an article which is:

(a) Completely safe. Faults of design or manufacture may lead to disaster.
(b) As comfortable as possible when it is something to be used personally by the patient.
(c) Easy to clean and free from inaccessible crevices. This applies with equal importance to the design of a milk jug and of a commode.
(d) As durable as possible. Apparatus which is continually going wrong is dangerous because of its unreliability. A faulty ward refrigerator or a hand-lamp with too short a flex, each constitutes a real danger to the patient.

It is not intended to give a full account of the innumerable items essential for adequate equipment for a surgical ward. Rather is it desired to point out the main features and uses of some of the basic items of equipment.

Hospitals in Great Britain all have central sterile supply services (page 311) and only rarely is any item of equipment sterilised at ward level. The use of disposable single-use syringes is universal. The nurse will receive instruction in the correct use of the particular CSSD, and the central service is responsible for 'topping up' supplies daily.

Ward design

While many wards used for surgical patients have been specifically designed for the purpose, there are unfortunately a great many hospitals where the surgical accommodation has been adapted from wards which were nothing more nor less than dormitories.

Each unit, in addition to providing well-spaced accommodation in an open ward, may have single or double cubicles for patients requiring isolation. The original purpose of the single side-room was to provide more suitable accommodation for the very ill patient requiring almost continuous nursing; it so happened that such a patient was frequently also a source of infection which would constitute a danger to patients in the open ward. Times have changed, infection is less prevalent, and the shortage of nursing staff has meant that in most circumstances it is better for the very ill patient to be in the open ward where he can be easily observed without requiring the sole attention of one nurse.

In addition to the sanitary annex, bathroom and ward kitchen, there is a surgical dressing-room to which patients are brought for their wound dressings. Such a dressing-room is essential for an ophthalmic ward and for a children's ward. In the former to provide for adequate lighting and delicate treatment: in the latter to avoid the curious or frightened gaze of other children. In most general surgical units however the dressing trolley is taken to the patient's bedside and the dressing-room is merely a preparation and sterilising room.

Many wards are subdivided by high partitions. This increases the bed accommodation by allowing centre rows and diminishes the risk of droplet infection spreading from patient to patient.

Furniture

Modern hospital furniture is mostly metal. Older-type wood furniture needs to be scrubbed regularly. The introduction of Formica plastic locker and table tops has eliminated the necessity for locker mats or detachable glass tops which are always liable to harbour the dirt.

All wheeled furniture requires regular attention in order that the fluff may be cleaned from the spindles and wheels. Bed and trolley castors should be oiled regularly unless they are of the sealed ball-bearing type which are packed with lubricant grease and require no attention in this respect. Broken castors should be reported as they damage the floor.

Beds

The modern hospital bed has a solid base and simple foam mattress which does not dip in the centre. It is adjustable for height, which makes it adaptable for patients of different build. Particularly the aged find it difficult to get into a high bed; people with stiff hips find it difficult to get out from a very low bed. The Ellison King's Fund bed is coming into general use and can be fitted with orthopaedic frames, side rails and an adjustable head rest (Fig. 16.1). A more sophisticated type of bed for intensive care in post-operative patients is the Manulift bed, the sectional base adding more adjustment of position. This also can be fitted with an orthopaedic over-head frame (Fig. 47.15). The advantages of a fully adjustable bed are that the patient can be tilted in either direction, and can be so adjusted that he will not require any foot rests or shoulder pillows. Both head and foot ends can be lifted off for intensive care or anaesthesia. Large wheels make moving the bed easy, but there must be a braking device to prevent the bed slipping away when the patient is getting in or out.

For patients who are nursed on the old-fashioned bed with spring under-mattress, solid fracture boards are necessary to place under the top mattress in order to give stability for those patients who are being nursed with extension apparatus or have injuries to the spine. Similarly bed elevators or blocks to raise either end of the bed are necessary with the old-fashioned bed.

In hospitals that are not equipped with modern furniture, work can be greatly reduced by the choice of a suitable height bed for a particular patient and by the use of a self-lifting pole at the head of the bed so the patient can to some extent lift himself.

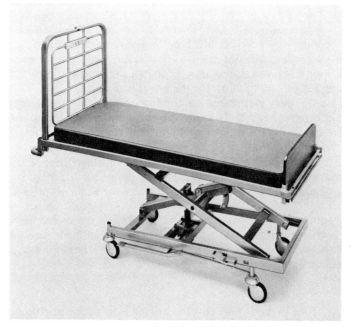

Fig. 16.1   The Ellison King's Fund general-purpose bed. Note the rigid base, detachable head and headboards giving ready access for resuscitation: variable height and tilt: large wheels with brake. (George Ellison Ltd.)

Bed blocks of various heights are available for lifting the foot of the bed in cases of shock, following lumbar puncture, for postural drainage and most commonly to prevent the propped-up patient from sliding down the bed. On certain occasions it is necessary to block the head end of the bed. Some hospitals have bed-tilting frames for the foot of the bed. A chair or wooden stool serves perfectly well in an emergency. Fracture beds usually have extending legs which may be pegged in position to eliminate the need for high blocks when the weight of the body is used for counter-traction.

Iron frames with wheels—**bed-jacks**—can be attached to the head and foot of the bed to facilitate transport to the operating theatre or other department.

Mattresses

The majority of hospital mattresses are made of hair and covered with strong ticking. The complete mattress can be sterilised by baking in a special steam oven. Some hospitals use detachable linen mattress covers over all their mattresses. Most wards have several rubber foam mattresses (Dunlopillo) for patients in whom pressure sores may be likely to develop. The very heavy and the very thin, the unconscious and the incontinent are particularly liable to develop such pressure sores. Rubber mattresses in their waterproof covers cannot be damaged by urine or faecal contamination. They are, however, apt to be rather hot for the patient because there is no ventilation. Excessive perspiration (and therefore increased risk to the skin) can be avoided by an adequate thickness of blanket on top of the mattress. The rubber covers of special mattresses can only be sterilised by wiping with antiseptics or fumigating with formalin or ethylene oxide. The frequency and necessity for sterilising bedding depends very much on local circumstances and local ideas.

Divided or sectional mattresses are used on fracture beds and for paraplegic patients (paralysis following fractured spine) in order to provide access to pressure areas without the patient being rolled, and to allow for the use of bed-pans.

Polyether plastic foam mattresses are coming into general use. They are cooler and very light. No turning is needed. They are, however, inflammable and if they burn, very toxic fumes are emitted. Other types of foam that comply with safety regulations are available.

The 'ripple mattress' (Fig. 45.16) is an air mattress in which there are two sets of small pockets. These are inflated alternately by an electric pump, ensuring that there is a constant change of the weight bearing area, to avoid pressure sores in paraplegic, elderly or very thin ill patients.

A 'water' bed[1] in which the patient lies on a taut Nylon sheet stretched across a tank of water kept at body temperature is used to nurse especially difficult paralysed or deformed patients, in particular those who have already developed a large pressure ulcer. Healing is greatly accelerated.

Bed rings

The purpose of the orthodox air cushion or ring is to allow the patient's weight to be spread around the buttocks, rather than taken on the ischial tuberosity. Bed rings are either inflatable or made of latex foam rubber. The aim of nursing should be a repeated change of the patient's position by his own activity or by being turned, and bed rings should therefore be used as little as possible.

Bed cradles

These are used to keep the weight of the bedclothes from the patient's legs. The ideal form of cradle is one which extends the whole width of the mattress and does not interfere with the movements of the legs. The method of arranging the bedclothes over the cradle depends on the circumstances. If the cradle is being used in the post-operative management of a lower limb amputation, the end of the cradle must be left open so that the stump bandages may be watched. For patients who are unconscious for a long time, the toes must be supported to prevent 'foot-drop'.

[1] Aquadorm, Medical Supply Assoc.

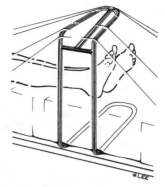

Fig. 16.2   Light-weight bed cradle to permit free movement of the feet and thus reduce the risk of calf vein thrombosis.

Toilet equipment

The importance of the patient's personal hygiene has already been stressed. Frequently the patient's greatest distress occurs over the use of bed-pans, and his inability to make the necessary journey to the privacy of the toilet. In recent years, patients are allowed out of bed within a day or so of operation. In the majority of surgical wards many patients are now able to visit the sanitary annex and do not require bed-pans. The accommodation is often totally inadequate. Constipation following operation and a period in bed is in itself liable to lead to the passage of a large hard motion and to the development of an anal fissure. This is much more liable to happen if the patient's visit to the toilet is hustled. The wheeled commode chair (Fig. 16.3) and the introduction of curtain partitioning in wards enables the patient to be delivered from the discomfort and insecurity of the bed-pan, and avoids the very real risk of the visit to the toilet annex being hurried. A bed-pan slides in beneath the orthodox toilet seat. Unless very carefully cleaned these commodes are a source of cross-infection; the fact that the bed-pan is disposable gives a false sense of safe hygiene.

The addition of large wheels as on a self-propelled chair is a great asset in convalescent or long-stay units. The patient can slide off his bed on to this chair (the arm is detachable) and wheel himself to the toilet annex: the closet doors need to be wide enough for him to reverse the chair over the pan. The independence of the patient not only gives more confidence, but eases the tasks of nursing.

Bed-pans are of various types and shapes and the only suitable material is stainless steel. Rubber bed-pans are occasionally used for incontinent patients and remain in position for long periods. Enamel bed-pans should not be used because they are difficult to clean when chipped. Disposable reinforced paper bedpans are increasingly used.

The ward annex may be equipped with an apparatus for cleaning bed-pans. Very few wards have **bed-pan sterilisers** though many are fitted with an automatic apparatus in which the pan is placed and washed with hot water under pressure. This type of bed-pan washer must not be confused with the true bed-pan steriliser in which the pan needs to be left under steam pressure for several minutes (page 302). Many hospitals use disposable bed-pans and have an installation for macerating the material which is channelled through the sewage system.

Urinal bottles for male patients are made of glass, earthenware, or unbreakable plastic polypropylene. Paper composition urinals are used in units having a disposable bed-pan installation. Each ward annex should have a hot water jet nozzle over which each non-disposable urinal can be held for washing, and some means of sterilising must be available, either by chlorine solution, Cidex, or heat.

A bed urinal may be used for a female patient who is unable to lift herself (for instance one in a plaster bed). One type has a long handle which allows the patient to be independent of nursing help. Other types of urinal are coming into routine use to replace the bed-pan in female wards.

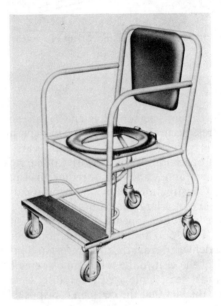

Fig. 16.3   Modern commode chair. For use with bed-pan or placing over the normal w.c. pedestal (Fig. 51.5). (G. McLoughlin & Co. Ltd.)

Treatment room

The ideal arrangement is for patients accommodated in open wards to be moved in their beds or chairs to a special room set aside for dressings. If such provision is not available the necessary equipment has to be wheeled to the patient's bedside, curtains drawn round the bed and the whole procedure carried out at some distance from the dressing store. This method has two disadvantages, one is the time taken to transport the necessary equipment and in many cases repeated journeys to fetch items which have been forgotten! Second, the drawing of the curtain around the bed creates a dust storm which encourages the spread of infection.

Two entirely separate systems are still in operation for the provision of dressings and relevant equipment. Modern hospitals depend entirely on the central sterile supply department (CSSD) which produces individual packs delivered to the ward wrapped in sterile paper or cloth. With this system there is no steriliser in the ward and all the items used are either disposable—to be thrown away—or are returned to the central depot for cleansing, sterilisation and re-issue. This system involves considerable storage space and very careful stock replacement to make certain that everything that is likely to be required on a particular ward is in fact immediately available.

The alternative system still in use in many hospitals where modern equipment has not yet been installed depends on the individual preparation of dressing trolleys for each patient. This work is undertaken by the ward nurses in a preparation room or sometimes even at the end of a large ward. Unless there is a CSSD service two sterilisers are necessary, one for small instruments and one for bowls and basins. These are electrically heated with an automatic cutout to prevent them boiling dry. In the dressing preparation station in, or adjacent to, the ward, trolleys are swabbed with Sudol or other antiseptic and the equipment for use at the patient's bedside is placed in order on a sterile paper or cloth sheet (depending on the particular system in use).

The Central Sterile Supply System is outlined on page 311.

Some hospitals combine the two systems, maintaining an individual instrument steriliser on each ward for certain specialised equipment and depending upon the central sterile supply for the majority of items. It is of course essential for the nurse to learn methods of sterilisation and preparation for dressings as the ideal Central Sterile Supply System is by no means universal.

Methods of sterilisation are described in Chapter 17. Each hospital will have its own particular schedule for the method of sterilisation to be applied for individual items of ward equipment.

Face masks. Masks are in fact sterilised by ordinary laundry processes but are taken from the ward container by unsterile hands. They lose protective value if worn for more than half an hour, or when they have been 'adjusted' with unclean hands. Although masks may not necessarily be worn for all dressings, disposable paper 'use once' masks are on hand for special cases or barrier nursing.

Ward oxygen equipment

Oxygen may be supplied in cylinders of various capacities each mounted on a stand with a pressure-reducing valve through which the flow rate is also controlled (Fig. 16.9). In many hospitals oxygen is now supplied to several bedside points in wards and to the operating theatres by pipe-line from a liquid oxygen store (Fig. 16.11).

Oxygen is used in the treatment of shock, and in the management of patients with respiratory or cardiac insufficiency. Oxygen administration by a funnel is useless: it is also dangerous since it gives the staff and patient a completely false sense of security. The purpose of oxygen administration is to achieve a concentration of oxygen in the air passages much higher than that of the atmosphere.

There are three main methods of administering oxygen which are fundamentally different in principle.

The first principle is to provide a stream of pure oxygen which is fed into the air passages through a special tube or mask. The flow is continuous, under very low pressure, and the oxygen is mixed with atmospheric air inhaled with each inspiration. During expiration, the oxygen flow is dispersed by the outgoing air. It must be administered through a proper fitting mask or by means of nasal catheters. Figure 16.4 shows a single effective apparatus. Sometimes a spectacle-frame type of fitting is used.

There is a risk that the patient may receive too much oxygen and not get rid of his CO_2. Also, his air passages become very dry. To overcome these difficulties a mask with a reservoir is used so that the patient rebreathes a mixture of expired air and oxygen. This conserves moisture. Lightweight polythene 'bag' masks (Fig. 16.8) are available which incorporate the principal features of the old type BLB mask which had a reservoir bag attached. The soft plastic transparent double pocket has a flexible wire in its upper border

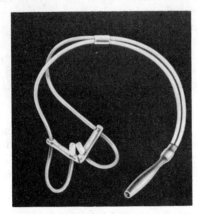

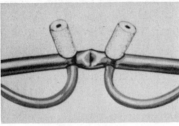

Fig. 16.4 Meredith oxygen cannula. Least frightening for the patient, safe and secure: double nasal catheters held in the nostrils by the rubber retaining strip which is guided to rest across the upper lip: the stream of oxygen is effective by entering the nasopharynx even if the patient breathes with open mouth. (Eschmann Bros & Walsh Ltd.)

and this is moulded around the patient's nose. Oxygen is fed into the bag between the two pockets. The inner pocket has two small holes which allow partial rebreathing into the bag while the exhaled air mostly escapes through two holes in the outer pocket. No humidifier is required and the flow is adjusted so that the bag is inflated during each expiration. The merit of this type of mask, in addition to its great comfort, is that it is inexpensive and can be destroyed after use; therefore no sterilisation problem is involved. As oxygen is very often needed after surgical operations for pulmonary infection the risks of transferring infection with other apparatus which cannot be autoclaved are thus eliminated.

The **Ventimask** (Fig. 16.6), which is a rigid plastic dome fitted over the mouth and nose, provides a reservoir from which excess expired air and oxygen escape through perforation in the dome. Moisture is retained in this way and further humidification is not needed. The oxygen concentration is regulated by the size of perforation in the mask, and three standard types are supplied.

The second principle is to place the patient in an atmosphere in which the oxygen percentage is raised. This is achieved by means of the oxygen tent (Fig. 16.10), or, in the case of a baby, by an incubator (Fig. 22.1) or an oxygen box. By this method the patient's respiration is unimpeded by the presence of masks and he is not disturbed by a nasal catheter. The method is of course more cumbersome, takes longer to apply and is only suitable for cases where oxygen treatment has to be continued for several hours or even days. The nursing of the patient is made more difficult, and in surgery the use of the oxygen tent (apart from its application in the surgery of infancy) is confined almost entirely to severe post-operative pulmonary or cardiac conditions. Patients who have had severe

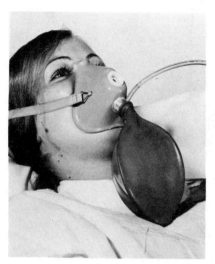

Fig. 16.5   Porton, similar to the former BLB re-breathing bag.

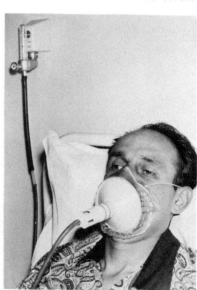

Fig. 16.6   Ventimask.

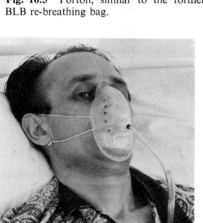

Fig. 16.7   Harris disposable rigid polythene mask which is very simple and compact.

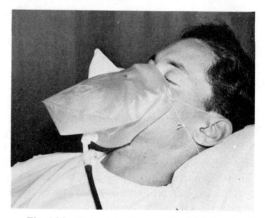

Fig. 16.8   Oxygenaire Pneumask with inflated cuff to conform to the patient's face.

operations on the chest, either for lung or heart disease, may be nursed in an oxygen tent or maintained on a respirator (see later) for the first few days following operation.

The third principle is the use of oxygen in combination with artificial respiration. This most commonly applies in the operating theatre where natural respiration is deliberately stopped by the use of drugs administered by the anaesthetist, in order that controlled rhythmic inflation of the lungs can be carried out. In certain conditions, paralysis of the mechanism of respiration occurs quite apart from operation. Poliomyelitis and myasthenia

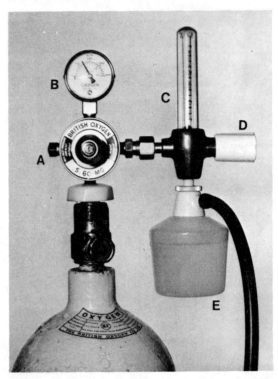

Fig. 16.9   Mobile oxygen unit. **A.** Pressure-reducing valve. **B.** High-pressure (cyclinder content) meter. **C.** Flow meter. **D.** Fine adjustment regulator. **E.** Nebuliser cup (e.g. for humidification or inhalation with antibiotic). (British Oxygen Co.)

gravis are two such conditions. Artificial respiration (page 178) can be carried on in various ways, manually or by mechanical ventilation (page 186).

Whichever method of oxygen administration is used, great care has to be exercised. Fire risk is greatly increased where there is a high oxygen concentration and no smoking can be permitted under any circumstances in the vicinity of an oxygen apparatus. Accidents have occurred with fatal results through another patient inadvertently approaching an oxygen tent while smoking a cigarette. Confused patients have even been known to reach out for a cigarette and strike a match, with disastrous results. Metal and clockwork toys, and torches, used by children in oxygen tents, have produced explosions.

Long-term administration of oxygen—that is through nasal catheters, mask or oxygen tent—requires also some control of humidity to prevent excessive drying of the lungs. In the nasal catheter method, oxygen is bubbled through a bottle of water, the humidifier, which may also act as a flow meter. With the plastic disposable mask the presence of the reservoir bag, by conserving some of the expired air, maintains the humidity: the use of an additional bubble-bottle may be dangerous as excessive water vapour will condense in the bag. The oxygen tent has attached to it an apparatus which controls humidity and temperature. Because of the increased insulation of the tent, the atmosphere needs to be cooled and a special ice-box is attached to many models.

Large-capacity oxygen cylinders are used, mounted in a trolley stand *to which a spanner key is tied*: the spanner is for tightening the regulator valve on to a new cylinder: the key is for controlling the flow tap.

The use of pressure-reducing regulators, humidifiers, and flow meters is described on pages 365 et seq. The identification and care of cylinders is described on pages 215 and 364. The ward nurse must be completely familiar with such apparatus: unlike the theatre nurse she will not be able to turn to the anaesthetist or theatre orderly in a crisis when oxygen is wanted.

Instructions for the use of oxygen tents

The tent itself is made of a transparent tear-resisting material, held above the patient by a metal support, draped round the bed and tucked in firmly under the mattress so that there is no leak. Oxygen is fed to the tent from a bedside cylinder supplied with pressure-reducing valve and regulator. The apparatus is so designed that the atmosphere in the tent circulates through the cooling chamber which also removes excess humidity. The rigid box-type of tent used for infants has a hinge-lid and stands on the cot mattress. It requires no cooling apparatus and the temperature is maintained by a hot-water bottle placed in a special rack: frequent changing of this is necessary.

The rate of flow of oxygen in tents varies, according to the requirements, between three and six litres a minute.

The following warnings must be observed in connection with tents:

(a) Before the patient is installed in an oxygen tent, the purpose should be explained carefully to remove anxiety and to obtain co-operation. Some patients feel quite unable to tolerate the 'shut-up feeling' of being in a tent.

(b) In no circumstances should oil or grease be used on the regulator, cylinder valve or any part of the tent equipment.

(c) Oxygen will not burn by itself but accelerates combustion of other items and a spark may cause a fire.

Therefore when an oxygen tent is used:

(i) It must be kept at a safe distance from open fires and naked flames such as spirit lamps.

(ii) No smoking on the part of staff or other patients must be allowed anywhere near the tent.

(iii) Electrical apparatus should not be used inside the tent. No electrical bell push, bed heater, inspection lamp, or radio equipment should be allowed. With children, great care must be taken to exclude all metal toys, especially those which may make sparks.

(iv) The patient should not be rubbed with oil or spirit whilst in an oxygen tent. If such treatment is necessary, the oxygen flow must be turned off and the tent temporarily removed.

Occasionally analysis of the air inside the tent is required to determine the oxygen concentration. This procedure requires special apparatus: It consists of a 'probe' sensor attached by a flexible wire to a small meter which gives a direct reading of the oxygen concentration.

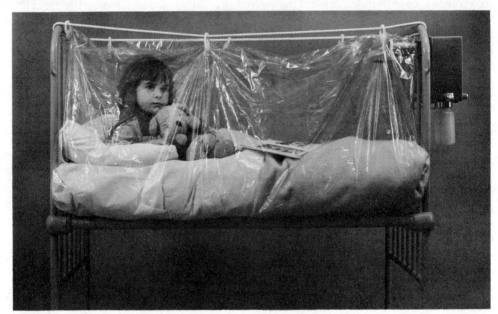

Fig. 16.10 Oxymist oxygen tent for use on a cot. A mist-producing unit is attached for humidification. Mechanical toys which might produce sparks should not be permitted. (Vickers Ltd., Medical Engineering)

Oxygen box incubator

This apparatus is used in the management of premature babies. Sometimes it is necessary in connection with the surgery of the new-born child (Fig. 22.1).

Suction

Modern units are provided with piped suction similar to the oxygen supply (Fig. 16.11). This provides for two types of vacuum, high and low. High is used in the ward for clearing secretions from the respiratory tract or vomit from the mouth. Low suction is used for continuous drainage, e.g. wounds and bladder. Low-pressure suction is provided by an electric pump such as the Robert's pump; high-vacuum suction can be provided by a device attached to the oxygen supply. The 3-bottle method of drainage for low-vacuum continuous drainage is described on page 663.

Atomisers

The simple spray used for applying anaesthetic solutions or antiseptics to surface tissues is a familiar part of ward equipment. This type of spray is however quite unsuitable for the administration of penicillin by inhalation, in the treatment of lung infections.

Antibiotics and 'detergent' chemicals which reduce the stickiness of respiratory tract secretions are administered with a nebuliser which is usually incorporated with some form of oxygen apparatus (Fig. 16.9E).

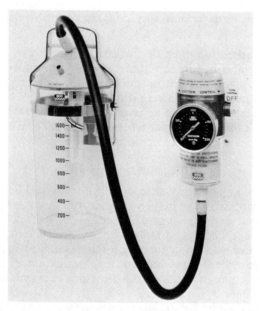

Fig. 16.11   Piped oxygen supply for suction. (British Oxygen Co.)

Emergency resuscitation equipment

Apparatus for cardiac massage, for resuscitation in shock and for dealing with asphyxia, needs to be instantly available in every ward. The occasions for its use will be discussed in other sections.

The essential equipment must include:

(1) Bed blocks.
(2) Emergency intravenous injection tray, which must be kept in the poison cupboard and used for no other purpose. This tray must contain:
   2 sterile syringes (2 ml)
   6 injection needles (2 each sizes 12 and 18 hypodermic and No. 1 serum)
   antiseptic (spirit or iodine), swabs
   2 each of ampoules for injection containing:
      adrenaline hydrochloride
      neostigmine
      digoxin
      nalorphine (Lethidrone)

hydrocortisone 100 mg (powder in ampoule to be dissolved with water for intravenous injection)

hydrocortisone 100 mg in 20 ml 50 per cent ethyl alcohol for use in infusion solutions

(3) For respiratory obstruction:

Equipment as in Fig. 16.12 including simple provision for positive pressure respiration (Ambu bag, Fig. 16.13; Brook airway, Fig. 10.5).

Sterile tracheostomy set (instruments and tubes), **including scalpel** (also page 803)

(4) Oxygen equipment, set up for emergency use as above, with Ventimask or Tudor Edwards apparatus.

It cannot be emphasised too often that when an emergency occurs from such conditions as pulmonary embolus, coronary thrombosis or respiratory obstruction, there is neither time nor staff to allow for a treasure hunt while the necessary apparatus is gathered together. Seconds, not minutes, lie between death and survival.

Warning.—Oxygen apparatus must never under any circumstances be connected to an intratracheal anaesthetic tube or to the side tube of an airway. There is no escape for the air, and over-inflation of the lungs leads to immediate death.

Diagnostic equipment

Gathered together on a large tray or separate trolley should be the various pieces of equipment which the medical officer may require in routine examination of the patient.

There are two general methods adopted by medical officers for conducting routine full examination of the patient. The first is to start with the head and proceed to the neck, chest and abdomen: the upper and lower limbs are then examined and finally the patient is turned on the left side with the knees drawn up for examination of the pelvis by palpation through the vagina or rectum. In addition the patient may be examined standing on a clean towel placed upon the floor by his bedside.

The variation on this method of examination is for the medical officer to concentrate on one system of the body at a time. For instance, he will examine the nervous system completely, working through the pupil, arm, abdominal and leg reflexes and investigating the skin sensation all over the body. The cardiovascular system may be examined separately —heart, peripheral circulation, blood pressure, and exercise tolerance tests.

The main items are enumerated in the order in which they are usually required in the course of examination.

Ward diagnostic tray

Torch. The requirements of a good torch are that it should shine the right type of light in the right place at the right time! Like all electrical diagnostic apparatus it should be tested daily by one member of the ward staff. The bulb and lens system must be such as to shed an even light. The type of torch which shows an irregular shadow and the outline of the filament is quite useless. Spare batteries must be available in the ward cupboard and a spare bulb for this and all other electrical lights on the trolley should be kept in a special box with this diagnostic apparatus.

Tongue depressor or spatula. Adequate examination of the pharynx is difficult with a straight tongue depressor and a metal angled one is very much better. Strips of white lint 12 × 5 cm, the corners rounded and each strip folded at its centre, are used to grasp the tongue during the examination of the mouth. Sterile throat swabs in tubes are at hand in case they are wanted at this stage.

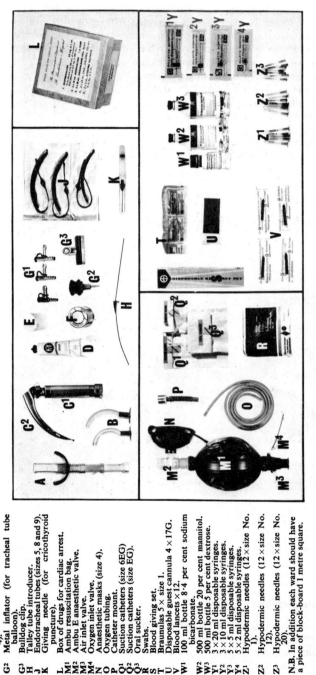

KEY

A   Brooke airway.
B   Foregger airways (sizes 2 and 3).
C^1 Laryngoscope and
C^2 detachable blade.
D   Tube of KY jelly.
E   2·5 cm cotton bandage.
F   2·5 cm waterproof strapping.
G^1 Cobb's suction unions (sizes 2, 3 and
     4).
G^2 Metal inflator (for tracheal tube
     balloon).
G^3 Bulldog clip.
H   Talley tube introducer.
J   Endotracheal tubes (sizes 5, 8 and 9).
K   Giving needle (for cricothyroid
     puncture).
L   Box of drugs for cardiac arrest.
M^1 Ambu resuscitation bag.
M^2 Ambu E anaesthetic valve.
M^3 Air inlet valve.
M^4 Oxygen inlet valve.
N   Anaesthetic masks (size 4).
O   Oxygen tubing.
P   Catheter mount.
Q^1 Suction catheters (size 6EG)
Q^2 Suction catheters (size EG).
Q^3 Oral sucker.
R   Swabs.
S   Blood giving set.
T   Braunulas 5 × size 1.
U   Disposable guest cannula 4 × 17G.
V   Blood lancets ×12.
W^1 100 ml bottle 8·4 per cent sodium
     bicarbonate.
W^2 500 ml bottle 20 per cent mannitol.
W^3 500 ml bottle 5 per cent dextrose.
Y^1 3 × 20 ml disposable syringes.
Y^2 3 × 10 ml disposable syringes.
Y^3 5 × 5 ml disposable syringes.
Y^4 5 × 2 ml disposable syringes.
Z^1 Hypodermic needles (12 × size No.
     1).
Z^2 Hypodermic needles (12 × size No.
     12).
Z^3 Hypodermic needles (12 × size No.
     20).

N.B. In addition each ward should have
a piece of block-board 1 metre square.

Fig. 16.12 Resuscitation equipment. Every ward has an emergency pack kept in a prominent position and containing everything necessary for the immediate treatment of collapse and respiratory failure. A typical schedule of equipment is illustrated here.

The patient's dentures should not be removed before the examination commences as the doctor will wish to see whether they fit correctly. A mug or dish must be handy into which the patient can then place the dentures. Nothing is more calculated to produce embarrassment to the patient, than a hurried search for a handkerchief in which to eject his teeth.

Thudicum speculum and head-mirror for examination of the nose.

Electric auriscope with two sizes of speculum.

Ophthalmoscope. Examination of the fundus of the eye is not always satisfactory unless the pupil has been dilated previously by atropine drops. These may be prescribed and a later examination of the fundus carried out.

Stethoscope.

Sphygmomanometer with an additional small-size cuff if children are in the ward.

Patella hammer, tuning fork, card of pins and pieces of cotton wool for examination of the nervous system.

Tape measure for neck, chest expansion, abdominal distension and limb lengths.

Receiving dish for the dirty speculum and tongue depressor.

Skin pencil.

Length of soft rubber tube (60 cm)—for tourniquet in varicose vein testing.

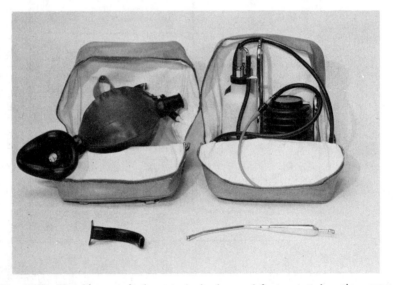

Fig. 16.13   Portable resuscitation set. Ambu bag and foot-operated suction pump.

Pelvic examination tray

'Pelvic examination' consists of a visual inspection of the perineum and a good light is essential: a bacteriological swab will be taken if there is vaginal or urethral discharge.

Disposable polythene gloves which can be used on either hand are preferable to rubber finger cots, but the latter should also be available, with paper cleansing tissues and a lubricant jelly (which should be self-sterilising). For the initial examination of new patients the following items are required:

>**Proctoscope,** preferably with self-contained light and battery box, or fibre-light source.
>**Non-toothed dissecting forceps** longer than the proctoscope.
>**Sim's vaginal speculum.**
>**Small cotton wool pledgets** for inserting through the proctoscope.
>**Large receiver** to take the soiled proctoscope or speculum.

Apparatus for special examinations

Sigmoidoscopy. This is a diagnostic procedure which can readily be carried out in a patient's bed. If a considerable amount of abdominal surgery takes place in the unit, the ward will have its own sigmoidoscopes (page 573) or will be supplied by CSSD (page 311).

Lumbar puncture. This is a common aseptic diagnostic procedure for which the apparatus needs to be specially prepared. It is described on page 863. In a neurosurgical ward, several complete sterile sets will be held.

Other surgical equipment

In a hospital in which the various special departments of the surgical division (page 6) have their own ward units, each will have apparatus designed for its particular work. In many hospitals the general surgical wards also accommodate patients under the various special departments. Whatever the organisation, the overlap between the requirements of the various specialties and general surgery is such that the basic equipment in all surgical wards, except perhaps those of the ophthalmic and throat departments, needs to be fully comprehensive.

These appliances may be grouped for convenience according to their use.

For gastro-intestinal conditions

>**Stomach tube** (wide bore).
>**Naso-gastric disposable tubes** (various).
>**Senoran's stomach pump** (Fig. 26.5).
>**Gastric aspiration tubes** (Ryle's).
>**Duodenal and intestinal aspiration tubes** (Miller-Abbott, Cantor; Figs. 24.5 and 24.6).
>**Anal dilators-metal conical** (page 557).

For Urological conditions (see Chapter 35)

>**Full range of urethral catheters,** plastic or latex, ready sterilised.
>**Bedside urine drainage bags.**
>**Straight and Y Nylon connectors** of various diameters.
>**Rubber drainage tubing and plastic tubing.**
>**Bladder syringe.**
>**Wardill's urethral syringe.**
>**Riches-Dukes type irrigator and stand.**
>**Tidal drainage apparatus with manometer and U tube** (Fig. 35.18) or proprietary Cystomat pack.
>**Suction apparatus** (Wangensteen gravity bottles or Robert's silent electric bedside pump).

There are various forms of suction pumps and whenever suction is used on drainage tubes there must be an air-leak or valve which prevents an excessive negative pressure; otherwise tissues get sucked into the mouth of the tube, which is then firmly plugged.

Splints, extension apparatus, and other orthopaedic equipment

This will depend on the amount of orthopaedic surgery undertaken by a particular unit. All wards require simple straight arm splints (used for intravenous infusion).

Fracture boards, where solid base beds are not provided.
Bohler-Braun leg cradle splint for support and elevation. The leg slings may be made of canvas or strips of flannel bandage (page 45).
Thomas 'knee' splints with **Pearson bent knee attachments** (Fig. 47.10) **and foot-piece** (Fig. 47.9) and other traction splints.
Extension cord, weights.
Splint clips.
Extension spreaders.
Extension adhesive strapping (the type commonly preferred is Elastoplast extension strapping which is rigid lengthwise but stretches sideways and is therefore moulded easily to the contours of the limb).
Overhead extension frame or Balkan beam with pulleys (Fig. 47.15).

Many hospitals have a splint room in which all this apparatus is kept and items are withdrawn by the individual wards when occasion demands. The use of this apparatus is described in Chapter 47.

HYPODERMIC EQUIPMENT

The term hypodermic embraces all procedures involving skin puncture whether in treatment or for diagnostic purposes. 'Hypodermic injection' is sometimes used to imply the same meaning as 'subcutaneous' injection, and because of the general customary use of the word hypodermic it is preferable to specify **subcutaneous** when it is intended that an injection should be given in the tissue immediately underneath the skin.

Perhaps the most frequently used surgical instrument is the hypodermic syringe. Injection equipment is often the least cared for and the most out-of-date apparatus in the ward's inventory.

Disposable syringes

Most hospitals now use factory sterilised disposable syringes. These are made of plastic with a rubber piston and are thrown away after one injection. For convenience and saving of labour they are excellent, but the piston does not move very freely and they are unsuitable for all purposes. Needles are packed separately, each in a plastic tube, sizes identified by colour code. Care must always be taken to ensure that the needle and butt of the syringe escape contamination by contact with the unsterile outside of the packet. On no account should a syringe or needle be used if the pack has been damaged in any way.

In many countries the repeat-use syringe will remain in general use for economic reasons, though it is now generally accepted that all needles should be of the disposable type, used once only.

Disposable syringes are available with various capacities, 1, 2, 5, 10 and 20 ml. Special syringes are available for particular purposes such as Mantoux testing where minute quantities of fluid have to be injected into the skin. Similarly, syringes are available marked with insulin unit dosage. The needle mount may be central or eccentric.

Special-purpose syringes

Syringes for special procedures such as paracentesis or the injection of haemorrhoids may still be kept in individual wards or departments, but in most hospitals these are supplied as individual items from a Central Sterile Supply and have been autoclaved in single unit packs; they are not disposable.

Many of the special-purpose syringes have glass barrels with individually matched glass pistons. These are sterilised by dry heat. Very few procedures now require the use of the original glass barrel and metal piston-type syringe; those used for the injection of haemorrhoids are still of this type (Fig. 16.14). The solution injected for the treatment of haemorrhoids is phenol in oil, which is self-sterilising and it is, therefore, not so important that the syringe itself should have been autoclaved.

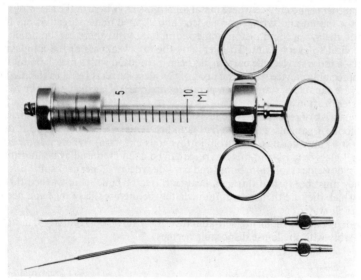

Fig. 16.14   Gabriel's haemorrhoid injection syringe with bayonet fitting needles: 5 or 10 per cent phenol in oil is used, and a lock-on needle is essential to withstand the pressure. A finger-grip wing on the barrel screws off to allow withdrawal of the barrel for cleaning. This syringe does not require autoclave sterilising as there is never any withdrawal of infected material into the syringe; it is only used for a phenol containing oil. Note the shoulder on the needles. This enables the surgeon to gauge the depth to which he has inserted the needle and to prevent excess penetration. The shoulder blocks the needle entrance point and prevents the immediate leak back of oil as it is being injected beneath the mucosa of the rectum. The angled needle is shown with its cleaning wire in position: the needle must be washed through with really hot water, autoclaved or chemically sterilised; it is not disposable. (Seward Surgical Instruments.)

To be satisfactory, 'non-disposable' hypodermic equipment needs to fulfil certain conditions.

(a) It must be robust and able to stand repeated and sometimes unskilled handling, without leakage, deterioration, or failure.

(b) It must be capable of rapid and complete sterilisation.

(c) It must be easily cleaned and readily prepared for re-sterilisation.

(d) As far as possible the various component parts should be interchangeable and standardised.

(e) It must be provided in sufficient quantity for the work to be carried out without lowering the standards of asepsis.

Sterilisation

Almost all commercially supplied disposable hypodermic equipment has been sterilised by gamma radiation. When a hospital has a syringe service of its own, autoclaving is the usual procedure—or the use of a dry oven.

For non-disposable syringes there is no doubt that the all-glass syringe is the safest pattern. It is lubricated with silicone and sterilised by dry heat or autoclave.

The weakness of the all-glass syringe is that the tip is readily broken. The great advantage of this type is that there is no crevice where metal joins glass anywhere in the assembly. The whole of the inside of the mount and syringe can be seen and cleaned under direct vision. If the piston is withdrawn and the syringe and piston immersed in antiseptic, there can be no doubt about the access of chemical to every point. To overcome the one weakness of the all-glass syringe—the brittle mount—a more serviceable pattern has been introduced with a metal mount for the needle: there is no appreciable crevice where the neck of the glass barrel is fused to the metal mount, and these syringes are capable of standing temperatures up to 250 °C, which is far above that necessary for absolute sterilization.

The principal risk of repeat-use syringes is the transmission of virus hepatitis from contamination by the blood of patients who have had jaundice. This can occur if blood is drawn into the syringe (i.e. testing on entering a vein from intravenous injection). Where it is necessary to re-use syringes, the all-glass or glass-and-metal syringe can be safely sterilised by boiling and then storing in glutaraldehyde (Cidex) solution, borax and paraldehyde, or 75 per cent spirit. If needles have to be re-used they must be washed through, heat-sterilised or boiled and washed through with the antiseptic in which they are then stored. Immediately before use the syringe and needle have to be rinsed with sterile water.

An individual patient requiring self-administration of drugs regularly can adopt this procedure, preferably with single-use disposable needles.

Needle mounts and adaptors

Size. The tip of nozzle of syringes varies in size and type of fitting. There are two sizes in common use. The **record** fitting is smaller; it is tapered and for many years has been the standard in general use. The **Luer** fitting has now been adopted as standard for all types of injection and infusion equipment. It is slightly larger than the record fitting and there will naturally be considerable confusion during the change over in the hospital service. The Luer fitting has been standard in America for many years. The difference in size is sufficient for the types to be easily recognisable.

Position. There are two positions for the tip. The central position is used on all small syringes while 5, 10 and 20 ml syringes are commonly supplied with an eccentric nozzle which simplifies intravenous injection. Where possible the eccentric type is therefore provided for venepuncture, for the withdrawal of blood, or where drugs are to be injected into the vein.

Method of attachment. Apart from the differences in size and position there are several varieties of fitting. The standard **taper** fit is not safe if very viscous or oily substances are being injected under considerable pressure. Even with thin watery solutions, it is not uncommon for the needle and syringe to part company and for the drug to be spilled. Various forms of locking device have been employed.

The **bayonet fitting** is standard on most syringes and needles used for injection of oily substances. It is found therefore on the Gabriel haemorrhoidal syringe used for phenol-in-oil injection treatment of piles.

The **'cam' fitting** is found on some haemorrhoidal syringes and outfits designed for the infiltration of solution into the tissues for local anaesthesia. The Labat syringe of the continuous-flow type is usually supplied with this fitting. A screw-on needle mount is fitted to some infiltrating syringes.

It is obvious that all such fittings require that the special needle should be available for use with the particular type of syringe.

The **Luer-lock** type and the needles for this pattern can be used on the ordinary taper Luer fitting. Although the Luer-lock mount on the syringe is more difficult to keep clean, it is a simple and safe method of attachment, and the inside of the injection channel is in fact free from crevices. Its great merit is the interchangeability of its needles with the ordinary standard syringe.

Special adaptors for matching varying types of syringe to special forms of needle and manometer are again usually prepared by the central sterile supply or syringe service, and the responsibility for ensuring complete sterility in this equipment usually lies with the hospital bacteriologist; the nursing staff is not involved.

Injection needles

These can be grouped into three main types:

(a) Hypodermic needles are fine needles used for subcutaneous, intravenous and intramuscular injection where free-flowing fluids are being given. These are described officially as being in the hypodermic range and the standard numbers are 0, 1, 2, and then 12 to 20; 0 is the thickest. 1 and 2 are identical in gauge but of different lengths and the nurse need not bother about the differences between these first three sizes. 20 is the finest with a standard length of 20 mm ($\frac{3}{4}$ in.). No. 12 has a length of 32 mm ($1\frac{1}{4}$ in.) and is a size in common use. There are many needles which do not comply with the special standards of length.

(b) Serum needles. These are thicker and more robust and are used for deep intramuscular injections, for the taking of blood from a vein if more than 5 ml is required, and for aspirating cysts or abscesses. The serum needles are numbered in Roman numerals O to VI, O being the thickest. Various lengths are supplied. Figure 16.15 gives a selection of standard sizes referring to thickness in particular.

(c) Special needles—usually of extra length, more flexible or with special mounts. Some of these are illustrated in Fig. 16.16. There are many patterns.

Needles and cannulae used for intravenous infusion are described on page 142.

Some of the special needles, for instance those used for entering the pleural cavity

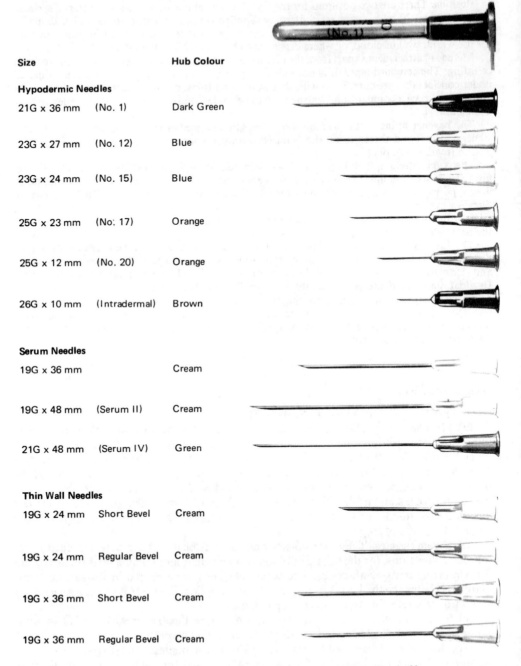

Size		Hub Colour
Hypodermic Needles		
21G x 36 mm	(No. 1)	Dark Green
23G x 27 mm	(No. 12)	Blue
23G x 24 mm	(No. 15)	Blue
25G x 23 mm	(No: 17)	Orange
25G x 12 mm	(No. 20)	Orange
26G x 10 mm	(Intradermal)	Brown
Serum Needles		
19G x 36 mm		Cream
19G x 48 mm	(Serum II)	Cream
21G x 48 mm	(Serum IV)	Green
Thin Wall Needles		
19G x 24 mm	Short Bevel	Cream
19G x 24 mm	Regular Bevel	Cream
19G x 36 mm	Short Bevel	Cream
19G x 36 mm	Regular Bevel	Cream

Fig. 16.15   Examples of needles in common use. (Gillette Surgical.)

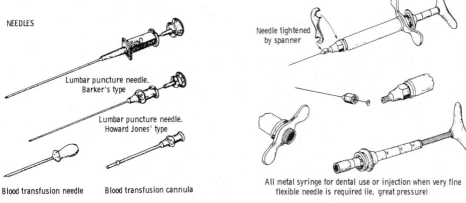

NEEDLES

Lumbar puncture needle.
Barker's type

Lumbar puncture needle.
Howard Jones' type

Blood transfusion needle   Blood transfusion cannula

Needle tightened
by spanner

All metal syringe for dental use or injection when very fine
flexible needle is required (ie. great pressure)

Fig. 16.16   Standard patterns of lumbar-puncture
needle: blood transfusion needle and cannula.

Fig. 16.17

(for pneumothorax or paracentesis) and those used for lumbar puncture, have a short bevel and a stilette which exactly fits the lumen of the needle. This strengthens the needle during its introduction and prevents the entry of any tissue into the narrow lumen as the needle is advanced. The head of the stilette has a locating pin to ensure the correct position of its bevel at the needle tip.

(d) Dental (Schimmel) needles. In dental surgery and sometimes in the injection treatment of birth marks, specially fine flexible needles are used. These have the Schimmel fitting, in which the small metal needle mount is compressed against the end of the syringe tip by a screw attachment. The needle is thrown away when it has been used once as the mount is destroyed in the fitting process.

Figure 16.18 shows a dental syringe with which disposable glass cartridges containing anaesthetic solution are used. The needle for this type of syringe has an extension inside the butt of the barrel and this pierces the bung in the cartridge when the piston is pushed home.

The care of needles

The amount of pain produced by an injection depends far more on the sharpness of the needle than on its size. Nearly all needles used in wards and out-patient departments are supplied sterile in plastic covers and are thrown away immediately after use. There are, however, many diagnostic procedures and special treatments which require the use of needles of a particular design. The maintenance of these needles may be undertaken by the syringe service of CSSD or by the ward staff where these special items are used. It is therefore important to know something of the requirements in the care of these needles.

Under no circumstances must a needle which has been damaged be used again. There are three points at which damage commonly occurs. First, the mount may be bent or distorted by careless previous use: it will not make a correct watertight seal with the syringe. Second, where the blade or needle shaft joins the mount, the needle may fracture. Very stringent tests are applied during manufacture to lessen these risks and the modern needles are much more flexible. Third, the point or bevel may become burred. The usual way in which the point develops this 'hook' is by its being stubbed against the bottom of a glass ampoule or solution bottle, inadvertently scraped on the side of a sterile dish, or dropped into a pot of antiseptic.

One of the great advantages of the fully organised syringe service is that every needle is tested individually by someone specially trained for the task.

After use, a syringe should be immediately rinsed and the water ejected through the needle. All needles which have been used should be put in a separate container and not returned to the sterile storage cabinet or jar. Once a day these needles are again syringed through and if necessary unblocked with cleaning wires. The nurse who performs this task must have a good light and inspect the inside of each needle mount to make certain that it is free from blood. A dirty mount is cleaned with a nail-brush. After thorough inspection and cleaning, the point of each needle is tested by drawing it across a piece of cotton wool to make quite certain that the point is not hooked. In the organised syringe service, blunt needles are re-sharpened by grinding and polishing but this is not a practical proposition for a small unit or department.

If during use or cleansing a needle shaft is severely bent, the needle should be thrown away to avoid the risk of fracture during subsequent use.

It should not be necessary to store needles with cleaning wires in place: occasionally short sections of cleaning wire, being left in the needle, have been injected into the tissues.

On every occasion the patency of the needle must be tested before the injection is given. This can be done without loss of any of the injection. The same rule must apply before any attempt at aspiration or venepuncture, and tests must be done likewise even on factory sterilised disposable needles which may sometimes be found blocked by metal dust.

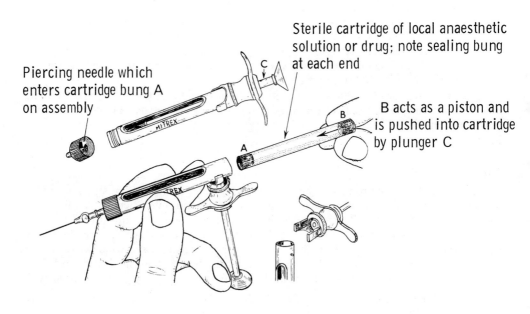

Piercing needle which enters cartridge bung A on assembly

Sterile cartridge of local anaesthetic solution or drug; note sealing bung at each end

B acts as a piston and is pushed into cartridge by plunger C

Fig. 16.18   Cartridge-type syringe.

Warning on the use of disposable equipment

Reference has already been made to the risk of contamination when withdrawing a syringe from a packet which is not in fact sterile on the outside. The majority of syringe packets can be opened by cutting across the plunger end and withdrawing the syringe while squeezing the packet from side to side to avoid the needle end touching the packet. After a packet has been cracked or torn on no account must the syringe be used. Disposable syringes after use should be put in special containers and it is advisable to break the piston or the needle butt off the barrel to avoid any possibility of the syringe being used again.

Needles are packed in different ways and are colour coded (Fig. 16.15). Care must be taken not to contaminate the butt of the needle when removing the cap of the tube. If the syringe is filled from an ampoule through the needle which is going to be used in the injection, then it is wise to replace the needle sheath carefully after filling until the moment of use. It is normal practice for injections to be checked by a senior nurse and therefore several minutes may elapse between the checking procedure and the injection. After use the needle should be bent at right angles on its butt by pressure on the side of a dish or some other hard surface to prevent possible second use.

17
Asepsis and Sterilisation

It is difficult to understand, amid the complexity and drama of modern surgery, that just one hundred years ago nothing was known of the significance, nor yet of the existence, of bacteria. John Hunter (1728–93) was a British surgeon who by his methods greatly advanced the pathology and surgical treatment of disease. He introduced the principle of the tourniquet—pressure on the main blood vessel of the arm or leg during an operation, which was usually an amputation: at that time the stumps of the limbs were cauterised by a hot iron or the traditional boiling tar. Hunter and his colleagues were unknowingly using antiseptic methods. Edward Jenner (1749–1823), who was a pupil of John Hunter, again without the knowledge of the existence of bacteria or viruses, demonstrated inoculation against small-pox in 1796. Vaccination was thus established but this had no influence on surgery. There was still no scientific knowledge to associate dirt and contamination with the development of infection in the tissues of the body. One of the earliest records of belief in this association claims that an Austrian doctor, Semmelweiss, with his assistants, washed his hands in chloride of lime solution (akin to Eusol) before undertaking surgical operations. He was dismissed for his stupidity! The American doctor and author Oliver Wendell Holmes (1809–94) also wrote of the association of dirt and disease.

Florence Nightingale (1820–1910) received part of her training in Paris and undoubtedly went to the Crimea War (1854–56) with some conviction that dirt played a part in infection, but still there was no knowledge of the existence of micro-organisms. Later, in his Paris laboratories, Louis Pasteur (1822–95) inaugurated the era of antisepsis by his discoveries that milk and wine were turned sour by organisms from the air. This knowledge was first applied to medicine in relation to rabies. Joseph Lister (1827–1912), an English surgeon, applied Pasteur's discoveries to the surgical wound. Lister became Professor of Surgery in Glasgow in 1860. He insisted on general cleanliness of all apparatus used in the operating theatre and instituted higher standards of sterilisation by using phenol. Upon this foundation of great men has been built a vast and complicated machinery to protect us from the ravages of micro-organisms.

Today, those who enter upon medical science in any of its branches are trained to be constantly and fully aware of the presence and importance of micro-organisms.

Asepsis and antisepsis

Asepsis is the condition of freedom from contamination by bacteria or viruses. Modern surgical procedures are aseptic. They are carried out under conditions in which the apparatus and environment have been rendered free from disease-causing micro-organisms. The personnel prepare and protect themselves so that they will not introduce infection. Asepsis and sterility are equivalent terms for all practical purposes.

Antisepsis is the destruction of organisms in order to sterilise or render an object aseptic.

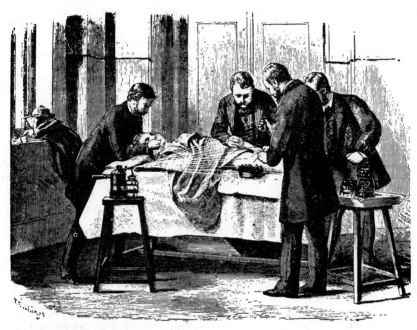

Fig. 17.1   The Lister carbolic spray in use. (Reproduced by permission of The Wellcome Museum.)

An **accidental** wound contaminated by organisms from clothing or from the object which has caused the wound, is treated by antiseptic measures: chemicals are applied to the wound and antiseptic substances (e.g. penicillin) are brought to the wound by the blood stream. A **surgical** wound is made under aseptic conditions: if there is reason to believe that contamination has taken place at the time of operation, antiseptics may be introduced as well. The aim in surgery is that every surgical procedure should be **aseptic**. The skin always contains germs and is therefore sterilised with an antiseptic before it is cut or punctured.

In the past much nursing time was spent in preparation of apparatus and in taking precautions to render procedures aseptic. Today the majority of this labour has been eliminated by the use of prepacked sterilised equipment supplied commercially or by a hospital CSSD. An appreciation of various measures adopted is the central part of a nurse's early training. Learning to live and work in an environment where every move is related to asepsis is a difficult task. Even the most experienced surgeon needs constantly to be vigilant lest he or a member of his team should err and introduce the risk of disaster through infection. Germs are at present everywhere, and in all surgical procedures there is a risk of introduction of organisms from the air. Such a risk is recognised, but the tissues fortunately deal with most of this airborne contamination without it becoming established as an infection. The 'hospital staphylococcus' is however a constant threat by cross-infection. The attack on organisms is threefold:

1. Measures to destroy recognised infection and prevent its spread: the burning of dirty dressings, and the prevention of spread of infection through environment—ventilation, isolation of contacts and other nursing methods (see Chapter 2).
2. Measures to increase as far as possible the patient's natural defence mechanisms so that the consequence of any infection may be limited.
3. Specific sterilisation and antiseptic methods to render everything used in surgery completely free from micro-organisms of any type.

The treatment of a plastic or rubber sheet with Sudol or Dettol illustrates the first of these principles. The sheet is hung on a rail, handled by the nurse and used on the new patient's bed; it is not free from bacteria but has been treated to prevent the spread of disease-causing organisms from other patients for whom it has been previously used. This is the prevention of 'cross-infection'. Asepsis is relative and incomplete in many nursing procedures, but when the skin is to be pierced (for instance, by injection), a catheter passed, a wound dressed or an eye irrigated, asepsis must be complete. Inadvertent contamination may mean that a complete instrument trolley will need to be reset. The nurse will find her conscience greatly tested on such an occasion.

Theoretical perfection and practice

In a busy general hospital with modern equipment the nurses are now taught the latest systems of sterilisation where almost everything requiring sterilising process is treated with a high-pressure autoclave. Supplies of sterilised equipment ranging from sigmoido-scopes to dressing towels and dressing dishes come from a central store whose stocks are being continually replenished from a central sterilising depot. This department is staffed by technicians with special training. In this way the simpler, less effective, sterilising methods in common use in wards are completely eliminated. Bulk supplies of disposable syringes, needles and catheters are sterilised by gamma ('atomic') radiation. Only by such a system can we eliminate almost completely the risk of cross-infection, or theatre infection, by the spores of tetanus and gas gangrene. Everybody who wishes can be protected against tetanus by active immunisation, and if this were done universally it would hardly be necessary to go to the lengths of reorganising hospital sterilisation methods to reduce the risk of tetanus. Gas gangrene organisms almost always come from the patient's own alimentary tract, and the risk of infection from this source is therefore not eliminated by any sterilisation method. It so happens, however, that the centralised system built up on the fear of these two infections is also very efficient and saves an enormous amount of nursing time which can be better utilised. When nurses are introduced to the system they may be puzzled as to how they will manage in domiciliary nursing, or away from centres of organised hospital services. In practice the very much simpler methods of sterilisation which have been used for years (e.g. boiling) are quite adequate if attention is paid to detail, but boiling will not destroy all viruses. It is thus essential that the nurse in training today must still be familiar with the simplest and most effective methods which she herself can apply with a reasonable degree of safety. Experience has shown that industrial disputes may cut power supplies or manufacture of essential goods and shortages of vital items occur for various reasons. A hospital must be able to maintain essential services and a knowledge of the more 'primitive' methods of sterilisation is essential.

Cleaning before sterilisation

All appliances must be thoroughly cleaned as sterilisation processes will not remove dried blood, mucus or other dirt. A wipe and a wash is insufficient; a soak and a scrub is essential. Soap or detergent solutions can be used on almost everything. Household detergents are not normally antiseptic (bacteria-killing) but are cheap and effective. Lissapol or Teepol, which are detergents, are better than ordinary detergent powders for ward-cleansing purposes since they do not contain the artificial frothing compounds present in the powders. Blood-stained linen or instruments can be soaked in such a solution with safety. Cetrimide (Cetavlon) is a powder made up as a solution of 1 or 2 per cent for similar purposes. It is a detergent which is now usually combined with 1 per cent chlorhexidine (Hibitane), and referred to as Savlon.

Brushes used for cleaning purposes (bottle brushes, nail brushes, etc.) must themselves be sterilised repeatedly, preferably by boiling or autoclave. **Nylon brushes must not be allowed to come into contact with phenol solutions or cresol as the Nylon dissolves in these chemicals.** Unfortunately, when autoclaved, Nylon nail brushes become very hard and the 'bristles' may tear the skin.

The majority of apparatus such as rubber, hardware and instruments is cleaned thoroughly after use and stored. The process of sterilisation takes place immediately before use.

Linen is virtually sterilised in ordinary laundering processes by boiling and again by ironing, but it is of course contaminated in the folding and subsequent handling.

Methods of sterilisation

Sterilisation is one of the most important tasks of surgery. Any method to be efficient must fulfil various criteria.

(*a*) It must destroy *all* forms of micro-organisms and their spores.
(*b*) It must not destroy or damage the article being sterilised.
(*c*) It must be simple and easy to apply.
(*d*) It must achieve its object in a definite known time.

Chemical methods depend upon the disinfectant solution reaching the bacteria: crevices and adherent matter on uncleaned apparatus prevent sterilisation by the immersion method. Simple boiling does not destroy spores of bacteria such as gas gangrene and tetanus, but it will do so if sodium carbonate is added to the water to make a 2 per cent solution. Boiling, however, depends upon the sodium carbonate solution reaching the spores as the temperature itself is not sufficient without the added chemical: a piece of rubber tubing firmly fixed to glass may trap such organisms and remain unsterilised.

Moist heat is the most certain method of destroying all organisms and spores if the temperature can be raised to 115 °C (240 °F). In practice this is achieved in steam pressure sterilisation with the autoclave.

In the description of sterilisation methods which follows, emphasis will be placed on the shortcomings of orthodox methods. Simple, safe and economic alternatives are indicated.

Antisepsis by heat

Autoclave sterilisation

The steam pressure steriliser works on the same principle as the domestic pressure cooker. By raising the pressure in the container, the temperature of the steam is also raised. To sterilise the contents of an autoclave, the steam must penetrate every crevice. Just as with the cooker, the air in the autoclave is removed by the first-generated steam, and the valve is not closed until there is a steady hiss of escaping steam. On large autoclaves the air is discharged by vacuum pump before the steam is introduced. The efficiency with which the air is discharged, determines the *real* sterilising power of the steam. A mixture of air and steam is not effective at low pressures.

The next essential is that the steam pressure is maintained for a predetermined safe time to ensure complete penetration of the contents.

Finally the sterilised articles (e.g. gowns or towels) must be dry. Complete drying is ensured by switching off the steam, removing any water that remains in the autoclave and then creating a vacuum. Any moisture held in the sterile material is thus evaporated by the vacuum and the contents are completely dried.

Every nurse should demonstrate this process for herself with a simple pressure steriliser.

Portable autoclaves for standing on a gas-ring or for use with electric heating are available for wards, special departments or private practice. In most hospitals, all auto-claving is undertaken centrally with a large machine equipped with electric vacuum pumps. In some operating theatres the routine instrument sterilisation is also undertaken by pressure autoclaves.

Summarised, whatever the pattern of machine, the procedure follows these steps.

(*i*) Packing.	Drums and loose packages must be placed so that steam can circulate freely round each: nothing must rest directly on the floor of the autoclave which should have a rack across it.
(*ii*) Autoclave door sealed. Heat on. Outlet or vacuum valve open.	Air is thus driven out by the incoming steam or drawn out by vacuum pump.
(*iii*) Outlet or vacuum valve closed. Steam pressure on.	Regulated so that full required pressure is held for the specified time.
(*iv*) Steam off. Outlet valve open to reduce pressure to zero. Water drainage tap opened to drain the chamber. The water tap must be closed immediately.	
(*v*) Vacuum produced for 20 min.	This occurs either from cooling of the closed cylinder or is produced artificially by a vacuum pump.
(*vi*) Outlet valve opened.	To allow pressure to rise to that of the atmosphere.
(*vii*) Unpacking.	Drums closed and sealed immediately.

In modern hospital autoclaves the whole apparatus is worked by superheated steam which has passed through an outer 'jacket'. The makers usually provide, with an autoclave, full instructions for its management and maintenance with details of the temperatures and pressures required.

The temperature actually reached within an autoclave depends not only on the steam pressure but on the amount of air discharge which has been possible before the steam is turned on. The effective pressure will therefore vary with different machines. Average times required are:

Soft goods and instruments including made-up apparatus such as
    irrigators and transfusion sets   .   .   .   .   .   .   25 lb per sq in. for 30 min.
Rubber gloves and latex articles   .   .   .   .   .   15 lb per sq in. for 20 min.
Pressures higher than 15 lb will destroy the elasticity of rubber gloves and make them unsafe, unless the initial air discharge is very efficient. If this is so, a pressure of 20 lb can be used on gloves. Less than 15 lb pressure is dangerously ineffective with the majority of autoclaves.

Except for endoscopic instruments, there are very few articles which cannot be autoclaved or boiled. Solutions for infusion and many glass ampoules containing drugs are also sterilised by autoclaving. The pressure in the autoclave overcomes the pressure within the glass bottle due to expansion and therefore prevents bursting. 'Plastic' goods may deteriorate when heated and should neither be boiled nor autoclaved unless made of heat-resisting material.

Preparation for autoclaving. Nursing staff may well have to make up packs or drums for sterilising in a central depot although in many hospitals all the packaging is done by non-nursing staff. To a large extent the metal sterile drums have been replaced by special wrapping paper through which the steam will percolate. Many depots use nylon film which has the advantage of being semi-transparent: it allows the passage of steam under pressure but will not permit the passage of water or bacteria. It is less likely to be damaged than paper. Even if equipment is supplied to wards in packets these packets themselves have to be placed in drums or other containers for sterilisation. Steriliser drums have perforated panels to allow percolation of the steam. These panels are sealed by a sliding band tightened over the perforations except during the process of sterilisation. Drums must be lined with porous cloth and white lint is normally used for this purpose. The lining should not extend upwards to form a flap over the contents at the top, since this would allow the covering material to fall over the edge of the drum when articles are removed and then to carry contamination back into the drum. The cover should be a simple disc of lint. Paper should not be used as it will stop the free passage of steam.

Linen (towels, gowns) must never be packed tightly: overcrowding means that steam may not reach the centre of the articles and the drying process may be ineffective. Small articles are autoclaved in lint or paper packets, each labelled and tied up. Pins should *never* be used on such packets; they rust and may get among surgical instruments and be lost.

The arrangement of drum contents varies with the unit's particular requirements and different sized drums may be available for different purposes. Gloves should always be packed in separate drums as the autoclaving requirements of pressure and temperature are different for rubber goods.

Autoclaving errors
There are three serious results from bad pressure sterilisation.
(a) The articles emerge damp or wet. This is caused by tight packing, or by insufficient vacuum after the sterilisation process.
(b) Decomposition of rubber goods. This is due to excessive pressure and temperature, with inadequate air discharge. Rubber goods become adherent if not adequately powdered before insertion.

(c) **Incomplete sterility.** This may only be discovered if infection develops in a patient on whom the apparatus has been used. If, however, articles emerge damp from the autoclaving process, it is assumed that sterilisation has been incomplete and the whole batch of drums must be rejected.

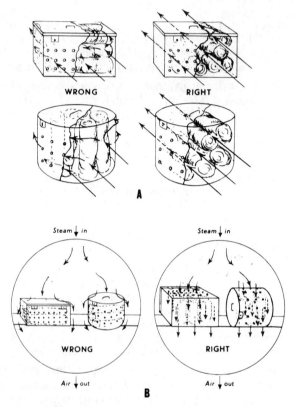

Fig. 17.2 A. Metal sterilising drums, still in use in many places, have an outer sliding metal shield which covers the perforations when sterilisation is complete. Whether in boxes or in drums, material must be packed loosely in such a way that the steam can penetrate freely. Items such as rolled gowns must be placed between the perforations, or vertically in boxes. **B.** When loaded into an autoclave, items again must be placed in such a way as to allow free passage of steam between and through the containers.

Autoclave testing

Regular testing of an autoclave is carried out either by hospital technicians or by the nursing staff. Control tubes which change colour when an adequate temperature is reached are packed in the centre of a specially marked drum. This method is not entirely reliable as the effectiveness of the apparatus depends not only on temperature but on penetration of the steam. Special indicator paper may be used on packages: this changes colour if the correct temperature was attained.

The most adequate method of testing is the insertion of a special packet of test organisms, prepared by the pathologist. Many hospitals arrange for the pathologist to carry out routine checks on all sterilisation procedures.

Boiling

Reference has already been made to the limitations of boiling in the destruction of spore-bearing organisms and certain viruses unless sodium carbonate is added to the water.

Surface sterilisation of steel operating instruments is probably attained in 1 minute after the water boils. Spores are destroyed by 5 minutes' boiling with sodium carbonate. There is no scientific basis for boiling instruments for longer than 5 minutes and nothing further is achieved. The nurse needs however to ensure that the timing is taken from the **point of boiling** and not from the point of immersion of the instruments.

Some simple rules for sterilisation by boiling are:

(*i*) Glass and breakable material must be wrapped in gauze or lint. The wrapping must be secured in such a way that it can be undone without the contents becoming contaminated (i.e. elastic bands are bad). Glassware should be heated in hot water before immersion, or the steriliser should be cooled by the addition of fresh water; small glass articles should be placed in a metal receptacle: large glass vessels should be sterilised alone to prevent impact with other things in the boiler.

(*ii*) All stainless steel instruments should be warmed in hot water immediately before immersion in the boiling steriliser. The sudden change of temperature may fracture the metal.

(*iii*) Needles and sharp instruments should be wrapped to prevent loss or damage.

(*iv*) The heat control is reduced during loading to prevent the nurse being scalded. Containers should be placed in carefully without splashing and those required first placed uppermost. It is ludicrous to have to turn the steriliser contents over like a clothes-wash, in order to retrieve the kidney dish which has been placed at the bottom, beneath all the instruments it is to receive.

(*v*) There is no merit in prolonged boiling and harm may be done to the apparatus.

(*vi*) Detachable scalpel blades, stainless steel scissors and sharp surgical instruments may be boiled with safety but not for more than five minutes.

(*vii*) The heat control should again be turned down while the instruments are being removed.

(*viii*) If the instrument rack is removed from the boiler, it must not be placed on an unsterile surface or on a glass trolley shelf.

(*ix*) Instrument forceps (Cheatle's) used for placing articles *in* the steriliser should *not* be used for removing them *from* the steriliser. Even if the forceps have been returned to a jar of antiseptic in the intervening period, the antiseptic action is not fast enough to sterilise the forceps. Two forceps in separate distinctly labelled jars should be kept beside the steriliser, one 'sterile—for removal only'. If the forceps used for the removal of sterile articles is dropped on the floor or otherwise contaminated, it should be boiled immediately.

Every time an article is placed in the boiler, the rest of the contents must be considered unsterile for a further 2 minutes.

(*xi*) When the sterilisation time is complete, the heat must be switched off.

(*xii*) Unwanted instruments should not be left in the steriliser indefinitely.

In order to obtain the necessary sodium carbonate strength, the capacity of the steriliser must be known and the necessary measure of sodium carbonate powder added each morning. Alternatively a special water jug may be set aside with the requisite stock solution in it for topping up during the day.

Sterilisers require descaling periodically. This is done with weak acid solutions (acetic or hydrochloric), **but under no circumstances must such acid be added when the steriliser is in use.** The steriliser must be washed out very thoroughly after descaling.

Sequestrine used regularly in sterilisers prevents scaling and powdery deposits on the instruments.

Dry heat

Sterilisation in a dry oven—simple baking—is used for substances which must not be exposed to moisture. Paraffin, bone-wax, paraffin-gauze dressings, sulphonamide and other powders are sterilised in this way. Also, syringes and needles, including lumbar puncture needles, are sterilised by dry heat. The syringes are of a special type to resist the high temperature.

The temperature for dry heat sterilisation is 160 °C for 1 hour. Jars, bottles and tubes for pathological specimens are sterilised by dry heat. Powder is sterilised in flat paper packets in amounts of approximately 5 G.

Metal instruments, trays, and lotion bowls are sterilised if autoclaving or boiling is not available, by flaming. A large tray may require 10 ml of methylated spirit. Only small quantities should be used owing to fire risk. The spirit is made to run over the surface to be sterilised and a lighted match applied. Great care must be taken that this is carried out away from towels or curtains, ether or spirit containers. The vessel, if large, should be tilted slightly during the flaming to ensure that the whole surface is scorched. Articles to be flamed must of course be absolutely dry. **More spirit must not be poured on while there is still a flame.**

It must be remembered that room has to be allowed for expansion when sterilising oil or wax, and therefore this cannot be done in sealed tins. A small open tin should be used unless special heat-resisting glass-ware is available. The bottle or tin is closed immediately after removal from the steriliser. Containers must never be filled completely to the brim or the oil will boil over.

Heat-resisting syringes, after thorough cleansing and drying, are lubricated with silicone and assembled. Each syringe is inserted in a special glass tube or metal canister in the bottom of which is a small cotton-wool plug. The appropriate needles are added to the tube. Alternatively the needle is affixed to the syringe before packing. Metal syringe tubes have slip-on caps while glass tubes are covered with brown paper and tied on with string. Reference is made to the sterilisation of syringes on page 292. Needles may be packed in individual tubes.

Chemical sterilisation

Many antiseptics destroy ordinary organisms but very few are effective against spores. It must be clearly understood that the following disinfectants, as commonly used in hospital practice, will not remove the risk of infection by spore-bearing organisms: cresol, phenol, spirit and mercury compounds. **Articles treated by such solutions are therefore only relatively sterile.** Preparations of chemicals recommended for sterilisation are shown in Table 14 and page 94. Chlorine solutions will kill spores and viruses.

Formalin vapour or formalin solution kills spores readily. Borax and formaldehyde solution[1] can be relied upon to destroy all ordinary organisms in 30 minutes' immersion, and spores in twenty-four hours. The borax is added to prevent rusting of the instruments. There is little doubt that this is the solution of choice for all immersion sterilisation. It is cheap and safe for the apparatus and for those who handle it.

For practical purposes, baths, wash-basins, rubber sheeting, ward furniture, bed-steads and lockers, after being cleaned with Sudol (1:20) on a mop, may be considered as sterilised (except for the spores) if the antiseptic has been left in contact with the article for **at least 2 minutes.** Sudol is a cresol-like coal tar derivative which is far less harmful to the skin and is therefore safe. Chloroxylenol (Dettol) is a safe alternative but is slower in its action: 1 in 80 Milton is far better.

The formalin cabinet

This is a gas-tight chamber with perforated shelves upon which are placed catheters, endoscopic bulbs, ampoules and other delicate articles which cannot be boiled. The for-malin gas is derived from paraformaldehyde tablets placed in the bottom of the chamber. The tablets are heated by an electrical element in the base of the cabinet or by a spirit lamp placed underneath. A small cabinet is sufficiently heated by placing it on a radiator. Four hours in strong vapour is regarded as a safe time for absolute sterility, but for most prac-tical purposes 30 minutes is sufficient. Sharp instruments such as knives used in ophthalmic surgery can be sterilised in this way.

Detergents

Fat-dissolving substances are known as detergents. In recent years many of these have come into general use instead of soap. Certain detergents are powerful antiseptics as well, although they do not destroy spores. The most widely used is cetrimide combined with chlorhexidine (page 308), which is innocuous and a satisfactory antiseptic for the skin or for instruments. It is used in 2 per cent solution; it has a 'soapy' feel and rapidly induces rusting unless an anti-rust chemical is included in the solution for instruments.

Roccal is another proprietary detergent antiseptic used for similar purposes.

Repeated use of detergents on the skin, for instance as a surgeon's or nurse's hand lotion, may produce dermatitis in sensitive individuals.

Alcohol and spirit

The most effective bactericidal strength of spirit is 75 per cent, but this will not kill spores. It is sufficient to destroy surface organisms in under one minute; hence it is used extensively as a skin antiseptic. Commercial spirit may actually contain bacterial spores and there is really no place for spirit in ordinary ward sterilisation techniques.

Chlorine compounds

Solutions which contain active chlorine are strongly bactericidal. Chloride of lime (bleaching powder) is used in large-scale disinfection, as for instance under military field-service conditions: 3 per cent solution is adequate for sterilisation of utensils, such as

---

[1] *Borax and formaldehyde solution:* borax 15 G, solution of formaldehyde 25 ml, phenol 4 G, water to 1000 ml. (The phenol is not essential.) A colouring agent should be added.

drinking vessels. Chlorine is also used in treatment of swimming baths. Similar chlorinated solutions are used for wound irrigation and the standard preparation is chlorinated soda solution BP (Dakin's solution). Eusol is similar but is unstable, and has to be used soon after preparation (see also Table 14).

Chlorocresol

This compound is in multidose containers for injectable solutions as a protection against moulds and other contamination. It is also recommended as an instrument preservative solution in combination with sodium benzoate which prevents rusting. The standard preparation for this latter purpose is sodium benzoate (1·5 G per cent) and chlorocresol solution (0·2 G per cent) BP.

Chlorhexidine (Hibitane)

This is now used extensively in spirit or water solutions for instruments, and in special soaps for hand cleansing: proprietary preparations combining it with cetrimide are Cetrex and Savlon

Glutaraldehyde (Cidex)

This is a powerful proprietary aqueous solution with a wide range of antiseptic activity. It has to be prepared fresh with an activator added.

The use of sterilisation methods

Although there is a wide variation in the methods used in different hospitals, the foregoing methods of sterilisation can be safely applied to different groups of apparatus according to the following pattern (page 96).

1. **Metal instruments**—autoclave or boil (in sodium carbonate 2 per cent).

2. **Sharp instruments**—dry heat, autoclave or store in borax and formaldehyde solution or chlorhexidine in spirit.

Note. A used instrument must not be returned to the tray of antiseptic from which other instruments are being used, unless it has been sterilised by boiling or immersion in a separate vessel.

3. **Ampoules and catgut tubes**—borax and formaldehyde, chlorhexidine in spirit or glutaraldehyde solutions; formalin cabinet.

Glass ampoules containing injectable drugs need to be sterilised on the outside only when they are to be handled by a surgeon or anaesthetist during the course of an operation or some procedure such as lumbar puncture. Such ampoules can be sterilised in a formalin cabinet.

It is wise that any antiseptic solution used for this purpose should be coloured since accidents have occurred by the fluid entering ampoules through tiny cracks. Particularly is this important in the case of drugs to be given into the spinal theca.

4. **Catheters, and plastic tubing**—formalin cabinet; boiling; immersion in borax and formalin; immersion in 1 per cent cetrimide with chlorhexidine *after heat sterilisation*. Endotracheal catheters are adequately sterilised by boiling.

Note. All new rubber catheters should be autoclaved initially, dried and inserted in the formalin cabinet for storage. There is no completely certain method of sterilising the inside of ureteric and other fine catheters except by syringing through with formalin solution. They are then rinsed with sterile distilled water and air blown through. They are again rinsed through with a syringe and sterile distilled water before use in order to remove all traces of formalin. All catheters and other instruments removed from the formalin cabinet should be similarly rinsed in sterile water before use. Almost all catheters are now disposable and are sterilised commercially by gamma radiation.

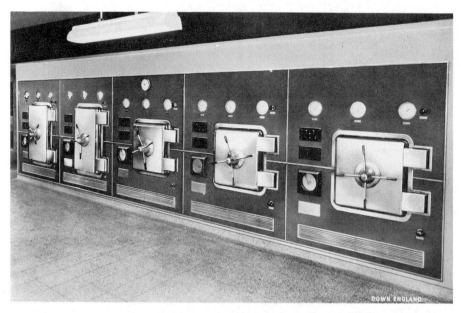

Fig. 17.3   Modern autoclave bank such as is used in central sterile supply department of multiple operating theatre suite. Cycling time is controlled automatically and recorded on a graph. There is thus a permanent record for every batch of material sterilised. (Down Bros.)

5. Ward utensils—Choroxylenol 5 per cent—30 minutes; Sudol 1 per cent—5 minutes. 1 per cent hyperchlorite solution.

6. Furniture, trolleys, wire mattresses, etc.—wipe with 1 per cent Sudol.

7. Bedding—Infected linen (depending on local conditions) should be soaked in 1 per cent Sudol for 6 hours and then laundered in the usual way. **Mattresses, blankets and clothing** are steam sterilised.

8. Destruction of excreta or sterilisation of heavily contaminated linen (e.g. from a case of gas gangrene). Formalin (40 per cent formaldehyde), 60 ml. Concentrated detergent solution (e.g. Teepol), 60 ml. Water to 1000 ml.

Such a method is necessary in military surgery where pressure sterilisation is not at hand. **Racasan** is a safe proprietary preparation of similar composition and eminently suitable for commode buckets, bed-pans, urinals and other utensils in domiciliary nursing.

9. Dirty dressings should be placed in paper containers (paper bags) initially and destroyed by burning.

10. Skin sterilisation (page 375).

Note. Surgical instruments are protected from rust by the addition of anti-oxidants to the sterilising solution. Borax is contained in the formaldehyde solution and sodium nitrite (2 G to 500 ml) is used with cetrimide.

Sterilisation of water

The ideal method of supplying sterile water for all purposes to wards and theatres is the provision of autoclaved litre flasks prepared in the central sterile supplies' depot or pharmacy.

In some old-fashioned operating theatres a 'still' is used for producing a constant supply of sterile water. This is steam heated and works on a similar principle to that of the autoclave, producing hot or cold water separately. Many such stills are unsafe as they are easily contaminated if the taps are not kept covered. They harbour pseudomonas organisms.

Commercial packaging

There is an ever-increasing flood of commercially prepared and sterilised articles of nursing equipment such as catheters, intravenous cannulas, needles for all purposes, dressings, feeding tubes, tracheostomy tubes, to name just a few.

The outside of all these packages is necessarily contaminated from the air and from cardboard boxes or packets in which they have been stored. There are on sale quite a number of items which have only one wrapping. If this envelope should be punctured accidentally then of course the whole content is rendered useless. We should only use articles which are doubly wrapped in such a way that the outer packet can be opened without any risk of dust or dirt falling from the lips of the envelope into the side of the package. Further, the inner packet should be capable of being ejected or withdrawn with a pair of forceps without touching at any point the cut or contaminated open edge of the outer container (Fig. 18.11). This warning applies particularly to hypodermic needles some of which are supplied in sterile envelopes instead of plastic sheaths. Some makes of catheter are correctly packed so that the outer envelope can be cut with non-sterile scissors or snapped off and the inner package withdrawn. This inside plastic sheath over the catheter is not sealed at the ends and the catheter can be inserted into the urethra with the fingers, using the sheath as a sterile protector. This is particularly convenient for domiciliary use as no preparation of instruments is necessary.

Many commercially packed sterile dressings cannot be removed from their envelope without the dressing being contaminated on the edges of the paper wrapper (Fig. 21.1). Cardboard has often been regarded as a source of tetanus infection and manufacturers of surgical equipment have to ensure that even the cardboard boxes are autoclaved before being sent to hospitals, where they may constitute a real danger.

The same principles of packing apply to all equipment assembled and sterilised in the hospital central depot.

Any package which has been punctured or damaged in any way must be rejected. Packets which have become wet from leaking pipes, or from condensation must be returned to the CSSD unused. The maintenance of the ward or department store for CSSD goods requires strictly disciplined oversight, to ensure 'rotation' of stock and correct placing of 'topping-up' supplies so that they are not used first.

There is inevitably some waste when using prepacked goods; for instance, several sizes of catheters may have to be tried before one is successfully passed. Clearly there must not be undue delay in carrying out a procedure because individual alternative items have to be fetched from the store, but nevertheless packets should not be opened until it is certain that the content is exactly what the nurse or doctor wants.

A few hours spent in the CSSD will familiarise any nurse with the apparatus available, and with its method of preparation and packing, and such a visit will help her to realise how dependent is the whole of patient care upon conscientious work in such service departments.

CENTRAL STERILE SUPPLY DEPARTMENT

The detailed organisation of a CSSD varies from hospital to hospital and is partly dependent on geographical considerations, available storage space and a variable degree of use of disposable material. Complete groups of hospitals are now being progressively supplied from one major CSSD.

Basically the material to be supplied to hospital wards and departments in a sterile condition are soft goods (gauze, cotton wool, dressing towels), hardware (bowls, dishes, trays, irrigators, jugs), instruments (forceps, probes, scissors), special items (manometers for lumbar puncture, biopsy equipment, diagnostic instruments, specula, sigmoidoscope etc.). The greater the number of these items which can be disposable—that is, used once and then thrown away—the less will be the load on the department, checking goods returned, cleaning, preparation and repair. In the field of soft goods, hospitals now use factory-made swabs and cotton balls. Large dressing towels have been almost completely replaced by non-wettable paper, and major items of this category which are returnable for laundry, repair and re-issue are towels and gowns used principally in the operating theatre. Most of the hardware traditionally used in dressing procedures has been replaced by aluminium foil containers which are cheap and of light weight. Many hospitals now issue disposable dressings forceps made of a plastic material or a cheap metal and the use of scissors for the removal of stitches has been replaced by the issue of a small disposable scalpel-type blade, **Seralet**, for cutting sutures. It is thus possible to provide a major ward dressing package containing everything required in disposable form which can be thrown away in a sealed paper bag at the end of the procedure (Figs 17.4 and 17.6).

Clearly the economic use of a CSSD depends on the degree of uniformity which can be established in the various departments so that a common basic pack is acceptable on all wards and in out-patient clinics. Individual items over and above the basic packs are supplied separately wrapped by the CSSD.

The packs are issued in outer paper or cloth wrappings, or in cardboard boxes. The only really safe method of packing is 'double wrapping' in such a way that the outer wrapper of paper or cloth is unfolded and discarded: the inner packet is then unfolded on a sterile or clean surface and the contents removed by sterile forceps or gloved hand, or 'decanted' on to a sterile trolley. Some CSS departments use **Bripac** cardboard boxes, but unless the contents are double wrapped these are not entirely safe. When the lid is drawn up a vacuum is created and contamination is drawn into the box from the air or from the surface on which the box is placed and from the exposed outer surface. A folded lining is sometimes used to protect the top of the contents but this has the same drawback as in the traditional drum. If the box is opened and the whole contents withdrawn it may be safe, but if the box is used as a 'reservoir' and opened more than once, it is unsafe. **Bripac** boxes are re-used several times and become torn at the corners. Figure 17.5 shows a **Bripac** box repaired with 'autoclave'-proof tape which develops stripes when the sterilisation is complete. Such a repair can be misleading even if the box is resealed with fresh tape on each occasion. The advantage of the box system is the ease of recording the contents in ink on the outside, with the date of packing and sterilisation.

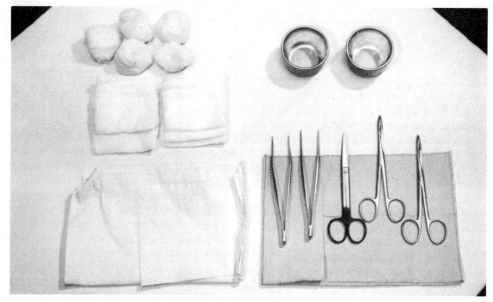

Fig. 17.4   Small dressing.

1 dressing towel	2 pairs dissecting forceps
2 gauze swabs	1 pair Vigo scissors
5 cotton wool swabs	1 handling tissue
1 2-oz gallipot	2 pair French pattern handling forceps
1 disposable foil gallipot	

This is a standard ward dressing collection. All these items are enclosed in two paper wrappings. The outer one is a bag which is clipped to the dressing trolley as a receptacle for disposable items and dirty dressings. The inner wrapper is unfolded and provides a sterile field on the trolley. The dressing towel and the instruments are returned to the CSSD and the rest of the items including the foil gallipots are placed in the outer wrapping bag for disposal. All CSSD scissors have blackened handles to discourage their removal and use for other purposes as they are easily identified.

Each ward has a store of its own which is topped up daily in a distribution round by members of the CSSD staff. Clearly at the initial establishment of a CSSD service there has to be a large purchase of non-disposable items so that there shall be an adequate reserve store to guard against a breakdown of sterilisers or shortage of labour.

'Disposable' items required in operating theatres and wards are being supplied increasingly already sterilised by the manufacturers by the use of gamma irradiation. Such items are usually packed in double wrapping (page 398). They may be issued direct from the Supplies Department to wards and theatres or on the other hand all these items may be issued through the CSSD.

Once a high degree of uniformity has been reached in the requirements of various wards and departments the numbers of different dressing packs required is very greatly reduced. Clearly the variety will depend upon the number of different specialties in the

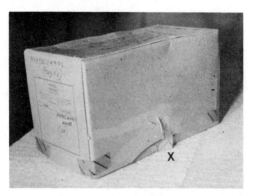

Fig. 17.5 Bripac cardboard box, widely used instead of drums but with many of the same disadvantages (see text). Each time the box is packed it is sealed at X with autoclave indicator tape in which the stripes only show after the correct heat treatment. The tape on the corners has been used for repairing the weak points. Boxes are convenient for storage but are not entirely safe.

hospital being supplied, but there will almost certainly be over a hundred different soft goods packs. These are major and minor dressings and complete equipment for such procedures as peritoneal dialysis, renal biopsy, tracheostomy, emergency thoracotomy and catheterisation. In addition to the large amount of material which is packed and sterilised in the Department there will be several hundred other items which have been supplied commercially pre-sterilised. The CSSD ensures that a safe method of packaging is used and acts as a distribution centre.

In some hospitals the operating theatres are supplied completely from the CSSD. This involves the purchase of very large numbers of instruments and the cost is enormous, particularly where special surgical departments are involved and every instrument must be duplicated, triplicated or supplied in even greater numbers to ensure that there is always one available. The majority of operating theatres are. however, supplied with their soft goods such as gowns, towels, and dressing materials from central depots and the work undertaken by theatre staff such as preparation of gloves and packing of gown drums and towels has been completely eliminated. Where standardisation between hospitals in a group cannot be achieved, theatre staff may still be called upon to prepare, check and count soft goods for sterilisation by autoclave in a central depot.

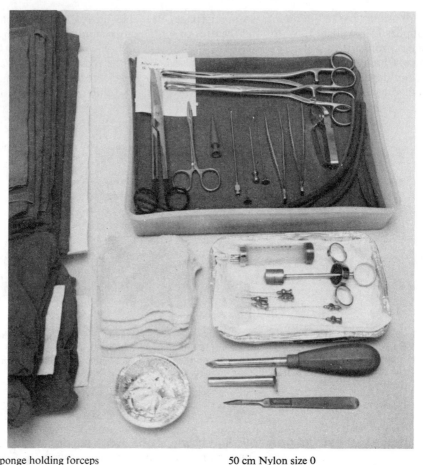

2 pr sponge holding forceps
1 pr straight artery forceps
1 pr toothed dissecting forceps
1 pr plain dissecting forceps
1 pr straight surgical scissors
1 Nelson trocar with cannula—26 English gauge
2 towel clips
1 10 ml Labat syringe
2 Labat needles 2 cm
2 ,, ,, 5 cm
2 ,, ,, 10 cm
1 modified government needle and 2 stilettes
2 fine straight needles

50 cm Nylon size 0
1 mixing cannula
1 scalpel handle and blade E
4 straight catheters—one each of size 8 : 10 : 12 :
    13 English gauge
1 spigot—medium
2 surgeon's gowns
2 hand towels
1 gallipot
3 large towels
4 medium towels
5 green Zobec swabs
2 6 × 6 gauze
1 24 × 2 gauze and wool

Fig. 17.6 Intercostal drainage set. This CSSD pack is for use in wards and casualty departments for removal of collections of pus or blood or air in the pleural cavity. The procedure is carried out under local anaesthesia and an intercostal catheter is placed in position through the trocar, later being connected to an underwater seal. Such a set could not be held in all wards but would be available on demand and included as a standard item in casualty departments and thoracic units.

The method of use of CSSD items and the particular system in use is taught to nurses in training at a very early stage of their course. Trained staff moving from hospital to hospital have to learn new systems, and may find the adaptation difficult.

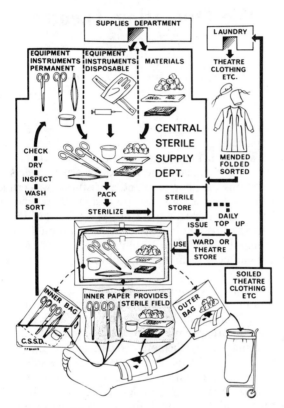

Fig. 17.7 Schematic representation of the supply and progress of CSSD items in a typical organisation. Note economy in containers. The outer unsterile pack cover is used for soiled dressings and disposable items. All processing undertaken in the 'enclosed' area is by non-nursing staff.

18

The Operating Theatre

In the minds of those unaccustomed to working in an operating team, the theatre and all that goes on within it is shrouded in mystery and awe. It is thought to be a place where the novice faints at the terrifying spectacle of bloodshed. This attitude has arisen in the history of surgery when amputations were common and anaesthesia was crude. The atmosphere of the theatre was made intolerable by a mixture of anaesthetic and antiseptic smells. In the modern operating theatre none of these horrors exist, but it is right, and in fact essential, that the theatre and its adjoining suite of rooms should always be treated with respect and the very highest sense of responsibility by all those whose duties take them there. Minor errors in conduct or technique may have major repercussions in disaster and death.

The purpose of this chapter is to outline the general principles behind theatre technique and management, to point out some of the dangers and hazards, and to give general guidance on important technical procedures. No attempt has been made to do more than outline theatre procedure in order that the junior nurse may become acquainted with the basic principles of operating routine, the potential dangers and the steps taken to diminish them. At the end of her general training, a nurse should be sufficiently experienced to make the necessary provision for minor operations. It is no longer assumed that every trained nurse is capable of accepting the duties of a theatre staff nurse without special experience and extensive training. The full training of the theatre nurse is achieved only in the hard school of practical experience.

An approach to theatre procedure has been made in previous chapters and references are given here for convenience.

The theatre suite

Accommodation and equipment in many surgical units is inadequate to provide the highest possible standards of safety and comfort for long operating lists. The less efficient the accommodation, the more skilled and disciplined the team must be.

Ideally, the minimum accommodation required includes:

1. Anaesthetic room. This room opens on to an approach corridor and has separate noise-excluding doors into the operating theatre. The room is sited so as to be free from extraneous sounds such as those arising from electric lifts and water-closet cisterns. It should be illuminated by wall lighting so that the patient is not dazzled by overhead lamps if he should reach the theatre still awake. The anaesthetic room is not a general theatre store where there is constant disturbance. All anaesthetic apparatus is available here. There must be a washbasin and small steriliser unless there is a full central sterile service supplying all theatre needs.

2. Operating theatre. One of the main objects in the design of an operating theatre is to provide really adequate space for the movement of the team in order to avoid contact with sterile trolleys, basins, and other apparatus. Ventilation is arranged in such a way that temperature and humidity are under control and as far as possible draught is excluded, to reduce the risk of infection being carried into the theatre atmosphere from surrounding rooms. There is direct access to the operating theatre from the anaesthetic room, from clean and dirty preparation rooms, and from the surgeon's scrubbing-up room. There should be no direct access from the outside corridor as this encourages casual visitors. There should be an intervening recovery room or corridor where the patient remains on a trolley or in his bed (brought from the ward at the end of operation) while awaiting return to the ward.

3. Sterilising room. Each theatre has in the past had its own complete set of sterilising apparatus. Sometimes theatres are constructed in pairs with a common sterilising room between the two. Such an arrangement is dangerous and unsatisfactory unless the sterilising apparatus is also duplicated so that the two teams can work independently. Boiling as a method of sterilisation is not wholly reliable and has been replaced by the provision of rapid-cycle autoclaves in the theatre suite. Progressively the provision of this system is itself being replaced by the use of a theatre sterile supply system in which every instrument and piece of equipment required for an operation is provided by the central department: there is thus no 'between case' sterilisation of instruments. The cost of providing many sets of instruments is enormous but theatre nursing staff are then no longer called upon to clean apparatus and prepare packs: a constant monitoring of sterilising procedure is possible. Where such a system exists there has to be a great degree of standardisation in making up sets of instruments, but this itself reduces the work load which has hitherto fallen on the theatre nurses and technicians.

If provision is made for pressure sterilisation of instruments, this room will contain the autoclaves and probably an additional boiler for quick sterilisation of instruments and bowls. A supply of sterile water is provided in litre flasks and sufficient bottles for operations in progress are stored in a temperature-controlled warming cabinet. No longer are stills used to produce sterile water in the theatre area. There must be table space, at least two sinks and adequate shelving. Ventilation must be sufficient to prevent condensation from steam.

4. Sluice room. This provides for the reception of all used apparatus at the end of an operation. Linen is sorted, instruments washed and cleaned, and used swabs disposed of. Many theatre suites have no separate provision for a sluice room and extreme care must be taken to separate the used and the unused instruments and equipment.

5. Store and work room. Table space is needed for the packing of drums, sorting and preparation of instruments, glove repairs and other procedures included in long-term preparation (see below).

6. Changing rooms. Adjoining the theatre suite must be a changing room for the surgical team with clothes lockers and toilet facilities. Similar accommodation must be provided for the nurses.

Modern theatres are designed with 'sterile' areas. Before entering these, all staff put on overshoes and then change top clothes and footwear in 'clean' changing rooms. No one is allowed in the sterile unit without having changed into theatre clothing.

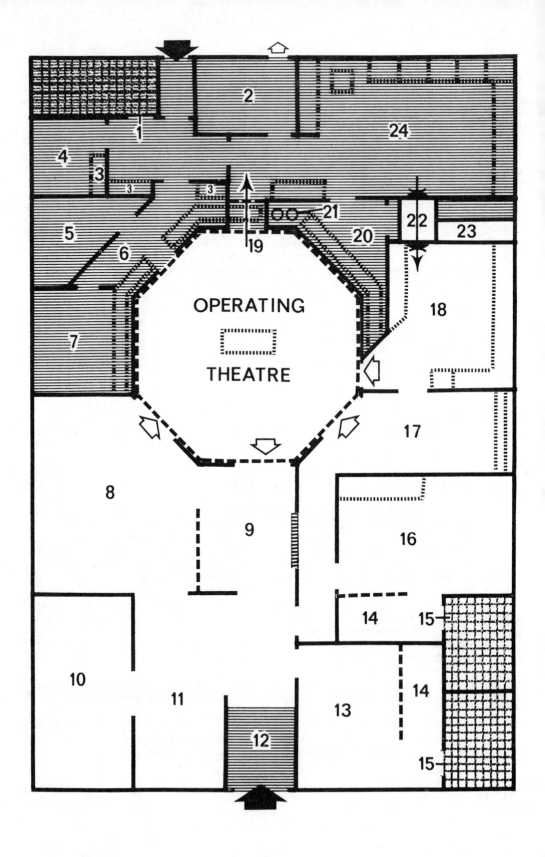

OPERATING
THEATRE

An extensive suite of the type visualised is designed to provide for operating lists of many hours' duration. In small units and in nursing homes elaborate facilities of this type are not required since operating sessions include only one or perhaps two cases. The risk of cross-infection is greatly reduced when the theatre is used for one case, and adequate time is given for cleaning before the suite is used again. Under these more simple conditions, single drums containing gowns, linen and swabs may be specially prepared for each operation and the tempo of activity is greatly reduced. There is closer individual supervision by fully trained staff at every stage in the preparation for and conduct of the operation. In the large and busy theatre, more people are at work and consequently the risk of error and infection is relatively great.

Ventilation. Elaborate systems of air conditioning have been devised but many of these are completely unsatisfactory. There are two factors to be considered. First, the temperature of the atmosphere should be capable of a steady control between 21 °C and 26 °C. Excessive temperature is unpleasant for the operating team and dangerous for the patient, particularly if the humidity is high. The second factor is one of humidity or moisture. The degree of humidity is indicated by the use of special meters. A very dry atmosphere is dangerous mainly from the point of view of explosion where ether or other inflammable anaesthetic agent is used. An excessively humid atmosphere is dangerous to the patient as it prevents the normal body temperature control. High humidity also leads to fatigue in the team. If the theatre temperature or humidity is high there is an increased danger from the use of plastic covers over the patient since these prevent heat loss. Death may occur from hyperpyrexia produced in this way. Children are particularly sensitive to overheating and it is wise to dispense with the use of rubber or plastic sheets over child patients (except babies), additional protection being given by a double layer of operating towels.

Moisture arises mainly from steam sterilisers. Air-extracting fans are convenient and economical but may be dangerous since the removal of air from the theatre leads to its replacement by air which is drawn under doors and through windows, thus introducing extraneous infection. Specially filtered air may be blown into the theatre and this system is used in conjunction with extractors to maintain both a constant temperature and humidity.

It is important to realise that the temperature at the operating table is more important than that recorded on the theatre wall. It is a nursing responsibility to see that the theatre temperature is correct at all times. This is particularly important in emergency operations at night-time when the normal outside temperature falls.

Fig. 18.1.—Typical operating theatre suite. This is planned round a standard theatre unit which has been used in various designs in new hospitals to comply with present conceptions of infection control with standard prefabricated units (the Honeywell System). The same system can be used to modernise some of the over-large and out-of-date operating suites in old hospitals. When the theatre is in use all staff in the unshaded portions are 'clean' with sterilised overshoes, which are put on at entry **12**. There is no movement of staff or patients into the theatre by any other entrance. At **22** equipment is placed in the autoclave on the 'dirty' side. Used equipment is returned through hatch **19**.

Key:
1. Toilet. **2.** Dirty linen. **3.** Instrument cupboards. **4.** Linen and drum storage. **5.** AC plant. **6.** Service corridor. Engineers attending to suction, diathermy and other apparatus do not enter the theatre. **7.** Storage. **8.** Anaesthetic room. **9.** Recovery room. **10.** Medical office. **11.** Entrance lobby. **12.** Entrance: stick mat and overshoes. **13.** Nurses' duty room. **14.** Changing rooms. **15.** Toilets and showers. **16.** Surgeons' room. **17.** Surgeons' scrub-up. **18.** Preparation room. **19.** Hatch. **20.** Servicing area. **21.** Suction bottles. **22.** Steriliser. **23.** Hot cupboards (sterile water storage). **24.** Sink room.

Lamps which emit ultra-violet irradiation are sometimes installed on the theatre walls. The rays are directed upwards away from the team and the ultra-violet light sterilises the circulating air: this is a relatively economical method of diminishing risks of infection where major structural alterations are not possible.

In an endeavour to reduce further the risk of wound infection at operation, particularly in procedures that involve exposure of a large area of tissue, a system has been devised in which the operating team is totally isolated from the non-operating members circulating in the theatre. Operation is carried out in a transparent plastic 'tent' into which is blown a supply of sterile air. The members of the operating team wear helmets with rigid face pieces. These are attached to the gown and an air extracting tube removes expired air and at the same time carries away organisms which are displaced from the body surface of the operator inside his gown. There is therefore during the whole procedure a constant downward displacement of air away from the patient's body—the so-called 'laminar flow'. The anaesthetist is outside the tent with the patient's head protruding through an opening. Instruments are passed through a special 'hatch' in the wall of the tent.

Noise and unauthorised entry. Noise is important to the patient during the induction of anaesthesia. Unless pre-medication has been sufficient to abolish consciousness, the patient is acutely aware of conversation and noise made by the careless handling of equipment.

However placid the surgeon may be in temperament, he too is susceptible to the noise of crashing bowls, banging doors, whistling or laughter in the adjoining rooms! Conversation between members of the team must be kept to a minimum and every effort must be made to eliminate unnecessary discussion. On the other hand, requests or instructions must be given clearly and in a normal speaking voice; whispering is particularly irritating.

The telephone is a nuisance in the operating theatre. **Telephone messages should be written and not communicated to the surgeon during the course of an operation.**

The entry of unauthorised persons to the operating suite must be completely barred. Some ophthalmic surgeons, during certain procedures such as corneal grafting, insist on the doors being locked to avoid any possibility of disturbance. Nurses, students and others who are spectators are properly gowned and instructed to remain at the side of the theatre until the operation has actually commenced. Clear and precise instructions must be given by the nursing staff to all such visitors to ensure that they do not touch any of the equipment or sterile trolleys.

The design of operating equipment is by no means standardised and when a nurse starts her theatre work, she must take trouble to be familiar with the major items of equipment and their mechanism. Her knowledge will be partly gained in the cleaning of this equipment.

Organisation and staffing

The team. Under normal conditions the operating team will include at least three nurses, two of whom should be fully trained. The theatre sister or charge-nurse must have had special theatre training and be familiar with the surgeon's technique.

The allocation of duties to individual members of the staff is a matter for the theatre sister. No attempt is made here to suggest how this is arranged, because the duties will depend on the relative experience of nurses who normally constitute the team, on the presence of a trained theatre technician or orderly, and to some extent on the arrangement of theatre accommodation. There must be a written programme of work so that the allocation is clear to all concerned, covering the period before, during and after operations.

Where a trained theatre technician is employed, his duties will include the movement of the patient from trolley to operating table, positioning the patient and making the necessary alterations and adjustments to the table in accordance with the surgeon's needs. It is probable that he will also be responsible for the surgical diathermy apparatus, suction pump and for the maintenance of the anaesthetic machine. Junior theatre nurses are changed frequently, while the theatre technician may remain with one team for many years. He becomes accustomed to the methods and foibles of anaesthetists and surgeons for whom he works and he is an invaluable member of the team. In many units, however, a porter is employed in place of a trained male technician and since such persons are not familiar with operating theatre procedure or aseptic technique their movements must be watched with great care. Untrained staff should not be allowed to remain in the operating theatre once the patient has been placed on the table.

Operating lists. A list of proposed operations should be available to the theatre sister at least twenty-four hours before the proposed starting time. She goes through the list with her staff so that each member understands the general procedure and is able to make the necessary preparations. Items of equipment may have to be borrowed from other operating theatres: packs containing special requirements may need sterilisation: drugs or injection solutions not normally held in the theatre stock may be required.

For emergency surgery there is no such time for preliminary preparations and operating theatres used for acute surgical cases must be kept ready for *immediate* action. Very few conditions require operation within an hour of admission, and there is usually adequate time for the sterilisation of instruments and the preparation of trolleys. There are occasions, however, when immediate surgery is required and it is therefore absolutely necessary that provisions be made in anticipation of such urgent need:
This may be achieved by having either:
  (a) A foundation set of instruments, for general surgery kept in a sterilised pack, or
  (b) a complete set of instruments required for abdominal surgery sterilised by auto-
      clave and left in the autoclave after drying by vacuum (page 302), so that it can
      be drawn and a trolley 'set up' without delay.

The operating table (Fig. 18.2). The reason for the great weight of the operating table is that it must be stable and rigid and yet be capable of being tilted endways or sideways without becoming unbalanced, however heavy the patient may be. The surgical team and the anaesthetist sometimes lean on the operating table and it must have a mechanism in its base whereby it may be locked to the floor to avoid unintended movement. Most tables are divided into three or four sections. The centre section or sections support the trunk and thighs while the two end sections support the head and legs respectively. The end sections are adjustable for angle. There are additional fitments which can be screwed into, or clamped on, the table so as to raise the centre of the trunk for kidney or gall-bladder operations, or the shoulders for operations on the neck. Some tables are designed to 'break' in the centre of the trunk section while others include special orthopaedic extension (traction) bars which support the legs in the abducted position, during operations upon the hip. In the latter case the centre section is constructed to be lowered, leaving the patient's sacrum supported on a pelvic rest or pillar. A lateral tilting mechanism and supports are needed for thoracic surgery.

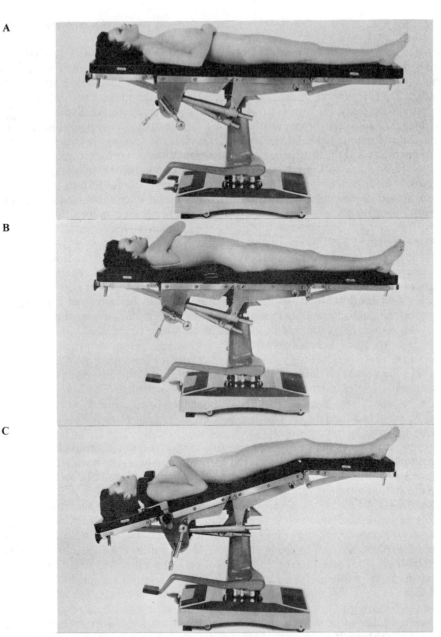

Fig. 18.2 Matburn operating tables. (Eschmann Bros & Walsh.)

A Modern four-section operating table: the controls are at the head end for the anaesthetist to adjust: the table tilts endways or sideways, and 'breaks' to give the desired angle: mattress sections can be replaced by radiolucent film carriers for angiography and other radiology during operation. Normal supine position, flat for most abdominal surgery: a pad is placed under the heels to take pressure off the calves, and arm protectors prevent the arms from falling.

B The back elevator raises the lumbar spine for upper abdominal operations—gall-bladder, adrenalectomy, porta-caval anastomosis, etc.; this cannot be used if operative cholangiography is required: a translucent radiographic cassette box is then inserted.

C Head-down tilt ('Trendelenburg' position): shoulder supports must be well padded. A steep tilt may cause excess pressure on the brachial plexus by the shoulder rests: this is avoided by using a rubber corrugated non-slip mattress and lowering the leg section.

D

E

F

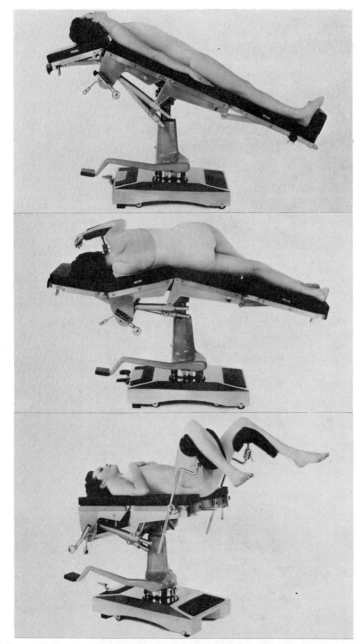

D Foot-down tilt (reverse Trendelenburg): foot-rest prevents slipping. Venous return from the lower part of the body is impeded—thrombosis is more likely: position used for thyroidectomy, neck and face surgery, as it diminishes venous congestion in the neck.

E Left lateral—for operations on the back, buttock or right kidney: the *left* knee may be flexed and elevated on a sandbag, with the right leg extended: this tips the pelvis back and improves the position for an approach through the loin to the kidney.

F Low 'lithotomy' position—(so called as this position was used in bygone days for cutting into the perineum to remove large bladder stones pressed down from above): the leg troughs are padded to prevent combined abdominal perineal operations: a head-down tilt helps to ensure that the feet are higher than the knees to discourage venous pooling. This table has a cut-away centre section to improve access to the perineum. For vaginal and anal operations and cystoscopy.

G

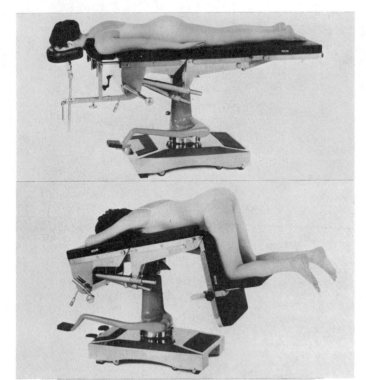

H

I

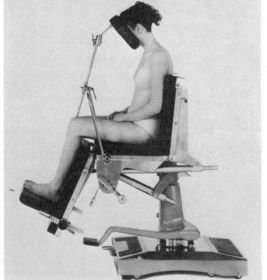

Fig. 18.2 (continued)

G Prone with head support—for operations on spine. The pelvis and upper chest should be raised on pads to avoid compression of the abdomen which interferes with venous return by pressing on the vena cava.

H Proctological position—rarely used: operations on sacral area: pudendal neurectomy, pilonidal sinus. Note that the abdomen is free from compression as it is over the cut-away centre section, and the weight is taken on the knees.

I Neurosurgical 'chair' position—for operations on posterior cranial fossa, or cervical spine: hypotensive anaesthesia may be used.

Additional fitments include lithotomy poles (stirrups) for holding the patient's legs in the vertical position during operations on the perineum. Special leg troughs are used to hold the lower limbs in the abducted position without interfering with the surgeon who is operating on the abdomen in combined procedures involving perineal and abdominal surgery (such as excision of the rectum).

The nurse must be fully acquainted with the exact method of attaching the operating-table fittings so that there is no delay or insecurity during an operating session. These fittings are kept on a rack in the theatre, each item having a particular marked position so that its absence can be noted at once.

The table is raised by a hydraulic pump. The mechanism may develop defects due to lack of oil or to improper adjustment. Periodic overhaul of the operating table is essential.

The illustrations (Fig. 18.2) indicate usual positions for patients undergoing various procedures and each position has its special risks and need for lessening these. No description of positioning can be adequate as so much depends on the build of the individual patient and on the exact nature of the operation. The theatre orderly or technician becomes accustomed to the particular wishes of each surgeon, but his knowledge does not absolve the nurse from her responsibility for the patient's protection against injury.

Instrument trolleys. Various shapes and sizes of instrument trolley are in common use. These are made entirely of metal with metal shelves welded in position. Glass or removable shelves are difficult to keep clean, and act as dirt traps. The wheels of the trolley must be kept clean. They have rubber tyres, the surface of which may become uneven from the attachment of pieces of strapping and the collection of dirt. Both the tyres and the spindle require cleaning and most patterns need occasional oil. Because of the risk of static electricity (page 358), the trolleys are earthed to the theatre floor, through tyres composed of 'antistatic' rubber which conducts electricity.

Trolleys which are used for sterile instruments are covered with a waterproof paper sheet which has been sterilised by autoclave. Sterile towels are thus kept from contact with the trolley shelf even if they become wet. The main instrument trolley has a rail or a ledge around three sides to prevent instruments falling on to the floor. A Mayo table is a tray on a movable stand which can be adjusted to the height of the operating table. This is placed over the patient and covered with sterile towels, to act as a receptacle for instruments which are in use by the surgeon.

Very great care must be taken to ensure that a contaminated used instrument trolley is not mistaken for one prepared for use. Confusion can arise in this way and lead to disaster by cross-infection. The author knows of one case of fatal tetanus which is thought to have arisen in this way when the theatre staff changed between two emergency cases. The first case was a compound fracture from a road accident. The wound was contaminated but the patient had been protected by routine anti-tetanus serum injection. The second case, one of appendicitis, became infected with tetanus and died. To avoid this risk the hanging edges of the towel are turned back over the trolley immediately the operation is over.

Drums and drum-stands. Cleaning, packing and sterilising dressing-drums is still one of the theatre nurses' principal duties in units which do not have a central sterile supply department. Various shapes of drum are used: small sizes for gloves and small items of haberdashery, the larger drums for gowns, towels and swabs. In busy theatres where the turnover of drums is very rapid it is unlikely that any single drum will escape sterilisation for more than a few days. In smaller hospitals there is more likelihood of drums remaining out of use after sterilisation for several days. There is little risk of infection entering the drum if it is stored in a cupboard and if the sliding bands which cover the perforations in its sides are a tight fit. It is unwise to rely on the sterility of drums of the ordinary type unless they have been autoclaved within a week. On the other hand, completely sealed containers such as those supplied commercially remain sterile indefinitely. Labels may be attached to drums indicating the time and date of the last sterilisation.

Sterilised drums should never be dropped or thrown as a dent may prevent the lid fitting correctly and allow the entry of infection.

With a full central sterile supply, all items will be packaged and labelled in the workroom and no drums will be used.

Waste buckets. Bowls or buckets mounted on castors are used to receive dirty swabs and dressings.

Swab racks. To facilitate the counting of packs and swabs a simple rack with hooks mounted in rows of ten or twelve is placed in the theatre in a position where it can be readily observed by the nurse in charge. Each swab which has been used is retrieved from the bucket and placed on a hook to ensure a constant check on the number of swabs in circulation. Swabs of each type are kept together, and hung in continuous sequence on the rack (Fig. 18.5).

Sterilisation

All these items of furniture require thorough cleaning and the particular antiseptic used for this purpose is a matter of local choice. Solution such as Sudol (a non-irritant cresol derivative) used on a sponge is safe and effective, or hypochlorite 1 per cent, but phenol should now never be used.

Lotion bowls. Bowls for sterile water are available throughout the operation for the surgeon to rinse his gloves and for the 'scrubbed-up' nurse to wash instruments or swabs. Sterile water is supplied to the theatre in sealed litre flasks. These are stored in a thermo-statically controlled hot cabinet; the nurses wear heat-resistant gloves to handle the bottles. The bowls are mounted on mobile stands with castors. Bowls must be sterilised by boiling or autoclave. During the operation, the water in these bowls is frequently changed so that the temperature can be maintained at between 50° and 55 °C. Every time the surgeon rinses his hands the water should again be changed. During major abdominal operations, where the hands become soiled with blood and fat, rinsing is more frequently required and twin bowl stands are essential, so that one bowl is always available. To avoid contamination of the surgeon's gown by contact with the drum stand, it is usual to place a sterile towel over the stand before placing the bowl in the ring. These lotion bowls are a potential source of danger in the operating theatre since the water becomes contaminated very easily from the air, particularly from the movement of theatre staff and spectators.

Wearing apparel. Ordinary uniform should not be worn in the operating theatre. It should be changed for a specially laundered short-sleeved overall to diminish the risk of dust and contamination from outside entering the operating area. Similarly, special footwear, either antistatic rubber boots or overshoes, should be worn by all those whose duties take them into the anaesthetic room, theatre or preparation rooms. No floor can be kept sterile, but the risk of infection in an operating theatre is always increased by any factor which introduces contamination and dust. Plastic waterproof aprons are provided for the surgeon and his assistant. These can for practical purposes be sterilised by washing with hypochlorite or chloroxylenol solution, but the apron is not regarded as sterile when in use. It diminishes the risk of infection passing through the front of the gown from the surgeon's clothes if the gown becomes wet from water or blood.

Rubber footwear must be scrubbed with soap and water after use.

Caps. The theatre cap has its origin partly in the traditional nun's cap from the association of nursing with religious institutions, and partly for the specific purpose of retaining long hair. It is extremely unlikely that infection will drop from the hair except on dandruff. The theatre cap should cover the hair completely. Theatre caps are sterilised for obvious reasons of hygiene but they are not regarded as sterilised items of wear such as gowns or gloves. The caps and masks can with safety be put on before the scrubbing-up begins. Many units use disposable caps.

The surgeon may require a turn of gauze roll inside the cap to absorb the sweat from the forehead during an operation. From the surgeon's point of view, it is essential that his cap should be comfortable and that his mask should fit.

Masks. Much controversy has centred round the efficacy of face-masks. Only if there is an impervious layer of paper or Cellophane can infection be prevented from passing into the operation field from the surgeon's nose and mouth. Even if such an impervious mask is used, the currents of air which escape at the side may also disperse infection. Most units use disposable paper masks. Masks should be changed frequently by all staff and after each case by the operating team, and never lowered to hang round the neck between cases.

Gowns. A theatre gown serves two functions. First for those who are scrubbed-up and part of the immediate operating team, the gown ensures a sterile operating field and prevents contamination by contact with the surgeon's clothing or skin. For those who are not scrubbed-up, the gown serves similarly as a further barrier to infection escaping from the clothes into the atmosphere but also acts as a protection for the nurse's own apparel. Procedure varies in different hospitals. The same type of gown may be used for both purposes, or operating gowns may be worn only by the scrubbed-up team, while the others wear a simple form of overall.

In some units where there is considerable movement during the operation (as for instance for operations on the hip joint) back-gowns are used to cover the surgeon's or nurse's shoulders and back where the ordinary gown has been tied across. A simple sterile towel may be used for this purpose, clipped to the shoulders with towel clips. Back gowns give a false sense of security and their use is not advocated.

Gowns are virtually sterilised by ordinary laundry processes but of course become contaminated in folding and packing subsequently. The purpose of a special method of folding is to ensure that the gown will unroll so that only its inner surface is handled by the surgeon as he slips his arms into it. Incorrect folding which necessitates turning the gown upside down after unfolding is very apt to lead to contact with unsterile objects, to wastage and subsequently to shortage of sterile gowns. All gowns must be inspected for holes in the front or sleeves before they are folded. Gowns used by those in immediate contact with the operation field should be made of special close-woven material and should preferably have double fronts, to diminish the likelihood of contamination passing from the surgeon's clothes or apron. Many hospitals still use gowns which are useless as a barrier to infection, being made of cheap, unsuitable material. The front of the gown in contact with the sterile drapes may be covered with a self-adhesive small plastic sterile apron (edge-adherent Steridrape).

Gloves. Disposable rubber gloves are used now almost universally. They may be supplied unsterile for packaging and autoclave sterilisation locally, or ready sterilised by gamma rays (radioactive cobalt) in a sealed packet. They are thrown away after use.

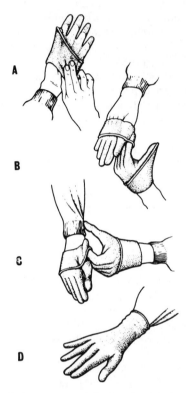

Fig. 18.3 Aseptic application of gloves. **A.** The left glove is picked up with the right hand and held by the turned back cuff, while the left hand is inserted. **B.** The left gloved hand is then inserted beneath the turned back cuff of the right glove into which the right hand is inserted. **C.** The right glove cuff is then turned up over the gown cuff, care being taken to avoid touching skin with the gloved left thumb. **D.** The left glove cuff is similarly turned over the gown cuff.

Although this sounds very wasteful and expensive the saving of nurses' time in cleaning, testing and re-sterilising gloves makes the use of disposable ones relatively cheap.

'Non-disposable' gloves are made of slightly better material and can be re-used several times. The cleaning, inspection and re-packing of gloves is then undertaken by theatre staff. Before packing for sterilisation all gloves, even if new, must be tested for punctures by the inflation method.

Gloves are packed with the cuffs turned back to enable the user to put them on without touching the outer surface at any time with an ungloved finger or the inner surface with a gloved finger. They are very lightly powdered before sterilisation to enable them to slip on without sticking. The hands may be powdered with a special sterile starch preparation or a quick-drying cream suspension, but care must be taken not to spill powder on the gown or create a 'dust' in the air with it. If the hands are dipped in spirit and allowed to dry it is not necessary to use additional powder as the inside of the gloves has a fine powder coating. The outside of the gloves has been coated with powder and this *must* be wiped off with a sterile wet swab before handling instruments. 'Starch' peritonitis and tissue reactions elsewhere (for instance, in the eye) occur if this precaution is not taken.

The common glove sizes are $6\frac{1}{2}$ and 7 for women and 7, $7\frac{1}{2}$ and 8 for men.

Towels. Sterilised towels are used to cover instrument trolleys and to surround the operation field in order to prevent contamination of instruments. No towel is a complete barrier against the passage of bacteria but for practical purposes, if certain additional precautions are taken, safety is ensured. The towel must be made from a close-weave material. On instrument trolleys and lotion-bowl stands, a layer of sterile wet-resistant paper or foil is used beneath the sterile towel and it is this waterproof layer which is the real bacterial barrier. As soon as an ordinary theatre towel becomes wet, it ceases to serve its protective function. A waterproof paper sheet is sometimes used to cover the patient, but more often the surgeon depends upon a double layer of towelling around the wound to guard against the introduction of infection. Pre-sterilised transparent plastic sheeting (Vidrape or Steridrape, Fig. 18.4) is now widely used. During the initial skin preparation

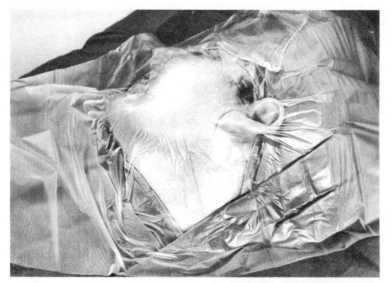

Fig. 18.4 "Steridrape" is one form of transparent drape, self-adhesive over the centre area. It is used here for operation on the parotid gland. The eye and the mouth which cannot be cleaned up in the skin preparation are visible to the operator, but are excluded bacteriologically from the operation zone. Thus when dissecting the parotid gland, the surgeon can see if the muscles of the face twitch, indicating risk to the facial nerve. The adhesive film fixes the towel drapes in position eliminating clips which make holes in the towels. "**Vidrape**" is not self-adhesive, but is applied after spraying the area with an adhesive solution.

a much wider area is cleaned than that which is finally exposed between the operating towels. Before being packed for sterilisation, all towels must be very carefully inspected by being held up to the light. Holes are produced by towel clips used to hold them in place where adhesives are not used, and repairs are therefore frequently needed. Different sized towels are available and in many theatres slotted large sheets are used to place over the operation area. For sterilisation the towels must be folded and packed loosely to ensure full penetration of the steam. Ready sterilised 'single-use' disposable sets of towel drapes are available commercially. The material is a type of paper of soft linen-like feel and is water repellent, and some have self-adhesive edges, to avoid the use of clips.[1]

Swabs. Skin cleaning, mopping of blood, packing of cavities and the protection of wound edges during operation all require the use of gauze swabs. Other terms are commonly used to describe them—'dabs', 'mops', 'wipes'. Whatever the size of shape of the swab, the gauze must be folded in such a way that no threads will become detached during use. Frayed edges must be entirely covered by folded surfaces. Each swab should be at least six layers of gauze in thickness. Large abdominal packs have sixteen or more layers. Many commercially prepared swabs are machine sewn round the edges and all swabs must contain one radio-opaque thread (Raytec). Various sizes are required according to the type of surgery being undertaken and in an operating theatre which serves several departments there may be considerable variation in the type of swab used. Large swabs used inside the abdomen frequently have a tape attached to one corner as an additional precaution against their being lost inside the peritoneal cavity.

Swab count

The 'lost swab' is one of the nightmares of surgery. The more difficult the operation the more likely it is that a small swab is left inside the operation site, hence the need for the radio-opaque thread. It may be a throat pack, a post-nasal swab, an abdominal pack or a small swab in the bladder. The following steps are taken in the preparation and use of swabs to prevent such loss.

1. All swabs are packed in bundles of ten or five according to local custom. Each bundle is tied or stitched to prevent any possibility of a swab becoming detached. Two persons should count the bundles before they are placed in the packet or drum for sterilisation.

2. The scrubbed-up nurse who assists at the operation is responsible for the swab count and must check the number in each bundle of swabs which is placed on her trolley. This count should take place in the presence of a second nurse.

3. The number of bundles taken from the drums and placed in service on the instrument trolley should be recorded on a blackboard or slate which is fixed in the theatre in such a position that it can be seen by any member of the nursing staff.

4. No swab should be cut in order to make a swab of smaller size. If for some reason during the operation the surgeon finds it necessary to cut a swab, the fact must be carefully noted and the pieces retrieved with certainty. It sometimes becomes necessary if a swab is inadvertently caught between a pair of artery forceps.

5. Used and rejected swabs should be thrown into a special bucket. During the operation the scrubbed-up nurse must watch the surgeon and his assistant constantly so that if any swab falls on the floor it can be instantly retrieved by a nurse or orderly and placed in the swab bucket.

[1] It is now known that cellulose fibres from these drapes enter abdominal wounds and may produce a form of peritonitis similar to that arising from glove powder (page 470).

6. The second nurse or orderly must be responsible for placing each swab on a counting rack—a simple frame with cup hooks arranged in rows of ten, or twelve (Fig. 18.5). The scrubbed-up nurse can then make an instant check of her swabs at any stage in the operation. The practice of spreading swabs on the floor for counting is both dirty and dangerous; the swabs should be confined to a small area.

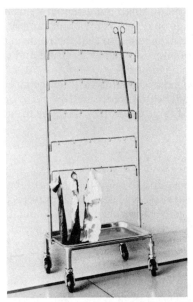

Fig. 18.5 Swab-counting rack. Used swabs are thrown into a bucket. They are then removed with Cheatle's forceps (shown on the rack), unfolded and sorted in the tray or on the rubber sheet in front of the rack. They are then placed on the rack as shown, different sizes being kept separate.

7. Swabs are not to be used for the final operation wound dressing. Special dressing packets containing cut gauze should be available as this is the only method of ensuring that no swab leaves the operating theatre. The dressing pack is not opened until the skin stitches are being. inserted. A second swab count is then carried out. There is then no further risk of a swab being lost.

8. If a gauze roll is used for packing, care must be taken that the unused portion which may have been cut off is removed to the swab rack. Under no circumstances should individual pieces be cut from a gauze roll during the operation.

9. It has become standard practice to use coloured (green) swabs in the anaesthetic room and to allow only coloured swabs on the anaesthetic machine or table in the theatre. This avoids any possible confusion by the introduction of uncounted swabs into the operating theatre.

10. If a swab is lost, the nursing staff must never assume that it cannot be in the patient, and a relentless search must take place until the missing item is found.

11. All swabs should contain a strand of radio-opaque material and in cases of doubt an x-ray photograph is taken on the operating table to ensure that no swab has been left in the wound.

12. Small items such as dental rolls or tiny swabs used in certain abdominal operations and neurosurgery must of course be checked in exactly the same way as the ordinary swabs.

13. When very small swabs ('Lahey dabs', 'peas') are used, they are clipped into pressure forceps or a length of tape is sewn to each swab to diminish the risk of its being lost in the depths of the wound.

14. It is the nurse's duty to inform the surgeon if a swab is missing and similarly to inform him as soon as she is certain that the swab check is correct, before the wound is finally closed.

Haberdashery. There are many small but essential items used for specific purposes— tape of various widths, special small swabs for brain surgery, etc. These should be made up in small packets each clearly labelled so that the name can be read. Such small items may be supplied out of a common sterile box or drum and care must be taken to avoid contamination of the remaining contents.

When packing a drum or other container with miscellaneous items it is essential that a standard arrangement should be followed. Small drums or boxes should be used to avoid unnecessary re-sterilisation of large quantities, since the drum should be autoclaved after each operating session.

Instruments

It is quite unnecessary for a nurse to know the names of the scores of instruments which are used in general and special surgery. There are, however, certain groups of instruments in common use and these together form the 'general foundation' set. Every theatre has a duplicated set of basic instruments of these types but special instruments may have to be borrowed from other units when it is thought that they may be required for an operating list.

The nurse must be conversant with the principal types of suture needle and ligature material used in simple surgery.

The exact method of sterilisation of instruments depends on the facilities, but the majority of items are prepared either by autoclave or by boiling. Sharp instruments such as scalpels, tenotomes, chisels and needles are kept in a rust-preventing powerful antiseptic (borax and formaldehyde, chlorocresol or glutaraldehyde), when an autoclave is not available in the theatre suite.

Table 33 shows, as an example, the instruments and sutures required for a simple hernia operation, in the order in which they will be used.

In the absence of pre-sterilised instrument packs, the 'foundation set' is usually kept sterile even when the theatre is not in use so that there will be the minimum delay in preparing for an emergency operation (page 321). If the instruments are sterilised by autoclave the set is dried by vacuum after sterilisation in the usual way, but the autoclave is left closed and the instruments are not drawn until they are required. No rusting occurs as the instruments have been dried hot and a 'vacuum' is present.

There are certain features common to the majority of surgical instruments. Almost without exception they are made from stainless steel but the nurse must at all times realise that surgical instruments are precision tools and must never be thrown about, dropped or strained during cleaning. Two-bladed instruments such as scissors and artery forceps may have screw-joints or box-joints. The advantage of the box-joint is that it does not become loose and the blades are then more likely to fit accurately. After being cleaned with a small nail brush, used instruments of this type should be decontaminated by boiling or autoclave, dried while hot, and the joint lubricated with a small brush. A heat-resisting silicone lubricant is more lasting than mineral oil. Even stainless steel will rust if neglected. Stiff-jointed instruments must be taken out of service as they have almost certainly been bent.

Table 33

Herniorrhaphy. A typical operation showing stage-by-stage instrument requirements. The 'scrubbed-up' nurse must learn to check her instruments in this way, so that there is no delay in handing them to the surgeon.

Skin cleaning—'Sponge holding' holding forceps (1 or 2 pairs) (page 375)

'Towelling-up'—5 towel clips (cross-action)

Skin incision—Scalpel handle No. 4. 2 blades (No. 20); a spare handle should always be available (Fig. 18.6); 10 or 20, pressure (artery) forceps, 12-cm, dissecting forceps, 2 pairs—toothed, 2 pairs—non-toothed. Plain catgut, thread, or diathermy may be required at this stage to deal with the bleeding points which have been clipped. Straight scissors for ligature cutting tetra towels (if used)

Muscle incision and dissection of hernial sac—Retractors, various, e.g. Czerney's and Langenbeck; curved Mayo scissors; tissue forceps (for holding spermatic cord), Littlewood's, 1 pair

Excision of hernial sac and tying of its neck by transfixion—Thread suture on Mayo catgut needle No. 5, or $\frac{1}{2}$-circle round-bodied needle No. 14; needle holder

Repair of inguinal canal—e.g. fascial strip from external oblique with curved scissors: attached to Gallie's needle by thread on a straight triangular needle: strip finally anchored by thread on small $\frac{1}{2}$-circle (page 343); No. 18 needle

Closure of muscle aponeurosis—Nylon thread or chromic catgut on cutting edge needle, e.g. Moynihan $\frac{5}{8}$-circle 70 mm.

Closure of subcutaneous fat—**Plain** catgut or Dexon on curved or $\frac{5}{8}$ needle as for muscle closure

Skin suture—Skin hooks (for assistant to hold wound ends); skin clips, rack and 'applying' forceps or straight 'triangular' needles with 'suture' silk or Nylon

---

Modifications of a standard type of instrument are found usually in the length of the handle, the weight, or perhaps the exact curve of the blade.

Artery forceps (haemostats, pressure forceps). Wells (Thomas Spencer, 1818–97) was an English gynaecologist whose name has become almost synonymous with the double-bladed clip designed originally for applying to the cut ends of arteries. Strictly, the Spencer Wells type has straight blades and an overall length of $12\frac{1}{2}$ cm. Many modifications of this forceps have been made, and these include the curved blade with fine grooves on the jaws (Dunhill, Cairns); small blades for plastic surgery or infants ('mosquito', Halsted); long handles with sharply curved blades (cholecystectomy, Moynihan); or heavier ones with terminal teeth used in orthopaedic surgery (Kocher).

When an artery forceps is held up to the light and closed on to the first ratchet of the handle, the tips of the blades should be evenly closed. On the second ratchet at least half the length of the blade should be closed. If light can be seen between the jaws when the handles are fully closed, the instrument should be rejected. Blades may become bent by incorrect use. One of the most common faults is to use a light haemostat as a marker on an abdominal swab. The instruments are designed for soft tissue and they should not be misused.

Every foundation set must include 20^1 ($12\frac{1}{2}$ cm) haemostats of the Spencer Wells, Cairns or Dunhill pattern.

Abdominal operations require in addition a range of longer instruments.

Dissecting forceps. These are toothed or plain (non-toothed). There may be two teeth on one blade and one on the other, three into two, or four into three. Variations include, in addition to the number of teeth, the size of teeth and the shape of the tips. Individual surgeons prefer forceps of a weight which best suits their own technique and the differences are particularly noticed in the strength of spring. Both toothed and plain forceps must meet evenly at the points and an instrument can be readily distorted.

After use the jaws must be cleaned by brushing. The most difficult place to clean is where the two blades are joined together. Toothed instruments become locked if one tooth is bent, and to prevent damage a piece of rubber tubing should be slipped over the end of each pair when the instruments are not in use. If the spring handles become weak after prolonged use, the instrument should be discarded or re-set.

Scissors. The type of scissors most commonly used by the surgeon are the Mayo dissecting scissors, curved or straight. These have specially contoured blades and narrow but blunt points. They are used for inserting into tissues, separating structures during dissection, and cutting the tissues. They are made in different lengths and weights.

Flat blunt-pointed scissors are used by the assistant or the nurse for cutting ligatures and dressings, and Mayo curved scissors should never be used for this purpose as it is essential that they be kept very sharp.

Scissors with pointed blades are used for stitch-removal but are very rarely used in the operation field, 20-, 25- and 30-cm scissors are used for thoracic surgery or pelvic operations and extremely fine scissors are required for ophthalmic surgery.

Scissors have screw-joints and failure to cut may be due to the blades being blunt or the joint being loose. Blunt scissors are a nuisance during an operation and may in fact be dangerous. Many surgeons prefer their scissors autoclaved, but in some hospitals it is the practice for the scissors to be sterilised in an antiseptic solution because it is thought they may be blunted by heat methods. This is a misconception: as has already been stated, bluntness is almost always due to misuse such as straining the joint by attempting to cut cotton wool or gauze with curved scissors.

If scissors are sterilised in an antiseptic solution, there is a very considerable risk that this antiseptic will be conveyed to the tissues, as it is impossible to rinse it from the joint unless the instrument is worked to and fro in water.

Scalpels and other knives. The original pattern of scalpel, made in one piece and sharpened after each case, is now hardly ever seen. The one-piece knife is more robust than the blades of the detachable type and special scalpels are sometimes used in orthopaedic surgery, especially in the removal of a cartilage from the knee-joint. These scalpels are not usually made of stainless steel and should be sterilised by antiseptic solution. When not in use they must be stored either in a rust-preventing solution or in the dry state, smeared with soft paraffin. The damp atmosphere of the theatre annex is far more likely to rust a scalpel than prolonged immersion in borax and formaldehyde.

The standard pattern of scalpel handle (Bard-Parker, Swan Morton, Gillette, etc.) is made in three sizes to fit a variety of blades (Fig. 18.6). Numbers 10 and 15 blade are most

---

[1] It has been customary to provide multiple instruments such as haemostats in dozens, but most theatres now prefer 5s or 10s as with swabs.

commonly used with the small handle, while 20, 22 and 23 on the large handle are used for the initial incision in the majority of operations. Handles are sterilised by autoclave or boiling. Blades are now supplied in double-wrapped foil packages, pre-sterilised by irradiation. If unsterile blades are provided they must be degreased and autoclaved or boiled but not left lying about in the damp, or they rapidly become blunt from rusting at the edges.

A **tenotome** is a special tiny blade on a long slender handle used for dividing a tight tendon through a small skin puncture, without open operation. Special knives for use in ophthalmic surgery have to be prepared with very great skill and are tested for sharpness immediately before use on a tiny drum of tightly stretched wash leather. Skin-graft knives also have to be specially sharpened but many plastic surgeons prefer to keep their own knife and hone it themselves. Skin-graft knives are available with detachable blades which are used for one or at the most two cases and then discarded without re-sharpening.

Probes, aneurysm needles. Various types of probe must be included in any foundation set of instruments and special probes are required for specific purposes such as exploring the common bile duct or probing the lacrimal duct. The ordinary straight probe has a slotted eye through which a piece of tape or a safety-pin is attached to prevent the probe becoming lost in the steriliser. Probes are usually made of a malleable metal so that they can be bent for exploring sinuses. The $12\frac{1}{2}$-cm malleable probe in common use is made of silver. A probe-pointed director has a grooved shank, down which a scalpel is passed to open a fistula track into which the probe has been inserted.

The aneurysm needle derived its name from its use in passing ligatures deep to an artery when the vessel was to be tied in the region of an aneurysm (pathological dilatation of an artery). The term 'ligature-carrier' is sometimes applied to this instrument which appears in various shapes and sizes with a right and left angle or a straight shank. The tip carries an eye through which the ligature is inserted before the instrument is passed. A straight and angled instrument must be included in each foundation set.

Needle holders. A surgeon becomes familiar with one particular pattern and may find it extremely difficult to use a different type. The needle holder becomes almost part of his hand and it is absolutely essential that the instruments should be free from faults. Needle holders designed for light work such as the Kilner and Gillies pattern are easily damaged if used on thick or heavy needles. Similarly if a heavy needle holder is used on a small needle, the needle will be broken. The MacPhail and Halsted types are particularly liable to puncture the surgeon's glove in its palm, and when these patterns are used particular inspection of the gloves is advisable.

Towel clips. These are used for attaching the draping towels around the wound, or for fixing a small tetra or side towel over the cut edges of the skin. The Doyen type is usually employed for skin towels in sets of four or six. The Backhaus pattern is also used for this purpose. Cross-action clips are used for attaching the surrounding towels and some surgeons have a habit of clipping the towel to the skin: two unpleasant punctures are then made which remain as sore places after the operation!

A minimum of six Backhaus or cross-action clips is required for any operation apart from those which may be needed for the tetra towels. Some surgeons avoid the use of towel clips by attaching the drapes with an adhesive mastizol painted along the edges of the area to be exposed. Commonly 'Steridrape' (Fig. 18.4) or other self-adhesive sterile protective sheet is used to cover the exposed operation area and this fixes the side towels.

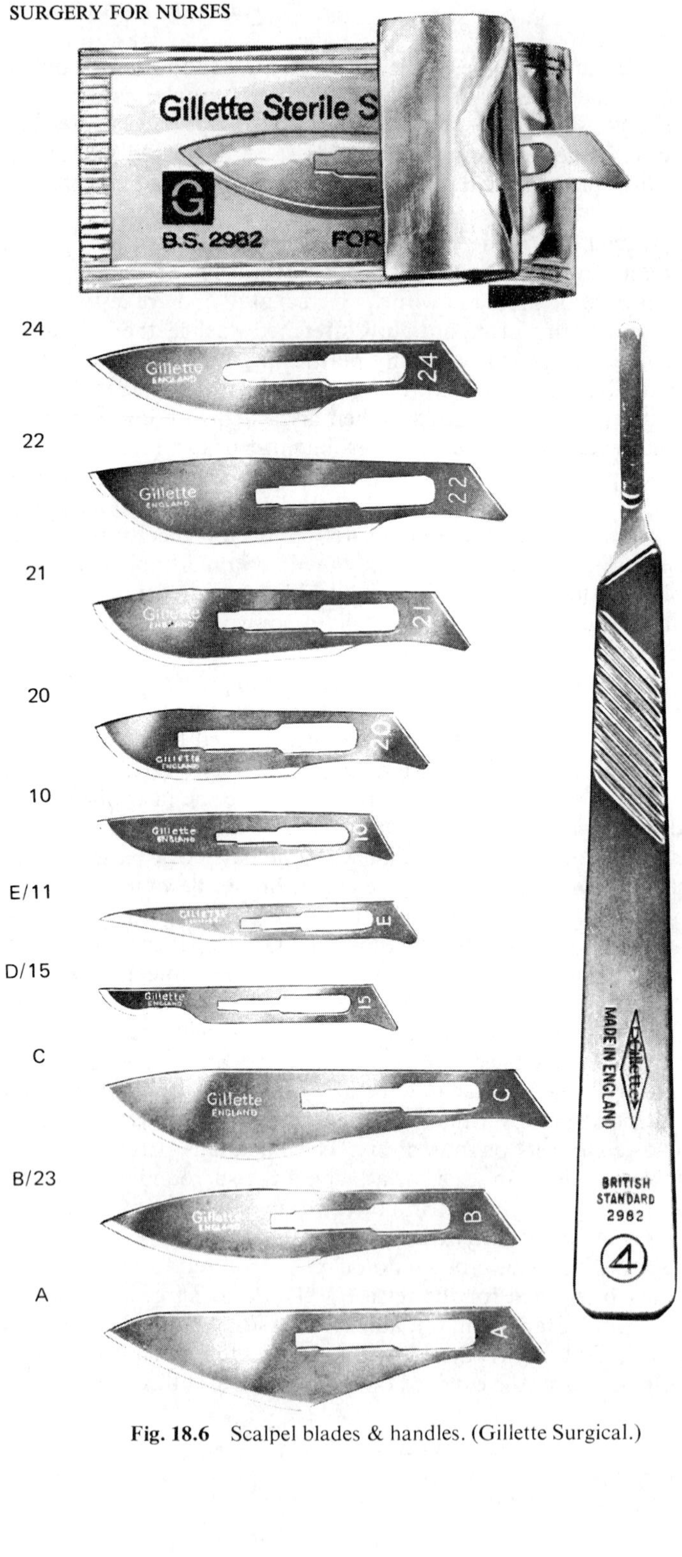

Fig. 18.6   Scalpel blades & handles. (Gillette Surgical.)

Tissue forceps. These are used for grabbing or holding tissues during dissection and every pattern has a ratchet handle. The varieties are distinguished by their jaws, which are illustrated in Fig. 18.7. The Babcock pattern is used in the majority of units for holding delicate tissues such as stomach or bowel; the Crawford or Allis pattern can also be used for this purpose, but is somewhat heavier. The Lane and Littlewood types are used for fat or aponeurosis such as the abdominal wall. The Duval type, originally designed for holding the lung, is also used on the intestine, liver or other soft tissue where the grip should be spread over a wide area. Care has to be taken not to strain the jaws as the teeth

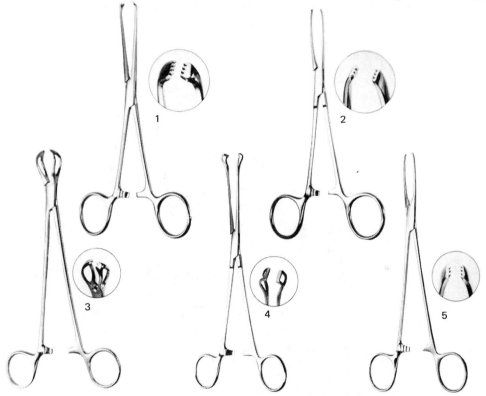

Fig. 18.7 An example of the variation to be found in surgical instruments. Five types of tissue forceps each designed for a specific purpose. Note the variation in the shape and gripping mechanism of the jaws. (Actual length 15–20 cm)

1. Allis'; for grasping fibrous tissue or skin that is to be removed; not suitable for delicate tissues. Note: 4 into 5 teeth. **2.** Similar, but with lighter jaws. Note 3 into 4 teeth. **3. Lanes';** very light springing; the jaws have no teeth. **4. Babcock's;** similar to 2, but longer. **5. Judd-Allis';** heavy pattern used for orthopaedic surgery in particular, or for grasping whole thickness of abdominal wall. (Seward Surgical Instruments.)

must be an accurate fit. After use the jaws must be scrubbed to ensure that no blood or tissue is embedded in the teeth.

Retractors. These are usually made of stainless steel with blades of various sizes, angles and curves. There are many varieties ranging from simple small hooks to deep retractors with 20-cm blades for operations in the depths of the pelvis. Some are double-ended while others have a single blade with a long handle. There are also several varieties of self-retaining retractors, the blades of which are attached to a frame which keeps them in place during use, whereas the ordinary retractors are held by an assistant. Malleable retractors usually made of copper are sometimes used, as these can be bent to the shape which the surgeon requires at any particular time during the operation.

Some self-retaining retractors are fitted with a light which is held in the depths of the wound. Every special department of surgery has its own particular variety of retractor. Eye, mastoid, thyroid, rib, abdominal, bladder and hip operations need special retractors.

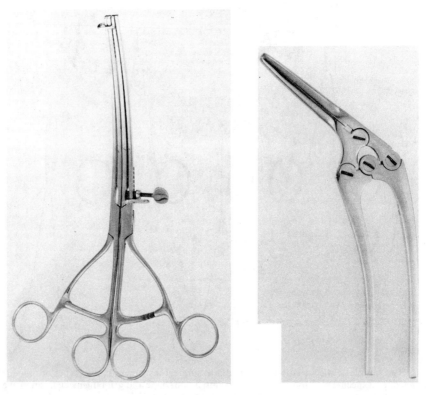

Fig. 18.8   Fig. 18.9

Fig. 18.8 Lane's twin clamp. This is the most commonly used instrument for holding together the width of the stomach and a loop of small intestine for anastomosis either following gastrectomy or in the construction of a gastro-enterostomy. Not only do the clamps hold the organs in accurate approximation but they control the bleeding while the sections are opened and the anastomosis formed. (Seward Surgical Instruments.)

Fig. 18.9 Payr's intestinal crushing clamp. The broad blades and great leverage ensure that a strip of bowel wall is crushed and sealed by pressure. It is then tied or oversewn to form a blind end. Such instruments, although made of hard stainless steel, require care, particularly in cleaning. (Seward Surgical Instruments.)

Various forms of clamps are used to hold sections of the gastro-intestinal tract during removal and reconstruction. Long-bladed clamps are applied parallel to the length of the stomach or bowel to be joined, thus preventing the escape of contents and controlling the blood supply (Fig. 18.8). When 'blind ends' have to be formed a straight clamp is used and the end to be closed is sometimes crushed and then oversewn to guard against haemorrhage and leakage (Fig. 18.9). A standard laparotomy set should always include a crushing clamp and two pairs of straight intestinal clamps. Special long-handled instruments are made for working in the depths of the pelvis in rectal operations.

Ligature and suture material

A **ligature** is a piece of material such as thread or catgut tied around a blood vessel or piece of tissue. The end to be tied may be held in an artery forceps or the ligature may be passed beneath the vessel or duct by means of an aneurysm needle. A **suture** is a stitch introduced on a surgical needle. Large blood vessels or pedicles of tissue are transfixed by a suture which is then tied round the piece of tissue as a ligature. During an operation, troublesome bleeding points are frequently under-run in this manner and if there is any likelihood of a simple ligature slipping, transfixion is used.

Surgical procedures are very rarely *absolutely* sterile. There is always the risk of infection in the wound and the ideal ligature material must produce the minimum of tissue irritation which would lower the resistance of the cells to infection. 'Monofilament' materials such as wire or Nylon are less likely to harbour infection than those made up of twisted multiple threads. Catgut is more irritant than other substances because it contains chemical by means of which it has been sterilised. Nevertheless catgut is absorbed by tissue digestion and, if infection should occur, a ligature or suture of catgut only acts as a foreign body for a few days. On the other hand a knot of thread or silk in an infected wound leads to the development of a persistent fistula or sinus and eventually the stitch may have to be removed.

Catgut is made from sheep's intestines. It is prepared commercially to British Pharmacopœia standards and is supplied in sealed packets (previously in glass tubes) which contain xylol or some other chemical used to keep the catgut in perfect condition, free from water.

The thickness of the catgut varies from 6/0 (extremely fine) to 4 (so thick that it is rarely used).

There are three degrees of hardness which determine the rate at which the catgut is digested by the tissues. As would be expected, digestion occurs very much more rapidly in the bowel and in the muscle than elsewhere such as in subcutaneous fat. **Plain** (unhardened) catgut is absorbed during the second week but it may lose its tensile strength and therefore its usefulness in four or five days. **Chromic** catgut (hardened by chromic acid) is used to sew muscles and muscle sheaths such as the abdominal wall where the strength of the catgut is required until the tissues have become firmly united; it is absorbed during the third week and retains its tensile strength for at least two weeks; sometimes chromic catgut knots can be found in a wound six weeks after an operation. **Intestinal** (extra hard) catgut resists digestion and retains its strength even in the bowel for seven days. During an operation it is essential that the surgeon knows exactly what catgut he is using and that he is not given plain catgut when he expects chromic. An error on the part of the theatre nurse may lead to a burst wound and subsequent fatality.

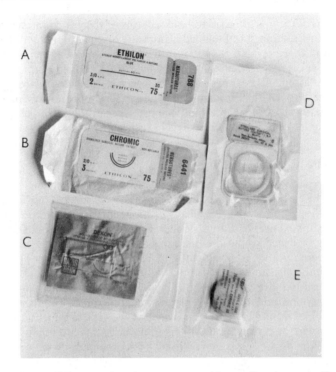

Fig. 18.10   Types of suture/ligature package in common use. Almost all packs are sterilised by irradiation with gamma rays, and there are variations in the manner of double wrapping. **A.** Foil and plastic outer packet: eyeless needle with non-absorbable polyamine suture: paper inner envelope (Ethicon). **B.** Chromic catgut suture: curved eyeless needle each end (for anastomosis of intestine): paper inner envelope (Ethicon.) **C.** Plastic 'see through' outer packet: golden foil inner envelope: catgut substitute synthetic absorbable suture: eyeless needle (Dexon, Davis & Geck). **D.** Foil and plastic outer packet: 'see through' inner packet: catgut ligature (Armour). **E.** Plastic outer and inner 'see through' packet: catgut ligature (Davis & Geck).

Catgut should not be exposed a long time before it is required as it must not be allowed to get dry. Most brands require a quick rinse in sterile water before use, but some makers recommend that the length of catgut should be passed through a wet swab and not immersed in water. Under no circumstances should catgut be soaked. If it is allowed to dry or become kinked some of its strands break and it is no longer reliable.

Most catguts are now available in overwrap pre-sterilised packets, packed in plastic or cardboard boxes. There is a foil or outer envelope, and a plastic or paper inner packet containing the ligature in fluid, or dry, depending on its type. The 'unscrubbed' nurse peels back the outer packet and ejects the sterile envelope to the sterile field of the instrument trolley. The scrubbed gloved nurse opens this as required. If it is not used, it may be made available for a subsequent case by storage in an antiseptic, or it may be thrown away, according to local rule.

Each packet contains a label showing the grade and manufacturer's batch number and these labels should be retained during the operation in case the surgeon wishes to check the grade or finds that the particular batch is faulty.

A synthetic protein-like material, Dexon, is used increasingly as a catgut substitute. It is less irritant and does not produce an inflammatory reaction in the tissues. There is thus less swelling in a wound. It is used for skin closure if a limb is to be encased in plaster, as these stitches usually dissolve and do not need removal.

Thread. Linen thread made from flax is a very popular ligature material as it is strong, cheap, easily sterilised and very reliable. Its disadvantage is that it may cause persistent trouble in the presence of infection. It is sterilised by autoclaving or boiling and sizes in common use are 100, 80, 60 and 40, 100 being the thinnest. Thread is used principally for ligaturing bleeding points. It is not used as a skin suture. It is loosely wound on spools and sometimes used from a metal perforated 'egg' which the surgeon holds in his hand. Some surgeons have coloured thread, different colours being used for different thicknesses. Thread is also supplied in pre-sterilised double-wrapped lengths.

Silk. Various forms of silk ligature and suture material are in common use. **Floss** silk is very thick but soft and is used for special purposes such as a ligature for a patent ductus arteriosus where there is no risk of infection, or for the ligature and excision operation for haemorrhoids where the silk is eventually extruded as healing progresses.

Chinese silk of various thicknesses 00000 to 5 is used for tissue repair where strength is needed. It is sometimes employed in intestinal anastomosis. It has been largely replaced by stainless steel wire when a strong suture is needed, as for tendon repair. **Suture silk** is specially manufactured for surgery and treated with special wax to prevent it harbouring infection or absorbing serum. It is relatively cheap, can be sterilised by autoclave or boiling, and for this purpose must be wound loosely on a large-diameter spool, or can be supplied in sterile packets. It causes practically no tissue reaction, and is used extensively for skin suture.

Nylon. This is supplied in various thicknesses distinguished by colour. Although it can be obtained in reels, it is usually supplied in hanks of approximately 51 cm in length. **Monofilament Nylon** is used for skin suture and increasingly now for muscle suture instead of chromic catgut. It is very dependable, does not encourage infection and is completely non-irritant to the tissues. As it has a slippery surface the knots are apt to slip. **Braided Nylon** is used for the suture of the chest wall and sometimes for special ligatures on the root of the lung and elsewhere. **Polypropylene** is similar to Nylon and is used particularly for suturing blood vessels.

Nylon is sterilised by boiling or by autoclave. It can be stored in borax and formalin solution, but for this purpose the standard solution must **not** contain phenol. Under no circumstances must any material or appliance containing Nylon come into contact with carbolic (phenol) in any form as the Nylon becomes spongy and eventually dissolves.[1]

Unused packets of ligature material which have been removed from the overwrap but not opened, may be re-sterilised in chlorhexidine spirit or alcohol solution.

Wire. Stainless steel and tantalum wire in thicknesses 25 to 40 standard wire gauge (SWG) are used in orthopaedic surgery for the repair of tendons and in general surgery for the suture of abdominal wall layers and for hernia repair. A lattice (filigree) is also supplied as a ready-made gauze. Fine **flexible** multistrand steel sutures are used for tendon repair (Flexon). Silver wire is occasionally used.

[1] Nylon nail brushes, which, though more expensive, are much more durable than bristle brushes, are completely ruined by immersion in carbolic solutions. Unfortunately they become very hard after repeated autoclaving and are then abrasive to the skin and nail beds.

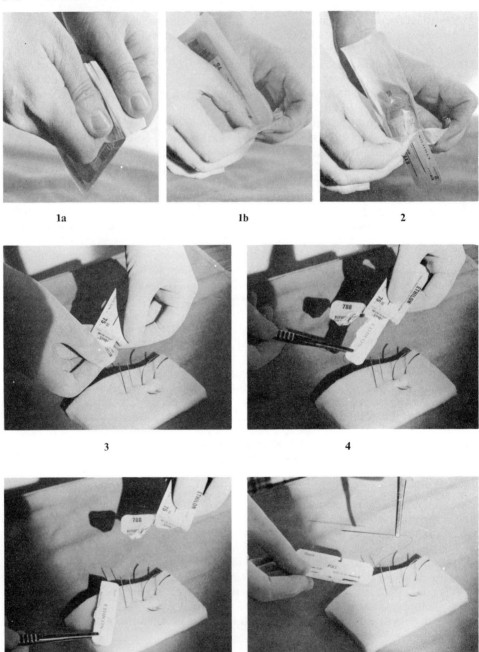

1a   1b   2

3   4

5   6

Wire is sterilised by boiling or autoclave and must be wound on a wide spool as it becomes readily kinked.

Clips. Clips for closing the skin are described on page 405 and are of two types, Kifa and Michel. They are available in various sizes from 9 to 14 mm, and single or double width.

Silver wire clips (Cushing) are used in neurosurgery and for such operations as lumbar sympathectomy. Short pieces of wire specially prepared on a rack are applied to the bleeding points with special clip-holding forceps. The silver is non-irritant and the clip remains in place permanently. Similar clips are made from tantalum wire. They are prepared by the theatre staff from a spool of wire. All metal clips are sterilised with the general instruments.

Fascia. Sutures of living fascia taken from the thigh (fascia lata) or from the external oblique aponeurosis are used for the repair of hernias and in certain orthopaedic reconstruction operations. The tissue is taken by the surgeon sometimes by means of a special fasciatome and is tied on to Gallie's fascial needles. Fascia lata is also available commercially and is then really a foreign body and is no longer living tissue. Kangaroo tendon has been used where great strength is required. This is also supplied already sterilised.

Surgical needles

There are many varieties in common use. The needles are made of special steel which does not break easily when a bending force is applied. The smaller needles are used in needle holders while the large types are held in the surgeon's fingers. Variations in the three portions of a needle, the eye, body, and the tip, are made to suit different purposes (Fig. 18.12). When the eye of a needle carries thick suture material, the bulk which is pulled through the tissue is considerable and makes a hole much bigger than the sharp body of the needle. For fine plastic work and for intestinal surgery, the suture material is attached to the end of the needle which has been made hollow to receive it: there is no eye and therefore no enlargement or rough portion to drag through the tissues. Needles with ready-fixed sutures of this type are **atraumatic** needles.

The body of a needle may be **round**, **flat** or **triangular**. The majority of surgical needles are flattened towards the eye to prevent them spinning round between the jaws of the needle holder during use. The part of the body nearest the tip sometimes has cutting edges to enable it to be pushed through thick tough tissue such as tendon or breast. In each pattern there is a range of sizes, and in most types the smaller sizes have the higher numbers. The needles illustrated are shown in their actual sizes, the numbers chosen being those most commonly used in general surgery.

Needles may be supplied in paper packets, greased to prevent rust; these must be cleaned with spirit or cetrimide or boiled initially. As many surgeons now use atraumatic sutures in which the suture is welded to the disposable needle, *packets* of ordinary needles

---

Fig. 18.11 Opening ligature/suture packets. **(1a)**. The outer envelope is opened by peeling back the free edges. The free flaps are gripped between the thumbs and index fingers and the hands rolled outwards thus avoiding any risk of contact with the inner pack: the 'scrub' nurse extracts the inner packet with forceps. Alternatively **(1b)** the 'unscrubbed' nurse peels up the flaps with her fingers and ejects the sterile inner pack onto the sterile field **(2)**. This method does not involve the 'scrub' nurse in diverting her attention from the operation. The 'scrub' nurse tears or cuts the inner packet **(3)** and extracts the suture **(4)**: this is placed on her needle/ligature (foam plastic) pad **(5)**. The suture is removed from its card when required **(6)**.

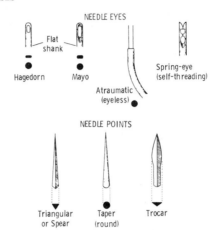

Flat
shank

Hagedorn   Mayo

Atraumatic
(eyeless)

Spring-eye
(self-threading)

NEEDLE POINTS

Triangular
or Spear

Taper
(round)

Trocar

Fig. 18.12   Distinguishing features in the eye and point of surgical needles.

are rarely supplied and most varieties are available in pairs, pre-sterilised. They may be stored in a dish of formalin instrument solution to which anti-rust chemical is added. If a particular type of needle is wanted urgently, sterilisation is easily achieved by boiling or autoclaving, the needles being attached to a piece of lint. When 'laying up' for an operation the nurse should ensure that there are at least four of every type of needle which the surgeon may require, so that while he is using one the second needle may be held already threaded, leaving two spare on the tray. Odd numbers are bad for checking. Nothing is more irritating for the surgeon than being requested to hand back his needle for it to be reloaded. When 'atraumatic' sutures are used, each packet from which the needle has come is preserved and the needle attached to it when the surgeon hands it back. Great care must be taken during an operation to ensure that no needle is lost and the needle check is as important as the swab check. Most types of needles are now available in pairs, prepacked, sterilised by radiation and disposable, as with ligatures.

Surgical needles do not last for ever. The points and the cutting edges become blunt. They should never become rusty if they are properly cleaned and kept in rust-preventive solution, or passed through anti-rust paper.

The needle holder must never be applied close to the eye of the needle as this is the weakest point. It should be placed one-third of the length of the needle from the eye.

If it is preferred to store the needles dry, sets of those required for routine operations may be prepared during quiet periods. A strip of lint with a complete set of needles is then sterilised with the other instruments by autoclave or boiler. Atraumatic needles are supplied already sterilised with the length of suture material attached, in foil packets in the same way as catgut is prepared.

Tubing and catheters

An assortment of drainage tubes of various types and sizes must always be available. Rubber is now rarely used though thin latex 'Paul's' tubing containing a strip of ribbon gauze is occasionally asked for. All tubes must be autoclaved. Various types are provided gamma-ray sterilised (e.g. corrugated Portex). Surgeons frequently use proprietary drainage tubes with suction provided to ensure constant drainage (page 402).

If single gamma-ray-sterilised double-wrapped items are not available, urinary catheters should be prepared in small bundles held together by elastic bands so as to avoid contaminating a complete set when only one catheter is required. Methods of sterilising urinary catheters have already been described (Chapter 17). They must be rinsed before insertion.

Dressing materials

The initial post-operative wound dressing is always of sterile gauze which should be taken from a distinctive packet to avoid confusion with swabs (page 331). The dressing packet must contain an adequate amount of sterile, high-quality wool. Sterile bandages are required in limb surgery, particularly if a plaster cast is to be applied; crepe bandages are frequently used and an adequate supply must be available, but crepe cannot be sterilised without deterioration.

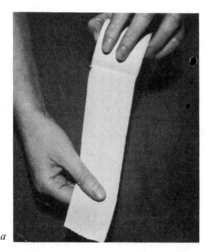
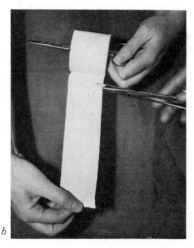

Fig. 18.13   The use of Elastoplast. Adhesive strapping must be kept clean and the adhesive surface should not be touched in taking it from the roll. (*a*) The incorrect method showing fingers unnecessarily applied to the roll. (*b*) The correct method. The roll is held quite easily on a pair of scissors, and the required length is pulled away by the surgeon and cut with **sterile** scissors.

The majority of dressings are anchored initially by adhesive strapping which should be kept in the theatre in tins, and not left on a tray exposed to the air and dust. Fig. 18.13 shows the right and wrong ways of handling a roll of adhesive strapping. For practical purposes the adhesive surface can be regarded as clean if not absolutely sterile. It must not be fingered except at the very end of the piece which is to be applied. Some surgeons prefer to seal wounds without a dressing by the spray application of a film of plastic (Nobecutane).

ENDOSCOPIC INSTRUMENTS

The care, assembly, testing and cleaning of endoscopic instruments calls for the utmost care and conscientious attention to detail. Some of the heavier instruments are boilable but all electrical apparatus must be detached during the sterilisation process. A formalin cabinet may be available in which even the long instruments such as the bronchoscope and gastroscope may be stored. Every time an instrument is replaced in sections in its wooden box, there is an additional risk of its being damaged. In preparation for endoscopic examination, particularly in urology, it is not known for certain which instrument will be used and several are prepared. For this reason it is much more convenient and economical to have a large formalin cabinet in which all these instruments are ready and from which they can be withdrawn and placed on the instrument trolley only as the surgeon requires them. In this way a great deal of unnecessary assembly and cleaning is avoided, with consequent reduction of damage.

Non-boiling instruments may be 'pasteurised' at a temperature below boiling point but sufficient to kill the common organism, but not spores. Cidex glutaraldehyde is a commercial product now widely used.

Many instruments have a lens system which is easily damaged by abrasion during cleaning (for instance, by an accidental scratch with the nurse's finger nail), by bending, or by a jar such as may be sustained if the instrument is placed sharply on a hard table. Exposed lenses may be cleaned with cetrimide: spirit should be avoided as it may dissolve the cement round the lens.

Many accessories such as rubber washers, spare bulbs and lighting flex should be sterilised with the instrument in the formalin cabinet and small items should be placed clearly labelled in a pill box or tin which has a perforated lid, to allow the free circulation of the formalin vapour (also page 307).

Fibre-optic Illumination

Glass fibres possess a property of conveying light along their length even when bent. A collection of glass fibres surrounded by an opaque tube acts as a flexible rod conveying light from a powerful projector lamp to the spot where it is needed. This principle has been applied to endoscopic instruments and eliminates the need for small bulbs which burn out very quickly and are individually expensive. Most operating theatres now, and many out-patient departments, are equipped with fibre-light illumination systems for all their endoscopic instruments. The 'light source' is a small quartz lamp as used in slide projectors. The light is collected into the end of a flexible cable made of glass fibre. The output end is locked into the instrument which itself contains another length of glass fibre arranged to give maximum illumination at the end of the instrument. There is no risk of the apparatus fusing, the bulb breaking, or of the instrument over-heating (see page 352).

Individual instruments and their use have been described in the appropriate chapters. Some of these are simple tubes with illuminated and very primitive lens systems, but the modern fibre-light flexible instruments also have a fibre-optical system and require very careful maintenance. Sigmoidoscopes and proctoscopes in many units are provided by the CSSD as required, or a single instrument may be kept on the ward or in a clinic, in which case it has to be cleaned and re-sterilised by the nursing staff. The special care required for urological endoscopes with very complicated lens systems applies to some extent to other types of apparatus.

Urological endoscopes

The female urethra can be examined with a simple tubular speculum resembling a miniature proctoscope, the 'Kelly's direct-vision female urethral speculum'. This instrument is in fact sometimes used for proctoscopy in children although it is a little narrow.

All other instruments used to examine various sections of the urinary tract contain a lens system arranged in such a way as to magnify and bring into correct focus the structures within the range of the end of the instrument. In addition to the lens system, the instrument must carry a light on the end. A third essential is that there must be some means of distending the urethra or bladder so that the mucous membrane is kept well away from the lens and the bulb. In the case of the anterior portion of the urethra, distension is achieved by air pumped in by a little hand bellows (cf. sigmoidoscopy, page 573): the posterior urethra and the bladder are distended with water.

Many endoscopic instruments have an extra channel through which can be inserted diathermy wire electrodes for cauterising or cutting structures in the bladder; long catheters may also be passed into the orifices of the ureters. Mounted on the head of the instrument may therefore be found irrigating taps, contacts for diathermy electrodes, contacts for the light, and tiny valves through which the ureteric catheters or operating instruments may be passed.

The insertion of instruments into the straight female urethra is a simple matter but the curve of the male urethra presents greater difficulty. Many endoscopic instruments are straight, but simple instruments for examining the bladder are frequently beaked to facilitate their introduction. Some of the curved instruments and all of the straight ones have an outer **sheath** and an internal **obturator** which is used for the introduction of the sheath to block up the eye, or opening at the end. Once the instrument is in position, the obturator is removed and the lens system and other accessories are introduced.

Urethroscopes

The anterior part of the male urethra is inspected by a short straight instrument consisting of an outer sheath (usually supplied in three sizes) which is closed with an obturator during introduction. The lens system consists of a simple eyepiece in the head to which is attached a light on a stalk. The urethra is distended by air introduced very gently by the bellows which is attached to the head of the instrument.

The posterior urethra is examined with an instrument which, like the cystoscope, has the lens system built into a tube or 'telescope', with a direct objective lens looking straight ahead. The posterior urethra needs to be distended with a continuous stream of water as the fluid will run straight into the bladder.

Cystoscopes

The simplest form of cystoscope is really a very simple telescope into which is built a light, and in which there is a prism at the tip to enable the field of vision to cover a wide area of the bladder wall (Fig. 18.16). Such a fixed telescope is sometimes used in tiny babies and the bladder is first distended with water injected through a catheter. The usual form of cystoscope, however, has an outer sheath from which the telescope is withdrawn after

English Pattern Cystoscope

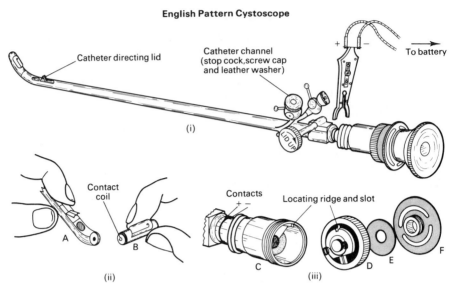

Fig. 18.14   Ringleb English pattern cystoscope with bulb lighting. This system is still in common use for routine cystoscopic work.

insertion into the bladder. Urine is then allowed to escape through the sheath. There is a flap valve at the head of the sheath and a cannula is passed through this so that the urine can escape. The bladder is then filled from a 250-ml syringe or from a gravity irrigator and the cannula withdrawn. The valve closes and retains the fluid in the bladder until the telescope is inserted. By rotating the instrument after insertion of the telescope, the surgeon can inspect the whole of the wall of the bladder.

An irrigating cystoscope is a similar instrument which carries in addition two valves on the head through which the irrigating fluid can be run continuously into the bladder, the inflow and outflow being controlled by taps (Fig. 18.15).

Catheterising cystoscopes

An instrument similar to the simple cystoscope but carrying one or two channels down which ureteric catheters may be passed, is used for the performance of 'retrograde pyelography'. The point at which the catheter enters the head of the cystoscope is made leak-proof either by a rubber teat with a small central hole or by a screw-down valve containing a leather washer. As the catheter is fed through the cystoscope the surgeon watches for its emergence at the tip of the instrument and then steers the catheter towards the ureteric orifice partly by movement of the whole instrument and partly by turning a small knob which controls 'bridge' or 'lid'. This is a tiny flap at the end of the instrument (Figs. 18.14, 18.15).

Larger instruments of this type are made to carry tiny knives or even scissors which by remote control may be used for operating on the ureteric orifice.

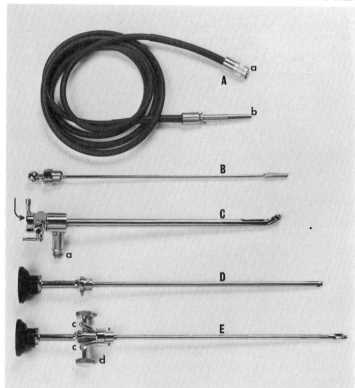

Fig. 18.15 Modern Brown-Buerger examination and catheterising cystoscope with fibre-light illumination. **A.** Light cable composed of thousands of fibre-glass strands. **B.** Obturator which is inserted into the main sheath **C** for the introduction of the cystoscope. It occludes the eye of the sheath, presenting a smooth surface to the urethra. **C.** The main sheath carrying in its wall a fibre-light bundle. The cable **A (a)** is attached to the light pillar **(a)**, the beam of light emerging from the beak of the sheath. The head of the sheath carries a rotating lock and two irrigating channels with individual taps. **D.** Examining telescope containing within the tiny tube a complex of lenses with a prism at the tip. **E.** Alternative operating telescope for catheterisation of the ureters or to carry a diathermy electrode. Tubes **(c)** are covered with rubber caps through which the catheter or electrode is passed, thus making a watertight seal. At the tip of the catheterising telescope is an elevating flap operated by a wheel **(d)** which enables the catheter or electrode to be directed to the appropriate point. **A (b)** on the fibre-light cable is plugged into the light source (Fig. 18.18).

Panendoscopes and resectoscopes

These terms are applied to the large instruments which are used mainly for operating on the prostate and bladder neck. The principles of their construction are similar but their sheaths may be made from insulating material and their diameter is very much greater. By means of a sliding wire loop, pieces of prostate may be cut out with diathermy or small portions of growth removed either from the bladder or prostate for biopsy. Such instruments need to have wide irrigating channels in order to remove the pieces that have been resected and in order that an adequate amount of fluid may be run through the bladder to absorb the heat generated by the diathermy current.

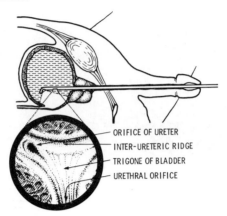

ORIFICE OF URETER
INTER-URETERIC RIDGE
TRIGONE OF BLADDER
URETHRAL ORIFICE

Fig. 18.16 Section through pelvis to indicate the field of vision in cystoscopy. By rotating the instrument the surgeon inspects the entire cavity. By altering the angle of the cystoscope and inserting it further, he can inspect any particular area more closely.

Care and maintenance of endoscopic instruments

All these instruments have to be treated with very great respect owing to their precision, their delicacy and their very great expense.

The telescope of a simple instrument may contain as many as sixteen lenses arranged in pairs along the length of a tiny tube. This telescope tube may easily be bent by a nurse inadvertently pressing on it on a trolley or pushing it hard during its insertion into the sheath. If the lens system has been distorted the field of vision will be elliptical (Fig. 18.17). A knock or a strain will disturb the lenses and careless cleaning will deface the eye-piece or objective prism. The cement with which the lenses are fixed at the ends may become damaged and water or air may gain access to the telescope inside. Cystoscopes should never be immersed in or cleaned with spirit as this may dissolve the cement. Before they are put away after use, and again before they are sterilised, all instruments should have their lens systems inspected by a competent nurse.

Telescopes should be cleaned with soap and water after use and wiped with great care. They should always be handled by the head end and particular care must be taken not to strain the joint between the shaft and the head. The instruments used for children are of course even more delicate because of their small size.

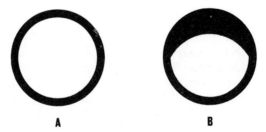

A   **B**

Fig. 18.17 The field of vision of the cystoscope should be a true circle (**A**). If it is elliptical (**B**), the telescope has been bent by careless handling.

Many hospitals have no duplicate instrument and if one which is needed is not serviceable, this fact must be discovered before the patient is anaesthetised. Such a warning may seem very obvious but instruments may be damaged easily in the hustle of preparing for a long list.

The sheath. This thin-walled metal tube can also be damaged very easily, particularly by picking it up with a pair of Cheatle forceps. Cheatle or bowl forceps should **never** be used on any part of a cystoscope because of the tremendous leverage which is produced by their long handles. Special types of cystoscope forceps are made but they are not recommended. The open end of the sheath may be very easily damaged by placing some other instrument on top of it. The inside of the sheath is cleaned by wool pledgets mounted on a special twisted probe usually provided with the instrument. The sheath must be thoroughly washed with a detergent or soap and water immediately after use, before there is any opportunity for debris or blood to become dried on the inside. The sheath usually carries also the wires for the light and has a detachable bulb at its tip. It is perhaps more convenient to describe the care of the individual components which are attached to this sheath.

The head valve. On the majority of simple cystoscopes there is a screw-on cap carrying a little metal flap-valve which is kept down by a small spring (Fig. 18.14, iii); if during handling this spring is nipped, then, when the telescope is inserted through the cap, the flap is raised and becomes jammed above the spring: when the telescope is next removed, the fluid rushes out of the bladder because the valve has not closed. This is a common and unnecessary fault with cystoscopes. The screw-on cap keeps in position a leather washer which itself has a small hole in the centre, making a watertight joint around the telescope. Leakage of water during use occurs if the washer is damaged or worn. If it is difficult to insert the cystoscope this may well be due to the cap being screwed up too tightly as it compresses the leather washer around the telescope. The cap should therefore be unscrewed a little during insertion of the telescope. This valve is not needed in irrigating cystoscopes as the bladder can be emptied with the telescope in position.

Catheter cocks. These may be of two types. The simple open tube type of cock is covered by a small rubber teat. If the instrument is being used without catheters or with only one catheter, the cock not in use is covered with a teat without a hole in the centre. If catheters are to be passed through these cocks, then punctured rubber teats are used. Spare teats must always be available. They are sterilised by boiling and the hole in the centre must be small enough to grip the catheter and prevent leakage of water. The second type consists of a minute leather washer which is compressed in a small cup by a screw-in cap in exactly the same way as the cap on the head of a cystoscope compresses the valve around the telescope itself. The type with the screw-on cap has in addition a tiny tap which can be turned so that there is no leakage when the catheter is not in position (Figs. 18.15, and 18.14, i, respectively).

Irrigating cocks. These usually have a type of bayonet fitting to which the irrigating tubes can be connected. It is of course essential that these tiny fittings should be undamaged and that the pair of plug-in connectors appropriate to the particular instrument should be available on the ends of the irrigating tubes.

The lighting system. The source of electricity is either a dry battery or a transformer from the main supply with an intervening variable resistance in each case. The surgeon's greatest risk is always the nurse who turns the resistance the wrong way and 'blows the bulb'! The lighting system of every cystoscope must be tested before sterilisation and again immediately before it is given to the surgeon. The connecting flex has two loose prongs which are attached to the terminals of the battery box or transformer. There is usually a claw type contact which fits on to the head of the cystoscope. It consists of strips of metal separated by an insulator and again it is essential that the correct flex must be available for each cystoscope. Sometimes these are interchangeable but usually there is a very slight difference in the size of the head of the instrument and to use the wrong connector is to run the risk of straining the instrument while pushing the connector into place. Panendoscopes and most American cystoscopes have a simple push-on terminal which is switched on and off by rotation. These connectors must be kept scrupulously clean, and if the wires become detached, they must at once be repaired by soldering.

The lamp. Two main types of lamp bulb are used. On some of the larger instruments the bulb itself is housed inside a screw-on glass-fronted cap. In the smaller instruments and almost all British instruments the bulb itself screws into the end of the cystoscope. The electrical contacts are made between the outer case of the bulb and the shaft of the instrument and between the very tiny coil spring at the centre of the bulb base and the corresponding fixed metal point in the tip of the cystoscope. Contact is maintained by the springiness of this tiny wire on the base of the bulb and when a new lamp is placed in position failure may be due to this little wire having been compressed too far. The bulb should therefore be removed and the wire lengthened a little. It must always be kept central so that it does not short-circuit on the side of the bulb case.

When endoscopic instruments are in use an adequate supply of spare bulbs must be available for each instrument. Bulbs become blackened with use, but a black bulb is not necessarily a useless one. The present-day cost of cystoscope bulbs is about 50 pence, but it is the inconvenience, even more than the cost, which should make the nurse extremely careful in the testing and care of these lights. A bulb practically never fails in use. If the cystoscope is sterilised with the bulb in position it follows that the instrument is no longer sterile if the bulb is removed for changing. This simple fact is not fully realised by nurses handling cystoscopes. If however the instrument is sterilised in a formalin cabinet with the bulb *not* in place in the inside of the bulb holder, then the inside of the bulb holder is of course sterile. Cystoscopes must not be sterilised in fluid with the bulb removed because it is not possible to dry out the bulb case sufficiently to prevent short circuit in use. Many cystoscope manufacturers provide a small rubber teat to slip over the bulb in order that one may grip it to unscrew or screw it up. Care must be taken not

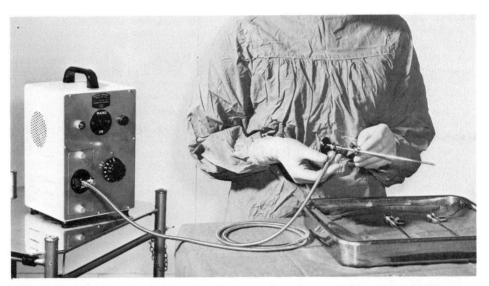

Fig. 18.18 Fibre-optic illumination for endoscopes. On the left is the light unit with a low-voltage quartz-halogen bulb similar to that used in slide projectors. The light is focused on to the end of a metal covered flexible fibre-glass cable which carries the illumination to the head of the instrument. A second bundle of glass fibres is built into the casing of the instrument and the light transmitted to the top of the endoscope. No heat is generated in the endoscope, there is no risk of bulb failure and there is no electrical connection to the patient. The instrument shown is a miniature infant cystourethroscope.

to insert the bulb with the screw thread crossed. If there is doubt about any particular bulb having fused, it may be tested very simply by touching its outer case on one prong of the flex connector and tiny base wire on the other prong. If it still fails to light the bulb could then be tested direct on the terminals of the battery, any metal instrument being used to connect one terminal to the base wire of the bulb. Rare instances have occurred of these bulbs bursting inside the bladder, but this is unlikely to happen unless the battery resistance is turned up too high.

Fibre-optic lighting is now being adopted generally for endoscopic instruments. This eliminates the use of a bulb on the endoscope itself (page 346).

The catheter elevating lid. This little flap on catheterising cystoscopes is pulled up and down by a tiny wire which passes up the sheath of the instrument to the control knob. Here again care must be taken not to damage this bridge or its control wire during cleaning operations when the cystoscope is put out for use; the action of this bridge must be tested. If the wire has become strained by careless use or cleaning, difficulty is experienced in shutting the lid right down. This limits the range of movement of the catheter when the surgeon is introducing it into the ureteric orifice or it may even prevent the introduction of the catheter carrier into the sheath.

Diathermy electrodes for resectoscopes. A nurse who has the care of such instruments will receive special instruction. The design of these more complicated endoscopic instruments varies considerably. The electrodes are made of special hard tungsten wire and care must be taken that they are not bent since the wire is brittle and will break. The electrodes have minute electrical contacts at one end and these too must be treated very gently.

The moving parts of a cystoscope such as the irrigating control taps, the screw-on or locking head valve, and the bulb carrier may be lubricated with special wax. Instrument manufacturers usually issue special instructions with their instruments and in many cases no lubrication at all is necessary. If for any reason abnormal stiffness develops, a trace of thin sewing-machine oil can be applied with a wisp of cotton wool or a tiny camel-hair brush. Fluid silicone is an excellent lubricant which can be sterilised by heat.

ELECTRICITY

Electric current is used for many purposes in the operating theatre and it is important that every member of the surgical team should be acquainted with the apparatus, its use, construction and maintenance.

Electricity in the operating theatre is considered under three headings:

(a) Low voltage used for illumination, of instruments from dry battery, accumulator or indirectly from the mains supply through a transformer.

(b) High voltage (main supply) for illumination—top light, mobile lights, x-ray screen illuminators; for suction and motor saws; for surgical diathermy; x-ray diagnostic apparatus; for cautery and low-voltage illumination through transformer units. Other special diagnostic apparatus such as an electrocardiograph may be used in the operating theatre.

(c) Static electricity.

Whatever the source or use of the electrical current there are certain inherent risks of its failure, its misapplication and subsequent danger to the patient or to members of the operating team.

Low-voltage electricity

Endoscopic instruments such as cystoscopes and illuminated retractors require a current usually between 2 and 10 volts. The current can be supplied from dry batteries, usually mounted in a box which contains a variable wire resistance so that the output voltage can be regulated to produce the desired degree of illumination. All instruments should be tested before use and care taken that the resistance is turned to zero when the apparatus is first connected. The control regulator should be turned up very slowly and if the lamp does not glow the control should be returned to zero and the circuit inspected for loose connections. Frequently a junior nurse is asked to turn the control knob up: no light shows when the control has reached its maximum, the surgeon or the sister moves some loose connection and the high voltage blows the bulb! Once the approximate desired intensity of light has been reached the resistance should not be moved and the light is then controlled solely by the surgeon with the switch on the instrument.

Electrical failure can occur through the battery being run down or through loose or corroded connections inside the box. Every operating theatre should possess a small voltmeter in order that the electrical circuits can be tested each day without the risk of damaging expensive instrument bulbs. There is a marked voltage drop in dry batteries before they fail completely. Daily battery testing is advised.

Low-voltage current may also be supplied through a mains transformer. The lead to the electric main must have a third wire for earth and 3-pin plugs are fitted to all theatre electrical apparatus.

Endoscopic instrument bulbs are best sterilised in formalin solution or preferably in a formalin cabinet. Some of the lamps have a small coil-wire contact which must not be damaged. The wire is brittle and if the contact is broken, the lamp is no further use. A blackened lamp is usually one which has become overheated, but it is not necessarily useless.

A cautery is a low-voltage hot wire loop in an insulated handle. It is used for haemostasis or destroying small tumours.

Electronic apparatus

With the increasing complexity of surgical procedures the variety of electrical apparatus used in the theatre is increasing. Low-voltage nerve stimulators with one wire connected to a pair of dissecting forceps are used when operations are being performed on peripheral nerves, or for instance in the dissection of the parotid gland to warn the surgeon if he is touching the facial nerve or its fibres. Pulse rate monitoring meters are usually battery powered. Electrical patient thermometers are supplied by mains electricity through transformers, or may be battery operated.

Oscilloscopes—like television screens—are electronic recorders for the continuous visualisation of electrical impulses in the body such as those produced by the heart-beat. These are very sensitive and can be put out of order by induced electrical currents from other apparatus in the theatre such as the diathermy.

The maintenance of all this electrical equipment is usually the responsibility of the theatre technician. Apart from the illumination of endoscopes and the use of diathermy, the majority of the other apparatus is controlled in use by the anaesthetist.

High-voltage mains electricity

In Britain the electrical mains supply is between 200 and 250 volts alternating current at 50 cycles per second. The supply voltage may vary between these limits and care must be taken that only suitable apparatus is used. A variation of 20 volts may make a very great difference in the working of an appliance or for instance of a mobile lamp. Diathermy and x-ray apparatus is usually equipped with a compensator to adjust for alterations of main voltage.

Illumination

The overhead operating lamp is usually suspended from the ceiling in such a way that it can be tilted in any direction. It can also be raised and lowered and in some cases traverses the theatre as well. The majority of lamps have a complicated lens system which produces a diffuse light from many angles so that the illumination of the operation field is 'shadowless' (Fig. 18.19). There should be no need for the nursing staff to interfere with this overhead lamp except for external cleaning. Most patterns have a focusing arrangement for the lamp and this is set by the engineer or whoever installs or replaces the bulb. Many operating lights fail to fulfil their function because someone has interfered with the focusing adjustment.

The main lighting usually has additional bulbs coupled with an auxiliary pilot supply which is switched on automatically if the main supply or bulb fails. The emergency pilot supply usually comes from storage batteries which are charged automatically by a 'trickle charging' plant. The emergency lighting must be tested regularly.

Mobile or spot lamps mounted on heavy-based trolleys are used as an accessory means of illumination and must be treated with the same care as the overhead lamp.

X-ray illuminating screens are usually wall-mounted with self-contained switches and require no maintenance except external cleaning.

Motor suction apparatus may be an independent unit or combined on a wheel-mounted trolley with diathermy and transformer units which provide the low-voltage current for endoscopic lights. The 'sucker' consists of a motor pump and one or two vacuum bottles. Some models have a pressure gauge and regulator. Many pumps have motors which are not totally enclosed and the sparks may cause an explosion if they are used at the same time as ether. Modern operating suites have the pump outside the theatre with a suction tap mounted on the wall. Various patterns of sucker nozzle are in common use. These and an adequate length of thick rubber pressure tubing must be sterilised with the instruments. A sucker is required for all abdominal surgery and must be available for operations on the nose, throat, ear, brain and chest. In fact, the sucker forms an essential item in every foundation set.

Immediately after use, sucker nozzles if not disposable and tubing must be washed through by a high-pressure jet from the water tap to prevent blood drying on the inside of the tube. It is insufficient merely to suck clean water through the nozzle and tube. Jars and fittings must also be cleaned regularly.

Surgical diathermy

By means of a special electrical apparatus working off the mains supply, a very-high-frequency current is used to cut or coagulate tissues in order to reduce bleeding, or to

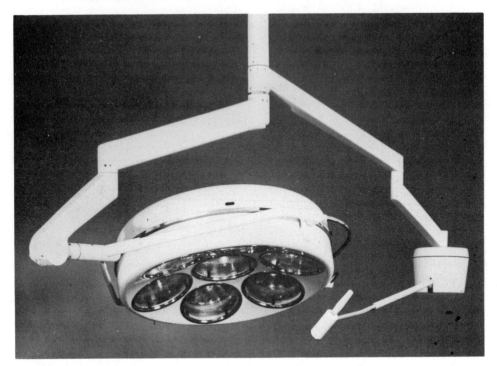

Fig. 18.19   Boston operating lamp. This is capable of movement over a large area: on the right, inde-pendently suspended, is a fibre-optic satellite providing an illuminating source for endoscopic instruments. (Sierex Ltd.)

destroy tumour cells. There are two types of diathermy machine. In the older pattern a spark-gap is used to produce the oscillations. The machine requires very little main-tenance, is extremely reliable, but lacks the fine adjustment of the more modern valve-operated circuits. The principle of the surgical diathermy is that when a high-frequency electric current is passed through the patient, the effect on the tissues depends on the path which the current takes. In the medical (short-wave) diathermy, electromagnetic waves are passed from one electrode to the other across the patient's tissues through a relatively wide area. In surgical diathermy one large electrode pad is used attached to the patient's leg or arm while the surgeon operates with a very fine pointed 'needle': all the energy (electric current) which is passing through the wide plate is dispersed over a broad surface and does no damage. At the other end of the circuit, the same energy is concentrated at the point of the needle which cuts through the tissues, sealing the blood vessels by coagu-lation. By varying the amount and type of current that is passed we can vary the degree of coagulation as well as the 'sharpness' of the cutting. Heat is generated by the diathermy and the chief risk in its use arises from improper application of the wide plate electrode, with the result that instead of being evenly dispersed the electrical energy is concentrated at one point and produces a burn. Unfortunately a diathermy burn is very indolent and slow to heal.

Diathermy apparatus does not have to be protected from the point of view of explosive risk, since the diathermy must never be used in the presence of any explosive anaesthetic agent and the anaesthetist's specific permission must be obtained in each case before the diathermy machine is connected. Most surgeons develop the habit of asking the anaesthetist immediately before using the diathermy needle. Apart from the maintenance of the apparatus, the nurse is concerned with two aspects of diathermy. The first is the application of the indifferent or plate electrode to the patient before the operation begins, and the second concerns the care of the active electrodes with which the surgeon operates.

The **indifferent electrode** consists of a soft metal plate to which is attached, by a screw clamp, one insulated wire from the diathermy machine. The **wet-plate** or **dry-plate** system may be used. With the wet method the plate (made of lead) must be **completely** enclosed in a bag or folded sheet of lint with at least two thicknesses over every part of the plate and with 5-cm overlap all round. Particular care must be paid to the corners of the plate, which may protrude through insufficient protection, and to the point where the terminal joins the plate. A thick bag made of turkish towelling into which the plate may be placed is perhaps safer than loose wrappings and the neck of the bag can be tied round the flex to ensure that the terminal is adequately covered. It is dangerous for this pad to be placed under the patient's buttock or sacral area if the diathermy is to be used for more than a few minutes, as the combination of pressure and diathermy may produce a sacral ulcer.

The indifferent electrode is moistened with strong saline (15–20 per cent) and the pad squeezed gently to remove excess of the fluid. The pad is then applied to a shaved portion of the thigh and bandaged firmly in position with a dry cotton or flannel bandage. A piece of waterproof sheeting should be bandaged lightly over the whole electrode to prevent any possible contact of the wet pad with the operating table or with any member of the surgical team. If these simple rules are followed there is unlikely to be any trouble from diathermy burn. The essential requirement is that the plate must be adequately protected and make even contact over as large an area as possible. The dry-plate indifferent electrode is so made that its edges are insulated to prevent high concentration of current at the corners. Very hairy skin should be shaved before application of the plate, which must be held firmly and evenly in position, usually on the thigh, by bandage or 'Velcro' bands.

Antistatic rubber which conducts electricity (page 325) is now used in the manufacture of theatre equipment. If the operating table mattress is made of this rubber, it is a source of danger if the patient's skin is in contact with it during the use of diathermy unless the area of contact is large. Care must be taken to protect the patient entirely or to ensure that the whole trunk is in contact with the mattress. Severe burns have occurred from local contact over a small area. On no account must any part of the patient be in contact with metal.

The **active electrodes** are attached to a sterile flex which has been prepared by formalin cabinet, by boiling, or by autoclave with the rest of the instruments. This flex is clipped in place on the operating table by means of a towel clip: care must be taken that the clip does not penetrate the flex or go through the operating towels into unsterile material underneath. On to the end of this flex is attached an insulated pencil-like electrode which carries a steel needle. A 'button' (small steel ball) electrode is used if the current is being used for haemostasis rather than for dissection.

The surgeon will give instructions as to the amount of current he requires.

By means of special cystoscopic electrodes the diathermy current is used for trans-urethral resection of the prostate and for destroying papillomas in the bladder wall. It is also used through other endoscopic instruments such as the thoracoscope.

Static electricity

Friction produces an electric change in certain objects. It produces the crackling sound which occurs when a cat is stroked, or when a silk garment is removed hurriedly. If a blanket is drawn quickly across a metal theatre trolley or operating table, a high voltage electric charge is given to the table if it is not properly earthed. This charge may jump to earth through an individual or piece of apparatus and in doing so it produces a spark. This phenomenon of static electricity is a very great risk in any dry atmosphere where there is explosive gas. In order to diminish the risk of static electricity as a cause of explosion and fires, all theatre furniture such as trolleys, drum stands, movable buckets, anaesthetic machines, and instrument trolleys, must be earthed by means of a chain dangling from their framework on to the theatre floor, or through antistatic rubber tyres specially made to conduct electricity. It is the nurse's duty to see that these earthing chains are present and actually reach the floor. If they are allowed to become rusty they may cease to be effective.

Antistatic rubber in Great Britain is distinguished by a yellow band: trolley wheels tyred with antistatic rubber are painted yellow.

The majority of explosions in operating theatres have occurred not from the use of some electrical apparatus but from static electricity induced by the sudden movement of blankets or apparatus.

An explosion can only occur if there is inflammable material present. Even if all explosive anaesthetic agents, such as ether and cyclopropane, are removed, there is still a risk of fire owing to the high concentration of oxygen present in the atmosphere immediately surrounding an anaesthetic machine. That is why the use of grease on gas and oxygen cylinder connections is absolutely forbidden (Chapter 12).

Many operating theatres have floors which themselves are not conductors of electricity. As these are usually in old buildings, the ventilation is also inadequate and the atmosphere in the theatre is very humid owing to the entry of steam from the sterilising annex. Humidity diminishes the risk of explosion but, as hospital authorities become aware of the hazard, conducting floor surfaces are being installed.

The risks of fire and explosion in the operating theatre can be diminished to a very low level by strict adherence to the regulations governing the installation and use of electrical apparatus, and by the adoption of recognised anti-static measures.

Nurses' uniforms made of Nylon are a particular risk, which is diminished by the use of a cotton overall.

X-ray and photographic equipment in the operating theatre

No x-ray apparatus is entirely spark-proof and explosive anaesthetic machines should not be used in the presence of an x-ray machine. It is now common practice for photographic apparatus to be used in the operating theatre. Flash bulbs and powerful floodlights may only be permitted if ether is not being used. This risk may well be overlooked owing to the intensity of interest which usually surrounds a procedure worthy of photography in the operating theatre.

Mishaps and hazards in the operating theatre

A recapitulation of the more serious mistakes and their consequences is justified by the frequency with which accidents still occur in operating theatres. The best recognised are those of fire and explosion. Many accidents have occurred from faulty equipment such as open-flame sterilisers or inadequately earthed electrical apparatus. Surgical diathermy has been responsible for many claims for damages.

Unfortunately many untoward incidents occur which have disastrous consequences. In spite of regulations concerning the identification of patients the wrong operation is still sometimes performed through changes in the order of the operating list. There are still errors in blood transfusion administration brought about by confusion of patient's names and numbers. Paralysis may occur from faulty positioning or the unskilled use of tourniquets on the leg or arm. Such matters are the responsibility of the surgeon, but he is very dependent on cross-checks by various members of the team.

There are, however, errors which can only be blamed on the irresponsibility of nursing staff.

All drugs and solutions must be double checked by a scrub nurse and another. Fatal poisoning may result from the use of wrong solutions, particularly from injections. Injectable fluids must never be placed in gallipots of the type used for antiseptic. Special graduated beakers have been standardised for the preparation of injection fluids to avoid any confusion.

Cardiac arrest may occur at any stage before, during or after an operative procedure and the whole theatre staff must be repeatedly drilled in the procedure to be adopted (Appendix II).

Asphyxia is most likely to occur at the end of an operation when the anaesthetist has left the patient to the care of the nurse, while he prepares the next patient. The nurse inadvertently leaves her post to do some other job and the patient's tongue drops into his pharynx. The unconscious patient must **never** be left, even while the telephone is answered or tea prepared.

In order to safeguard both the patients and the hospital there is in every unit an agreed procedure for checking swabs, packs, instruments and needles. It is the joint responsibility of the surgeon and the charge nurse or sister to see that this procedure is followed in every detail. Nevertheless, every member of the staff, however junior, provides a link in the chain and double checking necessarily involves dependence on junior staff.

Infection is an obvious hazard and is most likely to occur in overcrowded, ill-equipped theatre suites, but the presence of one disinterested or careless nurse may invalidate the labours of the whole surgical team, no matter how modern or lavish are the facilities.

With frequent changes in members of a team it is inevitable that at times there will be disharmony. Nurses during their initial period of training in theatre technique are often apprehensive and easily confused and it takes some time to become accustomed to the routine. Specialisation within the field of surgery has meant the development of widely varied techniques and the more surgeons or special units using any particular theatre the more confused the situation becomes.

If conditions are poor the staff is easily fatigued and errors are more likely. The provision and maintenance of a safe and proper environment for the surgical team is the responsibility of the hospital administration.

ANAESTHETIC APPLIANCES

Reference has already been made to inhalation anaesthesia. By means of specially devised appliances which mix and measure the gases the desired level of unconsciousness is reached and maintained either by the patient's natural respiration or by externally applied rhythmic pressure. In the majority of hospitals the care of these 'machines', as they are called, is part of the duty of the theatre nursing staff, but in large units a specially trained mechanic-technician is employed for this particular purpose. During the course of her training and in the practice which follows, the nurse will meet many different varieties of machine; it is essential that she should be familiar with the basic principles upon which they work and with the design and care of some of the more important component parts. Before an anaesthetic is administered the anaesthetist himself is responsible for checking the apparatus, but he must be able to depend upon the care and watchfulness of the theatre staff in keeping the apparatus clean and in working order.

Anaesthetic vapour mixed with an adequate supply of oxygen and perhaps nitrous oxide, has to be supplied to the patient at a rate which will fill his lungs as he expands them: the gases must be discharged from the lungs during expiration without the patient having to exhale forcibly (which of course he cannot do when he is unconscious). The exception to this rule is found in the technique already described as 'controlled respiration' where the patient's own ability to breathe is removed by the use of some relaxing drug such as tubocurarine, respiration being carried on artificially by the anaesthetist who pumps the gases

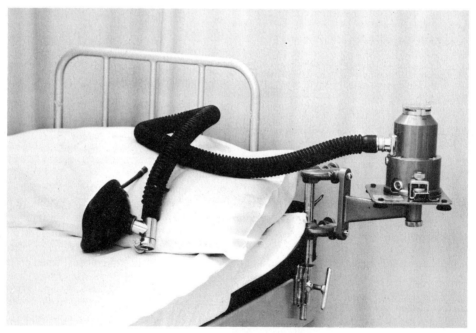

Fig. 18.20 *Takota Inhaler* for self-administered Penthrane or Trilene. Air is drawn over the anaesthetic liquid and vapour carried over in a regulated strength.

into the lungs rhythmically; the elastic recoil of the chest expels the breath at the end of each movement (page 178).

The simplest anaesthetic machine is one in which the patient *sucks* air through a container which holds an evaporating liquid such as ether, chloroform or Trilene. In practice Trilene inhalers are the most commonly used and are designed in such a way that the patient is unable to obtain excessive amounts. This makes it possible for a woman during child-birth to hold the machine herself and inhale the anaesthetic agent as fast as she likes: as soon as she becomes unconscious the flow of gas is automatically cut off as her hand slips from the valve; the depth of unconsciousness is thus regulated automatically. (See also page 212).

Figure 18.20 shows a Takota inhaler for self-administration of Trilene or Penthrane. The apparatus is clamped firmly to the bed. The patient holds the mask in position and draws air over the anaesthetic liquid in the container. As she becomes drowsy she relaxes the mask and the flow of anaesthetic vapour ceases.

Figure 18.21 shows a Penlon 'vaporiser' for use with ether. After induction with intravenous thiopentone, anaesthesia is maintained by the patient's natural respiration. The concertina rubber reservoir is expanded by an internal spring during expiration: this fills it with ether of a regulated strength which the patient then inspires. By pressure on the reservoir the anaesthetist can assist inspiration. This is a simple safe machine for use in 'field service' conditions where cumbersome apparatus and cylinders are not available. There is a wide safety margin with ether and it is a good anaesthetic agent, though explosive.

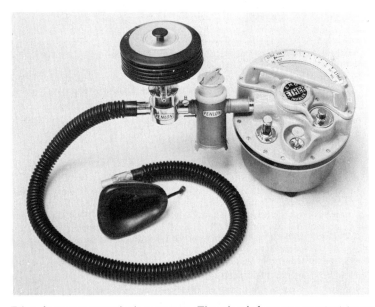

Fig. 18.21 Ether draw-over anaesthetic apparatus. The ether is kept at a constant temperature by the construction of the container where it is surrounded by special chemicals. The rubber cylinder is expanded by a coiled spring after each inspiration has emptied it. This may be used by normal or controlled respiration.

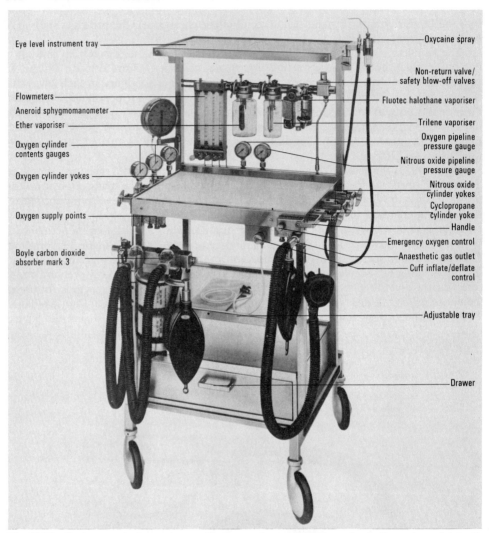

Eye level instrument tray

Oxycaine spray

Non-return valve/
safety blow-off valves

Flowmeters

Fluotec halothane vaporiser

Aneroid sphygmomanometer

Ether vaporiser

Trilene vaporiser

Oxygen pipeline
pressure gauge

Oxygen cylinder
contents gauges

Nitrous oxide pipeline
pressure gauge

Oxygen cylinder yokes

Nitrous oxide
cylinder yokes

Cyclopropane
cylinder yoke

Oxygen supply points

Handle

Emergency oxygen control

Boyle carbon dioxide
absorber mark 3

Anaesthetic gas outlet

Cuff inflate/deflate
control

Adjustable tray

Drawer

Fig. 18.22 Boyle anaesthetic apparatus. Gases may be supplied through pipelines plugged into the machine, or by cylinders suspended from the yokes shown on each side. The tyres on the wheels are made of special rubber which conducts electricity to diminish the risk of sparks from static charge. Older type machines may have an earthing chain hanging from the lower shelf. (British Oxygen Co.)

Instead of the patient simply sucking air over these liquids, he may be supplied with oxygen and nitrous oxide, perhaps with other gases, from storage cylinders. The gases are supplied in cylinders at a pressure (over a 100 lb per sq in. in the case of oxygen) which is far too high to connect direct to the tube which goes to the patient. There would be a risk of bursting his lungs, however carefully the valve were opened. The cylinder therefore has to be fitted with a pressure-reducing valve which screws into the head of the cylinder above the main valve. This reducing valve is a safety device. The gas is then fed through a thick-walled rubber tube into the machine itself where there is a further controlling tap which regulates accurately the amount of gas passing to the patient.

On the earliest form of anaesthetic apparatus the rate of flow of each gas was measured by passing it down a tube submerged in a bottle of water. There are holes in the side of the tube and the number of holes through which the gas bubbles indicates the amount which is passing at any particular time. This simple flowmeter although not particularly accurate, cannot go wrong and requires very little attention. Such water flowmeters are still used occasionally. More sophisticated and accurate flowmeters (Fig. 18.24) with rotating bobbins are fitted to modern apparatus.

The next stage is to pass the gases through one or more evaporating chambers which contain the liquid anaesthetic agents. All the gases are then passed into a wide corrugated rubber tube connected to the 'mask' or 'facepiece'. Attached to the side of this final tubing there is always at one point, a rubber bag which acts as a reservoir which expands and contracts in rhythm with the breathing, thus preventing excessive pressure being passed on to the lungs while they are attempting to expel the used air. Finally at the patient's end of this delivery tubing is a valve known as an 'expiratory valve' and this opens as the patient breathes out allowing some of the exhaled air to be blown off into the atmosphere. By adjusting this valve the anaesthetist regulates the pressure against which the lungs contract to expel the air.

All anaesthetic machines are designed to cover these various phases in the mixing and supply of gases. Arranged in this way they are described as having an 'open circuit'.

A **closed circuit** apparatus is one in which the exhaled gases instead of being blown off into the atmosphere, are passed back through a separate tube, purified and re-introduced into the delivery side of the circuit. Carbon dioxide is the gas which needs to be removed constantly from the exhaled vapour and this is done by passing the expired air through a container filled with 'soda-lime' granules. In the closed-circuit system, far less anaesthetic

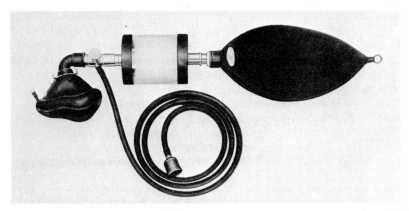

Fig. 18.23   Waters 'to-and-fro' carbon dioxide absorber. The anaesthetic gases are rebreathed from the bag, carbon dioxide being absorbed by soda-lime granules in the transparent container. A maintenance oxygen supply with additional anaesthetic vapour is fed in through the narrow bore tube as required. (British Oxygen Co.)

agent is used as it continues to re-circulate in and out of the patient: thus a more constant level of anaesthetic agent can be maintained and far less water vapour is lost from the patient's lungs. Figure 18.23 shows a Waters' soda-lime canister apparatus. In this the expired *and* inspired air passes to and fro through the canister: fresh nitrous oxide and oxygen is fed into the facepiece and at the end of each expiration some expired air is blown off into the atmosphere. In the 'closed circuit' absorber shown attached to the trolley in Fig. 18.22 the gases travel round a complete circuit, with oxygen being fed in as required. This is of particular value when cyclopropane is used.

Several of the substances used in inhalation anaesthesia are extremely explosive and inflammable. A very tiny spark produced by an electrical current, by a contact of two metals, or by static discharge from cloth or Nylon fabrics, is sufficient to cause a devastating explosion, and in the design and maintenance of anaesthetic apparatus great care has to be taken to eliminate the risk of fire and explosion of this type (page 358).

The main components of anaesthetic machines will be described in order that the nurse may be familiar with their purpose and care.

Cylinders

Oxygen, carbon dioxide, nitrous oxide and cyclopropane are the four main gases used in anaesthesia. The first three gases are sometimes supplied to the operating theatre through pipelines from a main cylinder store so that the nurse is relieved of the responsibility of handling cylinders. The majority of anaesthetic machines carry one or two oxygen cylinders, two cylinders of nitrous oxide, one of carbon dioxide and one of cyclopropane. Reference has already been made to the distinctive colouring of gas-containing cylinders which makes their recognition quite certain. Many fatal accidents have occurred through cylinders having been placed in the wrong position on the anaesthetic apparatus. All cylinders have a master control valve for which a special key spanner is required. This spanner forms a vital part of the anaesthetic equipment and one must always be attached to every oxygen cylinder trolley. It is a nurse's duty to see that the spanner is present.

Some cylinders have an end connection into which the reducing-valve screws; others have an end which is threaded externally so that the reducing valve screws over the top.

The amount of oxygen remaining in a cylinder is shown by the pressure gauge which is always attached with the pressure-reducing valve. Nitrous oxide, carbon dioxide and cyclopropane are, however, in liquid form in the cylinders and therefore the pressure remains constant, even though there is only a very small amount of liquid left in the cylinder. Pressure gauges are consequently useless and the only way to estimate the amount of gas left is by weighing the cylinder; the empty weight of the cylinder is stamped on the side but in practice this method is rarely used. Spare cylinders must always be kept at hand.

The following rules must be observed in the care and use of anaesthetic gas cylinders.

1. Before a new cylinder is attached to the anaesthetic machine care must be taken to blow out any grit or dust present in the nozzle of the cylinder, by momentarily opening the high-pressure valve.

2. Cylinder valves should never be opened unless the cylinder is in an upright position with the valve uppermost. The only exception to this rule is when carbon dioxide is being used for making 'snow' or when nitrous oxide cylinders are put horizontally in a dental gas apparatus.

3. Oil or grease of any kind must not be used for lubricating cylinder valves, gauges, regulators or other fittings; neither white lead nor paint may be used for fixing them.

4. When putting a cylinder into use the valve should never be opened suddenly.

5. Cylinders should not be exposed to any violent usage.

6. Cylinders must not be exposed to fire or excessively high temperature. They should be stored in a cool dry place in such a way that dirt and grit are not allowed to enter the outlet valves.

7. The valve of every cylinder should be tightly closed immediately after use, and should be left in a closed position when the cylinder is exhausted. Empty cylinders must be immediately removed from the operating theatre or ward and stored in a place apart from the full cylinders so there can be no confusion. It is a wise rule to chalk 'empty' on the side of the cylinders as soon as they are removed from the anaesthetic apparatus.

8. Metal hammers must never be used to tighten the wing nuts of reducing-valve containers and if the spanner is not sufficient then a wooden or hide mallet may be used. A spark from a metal hammer may produce an explosion.

Pressure-reducing regulators and fine adjustment valves

In addition to the master valve on the cylinder, a fine adjustment regulator has to be attached to give a safe control over the high cylinder pressure. Nitrous oxide cylinders are usually connected through an automatic valve regulator which controls the pressure at 5 lb per sq in. and oxygen cylinders on anaesthetic machines usually have a similar automatic constant pressure valve. They must never be tampered with or a dangerous pressure of gas may be passed. Valves and regulators are attached to the cylinders by a threaded nozzle and the lock nut must be very securely tightened (rule 8 above), a fibre washer being used in the joint on some types.

The flow of gas from the low-pressure side of the reducing regulator is controlled entirely with small valves on the anaesthetic machine. In the case of oxygen, where the oxygen itself is being delivered to the patient without the use of an anaesthetic machine, a different type of regulator incorporating a fine adjustment valve is used; this pattern is usually found on the ward oxygen apparatus.

It is the nurse's duty then, when she changes the cylinder to make quite certain that:

(a) the cylinder is of the right type.
(b) the cylinder which she is putting into position is a full cylinder.
(c) there is no dust in the coupling.
(d) the pressure-regulating coupling is not cross-threaded.
(e) the fibre joint washer is present and undamaged.
(f) the coupling on each cylinder is checked for tightness before the anaesthetist arrives.
(g) the special clip-on labels are in position on the cylinders indicating which one has the master valve open and is in use and which is untouched and in reserve.

Flowmeters

The simplest device for measuring the flow of gases, the water flowmeter, has already been described. This was used mainly in connection with oxygen apparatus in the wards. It has the additional advantage of moistening the oxygen but great care must be taken to make certain that the connections are not made the wrong way round resulting in water being blown into the patient.

The **dry-bobbin** flowmeter (Rotameter) consists of a specially graduated glass tube in which floats a grooved, very light metallic bobbin. As the gas rushes up the tube from below, the bobbin is made to float upwards and at the same time is set spinning. This rotation prevents it sticking to the side of the tube and the height to which it rises indicates the rate of flow of the gas in litres per minute. This type of flowmeter is extremely accurate and is used on all modern anaesthetic machines. Different coloured bobbins are used for different gases: it is not possible to use an oxygen flowmeter for nitrous oxide or vice-versa as each gas needs its own particular weight of bobbin. In Fig. 18.24 it is seen that the oxygen and nitrous oxide meters pass up to 10 and 12 litres of gas a minute: the cyclopropane (C_3H_6) and carbon dioxide quantities required are much less and the regulators prevent excess volumes being given.

The dry-bobbin flowmeters have a fine adjustment valve to control the rate of flow; this valve is an extremely delicate piece of mechanism which is frequently damaged by careless use. It depends for its accuracy on the screwing down of the fine metal cone into a small conical metal seat, and if force is used in closing the valve the cone will be damaged and the valve will become inefficient. Generally speaking, the nurse should not interfere with or make any attempt to take to pieces these delicate parts of the apparatus. In the

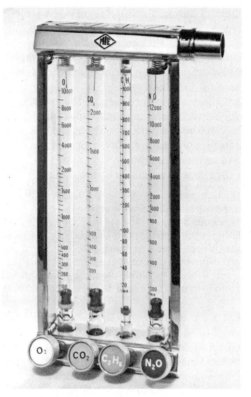

Fig. 18.24   Standard bobbin flow-meter. (Medical and Industrial Equipment Ltd.)

ward type of flowmeter care must always be taken to make sure that the tube is upright and that the coupling nuts are not overstrained on tightening.

The third type of flowmeter is the dial pattern frequently found in use with oxygen tents or other ward oxygen equipment.

If the tubes on the anaesthetic apparatus become soiled with blood or vomitus as sometimes happens, they can either be cleaned *in situ* with soap and water, or detached for the purpose. If they are removed, great care must be taken that they are hung up to dry so that no water remains in them when they are replaced on the anaesthetic machine. If this precaution is not taken, water may be carried through to the flowmeter and will render it completely useless thus endangering the patient's life. The pressure connecting tubes are coloured to correspond with the cylinders and should have non-interchangeable connectors to prevent their being attached to the wrong points on the machine.

Chloroform and ether containers

The common types of anaesthetic apparatus have two bottles for volatile anaesthetic agents; the first in series being labelled 'ether' and the second for Trilene. A further vaporising container is for Fluothane. These bottles screw into position and are held by their metal caps. There is sometimes a filling aperture in the apparatus over the bottle and when the cork is removed a funnel is inserted and the necessary anaesthetic agent poured in through it. It is a golden rule that a nurse should never put an anaesthetic liquid into the machine and at the end of every operating list the anaesthetic agent remaining in the bottle should be thrown away to avoid any risk of confusion. Before the introduction of the more modern methods of anaesthesia it was common for mixtures of ether and chloroform to be used; both these liquids were colourless. There is less risk of confusion now that the main agents in use are Trilene which is blue and ether which is clear with an unmistakable smell. Most anaesthetists prefer that the bottles should be left empty and dry and that they themselves should pour the necessary liquids into the bottles.

When ether evaporates it produces cooling of the remaining fluid and a frost may develop on the outside of the bottle. Because of this cooling the rate of evaporation is reduced. The ether bottle is equipped on some machines with a metal water-jacket which is detachable and is filled with warm water.

Breathing (delivery) tubes

The machine is connected to the patient through a wide-bore corrugated rubber tube which in turn is attached to the facepiece by a special metal connector or to the endotracheal tube by a short rubber intercepting tube with special connectors. The expiratory release valve is usually mounted on this final meter connector. [In the closed circuit apparatus there is a second tube returning from the mask to the anaesthetic machine. An exception to this is with the simple form of carbon dioxide 'to-and-fro' absorbing unit, the Waters canister (Fig. 18.23). This is inserted in line with the delivery tube.]

The rubber re-breathing bag is usually attached to the side of this delivery tube by a metal T-piece.

All tubing connectors and fittings have to comply with a British Standard: they are designed so that the gases flow from a cone (male) fitting into a socket (female). Fittings with one-way valves cannot therefore be applied the wrong way round.

Since exhaled air passes into the re-breathing bag through both the delivery and return tubes, these become contaminated and require cleansing after every case. Corrugated tubing should be washed through and its whole length passed through the closed hand as the water runs through it. Some people consider that this is unnecessary but it is certainly advisable, and after any case of known chest infection the bag and tubes must be completely sterilised by boiling for three minutes. The bag should be washed inside and out with soapy water, rinsed and boiled for three minutes and left hanging up to dry. There is a rubber loop attached to its end for this purpose. Punctured bags must be discarded but can be repaired in emergency by adhesive surgical strapping. (Page 308 for sterilisation.)

Masks or facepieces

In the simplest 'open' method of anaesthesia the volatile anaesthetic liquid such as ether or chloroform is applied to a piece of lint or gauze on a wire-framed mask (Fig. 18.25, Schimmelbusch mask.) This frame is bandaged round in figure-of-8 fashion with a 5-cm roll applied in such a way that the edges are padded, and the upper surface covered by several layers of gauze to provide a good pad for the liquid. Alternatively the anaesthetist may prefer to use an oval piece of 'gamgee' tissue on the mask. He may also wish to place such an oval piece of gamgee (with a hole cut in the centre for the mouth and nose) between the facepiece and the face to make a comfortable airtight joint, and to protect the eyes and skin from burning and pressure: ovals or 20-cm squares of gamgee tissue (cotton wool/gauze pad) should be available.

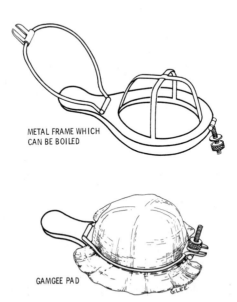

METAL FRAME WHICH
CAN BE BOILED

GAMGEE PAD

Fig. 18.25 Simple metal frame open mask for use with volatile inhalation anaesthetics such as ether, chloroform or Trilene.

When the anaesthetic is administered from an inhaler or other apparatus a rubber facepiece is used. There are several types and shapes graduated in sizes to fit babies, children and adults. Some are oval and fit across the chin and the bridge of the nose, while others have a special shaped upper lip for fitting over the nose nearer its tip—thus avoiding pressure on the eyes. The 'cushion' is either made of sponge rubber or is inflatable. The latter type has a small side tube with a screw stopper through which air is blown into the mask to the desired pressure, or the side tube may need to be tied off with thread after being doubled back on itself, like the neck of a toy balloon. The nurse must always make certain that there is an adequate range of facepieces, and that the metal angle pieces by which they are connected to breathing tubes are of the right type and size. She can only be certain of this by fitting them herself while the anaesthetic trolley is being prepared. Facepieces in which the rubber has deteriorated or which have become damaged in such a way that the metal connector will not fit must be discarded.

Head harness (Fig. 18.26)

In order that the anaesthetist may be free to carry out his other duties, such as intravenous injection, during the course of the operation, various appliances have been devised for holding the mask in position on the patient's face. Most types consist of a rubber head piece which passes underneath the head and is stretched to hook onto a detachable metal

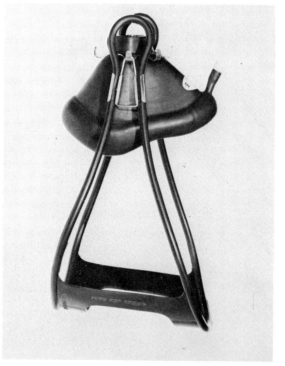

Fig. 18.26 Connell harness. This is used to hold the anaesthetic mask snugly against the patient's face. The airway holds the tongue forward and no endotracheal tube is used. (British Oxygen Co.)

ring which itself is placed over the face mask before the breathing tube is connected. The harness must of course be washed after use as it frequently becomes contaminated with saliva, vomitus or blood.

Other forms of elastic head band are in use to hold the delivery tube and take its weight when the endotracheal intubation method is used.

Sterilisation of anaesthetic equipment

Periodically the machine circuits and tubes are sterilised with ethylene oxide gas as are respirators, but this is undertaken in a special department. The gas chamber may use formaldehyde released from formalin instead of ethylene oxide. Shelves, trolley tops and the non-working parts of apparatus should be sprayed with Sudol solution after each list.

Many tubes—airways, endotracheal catheters, suction catheters and suction end-pieces—are disposable, and are placed in a waste bin.

Masks, airways and bags all require thorough washing and sterilisation. These items ideally are discarded after each case and collected for central sterilisation at the end of a list. Harness and corrugated tubing is sterilised at the end of a list or after any case in which it has been obviously contaminated.

Some apparatus is boilable but as the organisms involved are easily destroyed 'pasteur-isation' for 3 minutes at 75 °C will render these safe. Complete sterility including destruction of spores is achieved by soaking in glutaraldehyde 2 per cent for 4 hours. Strong antiseptics and any containing phenol (e.g. Sudol, Lysol) must not be used on rubber. Clearly thorough rinsing is essential after sterilisation, especially for face masks.

19

Pre-operative Preparation

The surgeon is entirely dependent on his nursing team for the essential preparation of the patient. There are many matters which require attention, both of an administrative and therapeutic nature. Forgetfulness or slipshod work in this phase of a patient's illness may add grave risks to the operation.

Much will depend on whether the case has been an emergency admission or one from the waiting list. A surgical emergency may have developed in a patient already in hospital for some other condition.

The date and time of an operation has to be fixed in relation to availability of the operating theatre, of the surgical team, and to the number of other cases waiting. There are very few grave surgical emergencies which require operation within an hour of admission to the hospital, but in all cases, whether they have been investigated as in-patients over a period of days or weeks, or whether they have been admitted only a few minutes previously, certain minimum pre-operative measures are essential.

We are concerned in this section with the general principles of such preparation in the period immediately prior to operation. This preparation may extend over three or four days or be telescoped into half an hour. Some of the items may appear unimportant—as for instance the administration of vitamins or instruction in breathing exercises. These are not exceptions, however, and if because of the urgency of the operation attention to these items has been omitted, it is all the more important that the omission should be remedied at the earliest possible time after operation. The patient who has had no pre-operative breathing exercises is the one most likely, because of this and because of the emergency condition, to develop collapse of the lung in the post-operative period. Similarly the patient who has not had adequate treatment for dehydration will be the one most likely to suffer from shock.

Patients who have been admitted from a waiting list may undergo operation within a day or so or may benefit from a period of rest and supervised diet before operation, even if full investigations are not required. The length of hospital waiting lists and subsequent demand for beds produces very often a situation of compromise in which the pre-operative time has to be shortened on economic grounds, to the patient's disadvantage.

Pre-operative preparation may be considered under the following headings:

1. Psychological factors.
2. Nutrition.
3. Hygiene and bowel action.
4. Respiratory exercise, mobility and smoking.
5. Urine test; blood tests.
6. Preparation of operation area (the side of operation in the case of limbs and hernia has to be marked by the medical officer to avoid errors in the operating theatre).
7. Special preparations, including provision of cross-matched blood, chest x-ray, electrocardiogram.
8. Organisation for post-operative care.
9. Immediate pre-operative measures:
    (*a*) identity,
    (*b*) consent form for operation and anaesthetic,
    (*c*) dentures and jewellery,
    (*d*) clothing,
    (*e*) bladder emptying,—time to be recorded,
    (*f*) pre-medication,—time given to be recorded.
10. Equipment and records to accompany patient.
11. Importance of communications.

1. Psychological factors

We have already seen that the patient needs to give consent to the operation. There is usually little difficulty over this, but some new anxiety may come to light when this formal consent is sought. The patient may be disturbed about relatives, perhaps about his work, perhaps by fear of the anaesthetic, of pain, or even of death. In non-emergency cases much of the patient's anxiety will be allayed by discussion with other patients and by seeing the return and recovery of other operation cases. Nevertheless, it always falls to the nursing staff, usually to the ward sister, to answer the many questions that are posed by the patient about to undergo operation. It is not enough for the nurse to say blithely and with repetition 'Don't worry; you'll be all right'! The nurse should not enlarge upon the horrors of an operation, but at the same time should not make light of any surgical procedure by describing it as 'only a minor operation' or 'just nothing'.

Fortunately for us all, the average patient has supreme confidence in those to whom he has trusted his life. Rosy promises of freedom from pain, of early recovery and rapid return to work or to 'mummy', are dangerous and out of place. The spiritual side of such a crisis as an operation must also be remembered; if there is a hospital chaplain he may well have an opportunity of seeing the patient before operation in his routine visits. It may cause great anxiety to the patient to be asked if he would like the hospital chaplain to be called or if he would like to see the priest! It is at this particular time that the personal faith of a nurse may enable her to give just the answers, just the encouragement, and just the peace of mind which the patient needs. The hours before an operation are most vividly remembered by a patient and every word that is uttered by those in close contact takes on great significance.

The skilful ward sister will, as far as possible, arrange the position of the patients in the ward in such a way that a particularly apprehensive patient is nearest to those who are least likely to upset him; nevertheless, it is sometimes a serious mistake to return the patient after an operation to a different position in the ward, so that he awakes to find himself in strange surroundings. Particularly is this so with children. In all of us there is certain instinctive claim to the piece of territory to which we have become accustomed. Even a hospital bed, a locker and a piece of wall becomes a familiar temporary home!

Adequate sedation the night before operation should be routine and the necessary pre-operative treatment must be arranged so that the patient is not being continually subjected to disturbance, prior to and after his pre-medication.

For an infant, baptism may be requested by the parents and very hurried arrangements may have to be made for this.

2. Nutrition

In the pre-operative phase the aim is a high calorie diet, easily digested with low residue. Major operations produce protein deficiency and vitamin supplement is also prescribed for the few days before operation. Operation may be deliberately postponed in order that the patient's general nutrition may be improved.

Dehydration has already been discussed (page 133), and infusion may be necessary in the pre-operative phase.

Severe anaemia (below 10 G haemoglobin), except in minor surgery, is usually treated by pre-operative blood transfusion.

There is great variation in practice concerning diet in the immediate pre-operative period. The healthy stomach empties in 4 hours, and this is the minimum period for withholding food and fluid. However, under stress and anxiety, digestion and motility of the stomach is reduced. It is probably wise to withhold solids for 6 hours and fluids for 4 hours as a general rule, to be varied specifically according to the type of operation. If the surgeon requires a really clear small intestine, solids may be withheld for a longer period. If an emergency operation is required and the patient has had a meal within the last 4 hours, the medical officer may request that the stomach should be washed out, to diminish the risk of post-operative vomiting.

The reason for withholding food must be explained to the patient and every conceivable step taken to see that apparently innocent items of diet like chocolate or an apple, are not consumed illicitly. Particularly this might seem important in children, but adults are equally ignorant when hungry!

3. Hygiene and bowel action

The general cleanliness of the patient is vital. Ambulant patients if they are otherwise fit should have a hot bath the night before operation: this also helps to induce sleep. During this bath male patients may shave the operation area if this is necessary. Attention must be paid to finger and toe nails and particularly to the cleanliness of the umbilicus. The teeth must be cleaned thoroughly. In units where cross-infection has been troublesome nasal swabs may be required as a routine, and nasal Hibitane (Naseptin) cream to eliminate particularly the penicillin-resistant staphylococcus is used regularly in some hospitals.

In the emergency case, there may be little opportunity for giving the patient a blanket bath, but as far as possible the same standard of cleanliness must be pursued.

Patients with recent injuries may require a great deal of preliminary cleaning up which needs to be done judiciously as opportunity arises, during the period of shock treatment (page 131).

A dose of castor oil the night before operation was for many years a routine in hospitals, but such drastic treatment is now never called for. We know that in the case of disease of the alimentary tract the use of laxatives may be dangerous and the nurse should never administer a purgative drug without specific instructions from the surgeon or his assistant. If there is to be an operation on the alimentary tract there will be a comprehensive pre-operative treatment programme for the bowel. In the case of children, an enema the night before operation is often advisable, especially if the 'basal anaesthetic agent' is to be administered by the rectal route. Some patients arrive in hospital with a stock of their own particular laxative and the nurse should be careful not to make light of this habit. It may be wise to let the patient continue with his routine, but this should, of course, only be done with the knowledge of the medical officer. If a patient has had no bowel action on the day preceding operation, suppositories should be used to secure an evacuation on the evening prior to surgery.

Morphine, codeine and other pain-relieving drugs are also constipating; except in abdominal cases, laxatives may well be required, and paraffin emulsion given before operation may avoid troublesome constipation later (page 81).

4. Respiratory exercise, mobility and smoking

Special attention is paid in the pre-operative period to the presence of any infection of the upper respiratory tract and if the patient has a cold or sore throat the operation may well be postponed. Except in emergency procedures, patients who are to have an operation under general anaesthesia should be taught breathing exercises before operation. This is the purpose of routine ward physiotherapy which has done a great deal to prevent the development of post-operative pneumonia. If the patient has learnt correct breathing before operation, it is very much easier for him to co-operate in purposeful chest expansion as soon as consciousness is regained. As far as possible patients should be kept active to diminish the risk of post-operative thrombosis, and to diminish general weakness.

Many people have a mild degree of bronchospasm due to sensitivity to drugs, dust, fumes (from stoves and chimneys), even if they are not recognised as being real asthmatics. Any tendency to spasm may be aggravated by anaesthetic and other drugs, and due precautions are taken. Known asthmatics have what is described as 'reversible airway obstruction'. Beta-adrenergic drugs which dilate bronchioles but have little effect on the heart are ideal: **terbutaline** (Bricanyl) and **salbutamol** (Ventolin) are used. (Page 697 for adrenergic stimulation and block.)

Smoking is a problem in the surgical ward and there is no doubt whatever that 'smoker's cough' causes post-operative chest troubles. Two or three cigarettes a day perhaps do very little harm, but smoking should be barred completely for any patient who is about to undergo a major surgical operation and if possible he should avoid smoking for at least a week beforehand. If the patient has a productive cough, the sputum will be sent for bacteriological examination.

5. Urine and blood tests

The urine must be tested for sugar and albumen some time during the day prior to operation. In emergencies, the first specimen which the patient passes after admission must be saved for testing. Blood is taken for haemoglobin estimation, as a relatively minor degree of anaemia in a patient who is having general anaesthesia may lead to serious anoxia.

6. Preparation of the operation area

Some surgeons insist that the patient's skin, where an incision is to be made, should be prepared with an antiseptic before the patient goes into the operating theatre. Others are content to carry out the whole preparation in the theatre. In either case a wide area must be free from hair.

Operations on the scalp or skull require the whole head to be shaved. Operations on the ear or mastoid require shaving an area at least 8 cm from the mastoid process. Eyebrows should not be cut unless special instructions are given. In ophthalmic operations the lashes sometimes need to be cut (page 842).

All operations on the breast, shoulder or arm, require shaving from the elbow, over the shoulder, to the mid-line of the back and to the nipple line on the opposite side. The axilla must of course be completely shaved.

For abdominal operations the whole abdomen and lower thorax must be shaved in *all cases*. The pubes, groins and upper thigh must be included. For hernia operations the whole abdomen below the costal margin, the upper thigh, pubes, scrotum (or labia) and perineum must also be shaved, but not the peri-anal area (also page 465).

It is not usual to shave patients who are only undergoing cystoscopy, but if there is a possibility of exploration of the bladder, then the full preparation must be completed.

An operation on the vagina, perineum or anus requires a complete pubic, perineal and peri-anal shave including the inner side of the thighs.

For an operation on the hip, the appropriate side of the abdomen, pubes, perineum and the whole of the thigh must be prepared.

Lower limb operations require preparation of the whole leg.

If a Gallie's operation (taking a fascial strip from the side of the thigh) has to be undertaken for hernia repair or for orthopaedic conditions, the thigh must be completely shaved, and the leg at least for 8 cm below the knee.

Who does the shaving? Many men, although they can shave their faces with impunity, are quite unable to shave any other part of their body, without producing scratches and cuts. (Such apparently trivial injuries constitute a risk from infection in the operation wound, and operation may therefore be postponed.) The hospital barber may be employed for all pre-operative shaving of the men, but it is still the nursing staff's responsibility to see that an adequate area has been prepared, in men and women patients. In the women the nurse will probably have to carry out the shave.

Sparse hair on limbs is best removed with a dry razor. Densely hair-bearing areas—axillary and pubic—require wet shaving using Savlon or soap and water, after the hair has been cut short with scissors. Ether soap should never be used for this purpose: if used on the head it gets in the eyes: if used on the abdomen it runs on to the scrotum or perineum and produces intense pain. A safety razor cuts long hair better if the blade is loosened.

Every ward should possess a pair of electric hair clippers which greatly reduces the difficulty.

The skin is thoroughly cleaned with soap and water in all cases.

Antiseptics commonly applied to the skin at this time are: 2% cetrimide with 1% chlorhexidine (Savlon), iodine in spirit; 75% spirit (sometimes with acetone).

Flavine has been used extensively but it may produce dermatitis. Iodine, in spite of the fact that a certain number of patients are sensitive to it, is still perhaps the most widely used antiseptic. To diminish the risk of iodine burns, the application must be allowed to dry completely before it is covered with any form of towelling or dressing.

The antiseptic is applied with cotton-wool swabs held in dressing forceps and the pre-pared area then covered with sterile towels. The towels are bandaged lightly in position. Adhesive plaster should never be used to anchor dressing towels to the skin, since traces of the plaster are difficult to remove with the ordinary skin antiseptics used in the operating theatre.

If the limbs are to be prepared with a coloured antiseptic, the fingers or toes should not be painted: these are left free in order that the circulation may be observed after the removal of a tourniquet or the application of plaster. The number of skin preparations and applications of antiseptics varies with the particular surgeon's wishes, but it is unusual for more than one application to be required. It has become the custom over the years for orthopaedic cases to receive special treatment in this respect, having a 'two- or three-day preparation'. It is true that infection if it enters bone may be devastating, but the same is true of the peritoneum. The advent of antibiotics and the better control of aseptic tech-nique has diminished the need for such extensive preparations. However, no operation which is non-urgent should be undertaken if there is any skin infection. Pre-operative preparation ensures that some one actually *inspects* the area involved, thus ensuring that the presence of any pustules is reported.

7. Special preparations

The specific pre-operative requirements of operations in different parts of the body are described under the appropriate sections.

Blood will have been taken for routine haemoglobin estimation: if transfusion is likely to be needed, availability of blood must be assured. If there is any history of abnormal bleeding or thrombosis, coagulation is estimated.

There is increasing evidence that a small dose of heparin pre-operatively (10,000 units, subcutaneously the night before operation) materially reduces the risk of post-operative thrombosis; It has been shown that the blood becomes particularly coagulable even before operation begins, associated with stress and fear. Subcutaneous heparin is then given daily for 10 days.

Many surgeons and anaesthetists insist on a routine chest x-ray and perhaps electro-cardiogram.

Operations on the intestinal tract require for 5 days the administration of an intestinal antiseptic—streptomycin or sulpha drug (Table 12). Operations in the pelvis require catheterisation of the bladder with the catheter strapped in position so that the bladder can be emptied immediately before the operation, or while the operation is in progress if necessary. Operations in the vagina require vaginal douching and probably the use of an antiseptic vaginal pack.

In general terms all major abdominal operations require the insertion of a naso-gastric (Ryle's) tube for aspiration.

8. Organisation for post-operative care

At this stage, provision has to be made for the immediate post-operative nursing care. For continuation of blood transfusion, the necessary pole on which to suspend the blood bottle must be attached to the bed before the patient returns. Infusion fluids must be at hand. Bedside drainage bottles may be required.

Particularly at night, when ward staff is reduced to a minimum, the bed which is to receive a post-operative patient *must* be placed in a position near the nurse's desk or observation point. If this precaution is not taken, sooner or later someone is left unobserved. A subdued light *must* be left beside any patient who has not recovered consciousness. A hand lamp,[1] independent of main electricity supply, *must* be readily available. Very few hospitals have organised recovery wards, therefore these precautions are life saving. A call bell or buzzer switch must be accessible to the patient. Some modern bedside nurse call panels are too complex for an ill or confused patient.

A special bed or mattress may be required; bed blocks, a cradle or traction apparatus may be necessary. All necessary charts (fluid balance, etc.) must be prepared before operation.

The whereabouts of relatives must be known so that they may be brought to the hospital if it is urgently necessary. If the relatives are waiting in the hospital, they must be accommodated in comfort and refreshment provided. There may be a special canteen for this purpose or this may be yet another duty for the ward staff. In any event care must be taken that the relatives are not kept sitting outside the ward as the unconscious patient is wheeled back from the theatre. The reputation of the hospital depends very much on the sympathy and kindness shown to the patient's relatives.

9. Immediate pre-operative measures

(*a*) *Identity*. There are many cases on record where the wrong patient has undergone an operation. Very often the anaesthetist has no opportunity of seeing the patient before-hand and it is the ward staff's duty to make quite certain that the anaesthetist knows the name of the patient and that there has been no mistake in the order on the operation list. All patients should wear an identity band on wrist or ankle with initials, name and hospital number. New-born babies are frequently identified with a tape-ring round the wrist: whatever the method, it must be followed meticulously. Before such operations as hernia where there may be some confusion as to the side on which the operation is required, this too must be checked to ensure that there is no mistake, and it is now accepted practice for the house surgeon to mark the skin of the affected side with ink. Errors such as these may at first mention seem incomprehensible, but the seemingly impossible is a frequent occurrence in many realms of medicine.

---

[1] A torch which has to be held in the hand is inadequate: the nurse's hands must both be free to deal with the patient.

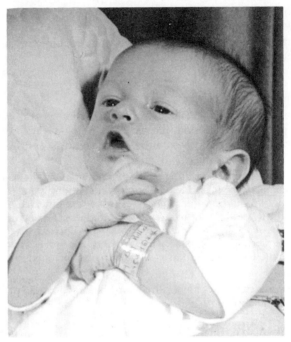

Fig. 19.1. Every patient, adult and child, wears an identification band, usually on the wrist: it must not be detachable (unless cut off) and must be impervious to moisture, and non-irritant to the skin.

(*b*) *Anaesthetic and operation consent form.* This completed form must accompany the patient to the operating theatre and must be attached to the clinical notes (page 249).

(*c*) *Dentures and jewellery.* There is unlikely to be any mistake about a patient with full dentures, but if he has perhaps a single artificial tooth, on a small gold bridge, this item may be overlooked and the anaesthetic may be commenced without the denture being spotted by the anaesthetist. Death can occur from the dislodgement of such a small bridge. The patient's teeth must be respected during his absence in the operating theatre: dentures should be washed and placed in a dry receptacle in the bedside locker. As a general rule all jewellery should be removed but there may be considerable resistance on the part of the patient, for sentimental reasons. Rings on the fingers are particularly dangerous as they may come into contact with metallic portions of the table and if diathermy is being used, a burn may occur. A patient's hands should never be placed under the buttocks during operation, but if this is done in the presence of a ring, the risk of gangrene of the finger is further increased. There is no doubt that whenever possible all rings should be removed from the fingers. If the patient refuses, then a piece of adhesive strapping must be placed around the finger to prevent the ring from slipping and to insulate it. Jewellery, money and other valuable property must be in safe custody while the patient is absent from the ward.

(*d*) *Clothing.* Special garments should replace the normal pyjamas or nightdress for several reasons. Cotton gowns should be used to cover the trunk and arms. Whatever the style, the garment must be removable from the front without the patient being turned to extract the arms from the sleeves. Under no circumstances must a gown be tied round the patient's neck. It was once customary for patients about to visit the operating theatre to be heavily clad in flannel gowns and long thick stockings as the journey often involved a trip through long cold corridors or even a spell out in the open. Overheating in the operating room was then recognised as a danger and the thick protective clothing was dropped. With modern air conditioning, operating room temperatures are lower and patients are again found to become hypothermic. The protective stockings and clothing are thus coming back.

Practice varies with regard to head covering. It is preferable for female patients to have some form of head-cap to hold the hair in position and lessen the risk of the hair becoming soiled with blood or vomit. This may be made with Tubegauz or Netelast. If the operation is upon the face or neck, the hair margin should be smeared with petroleum jelly to prevent hairs straying into the operation field during the 'towelling-up'.

It is quite unnecessary for a severely injured patient to be undressed before being taken to the operating theatre. The clothing may be removed more easily when the patient has been anaesthetised.

Cosmetics should not be allowed. This must be explained tactfully to appropriate patients. Intense perfume is obnoxious to the surgeon operating on the neck or face, while lipstick and other cosmetics irritate and mislead the anaesthetist.

(e) *Micturition.* Before the pre-operative drug is administered, the bladder must be emptied naturally or, if necessary, by catheterisation. The only exception to this rule is when the patient is about to undergo urethral instrumentation: in such cases the practice varies according to the wishes of the surgeon.

The rule is frequently broken in the case of children since a child should only be catheterised on express instruction from the medical officer. If pre-operative catheterisation is necessary it is likely to be postponed until the child is unconscious.

If the operation is in the lower abdomen or pelvis the catheter is left in for the duration of the operation to prevent filling of the bladder, which will probably be squeezed by a retractor. A full bladder may be injured during the incision through the abdominal wall.

The time when urine was last passed, and the volume, must be noted on the pre-operative record slip. If urine has not been passed this fact must be specifically stated.[1]

(f) *Pre-medication.* It is not always realised by the nursing staff that the time interval between the administration of a pre-operative drug and an operation is of vital significance. **It is exceedingly dangerous for barbiturates or drugs of the morphine group to be administered late in this pre-operative period.** If given subcutaneously these drugs do not become fully effective for at least one hour. Pre-medication injections are best given intramuscularly to ensure maximum action. If the drug is not given until 30 minutes before the start of the anaesthetic, the maximum effect will be reached after the operation has commenced and difficulty may be experienced in maintaining adequate respiration if the anaesthetic is not being given by the positive pressure method. It is impossible for the anaesthetist

---

[1] Conventional abbreviations are PU = 'passed urine', HNPU = 'has not passed urine'. The author has a vivid recollection of finding in a ward report book HNPUDNT. Enquiry revealed that the additional letters indicated 'did not try'—a vitally important but sometimes concealed observation! Patients must not be allowed to becomes overdistended merely because they are not uncomfortable: after pelvic operations the bladder is sometimes insensitive.

to ensure correct dosage of drugs such as thiopentone if he cannot rely on the pre-operative medication. **If for any reason the pre-medication drug has been overlooked and delayed, the medical officer must be informed before the injection is given as it may then be desirable to omit the injection, or for him to give it intravenously.** 'Better late than never' is a dictum that may well prove fatal in the administration of pre-operative drugs.

With planned operating lists, the first case usually receives the injection at least an hour before the list is due to begin: subsequent cases receive their injections on instruction from the anaesthetist, when he is able to assess the probable duration of the previous operation. Most pre-operative drugs have an effect which lasts approximately three hours and if for any reason there has been unforeseen delay it is a simple matter for the anaesthetist to give an additional dose of atropine.

The time, site and route of injection must be entered on the pre-operative record slip with the dose and the initials of the person who administered it (page 253).

10. Equipment and records to accompany the patient

Practice varies in different hospitals. A simple routine is for each patient to be accompanied by a small linen bag which contains a vomit bowl, tongue forceps, swab holder, mouth gag, anaesthetic airway, and distinctive swabs (coloured to avoid confusion with operating theatre swabs). This bag remains in the anaesthetic room with the patient's clinical notes and x-rays. The bag has a carrying loop which can be attached to the trolley for the return journey. A special pack may be provided by the CSSD.

Attempts to carry these individual items in a dish usually result in some of them being lost or forgotten. The nurse accompanying an unconscious patient returning from the theatre must have both hands free and therefore must not attempt to carry any item of equipment or the notes. In the course of visits to many hospitals, one has seen so often on this trek down a long corridor, the ward nurse carrying the blood bottle in one hand and balancing in the other a dish of essential instruments upon a bunch of notes and x-rays. Such a situation is perilous to say the least. She has no free hand to deal with asphyxia.

There may be additional items to go to the operating theatre—recent unreported x-ray films, bottles of cross-matched blood, or special splints.

11. Importance of communications

Reference has already been made to the procedures for identifying patients who go to the operating theatre. The busier a surgical ward becomes the more likelihood there is of error, particularly when instructions are given verbally instead of in writing. A common source of trouble is an alteration of the order of an operating list. This has been known to lead to blood prepared and cross-matched for the first patient on the list being given to the second patient in spite of all the rules concerning cross-matching and double checking on labels on blood bottles. The house surgeon is the person responsible for making absolutely certain that the ward and theatre staff and in fact everyone concerned are informed of any proposed changes in the order of operations, but no nurse can escape responsibility if she accepts a verbal message which is not absolutely clear or if she forgets to pass on such a message. There is no substitute for written instructions concerning post-operative treatment and, for her own protection as well as that of the patient, the nurse must insist on written prescriptions of drugs and intravenous fluids.

Similarly in time of crisis action to keep the relatives of a patient informed may be forgotten. It is now standard practice for individuals working in hospitals to wear a personal identity label and this materially reduces the risk of messages given or taken by wrong individuals. The 'bleep' system enables house officers and other key personnel in hospital service to be called immediately if they are wanted on the telephone by means of an individual transistor pocket receiver. However, the ward telephone remains the vital link. Unnecessary use of the telephone and long inconsequential calls result in delays and even in disaster. With modern telephone systems it has become increasingly common for important 'outside' calls to be lost through careless use of the call transfer mechanism when the individual who is required is not present in the ward first called.

Much has been done to relieve the burden of answering telephone calls from enquiring relatives by the installation of mobile instruments where the patients may themselves telephone to their friends and relations.

The reputation of a hospital and the efficiency of its service to general practitioners are very dependent on good communications within the hospital and to those outside.

Conclusion

Efficiency of a surgical nursing team is readily assessed from the reliance which can be placed upon the pre-operative treatment and preparation. The nurse in her training will do well to study the details of this most important phase of surgical treatment. Fortunately an omission, if recognised, can in all probability be remedied by one of the surgical team at some stage: even so, the nurse responsible must realise that she has added to the risk which exists in all surgical procedures. She may well have added also to the probability of post-operative complications.

Cock-pit check before 'take-off' for the theatre.
Have you seen the operation site? Is it shaved, clean and free from pimples?
Is the consent form signed?
Has the correct side or limb been marked?
Have you noted the telephone number of the next of kin?
Are documents—notes, blood-group card, x-rays—ready?
Has the patient passed urine?
Has he been told where he will wake up (if not in the same bed)?
And finally has his wrist identity band been checked with his 'boarding card'—i.e. the notes and the request from the theatre?

20

Post-operative Complications

The evolution of modern surgery has meant the waging of war against disease along many fronts. Surgical progress occurs only when new battles are won and new barriers crossed. The surgeon's skill is a combination of judgement, technical ability, and anticipation, whilst the severity of an operation from the patient's viewpoint is measured in terms of the complications which may arise. Technical achievement is useless of the patient succumbs to some complication which might have been prevented.

Thus a considerable part of nursing technique, which at the time may seem to have no purpose, is in fact routine preventive treatment, without which the operation may fail. However trivial an operation may appear, a patient is still liable to complications of great variety, whether the anaesthetic has been general or only local. 'He has come through all right'! How often is that phrase upon the lips of anxious relatives of those who have undergone surgical operation! The relatives' relief and jubilation are sometimes, unfortunately, too hasty.

Figure 20.1 indicates the complications which may arise after virtually any operation. In addition to these **general** or non-specific complications, there are **specific** disorders which may arise in relation to the particular operation which has been performed. For instance, a biliary fistula may persist after the removal of gall stones or a troublesome anal fissure may remain after the removal of haemorrhoids. These specific complications are almost always related to surgical technique or perhaps to errors of nursing management, and they are described in the succeeding sections in relation to particular fields of surgery.

General complications may arise directly from the anaesthetic, whether local or general, or may be the direct result of the surgical procedure. Often it is impossible to say what has led to the development of a particular complication and the patient's constitution plays a very big part in a smooth uninterrupted convalescence. Sometimes operation only precipitates an event which would have occurred sooner or later even if there had been no surgical intervention.

A child of seven was about to undergo a lumbar sympathectomy to improve the circulation in her leg. It was known that she had a minor degree of hemiplegia (weak arm and leg) and that this was probably due to an injury of the brain at birth. She died under anaesthetic before the operation had started. There seemed no explanation and there had been no difficulty with the anaesthetic. Post-mortem examination revealed that the child had a large cyst in the brain. It seemed clear that a minor injury at play or any sudden movement might have caused instant death apart from operation.

Such hazards cannot be foreseen, but we know that the strain of undergoing a surgical operation brings about alterations in physiological behaviour of the various systems, and the consequent development of unexpected complications.

Asphyxia. The maintenance of normal respiration in the unconscious patient is the first and foremost duty of the nurse in charge (see Chapter 10). Special attention is called to preventive preparation on page 173.

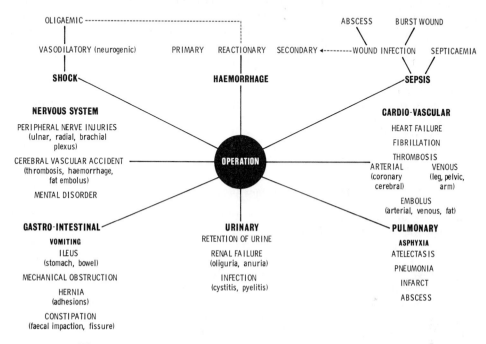

Fig. 20.1   The principal groups of general post-operative complications.

Shock and haemorrhage. In the immediate post-operative period, almost every patient exhibits some degree of shock. This might be very slight neurogenic shock shown by pallor, slow and probably deep respiration, and a slow pulse. Severe post-operative shock rarely develops unexpectedly unless there has been some operative mishap or heavy loss of blood. When shock is anticipated, blood pressure readings will be recorded at frequent intervals and the onset of shock will therefore be detected. The primary duty of the nursing staff is to make observations of pulse rate and blood pressure in all cases, so that any change which occurs in the patient's condition can be reported to the medical staff. In adults, systolic blood pressure readings of under 90 mm Hg must be reported to the medical staff at once. A pulse rate which continues to rise later than 1 hour after operation should also be reported. It is very difficult to estimate the amount of blood which comes from a drainage site in a wound or for instance from a catheter after operation on the prostate or bladder. After modern surgical procedures, if blood soaks through the top dressing which the surgeon has placed upon the wound in the operating theatre, it should be regarded as excessive. Such blood loss may be inevitable, but if it occurs it is likely that transfusion will be necessary.

Factors which may lead to post-operative bleeding by interfering with the normal clotting mechanism are described in Chapter 5, and the effect of shock and haemorrhage in Chapter 8.

Sepsis. During operation, infection may enter a wound from inadequate skin preparation or faulty operative technique. Sterilisation procedures may have been inefficient.

The formation of haematoma in a wound frequently leads to infection and subsequent breakdown of the wound margin. A deep abscess may arise or the infection may gain entry to the blood stream setting up metastatic abscesses elsewhere by septicaemia. Infection is the cause of secondary haemorrhage. Reference has already been made to bacteraemic shock (page 115).

Pre-operative measures to prevent infection have been discussed in Chapter 19 and the care of the wound is described in Chapter 21. Factors which delay the healing of the wound have been outlined in Chapter 3.

Immediate post-operative management

In the less dramatic aspects of shock treatment, the nurse will be taught the simple theatre and ward routine. Patients who have undergone a severe major operation should be transferred from the operating table directly into a warmed bed, so as to avoid the unnecessary second move which occurs when a theatre trolley is used. There should be special bed jacks with large-diameter wheels (page 275) so that the bed can be moved easily and smoothly while a head-down tilt is maintained. A stand is attached to this bed so that the blood transfusion bottle may be clipped in position in such a manner that it will not swing. It is not satisfactory for the nurse in charge of the patient to be the one who has to hold the transfusion bottle during this journey from the theatre to the ward. Her primary duty is to maintain the patient's airway.

Each hospital has its own particular post-operative ward routine, and much will depend on the lay-out of the ward, and the time of day or night and the number and experience of the nursing staff available.

The care of the unconscious patient is described in Chapter 11, but from the point of view of shock prevention, detection and treatment, there are certain minimum requirements.

(*i*) The foot of the bed must be raised on blocks or on a chair or ward stool. The purpose of this is to increase the blood flow to the brain; it also encourages the return flow of blood from the legs and thus lessens the chance of thrombosis, during this period of post-operative hypotension. If vomiting occurs, there is less likely to be aspiration of the vomitus into the larynx, with a head-down tilt.

(*ii*) Any transfusion apparatus must be correctly suspended and the limb to which the tubing is attached must be left outside the bedclothes, and suitably immobilised until the patient is conscious. If this measure is omitted, a sudden movement of the patient may result in a haematoma and a blocked transfusion.

(*iii*) A blood-pressure cuff must be applied evenly to the upper arm not in use for infusion. Readings of blood pressure should be recorded every 15 minutes if there is any suspicion of shock being or becoming severe. It cannot be too strongly emphasised that the volume of the radial pulse as estimated by palpation is a very crude and unreliable guide. The significance of the pressure readings has to be considered in relation to the patient's normal blood pressure if this is known. If the systolic pressure falls below 90 mm Hg, the nurse should report this fact to the medical officer.

The pulse rate must be recorded at the same time. Respiration rate and temperature are less important. If the respiration falls below 10 per minute, it is likely that the patient has had an excessive amount of narcotic. The temperature is of little importance, but a persistent low level of 36 °C or less is an indication that shock is still present. Any measure directed to raising the temperature artificially by hot bottles and electric blankets may actually result in a further lowering of the pressure. This does not mean that the patient should be exposed nor that it is unnecessary to warm the bed.

(*iv*) Any drainage tubes or catheters which need connecting to appropriate bedside bottles must be attended to within a few minutes of the patient's return to bed. If a catheter is spigotted (plugged) for as short a time as five minutes, sufficient blood may have accumulated in the bladder to cause blockage. Similarly if a caecostomy or nephrostomy tube is left clipped off for half an hour before the necessary tubing and collecting vessel can be obtained, sufficient pressure may be built up to produce a leak.

(*v*) Oxygen should always be available but should not be used enthusiastically. Its use can cause unnecessary alarm for other patients, for visiting relatives, and for the victim in particular if he is conscious. The presence of a mask on his face as he is regaining consciousness may be extremely worrying. Oxygen is, however, essential in severe shock and must not be withheld.

A slow respiration rate with cyanosis calls for oxygen. It may be administered through a special mask or with double nasal catheters carried on a spectacle frame (Fig. 16.4). If respiratory effort is very feeble the doctor may decide to use positive pressure artificial respiration with mask and bag for a while to ensure adequate oxygenation.

In the majority of surgical cases shock is usually well under control within 4 hours of the end of a major operation. The critical period is the first hour. Shock may of course return if post-operative bleeding is severe. It is likely to persist if there has been appreciable blood loss at the operation, and inadequate replacement by transfusion. Bacteraemic (endotoxic) shock is suspected if sudden collapse is accompanied by fever (page 115).

With good anaesthesia and generous supportive therapy by blood, saline and dextran infusion, oligaemic shock is very rarely serious in the post-operative period. If blood pressure falls or refuses to rise after 4 hours, it is likely that there is either continued internal bleeding, or that the initial shock and hypotension has been sufficiently severe and prolonged to produce tissue anoxia and capillary damage. Peritonitis occurring as the result of perforation of a viscus, from infection, or leakage of an anastomosis of bowel leads to a similar collapse of the circulation from toxaemia.

Cardio-vascular complications

Primary heart failure from shock may occur in the post-operative period. Coronary thrombosis is a grave risk in elderly patients who have shown previous evidence of arterio-sclerosis or who have anginal attacks (page 116). Oxygen must be used if there is the slightest suspicion of cyanosis or if the blood pressure is abnormally low.

Irregularities of rhythm occasionally occur following operation.[1] There is no particular nursing treatment, but the discovery of an irregular pulse should not be mentioned to the patient. It should be reported at once to the medical staff even if subsequent examination reveals that the pulse has returned to normal rhythm. Particularly is this important after operations on the thyroid gland.

Distension of neck veins if the head is higher than the heart indicates a raised central venous pressure (page 134) and inability of the right side of the heart to cope with the returning blood flow. Over-transfusion or right-sided heart failure must be suspected.

Venous thrombosis occurs spontaneously in veins which have been damaged by infusion or pressure or in which there has been stagnation during the operative period. Adequate exercise and movement of the patient before and after operation, and protection of the calves of the legs during the period on the operating table, are essential measures. The first sign of thrombosis is usually pain and tenderness in the calf, followed by oedema of the foot or shin.

In 'high-risk' patients (e.g. those undergoing pelvic surgery such as hysterectomy) infusion of dextran 70 at operation reduces the incidence of thrombosis. Pre-operative heparin, insufficient to affect haemostasis at operation, is sometimes given to counteract the over-coagulable state of the blood around the operation period. It is given subcutan-eously and repeated daily for the first week. The diagnosis and management when throm-bosis is suspected is described in Chapter 5, page 64. The condition occurs frequently apart from the post-operative phase.

Embolus may arise from venous thrombosis and will block the pulmonary artery or one of its small branches (Fig. 5.4). In patients with mitral stenosis or long-standing auricular fibrillation, clots may be dislodged from the auricular appendage of the heart and produce arterial embolus in the brain or limbs. Fat embolism may occur from fractures (page 924).

Arterial thrombosis occurs in patients with arteriosclerosis. Cerebral and coronary arteries are particularly liable to blockage, but occasionally the main arteries of the lower limb may become involved. Arterial embolus may occur from the detachment of an atheromatous plaque in the aorta or iliac vessels. Sudden pain is experienced in the leg. Embolectomy with a Fogarty catheter may be needed (page 67).

Gastro-intestinal complications

Vomiting may be due to inadequate pre-operative starvation. Apprehension is sometimes responsible for pyloric spasm which prevents food which was taken as long as six hours before operation, from passing on into the duodenum. Certain anaesthetic agents such as ether and ethyl chloride tend to produce post-operative vomiting. One common cause of troublesome persistent vomiting is sensitivity to morphine which has

[1] A description of relevant cardiac irregularities is given on page 769.

been given as pre-medication and probably repeated after operation. Vomiting later than twenty-four hours after operation may be due to paralytic ileus affecting either the stomach (acute dilatation of the stomach) or the intestinal tract. Treatment is by absolute rest of the alimentary tract, and by aspiration through an indwelling naso-gastric tube, or temporary gastrostomy by a Foley catheter. Mechanical obstruction due to internal herniation of the bowel, volvulus, or adhesions may occur at any time after operation. It is distinguished from ileus in being accompanied by colicky pain and audible peristalsis. Particularly after abdominal operation, but in any other case when ileus is suspected, a stethoscope is used to listen for signs of intestinal movement. The surgeon can distinguish between normal healthy bowel sounds and the high pitched 'tinkle' of weak movements of distended loops of gut, which are partially filled with fluid. Mechanical intestinal obstruction may be treated by further exploration of the abdomen or by the use of Miller-Abbott or Cantor intestinal aspiration tubes (pp. 474 et seq.), though these are seldom used.

The management of these conditions is described in Chapter 24.

If there is no evidence of ileus or mechanical obstruction and the vomiting is thought to be due to morphine sensitivity or to the anaesthetic agent, cyclizine, or some other anti-emetic drug is used (Table 34). If there is no contra-indication, alcohol by mouth is sometimes effective but other old-fashioned remedies such as sodium bicarbonate are dangerous as the electrolyte balance is further deranged.

Table 34   Anti-emetic drugs (adult doses)

Cyclizine	50 mg IM injection
(Valoid)	100 mg suppository
(Marzine)	
Chlorpromazine	25 mg IM injection
(Largactil)	100 mg suppository
Prochlorperazine	25 mg suppositories
(Stemetil)	
Metoclopramide	10 mg IM or IV
(Maxolon)	

For patients known to be morphine sensitive or to suffer from post-anaesthetic vomiting, these drugs may be given pre-operatively as a preventive.

Perphenazine (Fentazin) is also used: it may produce severe side effects with intense neck pain and retraction, like meningitis. This requires urgently diazepam (Valium) 10 mg, intravenously, for an adult.

Hiccough is occasionally a very troublesome post-operative complication. The intermittent spasm of the diaphragm which is responsible for it may be provoked by a distended stomach, but usually there is absolutely no explanation. Inhalations of carbon dioxide and oxygen to promote deep regular respiration are sometimes effective. Occasionally this complication is so severe and persistent that the patient becomes exhausted. In extreme cases, artificial production of respiratory arrest by the use of anaesthetic relaxant agents is necessary. A mechanical respirator is used (e.g. Cuirass type) to continue respiration artificially for a trial period of several hours. The phrenic nerve may be blocked by anaesthetic injection.

Constipation is a very common and troublesome post-operative disorder. It should not be allowed to occur, since a period of several days without a bowel action is then followed by the passage of a very large hard stool, and by the development of troublesome anal fissure. Because he is so pleased to have recovered from a major operation, the patient puts up with what may seem to be the minor inconvenience of anal pain and therefore receives no treatment for his fissure, which later on becomes a major disability. The use of paraffin emulsion *before* operation (except in intestinal and gastric cases) lessens the risk of this unpleasant complication. The nurse must not regard as normal the use of enemas or stimulant laxatives after simple straightforward operations. It results from mismanagement.

Occasionally, faecal impaction becomes so great that the patient requires an anaesthetic in order that the mass of hard faeces may be evacuated from the rectum by manual removal. Incontinence of faeces after a bout of constipation is probably an indication that there is a large mass of faecal material in the rectum, and the fluid stool which has been produced by laxatives is running past this mass producing what is in fact 'overflow incontinence'.

Constipation and straining after operation may bring on 'an attack of piles' accompanied by rectal bleeding. The presence of blood on the stool or in the bed-pan must always be reported.

Urinary tract complications

Acute retention of urine is particularly common after operations for hernia or other operations on the abdominal wall. Retention is often precipitated by pethedine given for post-operative pain. Similarly propantheline given to relieve colic may cause retention. The patient is unable to strain to start micturition and there seems to be an additional reflex inhibition of bladder emptying. If urine has not been passed naturally within 12 hours after operation the abdomen is examined to decide whether the bladder is distended. If there is no suprapubic dullness to percussion and the bladder cannot be felt, no further action will be taken for perhaps another 4 hours. If however the bladder is distended, then it is usual for the patient to be given an injection of carbachol, which acts as a direct bladder stimulant. This of course must not be given if there has been an operation on the urinary tract. Various other measures such as running taps, or a spoonful of boracic crystals by mouth, are tried from time to time, with diverse effects. Occasionally an enema will stimulate micturition as well as bowel action.

If these measures are ineffective, a catheter must be passed under the strictest aseptic conditions.

Persistent retention of urine due to prostatic enlargement is sometimes precipitated by a surgical operation and this is a particular risk in major pelvic operations in elderly patients. Transurethral resection of the prostate may be necessary to avoid the prolonged use of an indwelling catheter if the patient is not fit for prostatectomy by enucleation.

Suppression of urine may be partial or complete but it is unlikely unless there has been severe shock or previous renal damage. If anuria (no urine formed by the kidneys) is suspected, the patient will have to be catheterised at intervals to watch for the return of urinary flow.

Pulmonary complications

Clearly the most important complication affecting respiration is that of asphyxia due to obstruction in the larynx or trachea. Reference has already been made to that on page 173. It cannot be stressed too strongly that mechanical obstruction in the upper air passages can occur at any stage due to a dropping back of the tongue or to laryngeal spasm following intubation or from inhaled vomit. Assuming that the upper respiratory passages are clear of obstruction, we can now consider the pulmonary complications which may occur following surgery.

Atelectasis (collapse of lung)

By this is meant the failure of a portion of the lung to expand on inspiration. It is almost always due to blockage of a small bronchus by a plug of mucus. Any pre-existing inflammation of the bronchial tree obviously encourages the secretion of excessive mucus. The part of the lung not aerated is nevertheless being perfused with unoxygenated and CO_2-enriched blood which then flows unchanged to the left side of the heart, mixing with the oxygenated blood. Large areas of atelectasis produce a very considerable 'blood shunt' in this way and result in central cyanosis—'blue' (mixed) blood passing into the aorta (page 112).

The factors which encourage the development of post-operative pulmonary collapse are many and varied.

Pre-operative factors

1. POOR NATURAL LUNG MOVEMENT

   (a) From limitation of rib movement:

   Spinal disease in which rib movements become limited (e.g. ankylosing spondylitis; structural scoliosis)
   Paralytic conditions (e.g. poliomyelitis)
   Emphysema
   Previous lung disease
   Pain from rib fractures.

   (b) Diminished diaphragm movement:

   Inflammation in region of diaphragm
   Injury to phrenic nerve
   Abdominal distension (from intestinal obstruction, ascites or tumour).

2. CHRONIC OR RECENT ACUTE LUNG OR PHARYNGEAL INFECTION

   Asthma
   Sinusitis
   Tonsillitis
   Excessive smoking
   Bronchiectasis
   Infected teeth.

Factors during operation

1. Very deep anaesthesia.
2. Inhalation of foreign material into the lung, e.g. blood from oral or nasal operations when the pharynx has been inadequately packed (after tonsillectomy); a tooth in dental extraction under nitrous oxide anaesthesia; vomitus.
3. Irritation of diaphragm or bruising of abdominal wall by use of heavy retractors in the upper abdomen, or air under the diaphragm.
4. Excessive drying of secretions by use of too much atropine or hyoscine.
5. Use of Trendelenburg or 'head down' position in pelvic surgery.
6. Use of relaxant drugs in anaesthesia (page 219), if not sufficiently counteracted at the end of operation.
7. Pneumothorax or haemothorax if the pleural space has been entered intentionally or inadvertently.

Post-operative factors

1. Dehydration.
2. Depressed respiration from the liberal use of morphine or allied substances, especially in elderly patients.
3. Inhalation of vomit, blood or foreign body due to bad immediate post-operative supervision.
4. Pain, especially in the thoracic wall, or upper abdomen.
5. Post-operative abdominal distension.

Many of these causes can be relieved by careful pre-operative preparation. Pain may prevent adequate physiotherapy. Sometimes a Trilene inhaler (page 360) is used so that the patient can take a few breaths to relieve pain and then some very deep breathing takes place assisted by the physiotherapist. In patients who have had chest injuries and where respiration is impeded by the pain from fractured ribs, an anaesthetist may be asked to insert a small polythene cannula to the extra-dural space of the spinal canal, in order that local anaesthesia may be placed around the nerves supplying the area of the fractured ribs. Narcotic drugs given to relieve pain may make matters worse by diminishing the desire to breathe, or by direct action on the respiratory centre (e.g. morphine).

It is quite clear that preventive measures are in the hands of the whole team and each individual plays his part—the surgeon by gentleness; the anaesthetist by avoiding excessive depth of unconsciousness; the nurse by attending to hygiene and by being meticulous in post-operative attention; the physiotherapist by her conscientious encouragement of cough and respiration.

If respiratory tract infection is present, the operation, whether thoracic or otherwise, is carried out under a pre- and post-operative antibiotic protective cover. The patient's infecting organism is tested for sensitivity to various drugs, and those appropriate are used for perhaps two days before and seven days after operation.

Diagnosis and management. The onset of pulmonary collapse is shown by a very sudden rise of temperature and a corresponding rise of pulse rate. If the whole of one lung or a single lobe has collapsed the patient becomes extremely ill. The suddenness of onset and rapid pulse with dyspnoea resembles heart complications (coronary thrombosis or pulmonary embolus, or paroxysmal tachycardia). Unless the lung tissue expands within forty-eight hours, inflammation and infection of the collapsed area supervenes. The area of pneumonia may become an abscess. As soon as atelectasis is diagnosed vigorous steps are taken. These include individually supervised breathing exercises, and the physio-therapist may be called upon to assist a patient to cough up the plugs of mucus which are probably blocking a bronchus. During deliberate coughing the chest is slapped vigorously over the area affected. Coughing may also be encouraged by the administration of a *hot* mixture containing ammonium carbonate (15 grains).

A violent fit of coughing may be followed by sudden rapid re-expansion of the lung and a dramatic fall in the temperature and pulse rate.

If all these measures have failed, bronchoscopy is performed and the obstructing material sucked from the bronchus under direct vision (see Fig. 34.7). Frequent re-blocking by excess secretion calls for tracheostomy to enable the nursing staff to suck the air passages dry at regular intervals. Spasm of the bronchial muscle commonly occurs from inflammation even in patients who have not had asthma previously. This can be recognised best by the presence of a wheeze during the *expiration* phase of breathing. Relief by the use of aminophylline suppositories is sometimes dramatic.

Whatever measures are taken to re-expand the lung, antibiotic therapy must be started to prevent or limit the development of serious infection in the collapsed lung tissue. If this complication is suspected and a mobile x-ray apparatus is available, radiographs will be obtained daily until re-expansion has occurred, and at weekly intervals until the lung tissue has returned to normal (page 618).

Bronchitis. Post-operative bronchitis is a common complication, particularly in patients with emphysema, and in heavy smokers. Its development is shown by the production of thick sputum sometimes rusty from the presence of blood and a gradual rise of temperature in the evenings during the first four or five post-operative days. During this period the purulent bronchial secretion may produce atelectasis and a patient with bronchitis must therefore receive even greater attention to encourage mobility and chest expansion (Table 35).

Table 35   Post-operative sputum

Post-operative sputum:	
Copious and frothy	Pulmonary oedema
Thick and green	Bronchitis
Rusty	Bronchitis
	Consolidation
Blood streaks	Irritation by naso-gastric tube
	Bronchitis
	Pulmonary infarct
Frank blood	Pulmonary infarct
	Neoplasm

Pneumonia. Pneumonia is usually the result of unrecognised atelectasis. The collapsed area of lung is liable to result in bronchiectasis of the lobe affected. Such a complication may not be discovered until years later.

Embolus and infarct. Pulmonary embolus leads to infarct of the lung (Fig. 5.3). The patient complains of pain in the side due to pleurisy, or the very first symptom may be the appearance of blood in the sputum. Severe bronchitis may also result in blood-stained sputum. The blood is usually bright in streaks, in contrast to the rusty sputum of bronchitis.

The only treatment for pulmonary infarction is the administration of protective antibiotic therapy to prevent the formation of lung abscess. The development of these symptoms may be the first indication that thrombosis is occurring in the veins of the leg or pelvis, and this will be treated by anticoagulant therapy (page 66).

Abscess. Lung abscess is now a rare post-operative complication and results from failure of treatment of one of the other complications.

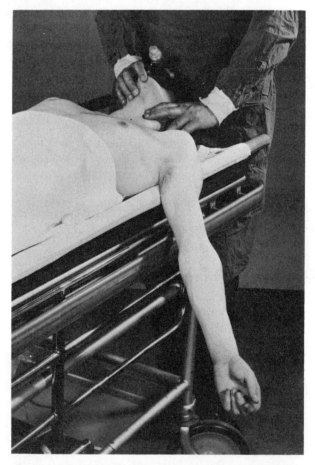

Fig. 20.2   One of the ways in which damage occurs to nerves of the brachial plexus, especially the radial nerve at the back of the arm. The arm is allowed to fall over the edge of the operating table or trolley. If an arm falls in this way it is an indication that the nursing staff are not alert.

Complications of the nervous system

Peripheral nerves

Injury may occur on the operating table. The brachial plexus is sometimes damaged by pressure from shoulder rests, when the patient is in the 'head-down' position, adopted for pelvic operations. Various methods have been devised for avoiding the use of shoulder rests: the most effective of which is the corrugated rubber top on the operating table. Injuries may also be produced to the brachial plexus by the arm being allowed to drop from the side during the transport of the patient or while he is on the operating table.

Similarly, the radial nerve is sometimes damaged by pressure against the side of the table, when the arm is allowed to hang down (Fig. 20.2). The ulnar nerve where it crosses the inner side of the elbow can be bruised by pressure against the edge of the table if the arm is not fully protected.

In the leg the peroneal (lateral popliteal) nerve is damaged where it winds round the neck of the fibula. This may occur from the pressure of plaster casts or the application of an Esmarch tourniquet (Fig. 47.28). The facial nerve to the muscles around the mouth may be bruised by vigorous pressure behind the jaw to hold it forward in an unconscious patient.

Cerebral vascular accidents

Cerebral vascular accidents due to thrombosis, haemorrhage or embolus are particularly liable to occur in elderly people. The only evidence may be a slight change in speech or behaviour. The same precautions are necessary as in the prevention of coronary thrombosis—namely, the avoidance of low blood pressure, the use of oxygen and early mobility.

Mental disorder

Surgical operation may precipitate severe mental disturbance especially if there has been a period of hypoxia. There may be previous history of a psychopathic condition, but a change of behaviour in the post-operative phase may be the first evidence. Mental confusion, shown by forgetfulness, incoherent speech or perhaps only by apathy, may be due to:

(*a*) incipient uraemic coma
(*b*) cerebral vascular accident
(*c*) fat embolism (page 924)
(*d*) narcotic overdose
(*e*) primary psychological disorder
(*f*) anaemia from blood loss or malnutrition
(*g*) unsuspected diabetic coma, or hypoglycaemia (insulin overdose).

Red eye

There are several causes of redness of an eye after operation under general anaesthesia:

(a) Injury by rubbing either inadvertently by the anaesthetist or by the patient when semiconscious.

(b) Abrasion to the cornea from head towels placed over the eyes, if the lids have not been fixed down with adhesive tape or tulle gras.

(c) Conjunctivitis—from anaesthetic gases or injury.

(d) Acute glaucoma (precipitated by atropine or hyoscine premedication).

Any suspicion of a lesion must be reported. A bacteriological swab must be taken *before* drops or ointments are used. If the eye is painful and the pupil dilated compared with the opposite eye, and not reacting to light, glaucoma is the likely diagnosis and this needs urgent treatment. Morphine constricts the pupil and may relieve the condition safely.

Diabetes

If glycosuria has been discovered by pre-operative urine test and it is found to be due to diabetes, the necessary insulin will be prescribed. Known diabetics who do not normally need insulin, but who are controlled by diet, always require insulin over the operative period. This is because of the increased metabolism and need for additional glucose.

Occasionally, diabetes is only brought to light by a slight or intermittent (and therefore undetected) glycosuria becoming severe in the post-operative period. Urine testing is essential in all cases in the post-operative phase, but is frequently overlooked.

Summary

A survey of the possible post-operative complications covers very many facets of surgical practice and nursing. Very few complications require urgent treatment, but the sooner the right corrective measure can be adopted, the less likely is the complication to be serious. Early diagnosis is largely dependent on nursing observations and these are frequently made during routine care such as washing and bed-making. Particularly important is the patient's colour, awareness of what is going on, his contentment or distress and the nurse must never ignore a patient's complaint of pain or other symptom however unrelated it may *seem* to be to the recent operation. A doctor patient, two hours after a hernia operation, complained bitterly about pain in his buttocks but was 'reassured', only to find later when he became more conscious that he was sitting on a vomit bowl.

Anticipation of a complication leads to suspicion; suspicion to watchfulness; watchfulness to discovery; discovery to diagnosis; diagnosis to treatment. The wider the nurse's knowledge, the more effective will be her powers of observation and the more successful will be her nursing in minimising post-operative complications.

21

Wound Care and Dressings

The natural protection of superficial wounds is the crust which forms from the drying of serous exudate. Healing is much more rapid in abrasions, scratches, and superficial burns if the wound is left exposed to the air than if dressings are applied which tend to keep the wound moist.

The purpose of the dressing is to ensure:

1. Protection of the wound from **contamination** and subsequent infection.
2. Protection of the wound from **friction** which would damage the delicate granulation tissue or new epithelium.
3. Protection from **movement**, for the skin and underlying tissues. Movement encourages haematoma formation and delays healing. Movement also produces pain.
4. The greatest degree of **comfort** for the patient. The dressing should not only prevent movement of the injured area but should also support the surrounding tissue to prevent drag.
5. **Adequate pressure**. Sometimes the specific purpose of a dressing is to exert an even pressure over a particular area, for instance to reduce oedema around an ulcer, or to prevent the formation of excessive granulation tissue in a burn, or to keep a skin graft in contact with its new bed.
6. The **absorption** of any discharge or exudate from a fistula or ulcer. The dressing then needs to be applied in such a way that the fluid is allowed to escape freely from the wound.

Types of wound

The nature of the wound will determine the appropriate type of dressing. From this point of view there are three classes of wound.

1. Primary suture. The wound whether surgical or accidental has been completely sutured, and healing is by 'first intention'.[1]

---

[1] If an accidental or surgical wound is likely to be infected, it may be left open initially, and sutured several days later when the risk of serious infection has passed: this procedure is **'delayed primary suture'**.

2. Open wound or ulcer. The base is covered with granulation tissue and there is a discharge of serum. The wound may be sterile or infected, but from the point of view of management the same aseptic precautions are necessary with an infected wound, to prevent the introduction of secondary and perhaps more harmful infection. Burns, healing abscess cavities, varicose ulcers and sutured wounds that have broken down, are included in this category. This is healing by 'second intention'.

3. The sinus or fistula with or without the presence of a drainage tube. Here the primary consideration is the absorption of the discharge; the fixation of the tube, the prevention of infection, and protection of the surrounding skin are also important.

Dressing materials

Skin does not tolerate constant moisture and whatever type of dressing is used it is preferable that it should provide ventilation to the underlying skin.

Gauze. This is made of cotton or Rayon in various qualities depending on the number of threads per cm. It is soft, absorptive and pliable. The gauze layer in a dressing provides a sterile porous barrier between the wound itself and the overlying wool, bandage or adhesive strapping. If gauze is placed round a drainage tube, it should be opened out and fluffed up, since layers of flat gauze do not provide a good medium for absorption. Gauze dressings should never be packed firmly into a wound as the pack becomes sodden and prevents the discharge of fluid exudate.

Gauze rolls. Surgical gauze is packed and sterilised in narrow folded rolls of 5, 7·5, 10 or 15 cm width. Their use is confined almost entirely to the operating theatre where they may be required for temporary packing to control bleeding or for use in the vagina or abdominal cavity during operation.

Ribbon gauze. Fine quality close-woven gauze of various widths (1·25 to 5 cm), is sometimes used as a light packing in cavities or to provide a wick-type of drainage. It is sterilised in small rolls with the appropriate length cut off as required.

Cotton wool. The purpose of this is essentially for padding and absorption. As supplied by the manufacturers it is firmly compressed. In the preparation of dressings the roll should be split in thickness. Cotton wool can only be torn evenly in one direction. The cheaper qualities of wool are harder and less absorptive. Special thin wool in rolls (draper's or tailor's wool) is used for padding under plaster casts and pressure bandages. The commercially supplied material is Orthoban.

Cellulose tissue. This is supplied in rolls in the same way as cotton wool. It is very absorptive and disintegrates when wet. It is a cheap and effective outer packing when large quantities of exudate or discharge need to be absorbed. It should never be placed immediately over the gauze layer, as bits of the fibre may become detached and enter the wound. Cellulose tissue in an outer covering of gauze is used for soluble diapers which may be disposed of in the sewage system.

'Gamgee'. This is a trade name for a layer of cotton wool enclosed in surgical gauze. In hospital practice, squares of Gamgee tissue are used for placing over large dressings as it does not become as lumpy as simple cotton wool. The material is also very suitable as clothing for tiny babies. Suitably shaped pieces are gently bandaged round the limbs and trunk.

White lint. This soft flannel-like material is not used extensively as dressings. It is suitable for such items as cut-out face masks or eye-shields to protect a burnt or ulcerated face.

Prepared non-adherent dressings. Cotton netting (like commercial net curtain material) is used widely for surface application to raw areas. The material, cut into 10-cm (4-inch) squares, is packed in tins with petroleum jelly (soft paraffin)[1]: it is sterilised by dry heat. This tulle gras, as it is called, can be prepared by the nursing staff, but the procedure is time consuming and not economical. It is supplied commercially under the trade names of Nonad Tulle, Optrex Tulle, etc. Other preparations are available with a gelatin instead of a paraffin base, and some makes contain in addition penicillin or other antiseptic. In the commercial packs, the squares of net are interleaved with grease-proof paper which ensures a more even distribution of the jelly, leaving the mesh-work open, when the dressing strips are removed.

The advantage of tulle gras is that it prevents the gauze adhering to the wound and allows the escape of exudate through its mesh. In subsequent changes of dressing, granulation tissue or delicate new epithelium is not damaged. Microporous plastic material is being used increasingly (Melolin, Smith & Nephew Ltd.). This allows the escape of moisture but does not become penetrated by growing granulation tissue; change of dressing therefore does no damage.

Packing and sterilisation of dressings

Various systems are in use for the provision of dressing materials from the CSSD. Scissors, dressing forceps and dissecting forceps in one packet together with dishes and 'gallipots' in a second packet, both contained in a double wrapped pack the outer paper of which acts as the sterile cover for the dressing trolley, with an additional paper drape to place alongside the wound to be dressed: a paper bag is provided for removed dressings and used disposable instruments, and a separate bag for utensils which have to be returned to the CSSD.

Items of special equipment such as probes, investigating appliances and ribbon gauze are usually packed individually.

Adhesive plasters and bandages

Various strapping materials are used to fix dressings and splints. Some are non-stretch, some elastic in length, others in breadth, some waterproof, some impervious to water but allowing moisture to evaporate from the skin.

Zinc oxide strapping. 2·5 and 5 cm widths; cheap; strong; used to fix tubes, large dressings and splints.

Elastic adhesive BPC. 2·5, 5 and 7·5 cm widths; Elastoplast-type two-way stretch elastic; for dressings, varicose veins, splints.

Elastic adhesive extension. 5 and 7·5 cm widths; extension-type, non-stretch lengthwise; for skin traction.

Plastic adhesive BPC. (waterproof)—to exclude contamination or to fix tubes or stoma appliances.

---

[1] The term paraffin has various meanings in medicine. 'Liquid paraffin' is a clear white lubricant fluid used also as a laxative: 'soft paraffin' is the official term for petroleum jelly.

Micropore (3M). 2·5, 5 and 7·5 cm widths; very adhesive; allows moisture to evaporate; non-stretch and should never be used across abdomen as distension may lead to skin being damaged.

Dermicel. 2·5 cm; expensive; for skins which are allergic to other types.

Blenderm (3M). Plastic, and stretches in both directions.

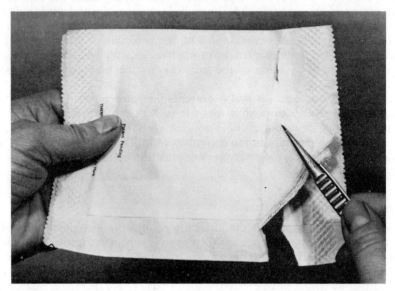

Fig. 21.1   This factory-packed sterile dressing is being contaminated as it is removed from the packet. There is no outer cover.

Sealed dressings

Many surgeons prefer to apply to a clean suture line an adherent seal which renders unnecessary the use of cumbersome and insecure dressings. Aerosol sprays of plastic waterproof varnish (Nobecutane or Octaflex) are used in some units, with no other dressing material.

Strips of single cut gauze may be placed along the length of the wound and moistened with Whitehead's varnish (**pigmentum iodoform co.**), **collodion, mastisol** or **Opsite.** Whitehead's varnish is the most satisfactory since it does not make the dressing completely airtight and the iodoform has a constant mild and harmless antiseptic action. **Nobecutane** transparent lacquer is used as a spray.

Sterilised Cellophane is sometimes used as a wound covering, the edges being sealed with adhesive tape. A window dressing of this type is manufactured commercially (Dalmas dressings).

Application of dressing

The initial wound dressing has usually been applied in the operating theatre. In all cases surgical gauze will have been placed next to the skin. If no discharge is expected, the dressing may have been sealed and the gauze covered with elastic adhesive strapping without the intervention of wool. This method has the advantage that the dressing is completely fixed, and if porous adhesive strapping is used, the underlying skin will not become moist: non-porous adhesive strapping should have a small hole cut in the centre to enable the dressing to 'breathe'. If the gauze dressing has not been sealed it may be lightly anchored by strips of adhesive plaster to prevent slipping. A subsequent layer of wool is similarly anchored or a bandage may be applied.

If there is a drainage tube in the wound, separate packing will be placed around the exit of the tube with an additional layer of wool and probably cellulose beneath the band-age. If the drain has come through a separate incision away from the main incision (usually in the abdominal wall) the main wound should be isolated by enclosing it completely with elastic strapping. The dressing around the tube may then be changed as necessary, without disturbing the main wound.

Immediate post-operative dressings are sometimes deliberately applied with pressure to prevent swelling and accumulation of blood. This applies particularly to the limbs. Elastoplast or crepe bandages are used for this purpose.

Subsequent dressings, particularly when frequent change is necessary, should be held in place by a material which is light and allows evaporation of moisture. The orthodox cotton bandage has been almost eliminated from nursing by the use of tubular elastic cotton materials such as Tubegauz, Tubigrip, elastic stockinette and netting materials which grip the body firmly but without causing unnecessary restriction of movement (Fig. 21.2).

Changing the dressing

The majority of clean surgical incisions heal by first intention and the wounds should not be disturbed until the clips or stitches are removed on the fifth, eighth or twelfth day according to the instructions of the surgeon.

Such a wound should only be inspected if there is otherwise unexplained pyrexia and the patient complains of more pain at the wound site than would normally be expected. When the dressing material has been removed the stitch line may be sprayed with Nobe-cutane and the patient may bath, but practice varies and there can be no very firm rules.

Drainage tubes should be moved at least every 3 days to prevent their becoming adherent in the depths of the wound. Rubber tubes can be rotated but corrugated rubber drainage can only be moved by withdrawing it slightly from the wound.

Wound drainage is used for two reasons. First it is a protection against the collection of blood in the depths of the wound. Tubes inserted for this purpose are usually removed within forty-eight hours of the operation, without intermediate shortening. Second, drainage may be to guard against the collection of urine, bile or other fluid in a deep wound: the tube should then only be removed by repeated shortening over a period of several days, the interval being determined by the surgeon. At the operation, drainage tubes and rubber strips are anchored with a stitch, and a large sterile safety pin is passed through the upper end of the tube to avoid the risk of its slipping inside the wound. If the tube has been moved or shortened at subsequent dressings and the anchor stitch has necessarily been withdrawn, a fresh safety pin should always be inserted into the projecting end of the tube.

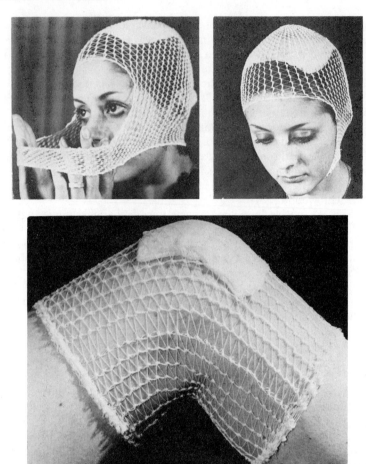

Fig. 21.2   Examples of stretch net material used to hold dressings in awkward situations without restricting movement. These are of particular value in the perineum and pelvic area as the dressing is retained in place but allows full ventilation in contrast to circular bandages which encourage sweating. There are two products of this type on the market in Great Britain with the trade names Surgifix (Armour) and Netelast (Roussel). (Armour Pharmaceutical Co. Ltd. and Roussel Laboratories.)

Constant suction, using one or two long plastic drains with multiple holes is achieved by the use of commercially supplied units. The Redivac (Fig. 21.4) is a glass bottle with rubber stopper. A vacuum is created in the bottle by means of a theatre or ward suction pump or the bottle is supplied by CSSD ready de-pressurised. The drains are inserted through a small stab wound away from the suture line. When the vacuum becomes insufficient as drainage proceeds two rubber tell-tale 'ears' on the stopper move towards one another. Either the bottle must be re-evacuated or a new one applied.

The Snyder-Hemovac (Fig. 21.5) supplied sterile is more convenient. Suction is provided by a group of springs which expand the plastic cylinder. Vacuum can be easily

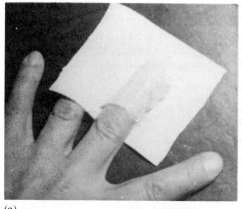

(a)

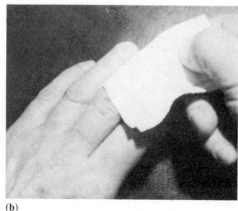

(b)

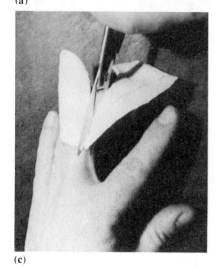

(c)

Fig. 21.3 Elastoplast finger or toe dressing. The smallest possible amount of dressing material is used. (a) A 10-cm strip of 7·5 cm wide Elastoplast is placed under the finger, slightly to one side of the centre, and sufficiently far up towards the finger web to clear the gauze. The seam is placed towards the back of the hand, but if it is not at the side of the finger it will split open when the finger is flexed. (b) The longer end is folded round the finger and the two flaps **pulled** and pressed together. (c) The cover is trimmed to allow only a narrow flange. If with use the strapping gapes it can be stretched further and nipped together.

restored when the container becomes full with blood or air. Care must be taken to ensure that the patient does not inadvertently compress the container, which should stand outside the bedclothes. If two drains are used, a Y-connector is needed. This type of suction carries a greater risk of infection than the Redivac, as the 'vacuum' has to be restored by opening the container.

Constant suction may be provided by a low vacuum electric pump, e.g. Roberts or Anderson (Fig. 21.6). To ensure continued drainage and to avoid the holes in the tube being blocked by contamination or other tissue as the suction builds up, a vented drainage tube is ideal (Fig. 21.7).

Disposal of soiled dressings

When a large dressing is 'taken down' the bandage and outer layer of cotton wool, if clean, may be re-applied over the new dressing. All soiled dressings should be placed immediately into a bin or paper bag. A large dirty dressing should not be balanced precariously on a small receiving bowl. Individual paper bags are undoubtedly the best receptacles as each may be screwed up and put in a bin without fear of the contents escaping. An incinerator may be provided in each unit for the immediate destruction of such dressings, or they may have to be taken to a central disposal point.

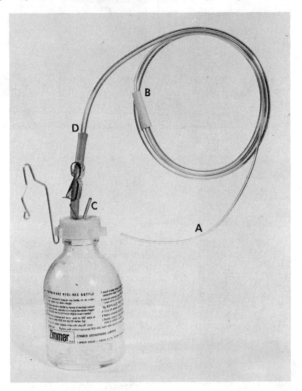

Fig. 21.4 Redivac continuous wound drain. The perforated PVC drainage catheter **A** is inserted in the wound and its outer end drawn through the skin flap with a special trocar. The bottle is evacuated with the 'sucker' through the wide PVC tube at **B**, clipped off and then connected to the wound drain. Negative pressure in the bottle keeps the rubber antennae **C** on the cap pointing outwards. When they no longer point outwards the bottle requires re-evacuating at connector **D**: the wound drain is clipped while this is done.

Most dressings can be performed by the '**no-touch technique**'. This implies that the fingers do not touch any sterile material at any time. The swabs, dressings and stitches or clips are handled entirely by forceps. The pair used for the removal of the soiled dressing is immediately discarded and a second sterile pair used for the rest of the dressing. A pair of scissors may be used in the opposite hand when necessary, if a third pair of dressing forceps is not available.

If the 'no-touch technique' is used it is unnecessary for the dresser to 'scrub-up'. She must first arrange the patient, the bedclothes and her trolley: the outer dressing if present

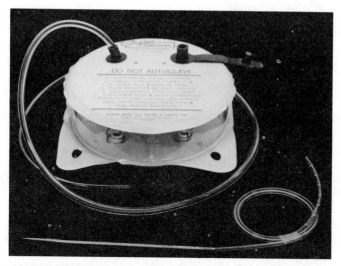

Fig. 21.5 Continuous suction device for wound drainage—Snyder-Hemovac. The trocar in front is pushed through the skin several centimeters from the edge of the wound leaving the perforated end of the tube lying in the area to be drained. The trocar is cut off and the open end of the tube joined to the rubber connector on the plastic tube leading to inlet **A**. The spring-loaded container is then compressed expelling the air and the attached bung is placed in opening **B**. Continuous suction is maintained by a spring which separates the two diaphragms. As necessary, **B** is opened, the container emptied and suction re-established by compressing the pump before replacing the bung. (Down Bros. and Mayer & Phelps Ltd.)

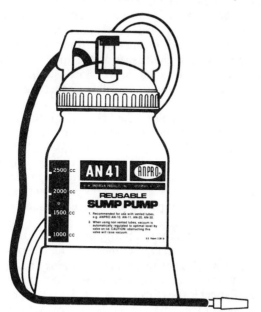

Fig. 21.6   Anderson electric suction pump. (H. W. Anderson Products Ltd.)

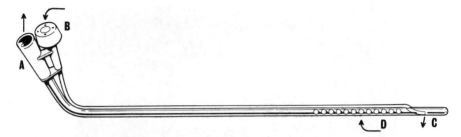

Fig. 21.7 Shirley wound drain (half actual size). Suction is applied at **A**. A constant flow of air passes through the side tube from the filter inlet **B**. The air escapes into the bottom of the wound at **C**, preventing tissue from being sucked into the drainage holes at **D**. As long as bubbling is seen in the tube there is no blockage at the lower end. (H. W. Anderson Products Ltd.)

is removed and all strapping or bandages released. She must then wash her hands in the normal manner before touching the sterile instruments with which she handles the dressing and stitches. Dressings performed in this way can be undertaken by one nurse without an assistant. When the CSSD system is used an exact dressing drill using the special packs is taught to all nurses.

Wound treatment

One of the most important points in the avoidance of infection during dressing procedures, is that the wound should be kept dry whenever possible. Thus if stitches or clips are to be removed, the wound should not be moistened. It is a common fallacy to swab the stitches with an 'antiseptic solution'. This procedure runs the risk of carrying infection in the fluid round to the points of exit of the stitch from the skin, and greatly increases the risk of conveying infection into the tissues as the stitch is withdrawn. Apart from iodine and spirit there is no antiseptic solution which will sterilise the skin with certainty under one minute, and in any case the solution will not penetrate small particles of blood clot around the stitches.

The gauze and blood clot present along the line of the wound is therefore picked off as gently as possible and the stitches removed, if this is the purpose for which the dressing is being undertaken (see below).

If the wound is an open one, the cavity is carefully cleaned with balls of cotton wool held in the dressing forceps. After any surface exudate or pus has been removed, the granulating area or surrounding skin is cleansed *very gently* with saline or Savlon. Spirit may be used to clean and harden the skin around a sutured wound, but must not be allowed to enter a cavity.

Wound irrigation may be necessary to remove debris from the depths of the cavity, and it is best carried out with a Wardill type syringe, or 20-ml disposable injection syringe with a catheter (page 661). An irrigating reservoir with tubing and catheter may be needed for a large cavity such as that remaining after excision of the rectum. The irrigating fluid may be saline or sodium hypochlorite (Eusol 1 part in 4, or Milton 1 part in 40).

Baths may be prescribed for the arm or foot for burns or extensive injuries where there are large areas of granulating tissue in need of cleansing. If 'hot soaks' are prescribed, normal saline is used and the temperature maintained as warm as the patient will tolerate. There is no standard temperature as individual tolerance is very variable. Occasionally hypertonic saline baths are prescribed, but the era of 'soaks' and fomentations, as common surgical routine, has now passed.

The procedure required for changing a dressing or tubes may be extremely painful and the patient is therefore given an injection or analgesic drug an hour before the dressing, or an 'on demand' short-acting inhalation anaesthetic is used such as Trilene or Entonox (page 213).

Removal of clips and stitches

Suture clips are of two common types. The Michel is a plain metal strip with rolled ends, each of which carries a tiny tooth. The clip is applied by the surgeon with special forceps and approximates the whole thickness of the skin edge. For removal, the centre of the clip is pinched by a special forceps, one blade of which is slipped underneath the apex of the clip: sometimes it is easier to grip the centre of the clip by passing a pointed scissor blade underneath: the metal is soft and it is unlikely that the scissors will be damaged. The Kifa clip is similar but has two small wings on its surface: removal is simplified: the wings are squeezed together with dressing forceps (Fig. 21.8). The Kifa clips become entangled more easily in the dressing gauze and when the initial dressing is applied by the surgeon, it is customary to place a small roll down each side of the wound, making a 'trough' which to some extent protects the wings of the clips from the dressing gauze. Care is necessary in removing the initial dressing. Clips are usually removed after 4 days, tension on the wound being taken by subcutaneous stitches.

Skin stitches are of various types. Fig. 21.9 illustrates the more common methods of suture. Skin stitches are not pulled tight when they are inserted because the skin edges swell and tend to strangulate: if this occurs small points of gangrene develop beneath the stitch. Any skin stitch which leaves a permanent mark across the line of incision, has been

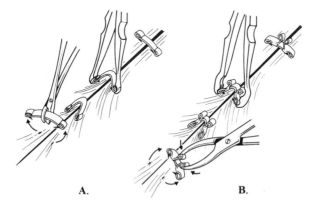

A.   B.

Fig. 21.8 Metal skin clips. **A.** Michel skin closing clips; removed by inserting special removal forceps blade beneath apex of clips. **B.** Kifa clips. Note 'wings' on apex of clip; removed by gripping together with any forceps.

pulled too tight and has produced a tiny line of necrosis. To prevent this, deep tension sutures are sometimes protected by threading over the stitch a small length of rubber which protects the skin from pressure. Alternatively double stitches may be tied each side of the wound over buttons.

Whatever method of stitching has been used, the suture is lifted by the knot and cut with scissors **at the point which is thus withdrawn from the skin puncture.** The stitch is then

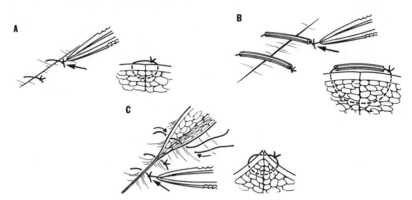

Fig. 21.9 Three common types of stitch. **A.** Simple stitch entered vertically through skin and subcutaneous tissue and tied loosely. For removal the knot is lifted and the suture cut with scissors or disposable knife blade at the point shown. It is withdrawn away from the incision thus avoiding separation of the healing edges. **B.** 'Deep tension' stitch, protected by thin rubber tubing to prevent it cutting the skin. This is used to hold subcutaneous fat and sometimes muscle, to prevent accumulation of blood. It is sometimes used to close a 'burst abdomen'. **C.** 'Vertical mattress' stitch, used to ensure eversion of the skin edges. If the suture does not cross over the healing edge of skin there is less tension on the edge: it must again be cut behind the knot.

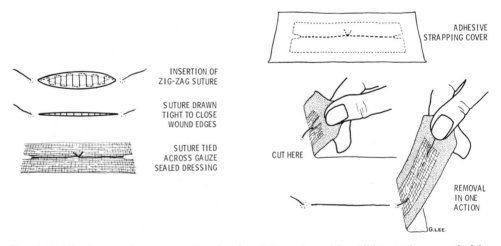

Fig. 21.10 Continuous subcuticular anchor dressing. Commonly used for children as the removal of the single stitch is simple and causes no discomfort. The dressing cannot be changed without removing the stitch. Dexon is also used for subcuticular sutures and does not require removal.

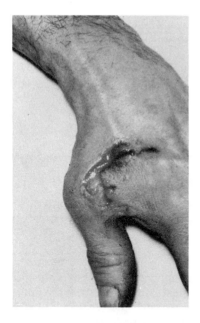
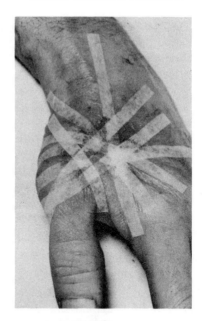

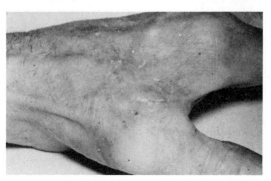

Fig. 21.11 Adhesive Steristrips used instead of stitches to close a lacerated wound.

pulled out **towards** the side on which it has been divided to avoid the risk of dragging the skin edges apart. Great care must be taken that the stitch is only cut once. It is very easy to make a mistake and leave a small portion of the stitch in the depths of the wound.

Most wounds can be left uncovered from the removal of the stitches, provided there is no drainage tube or sinus. Before the final dressing is applied, all traces of previous adhesive strapping must be removed with ether, acetone, or Trilene.[1]

[1] Trichlorethylene (Trilene) is far the best solution for this purpose: its smell is less offensive: it is non-inflammable: in its commercial form as a dry-cleaning agent, it is cheaper than ether. It is not necessary to use the purified preparation supplied for anaesthesia. All these solvents may burn the skin if used in excess and not allowed to evaporate fully, or if allowed to trickle into folds of skin, e.g. umbilicus, groins, axillae.

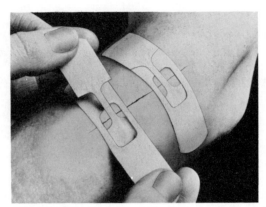

Fig. 21.12 Application of interlocking Neatseal which eliminates the need for sutures in superficial wounds. (Robinsons of Chesterfield.)

Wound closure with adhesive tape

Two common types are in use. Steristrips are supplied in several sizes attached to cards (Fig. 21.11); these are made of 'micropore'. Neatseal skin closure strips are similar and are extremely useful for first aid and casualty work to avoid the necessity of stitching (Fig. 21.12). As there is no supporting suture in the underlying tissue the strip must be left for at least 12 days.

Preparation of the patient

Large dressings are painful and where possible should be performed under general anaesthesia, particularly if they are to be repeated.

A short-acting inhalation anaesthetic is preferable and this can be administered by the patient himself, using a Trilene inhaler (page 360). This method is particularly useful for dressings after operation on the anal canal. Ketamine or nitrazepam may be used instead of general anaesthesia. Alternatively an injection of morphine or pethidine an hour before the dressing may be adequate.

Conclusion

The majority of surgical wounds require very little attention—in fact the less they are disturbed the better. On the other hand, extensive open wounds demand the most careful and rigid supervision. The changing of the dressing, whether great or small, is the patient's first opportunity of seeing the cause of his suffering, if indeed he can see it. To the medical or nursing student, 'doing a dressing' is an exciting and satisfying experience, and one which can bring great comfort to the patient. To all who have the care of wounds is given the warning:

keep your fingers off,
protect from dust,
avoid tight packing,
make the dressing secure,
never 'peep' at a wound by lifting the edge of the dressing.

22

Surgery in Infancy and Childhood

The importance of children's nursing

On account of the earlier age of entry upon training, many nurses start their career in a children's hospital. By the time general training commences, they are already familiar with the particular requirements of the child patient. The successful nursing of the sick child requires the combined art of the mother, the nurse and the veterinary surgeon. The infant, like the sick animal, is unable to talk and has but simple means of indicating discomfort or pain. Alike they respond to sympathy and affection, and their recovery brings joy and encouragement to all around. While, in many respects, it is clearly advantageous for children in a general hospital to be segregated in special wards, the presence of a child patient in a men's or women's ward frequently has a most stimulating effect on the morale of the adult patients. Very rarely is the presence of a child resented and in surgical cases he seldom demands more than his share of nursing attention.

Children of all ages require treatment in the various special departments of a large general hospital and the care of children is therefore an essential part of the training of every nurse.

As in other special fields of medicine and surgery, great advantage has accrued from the development of children's hospitals, but there are very few in which the various subdivisions of surgery are able to have self-contained specialised ward units. In recent years much greater attention has been paid to the particular problems of paediatric surgery and technical success has been largely due to increased knowledge in the control of infection and the management of fluid balance in the baby. It is only possible here to touch briefly on the important differences between nursing the young surgical patient and the care of the adult. Surgical nursing in childhood, and especially in infancy, is a combination of the skill acquired in the special care of babies and a really sound understanding of general surgical principles. Though many of the conditions which occur in adults also affect babies and require similar surgical treatment, there are certain disorders peculiar to the first few years of life. Although there are some factors which require special knowledge and skill, the general principles of surgical management are the same as with the adult, even in these conditions peculiar to the young child.

Everything tends to be 'speeded up' in the young patient. The onset of disease is sometimes extremely rapid. Appendicitis, for instance, may become a grave and serious illness in an hour or so with no previous symptoms. Diarrhoea, arising after an operation for some quite unconnected condition such as hernia, may produce rapid and fatal dehydration. On the other hand, the healing and recovery processes are equally accelerated in comparison with the adult.

Attention has already been drawn to the fact that one of the most important functions of a nurse is to watch for signs of impending complications which may arise in the course of surgical management. It would be wrong to suggest that greater vigilance is required in one branch of surgery than in another, since the best possible standards must be maintained on every occasion. In the care of children, however, seemingly trivial neglect on the part of one nurse, is much more likely to have serious or even fatal consequences. The special hazards are described below.

Age groups

The first month of life is the **neonatal** period. The general vitality of the new-born child is very great unless he has been born prematurely. Certain gross congenital abnormalities may arise which are incompatible with life and which cannot be treated by surgical operation. There are however many conditions for which surgery is urgently needed during the first few days of life. Other congenital abnormalities may come to light during **infancy** (the first year of life) or during the **toddler** stage (up to the age of five years). The older child has very few surgical conditions which are different from those found in the young adult and there is very little difference in surgical or nursing technique.

Special hazards

Physiological immaturity. Many physiological functions are under-developed at birth and the younger the child, the less he is able to adapt himself to changing environment, so much so that babies born prematurely are cared for in specially heated nurseries. Temperature control is extremely poor in the baby and he is therefore liable to suffer from exposure to cold or excessive warmth. This inability to adjust to the temperature of the environment is so serious that a febrile illness in a baby may be fatal merely on account of the rise in temperature. The baby is unable to sweat and lower its temperature and may have convulsions. A baby born with spina bifida has a varying degree of paralysis of the lower limbs and is even less able to generate heat by muscle movement than the normal baby. It is absolutely essential that such a baby should be put in a heated incubator at the earliest possible moment and should not be allowed to cool down to room temperature. Babies with congenital defects such as this, needing urgent surgery, have to be moved to special neonatal surgical units; they are very often sent quite wrongly in unheated oxygen boxes, or even wrapped up in plenty of shawls in an unheated ambulance, in the hope that insulation will warm the baby! If a baby reaches hospital with a temperature of 35 °C or less it is not fit for surgery for several hours. Nursing action has therefore to be taken quickly.

The modern surgical incubator (Fig. 22.1) is really an isolation unit of its own with complete temperature and humidity control, fully air-conditioned with fresh filtered air which is raised to the required temperature as it circulates. The provision of such equipment as this has increased the success with which new-born babies can be treated and clearly if this equipment is not available the chances of a baby surviving are very much less. The intensive care of seriously ill babies is highly specialised and whilst the incubator provides a reasonable environment it is not ideal when technical procedures such as blood sampling and intravenous therapy are required. Figure 22.2 shows a special infant care unit.

An active new-born baby has a very high rate of metabolism and as he is so small all changes in the chemistry of his blood are relatively great. His kidneys are very immature and are less able to deal with severe disturbances of electrolyte balance than the normal adult kidney. Particularly the renal tubules lack the power to concentrate the urine.

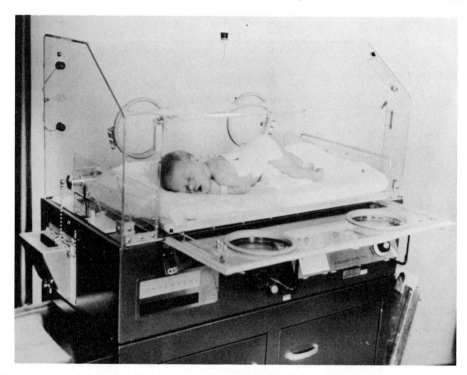

Fig. 22.1   A modern incubator designed primarily for neonatal surgery. The drop front enables the baby to be withdrawn on the tray for special procedures and x-ray examination. Routine nursing is carried out through the ports. The incubator is fully air-conditioned with a constant flow of fresh filtered bacteria-free air. The risk of cross-infection is greatly reduced and several of these incubators may be used in the same room. Automatic control of temperature can be arranged by attaching to the baby's skin an electric thermometer which regulates the temperature of the incubator according to the baby's needs.

Thus if insufficient fluid is available, the kidneys are unable to dispose of the urea and other waste products and the child becomes uraemic. This happens even more rapidly if the kidneys are inflamed. Dehydration from gastro-enteritis or other cause, rapidly produces uraemia (Fig. 22.3). One of the most important aspects of nursing small babies is the maintenance of an adequate fluid intake.

Suffocation. Babies may be suffocated by burying their faces in a soft pillow. Pillows are unnecessary, and to place a baby on a pillow is courting disaster. Similarly, infants

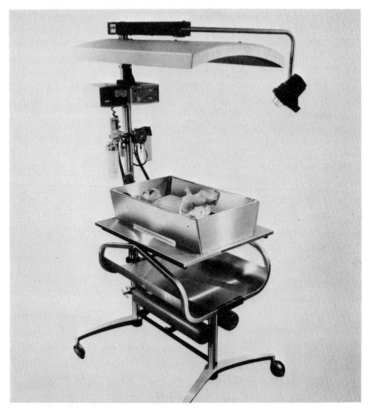

Fig. 22.2   Infant Care Centre. The baby is kept warm during handling for technical procedures by a 'black heat' overhead unit. Monitors for respiration and pulse rate, oxygen and suction equipment are provided and the baby's temperature is maintained by a thermostat controlled by the baby's body temperature. (Becton, Dickinson U.K. Ltd.)

drown easily by inhaling a vomited feed. This is a particular risk in weak babies who have undergone operation in the neonatal period. To prevent such accidents the baby is therefore kept on his side with a head-down tilt, and all the precautions taken as with an unconscious patient (Chapter 11). Mechanical suction pump, aspirating catheters (sterile), mouth gags and bronchoscopic outfit (page 620) must be available for *immediate* use. The risk of respiratory arrest in ill babies is very great and special monitoring equipment is used (Fig. 22.4).

Digestive disorders. The baby's alimentary tract is intolerant as digestion is weak. Slight alterations of diet may completely upset his routine and lead to dehydration by vomiting or diarrhoea. The baby has no nutritional reserve and even a short period of fever, infection, or reduced feeding, leads to rapid deterioration.

Convulsions. Children are particularly liable to convulsions during the course of any severe illness, particularly if it is accompanied by pyrexia: tepid sponging is required as a preventive measure in a feverish child who has had convulsions on some previous occasion.

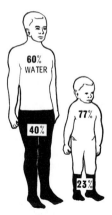

Fig. 22.3   The water content of the child is very much greater in proportion to the solid tissue than in the adult. Dehydration can occur very rapidly. When severe it is very difficult to control.

Gastro-enteritis. However short the stay in hospital there is the ever-present risk of the child contracting some other infection such as gastro-enteritis. Neonatal cases are preferably nursed in single cubicles with the strictest possible precautions and full barrier nursing technique (page 26).

Infectious disease. Acute infective disorders such as measles and chicken pox spread rapidly in a children's ward and such 'cross-infection' is an ever-present additional risk in the surgery of childhood.

Mental reaction. Most children respond very well mentally and morally to the care they receive in hospital. It is an exception to find a child with difficult behaviour, but the nurse must always be conscious of the psychological strain which has been placed upon the child by his admission and separation from parents, brothers and sisters, and home.

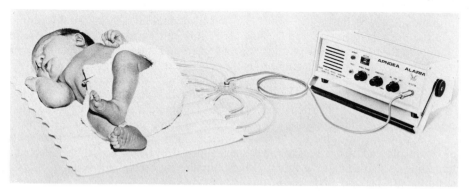

Fig. 22.4   Newborn babies are prone to respiratory arrest: this air-filled tubular mattress registers every respiratory movement; if there is no impulse for longer than the selected number of seconds the alarm sounds and the light flashes. This is a vital safeguard in special baby care units. (Vickers Ltd., Medical Engineering.)

For routine surgical operations such as appendicectomy or the treatment of hernia, the stay in hospital is very short and the child recovers much more rapidly than the adult with a similar condition.

Self-inflicted injury. In addition to the hazards of disease there are additional risks of injury. Children need to be protected from themselves, from falling out of bed, from injury by mechanical toys, from fire and from poison. Medicines and thermometers must never be left within reach of a child in hospital. In Great Britain special standards have been adopted in the manufacture of cots to ensure that the bars are sufficiently close to prevent the child wedging his head between them.

Gangrene and thrombosis. Although these two conditions are most commonly associated with old age and arterial disease, the newborn baby is occasionally afflicted. At birth, changes occur in the heart which leave an unused channel—the ductus arteriosus—between the aorta and pulmonary artery (Fig. 34.8). It becomes blocked by thrombosis, which is a normal process here,[1] but fragments of the clot may break off and travel into the arteries. Infarction of a kidney may occur in this way. Similarly arteries running to the umbilicus from the iliac arteries in the groins become blocked after the umbilical cord has been separated. The thrombosis may spread into the iliac vessels and emboli may go to the legs. Septicaemia leads to the production of infected emboli and localised patchy gangrene.

If during routine nursing of a baby, any suspicious area of discoloration is seen in either leg or buttock it must be reported to the medical staff at once so that anti-coagulant therapy can be started to limit the spread of the thrombosis from the site of embolism (Chapter 5).

Bladder and bowel function

The new-born baby passes urine approximately every hour. The frequency diminishes as the child increases in size and as the bladder control becomes more regulated (Table 36). Incontinence of urine adds to the difficulties of nursing but rarely leads to trouble with surgical wounds. It is most important that the incontinent child's diaper should be changed frequently as the urine rapidly decomposes with bacterial action and warmth, liberating free ammonia which burns the skin. The so-called napkin rash is usually ammonia dermatitis, probably with secondary infection: this can be avoided by very frequent changing and the use of boracic powder or some other mild antiseptic. Complete voluntary control of micturition should be present by the age of four, but under the stress of hospital conditions some children develop enuresis (bed-wetting), which may persist after their return home. Shyness may prevent a child asking for the chamber and may be the sole cause of apparent faecal or urinary incontinence. To obtain a specimen of urine from an infant for laboratory investigations requires great care and patience, and the child must not be upset by the procedure. A 'clean catch' specimen may be obtained from children from 3 years old and upwards as for adults. Specimens from babies must be collected into a sterile self-adhesive bag or by suprapubic puncture by needle and syringe; this latter procedure must be done by the medical officer.

---

[1] Failure of this process leads to the congenital heart condition of 'patent ductus' (page 625). Other congenital heart defects may be present in addition, giving rise to the baby being 'blue' from mixing of oxygenated and unoxygenated blood.

Table 36 Normal urine output in childhood

Age	Weight	Frequency of micturition in 24 hours	Output of urine in 24 hours	Bladder capacity
	kg		ml	ml
1 wk	3·4	30	250	45
2 m	4·5	20	350	105
6 m	7·3	16	420	120
1 yr	9·3	12	500	180
2 yr	12·0	10	550	240
4 yr	16·0	9	660	360
6 yr	21·0	8	780	540

Owing to the grave risk of gastro-enteritis, a most careful watch must be kept on bowel action. The infant stool is at first mustard-coloured and semi-solid. Pale constipated stools develop in some bottle-fed infants and constipation leads to the development of anal fissure. Admission to hospital limits the activity of the older child and the alteration of habit may again lead to constipation, with the development of a troublesome fissure. The pain of defaecation then frightens the child and may completely upset the management of his condition.

The glycerin suppository is a convenient way of stimulating bowel action without causing distress or provoking diarrhoea. Enema quantities need to be reduced according to the child's age: 30 ml (one ounce) for each year of age is a safe quantity. A Higginson syringe must never be used.

Particular attention must be paid by the nursing staff to the child's cleanliness after bowel action, and if peri-anal soreness develops, a barrier cream (page 469) is useful: **thrush** (fungus infection) sometimes affects the rectum and anus: the visible area is then painted with 2 per cent crystal violet solution twice daily, or nystatin which is also given by mouth.

Incontinence of faeces is usually the result of diarrhoea, or extreme constipation leading to overflow. In the latter, rectal examination will reveal the presence of the hard mass of faeces which may require removal under anaesthesia. Hard rock-like lumps may be softened by retention enemas of molasses or bile. In these cases the rectum is usually insensitive and retention of the fluid is unlikely to be difficult: it should remain in overnight and a simple enema again tried in the morning (page 81, enemas).

Diet

Infant feeding is a matter requiring special knowledge. During the first few months of life a baby's requirement is calculated in relation to the expected weight of a baby of the same age. The total daily calorie requirement is distributed throughout the 24-hour period. Attention has to be paid to the proportion of the carbohydrate, fat and protein in each feed and to the fluid requirement. Vitamin C is usually added to the feeds. While the healthy baby needs no feed during the night hours, extra feeds may be necessary for a sick child or in the post-operative period. The plan of the infant's diet is the 'feeding schedule' and this will be prescribed by the medical officer.

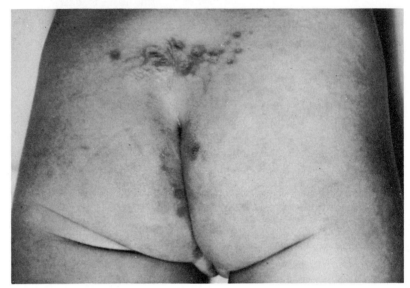

Fig. 22.5   Ammonia burns of sacral area in a child with incontinence of urine from a spinal cord abnormality.

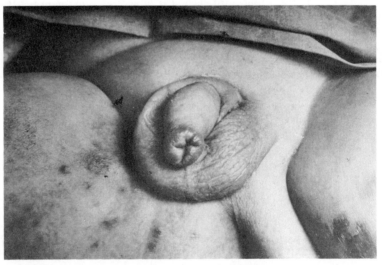

Fig. 22.6   This baby has balanitis (inflammation of the foreskin) caused by burning with ammonia which has also produced blisters of the skin on the thighs. Note the thick scaly scrotal skin. This condition is due to lack of nursing care, and very easily becomes infected.

The majority of babies in hospital are artificially fed and the same precautions must be taken with feeding bottles and teats as with surgical instruments. Thorough cleansing and complete sterilisation must be assured. Many hospitals use 'disposable' plastic feeding bottles. In a children's hospital it is usual for all bottle feeds to be prepared in a special milk kitchen to avoid the handling of milk by untrained persons. The requisite number of feeds are delivered to the ward for each baby. The organisation is similar to that of a syringe service. Weak and premature babies are sometimes unable to suck and very careful feeding by a dropper pipette or a disposable syringe with a catheter attached. Sometimes tube feeding is necessary; a sterile plastic catheter is passed into the stomach and any residue aspirated before the feed is injected down the tube. The tube is inserted through the nose if possible, because oral tubes are ejected by constant chewing movement. If the tube is to be left in position between feeds, it must have a spigot to block the funnel end.

Whenever it is necessary to admit a breast-fed baby to hospital for surgical treatment the mother should be admitted as well to ensure a continuity of feeding. The mother is thus also able to help in the nursing care of the child, and the instruction which she receives at this stage may be a very important factor in the baby's recovery.

Alternatively the breast-fed baby may be supplied with expressed breast milk obtained from his own mother, or surplus milk from another mother.

The normal infant requires 30 ml of fluid per kilogram of weight and approximately 20 calories per kilogram for every 24-hour period. In illness, particularly, if there is fever, both the fluid and calorie requirement will be considerably increased. Dehydration is estimated by examination of the anterior fontanelle of the skull which becomes sunken. Constipation may be the first evidence that the child is having insufficient fluid. Fever can arise solely from dehydration.

The expected daily output of urine at different ages is shown in Table 36 and this must be a guide to fluid requirement.

The average toddler or older child has developed firm likes and dislikes in relation to food, or has at least become accustomed to certain items of diet and methods of preparation. Hospital diet, however nutritious and presentable, may be something new and strange. One child may regard this as a special treat while another may regard the change with great suspicion and refuse to eat. The nurse must not be intolerant and in this particular compartment of the child's life, tact and firmness are essential.

If any child is 'choosey' over food it is very difficult to estimate how much he has consumed in the 24 hours. The ward sister needs to keep a watchful eye on the 'left-overs'. The calorie requirement in the form of sugar can usually be successfully introduced with drinks. In view of the difficulties which may arise particularly in the immediate postoperative period, it is as well for the nurse to discover from the child's mother what are his favourite forms of food.

Management of dehydration

If ordinary feeding is disturbed or dehydration has occurred from excessive loss from the alimentary tract, it may be necessary to institute parenteral feeding. This is usually possible by the subcutaneous route, but sometimes a 'cut-down' intravenous infusion is necessary.

The risk of disturbing electrolyte balance by excessive chloride infusion is very great in infancy, but babies who have been vomiting severely may have chloride depletion. A marked swing to acidosis or alkalosis interferes with renal function and uraemia develops as a direct result of dehydration. Biochemical blood examinations are essential in severe cases.

The risk of over-infusion and oedema is also considerable. Intravenous infusion in babies is difficult and spasm of the tiny veins frequently interrupts the flow. The usual site for a 'cut-down' is the saphenous vein immediately in front of the ankle. With a fine

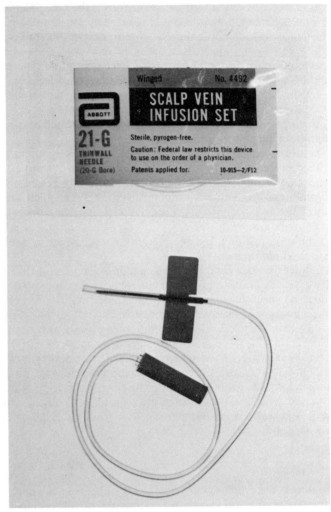

Fig. 22.7 Gamma-ray sterilised disposable scalp vein needle. The wings enable it to be strapped firmly to the skin.

'butterfly' needle (page 143) it is often possible to cannulate a scalp or wrist vein and avoid a 'cut-down'. The leg is attached to a wooden splint which protrudes at least 15 cm beyond the foot. The control of the rate of flow is far more important than with the adult as the infusion must be given *very slowly*. To ensure accurate control of the amount of intravenous infusion a 'burette' interception chamber is used. If for instance the amount to be given is 20 ml per hour, that amount is run into the burette from the main bottle which is then clipped off. The nurse can regulate the outflow accurately to ensure that the correct amount is given in the hour.

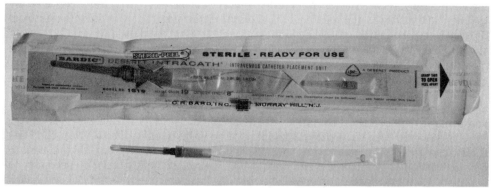

Fig. 22.8 Nylon 'Intracath'. A very fine Nylon tube is introduced through an intravenous needle which is then slipped out and discarded. The illustration shows a double sterile wrapping. This same instrument is used to obtain an uncontaminated urine specimen from a baby, by direct bladder puncture.

A 15-cm length of fine polythene may be used but this method is rarely possible in tiny babies without a 'cut down' to expose the vein. Nylon intravenous catheters are available in various sizes and with metal trocar introducers (similar to the Bateman needle in principle). The catheter is passed through the needle which is then withdrawn from the vein, and slipped over the catheter.

Pain

Pain is a mental process produced by physical disorder. The perception of pain is much more acute if there is fear or worry as well. Once the average child has settled down in hospital, he is extremely tolerant and he appears to suffer far less pain than the adult with a comparable condition, even after a major surgical operation in the abdomen. He does not worry about the nature of his illness, the success of failure of the operation, or the possible consequences.

Many infants are quite prepared to stand up in their cots or crawl around on the day after operation. Pain-relieving drugs are rarely required except for the first 24 hours of a post-operative period, but fever produces restlessness, especially at the toddler stage, and a sedative such as syrup of chloral may be required at night.

On the whole, children are very accurate in indicating the site and nature of pain and the nurse must learn to interpret the child's reactions. A baby with colic will flex his knees on his abdomen and the older child will almost always curl up on his side.

Discipline and restraint

To instruct nursing staff in the discipline of child patients is impossible, since the handling of both healthy and sick children is so often a matter of personalities clashing, or of sympathy and mutual understanding. Children are very astute and soon discover the weak points in ward organisation and the nurse who does not know her job. Conversely, they will very soon develop affection for, and confidence in, an efficient and kind nurse who understands them.

A child patient must never be smacked or threatened with smacking, however great the temptation may be. Such action is cruel and a complete betrayal of the trust which the parents have placed in the nursing staff. Conditions in hospital are quite different from those at home, and although the child may be used to corporal punishment in the normal course of family life, any such suggestion in hospital will destroy confidence. Silent firmness in carrying out nursing routine is perhaps the best method of dealing with the resistant child. Comfort and affection are essential at the same time.

Children should be warned of any change which is to take place, such as a visit to another department. They must never be taken by surprise. Bribes are rarely called for and promises which cannot be fulfilled are as dishonest as they are useless.

Conversation with child patients should not be in 'baby talk'. The average child has a very good understanding of what takes place in the ward, and the nurse should learn to regard every child as intelligent and reasonable. It is of course occasionally necessary to restrain a child by physical force if he is objecting to a penicillin injection, or some such treatment. When such restraint seems essential, the nurse should ask herself whether perhaps unnecessary pain has been produced by bad technique on a previous occasion.

To prevent a child patient from interfering with dressings, these should be sealed with adhesive strapping and if necessary the arms may be splinted without risk. This is done by bandaging a piece of corrugated paper lightly around the arm from the axilla to the wrists (Fig. 22.9). The author has known a child of three to pick all the stiches out of her abdominal wound so that the surface layer gaped widely open. She was in no pain and was very interested!

One of the most difficult problems of restraint arises in the healing stage of burns when intense irritation develops. Heavy sedation with drugs may be the only way to prevent scratching.

After abdominal surgery or the repair of hernias, no particular position is required and the child may safely be allowed to do what he likes within the confines of his cot, as soon as he recovers from the anaesthetic.

Administration of drugs

As far as possible injections should be avoided. Effective oral preparations are available for almost all antibiotics.

Many children have difficulty in swallowing tablets, and drugs such as sulphonamides are better administered as a suspension. Capsules (such as those used for Seconal and Nembutal) are more readily swallowed. They should be punctured at each end to ensure rapid solution of their contents and each capsule may be given in a small spoonful of jam. Very great care should be taken with hypodermic injections and the hand which holds

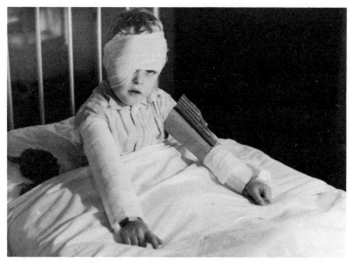

Fig. 22.9   Corrugated paper splints to prevent interference with dressings. Restraint may seem unkind but it is essential to prevent interference with dressings.

the syringe should always rest against the child's body as the injection is being made (Fig. 7.4). This will ensure that should the patient move, the syringe and needle will move in the same direction. The modern hypodermic needles are flexible and breakage is extremely rare. The greatest danger is that the injection is given too superficially and may produce an abscess: particularly is this likely to happen if 'intramuscular' injections are given into the front or side of the thigh in a child whose muscles are wasted or replaced by fat (as in paraplegia).

Preparation for operation

Infants require no pre-operative sedative but may be given atropine. Many anaesthetists prefer to avoid the use of sedatives under the age of two owing to the risk of interference with respiration. Over this age, however, the aim should be that every child reaches the anaesthetic room already asleep. This ideal is readily attained if there is adequate co-operation between the theatre staff and the ward. Much will depend on the type of basal narcotic drug which has been ordered. **Vallergan** (trimeprazine tartrate) 2–4 mg per kilo body weight is widely used, by mouth two hours before operation. Prejudice against the use of morphine has now largely disappeared. The use of **ketamine** is described on page 218 and is particularly valuable for children.

One of the nurse's principal duties in the pre-operative period is to make absolutely certain that the child has no access to sweets or other food. A hungry child will not be restrained from seeking to satisfy his craving by the knowledge of an impending operation.

As the child's skin is delicate and of a finer texture than that of the adult, pre-operative preparation of the operation area with antiseptics is not essential. Methylated ether should never be used owing to its offensive smell.

It is preferable that child patients should wear some form of head-cap (e.g. Surgifix, page 400) as they are likely to vomit and the hair may easily become soiled, but babies should not wear bonnets as these invariably come adrift and hamper the anaesthetist.

When anaesthetists with special skill in the management of tiny babies are available, abdominal operations are best performed under general anaesthesia. There are, however, still many occasions when such skill is not available, and local anaesthesia is very satisfactory for such procedures as pyloromyotomy for congenital pyloric stenosis, or suprapubic cystotomy. In such circumstances, the child is fixed (in the ward) to a padded 'crucifix', the arms and legs being surrounded with Gamgee tissue and a larger square of Gamgee placed over the trunk as a blanket. This ensures that the child is in the correct position and is kept warm while exposed on the operating table (Fig. 22.10).

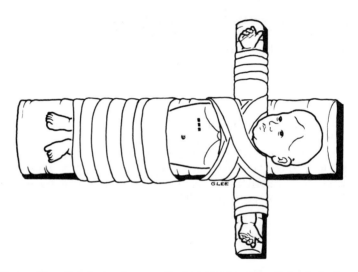

Fig. 22.10 The crucifix splint. Laparotomy, as for instance for congenital pyloric stenosis, performed under local anaesthesia is greatly facilitated by the infant being attached to a simple padded wooden cross. After toilet and skin preparation the infant's limbs are bandaged lightly with wool padding or Gamgee tissue. The infant must be firmly fixed to the splint with additional padding and bandages as shown. Care must be taken to leave the neck free from restriction, and the bandage round the chest must leave the lower ribs exposed; this is essential not only for access to the upper abdomen but because the baby's respiration is mainly with the lower ribs and abdomen. The pelvis also must be firmly fixed but the bandage must not come above the pubic crest. A subcutaneous infusion may be required and the outer side of the thigh is a convenient position for this, the tubing being attached to the splint as shown. The over-blanket of Gamgee is now applied and remains in position until the surgeon is ready to begin the operation. The diagram shows the position of the usual incision for congenital pyloric stenosis. The splint and its covers should be autoclaved after use and stored in a linen bag or pillow case.

A special restraining tray is available commercially. It has a Velcro base and a series of padded Velcro self-fixing straps which can be applied to limbs and trunk.[1]

[1] St. Mary's Hospital Pattern Infant Immobilising Board (Down Bros.).

Recovery period and convalescence

Children recover very rapidly after simple, or even quite severe, operations. A toddler will be running round on the day after a hernia operation, and if his home is not far from the hospital he will probably return there on the second day.

For children who are allowed out of bed there must be adequate provision to find full and safe occupation. Many children's units provide a playroom in the charge of a ward orderly or nursery-trained nurse. In addition a school teacher is appointed for units where there are perhaps more than twenty children so that the child's interest in learning can be maintained, particularly if the stay in hospital is likely to be prolonged for more than a month. Repeated interruptions of education in the early years of school life sometimes have a permanent effect on the child's ability to learn, and this aspect of child care must be provided for wherever there are sick children. Nurses need to co-operate with the school teachers so that each may understand the others' problems, with the maximum benefit to the child.

Common surgical conditions

The surgical treatment of congenital abnormalities extends to most branches of surgery. Remnants of the branchial apparatus—cysts and fistulae—are removed from the neck. The ophthalmic surgeon corrects congenital squints and the plastic surgeon is called upon to correct hare-lip, cleft palate or bat ears. The thoracic surgeon undertakes operations on congenital abnormalities of the heart and great vessels. Congenital atresia (blockage) of the oesophagus requires operation within the first four days of life. There are errors of development of the spinal cord and brain, some of which are treated by surgical operation. Club feet should be manipulated during the first day of life if the best results are to be obtained, and there are many other orthopaedic conditions arising from errors of development of the skeleton. Some of these have been caused by the mother taking certain drugs during her pregnancy. Thalidomide, taken as a tranquilliser, resulted in several thousand babies being born with short, deformed or absent limbs (Fig. 7.1).

There are many congenital abnormalities in the urinary tract such as double kidneys, fused or horse-shoe kidneys, and serious disorders of the bladder mechanism. The study of these urological conditions alone is quite a large subject.

Circumcision (the removal of the foreskin) of male infants is a Jewish and Moslem religious ritual but is occasionally required on medical grounds.

In the abdomen, congenital **hypertrophic pyloric stenosis** is a condition which only occurs during the first few weeks of life and is treated by a surgical operation which divides the muscle of the pyloric sphincter. This operation is usually performed under local anaesthesia. Errors of development of the umbilicus and the intestines also require surgical operation in the neonatal period. **Intussusception** is a peculiar condition almost entirely confined to childhood. The bowel swallows itself. The condition usually starts at the end of the ileum which travels inside the caecum and colon, like a sleeve of a coat as the arm is withdrawn. Blood is frequently passed from the rectum and surgical operation is urgent to relieve intestinal obstruction (Fig. 27.1).

Appendicitis, hernia, urinary infections and stones all afflict the young, but the nursing care is similar to that required in the adult.

Many children have to undergo the removal of tonsils and adenoids. Because of the large numbers waiting to be done, arrangements in some hospitals are far from perfect. This applies particularly to pre-operative preparation and anaesthesia, owing to shortage of time, and the utmost care is necessary on the part of the nursing staff to ensure that the child is not scared by the rush and unpleasantness of a large 'tonsil session'.

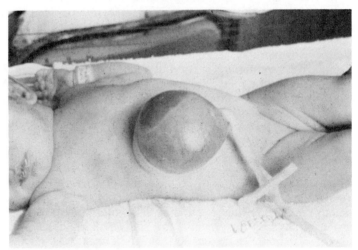

Fig. 22.11 A new-born baby with protrusion of bowel and liver—exomphalos. This condition requires immediate surgery and is often fatal.

Children are particularly liable to burns and scalds. They become very easily shocked and plasma or dextran infusion is frequently called for, because the area involved is usually large in relation to the child's total surface (page 961). The child has also been frightened by fire, and fear plays an important role in the development of shock.

Particular forms of malignant disease occur at various sites in the infant. The brain, the eye, the suprarenal glands and the kidneys are the organs most commonly affected. The growths are usually extremely malignant and survival is uncommon in spite of early surgical treatment. On the other hand the response of large tumours to radiotherapy or chemotherapy is sometimes dramatic.

Many metabolic disorders occur in childhood but few require surgical intervention.

Long-stay hospitals

Conditions such as tuberculosis of the skeleton, poliomyelitis, and congenital defects of the spine with paralysis require repeated or prolonged hospital treatment. In order that this shall not interfere with education, special long-stay hospitals are provided where a full school curriculum is carried on. In Great Britain there are hospitals of this type which were founded in the early part of this century by men and women of great vision and courage, in order to salvage the crippled child and give him an opportunity of becoming a useful citizen. The Robert Jones and Agnes Hunt Hospital at Oswestry, the

Table 37   Common surgical disorders of infancy and childhood

Disorder	Common age for onset	Clinical features	Principal treatment	Page reference
Oesophageal atresia with tracheo-oesophageal fistula	at birth	cyanotic attacks	thoracotomy and end to end anastomosis of oesophagus	497
Intestinal obstruction atresia, volvulus, malrotation, etc.	1st few days of life	bile-stained vomit	immediate operation	516 533
Exomphalos	at birth	herniation of bowel and sometimes liver through umbilicus	immediate operation	424
Congenital hypertrophic pyloric stenosis	1st month	projectile vomiting; palpable pyloric tumour	pyloromyotomy (Rammstedt's operation)	423
Hirschsprung's disease	early weeks	gross distension from rectal paralysis and obstruction	removal of affected rectum and colon; temporary colostomy	548
Intussusception	9–12 months	colic, vomiting and blood clot stools (red-currant jelly)	immediate operation	423 534
Heart—patent ductus	hereditary: onset infancy or childhood	circulatory disturbance	operation in due course	625
Meningomyelocele (spina bifida)	at birth: protrusion of spinal cord open on surface	spinal defect: hydrocephalus: paralysis	immediate operation	869
Hydrocephalus	at birth or infancy: may be secondary to meningitis or tumour	enlargement of head	dependent on cause: insertion of Holter valve: ventriculo-atrial (brain to heart) shunt	854
Congenital dislocation of hip	at birth	found on routine neonatal examination	splints: plaster cast: operation later	—
Club foot, talipes	at birth	deformity of feet	manipulation and plaster cast or splint	—
Cleft (hare) lip and palate	at birth	deformity: difficulty in feeding	surgical repair in 1st year	957
Hypospadias Epispadias	at birth	deformity of penis and urethra	surgical repair age 3–4	717 718

Table 37—*continued*

Disorder	Common age for onset	Clinical features	Principal treatment	Page reference
Eyes—squint	infancy	obvious defect	surgical correction, adjustment of lengths of eye muscles	831
Cancer nephroblastoma (Wilm's tumour)	at birth and in infancy	mass in abdomen: haematuria	radiotherapy: nephrectomy: chemotherapy	683
neuroblastoma and ganglioneuroma	at birth and in infancy	mass in abdomen or pelvis	radiotherapy: chemotherapy	832
retinoblastoma	hereditary: onset infancy or childhood	visual disturbance	removal of eye: radiotherapy	

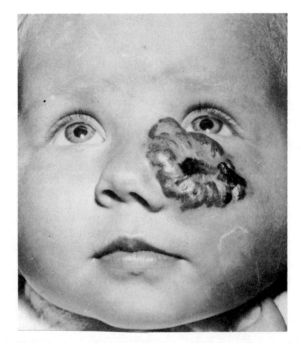

Fig. 22.12 Congenital haemangioma. A benign neoplasm of blood vessels, one of the well-known 'birth-marks'. This has been treated by repeated injections of boiling water to produce aseptic thrombosis of the vessels which compose the tumour. The scar will be only slight (page 934).

Lord Mayor Treloar Hospital at Alton (where Sir Henry Gauvain was the first superintendent), and the Chailey Heritage in Sussex, are three such notable hospitals. The care and devotion of medical and nursing staffs in these pioneering hospitals has played a very great part in the development of a high standard of orthopaedic nursing and surgery for which Great Britain is rightly famous. These hospitals were faced with the seemingly hopeless problem of advanced tuberculosis of a degree which has now been eliminated

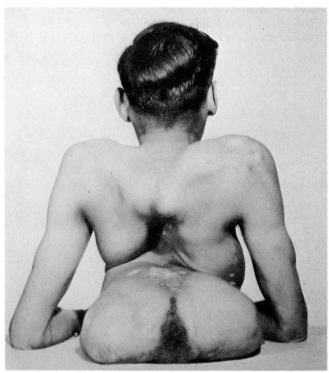

Fig. 22.13 A problem of long-term nursing. Gross congenital defect of the spine; a highly intelligent boy, with complete paralysis below the waist, and double incontinence. The prevention of pressure sores and urinary infection is a continuous problem. He received full secondary education in a hospital school and in spite of his disability became self-supporting.

almost completely from Great Britain. Similarly with the nation-wide immunisation service anterior poliomyelitis has been so greatly reduced that very few new cases are requiring prolonged hospital treatment. On the other hand, many babies with severe congenital disorders of the nervous system or skeleton now survive the hazards of infancy and during their childhood require continuous hospital care and repeated orthopaedic admissions.

As these long-stay orthopaedic hospitals, mainly for children, are not recognised as complete training schools for nurses they are staffed at a junior level by nursing auxiliaries and cadet nurses who may be waiting for their full training at a teaching centre. Special orthopaedic experience and training in child care is an excellent preparation for a full nursing course.

In addition to the hospital schools there are many special residential schools for children with particular types of physical handicap. In Great Britain many of these belong to charitable organisations while others are the responsibility of the Local Education Authority. Densely populated areas also have day schools for physically handicapped children where there is additional nursing supervision. There are among others, special schools for the blind, the partially sighted, the deaf and for those with severe orthopaedic deformities. Most of these children are under continuous medical supervision.

23

Neoplastic Disease and Radiotherapy

It is convenient to consider these two subjects together because many patients with malignant disease undergo some form of radium or x-ray treatment, probably in addition to surgical operation. Radiotherapy is also used for a number of non-malignant conditions but the dosage in such cases rarely demands special nursing techniques.

The study of neoplastic tumours is **oncology.** Malignant disease is also commonly treated by some form of chemotherapy and the whole programme of treatment by surgery, radiation and drugs has to be carefully co-ordinated. Development of these special treatment 'protocols' has led to the establishment of combined departments of oncology, where the varied skills are available.

NEOPLASTIC DISEASE

Pathology

Neoplastic disease forms one of the main groups of disorder requiring surgical treatment (page 11). It arises at any age, in any site of the body. Both **innocent** (benign) growths and those which are **malignant** (non-benign or cancer) can arise from most tissues and their cell structure resembles that of the tissue of origin.

An innocent growth causes disease by its size; it grows slowly and may remain stationary in size for many years. It may be brought to the patient's notice by the appearance of a visible lump or by symptoms from pressure on some other organ or tissue. It does not eat its way into other tissues by 'invasion'. It does not recur if it is removed, and it does not spread by a process of seeding.

A malignant growth, on the other hand, increases at a variable rate but relentlessly. It erodes and invades surrounding tissue, forming ulcers, craters, abscesses and, in bone, fractures. Malignant disease by its attack on blood vessels frequently presents as severe haemorrhage. It spreads to neighbouring lymph glands; by the blood stream it is seeded to other parts of the body. It affects the whole patient, produces debility, anaemia and ultimately death.

Innocent tumours may change their nature and become malignant after many years of lying dormant. This risk is a good reason for the removal of apparently harmless tumours.

Neoplasms are parasites. They live at the expense of their host and serve no purpose. Certain tumours produce cells which can function like their parent cell, as for instance in producing hormones. A tumour of the pituitary or pancreas may so alter the patient's metabolism that the endocrine change is the first feature to arouse suspicion that a neoplasm is present.

Treatment

The clinical features and management of neoplastic disease are included in the appropriate sections on regional surgery. There are however general factors common to the treatment of patients with innocent or malignant tumours. Sometimes the complications, such as intestinal obstruction or anaemia, require treatment before the underlying growth can be tackled (page 483).

Innocent growths are usually removed by simple surgical operation. The difficulties involved depend upon the site and size of the particular neoplasms. For instance, a papilloma of the tongue is completely removed under local anaesthesia. On the other hand, an innocent brain tumour requires a major surgical operation involving considerable risk.

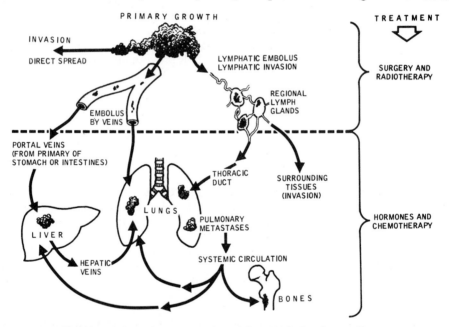

Fig. 23.1   Schematic representation of the spread of malignant disease.

Malignant growths frequently involve very large and disabling operations. The treatment of a malignant neoplasm necessitates also the treatment of the regional lymph nodes to which it may have spread. The principal difficulty is that we never know exactly how far the spread has extended, so that our surgery has to be planned to pursue the growth along the lines which it may have followed. The operations required in malignant disease usually involve heavy nursing responsibility.

Radiotherapy is used in some cases as an addition to surgical operation to cover those areas which the surgeon has been unable to excise. On the other hand radiotherapy may be used to treat recurrence when further operation is impossible. The modern treatment of cancer involves very close co-operation between the surgeon and the radiotherapist who together plan the best treatment for each particular patient, bearing in mind the age, the type of growth, its site and stage of development. Sometimes the course of treatment is not decided until a small piece of the tumour has been removed (biopsy) for histological examination. Table 38 contains the names and tissues of origin of common growths.

It is the aim of medicine that all cases of cancer shall be discovered at a stage in their progress when treatment can provide a really practical chance of cure. Many patients, however, through fear or ignorance conceal their symptoms or their growth until it is too late to offer any hope of cure. On the other hand, certain growths, especially those of the intestinal tract, may grow with such rapidity that the patient is overwhelmed in a very short time.

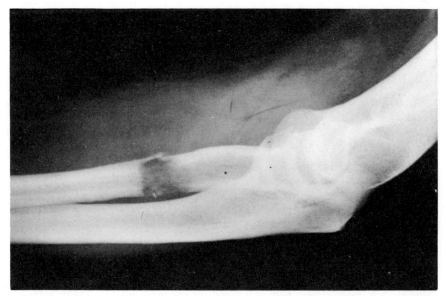

Fig. 23.2   Spontaneous fracture in radius from secondary deposit of carcinoma in the breast.

Nutrition is a very important feature in the nursing management of malignant disease for several reasons. In disorders of the alimentary tract there may well have been inter-ference with feeding and digestion and this will have led to malnutrition. Ulcerative conditions of the mouth discourage eating because of pain and discomfort. Growths of the stomach cause the patient to lose his appetite. Cancer of the bowel produces intestinal obstruction of an acute or chronic form. If malignant disease is widespread, the patient loses weight very rapidly and becomes anaemic.

Particular attention needs to be paid to the protein and vitamin intake and a great many patients require treatment for **anaemia**. From every point of view, diet arrangements in wards dealing with malignant disease must be of a very high order. Food should be appetising, attractively presented, well cooked and of high nutritive value: partly because

Table 38   Common neoplasms

(A) Neoplasms arising from epithelial tissues

(*i*) SURFACE EPITHELIUM

    skin
    tongue
    mouth
    pharynx   *innocent*—papilloma
    nose sinuses
    larynx and air passages
    oesophagus   *malignant*—epithelioma
    renal pelvis, ureter, bladder
    vagina and cervix
    anus

      Rodent ulcer is a special form of carcinoma of the skin which never shows distant spread by metastasis.

(*ii*) GLANDULAR EPITHELIUM—

    alimentary tract—stomach,
                     colon,   *innocent*—adenoma
                     rectum
    liver, gall-bladder, pancreas
    kidney
    breast, prostate   *malignant*—carcinoma (adenocarcinoma)
    thyroid, adrenal

(B) Neoplasms arising from connective and skeletal tissue

                  innocent   *malignant*
    fibrous tissue   fibroma
    bone   osteoma   sarcoma
    cartilage   chondroma
    muscle   myoma

(C) Neoplasms arising from nervous tissue

    nerves   —neuroma
                     neurofibroma *innocent* but may become *malignant*
    meninges   —meningioma—*innocent*
    brain and   —glioma   —*innocent* or *malignant*
    nerve cells
    Glioma may arise in the nerve cells of the retina.

(D) Neoplasms arising from the reticulo-endothelial (lympho-glandular) system

    Various forms of reticulosis—Hodgkin's disease,
                              lymphosarcoma
                             leukaemia

(E) Neoplasms arising from special cells in the reproductive system

    dermoid cysts (ovary and testis)—*innocent*
    teratoma (ovary and testis)
    chorionepithelioma (testis: or pregnant uterus) *malignant*
    seminoma (testis)

of the material requirements of the patient and partly because it is vital to maintain a high standard of satisfaction and morale.

Hormone therapy

There is no known drug which *cures* cancer, but some growths are influenced by treatment with certain chemicals, including hormones. The most successful application of this method is the control of carcinoma of the prostate with widespread metastasis in bones, by the administration of stilboestrol. Testosterone (male hormone) is sometimes used in recurrent carcinoma of the breast, and both ovaries may be removed to eliminate the effect of ovarian hormone in supporting the growth of malignant cells. To avoid repeated hormone injections, tablets are implanted in the rectus muscle sheath or subcutaneous tissues to provide prolonged absorption over several months.

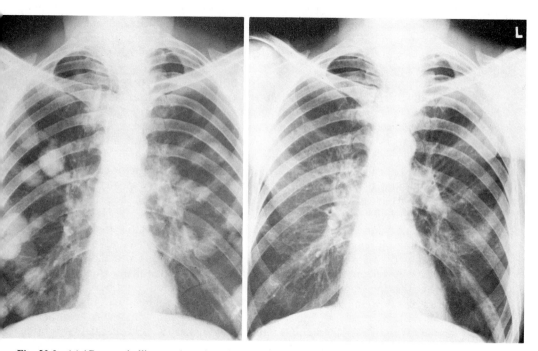

Fig. 23.3 (*a*) 'Cannon ball' secondary deposits in both lungs from carcinoma of the breast in a man. (*b*) The metastases have disappeared after castration and 7 months' hormone treatment.

There is no doubt the 'host resistance' of patients to an invading cancer plays quite a large part in halting the advance of disease. It is thought that this depends to some extent on the rate of metabolism of the parent tissues. If the cells are in a state of robust good health—anabolic—the disease is less likely to spread than if the tissues are in a state of decay—catabolic—such as occurs with vitamin deficiency and malnutrition. The male sex hormone, testosterone, is anabolic in its effect on the body, but there are now many synthetic chemicals which have a much more powerful anabolic effect without the unpleasant side effect of producing masculinising changes such as abnormal hair growth. Durabolin and the longer acting Deca-Durabolin are such hormones and are given by injection at intervals to boost the patient's general metabolism; the effect seems to be sometimes quite dramatic, particularly in the treatment of bone metastasis. Other corticosteroids are used in metastatic disease: their mode of action is uncertain: betamethasone and prednisolone are given to suppress adrenal function instead of adrenalectomy for carcinoma of the breast.

Cancer chemotherapy

Reference has already been made to the use of steroid anabolic hormones and to the effect of the sex hormones in certain types of growth. Apart from hormones and hormone antagonists other chemicals have been discovered which affect the vitality of, and may in fact kill, malignant cells. The main use of such drugs has been in the treatment of leukaemia and similar diseases of the blood-forming cells which are not amenable to radiotherapy as such large volumes of tissue in the bones are affected. These cytotoxic ('cell poisoning') drugs are divided into two main groups. The first includes the so-called alkylating agents which are direct tissue poisons altering the essential chemical constituents of the cell. Drugs commonly used in this group are thiotepa and nitrogen mustard and its derivatives melphalan (phenylalanine mustard) and cyclophosphamide (Endoxana). The second group of chemicals act in a rather different way. Since they are chemically closely allied to essential substances which cells need for their metabolism they are mistaken for these ingredients by the rapidly developing tissues and become incorporated in their structure. They act as a sort of 'fifth column' or underground movement within the cells and prevent the proper functioning of each cell. 5-Fluouracil and methotrexate are in this group. The effectiveness with which any chemical will attack cancer depends on the rate at which the malignant cells are dividing. The more virulent a growth the more rapidly is it using up the essential chemicals required for development. Unfortunately, healthy tissues which are multiplying and developing at a rapid rate may be similarly affected and in consequence the blood-forming tissues—bone marrow—the gastro-intestinal mucosa and the skin may be affected to such an extent as to prevent the continuation of treatment. During all forms of cancer chemotherapy regular weekly checks of the white blood count have to be undertaken and full blood examinations done periodically. If the white count falls below 2000 cells per cubic millimetre, or the platelets below 100,000 per cubic millimetre, treatment is usually suspended until the blood count returns to a higher level. Fortunately it is often possible to repeat courses of chemotherapy and although this treatment is very rarely a cure metastatic deposits in bones and other tissues sometimes disappear dramatically. Perhaps the most valuable effect of chemotherapy is to reduce the activity of a growth and in consequence relieve pain. (Additional side effects as well as anaemia are the production of rashes, severe nausea and even vomiting and perhaps diarrhoea. Gastro-intestinal haemorrhage or the development of purpura is an indication for the immediate suspension of treatment.)

The drugs may be given by mouth as tablets and Endoxana (cyclophosphamide) is usually given in this form. Alternatively a larger dose may be given intravenously at the time of operation in the hope of destroying any circulating cancer cells that have been displaced into the blood stream during manipulation of the tumour at operation. It is known that a relatively large number of cells escape into the blood stream in this way but it is also certain that only a relatively small number of these circulating cells in fact become implanted in the tissues and grow as secondary deposits.

If a malignant tumour is in the arm or leg regional perfusion is used (Fig. 48.13). The main vessels to the limb are occluded by a tourniquet and fluid containing the cytotoxic chemical is injected into the artery and allowed to remain in the tissues for a short time, being subsequently washed out through the vein before the tourniquet is released. Only

Table 39   Cancer chemotherapy

ROUTES: oral; intravenous; arterial infusion; limb or regional perfusion; intrapleural (for malignant effusions); intralymphatic

DRUGS: **Alkylating agents**—cell poisons:
        chlorambucil (Leukeran)
        cyclophosphamide (Endoxana)
        mannomustine (Degranol)
        nitrogen mustard (mustine)
        phenylalanine mustard (melphalan)
        thiotepa
        Antimetabolites—essential tissue component 'substitutes'; folic acid blocking agents:
        actinomycin D
        adriamycin
        asparaginase
        daunorubicin
        5-fluouracil
        6-mercaptopurine (Mercaptan)
        methotrexate (Amethopterin)
        thioguanine
        vinblastine (Velbe): vincristine (Oncovin)
        Anabolic supplementary hormones:
        Durabolin; Deca-Durabolin; Dianabol; testosterone; Masteril; norethisterone

Side effects: gastritis; enteritis; intestinal obstruction; depression of white count; anaemia purpura; haematuria; loss of hair.
        Any of these symptoms must be reported at once.

a small amount of the poisonous substance therefore gets into the general circulation whereas a high dose is delivered to the affected limb. An alternative method of delivering a high concentration of the drug to a local area of tissue in a limb or for instance in the liver, or to a growth in the pelvis, is to put a small plastic catheter into the main artery supplying the part concerned and injecting the drug at that point. The force of the injection obviously has to be very considerable to overcome the arterial pressure and the usual way of achieving this is to have the arterial catheter connected to a 'drip' apparatus on a stand at least 3 metres high. The height of the infusion bottle has to be adjusted to prevent regurgitation of arterial blood into the transparent catheter. The necessary quantity of fluid is allowed to flow in at set time intervals of several hours. This method has been used extensively in the treatment of advanced malignant disease in the head and neck.

The control of the complicated techniques for giving intra-arterial chemotherapy is very specialised and it is unlikely that the nurse will come across this treatment except in well-organised cancer units.

Cytotoxic drugs lower the resistance of a patient to infection as do immuno-suppressive drugs used in transplant surgery. Avoidance of contact with relatives and friends who have infectious disease is essential, and any infection that arises must be treated vigorously with antibiotics.

Special hazards in malignant disease

Apart from the dangers of spread, there are certain other complications which are especially liable to arise in patients with cancer. Venous thrombosis and anaemia to some extent go hand in hand, but both are particularly liable to develop in elderly people with malignant disease. It is therefore important that such patients should be kept mobile, given exercises, and treatment for anaemia. Blood transfusion is frequently used as a pre-operative preparation.

The surgical wounds are less inclined to heal and the tissues are more liable to infection.

Although these features may be partly due to malnutrition there seems to be some other factor in the patient with malignant disease which interferes with health and the repair processes of the body.

Convalescence

Particular attention is paid to the recovery period of patients who have been treated for malignant disease. Anxiety and perhaps the strain of a prolonged period of treatment involving x-rays or radium will have sapped the patient's strength. It is of course extremely important that those who are able to do so should return to their normal occupation in order that they may not become discouraged and depressed, but the knowledge that a patient has malignant disease may have such a profound effect on his household that it is wiser for him to spend a period of convalescence away from his home.

Ethics and the cancer patient

There is always an element of insecurity surrounding the patient with a malignant growth.

First, there is the fear in his or her mind that the symptoms or lump in question are due to cancer.

Second, there is perhaps a period of uncertainty during investigation before the true nature of the disease is determined.

Third, there is the atmosphere of tension and difficulty that arises when a decision is to be made as to what to tell the patient with proved malignant disease.

Fourth, whether a true or evasive statement is made, there still remains the difficulty and suspicion that only the half-truth has been told.

Fifth, there is the impossibility of giving an absolute assurance that the malignant disease has been cured. For practical purposes we can in many cases give an honest opinion that we regard the patient as cured, but there are others where we know the chance is slight and yet others in which we know our treatment has only added a few months to the expected duration of life.

Sixth, there is the repetition of all these problems if the disease recurs after having been apparently cured.

During training, it is inevitable that both medical students and nurses themselves experience considerable doubt as to what must be their part in the miniature drama which arises when a patient is in fear, and in fact in danger, of a killing disease. No rules can be written on such a complex problem. The surgeon in charge determines from his experience what is the correct approach. Both medical students and nurses need to cultivate an ability to answer enquiring patients without hesitation, for hesitation only adds to suspicion. They must say quite frankly that they are not competent enough to express an opinion. All nurses must be informed when they join a surgical team as to what is the particular attitude of the surgeon-in-charge, to these problems. The experienced ward sister will regard this as a primary duty of instruction to her nurses so that neither they nor the patients will be embarrassed when the natural fears and doubt arise.

Reference to the plan of hospital organisation (Fig. 1.1) will show clearly that many persons are involved in the management of one patient. All must learn the same degree of caution when dealing with cancer patients. Perhaps the only rigid rule is that a nurse or medical student who is tackled by a patient on the question of malignancy or its outcome, must at once inform the ward sister so that there may be no confusion. The sister or medical officer will then be in a position to deal with the patient's query and perhaps counteract any false impression which may have been given. Fortunately many patients with cancer are aware of their condition and, believing themselves curable, are consequently easy to deal with. Others fear that they have cancer but never ask and therefore there is no opportunity of discussing their problems. A patient whose course is known to be rapidly deteriorating may be planning some future action such as moving his home or getting married. In such an instance, the surgeon may feel it is his duty to break the cruel news of impending disaster. This is a most difficult task and one which is, in practice, rarely called for.

Cancer patients, many of whom undergo radiotherapy at some stage, consequently attend a special follow-up clinic. Here they have contact with other sufferers from malignant disease and soon discover the true nature of their condition. Fortunately there are many who return to full normal activity, 'cured' and healthy. These patients are an encouragement to those who face their initial treatment and convalescence.

As a contrast to the calm and logical cancer sufferer who has complete confidence in his treatment, there is the problem of the patient with **'cancer-phobia'**. This dread of cancer, sometimes because there is a family history of malignant disease, is often present without any growth. Symptoms may arise from some other problem, or may be psychological in origin. Extensive and expensive investigation may be required before the patient or his relatives can be reassured. The nurse may discover by casual conversation that a patient's main worry is cancer-phobia although he is in hospital for some completely different condition. This information must be passed to the medical officer.

The nurse should never be in the position of having to break the news, to a patient or his relatives, that the patient has cancer. This is the duty of the medical staff because there arise at once in the minds of the patient and his relatives, questions which cannot be answered without the fuller knowledge which medical training and experience provide. Frequently, as doctors, our replies are evasive and unsatisfactory, but it is the author's belief and experience that in most cases, if the patient should ask, it is better for him to be told the true nature of his disease. Continued confidence and co-operation is not possible if the patient feels or knows that he has been deceived. It is usual to inform some close relative if we find that the disease is incurable.

Evidence of recurrence

Every patient with malignant disease should be weighed before leaving hospital. Continued loss of weight is an indication that the disease is progressive. Growth may return at the site of surgical removal or irradiation and is particularly liable to develop along the surgical scar. Enlargement of lymph glands which drain the area may be the first sign of recurrence or the patient may return with a pathological fracture due to blood-borne metastasis.

The lungs are very commonly the site of growth which may be discovered there by routine chest x-rays taken during the follow-up period. The pain of pleurisy, an attack of pneumonia, or haemoptysis may be the first evidence of pulmonary metastasis.

Liver enlargement, distension due to **ascites**,[1] and rapid loss of weight are the main features of abdominal recurrence.

Dermatomyositis occurs with various forms of cancer and may be present before the primary growth is detected. There is widespread thickening and erythema of the skin, with weakness of the muscles especially of the shoulder girdle. It is thought to be due to toxins arising from the malignant tissue.

Herpes zoster also commonly heralds the recurrence of cancer. Herpes is due to reactivity of chickenpox virus present in the body.

Malignant disease of the organs which normally occupy the pelvis—the rectum, bladder, uterus and vagina or prostate—is almost always treated by surgical removal initially. Recurrent disease in this area or the primary disease which has become very advanced is invariably the source of extreme pain and distress on account of involvement of the pelvic nerves. To avoid this, extensive surgical operation is frequently undertaken for cancer in this region even if there is no hope of permanent cure.

In many cases of malignant disease in various sites, the advanced stages of the condition are much more distressing if the primary growth cannot be removed. There is thus a very large place for palliative treatment in the management of cancer, perhaps to avoid involvement of nerves, ulceration or obstruction to the bowel by the unchecked primary growth. The last few months of life are then more tolerable as the general health is failing from widespread metastasis.

RADIOTHERAPY

Electromagnetic waves are emitted from many natural sources. The distance between the peaks of the waves, like the ripples on a pond, is the 'wave-length'. The sun emits waves of many different wave-lengths. There are also sources of this 'radio-activity' to be found in the

[1] ascites = collection of free fluid in the peritoneal cavity (page 492).

earth; radium and uranium are those most used. Electromagnetic waves can be produced artificially and play a large part in our daily lives. The very long waves are used for sound broadcasting, shorter waves for television and radar, and yet shorter ones, the infra-red rays, are used in medicine. Coming down the wave-length scale there is next the visible light spectrum from red to violet, followed by the ultra-violet irradiation which is again used in medicine. The greater waves are measured in hundreds of kilometres between their peaks; the length of light rays is so small that special units are used, smaller than a thousandth of a millimetre. Of a wave-length yet smaller than ultra-violet light are x-rays which have the property of penetrating solid matter and affecting a photographic plate. Very specially produced x-rays of extremely short wave-length have a damaging effect on living cells and this is used in the treatment of cancer. Even shorter waves are produced by radium from the gamma rays which are emitted. Unfortunately radium also emits entirely different types of rays which are more destructive—alpha and beta irradiation. γ (gamma) rays are electromagnetic. An α (alpha) particle is a nucleus of a helium atom, β (beta) rays are electrons and penetrate tissues only to a depth of 1 cm. Radioactive cobalt and radioactive caesium are now used extensively in therapy.

Effect of irradiation with x-rays and radium

Just as the sun burns a delicate skin exposed too long to its rays, so the artificial forms of radiation produce burning and death of tissue (page 958). The rapidly budding cells of cancer are however far more easily damaged by these penetrating rays than are the normal cells of surrounding tissue. The whole process of radiotherapy is therefore bound up with directing the rays, calculating the necessary amounts required, and protecting surrounding tissue from damage.

Radiotherapy has an effect which varies with the particular type of growth being treated. Some growths are completely resistant while others melt away with great rapidity. From experience the pathologist and radiotherapist can judge which types of growth are most likely to respond to this form of treatment.

As well as the local effect in killing growth, producing inflammation of surrounding tissue and perhaps burning the skin, exposure of the patient to these rays lowers vitality, and produces anaemia by interfering with the production of red blood cells in bone marrow. Tissue which has been exposed to x-rays heals very badly for several weeks after a course of treatment.

Types of treatment

Radium

Radium is a solid substance which for all practical purposes is everlasting and continues to emit its powerful rays indefinitely. For use in surgery, minute quantities of between 1 and 5 mg are contained in hollow needles made of platinum. The effect of the platinum shell is to prevent the escape of the damaging alpha and beta rays but to permit the passage of the useful rays. These radium needles are inserted into the growth or surrounding tissue for periods up to one week and the exact pattern with which the needles are placed is carefully calculated beforehand in order that there may be an even distribution of rays. Each needle has a silk thread attached to it, so that it cannot be lost. The thread is stitched to the skin or otherwise anchored. Very great care needs to be taken during the period of treatment so that the needle shall not be dislodged and rigid precautions are observed to guard against the loss of a needle in dressings (Fig. 23.4).

Radium is also used on the surface of the body or elsewhere where it can be conveniently placed, such as the vagina. For this purpose, needles or tubes containing radium are incorporated in a 'special mould' or appliance which ensures the correct spacing and keeps the needles together. This applicator is held against the surface to be treated for several hours or days according to the dose required.

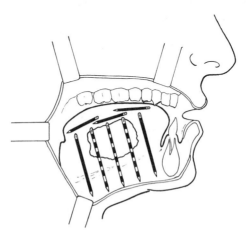

Fig. 23.4 Radium needle implant for carcinoma of the side of the tongue. Plan of needle positions. Duration of treatment—7 days. (Paterson, *The Treatment of Malignant Disease by Radium and X-rays.*)

Radon gas is emitted by radium and this is also radioactive. The gas is contained in tiny glass or gold beads which are implanted in the tissue at operation. The activity passes off in a few days, and the beads may be left in position, being then quite harmless.

A large block of radium, weighing several grams, is described as a **radium bomb**. It is placed in a ray-proof container in which there is a small opening like the lens of a lamp. Thus the rays can be directed in much the same way as x-rays.

Caesium is also used in applicators and platinum-coated radioactive gold 'seeds' are implanted into the bladder and other sites. Gold seeds lose their activity very quickly and these grains do not have to be removed. Other applicators and needles are only in contact for strictly measured periods. Radioactive wire is used similarly, as needles.

Needles and applicators are of particular value in treating carcinoma of the uterus (page 741).

X-ray therapy

The therapy rays are referred to as 'deep' x-rays, because of their greater power of penetration than the rays used in x-ray photography. These rays are produced by very expensive apparatus which involves the use of extremely high-voltage electric current.

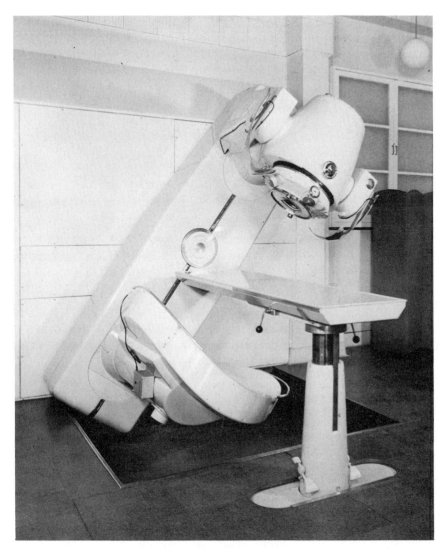

Fig. 23.5   Radioactive cobalt unit installed at the Middlesex Hospital, London.

The higher the voltage available, the shorter the wave-length and the greater degree of penetration of the resultant waves. Thus as cancer treatment advances, more and more powerful x-ray plants are being installed.

X-ray treatment requires the use also of a special department, as a patient cannot be treated in his home, in the operating theatre or in the ward. A course of x-ray treatment may extend over several weeks and has to be planned with all the precision possible.

The principle of x-ray treatment is to deliver a lethal dose to a deep-seated growth:

it is necessary to direct the beam from several different angles in order to reduce the damage to overlying tissues through which the rays pass. Figure 23.6 indicates how x-rays may be directed at a growth of the oesophagus from four angles, thus concentrating the dose in the growth but exposing the lung and each skin area to only a fraction of the total radiation.

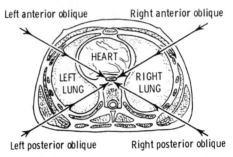

Fig. 23.6 Transverse section through thorax to show cross-fire method of x-ray therapy in the treatment of carcinoma of the oesophagus.

However careful and precise the treatment has been there will inevitably be an inflammatory reaction in all the tissues through which these waves have passed. It is this reaction which demands special nursing methods and great care. Sometimes the discomfort and distress which the patient experiences as the result of treatment, seem almost worse than the disease itself, but since cancer untreated is fatal, aggravation of the patient's immediate distress has to be accepted as inevitable.

Cobalt 'bomb'

Radioactive cobalt has largely replaced radium and ordinary x-ray therapy. Its use in treatment is similar to that for the radium 'bomb' and the resultant radiation is beamed to the patient with a special machine. There is far less skin reaction and a greater degree of accuracy than with radium x-ray treatment.

Mega-voltage therapy—linear accelerator

To reach higher voltages a different system is now in use whereby radio waves are used to assist in the production of the beams. This is done in a 'linear accelerator', and in Great Britain the standard apparatus reaches 6 million volts. At St Bartholomew's Hospital an accelerator is used producing the equivalent of 15 million volts, from which various types of radiation can be used.

Clinical complications and nursing care

It must be remembered that most patients undergoing radiotherapy have malignant disease. The psychological factors have already been discussed and these are of particular importance, owing to the nature and extent of the reaction which may occur during and after radiotherapy. **Radiation sickness** is one of the principal general complications which depends more upon the extent of treatment than on its location. The patient loses all appetite, develops persistent nausea, and becomes extremely depressed, dehydrated and starved unless special treatment is introduced. Fortunately with modern technique, radiation sickness rarely goes beyond the stage of nausea. It is more likely to occur if heavy dosage is used at the beginning of treatment. If the symptoms become troublesome the amount of radiation given each day is reduced. Many medical remedies have been tried; chlorpromazine and promethazine are often helpful. Radiation sickness must of course be distinguished from nausea and vomiting due to obstruction or any other cause, such as cerebral irritation from a metastasis in the brain.

Anaemia is sometimes very severe and weekly blood examinations are made during treatment. If radiotherapy is applied to the thorax, which contains in the ribs a large amount of red bone marrow, the generation of blood cells is reduced. Increased activity on the part of other bones will make up for any area which has been irradiated if the treatment is not too rapid. Nevertheless many patients undergoing prolonged radiotherapy require blood transfusion.

Hyperbaric oxygen

Some types of malignant cells are more sensitive to radiation if they are in high oxygen concentration. By placing a patient in a closed tank into which oxygen is fed at a pressure higher than that in the atmosphere, the blood stream is made to carry an abnormally high concentration to the tissues. This method of treatment is sometimes used in the management of patients with ischaemia, and in gas gangrene (page 34). With mega-voltage therapy apparatus the patient can be treated for malignant disease while in such a tank. The radiation effect is enhanced and, in consequence, for the required exposure there is less harm to the normal tissues.

Skin reaction

In the normal course of x-ray treatment or after the application of radium, the skin through which the rays have passed becomes increasingly red from about the tenth day after the start of treatment. This erythema resembles sun-burn and is followed by shedding of the surface epithelium. If the reaction is severe, the skin becomes raw and moist. It is then extremely painful and requires several weeks for recovery and return to normal. Skin which has been irradiated frequently becomes pigmented and rather inelastic.

Care of the skin

Tolerance varies considerably with different patients and in different sites of the body. The trunk is more tolerant than the distal parts of the arms and legs. Feet and hands are particularly liable to brisk skin reaction. Vascular skin is more tolerant than pale and relatively avascular areas. Certain precautions are taken to diminish the likelihood of brisk reaction, and as far as possible the area to be treated is left exposed to the air, rather than wrapped in bandages. **On no account must adhesive plaster be attached to any area which is to be irradiated.** Usually radiotherapists prohibit the shaving of any area which is

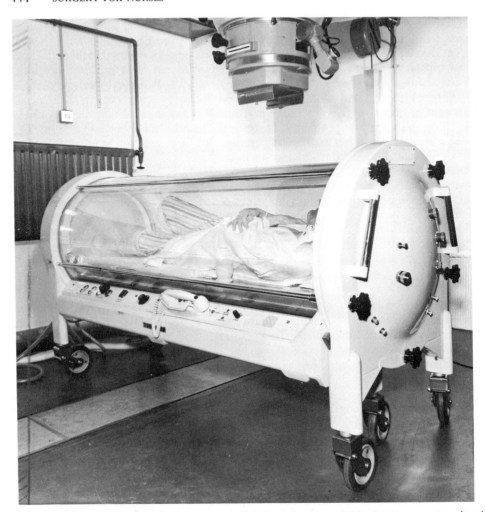

Fig. 23.7 High-pressure (hyperbaric) oxygen tank. The patient is sealed in the transparent tank, with telephone communication, and is undergoing super voltage radiotherapy.

being irradiated, but x-ray treatment causes the hairs to fall out. Hot baths or hot water for washing should not be allowed but opinions differ as to the use of soap. If the particular department permits the use of soap, care should be taken that only good quality soap, free from soda, us used. On no account may 'bath salts' which contain soda be allowed. The most important thing is that the skin must not be rubbed or scrubbed: it may only be cleansed lightly.

Irritation may be the first symptom of reaction and a simple starch dusting powder may be used, but this must not contain zinc or bismuth as the heavy metal interferes with the passage of the rays. It may in fact increase the damage to the skin. No grease, lotion or ointment should be applied if it can possibly be avoided. When the treated area becomes moist as the surface epithelium is shed, a dry covering of sterile gauze or preferably lint may be required. Padding with cotton wool and the application of bandages should be avoided in order that the raw areas should be as dry as possible. Infection cannot be prevented in certain areas like buttocks and perineum, and pieces of lint soaked in sodium hypochlorite solution (Milton) may be applied to the weeping areas. Crystal violet solution is also used sometimes to encourage the formation of crust as in the treatment of burns elsewhere (page 960). When the course of treatment has finished zinc cream is commonly prescribed. All applications of this type must be applied very lightly and the skin must never be rubbed either in cleaning or in applying ointment.

Even minor injury after treatment, when the reaction seems to have subsided, may cause severe return of the reaction and ulceration. To the nurse, the principal warning is to avoid adhesive plaster, chafing and pressure from bandages.

Because of the discomfort from the skin reaction, the patient undergoing radiotherapy will probably require the regular use of hypnotics to ensure a good night's sleep.

Care of the mouth and pharynx

If radiotherapy is applied to the tongue or mouth or to any structure in the neck, the mucous membrane undergoes changes similar to that seen in the skin. Particular attention must be paid to oral hygiene and great difficulty is experienced with swallowing. Bland thickened fluid feeds with high calorie and high protein value are given frequently. Aspirin-containing gargles or anaesthetic lozenges (page 242) may be given before the feed to make swallowing more comfortable. If the reaction is severe, feeding may have to be continued through nasal tubes. Surface anaesthetic agents do not work well in inflamed skin or mucous membrane, but the use of a spray containing 1 per cent lignocaine may be tried.

If the salivary glands have been included in the field of irradiation, the patient's mouth will be extremely dry and therefore more liable to infection. Small pellets of butter or peanut butter may be a help, and dry foods such as bread or biscuits should not be given.

Dental sepsis has to be dealt with before radiotherapy is used in the mouth.

If radium needles are to be used in the tongue or mouth, the patient must be warned about this before the operation to implant the needles, and the nurse must remain at the patient's side until he is fully conscious and has realised that the object in his mouth must not be ejected. Radium needles are attached to the mucous membrane by a silk stitch. They are removed, sometimes without a further anaesthetic, at the end of the requisite time: the procedure is not normally painful as the needle tract has been rendered insensitive.

If the pharynx has been affected, as for instance in the treatment of glands in the neck, the larynx will also be involved and the patient may have a very troublesome and painful cough. A sedative cough mixture may be prescribed, but the principal danger is one of pulmonary atelectasis or broncho-pneumonia from a downward spread of infection, combined with the patient's inability to cough adequately. This is yet another example of team work in nursing, and these patients require particular attention to general mobility and breathing exercises. It is a general rule in many units that a patient with radium needles in position is not allowed to leave his bed except to use a bedside commode. Such a precaution is vital to prevent the accidental loss of a needle.

Good nursing, combined with cheerful encouragement, may enable a badly distressed patient to tolerate a course of x-rays or radium which might otherwise have to be shortened.

Intestinal reaction

Neoplastic disease within the abdomen, particularly when the lymph glands on the posterior abdominal wall are involved, necessitates the exposure of the bowel to the rays during radiotherapy. The reaction of the mucous membrane is similar to that in the mouth and to that of the skin. Diarrhoea occurs and may become distressing. Constipation may be encouraged artificially by the use of simple mixtures containing codeine or kaolin. If the diarrhoea is accompanied by mucus or blood, x-ray treatment is usually suspended. The stools become pale from the accelerated progress of food through the intestinal tract, and from interference with digestion. **Three to six weeks may elapse before the patient's bowel action again becomes normal and patients must be warned.**

Careful regulation of the diet is therefore essential and again frequent small meals with high protein and high calorie content are necessary together with a vitamin supplement. A complete record must be kept of the calorie and protein value of the food which has been taken, so that the radiotherapist may be aware of any impending nutritional deficiency.

Rectum and urinary bladder

Radium placed in the vagina is sometimes used in the treatment of carcinoma of the cervix and x-ray treatment is employed in palliative treatment of carcinoma of the bladder or rectum. Patients who are submitted to irradiation in the treatment of one of these pelvic conditions are usually already in an advanced state of disease which has rendered radical surgery impossible. It is inevitable that both the bladder and rectum are affected by the radiation and the reaction may sometimes be severe. Painful and troublesome cystitis, with intense frequency of micturition, will almost certainly require the use of sedative drugs. There is no effective local treatment unless the urine becomes infected and very thick with pus and mucus: antiseptic bladder wash-outs may then be ordered.

Inflammation of the rectum produces a frequent but ineffective desire for defaecation (tenesmus). The subsequent straining may aggravate haemorrhoids if these are present.

Very great care must be taken to see that the anal area is kept clean and every bowel action must be followed by nursing attention to the perineum, in order to diminish the risk of infection.

In a case of rectal cancer, radiotherapy will probably be employed in order to diminish the discharge of blood and mucus which distresses the patient by causing frequent defaecation and tenesmus. The inconvenience of the treatment is then more than balanced by an improvement of the symptoms arising from the growth itself.

Similarly treatment of advanced carcinoma of the cervix leads to a lessening of the foul vaginal discharge (page 742).

Application of radiotherapy in the treatment of neoplasia

X-ray or other radiation may be used in the treatment of the primary tumour. A course of x-ray therapy may precede surgical excision. Alternatively, as used in many cases of carcinoma the breast, x-ray therapy may be given after removal of the primary tumour, in order to deal with the areas of lymphatic drainage. If surgical excision is not feasible, radiotherapy may be employed as the sole method of treatment. There are certain growths for which radiotherapy is used again on the area of recurrence.

There is a group of diseases which affects the reticulo-endothelial system including lymph glands, the spleen and bone marrow. In this group is included Hodgkin's disease (lymphadenoma), various forms of leukaemia, and certain rare tumours such as plasmo-cytoma. The main feature of these 'reticuloses' is that the various tumours which arise are not seedlings as in carcinoma or sarcoma, but are separate centres, each being in effect a primary growth. The condition is a generalised one affecting the whole system. Some forms of this disease are sensitive to x-ray treatment which has to be widespread. There is therefore a severe general reaction and it is in these cases that radiation sickness is most likely to occur.

Other uses of radiotherapy

Apart from the treatment of neoplastic disease, radium or x-ray therapy is employed to diminish tissue activity in organs which are known to be sensitive. The sex cells in the ovary and testis are particularly liable to damage by x-ray or radium; radiotherapy is therefore used to produce an artificial menopause, particularly in women who are affected by very heavy menstrual loss in middle age. In such cases, the amount of treatment required is not sufficient to produce any significant radiation reaction.

The thyroid gland in cases of thyrotoxicosis may also be treated by x-rays, but it is usual to reserve this method for cases which have recurred after surgical operation.

X-ray treatment is sometimes given to patients with painful chronic mastitis to diminish the activity of the breast and thereby relieve pain.

Birth marks, keloid scars, and certain skin diseases are treated by x-rays or radium, but again the dosage involved is insufficient to provoke a severe reaction.

Radioactive isotopes

The figures on the luminous dial of a watch or clock continue to be visible in the dark for a certain time after exposure to bright light. Similarly certain simple chemicals after exposure to powerful sources of atomic energy, themselves become radioactive and continue to emit rays or particles without having any alteration at all in their chemical property. These rays are detected by special apparatus known as a Geiger counter. It has thus become possible to use simple chemicals such as phosphorus, iodine and zinc, in biological experiments, and trace their path through a growing plant or animal into whose tissues the chemical has been incorporated. The thyroid gland uses iodine in the manufacture of thyroxin. Iodine is one of the elements which can be made radioactive, and if a patient is given an injection of this special iodine, the presence of the marked atoms can be detected in the thyroid gland a few minutes later by means of the Geiger counter which 'listens-in' over the neck. Thus the degree of activity of the thyroid gland can be measured.

If, however, a larger dose of radioactive iodine is administered, the special atoms emit so much radiation in the gland that they destroy the epithelium and thus reduce the activity of the gland. Sometimes carcinoma of the thyroid manufactures thyroxin like the parent gland and therefore takes up iodine from the blood stream. Radioactive iodine can then be used in treating secondary deposits, because these metastatic tumours kill themselves by picking up radioactive iodine.

These radioactive substances are called **isotopes** and they have chemical properties exactly the same as the simple element, in spite of the fact that they are shooting off radioactive rays.

Just as the luminous clock face loses its power, so radioactive substances become weaker with the passage of time, but the rate of decline of their power is very variable. Radium loses its activity so slowly that the loss is for practical purposes negligible, and a milligram of radium is just as dangerous and just as useful each year. The loss of power is described in terms of 'half-life'. Radioactive iodine (^{131}I) has a half-life of eight days which means that at the end of each eight-day period only half the activity remains. There is thus no continued effect. ^{60}Co, the cobalt source of teleradiation, directed as a beam, has a half-life of 5 years and the 'bomb' used in the treatment machines has to be renewed at approximately 4-year intervals, the dose time being increased as the plant ages.

^{137}Cs, caesium, used in tubes and applicators, has a half-life of 37 years and radium 1600 years. The half-life value thus affects the precautions taken when radioactive substances are used in diagnosis or treatment by injection or oral administration.

Most radioactive isotopes are used in liquid form, and when one of these substances has been administered to a patient, the faeces, urine, and sputum may all contain radioactive chemicals. If the excreta are spilt, very serious consequences arise from the presence of radioactive substances in the bedding, on the floor or on the furniture. During a period of investigation or treatment with isotopes, special precautions have to be taken to ensure that no radioactive substance finds its way into the sewage system. Nursing staff must take great care that they do not contaminate themselves with any substance which might be active. (See below for technetium.)

Nurses will be specially instructed when these substances are used and the supply of isotopes is very carefully controlled because the consequences of wide distribution of radioactive substances are not known. No patient to whom radioactive isotopes have been administered must be allowed to leave the ward until permission has been given by the medical officer responsible for the special treatment or investigation.

Scannograms

Radioactive isotopes are used for diagnosis and research purposes and the area being investigated is scanned by a counting detector mentioned above. This is usually coupled to an apparatus which 'writes' the activity as a map in different colours. This map indicates the shape of the organ and areas of activity or defects where, for instance, there is a malignant growth. The map so produced is a **scannogram.**

Radioactive hippuran is used to examine renal function. After an intravenous injection the isotope is concentrated in the kidneys and the relative function of the two kidneys can be determined very quickly by a scanning 'Geiger' counter over each, posteriorly. It is extremely useful if a patient has failed to pass urine, the bladder is empty, and it is not known whether the kidneys have stopped secreting or the ureters are blocked.

Phosphorous isotopes are used to localise brain tumours, and certain other neoplasms concentrate phosphorous compounds.

Radioactive chromium is used to 'label' a measured quantity of red blood cells which are put back into the circulation. If there is a leakage of blood into the gastro-intestinal tract it is then possible to determine the site of the leakage when other methods have failed. The life of red cells can also be measured in this way.

Technetium is a synthetic compound which has now replaced other isotopes as it is concentrated by glandular tissue. It has a half-life of 6 hours and therefore loses its activity very quickly. The very small amount given for scanning does not produce sufficient radioactivity to require isolation of the patient. Figure 23.8 shows a typical liver scannogram. In this case the outer zone of the enlarged liver does not concentrate the isotope. A clear zone in the centre of the liver would indicate one large metastasis.

The results of isotope examination are sometimes expressed merely in percentages of the substance that has been given.

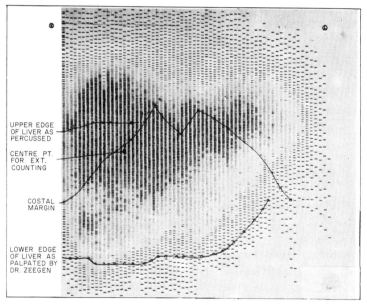

Fig. 23.8 Scannogram of liver after intravenous injection of antimony sulphide 'labelled' with radioactive technetium. This is concentrated by healthy liver, mapped out by the 'detector'. The healthy dark area is surrounded by a pale zone which extends to the edge of the liver as felt on examination. This part is non-functioning and filled with secondary carcinoma.

Doses of isotopes are measured in terms of radioactivity, the unit being a millicurie (mCi) or microcurie (1/1000 of mCi) expressed by Greek 'm' (μCi).

When isotopes are used for **diagnostic** purposes as tracer substances, only **micro**curie amounts are used. In therapy the amounts given are in millicurie dose and the risks are consequently greater. Table 40 gives the isotopes in regular use for diagnostic and therapeutic purposes. Special preparation of the patient is required on most occasions. For instance, if any iodine compound is to be used other than for thyroid testing, 60 mg potassium iodine is given first to saturate the thyroid gland and prevent it taking up the radioactive drug: if it did so the test would be invalidated and the thyroid damaged.

Table 40   Isotopes used in diagnosis and treatment

For diagnosis

Isotope	Investigation
Iodine^{131}I, ^{132}I, or ^{125}I	Thyroid function
Chromium ^{51}Cr	Red-cell survival time
Iron ^{59}Fe	Study of iron metabolism
Hippuran labelled by ^{131}I	Renal function (renogram) and residual urine volume
Selenium-labelled methionine ^{75}Se-methionine	Localisation of pancreatic and para-thyroid tumours
Technetium Tc^{99} with human serum	Albumin
Technetium Tc^{99} with antimony sulphide colloid	Liver scan
Cobalt ^{58}Co (vitamin B$_{12}$)	Absorption test

For treatment

Isotope	Disease
Iodine ^{131}I	Thyrotoxicosis or carcinoma of thyroid
Phosphorus ^{32}P	Polycythaemia
Gold ^{198}Au	Malignant pleural effusion
Iodine ^{131}I-labelled lipiodol	Treatment of lymphatic glands by injection into lymph vessels

Protection against irradiation

Because of the dangers of x-rays or gamma rays from radium, special arrangements are made for the protection of those who supervise the treatment. X-ray therapy rooms have walls through which the rays cannot penetrate, and while treatment is in progress, the operator sits at a control desk outside the room and is able to observe the patient through a window or periscope. The parts of the patient which are not being treated are screened with lead sheets.

Radium is stored in special containers made of lead which prevents the spread of the gamma rays. Radioactive needles and applicators are conveyed from place to place in the hospital in one of these special containers (Fig. 40.10). The effect of radium is cumulative, so that day-to-day contact with radium needles, even though it is only for a few minutes, will have an effect similar to intensive treatment for a short period. Special instruments are therefore used for the introduction of the radium, in order that the surgeon exposes his hands as little as possible to the harmful irradiation. If during treatment a radium applicator or needle should become dislodged, it must be handled with forceps and immediately returned to the radiotherapy department, not only because of its great value but because wherever it may be placed it may do harm.

Mention has already been made of the fact that the sex cells are particularly sensitive to electromagnetic waves (x-rays or radium gamma rays). It is known that exposure to small amounts of irradiation, insufficient to destroy these cells, may yet have sufficient effect to change the nature of the genes and so produce certain hereditary defects which may not show for several generations. This 'mutation' as it is called may have a very serious and far-reaching effect. Even repeated x-ray photography of the abdomen may well be dangerous in this respect and x-ray workers are in particular danger if they are careless.

When using irradiation we are handling an unknown power and far more knowledge has yet to be obtained about the biological effects of radioactivity.

Most hospitals have a radiation protection officer who is responsible for regular surveys and for controlling the use of radioactive substances.

Radiographers, nurses and others who come in close contact with patients receiving isotope treatment or other form of radiation exposure have to wear a radiation detector badge: this is a small photographic film in a screened container and indicates the amount of scattered irradiation the radiographer or nurse may have received in a week, for instance.

Whenever isotopes or any other radioactive substance is used strict routine is prescribed by the Radiotherapy or Isotope Department, and the basic principles are given in Appendix I.

SECTION VI

24

The Principles of Abdominal Surgery

All surgical conditions which involve operation on the peritoneal cavity and the abdominal viscera carry with them certain risks and possible complications, irrespective of the exact nature of the particular disease or operation. The nurse needs to be familiar with the general principles of abdominal surgery in order to understand and apply the details of pre-operative and post-operative technique. Without such an understanding she will become confused and even dangerous, in attempting to follow routine measures.

Abdominal disorders and their treatment form a large proportion of general surgery. There are three main reasons for which patients with abdominal disease may require admission to hospital.

(a) **The emergency.** Such a case is known colloquially as an 'acute abdomen'. The patient may be extremely ill, or relatively fit except for severe pain. The diagnosis is often in doubt. The surgeon has to decide whether to operate immediately or to wait. Sometimes he may decide to open the abdomen without having made a precise diagnosis. The nurse plays a vital part in the diagnosis by her observations and in pre- and post-operative treatment.

(b) **The 'waiting-list' case.** Here the patient's symptoms have led to a clear-cut diagnosis made at an out-patient consultation or home examination. Most probably x-ray and other investigations have already been completed and the patient has come in for a planned operation. Many such cases have a straightforward convalescent period and very little nursing attention is required. These patients, having had time to brood over their forth-coming operation, are often filled with anxiety. The nurse by her sympathy and under-standing can do much to allay their fears.

(c) **The case for investigation.** The degree of specialised examination which has been possible before admission depends on the type and quality of the hospital out-patient service. However thorough this investigation may have been, a certain number of patients require further investigation procedures and observations before operation is contem-plated. Patients are sometimes irritated by what seems to them an unnecessary delay before the great day comes for operation to bring what they hope to be complete relief from their troubles.

Principal types of operation

Very broadly, abdominal operations can be grouped into those in which the peritoneal cavity is necessarily opened, and those operations which are performed upon organs which normally lie outside the peritoneal cavity. With certain exceptions, these groups correspond to the alimentary tract in the first place, and the urinary tract in the second place, together with some structures on the posterior abdominal wall, such as the sympathetic nerves.

Intraperitoneal operation

In the first group, disorders of the alimentary tract come to light usually on account of some specific complication. The underlying condition—for instance a growth in the colon—may have been present for months before an acute 'event' occurs to bring the patient for treatment. Such complications are:

(a) Perforation. The stomach, duodenum, small or large bowel may, as the result of ulceration or injury, undergo a perforation of the wall with consequent leakage of its contents into the peritoneal cavity.

(b) Peritonitis. Infection of the peritoneal cavity can occur from perforation of the hollow viscus, by the introduction of infection from outside the body, or from abdominal operation. The risk of its development is always present in abdominal disease.

(c) Obstruction. Either from inflammatory disease or growth, the lumen of the alimentary canal may become obstructed. Adhesions, kinks and twists of the bowel will also produce obstruction to the lumen. Paralysis of the bowel occurring in the course of peritonitis or as the result of injury (page 473) has a similar obstructive effect and is sometimes referred to as **physiological obstruction.**

(d) Haemorrhage. Bleeding occurs from ulceration or injury in the bowel and in the course of certain 'bleeding' diseases. The blood usually pours into the lumen of the bowel and may appear clinically as haematemesis or melaena. If the blood loss has been great and sudden the patient will collapse and be admitted to hospital as an acute abdominal catastrophe. On the other hand, if the blood loss is continued over a long period of time and in lesser amount, a serious degree of anaemia with its own train of symptoms may be the condition which has brought the patient first to hospital.

Haemorrhage may also occur into the peritoneal cavity. It may follow abdominal operation or injury either to the intestinal tract or to any of the solid viscera which project into it, i.e. the liver, the spleen and the kidneys. Following operation or injury extensive bleeding may also occur into the loose tissues *behind* the peritoneum on the posterior abdominal wall: the peritoneum is then stripped off the muscles and a severe degree of shock arises.

Perforation, peritonitis, obstruction and haemorrhage are similarly potential postoperative complications when the alimentary tract has been operated upon.

Diseased sections of the abdominal digestive tract—stomach, small or large intestine—are removed **(resection)** and the ends joined **(anastomosis)** to restore continuity. Sometimes anastomosis is performed between stomach and bowel, or between two loops of bowel, without resection; this is known as 'short circuit' operation.

Extraperitoneal operations

The second group of abdominal operations includes those which are performed on organs which can normally be approached without the peritoneal cavity being opened. The kidneys are operated upon through the loin and a similar approach is made to the lumbar sympathetic ganglia, to the ureter and suprarenal glands. Operations upon the uterus and ovaries are undertaken through the peritoneal cavity. Operations on the bladder are usually performed by pushing the peritoneum upwards to avoid the risk of contamination of the peritoneum, but if a major part of the bladder is to be removed the peritoneal cavity will be opened. The prostate is extraperitoneal.

Inguinal and femoral hernia operations do not involve formal opening of the peritoneal cavity unless there is strangulation, though the hernial sac is itself a protrusion of peritoneum. There are usually no abdominal complications from hernia operations. If the hernia has become obstructed or strangulated (page 486) a piece of bowel may have been involved or even resected. All the hazards of an intestinal disorder and operation are then present (Chapter 27).

Although it is convenient therefore to talk of operations as being intraperitoneal or extraperitoneal and although the peritoneum does not become involved in the latter group, from the nurse's point of view all the risks of intraperitoneal operations are present whenever there is an operation upon any organ or structure adjacent to the peritoneum. The exact nature of any particular operation is of less importance to the nurse than the detection and management of each particular complication which may arise.

Investigative procedures

The diagnosis of abdominal disease is frequently extremely difficult. There are very few conditions in which the clinical picture is so clear cut that no pre-operative investigations are required. Acute appendicitis is perhaps the most common of these conditions in which the diagnosis can be made with a fair degree of certainty. Other emergency conditions such as perforated peptic ulcer and intestinal obstruction are also typical in their presentation, and the surgeon is able to make an immediate diagnosis and proceed with an emergency operation. Frequently, however, in such cases he is only able to carry out an emergency procedure to save life. Investigations have to be performed at a later date and subsequent operations may be needed to deal with the cause of the intestinal obstruction or prevent a recurrence of the perforation of the ulcer.

There are many ways of investigating the condition and behaviour of abdominal organs.

(a) Radiology

X-ray examination of the abdomen in its simplest form is by what is known as the 'straight film'. This is a simple x-ray of the abdominal cavity from which considerable information can be obtained for two reasons.

First, the accumulation of gas in the stomach or intestinal tract is abnormal in cases of intestinal obstruction and the distension of certain loops of bowel which have been obstructed results in the accumulation of fluid within those loops. 'Fluid levels' are seen on the x-ray and their presence, together with the particular pattern of gas distribution, may enable the surgeon to make an accurate diagnosis in cases of intestinal obstruction.

Second, the outlines of solid organs such as the kidney and the spleen and in some cases the outlines of solid tumours may also be seen on the plain x-ray film which reveals their shape and size. Tissues in which there is an abnormal amount of calcium will also show up on the x-ray. Calcified tuberculous glands, calcification in new growths, stones in the gall bladder or the urinary tract, and rarer findings such as calcification in hydatid cysts, and teeth in ovarian dermoid cysts, all add to the diagnostic value of the plain x-ray film.

Alimentary tract. The whole of the intestinal tract can be examined by giving the patient a fluid containing barium compounds. The radiologist watches on the fluorescent x-ray screen the passage of barium through the patient's oesophagus, stomach, duodenum and intestinal tract. At certain times during this examination photographs are taken and further information is obtained from the examination of these x-ray photographs. The barium meal can be followed in its passage through the whole of the intestinal tract, but because of the accumulation of digestive juices and secretions from the bowel wall, the outline of the large bowel is not shown with sufficient accuracy in this examination which is known as the 'barium follow-through'. The rectum and colon are therefore examined more adequately by a 'barium enema' and again the radiologist examines the patient under the x-ray screen while the barium is actually flowing in. Subsequently photographs are taken before and after evacuation of the enema and abnormalities of structure and function of the bowel are thus revealed.

The nurse is concerned in preparation for these examinations by x-ray and the exact requirements vary between different hospitals. Details of the preparation for barium examinations are given on page 267.

The gall bladder. The gall bladder is examined by means of the plain film for the presence of stones or calcification in its walls. The patient is given a special compound by mouth and this is absorbed from the intestinal tract and excreted by the liver. Bile, and therefore the dye, is concentrated by the gall bladder whose outline is thus shown up on the x-ray. If the dye fails to appear in the gall bladder it is an indication that the power of concentration has been lost and that the gall bladder is diseased. On the other hand, there may be gaps in the shadow of the dye showing the presence of stones in the gall bladder. When the gall bladder is outlined the patient is given a fatty meal which causes the gall bladder to empty itself so that its function may also be observed on the x-ray. Sometimes following operations on the gall bladder and biliary passages, dyes opaque to x-rays are injected into the bile duct to show its size and shape. (For preparation, page 267.)

The **urinary tract** is similarly examined by plain 'control' film which may show the presence of stones. A contrast medium (Table 32) is given by I-V injection: this is excreted and outlines the pelvis, ureters and bladder.

(b) Endoscopy

By means of specially designed instruments, we can peer into and examine many parts of the body which cannot be seen with the naked eye.

The simplest method of instrumental examination is that employed for the anal canal and rectum. A 'speculum' (**proctoscope**), which is in fact a simple tube with a handle, is introduced through the anal canal and the surgeon examines the rectal wall through the tube. To facilitate the introduction of the instrument, there is a shaped conical stopper which is known as the 'obturator'. This same principle of a shaped introducer is used on many instruments which have an open tubular end.

Sigmoidoscopy is the examination of the upper regions of the rectum and the sigmoid or pelvic colon with a longer tubular speculum. Because the folds of mucous membrane fall against the end of the instrument and obstruct the view, air inflation is used for the introduction of the **sigmoidoscope** so that the lumen of the bowel is distended. The surgeon inserts the instrument under direct vision, inspecting the wall of the bowel as far as 25 cm from the anus. A larger flexible illuminated **'colonoscope'** is used to examine the whole length of the colon, which must of course be adequately emptied and cleansed before the examination is undertaken (page 83, Veripaque enema).

The **oesophagoscope** is a similar instrument passed down the oesophagus through the mouth, thus enabling the surgeon to inspect the whole length of the gullet. The inside of the stomach and duodenum are examined by the flexible **gastroscope** using air inflation.

Biopsy of the lining epithelium of the duodeneum and upper intestine can be obtained by a special flexible tubular instrument passed through the mouth (page 540, Crosby capsule).

Through a very small incision in the abdominal wall the surgeon may introduce another viewing instrument, the **peritoneoscope (laparoscope)**, and with this he may inspect the inside of the peritoneal cavity and obtain information to enable him to reach a decision without open operation. In order to separate the coils of intestine from one another and allow the satisfactory inspection of the viscera, the peritoneal cavity is inflated with nitrogen or CO_2 gas through a separate cannula. This is of particular use in gynaecology, for examination of the ovaries and tubes (page 752).

Endoscopic instruments, except for the simpler forms of proctoscope, carry their own miniature lamps which draw electric current either from a battery or the mains through a transformer to reduce the voltage or have adapters to connect to a glass fibre light core.

The bladder and urethra are inspected with the **cystoscope** and **urethroscope**. These instruments are described in Chapter 18. The urinary tract is distended with water instead of air for the inspection, but air inflation is sometimes used for the lower part of the urethra.

Various forms of speculum are used for the vagina and these are usually illuminated by direct light, although some forms carry a light source of their own (Chapter 40).

Operations for the removal of tissue for microscopic examination (biopsy) are performed through some of the tubular instruments, and for this purpose there are special long forceps and diathermy electrodes.

Examinations carried out with endoscopic instruments may be made with local or general anaesthesia and, in the case of the rectum and colon, without anaesthesia.

Preparation for endoscopic examination is described in each case under the sections appropriate to the particular types of disorder.

The care and maintenance of endoscopic instruments is described on page 350.

(c) Function tests

By the use of a naso-gastric tube passed to any level in the alimentary tract, secretions can be aspirated and tested chemically and examined microscopically for abnormal cells.

Tests for gastric secretion are described on page 258. These are usually required in cases of suspected peptic ulcer.

Stool examinations, not only for blood but for undigested meat fibres and recognisable food particles, give clues to digestive disorders.

Fat digestion tests require collection of stools over a 3-day period on normal ward diet.

The **carmine dye** test is a simple method of determining the speed of passage through the alimentary tract without the need for x-ray. 0.3 G is given by mouth for a child and 0.5 G for an adult. The dye should be cleared from the stools in 2 days. Prolonged retention means very marked constipation or obstruction.

Abdominal pain

The diagnosis of abdominal disorder, whether as a primary condition or occurring as a complication of some known disease or operation, depends largely upon the patient's description of the pain, its site, its character, its duration, and its intensity. The nurse in her close contact with the patient is best able to form an estimate of the degree of pain which a patient is suffering. Individuals vary greatly in their reaction to pain, and constant observation by the nurse will enable her to indicate to the surgeon features of the pain which the patient may not have described.

The nurse must know the meaning of various types of pain, their importance, and what action she should take. Pain fundamentally is protective and is largely a warning that something has gone wrong. The experienced ward sister is able to detect post-operative complications such as intestinal obstruction or peritonitis at a stage when they can be rectified. No feature of the patient's pain is too small to report. Frequently when one is unable to explain the meaning of a particular pain to the patient, one merely has to give him the rather unsatisfactory excuse that 'it is to be expected after operation and will not last long'. One must not destroy his confidence by showing that the cause of the pain is a mystery, unexpected and worrying! Pain-relieving drugs may only be given in abdominal disorders when the diagnosis is certain. The use of narcotics when we are uncertain of the cause of the pain will mask any changes and symptoms and may lead to disaster.

Abdominal pain may be described under four headings:

The pain of muscular spasm.
The pain of inflammation (peritonitis).
The pain of distension.
Specific visceral pains (localised).

Frequently, of course, a patient is suffering from pain of more than one type, but it is important for us to try and pick out the individual features of his pain and make a note of any subsequent changes. Different drugs are appropriate for different types of pain.

The pain of muscular spasm

Most people at some period of life, usually in childhood, have suffered from intestinal colic, and so the term colic has come to be used in describing all similar forms of pain due to muscle spasm. It is a gripping, griping pain which may cause the patient to double up with his thighs drawn up to his abdominal wall and his spine flexed. Sometimes the pain is so severe that he feels quite unable to move. The suddenness of the pain, its intensity and the fear which it produces results in shock, sometimes of a severe degree. Colic can occur in any muscular tube and we can recognise, usually from the patient's description, which organ is producing the pain. The stomach, the small bowel and the colon, if irritated by inflammation or obstruction, produce this violent colic. Sometimes the patient is able to localise this colic to one particular area but in cases of intestinal obstruction, in which colic is the earliest feature, the pain travels around all over the abdomen as various segments of bowel undergo these violent contractions. Gastric colic usually results in the stomach expelling its contents as vomit. The pelvis of the kidney and the ureter are similarly sent into spasm by the presence of stone or blood clot. Renal colic is described by the patient as being in the loin and travelling round to the front and down into the groin. As the spasm passes down the ureter so the pain passes lower down in the iliac fossa and into the perineum. Gall-bladder and bile duct colic occurs with stones and the patient is able to point to the region of the gall-bladder as the seat of the pain. The appendix, as part of the intestine, produces a violent type of colic frequently confused with other forms.

The pain of colic is usually intermittent—that is, it comes in attacks. While there may be complete freedom of pain in the intervals between attacks there is frequently the sense of dull aching pain sustained from one attack to another. Thus we have to determine not only whether the pain comes and goes, but whether it is varying in intensity although present in some degree all the time.

The pain of inflammation

Most of us are familiar with the dull, aching, boring pain of inflammatory disease, such as the pain of mumps, of an infection of the ear, or of a septic finger. In the abdomen, inflammation, usually due to infection, produces pain largely by spread to the peritoneum which covers the individual organs. The lining of the bowel is insensitive—we are not conscious of the passage of food through our intestine. The muscular wall of the bowel transmits sensations of muscle contraction and thus we are conscious of gross intestinal movement and particularly of spasm. The peritoneal membrane is, however, extremely sensitive, and when the inflammatory process reaches the covering peritoneum, particularly the layer lining the abdominal wall, then the intense pain of peritonitis is experienced. This is constant, unremitting, and is accompanied by a varying degree of shock and by a rise of temperature (page 461). The pain of inflammatory disease is a combination of muscular spasm, peritonitis and discomfort which arises from disordered function such as distension.

The pain of distension

The bowel is particularly sensitive to **stretching** of its muscle wall, just as it is sensitive to **contraction**. The accumulation of abnormal amounts of gas or fluid inside the bowel produces the discomfort of distension; it may be generalised, involving the whole of the abdomen, or confined to one particular loop of intestine which may be obstructed. The pain of distension is sickening, constant, and depressing, it is perhaps the most common cause of post-operative distress in abdominal surgery—the accumulation of gas in the intestines before the bowel function is restored. Again, most of us have experienced the feeling of distension of the stomach when we have eaten some food that causes gastritis; the pylorus has gone into spasm, and the stomach becomes blown up with food and its own secretions. The pain of distension is usually accompanied by nausea, loss of appetite, and frequently by vomiting. Added to this there may be the additional pain of intestinal colic if the cause of distension is mechanical obstruction to the bowel. In cases of paralytic ileus where the discomfort of distension is very great, the addition of colicky pains is a sign for rejoicing, for it is an indication that the bowel movement has begun again. Generalised abdominal distension occurs from bowel obstruction, distension of the upper abdomen when the stomach is over-loaded, and dull aching suprapubic pain arises from distension of the bladder. The peritoneal cavity may be distended with free fluid—ascites —from malignant disease or chonic peritonitis. The pain is very much less severe, sometimes almost negligible, for the intestinal wall is not being stretched.

Ileus, from handling of intestines at operation, occurs to some extent after almost every abdominal operation. Bowel function is resumed spontaneously in most cases and the period of painful distension is short (24–48 hours). One of the great advantages of early mobilisation of the patient following abdominal operation is that, by getting out of bed and walking round the ward, he is far less likely to suffer from distension, so that any apparent 'unkindness' in persuading a patient to rise from his bed so soon after a laparotomy is more than outweighed by the relative freedom from discomfort during the succeeding days.

Specific visceral pains

Whether occurring as one of the foregoing types or as a combination, pain coming from a particular organ is distinguished by

(a) The site of the pain.
(b) Any associated symptoms—such as a feeling that the bowels want to move, or an urgent desire to pass water.
(c) The knowledge that certain actions bring on the pain or relieve it: for instance, the pain of cholecystitis is typically precipitated by the patient taking a fatty meal, or the pain of duodenal ulcer is usually relieved by drinking a glass of milk.
(d) Other clinical findings which may lead to a particular diagnosis, the site and character of the pain being added confirmation: for instance, an 'appendix mass' may be discovered in the right iliac fossa in the patient who is obviously ill and feverish: on close questioning he admits that perhaps a week previously he has had pain typical of appendicitis; this history of typical pain confirms the diagnosis.

Abdominal pain of any sort is very wearing for the patient, and of all the types of pain that of intestinal obstruction and distension is the most tedious and difficult. Large-bowel distension is felt mainly in the flanks, and small-bowel distension produces more central pain.

Referred pain

Colic, inflammation or distension may be responsible for pain 'referred' to some other site. As we so rarely experience sensations of pain from our internal organs the brain frequently makes mistakes when interpreting the origin of pain impulses. Each organ is supplied by nerves which come from the same part of the spinal cord as those nerves going to various areas of skin, in the abdominal wall or elsewhere. The brain misinterprets the visceral pain as coming from the skin. Thus gall-bladder pain, in cholecystitis, is frequently referred to the right shoulder because the phrenic nerve arises in the neck and supplies the peritoneum covering the gall-bladder area! The nerve to the skin over the shoulder arises from the same part of the spinal cord and the brain misinterprets the impulses. In the left side of the upper abdomen, inflammation or injury to the spleen produces referred pain in the left shoulder for a similar reason. When, therefore, a patient complains of abdominal pain in any particular place the surgeon has to consider not only the structures at the site of the pain, but the structures which have the same nerve supply as that area and which may be involved in disease. Localisation of the disease may be helped by the presence of pain outside the abdomen, e.g. in shoulder, back or testis.

Post-operative pain

Persistent violent abdominal pain always indicates trouble. It is not normally present after the first 2 days, and if it is, it means most probably that there is peritonitis or intestinal obstruction. Post-operative pain arises from various causes.

The wound. Following abdominal operation there is of course always pain in the region of the wound and this is made worse by the use of deep tension sutures or skin stitches which have been tied too tightly: the occurrence of post-operative distension further tightens these stitches and adds to the pain. Post-operative abdominal pain discourages the patient from moving his abdominal wall and therefore prevents him from taking deep breaths. Chest complications are then most likely to arise. It is possible to alleviate wound pain by injection of a long-action local anaesthetic agent (bupivacaine), not into the wound but as a field block (page 240). For instance after an inguinal hernia repair a 'block' at the anterior iliac spine will enable the patient to cough without pain. Wound pain is increased by bandages encircling the abdomen, as there is movement of the dressing with each respiration.

In her initial training the nurse will have learnt how to move a patient who has had an abdominal operation in such a way that the patient is not called upon to strain the abdominal muscles. Patients sometimes fear that the wound will come undone and they therefore hold their muscles tight, producing more pain for themselves and more difficulty in breathing. Pre-operative abdominal exercises, especially in relation to breathing, help to produce this post-operative relaxation which is such an asset to recovery.

The sudden recurrence of pain in an abdominal wound after the first 48 hours, indicates either bursting of stitches (probably tearing of the peritoneal layer—page 469), the occurrence of a haematoma, or the onset of infection. Such pain must never be regarded lightly.

Pneumoperitoneum

When the peritoneal cavity is opened, air enters, and if at the operation the liver and upper abdominal viscera have been disturbed, air may have collected under the diaphragm. This **pneumoperitoneum** impedes the action of the diaphragm by interfering with the 'suction' normally produced by the weight of the liver. The presence of air also produces severe pain in the diaphragm area, further interfering with deep breathing. The presence of the air pocket can be demonstrated by x-ray examination and it is sometimes the explanation of troublesome pain and limited movement in the first few days. There is no treatment except to relieve the pain by drugs: the air is absorbed naturally.

Pain of peritonitis

Persistent ileus or persistent severe abdominal pain indicates peritonitis. The pulse rate rises progressively unless the infective process is localised, as for instance in the development of pelvic abscess following the perforation of the appendix. The pain will also be localised to the area of the abscess: subphrenic abscess produces shoulder pain (page 481).

Mechanical obstruction

The onset of severe colic after laparotomy may be due to coincident gallstones, renal calculus (or passage of blood clot in the ureter, page 635), but its occurrence always gives rise to the suspicion of mechanical intestinal obstruction from adhesions, kinks, or internal herniation. The bowel sounds are particularly loud. Distension may not occur early, and if the obstruction is intermittent, the bowel actions may be normal.

Bacillary dysentery or other form of food poisoning may occur in this post-operative phase and give rise to difficulty in diagnosis. The occurrence of other cases of diarrhoea in the ward adds weight to a diagnosis of intestinal infection. Bacteriological examination of the faeces is required.

Bladder pain

Retention of urine may be the cause of severe post-operative pain and this is particularly liable to occur in elderly gentlemen from unsuspected prostatic obstruction or in women after gynaecological operations. Some urine may be passed naturally at regular intervals and the distension (retention with overflow, page 633) is then overlooked. Painful retention may readily be unnoticed if a patient is delirious (for instance after injury).

The relief of abdominal pain

Warning has already been given about the use of narcotics before a diagnosis has been made because when pain is abolished valuable physical signs which the surgeon might otherwise find, will have disappeared.

Generally speaking, the most effective drug for abdominal pain of any sort which is believed to be due to muscular spasm is **pethidine**, given either intramuscularly or by mouth. The effect of this drug is to relieve spasm and consequently the pain passes off spontaneously. It has also a definite pain-killing effect so that it is effective even in the pains of inflammation and distension. The pain of peritonitis is usually only relieved by large doses of morphine or its derivatives. A remarkable feature of peritonitis is the way in which the devastating pain which occurs at the onset is dramatically relieved by laparotomy and drainage of the peritoneal cavity.

Most patients who have a major abdominal operation require at least one post-operative dose of pethidine, morphine or papaveretum, and some surgeons prefer an analgesic given 4- or 6-hourly for 2 days, without waiting for an 'on request' administration. After the first post-operative day, pain is most commonly due to distension which itself arises from a mild degree of ileus. A stethoscope is applied to the abdominal wall, and if bowel sounds can be heard, indicating the presence of bowel activity, the patient is usually given a suppository, or if that fails an enema, to relieve distension of the colon. Post-operative distension of this type is more likely in patients in whom pre-operative preparation has been inadequate or in those who, because of dehydration or starvation, have become constipated. The administration of a glycerine suppository or the simple passage of a rectal tube may be sufficient to cause an evacuation of gas from the lower colon and rectum. If a simple enema is ineffective, enemas containing ox bile, or molasses are used to stimulate the sluggish or overloaded colon. It is far better for the initial post-operative bowel evacuation to be induced by an enema than for the patient to be given drastic aperients. If at operation neither the stomach nor any part of the intestinal tract has been opened, then it is safe for the patient to have 30 ml (1 oz) of **liquid paraffin emulsion**, on the second post-operative evening and each subsequent evening until the bowels move. Cascara and other strong laxatives should be avoided, unless the patient has been in the habit of taking such drugs and his reaction to a certain dose is known. Some patients are particularly sensitive to the use of laxatives and post-operative diarrhoea is as distressing as distension. If there has been a large-bowel anastomosis, enemas are not used or a flatus tube passed for at least a week.

Ileus occurring in the post-operative period (page 387) is treated by gastro-intestinal suction as in peritonitis (page 474).

The amount of pain which a patient has after an abdominal operation depends upon many factors. The skill of the anaesthetist in producing adequate relaxation allows the surgeon to avoid the heavy use of large retractors. Good pre- and post-operative nursing technique prevents or relieves distension and diminishes fear and avoids dehydration. Finally, much depends upon the make-up of the particular patient. Nevertheless, some operations are essentially more pain-producing than others. Pelvic operations seem to produce far less post-operative pain than operations in the upper abdomen. Operations on the kidney are frequently followed by severe pain largely because, in the approach to the kidney, the surgeon cuts across the thick muscles of the abdomen wall and loin. Bladder operations are followed by considerable discomfort mainly because of the presence of tubes and catheters, with associated embarrassment.

Nursing observation in abdominal surgery

In the care of any patient with suspected abdominal disease, there will of course be all the routine examinations and observations on the patient's admission to hospital. If the diagnosis of an acute disorder is in doubt, there may well be a period of observation, for several hours. During this time half-hourly pulse records will be necessary as a rise of pulse rate is frequently the earliest sign of developing peritonitis. If there is doubt as to the presence of distension the nurse must *measure* the circumference of the patient's abdomen at the level of the umbilicus. This is the only way of noting with any degree of certainty the progress of distension before or after operation.

Particularly in relation to the abdominal case, the nursing staff needs to consider the diet, to plan the fluid intake and nutrition, to examine the stools and urine, and to pay particular heed to maintaining the patient's general muscular activity as far as possible.

If conditions make it possible, it is always preferable for a patient to spend at least two days in hospital before any major abdominal operation, even though all the necessary investigations have been carried out in the out-patient department. It is then possible for the nursing staff to assess his personality and habits so that there will be a far greater understanding after operation. It is a mistake for patients to be transferred from one ward to another on the day of operation.

During the period of observation and investigation, the nurse must be very careful not to reveal the results of these various tests, unless she has been instructed to do so. A patient may obtain a very false idea and suffer considerable anxiety if he is given inaccurate or ill-timed information. The less experienced the nurse, the more liable she is to be interrogated by the patient, since it is usually the junior nurse who performs the chores of toilet and bed making, and who therefore has the most personal contact.

Ward records in all cases of abdominal disorder, except uncomplicated hernia cases, must include four-hourly temperature, pulse and respiration charts; urinary output, fluid intake and bowel actions must be charted and if an aperient is given or enema administered the facts must be entered. The method of charting other relevant data varies greatly in different hospitals, but it is usual to record on the temperature chart any important investigation procedures, such as x-ray examination or sigmoidoscopy as this simple record of events is then immediately related to the TPR record which the doctor looks at. He may not inspect every Kardex entry (where of course a record has been made as well). The nurse needs to remember that a house-surgeon or consultant has many patients to care for, and the ready presentation of all the information about each patient makes a tremendous difference to the smooth and efficient working of a busy unit.

Weight records should be made on the day of admission and the day of discharge, *without fail*, and once every week when this is not prevented by the patient being confined to bed. Bedside weighing machines should be available in every ward, the routine weighings should take place at the same time of day on each occasion. If through forgetfulness, the patient is not weighed on admission, there will be no useful post-operative comparison of weight. Drug dosage, too, is frequently calculated in relation to body weight.

Pre-operative preparation

(Also Chapter 18)

Sometimes in the surgery of abdominal disaster, such as the perforation of an ulcer or in severe abdominal injury, there is little time for pre-operative preparation. Nevertheless, in such cases the success of operation may be dependent on adequate pre-operative treatment, and as far as it is humanly possible the nurse must endeavour to follow the routine which has been established in the unit in which she works—for instance, emptying the bladder.

All 'list' surgical cases are prepared for operation on well defined principles though there is wide variation in detail from specialty to specialty: surgeons have individual preferences.

Nutrition. Many patients awaiting operation for abdominal disorder are under-nourished. The sequel to malnutrition—involving anaemia, lack of vitamin C, and lowered resistance—is that the patient's fitness for operation is greatly reduced.

Where there is no contra-indication the pre-operative diet in abdominal disorder needs to provide a high calorie intake, a high protein intake and to be sufficiently mixed to provide adequate minerals. When there has been gastric or intestinal disease it is likely that the patient will not be able to consume sufficient of the ordinary full ward diet to meet his nutritional requirements. The added supplement must include vitamins A, B, C, and D and various fractions of the B vitamin group (Chapter 7). Patients called in from a waiting list should have already received instruction on diet, so as to lessen the length of pre-operative stay.

If malnutrition has been prolonged and oral feeding is possible, a high protein supplement should be added, such as Casilan (page 84); if the blood protein estimation shows a reduction, the surgeon may order the administration of intravenous protein concentrates such as protein hydrolysate, Aminoplex, Aminosol or Trophysan (page 139). In order to utilise (metabolise) these amino-acid solutions from which to build body protein the patient requires *additional* calories, and a suitable combined solution is 'AFE':[1]

$$1 \text{ litre} = 875 \text{ calories} \begin{cases} \text{Aminosol } (3 \cdot 3\%) \text{ 100 calories} \\ \text{Fructose 600 calories (or glucose)} \\ \text{Ethanol (alcohol) 175 calories} \end{cases}$$

(Aminosol 10% alone gives 310 calories per litre.)

The method of presentation of food is extremely important. Patients with abdominal disease are frequently disinterested in food and have formed fads. They have often discovered that certain items of diet upset them, such as onions or pastry, and the nurse must not attempt to show her authority by ignoring the patient's views on the subject of diet.

Generally speaking, patients who are to undergo operation on the alimentary tract receive a diet which will produce a low intestinal residue. Coarse vegetables such as roots and the cabbage family should be omitted. This is partly to rest the intestinal tract and partly to diminish the amount of wind which collects in the bowel after operation.

Hydration—fluid balance. The amount of fluid requirement in the pre-operative phase depends largely upon whether there has been any vomiting or diarrhoea before admission to hospital. Especially in the presence of fever the patient may easily become dehydrated because we tend to pay too little attention to fluid balance until *after* operation. The fluid intake should therefore be increased and records kept for at least three days prior to operation in all but the minor cases. If because of intestinal obstruction or pyloric stenosis the patient is unable to take an adequate amount of fluid by mouth then it must be given rectally or intravenously. In the case of a baby, fluid loss may be gauged by weight. The baby's greatest normal weight is usually known: loss of one pound is equivalent to 450 ml of fluid and most of the weight loss in acute illness in babies is a water loss.

There is again of course the personal factor. Some people's natural fluid intake is very low, and if there is likely to be any need in the post-operative phase for increased fluid intake it is as well for the patient to become accustomed to this increased intake in the pre-operative phase.

Evacuation of the bowel. The days of drastic purgation have gone. It is nevertheless

[1] See page 139 for danger of fructose.

essential that a patient who is undergoing operation in the abdomen, whether the intestinal tract is to be opened or not, should by the time of operation have a bowel that is as near empty as can be managed. Patients who have been dehydrated are also constipated (unless the dehydration has occurred as the result of diarrhoea, which is extremely rare in surgical conditions). Liquid paraffin in any form should not be used in the pre-operative phase for reasons which have already been given, namely, that paraffin will seep through the intestinal suture holes, and may well produce peritonitis. If there is no suspicion of intestinal obstruction, it is usual for the patient to receive a mild aperient eight hours before operation. Care must be taken that a patient who is to undergo an operation in the afternoon, does not have to spend the morning in repeated visits to the toilet; similarly, if his operation is to take place in the morning, a good night's sleep is essential.

If a patient is not used to taking laxatives at any time, then a small dose of Senokot may be given. If this is ineffective, then a simple enema may be given 12 hours before operation.

Before emergency abdominal operations there is no opportunity for this evacuant treatment, but enemas will in all probability have been given in cases of suspected intestinal obstruction for diagnostic purposes. It is therefore best if the patient has had no bowel action in the 24 hours prior to operation to insert one or two glycerine suppositories. If this is still ineffective, a small simple enema should be given.

The particular preparations required for operations upon the bowel are described on page 551. Some surgeons are very strict over the treatment they wish the patient to receive before operations such as haemorrhoidectomy.

If there is the possibility that the intestinal tract will be opened, drugs are given to 'sterilise' the intestinal contents, and in addition an antiseptic retention enema may be ordered containing a drug of the sulphonamide group (page 89). Neomycin is sometimes given by mouth two days preceding operation for a similar purpose.[1] This sterilisation of the intestine which is now possible has greatly reduced the risk of peritonitis: it is probably not complete but diminishes the intestinal bacteria to insignificant numbers.

Skin preparation. In some units, no pre-operative skin preparation is performed except for the removal of abdominal and pubic hair. All cases for operation on the genitalia, perineum or sacral area must have a complete 'through shave'. This particular part of the pre-operative preparation is frequently a source of great embarrassment and discomfort to the patient. The majority of patients are able to carry out the process themselves, but need supervision in order that it may be adequate. In some hospitals the visiting barber deals with the male patients and the nurse with the female patients.

The particular type of antiseptic used on the skin depends on the preference of the surgeon concerned. The most important point, however, is cleanliness rather than antisepsis, and particular attention should be paid to the creases of the groin and the umbilicus; the latter needs cleaning with small pledgets of wool on a pair of forceps and there is absolutely no excuse for the nurse who allows the patient to reach the operating theatre with a dirty umbilicus. **If the patient is quite unable to tolerate cleansing of the umbilicus, then it is the nurse's duty to inform the theatre staff, so that the cleansing may be completed in the anaesthetic room when the patient is unconscious.** An antiseptic detergent solution such as 1 per cent cetrimide with chlorhexidine applied with cotton-wool balls is the best

[1] Neomycin is not used if there is a likelihood of absorption from an ulcerated area (e.g. colitis): it produces deafness.

agent for skin cleansing, followed by an antiseptic. Not only is the dirt removed but also the thin film of sweat, so that the antiseptic used subsequently in ward preparation or in theatre is applied to a fat-free surface and is therefore more effective. Chlorhexidine in spirit is most commonly used as a skin antiseptic.

After the skin has been cleansed and (if required) the antiseptic solution has been applied, the abdomen should be covered with a sterile linen or paper drape held in place by a bandage. **Skin preparation towels should never be anchored to the skin with adhesive strapping.**

A word of warning is necessary about the use of antiseptics on the abdominal wall. While the skin is being painted a piece of sterile wool should be held below the pubis and so used to prevent the antiseptic fluid trickling down between the legs. It may produce great discomfort on the sensitive skin of the perineum or scrotum. It is not necessary to use ether in any form to cleanse the skin except to remove adhesive strapping marks: but if it is being used extreme care must be taken to see that it is not spilled on to the scrotum as it produces intense pain.

Abdominal incisions

There are certain common incisions used in abdominal section (**laparotomy**). Their positions are shown in Figs. 24.1, 24.2 and 24.3, with some of the operations most commonly performed through each. The surgeon's technique in opening the abdomen makes a considerable difference to the patient's post-operative comfort. A speedy rough surgeon produces bruising and much after-pain; a gentle and precise surgeon will be rewarded by the relative absence of post-operative wound pain. Pain in the wound leads to limited abdominal movement and limited breathing which, in turn, may lead to trouble with the lungs.

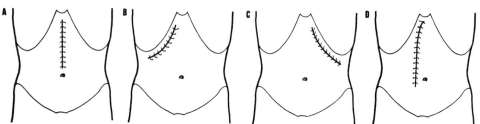

Fig. 24.1 Upper abdominal incisions. **A.** Upper midline—for stomach and duodenum, especially emergency operations, e.g. perforated ulcer, injury to intestine. **B.** Right subcostal—for gall-bladder or bile duct. **C.** Left subcostal—for spleen. **D.** Right paramedian—for stomach, duodenum, biliary apparatus or transverse colon.

Drainage tubes are sometimes introduced and they may be brought out through the main wound or through a special 'stab' incision away from the wound. Sometimes this may become infected. An infected wound haematoma is commonly described as a 'stitch abscess' and its presence may lead to a burst wound.

The abdominal wall is sewn up in layers:

(a) The peritoneal layer or inner layer. This is a fragile sheet of peritoneum but it heals quickly and seals the cavity from infection: it is absolutely vital that this layer should be

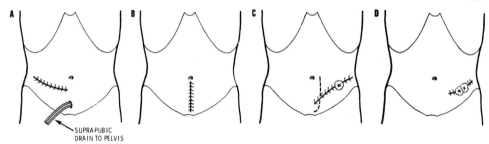

SUPRAPUBIC
DRAIN TO PELVIS

Fig. 24.2 Lower abdominal incisions. **A**. Transverse right iliac—for appendix, or right ureter: if used for appendicitis with peritonitis, a suprapubic 'stab' drain may be used. **B**. Lower midline or suprapubic —for any pelvic operation: bladder, prostate, ovaries, uterus. **C**. Oblique left iliac—for left or pelvic colectomy; a terminal colostomy is shown. It is more usual for the main incision to be paramedian with the colostomy performed through a small separate incision. **D**. Transverse left iliac—for colostomy.

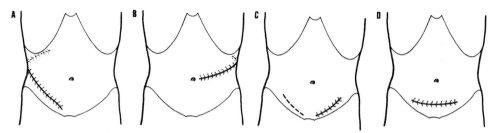

Fig. 24.3 Extraperitoneal abdominal incisions. **A**. Oblique lumbar or lateral—for kidney or right colon; the 12th rib may be removed to give better access to the kidney. **B**. Lumbar transverse—for sympathectomy ureter or colon (right or left). **C**. Inguinal—for hernia (femoral or inguinal) or orchidectomy. **D**. Transverse suprapubic—for pelvic operations (bladder or gynaecological).

completely closed. It is normally sewn together with catgut, and the abdominal wall needs to be really relaxed while this is done.

(b) The muscle layer. The abdominal muscles on either side of the midline are encased in tough fibrous fascia and this is sewn up to provide strength to the repair. Hardened (chromic) catgut is used for this or some material which is not digested by the tissues— silk, linen thread, stainless steel or tantalum wire. This closure may be with interrupted single stitches or with one continuous suture. The muscles or their sheaths may be sewn in one or two layers, depending on the site of the incision.

(c) The subcutaneous fat. Sometimes this layer is closed separately to reduce the risk of blood collecting under the skin. Plain catgut or Dexon[1] is used here.

(d) The skin. Non-absorbable sutures of silk or Nylon are inserted as single stitches. Silkworm gut is also used though it is not as reliable as Nylon. Occasionally the wound may be sewn up with a continuous stitch, or metal clips of the Kifa or Michel pattern are used (Fig. 21.8). Clips are usually removed on the fifth post-operative day as they produce inflammation when they are left longer. Stitches are removed between eight and twelve days. In children and in short incisions in adults a continuous subcuticular stitch of Nylon may be used as this simplifies the removal and enables the dressing to be tied on at the same time (see Fig. 21.10).

[1] A synthetic substance (polyglycollic acid) which causes no tissue reaction.

(e) **Deep tension sutures.** Some surgeons use a few deep silk or nylon stitches going through the whole muscle layer and the skin. Occasionally, as for instance in the repair of the 'burst' abdomen, these take in the peritoneum as well. Deep tension sutures are usually protected to prevent them cutting into the skin, either by tying them over a button or rubber tube or using a layer of gauze over which the complete row of deep tension sutures is tied. These stitches have the disadvantage of producing more abdominal pain by keeping the wound 'tight' and preventing free action of the muscles.

Dressings

Discomfort is produced by movement of the dressing over a wound. The routine use of adhesive dressings has much to commend it. Infection of a wound is uncommon and dressings rarely need to be changed until the stitches are removed. Bandages and cotton wool are unnecessary unless drainage tubes are present. Commonly the wound is sprayed with a sealing varnish and no other dressing applied unless there is a drainage tube. Dressing technique has been discussed already (Chapter 21). The old many-tailed bandage tightly applied to the abdomen is quite unnecessary and is dangerous in that the movement of the abdominal wall and lower ribs may be severely limited, making breathing more difficult and leading to post-operative chest complaints. Rarely is any form of abdominal bandage required, except if an abdominal wound has burst (page 469).

When drainage tubes are inserted it is best to wall off the main incision with some such seal as has been described. A barrier of adhesive strapping is built up to keep away any discharges that may come through the tube, and to simplify re-dressing. The tube itself should be surrounded by unfolded fluffed-up gauze which will absorb far more moisture than a folded pack. A square of cotton wool should be fixed over the tube and gauze with strapping or a lightly applied bandage. Very often a drainage tube has to be connected to a long plastic or rubber tube so that the discharge may be collected in a bedside bottle and measured: the adhesive strapping over the wound must then also fix the tube which goes through the abdominal wall so that it cannot possibly be dragged by the connecting tubing. The two tubes need to be joined by a short Nylon connector, which must be cylindrical and not tapered to a point which will very soon become blocked: the use of such *tapered* glass connections is a common cause of trouble with drainage tubes and injury to nurses' fingers.

The drainage of the peritoneal cavity for peritonitis or the drainage of an abscess is usually maintained by an 'open' tube or strip of rubber covered with dressings. The drainage rubber is held in place with one stitch, a sterile safety pin being placed through the end of the tube or strip to guard against the possibility of it getting drawn into the peritoneal cavity if the stitch should give way. The tube will only be moved at the direction of the surgeon; when draining an abscess cavity, for instance in the pelvis, the tube should never be left in exactly the same place for more than 3 days because it may become stuck to the tissues at the bottom of the cavity. It is usual to cut the anchoring stitch and to shorten the tube by perhaps 2 cm each day, according to the amount of discharge and the improvement in the patient's condition. If the open drainage tube has been placed in position to guard against the collection of blood, it has usually performed its task in 2 days, and then should be completely removed and not shortened. As will be seen later, in operations on the urinary tract, such as on the pelvis of the kidney, an open drainage tube is placed in the kidney bed in case urine should leak. Here again the tube is usually removed by daily shortening.

The management of tubes introduced to drain off the contents of structures such as the bile duct, the bowel, or the bladder, is a completely different matter. In order to keep the patient clean and so that the quantities discharged may be measured these tubes are led into bedside containers. Various types of plastic disposable bags are in use each with a length of plastic tubing attached, and sterile. These bags must never be allowed to fill more than two thirds of capacity as the pressure builds up in the bag and prevents drainage from the tube.

A discharge of pus, and more especially of urine, bile or intestinal contents, very soon leads to ulceration of the skin surrounding the tube. The skin can be protected against discharge in several ways. Before ulceration has occurred, a barrier cream containing 20 per cent **silicone**[1] can be smeared around the opening: this waterproofing cream is applied daily. If the skin is already excoriated, especially if the discharge contains digestive juices, aluminium paste is very effective: its protective action is due partly to its absorptive action with the enzymes. Antiseptic neutralising jellies of various types have been used and Hirst's paste containing powder aluminium is occasionally prescribed. The skin may be protected by spraying with a plastic paint such as Nobecutane, Octaflex or Opsite.

Very often an adhesive disposable bag over the opening and tube is the best way of excluding infection and limiting excoriation of the surrounding skin.

The burst abdomen

In spite of all care and attention in closing the abdominal wall, occasionally a wound breaks down. This usually commences by the peritoneum giving way, but the burst may affect only the skin, or the skin and muscle. Distension of the abdomen after operation and malnutrition with general debility from malignant disease, or chonic infection, are all factors which delay adequate healing and may therefore be responsible for a 'burst abdomen'. The burst may be heralded by the escape of peritoneal fluid or serum; if a wound dressing which has hitherto been dry, suddenly becomes really wet, an impending burst should be suspected. The usual precipitating cause is infection or blood in the wound. This catastrophe may occur at any time after operation but it is usually about the end of the first week. If catgut has been used for the suture of the abdominal wall it may have been faulty and become digested too soon. Sometimes the patient reports that he feels something has given way. The nurse must avoid lifting the dressings up to have a peep, and a fully equipped trolley with sterile dressings and towels should be obtained immediately. In the case of real emergency when the abdominal contents have already escaped, a clean linen hand towel, sheet or pillow case should be immediately placed over the wound and a many-tailed bandage applied.

In the lesser degrees of burst, when simply skin or skin and muscle are involved, an inspection of the wound (with the dressing trolley near at hand) will show an intact deep layer; it may be possible to sew up the superficial layers while the patient is still in bed,

---

[1] Silicone-Vasogen (Lactagol Ltd.) is a suitable water-repellent protective barrier cream. It is available containing also cetrimide as an antiseptic. Siopel (Imperial Chemical Industries) cream spreads rapidly.

with the use of a local anaesthetic (**secondary suture**). The nurse may temporise by using long strips of non-elastic adhesive strapping to pull the sides of the wound together.

In the more severe cases and in any case where the peritoneum has given way even for a small length of the wound, the patient has to be returned to the operating theatre as soon possible, to have the whole abdominal wound repaired. The surgeon may find great difficulty in identifying individual layers and therefore, especially if the patient is very ill, he will use what are called 'through and through' sutures of strong material which bring all layers of the abdominal wall together. The repair of a burst abdomen is a very difficult procedure and unfortunately this occurs most commonly in those patients whose post-operative course has not been smooth and who may have peritonitis.

If the nurse discovers that an abdominal wound has burst she must act promptly, calmly and deliberately in order to fortify the patient whose confidence will have been completely shattered. If medical help is not immediately available she must treat the patient for shock, by lying him flat and covering the exposed viscera as already described with a clean towel or sheet. The waterproof wrapping paper from sterile packs is safe and will not fragment. Its inner surface can be regarded as sterile for this purpose. Pre-medication drugs may be ordered and an intravenous infusion required, with dextran if the patient is shocked. Under no circumstances should single pieces of gauze or wool be applied as they may enter the abdominal cavity and be lost. No attempt should be made to replace loops of bowel which have escaped through the wound. (*N.B.* The inner layers of recently laundered sheets may be virtually sterile, from the ironing process.)

PERITONITIS

The peritoneum is the membrane which lines the abdominal cavity and surrounds the stomach, the intestine, and other organs which protrude into the abdominal cavity.

The prevention, detection and treatment of peritonitis constitutes the central problem of the nursing of abdominal cases. Congenital disorders, infections of the intestine, malignant disease and perforations all take their toll by peritonitis. Acute peritonitis leads to paralysis of the intestinal tract (ileus), to adhesions and mechanical obstruction of the bowels. The grave toxaemia which occurs is accompanied by dehydration from vomiting; heart failure ensues.

Whatever may be the cause of peritonitis, the manifestations and effects are similar. In treatment, the use of antibiotics and sulphonamide drugs has brought a great advance, but in every case the patient depends for his survival on skilled and conscientious nursing.

Causes of acute peritonitis

Irritation and inflammation of the peritoneum can occur without infection, though infection may be added in the later stages. For instance, the mere handling of the intestine at operation produces patches of peritonitis which usually are of no consequence. It is known that minute quantities of prepared starch used for surgical rubber gloves may produce areas of inflammation inside the peritoneum which later give rise to serious

Table 41   Surgical sources of peritonitis

Acute abdominal infections:
  Appendicitis
  Meckel's diverticulum
  Diverticulitis
  Regional ileitis
  Cholecystitis and Empyema of the gall bladder
  Salpingitis (uterine tube)

Perforations:
  Gastric ulcer
  Duodenal ulcer
  Diverticulitis or typhoid ulceration of the colon
  Malignant disease of the bowel
  Foreign body (e.g. swallowed fish-bone) in the bowel

Gangrene of the bowel:
  Strangulated hernia
  Mesenteric thrombosis
  Volvulus

After operations:
  Any operation in which the bowel has been opened and an anastomosis performed,
    by spillage at the time of operation or from leakage at the joint e.g. Gastrectomy,
    Colectomy. Glove powder.
  Any other operation in which the peritoneum may have been contaminated
    from outside.
  In operations on the bladder.
  Removal of uterus (the vagina is opened).

After injury to the abdominal wall:
  'Closed' injury with rupture of internal viscus (e.g. crush injuries).
  Penetrating wound from stab or gunshot.

  to the colon by:
    enemas
    sigmoidoscopy, colonoscopy

  to the vagina or uterus by:
    curettage or uterine biopsy
    criminal abortion

---

trouble from peritonitis.[1] Similarly, cellulose fibres detached from disposable paper surgical drapes and gowns can cause a non-infective peritonitis. Blood escaping into the peritoneal cavity sets up peritonitis.Leakage of bile (after operations on the gall bladder or common bile duct) leads to biliary peritonitis and similarly the leakage of urine from

[1] Starch peritonitis is sufficiently common and serious to require very thorough removal of starch from the outer surface of the gloves of all the members of the surgical team. This cannot be achieved by a quick dip in a bowl of water: careful wiping of each gloved hand with a cotton swab moistened with dilute Savlon is now the recommended procedure.

injury to the bladder, ureter or kidney produces yet another form of chemical peritonitis. The escape of acid juice from the stomach through a perforated gastric ulcer, or of alkaline duodenal contents from a duodenal ulcer, sets up immediate chemical peritonitis which is so severe that collapse occurs as the peritoneum becomes rapidly contaminated.

On the other hand, the peritoneum can be affected by organisms such as the staphylococcus or the pneumococcus, and infective peritonitis complicates such acute infections of the intestinal tract as appendicitis or diverticulitis. Perforation and faecal peritonitis occur in typhoid and other forms of dysentery. Peritonitis may complicate infections of the gall bladder or uterine tube (salpingitis) or the infection may gain entry into the abdominal cavity at the time of operation.

The spread and results of peritonitis

If the source of infection or leakage is small at first, the peritoneum has time to defend itself by local inflammation: fluid is exuded from its surface and sticks the omentum and various viscera together in an attempt to shut off or localise the infection. An inflammatory 'mass' develops (e.g. in some forms of appendicitis). Though this mass is often referred to as an abscess, the term is sometimes incorrect as pus does not necessarily collect and the whole inflammation may subside. Such a condition is referred to as **local** or **focal peritonitis**. If, however, the peritoneum is suddenly showered with a large quantity of infected fluid, escaping from the perforated appendix or other part of the intestine, there

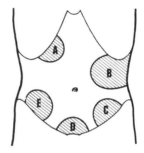

Fig. 24.4   Common sites for abdominal (peritoneal) abscess or inflammatory mass.

is not time for such local 'walling-off' processes to occur, and **diffuse** or **general peritonitis** results. Local peritonitis may become generalised as the infection leaks beyond the wall of defence, and so from the nurses' point of view, similar treatment is pursued for all forms of peritonitis, unless clear orders are given to the contrary.

Old age, malignant disease and obstruction to the intestinal tract are all factors which increase the likelihood and risks of peritonitis following abdominal operations.

The peritoneum has great powers of recovery and repair. Its first action on being irritated is to ooze serous sticky fluid. The amount of fluid may be considerable: this condition of excess free fluid in the peritoneal cavity is known as **ascites** (page 490). The fluid, kept warm by the blood, makes an excellent medium in which germs may thrive so that pus forms very quickly. The surgeon decides at the time of operation on a case of established peritonitis whether the quantity of fluid demands that he should leave a drainage tube in the peritoneal cavity. If a tube has been left in, a large quantity of fluid may pour from the tube during the twenty-four hours following operation. This 'peritoneal exudate' becomes sticky and glues the intestinal loops together thus forming adhesions. The bowel may become mechanically obstructed by these adhesions. As the body overcomes the infection, it tries once again to wall off the pus into certain areas where the intestinal movement is diminished and where the fluid tends to gravitate when the patient is lying in bed. The pus tends to collect in certain pockets between the liver and the diaphragm forming **sub-phrenic abscesses** (page 589) or in the pelvis (**pelvic abscess**, page 481). These abscesses have to be drained by surgical operation or aspirated with a needle. Sometimes a pelvic abscess will burst into the vault of the vagina or into the rectum, and discharge (Fig. 24.8). When the infection subsides and collections of pus have been adequately drained the peritoneum may return to normal so that the coils of intestine slide freely once more over one another. On the other hand, permanent adhesions may result. Peritonitis therefore always leaves a risk of later intestinal obstruction from the development of bands or kinks. It is not only infection which leads to such permanent adhesions. One loop of bowel may become stuck to another loop, or to the anterior abdominal wall where the peritoneum is sewn together at the end of the operation.

Infective ileus

The poison from the infected peritoneal fluid 'paralyses' the intestines. In fact there may be some bowel activity but it is inco-ordinated and therefore ineffective—for practical purposes paralysed—and this term is used widely to indicate the absence of effective peristalsis. The whole of the bowel may be involved (complete ileus) or perhaps only one or two loops which may be in the pelvis surrounded by pus. This latter condition is called **ileus duplex**. The affected segment of bowel acts as an obstruction since it has no peristalsis. In general paralytic ileus, bowel sounds will not be heard when a stethoscope is applied to the abdomen, but in ileus duplex peristalsis may be vigorous from the healthy bowel in its effort to overcome the obstruction produced by the paralysed loop.

Illeus may occur without infection or peritonitis and spontaneous recovery is then likely (pages 480, 872).

The nursing treatment of peritonitis

The nursing technique adopted for post-operative care in major surgical conditions is directed largely to the prevention of peritonitis and its consequences. These measures follow certain established principles.

1. The administration of antibiotics and chemotherapy by intramuscular or intra-venous routes.
2. The effective removal of gastric and intestinal contents by aspiration through a nasal or oral tube to prevent putrefaction and thus to avoid distension of the bowel or stomach.
3. The maintenance of adequate fluid, calorie and mineral intake, with especial attention to chloride and potassium salts and adequate vitamins.

4. The attendance to general hygiene (mouth and pressure points particularly).
5. The restoration of normal gastro-intestinal function, the return of normal bowel habit and the return to normal diet.

After an abdominal operation when there is any reason to suspect development of peritonitis or indeed if the operation has been one in which peritonitis is a particular hazard, nursing methods are largely governed by the rule that nothing must be given by mouth until specific instructions are given by the surgeon. This means that no sedatives, no chemotherapy, no antibiotic capsules, no nourishment—in fact, absolutely nothing—can be given except by injection. A good deal of difficulty can be avoided by forethought in the adequate preparation of the patient before operation. Even if the patient has not been dehydrated before operation, and even if adequate vitamin intake has been possible right up to the time of operation, every single factor needs attention.

The administration of antibiotics and chemotherapy

Antibiotic which is given intramuscularly should be injected into the lateral muscles of the thigh, care being taken to avoid areas upon which the patient wishes to lie. Usually, however, it is administered through the intravenous infusion line which is an essential part of the treatment. After insertion of drugs into an established infusion delivery line the infusion is then run fast for half a minute to wash the antibiotic solution into the blood stream and lessen the risk of thrombosis (page 99). Many drugs given intravenously are incompatible with one another and with infusion fluids: tables showing incompatability are available.

Aspiration of gastric and intestinal contents (gastric suction)

Even though no fluid is being administered by mouth, the stomach and bowel does not remain empty. There is always a certain quantity of saliva, of gastric juice, of duodenal and intestinal secretion together with bile and pancreatic secretion; all this accumulates in the upper small intestine. If there is any degree of obstruction to the large or small intestine, the fluid will become banked up behind the obstruction. Putrefaction takes place and the distension of the bowel becomes great by accumulation of fluid and gas. This distension and decomposition further damages the wall of the bowel, stretches and poisons it, and increases the likelihood of persistent ileus. As the pressure rises in the distended bowel, the contents will flow back into the stomach and eventually vomiting will occur. Vomiting is distressing for the patient; it produces fear and exhaustion as well as pain from the straining of abdominal muscles. The greatest risk, however, is that some of the vomitus may find its way over the epiglottis into the trachea and lungs, setting up an aspiration pneumonia. Many patients died of this condition following major abdominal operations before sufficient attention was paid to the routine aspiration of stomach contents.

The simplest method of protecting the patient against this overflow vomiting and the subsequent risk of aspiration into the lungs, involves the passage of a thin tube through the nose or mouth into the stomach. The weighted end of the tube prevents it from floating on the stomach contents and by means of a syringe the stomach is emptied every hour. The metal insert in the tube also acts as a radio-opaque marker, enabling the position to be checked by x-ray. In a great many cases this is quite adequate to keep the stomach empty, as, for instance, following a partial gastrectomy, when the repeated aspiration also gives an indication of any untoward bleeding. Such a method will not, however, deal satisfactorily with the back-wash that occurs into the stomach in cases of intestinal obstruction when retrograde peristalsis may be quite vigorous. As a more efficient method, therefore, continuous suction is applied to the tube by means of a simple hydraulic bedside apparatus—Wangensteen suction—or by the use of a small bedside electric motor. The three-bottle hydraulic suction apparatus is adequate and requires no special equipment: every nurse must be familiar with the method of setting it up (page 663; Fig. 35.19).

In cases of intestinal paralysis or obstruction, the most effective method is undoubtedly to use a very much longer tube which is guided through the pylorus and is carried onwards down the intestine by any normal peristalsis which may be taking place. The method is of particular use in low intestinal obstruction. These intestinal tubes are fitted with a bulb or balloon near the tip which is distended inside the small bowel and so prevents the rush of fluid past it. Some of the tubes have suction holes in the tip beyond the balloon while others only have aspiration holes in the side of the tube proximal to the balloon. By means of one of these long intestinal tubes the bowel may be blocked so that back-wash is prevented, and the bowel can be kept continuously and completely empty, proximal to the tube.

Various types of tube are in common use, and each pattern has its own particular advantages.

Gastro-intestinal tubes

Ryle's duodenal tube is made in several diameters and varying lengths. The standard lengths are 76, 92 and 107 cm (30, 36 and 42 inches). The tubes are also made in various diameters and an average useful gauge is 15 Charrière (0·5 cm diameter). There are various modifications of the original Ryle's tube. Some of them are opaque to x-rays so that the level to which they are passed may be determined by x-ray screening, but most of those found in hospital wards are not opaque to x-rays.

Einhorn's tube. Various methods of inducing the tip of an aspiration tube to pass through the pylorus, so that the duodenum can be aspirated, include the fitting of bulbous tips and weights. The Einhorn's tube has on the end a little perforated metal bobbin which is directed towards the pylorus by lying the patient on his right side. This particular pattern of tube is useful for obtaining specimens of duodenal secretions (e.g. bile, pancreatic juice).

Maurice Lee tube. This is a PVC double-lumen tube. It consists of a Ryle's tube with a second narrower tube welded to its side and extending 20 cm further. The main tube stays in the stomach with the prolonged end extending into the duodenum. The purpose of this is to enable drip feeding to take place into the small bowel while at the same time keeping the stomach empty through the large tube. Gastric ileus often persists after the duodenum and small bowel have started to work. This tube is of particular value after vagotomy or pyloroplasty.

Miller-Abbott's tube. This type of tube is made in various lengths up to 312 cm. It has an inflatable rubber balloon, near its tip (Fig. 24.5), and two channels, one of which is used for blowing up the balloon and the other, passing through the balloon, for sucking out the intestinal contents. The purpose of the balloon as already mentioned is to prevent back-wash and to give the bowel something to push by normal peristalsis in order that the tube may be carried right down to the level of obstruction.

Cantor's tube (Fig. 24.6). This is for intestinal aspiration but the balloon does not block the bowel. The balloon is weighted with mercury, so that its course may be directed round the duodenum by positioning the patient even if peristalsis is deficient. The mercury is injected with a syringe through the last eye in the tube and the neck of the balloon then tied off firmly with thread. The balloons are replaceable if they get damaged. There are two sets of aspiration holes extending for several inches from the balloon.

The standard length is about 305 cm, 15 Charrière gauge (0·5 cm diameter).

There have been various modifications of these tubes, mainly concerned with placing of the eyes or the shape of the balloon, but the Ryle's tube for gastric suction and the Cantor's tube for intestinal suction are those in most general use.

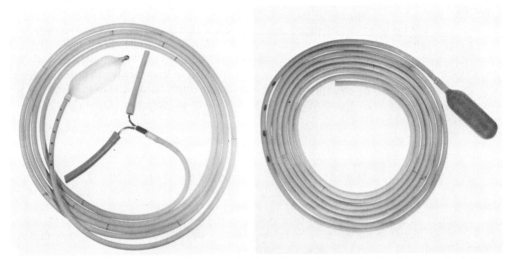

Fig. 24.5   Miller-Abbott tube for intestinal aspiration with openings proximal and distal to the balloon.

Fig. 24.6   Cantor intestinal aspiration tube. The balloon is filled with mercury, and by positioning the patient it may be guided through the pylorus.

Technique of gastric aspiration

This procedure frequently has to be carried out in preparation for abdominal operation, in the course of a fractional test meal, or as a post-operative measure.

To induce the patient to swallow the tube without vomiting calls for great skill and patience and the nurse can only learn how to do this from her practical ward experience. It is necessary to explain to the patient what is to be done. His position is made as comfortable as possible, sitting upright with adequate support from pillows. A large towel is draped round his shoulders, but it is quite unnecessary to scare him by surrounding him with mackintosh sheets. A vomit bowl must be at hand and some swabs. A 'feeder' containing water or saline should also be at hand as a sip of water now and then may facilitate the passage of the tube and will do no harm. The tube is lubricated with an analgesic jelly and introduced over the back of the tongue or through the nose with very great care. The patient is asked to swallow repeatedly, and if he feels he is going to vomit, he should stop swallowing, open his mouth and take deep breaths. The majority of patients tolerate intubation very well provided there is no atmosphere of hustle. Care has to be taken that the tube is not coiling up in the pharynx, which is almost certain to happen if the nurse pushes it too fast.

Standard marking rings on a 92-cm naso-gastric tube are placed at the following approximate positions.[1]

One ring at 38 cm corresponds to cardiac sphincter of stomach
Two rings at 54 cm corresponds to pyloric sphincter
Three rings at 72 cm corresponds to entry of bile duct to duodenum
Four rings at 82 cm corresponds to duodeno-jejunal junction

The tube should be passed so that the nostril or incisor teeth are just short of the second ring, at about 50 cm. If the pharynx is sprayed with 0·5 per cent lignocaine or 1 per cent amethocaine, the passage of the tube will be greatly simplified, but because of the risk of overdose, this spraying should only be done by a medical officer.

If great difficulty is experienced in the passage of the tube, swallowing may be stimulated by the use of small quantities of brandy, given to the patient on a moist swab. Bland substances such as liquid paraffin and lubricant jellies discourage the swallowing reflex rather than stimulate it and the use of something tasty is often of very great assistance. Sometimes of course the tube will have been passed into the stomach by the anaesthetist and will already be fixed in position when the patient returns to the ward from the operating theatre, but usually in operations upon the stomach or intestines the tube has to be passed before the patient goes to the operating theatre.

The end of the tube is taken round the side of the face (Fig. 2.11) and strapped to the temple. A 20-ml syringe is used to aspirate the stomach contents and it will be necessary from time to time to squirt a little air down the tube if it becomes blocked. When all the fluid has been withdrawn, a continuous suction apparatus is connected, with an interposed collection jar. If intermittent suction only is to be used, a small spigot should be placed in the end of the tube, and the aspiration repeated every hour. The amount which has been withdrawn must of course be recorded on the patient's fluid balance chart, its colour and consistency also being noted. If in the immediate post-operative period the naso-gastric tube is ejected, it may be necessary to use an oesophageal tube or plastic semi-rigid tube, as it is difficult to pass the small soft tube while the patient is unconscious.

Technique of gastro-intestinal suction. The purpose here is to pass the tube *beyond* the pylorus into the small intestine.

(a) **With the Miller-Abbott tube.** The tube is smeared with a non-oily jelly and placed over the back of the patient's tongue. If the patient is unconscious (the technique is sometimes used in concussional states or in coma from any cause) the tube may then be pushed on gently into the stomach. If the patient is conscious, swallowing naturally has to be encouraged, and as the tube is somewhat larger than a simple naso-gastric tube, there will be considerable retching. The use of an analgesic spray in the pharynx will help considerably. Approximately 75 cm should be passed initially and the balloon slightly inflated with water, the quantity having been determined experimentally with the balloon beforehand,

If the balloon is inflated with air, it will float on the stomach contents. The tube is then withdrawn until the bulb is felt to come up to the cardiac sphincter of the stomach. It is then pushed in

[1] Varied from different manufacturers: usual length 107 cm.

again for a distance of 25 cm and the balloon deflated. The stomach is then emptied by syringe and the patient left lying on his right side for half an hour.

The material aspirated from the stomach should be tested with pH indicator or litmus paper.[1] If there has not been much regurgitation of intestinal contents, the stomach contents will be strongly acid. The tube is aspirated again each half-hour and if the contents are alkaline or contain bile then it is likely that the balloon has passed through the pylorus. The balloon is again inflated and the remaining length of the tube is then passed slowly down the oesophagus. If possible, an x-ray photograph is taken to show the position of the tube if it is a radio-opaque one. Continuous suction is now applied and may need to continue for several days.

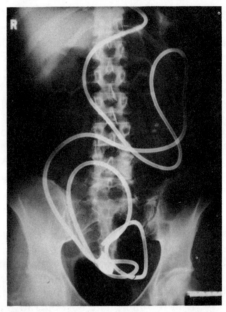

Fig. 24.7   Cantor tube in position. The tube took 24 hours to reach this position and completely relieved the patient's obstruction which was due to kinking of the small bowel by adhesions.

(b) **With the Cantor's tube.** The procedure should be similar but as the end of the tube is weighted with mercury, the positioning of the patient is even more important. It cannot be deflated of course while in position. Its weight causes the pylorus to relax if positioning is correct. When it has reached the duodenum, the patient is made to sit up for about 20 minutes; he is then placed on his left side, slightly over on his face, to direct the heavy tube across the transverse portion of the duodenum: after a further 20 minutes he is propped up again in the hope that the balloon has passed the duodeno-jejunal flexure. The position is checked radiologically, and the tube should continue to travel down the small intestine even if peristalsis is absent or feeble (Fig. 24.7 and Fig. 26.1 for anatomy).

Any patient who has an indwelling gastric or gastro-intestinal suction tube, is liable to develop ulceration of the pharynx or the oesophagus, particularly if he is dehydrated. It is therefore wise, unless instructions have been given to the contrary, for the patient to be allowed at least half an ounce of water (15 ml) every hour, this amount also of course being recorded on the fluid balance

[1] Indicator test paper: page 640.

chart. Provided fluid is not given in quantities larger than two ounces at a time, it is very unlikely to stimulate peristalsis and the patient will derive great benefit from being allowed to moisten his mouth and throat. In assessing the significance of the amount withdrawn, allowance must be made for swallowed saliva: it may be as much as 500 ml in 24 hours in the post-operative period.

In cases of peritonitis and intestinal obstruction, vast quantities of fluid may be removed from the stomach and intestines; this fluid and salt loss has to be made good by the administration of water glucose, sodium, potassium and chloride salts subcutaneously or intravenously (pages 133–137).

The course of acute peritonitis

When infective peritonitis has followed the perforation of an acutely inflamed appendix, the recovery is very often extremely rapid. Post-operative progress depends mainly on whether the infection had become really established in the peritoneal cavity before operation. Because the outcome of drainage is never certain, every case has to be treated without compromise; that is, we must expect the worst and go very slowly with return to normal feeding.

In assessing the patient's progress we depend upon certain observations. First, we expect the temperature to be elevated, perhaps to 38 °C or 39 °C for several days after operation, but it should have reached the normal base level by the end of the first week. The pulse rate will be correspondingly raised, but if it starts to climb, either the infection is not being adequately controlled or the patient is receiving too much intravenous fluid. Post-operative distension will produce distress and a rise of pulse rate. Hiccough is sometimes a distressing feature of peritonitis and is frequently a bad sign.

It is usual to allow nothing except sips of water for 48 hours following operation, if gastric aspiration has been instituted. At the end of that time if peristalsis can be heard when a stethoscope is applied to the abdominal wall, and providing that the quantities being aspirated through the naso-gastric tube are less than the small quantities being taken by mouth, it can be assumed that intestinal activity has been restored. The surgeon may then give instructions for the aspirating tube to be removed and for oral feeding to commence: alternatively feeding may be increased and the tube retained for twenty-four hours so that intermittent aspiration will reveal if there is still any ileus or 'hold-up'. The nurse must be extremely vigilant if the patient complains of a return of the feeling of distension or nausea, or if abdominal distension is apparent. If vomiting recurs the tube must be at once inserted again and the stomach emptied.

In a severe case of peritonitis it may be necessary to continue gastric aspiration for several days and it is not possible to lay down any strict routine method of nursing. Each case has to be judged on its merits and if there is any doubt about the restoration of bowel function, continuous aspiration is stopped and intermittent suction resumed (gradually increasing the intervals between aspirations from one to 4 hours).

If the gastro-intestinal suction is working satisfactorily, the patient will not become distended except by the accumulation of gas in the large bowel. This is relieved by an enema or the passage of a flatus tube.

As has already been mentioned, mechanical obstruction due to adhesions can occur during the recovery stage after acute infective peritonitis. Return of distension, recurrence of vomiting, sudden rise in the patient's pulse or temperature must be taken as an indication to stop all food and fluid by mouth, and it will probably be necessary to return to suction.

It is only by such prompt measures that episodes of obstruction of a minor nature can be limited and prevented from becoming serious. Severe colic may be the first symptom (page 461).

Morphine in peritonitis. It is important that patients who have peritonitis should be rested both physically and mentally, and there is no doubt that morphine and its derivatives achieve this very satisfactorily. Morphine was sometimes given and repeated at 4-hourly intervals whether the patient appeared to be in need of sedative or not, as it was thought that the regular use of the drug prevented intestinal movement and therefore rested the bowel. It is probably more correct to say that morphine relaxes spasm of the bowel but does not stop peristalsis. Its repeated use may have other untoward side effects such as depression of respiration, and actually encourage unwanted peristalsis in the early stage after anastomosis. It is therefore now considered better to use pethidine for the relief of pain and to depend upon gastro-intestinal suction for resting the intestinal tract. Pethidine is not as good a 'sedative' as morphine and many surgeons reinforce its effect with intramuscular phenobarbitone.

Gastro-intestinal recovery and ileus

The peritoneum has a remarkable power of recovery. Though the bowels have been bathed in pus and poisoned to the point of paralysis (page 473), yet within a few days normal peristalsis may be resumed, and the infected exudate in the peritoneal cavity may be completely absorbed. There still remains the risk of mechanical obstruction from adhesions and, if localised pockets of pus have formed in the pelvis or elsewhere, recovery will be delayed. In acute peritonitis, progress is assessed by listening for peristalsis with the stethoscope applied to various areas of the abdominal wall. After a major abdominal operation, even though there is no infection in the peritoneal cavity, we do not expect to hear vigorous peristalsis for the first 24 hours. Just as the disappearance of bowel sounds indicates the onset of infection, so the reappearance of bowel sounds is an indication to increase oral feeding and discontinue intestinal and gastric suction. The passage of flatus may occur spontaneously without the use of suppositories or rectal tubes. If distension is occurring in the presence of adequate bowel sounds, an enema is given. There may be considerable difficulty in producing a successful first evacuation, especially if there was no opportunity for preparing the patient adequately before operation. Such difficulties may be encountered if, for instance, the patient has been admitted with a perforated peptic ulcer and has subsequently developed peritonitis. Neostigmine (2·5 mg) may be given intramuscularly 20 minutes before the enema. It used to be common practice in cases of 'paralytic' ileus and peritonitis to give neostigmine repeatedly in order to restore peristalsis. This was 'whipping a tired horse'; it is unwise to give neostigmine until bowel sounds are audible and it will not be prescribed for at least a week after an anastomosis. The drug acts by augmenting movements which are present but feeble. It is of value in patients who have been by habit constipated and who tend to accumulate large quantities of gas in their bowel during this recovery stage.

If ileus continues, with increasing distress and distension, it has been found that the use of guanethidine[1] (which blocks sympathetic nerve action) in a slow IV drip (20 mg in

[1] Guanethidine is a 'beta' blocking agent. Bethanechol, another parasympathetic acting drug, may be used instead of neostigmine (page 697).

40 minutes), followed by neostigmine as soon as bowel sounds are audible, may be dramatically effective.

When the crisis has passed and at the stage when normal feeding has been resumed, abdominal exercises should be instituted. The patient should be discouraged from taking laxatives when he is discharged from hospital. Patients who have had acute peritonitis lose an excessive amount of weight and usually require prolonged convalescence.

Subphrenic and pelvic abscess

Reference has already been made (Fig. 24.4) to the localised collections of pus which may occur during the course of acute infective peritonitis.

The presence of such an abscess is to be suspected if the fever which accompanied the original peritonitis, having subsided, now returns, although the general abdominal condition seems to be satisfactory. 'Satisfactory' in this connection indicates that the general abdominal distension has subsided, that peristalsis has been restored and the patient is able to take at least fluids, by mouth. Bowel action will have returned. Before the introduction of powerful antibiotics, the return of the swinging temperature invariably accompanied the development of localised collections of pus within the abdomen. Now such abscess formation may be completely masked at first. There may be no fever and in such cases we are led to suspect the presence of an abscess by the delayed recovery of the patient's general condition, by pallor and malaise. Weekly blood counts should be routine in the management of cases of peritonitis: increasing anaemia, together with a rise in the white blood cell count, will point to the development of a localised collection of pus. Subphrenic abscess produces very little in the way of physical signs or symptoms. On the other hand, a pelvic abscess causes a patient to have some difficulty with micturition and to develop mucous diarrhoea with a feeling of fullness in the rectum. The development of a pelvic abscess may therefore be detected by careful nursing observation and its presence is confirmed by rectal examination performed by the surgeon.

Subphrenic abscess now rarely requires open operation with drainage but occasionally this is necessary. The abscess can usually be evacuated by aspiration.

The inflammatory mass which develops in the pelvis in some cases of general peritonitis consists mostly of coils matted with inflammatory exudate rather than there being a true abscess. In this stage of peritonitis the condition can often be resolved by the use of hot rectal irrigations. At least 3 litres should be used on each occasion twice a day, the hot water or saline being run in and out approximately half a litre at a time. Tepid water is useless and it should be initially at least 50 °C in the irrigator reservoir: the stream of water as it leaves the catheter should be tested on the back of the hand. Even if a true abscess is present, this treatment will aid its resolution and, in the majority of cases, such pelvic abscesses discharge themselves spontaneously into the rectum, and heal rapidly.

If spontaneous discharge does not occur it is drained either by a suprapubic incision made under general anaesthesia or by means of a stab incision through the anterior wall of the rectum into the abscess. This latter manœuvre is performed by using an ordinary scalpel inserted under direct vision through an anal speculum. In a female patient, the abscess may be drained through the vault of the vagina. In many cases the abscess may be simply punctured by a sinus forceps introduced through the anal canal alongside the examining finger. Figure 24.8 shows a barium enema examination of the rectum after the discharge of a pelvic abscess resulting from appendicitis. The barium has flowed into the abscess cavity which subsequently healed without any further trouble. If a pelvic abscess has been suspected, every stool which the patient passes must be examined by the nurse for the presence of blood or pus.

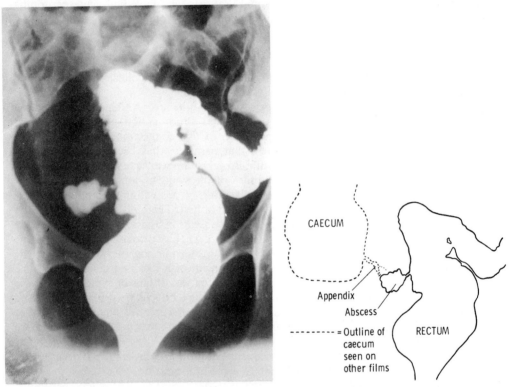

CAECUM

Appendix

Abscess

- - - - - - - - = Outline of   RECTUM
caecum
seen on
other films

Fig. 24.8 An appendix abscess has formed. No operation was undertaken and the abscess discharged spontaneously into the rectum. Barium enema examination a few days later showed the connection with the abscess cavity which was in close contact with the appendix. Fortunately a fistula between the appendix and the rectum did not develop and the appendix was removed at subsequent operation.

Phlebitis and thrombosis of the portal vein

Infection within the abdominal cavity may lead to thrombosis of veins in the mesentery. These are tributaries of the portal vein and, should they become infected, septic emboli may be carried to the liver where the portal vein terminates. This condition is known as **portal pylephlebitis**. It is an occasional complication of acute appendicitis. It is treated by antibiotics, but it now rarely arises owing to the widespread use of antibacterial measures in the treatment of all abdominal infections. The condition may of course already be established by the time the patient comes for treatment of the underlying disorder, such as appendicitis. Rigors and collapse suggest the occurrence of this condition and of septicaemia (page 56).

Mesenteric vein thrombosis may arise from other causes and gives rise to an acute abdominal emergency. Removal of the affected segment of bowel is usually necessary but sometimes the length involved makes resection impracticable.

Thrombosis of the portal vein or its splenic tributary may occur apart from any acute abdominal emergency, and the resulting venous back-pressure in the portal system is **'portal hypertension'**. The spleen enlarges and ascites develops. The surgical treatment of this condition is described on pages 591, 595.

INTESTINAL OBSTRUCTION

The normal flow of food through the gastro-intestinal tract may be disturbed in a variety of ways. The simplest form of obstruction is by something which is passing along in the lumen but is too big to pass through certain narrow sections of the canal such as the pylorus or the ileo-caecal valve. Occasionally the oesophagus or the pylorus or small bowel becomes blocked by a swallowed foreign body, and the large bowel becomes obstructed by a large dry mass of faeces. Whatever may be the cause of intestinal obstruction, the effects are similar though they vary greatly in degree.

If the onset of obstruction is sudden, the symptoms and resulting clinical condition will be dramatic—a condition which we describe as **acute intestinal obstruction**. As a result of gradual increasing obstruction, such as occurs when cancer is growing in the wall of the bowel, the onset of symptoms will be very much more insidious, and the prolonged interference with normal intestinal function results in great loss of weight and malnutrition. This latter condition we refer to as **chronic intestinal obstruction**. Chronic obstruction is of course incomplete—that is the bowel has been working against increasing blockage but its contents have been passing the site of obstruction, though the flow has been small and perhaps intermittent. As the result of further pathological change in chronic intestinal obstruction, the block may become complete so that the clinical condition now becomes acute. Many patients who come into hospital as cases of acute intestinal obstruction are found on interrogation to have been suffering from increasing constipation and perhaps distension for a considerable time before the acute crisis has developed.

Acute intestinal obstruction is always a surgical emergency and the primary purpose of treatment is to save life. Sometimes in relieving the obstruction the patient is at the same time cured of the disease which has caused the block. On the other hand, occasionally an emergency opening has to be made into the bowel to allow free drainage of its contents and the primary cause of obstruction is dealt with at a later date (page 489).

A patient with chronic intestinal obstruction is not submitted to immediate operation. Sigmoidoscopy, x-ray examination by barium meal and barium enema is used whenever possible in order that the surgeon may determine the exact site and nature of the disease which is producing the obstruction. The removal of the cause of obstruction is often a very serious operation and a considerable amount of nursing preparation takes place, in order that the patient's resistance may be built up and the risks of operation diminished.

Causes of intestinal obstruction

Congenital. During the development of the bowel in the embryo, the formation of the tube may be incomplete. The baby is born with a gap in the continuity of the bowel; there may be several such gaps, so that the intestine consists of a series of closed segments.

This obstruction is complete. There may, on the other hand, be a mere narrowing of the bowel at some point, which will lead to chronic obstruction. Symptoms develop immediately or very soon after birth; operation is urgent and the outcome is frequently fatal.

Inflammatory. Inflammation due to infection, anywhere within the peritoneal cavity, may subsequently involve the wall of a section of intestine. The thickening and swelling which result cause blockage. Regional ileitis and diverticulitis are two such conditions.

Traumatic. Injury is rarely a cause of intestinal obstruction except indirectly as a result of stricture formation at the site of previous operation on the bowel. Gun-shot wounds of the abdomen frequently involve coils of the intestine and the repair of the holes in the wall of the bowel may lead to obstruction.

Neoplastic. Malignant growths are by far the most important causes of intestinal obstruction. Growth may start in the wall of the bowel and protrude into its lumen or it may produce obstruction by causing a ring constriction of the bowel. The growth may start in another organ and spread to the wall of the bowel which becomes stuck to it and later obstructed. The large bowel is a common site for growths and cancer of the large bowel is usually diagnosed on account of symptoms of obstruction.

Other causes. As the result of inflammation of the peritoneum, adhesions form. Loops of intestine may become stuck to one another. These adhesions form bands across parts of the peritoneal cavity, and with their constant wriggling movements the intestines may become twisted around these bands and thus obstructed. When a coil of small or large bowel becomes twisted on its mesentery, the condition of **volvulus** (Fig. 24.9) is present. A loop of bowel may slip into a hernial sac where it becomes obstructed or strangulated (page 723). Another form of mechanical obstruction occurs in intussusception (page 423), where the bowel gets folded into itself rather as a stocking may be turned inside out. In adults, this condition usually arises from a growth in the wall of the bowel: the lump is carried on by the peristalsis and drags the bowel wall along with it.

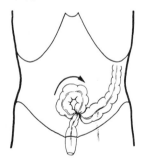

Fig. 24.9   Volvulus of pelvic (sigmoid) loop causing intestinal obstruction.

Paralytic obstruction

In all the conditions so far described as causes of intestinal obstruction, the bowel is still active and capable of muscular activity which becomes greatly increased in the phase of obstruction. If, however, the wall of the bowel, from fatigue and from poisoning, becomes paralysed, the condition of paralytic ileus exists, as it does in cases of peritonitis. This paralysis of the bowel is a form of intestinal obstruction. The features of paralytic ileus have already been described (pages 473 et seq.). The management is by parenteral feeding, gastro-intestinal suction and other measures as for peritonitis and other forms of obstruction (page 474).

Acute intestinal obstruction

Colic, sometimes very severe and persistent, is usually the first symptom of acute intestinal obstruction. The bowel in its violent efforts to overcome the obstruction produces greatly increased movements, sometimes in the reverse direction. Vomiting is a constant feature, especially if the obstruction is in the small intestine. The abdomen becomes distended from the accumulation of gas in the obstructed loops. If the obstruction is very high in the small bowel towards the duodenum or actually at the pylorus, then of course there will be very little distension. Constipation occurs, although the patient may have one or two bowel actions after the onset of obstruction. If the condition is not treated urgently, vomiting leads to severe loss of fluid and chloride, the patient becomes rapidly ill from dehydration and absorption of toxins from the dilated intestines. Unfortunately acute intestinal obstruction sometimes follows abdominal operations when it is least expected. This is usually the result of adhesions which have developed in the days following operation or from a kink. The nurse who is caring for abdominal cases needs to be on constant watch for the development of acute intestinal obstruction. If the condition is not relieved immediately, a patient who is already ill from a previous operation will rapidly reach a stage from which he will not recover.

Nursing management of acute intestinal obstruction

Much will depend on whether the condition is one of primary acute obstruction or whether the condition is superimposed upon chronic obstruction. In either case the patient will be dehydrated and the replacement of fluid and chloride is of prime importance. When the patient is admitted the surgeon will almost always require that an enema be given, followed by a second enema an hour later to determine whether any intestinal contents are in fact reaching the large bowel. This 'two enema test' is not entirely reliable and only really serves to confirm the presence of acute obstruction when the site of obstruction is in the large bowel. An x-ray film of the abdomen is usually obtained with the patient sitting up, and fluid levels may be seen in loops of distended intestine. Preparation for operation consists of the immediate introduction of a gastric tube so that the stomach contents may be aspirated completely and the aspiration repeated at half-hourly intervals. If acute obstruction has developed in the course of recovery from another operation, further operation may sometimes be averted by constant gastro-intestinal suction. The deflation of the distended intestine allows the coils which have got twisted to undo themselves. The surgeon will indicate whether he wishes gastric suction or intestinal suction instituted and this process must be carried out exactly as for cases of peritonitis (page 474).

Even if the patient is not severely dehydrated, intravenous infusion is essential to maintain an adequate fluid and electrolyte balance after operation, before oral feeding is resumed. Potassium salts will be added to the infusion to lessen the risk of ileus (page 137). The nurse must assume that every case of intestinal obstruction will be treated as a matter of urgency by gastric or gastro-intestinal suction and by intravenous infusion. If it seems that the acute obstruction has followed chronic obstruction of considerable duration and the patient is undernourished, blood transfusion may be required as a pre-operative measure followed by infusion of amino-acid solutions (page 139). Intravenous or intramuscular antibiotics may also be started at once to diminish the risk of subsequent peritonitis.

Surgical treatment of acute intestinal obstruction

The cause of the acute obstruction will be obvious in such conditions as strangulated hernia or growth at the upper end of the rectum where it can be felt by digital examination. The surgeon will be able to decide beforehand what operative procedure will then be necessary. In the majority of cases of intestinal obstruction, however, the nature of the underlying disease is only determined at laparotomy. If the obstruction is a simple mechanical one, by volvulus, by bands, by intussusception (page 423) or by hernial strangulation, the surgeon will be able to deal with the primary cause at once; the relief of obstruction is straightforward; the abdomen is closed without any further measures being necessary. On the other hand, the condition which has caused the obstruction may also have interfered with the blood supply of the bowel and gangrene may be present: a section of bowel will then have to be removed and an anastomosis performed immediately. Occasionally, even in the presence of growth as the cause of obstruction, a surgeon may be able to remove the growth at the initial operation. The patient's treatment from the operative point of view is thus completed with one procedure.

The patient's condition at the time of operation, especially if the acute obstruction has followed a chronic obstruction, may however be so poor that any major surgical procedure such as removal of bowel is out of the question. A 'safety valve' has then to be made above the level of intestinal obstruction to allow the escape of intestinal contents. Transverse colon colostomy (artificial anus in abdominal wall) may be performed with safety as a life-saving measure in a case of carcinoma of the sigmoid (pelvic) colon which has produced acute obstruction; any attempt to remove the primary growth at the initial operation will involve too great a risk. In some cases, where the surgeon has been compelled by necessity to remove bowel and perform an anastomosis, an additional safety valve drainage may be provided to prevent any stretching of the anastomosis until it has healed.

Ileostomy, caecostomy, transverse colostomy or left iliac colostomy may be performed for acute intestinal obstruction as a temporary measure.

Two abdominal incisions may be made in the initial operation. The first, usually a midline or paramedian incision, enables the surgeon to examine the whole of the abdominal cavity and determine the nature and extent of the disease. If a safety-valve operation such as colostomy is necessary, the lumen of the bowel is brought to the surface through a separate incision so that the bowel may be opened and allowed to drain immediately. The second incision is a small one and by keeping it away from the large midline or paramedian wound there is far less risk of infection of the abdominal wall. An additional reason for a separate incision is that the surgeon may need to open the abdomen at a subsequent operation and he will therefore wish to keep the colostomy or ileostomy as far as possible from the site of his later operation.

Post-operative treatment of acute intestinal obstruction

On general lines this is the same as the nursing management of general peritonitis (pages 473–480). Continuous or intermittent gastro-intestinal suction, intravenous infusion, a complete record of fluid balance and the treatment of distension are the essentials. In addition, there may be the care of a colostomy or other form of drainage.

There must be a daily measurement of the abdomen to assess distension and the stethoscope will be used repeatedly to listen for the return of peristalsis. Bowel evacuation will be delayed for several days as the whole intestinal tract will probably have been emptied by vomiting and aspiration.

The surgeon will decide when aspiration will be discontinued and oral feeding resumed. While some cases are absolutely straight-forward after the relief of obstruction, others have an 'up and down' course with crises in which the surgeon may suspect that obstruction has recurred.

Acute intestinal obstruction produces both a physical and a mental crisis in the patient; the whole scene is frequently one of anxiety and drama. The nurse needs to be calm, efficient and tactful in her handling of the patient who has been precipitated into a grave illness and perhaps finds after the operation that his bowel is now discharging through the abdominal wall. Sympathy and gentleness are absolutely vital in dealing with such patients and the hearty disciplinarian nurse is not welcome. The pain and discomfort of distension, the worry of the gastro-intestinal suction, and lack of sleep add to the patient's difficulties. Except in the more straightforward cases of obstruction due to bands, volvulus or strangulated hernia, anxiety continues for several days or even weeks and convalescence is frequently prolonged. Especially is this true if peritonitis accompanies the initial obstruction.

Chronic intestinal obstruction

Obstruction of the gastro-intestinal canal may occur as an acute episode appearing 'out of the blue' without any previous obstruction. It may, however, occur as an episode in a disease which has produced gradual progressive obstruction over many weeks or months. There may, on the other hand, be no acute obstruction and the patient then seeks medical advice because of increasing indigestion, discomfort and perhaps distension. The management of chronic intestinal obstruction differs from that of acute obstruction in several respects.

As the result of long-standing interference with normal peristalsis, the bowel becomes greatly thickened from hypertrophy in its effort to overcome the block. Consequently huge loops of thick and inflamed bowel develop. In this stagnant intestine, abnormal bacterial fermentation occurs which produces indigestion, toxaemia and anaemia. The feeling of discomfort leads to anorexia and the patient, both from distaste and fear of pain, reduces his diet to such an extent that wasting occurs.

In long-standing obstruction, the abnormal fermentation results in ulceration and inflammation of the wall of the bowel. Liquefaction of the constipated faeces, in the case of the colon, supervenes and an 'attack of diarrhoea' follows. Some of the diseases which produce chronic intestinal obstruction, such as diverticulitis or carcinoma of the large bowel, also produce blood and mucus which trickle into the bowel beyond the obstruction. The patient then complains of diarrhoea but at the same time of distension and inability to pass normal stools. The passage of blood and slime under these conditions is termed **'spurious diarrhoea'**.

When a case of chronic intestinal obstruction is admitted to hospital, there will in all probability be a preliminary period of observation and investigation. During this time particular care must be taken to watch the stools for the appearance of blood, mucus or alteration in colour. On no account must laxatives or enemas be given unless they are specifically prescribed by the medical officer.

Most of these patients are suffering from malnutrition and a high calorie diet with low residue is required, to which there is an added vitamin supplement. Owing to loss of appetite, difficulty may be experienced in tempting the patients to eat sufficient for their nutritional requirements. Sympathy and skill in the preparation and presentation of food is then of great importance. A record should be kept of the amount of food consumed, as operative treatment may have to be delayed until there is an improvement in the patient's general condition. The removal of the cause of obstruction (it may be a carcinoma of the colon) will probably involve an operation of considerable magnitude, and a few days spent in pre-operative preparation may reduce the risk of complications considerably.

Between frank acute obstruction and chronic obstruction there are intermediate degrees. The patient may for instance be suffering from bouts of intestinal colic and vomiting which may be sufficient to interfere with nutrition; in the intervals between attacks, normal bowel action may be taking place.

As in cases of acute obstruction, operation will be performed sometimes before a clear-cut cause of the chronic obstruction is revealed. The extent of the operative procedure will therefore not be known beforehand. Because of this uncertainty of the nature of the condition and the required treatment, the pre-operative preparation must be as complete as possible. This may be summarised:

(a) High calorie, low residue diet: vitamin supplement.
(b) Evacuation of the bowel distal to obstruction by enemas or high colonic wash-outs.
(c) Decompression of the bowel proximal to the site of obstruction by
   (i) gastric or intestinal aspiration tube (Cantor or Miller-Abbott, page 476; Fig. 24.5; 24.6)
   (ii) preliminary decompressive operation such as caecostomy before resection of the large bowel for malignant disease in the left half of the colon. Such preliminary operation enables normal gastro-intestinal function to be restored, before the major operation for resection of the growth is undertaken.
(d) Sterilisation of the intestinal tract by oral sulpha drugs or antibiotics.
(e) Parenteral administration of fluid to combat dehydration: transfusion of blood is usually required if the haemoglobin is under 60 per cent.
(f) During the preliminary period of observation, an assessment of renal function is made and particular attention is paid to any difficulty of micturition which may be present (for instance, due to prostatic obstruction) and may lead to post-operative retention.
(g) As chronic intestinal obstruction is frequently due to malignant disease, x-ray examination of the chest before operation is essential in case pulmonary metastasis is present. If the disease is found to have spread to the liver, to the lungs, or elsewhere inside the abdomen, this knowledge may lead the surgeon to undertake an operation merely for the relief of obstruction without the removal of its cause, in the full knowledge that whatever he does will only be palliative and not curative.

The objective of operation

The purpose of operation in chronic intestinal obstruction will be to restore gastro-intestinal function as soon as possible with the minimum risk to the patient. This will be achieved in one of four ways.

1. By the establishment of a safety valve, as already mentioned—for instance, caecostomy in large-bowel obstruction, ileostomy in small-bowel obstruction, though this is uncommon. Such relieving operations are usually only undertaken for acute intestinal obstruction which has supervened on a chronic condition, but if the patient's nutrition and general condition are poor, a period of several weeks with temporary external drainage of the intestine may be necessary. The colon, usually in its pelvic loop, develops pockets in its walls. These diverticula become inflamed and the surrounding tissues mat together to form a large hard mass. The surgical removal of this tumour may be impossible because of the risk of peritonitis: peritonitis may in fact already be present. In such a case a temporary transverse colostomy diverts the stream of faeces from the inflamed area. The inflammation around the colon subsides and the infected piece of bowel may be resected with safety at a later date. An end-to-end anastomosis is then performed so that the colostomy can be closed by a third operation. (See Chapter 29.)

2. Palliative short-circuiting operation where the obstruction cannot be removed. Tuberculosis sometimes affects the caecum and produces complete obstruction of the ileocaecal valve as does Crohn's disease. A portion of the small bowel is then joined to the transverse colon thus by-passing the obstructed ileocaecal junction. Carcinoma in the ascending colon may be similarly treated by an ileo-transverse anastomosis. A growth occurring in the colon beyond the middle of the transverse colon, and which is irremovable because of its spread, is by-passed by joining the terminal ileum to the loop of the pelvic colon.

3. By removing the cause in intestinal obstruction of extrinsic origin—for instance, division of bands or adhesions from former peritonitis or congenital malformation.

4. By removing the segment of the bowel which contains an intrinsic obstruction such as a growth. In the majority of cases this operation will include the restoration of continuity of the bowel or anastomosis of the two cut ends (page 552). Clearly this is the ideal method of dealing with chronic intestinal obstruction where the disease is within the bowel, since only one operation is necessary.

Whatever type of operation has been performed, if the surgeon is anxious about the condition of the bowel or the security of an anastomosis, he may establish a temporary safety valve such as caecostomy to prevent the risk of distension and subsequent leak with peritonitis.

Post-operative care

The general management is exactly the same as that for acute intestinal obstruction, since the main risks are identical—ileus, peritonitis, recurrence of obstruction from adhesions. The detailed management will depend upon whether an external fistula (ileostomy, caecostomy, or colostomy) has been established.

The bowel which has been obstructed for a long period has become accustomed to distension, and although active peristalsis may be restored, pooling and stagnation of large quantities of intestinal secretion may occur and distension may be troublesome. Restoration of normal bowel function may therefore take a considerable time after the relief of chronic obstruction.

There is usually little difficulty in feeding once the hazard of ileus has passed, because the relief from distension and discomfort completely changes the patient's outlook and brings with it the risk of over-eating before the intestinal tract and digestion has settled down. This is particularly true if the obstruction has been high in the small bowel or at the pylorus. This 'intestinal hurry' which follows gastric operations is described on page 528.

INTERNAL HAEMORRHAGE

The likely sources of severe internal abdominal haemorrhage are given in Table 18 (page 122). The three most common causes of severe internal bleeding which prove rapidly fatal if medical assistance is not immediately available, are

(a) rupture of spleen, liver or kidney due to injury. Football injuries, a kick by a horse and crush injuries are likely causes. If a motor-car wheel passes over the abdomen there may be no external injury but very severe damage to the viscera.

(b) ruptured ectopic gestation. Here the fertilised ovum remains in the uterine (Fallopian) tube instead of migrating into the uterus. It usually continues to grow in the tube where it obtains a very rich blood supply, and after approximately 6 weeks from fertilisation it bursts into the peritoneal cavity. There may be a preliminary period of pelvic pain for several days or only a few hours before the final rupture occurs. There is then torrential haemorrhage into the peritoneal cavity. Operation is a matter of desperate urgency and blood transfusion is essential.

(c) haemorrhage into the gastro-intestinal tract from gastric, duodenal or intestinal ulceration. The rupture of an artery in the base of an ulcer, especially if this is in stomach, leads to profuse haemorrhage with collapse. There may have been no previous symptoms of the presence of an ulcer.

There are many other sources of bleeding both into the intestinal tract and into the peritoneal cavity. Chronic blood loss from the bowel occurs in malignant disease and especially in ulcerative colitis (page 548). Recurrent daily bleeding from haemorrhoids may also lead to severe anaemia of such a degree that transfusion is required.

Apart from these principal sources of bleeding, internal haemorrhage is a possible complication after every abdominal operation, especially after those in which an organ or part of an organ has been removed—cholecystectomy, gastrectomy, nephrectomy, etc. Operations involving resection of part of the intestinal tract are sometimes followed by severe haemorrhage into the lumen of the bowel or stomach.

Bleeding into the peritoneal cavity occurring post-operatively is usually due to the slipping of a ligature round some important blood vessel. The abdomen will probably be re-opened in order to locate and deal with the source of haemorrhage. Bleeding into the lumen of the stomach or bowel usually stops spontaneously and further surgical intervention is rarely required.

Symptoms and signs of internal haemorrhage

(a) Bleeding into the stomach or bowel stimulates peristalsis and the first indication is therefore vomiting, colic or diarrhoea. Bleeding into the stomach generally results in the production of 'coffee ground' vomit. This appearance is due to the alteration of the blood by the action of the acid gastric juice, but if the haemorrhage has been severe the patient may recognise the vomit as containing blood. Duodenal haemorrhage or bleeding in the upper part of the intestinal tract stimulates peristalsis but the first subsequent action of the bowel will result in the evacuation of a normal stool. The black tarry stool which is characteristic of intestinal haemorrhage, will not appear for several hours after the commencement of the bleeding. Gross haemorrhage from the large bowel is uncommon but occasionally occurs as a complication of the injection treatment for haemorrhoids or from haemorrhoidectomy. The patient then passes large quantities of bright blood.

Accompanying these symptoms of gastro-intestinal disturbance will be a feeling of faintness, sweating and extreme pallor. Reflex vomiting may occur from disturbance of the colon without there being any disease of the stomach or duodenum. It is unlikely that there will be severe abdominal pain.

(b) Haemorrhage occurring into the peritoneal cavity produces rather different symptoms. If there has been a minor leak of blood following injury to the liver, spleen or intestine, the patient will have very severe but poorly localised abdominal pain from irritation of the peritoneum. It is probable that at this stage the patient will seek medical advice. There may be the history of a recent injury in the left loin and tenderness over the lower ribs suggests that the spleen has been injured. There may be some haematuria indicating that the kidney has been damaged (page 679). Under such circumstances the patient will probably be admitted to hospital for observation as it is known that minor tears of the spleen subsequently burst and require emergency splenectomy, and an injured kidney may need to be removed.

In a woman patient, there may be the history that one period has been missed or has been slightly abnormal. Pain in the right or left iliac fossa with associated tenderness will probably be accompanied by pain referred to the shoulder on the appropriate side. There is then the immediate suspicion that a tubal or ectopic pregnancy is present, the pain in the shoulder being due to blood tracking up beside the colon and irritating the peritoneum in the region of the diaphragm. Vaginal examination may reveal the presence of a swelling in the broad ligament beside the uterus. Operation for the removal of the ovum and tube is then possible before severe haemorrhage occurs.

Unfortunately there may be no such preliminary warning by pain. Collapse with pallor, sweating, 'air hunger' and loss of consciousness may be the first indication of trouble. Death may supervene in a few minutes from either of the causes mentioned as examples, and this type of internal haemorrhage constitutes one of the gravest surgical emergencies, for which every hospital must be prepared at any time of the day or night. Such conditions are among the very few which require operation so urgently that the patient may be taken immediately from the admission room to the operating theatre without any preliminary formality, such as the signing of consent forms or the filling in of hospital records. Unfortunately hospital organisation is not always such that an emergency of this type can be effectively dealt with. Such delays as inaccessibility to an electric lift or the fact that basic instruments for emergency surgery are not held ready sterilised, may make it quite impossible for a surgeon to save the patient's life (page 321).

In patients who are known to have bled internally one great problem is to decide if bleeding has stopped and to detect if it restarts. Observation of the central venous pressure helps and a fall will be seen before a rise of pulse or fall of *arterial* blood pressure calls attention to the further bleeding (page 134).

ASCITES

Under normal conditions the abdominal viscera are lubricated by a thin layer of serous fluid which fills the interstices between the loops of the intestine and the solid viscera. This fluid is produced by the peritoneum. Inflammation of the peritoneal surface leads to an increased production of this fluid and to clotting on the surface; this in turn leads to adhesions between the inflamed surfaces.

Under certain pathological conditions there is a great increase in peritoneal fluid, to such an extent that the abdomen becomes distended, with subsequent impairment of diaphragm movement and respiration. This is the condition of ascites, occurring quite apart from inflammation of the peritoneum, and it arises perhaps more commonly in patients in medical wards than in those undergoing surgical treatment.

Ascites is usually the symptom of serious disease. There are five main causes.

1. Systemic venous back-pressure. Its appearance is common in heart failure, particularly with disease of the lung where the main strain falls upon the right side of the heart. The subsequent back-pressure through the right auricle and vena cava leads to oedema of the lower limbs, enlargement of the liver and ascites. In cases of severe pericarditis the heart's activities are interfered with and ascites may occur from back-pressure.

2. Renal failure may also lead to back-pressure ascites, occurring with associated heart failure or as the result of severe nephritis where there is generalised oedema.

3. Abdominal malignant disease. Carcinoma of any abdominal organ ultimately reaches its peritoneal covering and spreads by seeding over the peritoneal surface. Severe ascites frequently accompanies this condition of malignant peritonitis (page 438).

4. Chronic inflammation. Acute infective peritonitis is accompanied by an increase of peritoneal fluid which forms **pus**. The term ascites is not usually applied to such an effusion. Tuberculosis produces **chronic** peritonitis which is invariably accompanied by a large effusion and is usually associated with active tuberculous ulceration in the bowel. Infection of the lungs or skeleton may be present in addition.

5. Portal hypertension. Various diseases of the liver result in fibrous tissue formation and consequent strangulation of the tiny branches of the portal vein within the liver. This 'cirrhosis' of the liver leads to back-pressure in the portal vein through which blood normally returns to the liver from the stomach, spleen and intestinal tract. Sometimes the splenic vein undergoes thrombosis and this further interferes with the return of splenic blood through the portal circulation. Subsequently gross ascites develops unless an adequate network of veins opens up in various sites in the abdominal wall where the systemic and portal systems link up (pages 506 and 591). Consequently this type of ascites is often associated with liver disease and an enlarged spleen.

6. Chylous ascites. This is due neither to inflammation nor to venous back-pressure, but to obstruction of the lymphatic drainage from the abdomen. The lymphatic vessels from the lower limbs and abdominal viscera join together to form the cisterna chyli which lies in front of the vertebral column at the level of the diaphragm. The development of malignant glands or other tumour in this area sometimes obstructs the flow of lymph, which then leaks into the peritoneal cavity.

7. Ascites in nutritional oedema. Vitamin B deficiency, especially with beri-beri, may lead to generalised oedema in which ascites develops. The loss of protein with the ascitic fluid aggravates the nutritional deficiency.

8. Polyserositis. There are in addition certain specific diseases which produce an effusion from all serous membranes simultaneously—pericardium, pleura and peritoneum. Ascites may thus be a symptom of this 'polyserositis'.

Ascitic fluid is usually clear yellow containing a large amount of protein (which clots when the fluid is heated), but in chylous ascites the fluid is milky.

Differential diagnosis

Very often the cause of ascites is readily apparent. The patient may be known to have a failing heart or may already have undergone an operation for abdominal malignant disease. There remain, however, a considerable number of cases in which the diagnosis is in doubt. Similar distension of the abdomen can be produced by the presence of a very large cyst arising from the pancreas, mesentery, or ovary.

When the cause of the ascites is not known various investigations may be required. These will probably include a barium-meal x-ray examination of the whole intestinal tract. Varicose veins (oesophageal varices) develop at the lower end of the oesophagus in portal hypertension because at this point the systemic and portal circulation is linked. These varicosities may be demonstrated by barium swallow examination or their presence may have been suggested by the patient suffering from haematemesis. Oesophagoscopy will be performed to look for such varices if portal hypertension is suspected. X-ray examination may reveal the presence of malignant disease in the stomach or bowel while x-ray of the chest may show secondary deposits in the lungs from an unknown primary focus.

Peritoneoscopy (laparoscopy) is sometimes used to investigate the cause of ascites of obscure origin.

Full clinical examination of the abdomen is difficult because of the presence of fluid, but by pelvic examination per rectum or per vagina the surgeon may be able to feel hard nodules of malignant disease in the pelvis. These may be metastases from stomach or other organ.

Treatment of ascites

In the majority of cases the underlying cause cannot be removed. When ascites is due to systemic venous back-pressure from heart or renal failure, removal of the fluid (paracentesis) may add greatly to the patient's comfort and relieve the strain on the heart produced by embarrassed respiration.

In advanced malignant disease, the presence of ascites may be the patient's chief worry. Paracentesis may then be performed at perhaps monthly intervals as a palliative measure to relieve distension.

Tuberculous peritonitis requires sanatorium treatment and the amount of fluid present is rarely sufficient to embarrass the patient's respiration. Chemotherapy, complete rest, and active treatment for any focus of tuberculosis elsewhere in the body are the main objectives. Intestinal obstruction from adhesions may occur at any time during the treatment. Since tuberculous disease of the bowel with ulceration is also present in some of these cases the problem of nutrition resembles that found in the treatment of ulcerative colitis (page 548) and anaemia develops from constant loss of blood and toxaemia.

In portal hypertension, due to cirrhosis, ascites varies considerably in its degree and from time to time there is a 'flare-up' which may have to be treated by paracentesis. During recent years operations have been undertaken to short-circuit the blood from the portal vein back into the systemic veins. This relieves the back-pressure and consequently allows the ascites to subside. The principles of these operations—porta-caval anastomosis, spleno-renal anastomosis—are described on page 591.

Chylous ascites is rarely amenable to treatment unless it has occurred from injury to a major lymphatic duct which can be repaired.

Nutrition. The serous peritoneal exudate contains large quantities of protein. If repeated paracentesis is necessary, there is then a considerable loss of body protein, as in a case of severe burns. The diet must therefore also be rich in protein. Liver damage due to cirrhosis impairs glycogen storage and the production of vitamin K. Extra carbohydrate and full vitamin supplement is required. If the liver is affected by disease the production of bile is inadequate and fat digestion is impaired. The diet should contain a minimum amount of fatty food, and cooked fats should be avoided.

If the ascites is a complication of heart or renal failure, restriction will probably be placed on fluid or salt intake.

Technique of paracentesis abdominis

This may be performed under local anaesthesia by means of a pneumothorax trocar-needle or a simple trocar and cannula such as is used for aspirating hydroceles (Fig. 24.10).

As the amount of fluid to be removed may amount to several litres, a collecting bottle is required with rubber tubing for attachment to the cannula, in order that drainage may take place over several hours. Except in cases of heart failure it is usual to remove the fluid as fast as possible and the surgeon may therefore decide to use a wide-bore cannula and trocar of the type used for suprapubic puncture of the bladder (Fig. 35.12).

Equipment required includes:

(*a*) sterile towels.
(*b*) (gauze) swabs.
(*c*) sterile wool. (A large piece of wool should be placed each side of the abdomen to absorb any fluid which leaks.)
(*d*) antiseptic for skin sterilisation.
(*e*) 20-ml syringe and needles for the injection of local anaesthetic solution.
(*f*) local anaesthetic solution (e.g. 2 per cent lignocaine).
(*g*) trocar and cannula.
(*h*) sterile test tube for collection of fluid for laboratory examination.
(*i*) fine sterile rubber tubing, connectors and bedside bottle for continuous drainage.
(*j*) adhesive strapping and Nobecutaine or collodion for final sealed dressing.

If a large trocar is to be used, a scalpel should be available to make an initial nick in the skin. In this case the surgeon may wish to insert a skin stitch at the end of the procedure.

The trocar is usually inserted in the midline below the umbilicus, or at the outer border of the rectus muscle. The bladder must be emptied immediately before the procedure.

Peritoneal dialysis

Although this procedure is unrelated to ascites the technique is similar to that of paracentesis and it is therefore convenient to include it here. In certain cases of renal failure and advanced uraemia, recovery of the kidneys can be expected in a matter of a

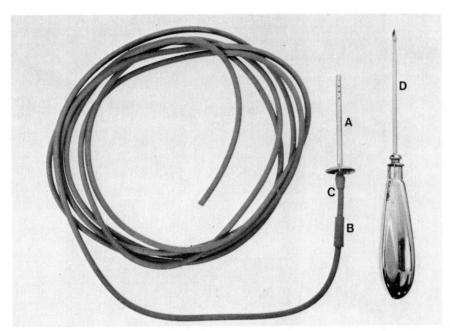

Fig. 24.10 Trocar and cannula for paracentesis abdominis or hydrocele drainage. The cannula **A** is provided by CSSD: attached above the flange is a length of narrow rubber tubing over which is a cuff of wider tubing **B**. The tube is folded over at **C** and the trocar **D** pushed through the rubber. The trocar and cannula are then inserted under local anaesthesia. Once the cannula is in position, the trocar is withdrawn and the rubber cuff **B** slipped over the puncture. This method eliminates the risk of contamination by back-flow through an open-ended cannula. (The rubber tube is connected to a bedside bottle.)

few days, if the patient's life can be protected from the effects of accumulating urea during the critical period. The function of the kidney can be imitated by irrigating the peritoneal surface with large quantities of sterile fluid. Urea and other products of metabolism are exuded from the peritoneal membrane and carried away in the irrigation fluid. The method is suitable for such cases as acute renal failure in shock (page 674) or following overdose with sulphonamide drugs.

The procedure consists of the insertion of a trocar in the left upper abdominal quadrant and a second trocar in the right lower abdominal quadrant. Catheters are passed into the peritoneal cavity through the trocars and irrigation continued from the upper to the lower catheter. Five or six litres of fluid a day may be used, the composition being determined by the patient's blood chemistry. From time to time the fluid escaping from the lower catheter is sent to the laboratory for analysis to determine the amount of urea which is being removed from the body. Both the inlet and outlet catheter drainage tubes must have a visible drip chamber so that the rate of escape can be watched: input must not exceed output rate. Alternatively, a single tube may be used, the fluid being run in and left for a set interval and then allowed to escape.

Infection may gain entry at the site of catheter insertion but organisms easily enter the dialysing fluid when bottles are changed, and for this reason it is now recommended that a bacterial filter be included in the in-flow line (Fig. 24.11).

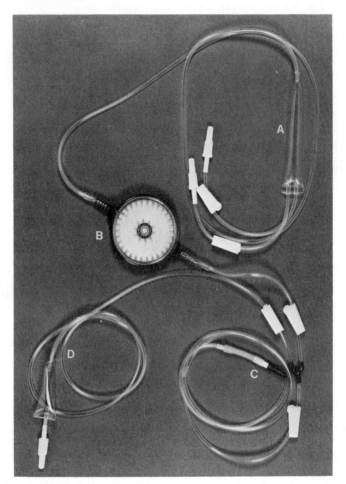

Fig. 24.11   Millipore peritoneal dialysis unit. **A.** Twin reservoir supply tubes. **B.** Filter. **C.** Peritoneal catheter. **D.** Outflow tube. (Millipore (U.K.) Ltd.)

The risk of such a procedure is naturally one of peritonitis and the patient must receive the protection of antibiotic treatment while this is in progress.

There must of course be strict and careful measurement of all fluid taken by mouth and of the input and output of the dialysation fluid. As renal function is resumed, urine will be produced. It is likely that an indwelling urethral catheter will be in place so that the progressive increase of urine flow may be detected.

Repeat peritoneal dialysis can be undertaken with suitable patients in much the same way as home haemodialysis. A Silastic pliable catheter is fixed in the abdominal wall by a dacron cuff into which tissue grows to create a seal at skin level. An automatic perfusion machine is used.

In some centres peritoneal dialysis is used increasingly instead of haemodialysis. It is a more simple procedure, less costly and with fewer risks.

25

The Oesophagus

Anatomy

The funnel-shaped pharynx is composed of voluntary muscle and converges to join, at the level of the cricoid cartilage, with the tubular oesophagus. This is composed of a thick muscle wall which is voluntary (striped) muscle in the upper part, and involuntary (smooth) muscle in the lower part. The oesophagus ends by joining the cardiac orifice of the stomach a little less than 4 cm (2 inches) below the diaphragm. It therefore has three parts. The **cervical** portion in the lower part of the neck lies immediately behind the trachea with lobes of the thyroid on either side. The **thoracic** portion lies, in the upper part, close to the back of the trachea in front of the vertebral column. In the lower part the oesophagus passes a little to the left and is crossed by the left bronchus, later lying immediately behind the pericardium until it pierces the diaphragm. The **abdominal** portion connects with the fundus of the stomach. Except during the passage of food, the oesophagus is flattened like a muscle strap but can distend to 2·5 cm (1 in) in diameter. With the exception of the pylorus it is the narrowest portion of the alimentary tract and the oesophagus itself has three constrictions where it becomes narrower than in the rest of its course. The first is at the upper end behind the cricoid cartilage; the second is at the level of the bifurcation of the trachea into right and left bronchus; while the third narrow point is where the oesophagus passes through the diaphragm.

Unlike the abdominal parts of the alimentary tract, there is no peritoneal coat on the thoracic and cervical oesophagus. Any perforation of its wall, whether by accident or from operation, is therefore far more likely to leak after repair as it is not immediately sealed by the peritoneal covering. Until the recent introduction of drugs which control infection, surgery of the oesophagus has been extremely dangerous because leakage led to spreading infection in the mediastinum or in the loose tissues of the neck.

Pathological conditions of the oesophagus

Congenital

In the developing baby, the oesophagus and trachea are formed from the same tube and occasionally at birth the two tubes communicate by a fistula. This leads to choking attacks every time an attempt is made to feed the baby, because food finds its way into the air passages. Sometimes this oesophagotracheal fistula is associated with 'atresia' or failure of development of part of the tube. There is then a blind upper end which overflows into the larynx when feeding takes place, while the lower end opens into the trachea. Sometimes the upper end opens into the trachea and the lower end is blind, opening only into the stomach below.

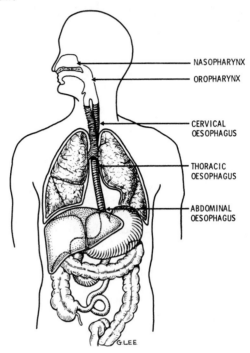

Fig. 25.1   The oesophagus showing its relation to other structures in the thorax and abdomen. The heart has been omitted.

This condition is diagnosed within the first 24 hours after birth by the occurrence of choking attacks. A catheter is passed down the baby's throat and the blockage is felt at the expected level of the fistula. Operation is undertaken immediately through the right side of the chest and the oesophagus is reconstructed. A very fine tube is left down the repaired oesophagus and through this the baby is fed. Sometimes an emergency gastro-stomy is performed at the same time to improve nutrition. The operation calls for very great skill both in surgery and in nursing and the baby requires nursing in an incubator (page 411).

Foreign bodies

Foreign bodies such as whistles, toys, small or broken dentures and hard pieces of food, occasionally become impacted at one of the narrow sections in the oesophagus, merely because they are too big to pass. Removal is an urgent necessity. Anaesthesia is required and special forceps are used through the oesophagoscope.

Occasionally sharp foreign bodies such as fishbones or pins become caught in the oesophagus and similarly require removal. If the wall of the oesophagus has been perforated, acute infection in the mediastinum may lead to death. The extraction of an impacted fishbone is therefore also a matter of urgency. Its presence may not be known until **mediastinitis,** with fever and pain, develops.

Injury

Cut-throat or knife wounds of the neck occasionally penetrate the oesophagus which requires immediate repair.

The swallowing of corrosive fluids accidentally by a child, or with suicidal intent by the adult, produces ulceration of the oesophagus. Temporary blockage from oedema occurs and may be followed later by a firm fibrous stricture. This is usually treated by repeated dilatation with special bougies. In the initial stage of acute inflammation and ulceration, the oesophagus is very liable to perforation from tearing. Tubes should not be passed unless specified by the medical officer. A temporary gastrostomy will probably be required to maintain nutrition. Healing leads to stricture formation. This has to be dilated repeatedly and if an appreciable length of the oesophagus is scarred a new tube is fashioned from intestine and passed up through the diaphragm and chest into the neck. The oesophagus may be ruptured by the sudden distension when a patient vomits. Pain in the chest simulates that produced by coronary thrombosis and a misdiagnosis ensues. Immediate transthoracic repair is essential to avoid fatal mediastinitis. Repeated minor tears occur in patients with gastric disorders (Mallory-Weiss syndrome).

Neurological

The nerve-muscle mechanism of the gullet may be affected in generalised nervous disorders (such as myasthenia gravis) or in certain forms of infantile paralysis. Fluid food runs to the stomach by gravity but regurgitation is common from peristalsis in the involuntary muscle of the stomach. The patient may be unable to swallow any solid or thick fluid food. Tube feeding may be necessary.

'Achalasia' of the cardia is a condition of spasm of the lower end of the oesophagus somewhat like congenital hypertrophic pyloric stenosis (page 515). The firm muscle sphincter refuses to relax and the oesophagus above dilates to such an extent that it may hold as much as a litre of decomposing food. The cause of the condition is unknown, but it is thought to be due to some form of neuro-muscular imbalance. It occurs mainly in young women in their twenties. There may be a psychological element in its development. By the time the diagnosis is confirmed (by barium swallow) the patient may be emaciated. In the past attempts were made to dilate the tight muscle with bougies but the standard treatment now is Heller's operation. The lower end of the oesophagus is reached through a thoracotomy incision, or the upper abdomen, and the thick muscle coat divided in a manner similar to that used in Rammstedt's operation for congenital hypertrophic pyloric stenosis (page 516).

Post-operative nursing problems are those arising from any thoracotomy. Infection through leakage may occur and lead to empyema or mediastinitis. Oral feeding is with fluids only for several days.

Neoplastic

Carcinoma of the oesophagus is of two types. Growths may arise from the squamous epithelium which lines the oesophagus for most of its length from the pharynx to the diaphragm, or an 'adeno-carcinoma' may grow from the gastric type of mucous membrane at the lower end, in the abdomen near its junction with the stomach. Unfortunately the growth spreads up and down in the wall of the oesophagus and extends outside to the adjacent structures without in fact blocking the lumen in the early stages. Consequently the symptoms of obstruction to swallowing do not appear until the growth is fairly far advanced. In the early stage the patient may complain of slight difficulty in starting to swallow at the beginning of a meal, but after initial difficulty swallowing improves and the meal is completed. Many patients are, however, wasted and have been on insufficient food intake for months before they come for treatment. The surgeon's first problem is to attempt an assessment of the extent of growth to decide whether there is any possibility of treating the patient with a view to 'cure', or whether he must abandon this objective and merely treat the patient's symptoms. These are essentially inability to swallow, constant saliva-tion, and malnutrition. The appearance of metastatic gland enlargement in the neck, or a very extensive growth shown on x-ray, makes it clear that only palliative treatment is possible. Diagnosis is confirmed by barium-swallow examination, and then sometimes by oesophagoscopy and biopsy.

When the growth is confined to a relatively short length of the oesophagus the usual procedure is to excise the growth if the cervical portion or the lower third are involved. Growths in the middle third behind the heart are treated by radiotherapy without operation. With improved surgical techniques more patients are being treated by excision. Frequently it is impossible to assess the feasibility of surgery until the chest has been opened so that the surgeon can examine the growth by direct vision. Alternative procedures are then:

(a) **Radical excision.** The affected portion of the oesophagus with a considerable length above and below is removed. The stomach is brought up into the chest to be anastomosed to the cut end of the upper portion of the oesophagus. Figure 25.2 shows a more radical method of treating the cervical portion by bringing the colon up from the abdomen. This 'colon swing' operation uses the transverse colon extended to the ascending or descending colon with the vascular pedicle in the meso-colon as its principal supply. The graft is brought up through the right side of the thorax or may be threaded through the medias-tinum into the neck without opening the pleural cavity. Occasionally, it is brought up under the skin. A length of jejunum may be used instead of colon.

(b) **By-pass operation.** If it is decided that the growth cannot safely be removed, a by-pass operation may be performed using again either the colon or a piece of jejunum, as after a radical excision. This will relieve the obstruction and allow oral feeding.

Nursing problems which may arise after a radical operation of this type are those of any thoracic operation, together with the complications of upper abdominal surgery. An inter-costal underwater seal drain may be left in place at the end of operation in case there is bleeding and to ensure full expansion of the lung. Mediastinitis or empyema may arise if leakage occurs from the anastomosis in the chest or peritonitis from the colonic anasto-mosis in the abdomen.

Whether or not the chest has been opened in the course of the operation, there will be restricted respiratory movement and great attention will have to be paid to post-operative physiotherapy.

A *gastrostomy* or 'feeding' jejunostomy may be performed at the time of the excision operation so that feeding may take place below the level of the anastomosis to maintain the patient's nutrition, and to allow the new conduit to heal without being disturbed by the passage of food.

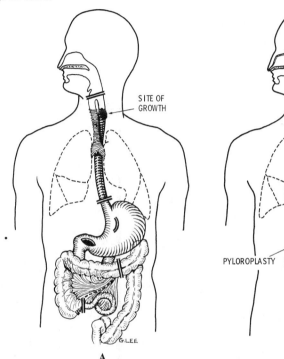

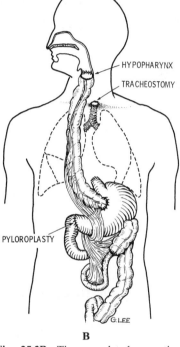

A

Fig. 25.2A. Surgical excision of the oesophagus when feasible may involve removal of part of the trachea and larynx. Pyloroplasty is essential to ensure emptying of the stomach as the vagus nerves are divided. The diagram shows lines of excision for isolation of the right colon for use as a pedicle graft.

B

Fig. 25.2B. The completed operation showing the tracheostomy, the upper end of the stomach closed and the colon graft attached from the stomach to the pharynx, with continuity of bowel restored between the ileum and splenic flexure.

(c) Intubation. If excisional surgery is not possible and a by-pass operation is similarly thought to be too hazardous, temporary relief of the obstruction symptoms can be achieved by passing a plastic tube into the oesophagus where it is lodged at the site of obstruction and maintains a reasonable passage for food. This may give complete relief of symptoms for several months, but in the end ulceration or occlusion of the tube takes place. Infection may spread into the mediastinum either from an increase in the growth or from pressure necrosis.

Various types of tube prosthesis are used. A Souttar's flexible tube made of noncorroding spiral wire was designed to maintain the lumen through the growth and thus prevent obstruction. The metal tube has been partly superseded by various designs of PVC and Nylon tube. The narrow portion of the oesophagus is dilated by the passage of bougies under anaesthesia and the tube inserted with a special introducer. The tube has an expanded upper end which prevents it being pushed on into the stomach. The Celestin tube (Fig. 25.3) is less likely to cause damage, as it is soft and fully flexible. This is threaded through the stricture from above and the tube is then pulled down into position by means of an open operation on the stomach. It is of particular use for growths of the lower end of the oesophagus but is very big and rigid.

The Mousseau-Barbin oesophageal catheter is another such prosthesis which has a long 'rat tail' at the lower end.

After the insertion of a tube, the patient must be warned against the danger of swallowing, perhaps inadvertently, large lumps of food which may block the tube. Food must be chewed very thoroughly. The healthy oesophagus invariably shifts such obstructions by vigorous contraction, but the rigid tube cannot play any active part in dislodging the food. In order to lessen the risk of impaction of food the patient is encouraged to sip an effervescent drink during his meals.[1]

In order to clean the crevices of the tube, it is recommended that the patient swallows a small quantity of dilute hydrogen peroxide at bedtime. This should be taken in sips. Hydrogen peroxide releases oxygen and by a frothing action breaks up decomposed tissue or food. It is supplied as '20 volume' and 10 ml of this with 30 ml of tapwater is sufficient.

(d) **Radiotherapy.** This may be used alone or in combination with a by-pass operation or the use of an intra-luminal tube. In the past, radium needles have been used on an applicator placed in the oesophagus, or radon seeds inserted into its wall at the site of the growth, but these have now been discarded in favour of carefully regulated external radiation from a cobalt source, or linear accelerator. The principle of this treatment is to use 'cross fire' radiation (page 442), aiming the beam through various fields so that the fields used on successive days cross at the point of the growth where the maximum growth causes necrosis of malignant tissue. The result is sometimes dramatic in the relief of symptoms and long time 'cures' can be obtained. There is, however, a risk of severe necrosis of the growth and the spread of infection in the mediastinum; sometimes obstruction occurs from scarring and subsequently regular dilatation is needed.

Patients who have radiotherapy develop oesophagitis and may be completely unable to swallow even though they were able to take fluids before treatment is started. Though gastrostomy may have to be performed until the oesophagitis has settled it is usually avoided except as a temporary measure as it prolongs life without relieving symptoms.

Oesophageal compression

The oesophagus may be pressed and obstructed by growths arising from other tissues. In the neck, swellings of the thyroid gland (goitre) may compress the cervical portion and impede its movement. Malignant growth of the thyroid gland may actually invade the oesophagus. In the thorax, mediastinal tumours, such as those arising from the thymus or lymph glands, may produce similar obstruction and aneurysm of the aorta may likewise

---

[1] 4 parts sugar, 2 parts tartaric acid, 2 parts sodium bicarbonate with lemon or other flavouring makes a suitable basic powder.

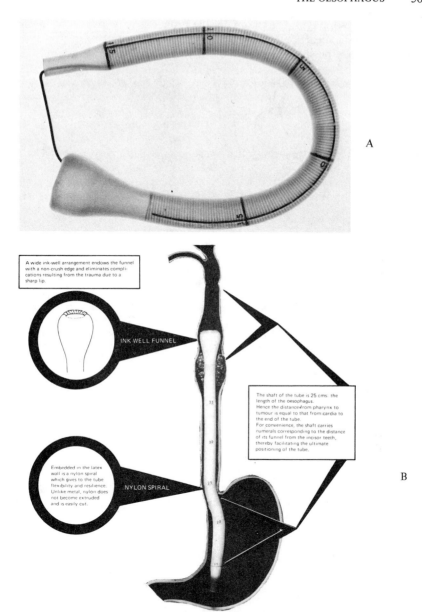

Fig. 25.3 Celestin oesophageal tube. **A.** This flexible silastic tube with nylon spiral in its wall is safer than more rigid tubes. The large size (S.IV A) allows the passage of chewed solid food: the smaller size in child (S. IV B) and adult (S. IV C) lengths allows fluid only. Its use as a temporary measure may enable a patient to be built up and regain a nutritional state fit for radical surgery, perhaps for benign stricture. **B.** This shows the principle of intubation. The tube is inserted with the aid of a special bougie. (Ambleletin Ltd.)

compress the oesophagus. Carcinoma of the bronchus may invade the lower portion and enlargement of the heart presses the oesophagus from the front in its lower third. All such constrictions may be shown by the barium-swallow x-ray examination.

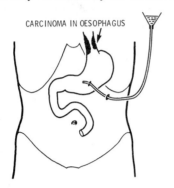

CARCINOMA IN OESOPHAGUS

Fig. 25.4   Gastrostomy for artificial feeding in oesophageal obstruction from growth or stricture (page 486).

Hiatus hernia

In this condition there is a hernia through the oesophageal opening in the centre of the diaphragm and part of the stomach comes upwards into the thorax (Fig. 25.5). The lack of sphincter action of the diaphragm muscle around the oesophagus allows acid to regurgitate

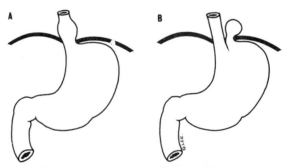

A   B

Fig. 25.5   Hiatus hernia. 'Sliding' type with short oesophagus and loss of normal junction with stomach, thus allowing reflux. **B.** 'Rolling' paraoesophageal type associated with pain rather than reflux.

into the lower part of the gullet where it may produce peptic ulceration. The condition is very common, especially in women past middle age. Symptoms are 'heartburn' or burning in the sternal region, especially at night when lying down, or stooping to work. The majority of patients with mild symptoms are relieved by having extra pillows at night or propping up the head of the bed. The patients are often obese and weight reduction helps. The development of an hiatus hernia alters the valvular mechanism where the oesophagus joins the stomach with the result that acid regurgitates into the oesophagus and causes chronic inflammation. This leads to ulceration, fibrosis and obstruction which may be very severe. Chronic loss of blood from this lesion leads to anaemia. Surgery may be required to relieve pain and obstruction, or to prevent haemorrhage.

Acid perfusion test will confirm that the symptoms are due to reflux: a naso-gastric tube is introduced to mid-thoracic level (checked by x-ray): dilute hydrochloric acid 0·1 mol/litre is dripped at 10 ml/min after an initial flow of saline. If no pain occurs the flow is increased to 20 ml/min. If acid reproduces the symptom pain it is then replaced by sodium bicarbonate which should give instant relief.

The principle of operative treatment is to reduce the hernia into the abdomen and at the same time to re-form the angle between the oesophagus and the fundus of the stomach so as to prevent acid regurgitation. Various types of operation are used. These may be performed either by an abdominal approach or through the 8th rib and the left plural cavity. Sometimes a combined abdomino-thoracic approach is required, particularly if the condition has recurred after a previous operation. In one method, the fundus—the bulky upper portion—of the stomach is folded around the lower end of the oesophagus, which it then grips. This operation is **'fundal plication'**.

Vagotomy may be added to reduce acid production. Full (truncal) vagotomy with pyloroplasty may allow bile to reflux into the stomach and aggravate the oesophageal condition. A simpler operation for hiatus hernia, in many cases very successful, is Boerema's operation in which the stomach is stitched to the anterior abdominal wall.

In post-operative care the complications are those of any upper abdominal operation. There will have been considerable retraction in the region of the diaphragm; post-operative basal pulmonary collapse is common and particular care has to be paid to immediate post-operative physiotherapy.

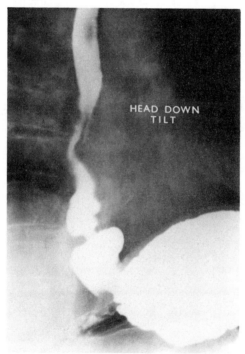

Fig. 25.6 Hiatus hernia. The patient has swallowed the barium and has been tilted into the head-down position. The oesophagus has refilled by flow-back from the stomach and is shown to be irregular from spasm and inflammation (cf. 25.5A.)

Oesophageal varices

Varicose veins at the lower end of the oesophagus develop in cases of portal hypertension (page 591) and are an attempt on the part of the circulation to increase the flow of
blood from the portal to systemic venous systems where there is normally only a fine
anastomosis around the lower end of the oesophagus. These varicosities occasionally
rupture, producing haematemesis. They may be demonstrated by barium x-ray examination and seen through the oesophagoscope.

Bleeding is often very severe and has to be treated by transfusion. To control the
bleeding a special oesophageal tube (Fig. 25.7) is passed into the stomach. The illustration
shows a three-lumen tube, one tail leads to an eye at the end of the catheter, for aspirating
the stomach; a second is used for inflating the small bag and a third for inflating the long
bag. Another type of tube has a fourth tail for aspirating the oesophagus above the long
bag through a side eye. When the distal end of the tube has reached the stomach the small
bag is inflated and the tube drawn back against the cardiac opening. The long bag is then
inflated to a pressure of 40 mm mercury: this pressure can be measured with a Y-connector
and a sphygmomanometer. Alternatively the tube which has been inflated can be clipped
and connected to the manometer tube in order to check the pressure. As the patient
cannot swallow, the oesophagus must be emptied regularly with a catheter; suction every
quarter of an hour can keep the oesophagus clear if the tube is one with a fourth tail.
The stomach can be aspirated if necessary but it may empty spontaneously and if so the
patient can be fed with fluid through the tube. The bag may be kept inflated for 24 hours

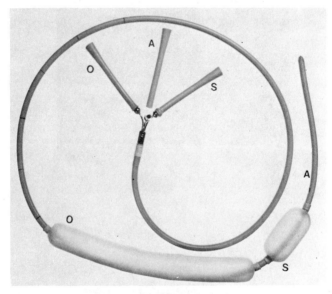

Fig. 25.7 Sengstaken tube. **OO** Inflation—oesophageal balloon. **SS** Inflation—stomach balloon. **AA**
Aspiration catheter, for suction or stomach washout. The balloon **S** is inflated first after passage of the
tube, which is then withdrawn so that **S** is tight against the cardia. **O** is then inflated to the required pressure
to control bleeding from the oesophageal varices.

and if bleeding recurs it may have to remain in place for several days being released and re-inflated at intervals. Laxatives are given to aid the evacuation of the stale blood. Neomycin is administered by tube to limit bacteriological decomposition of this blood. The nitrogenous breakdown products of the blood in the bowel are not dealt with adequately by the damaged liver and hepatic coma may follow (page 592). Repeated bleeding may lead to the necessity for a shunt operation or even removal of part of the oesophagus. Gastrostomy may be required.

Oesophageal symptoms

Difficulty in swallowing (dysphagia) may be due to disorders of the teeth, mouth, tongue or pharynx. Perhaps the most common cause is tonsillitis. When all these more obvious reasons for dysphagia have been eliminated, it is then likely that the symptom is produced by some obstruction or inflammation in the oesophagus. The gullet occasionally becomes involved in generalised inflammation of the pharynx or other parts of the alimentary tract. This oesophagitis may be produced by drinking excessively hot fluids or may result from a reaction to penicillin which has been taken by mouth. Oesophagitis produces a burning feeling in the throat and pain behind the sternum during swallowing. Oesophageal pain is also referred to the upper abdomen, to the region of the heart, or to the root of the neck.

In conditions where the obstruction has been prolonged, such as in achalasia or stricture from ulceration, there is gross dilatation of the oesophagus above the obstruction. Food decomposes in this reservoir and the mucous membrane becomes very inflamed. The patient complains of a foul taste in his mouth, eructation of unpleasant gas and vomiting of large volumes of unchanged food, the constituents of which are recognisable. When tested with litmus paper the vomit is found to be alkaline (from the saliva). If the obstruction has been due to carcinoma, it is unlikely that there is very much dilatation and the amount of vomitus will be considerably less (e.g. 100 ml compared with perhaps 400 ml from achalasia). It is also more likely to contain blood.

In all cases of oesophageal obstruction, the patient very soon loses his appetite and gross loss of weight and emaciation follow.

Investigation procedures

The first investigation in cases of dysphagia not originating in the mouth is a **barium-swallow x-ray screen** examination. This locates the site of any obstruction, and determines the size of the remaining lumen, if any. It will also show the extent of a carcinoma if this is the cause of the obstruction, since the outline of the barium shadow will be irregular where the growth has spread along the wall of the oesophagus.

Oesophagoscopy is performed usually under general anaesthesia. A direct-vision instrument is passed down the whole length of the oesophagus (Fig. 25.8) or a fibre-optic flexible instrument is used (Fig. 25.9).

Before barium-swallow examination or oesophagoscopy, if there has been real difficulty in swallowing, or if there has been vomiting, a naso-gastric tube should be passed down to the obstruction and the oesophagus gently irrigated with saline to remove mucus and particles of food (page 476). This is necessary not only as preparation for investigation, but also as part of the treatment where there is gross dilatation of the oesophagus such as in cases of achlasia. If this preparation is not carried out it is likely that the oesophageal contents will regurgitate into the throat during anaesthesia for oesophagoscopy and this in turn may produce pneumonia by aspiration.

Technique for oesophagoscopy[1]

If this is to be carried out under general anaesthesia, an endotracheal tube will have been inserted. Local anaesthesia may be used if the surgeon is experienced in this particular technique (page 514). Relaxant drugs of the curare type are used to prevent spasm and avoid very deep anaesthesia. Obstruction may be such that dilatation is needed before the instrument is passed. This is done with flexible plastic bougies. When a fibre-optic instrument is used, a guide wire is passed down the biopsy channel, the scope withdrawn

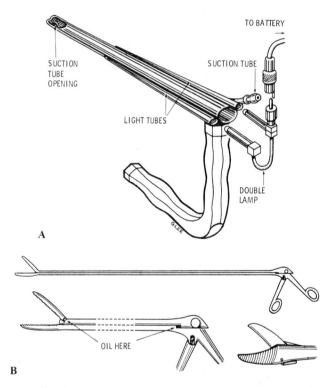

Fig. 25.8   A. Oesophagoscope. **B.** Alligator forceps and scissors (for oesophagoscope).

[1] Gastroscopy is similar (page 514), but the latter procedure is performed on patients in whom the oesophagus is normal, elastic and less liable to injury. Oesophagoscopy requires more relaxation and is more disturbing for the patient.

and Eder-Penstow dilators threaded over the wire. The oesophagus is very easily injured by the passage of instruments. Various types of oesophagoscope are in common use and they differ mainly in the method of illumination. The rigid Chevalier-Jackson pattern has lights at the lower or distal end and the Negus instrument has the lights incorporated in the proximal end of the tube. The oesophagus is normally curved, as it follows the curvature of the spine. For the passage of a straight instrument it is therefore necessary to straighten the head and cervicothoracic spine as far as possible to lessen the risk of injury to the walls of the oesophagus. Fibre-optic lighting is used with modern instruments. For diagnostic and biopsy purposes a longer flexible instrument in which the lens system ' is also fibre-optic is used for the oesophagus and stomach, and photographs may be taken with this instrument (Fig. 25.9).

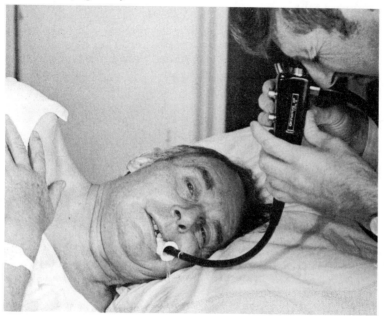

Fig. 25.9 Flexible gastroscope. The advance of flexible fibre-optic endoscope instruments has made possible visual examination and biopsy of the whole of the alimentary tract into the duodenum, and from below as far as the caecum. Above is shown a flexible oesophago-gastroscope which carries its lighting lens system, water injection and suction tube. This is used with local anaesthesia or neuro-leptanalgesia.

Oesophagoscopy is required for:

(*a*) removal of foreign bodies from the pharynx, or oesophagus.
(*b*) diagnostic investigation and biopsy in cases of suspected oesophageal obstruction.
(*c*) dilatation of strictures.
(*d*) treatment of carcinoma by the insertion of radium or Souttar's tubes.

A suction tube is used to remove secretions. Various forceps are available with which the surgeon can take small pieces of tissue for biopsy or extract foreign bodies. There is also a special pair of nibblers for breaking up pieces of dental plate which become stuck in the oesophagus.

The apparatus required for any particular case will depend upon the reason for which oesophagoscopy is being performed but in all cases there must be at least the following:

1. Oesophagoscope of the size to be determined from the surgeon by previous enquiry.
2. Set of sterile gum elastic oesophageal bougies.
3. Efficient suction apparatus.
4. Narrow-bore oesophageal tube and 20-ml syringe for aspirating fluid or pus for examination in the laboratory.
5. Adrenaline hydrochloride solution (1:1000) which may be used on pledgets of wool to diminish the oozing of blood from the surface of the oesophagus.
6. Ancillary instruments for the extraction of foreign bodies, insertion of Souttar's tubes or other special procedures.
7. Small specimen bottle containing formol-saline for biopsy fragments.
8. Lubricant.

As the procedure is entirely dependent on efficient lighting the illumination of the instrument must be thoroughly tested beforehand. The procedure may be prolonged and spare batteries should be available if the source of electricity is not from a mains transformer.

Post-operative nursing following oesophagoscopy

There is no particular feature in the nursing except that associated with the care of the unconscious patient and particularly with the prevention of regurgitation of oesophageal contents which might be aspirated into the lungs. The patient should be nursed on his side with the head lower than the shoulders, in the 'tonsil' position until consciousness returns fully. No fluid or food should be allowed for 3 hours after the operation. Some surgeons prescribe the administration of a paste containing 3 G of sulphathiazole to be swallowed when consciousness returns, to diminish the risk of infection in case there has been injury to the wall of the oesophagus. A similar procedure is adopted after gastroscopy.

In elderly patients with arthritis of the cervical spine it is difficult to straighten the neck for the passage of the instrument. There may be severe pain in the neck after the investigations. Pain and tenderness in the front of the neck suggests that a tear of the oesophagus may be present and x-ray will show air in the tissues; immediate surgical repair may be needed.

Nursing problems in oesophageal disorders

In diseases of the oesophagus which require surgical treatment, nursing calls for considerable skill. The patient is usually suffering from severe malnutrition and these conditions occur most frequently in the elderly. Much care and patience is required in feeding, and if oesophageal obstruction is complete, an emergency gastrostomy and parenteral administration of fluids may be necessary.

The greatest possible attention must be paid to oral hygiene, particularly to teeth. Infection of the parotid gland is a serious and distressing complication of these debilitating digestive disorders, if oral infection is present. Monilial infections (thrush) are common.

Soon after admission to hospital the nursing staff will discover whether the patient is in fact able to swallow any fluid at all. It is quite likely that if the dilated oesophagus is gently washed by the repeated injection and immediate re-aspiration of small quantities (20 ml) of saline or bicarbonate of soda, the inflammation of the lining mucous membrane will subside and, even in cases where the obstruction was thought to be complete, the swallowing of thin fluids may again be possible. After this initial period of local toilet, oesophagoscopy is likely to be the next procedure if x-ray examination has been carried out before admission to hospital.

It is not possible to give detailed directions for the post-operative care of various operations performed on the oesophagus as these differ greatly according to the site and type of operation. There are, however, certain principles common to all operations in which the oesophagus is exposed and opened or resected.

First, there is the risk of post-operative infection and therefore the wound is invariably drained. The drainage tube is left in position until specific instructions are given for its removal, which will probably be 2–4 days after operation. After operations on the thoracic portion of the oesophagus the surgeon may close the pleura completely or establish an under-water seal drainage (page 603). Alternatively he may leave a rubber strip extra-pleural drain down to the site of operation. Normal feeding will be suspended completely in the immediate post-operative period. Antiseptic or antibiotic mouth wash may be pre-scribed, specifically to be swallowed, to limit the infection at the site of operation, but the patient must be prevented, as far as possible, from swallowing saliva, sputum, or other mouth wash. A gastric tube may be left in position through the oesophagus for aspiration and feeding.

Mediastinitis from leakage is shown by progressive rise in temperature and pulse rate. Antibiotic treatment, given as a preventive measure, may mask these symptoms and the later onset of a 'swinging' temperature indicates the presence of a mediastinal abscess or empyema.

All operations through the thorax have the additional risks of thoracotomy (Chapter 34), of which **persistent atelectasis** of the lung, **haemothorax** or **pleural effusion** are the most common. Breathing exercises are therefore a vital part of the pre-operative and post-operative nursing care.

Operations on the lower end of the oesophagus where the abdomen has been opened either directly or through the diaphragm from the thoracotomy approach, carry the additional risk of paralytic ileus and peritonitis (Chapter 24).

The magnitude of these operations involves the risk of severe shock which is increased by impaired lung expansion after thoracotomy and impaired diaphragm movement if there has been a combined abdomino-thoracic operation. There may also have been considerable blood loss and transfusion will certainly be required in these procedures.

It will be apparent that the nursing of such cases constitutes one of the greatest problems of surgery and involves strict observation of the basic principles of both thoracic and abdominal nursing procedure. The patients upon whom such operations are performed are from the very nature of the disease among those least fit for any surgical procedure.

26

Stomach and Duodenum

Anatomy

The stomach lies in the upper abdomen and is principally on the left side of the body, its upper portion being covered by the lower ribs. Figure 26.1 indicates the names applied to the various parts of the stomach. The cardia is in close proximity to the heart, separated only by diaphragm and pericardium. On the left, along the upper part of the greater

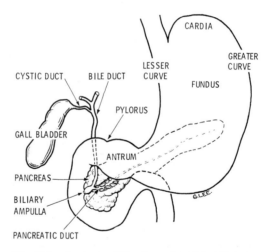

Fig. 26.1 Anatomy of the stomach and duodenum.

curvature, the stomach is attached to the spleen, and some of the principal arteries of the stomach pass through this attachment which is a double layer of peritoneum. Continuous with this 'gastro-splenic' ligament along the rest of the greater curvature, is the great omentum behind which, close up against the greater curvature of the stomach, lies the transverse colon. Along its lesser curvature, the stomach is slung from the undersurface of the liver by the lesser omentum, in the free edge of which runs the bile duct. The outlet to the duodenum is surrounded by the pyloric sphincter muscle. The first part of the duodenum passes backwards. The duodenum then lies behind the peritoneum of the posterior abdominal wall, and remains as an extraperitoneal organ until it turns forwards again on the left side of the vertebral column, to become the first part of the jejunum. In this U-shaped loop of duodenum lies the head of the pancreas through which the bile duct passes to open into the vertical portion of the duodenum.

The stomach may be small and therefore high, or it may be very large from chronic pyloric obstruction; it then comes to lie quite low in the abdomen, being stretched by the weight of its contents. Behind the stomach is a pocket of the peritoneal cavity known as the lesser sac.

The stomach is thus completely surrounded by peritoneum on all its surfaces. If it is opened or divided at operation, the repair-line is sealed and made safe by closure of this peritoneal or 'serous' surface.

On the other hand, the duodenum, except in its first part, is not completely surrounded by peritoneum, and if it is opened at operation or torn by abdominal injury, leakage and subsequent spread of infection in the loose tissues of the posterior abdominal wall is a serious risk.

As the pancreas is so closely attached to the duodenum, surgical removal of the pancreas for growth entails also removal of the whole of the duodenum (page 599).

The veins of the stomach go into the portal system and the liver. The main lymphatic glands are grouped around the pylorus and on the undersurface of the liver.

Physiology

The stomach is a muscle and its contraction waves pass along the greater curvature from left to right. In a baby with congenital pyloric stenosis, these waves of peristalsis can be seen raising the abdominal wall in their progression towards the pylorus.

In addition to the storage and transport of food the stomach has several distinct functions. The production of hydrochloric acid and pepsin for the digestion of protein depends upon the mucous membrane lining. Sometimes this is very thick and hypertrophied with a rich blood supply. This **'hypertrophic gastritis'** is associated with excessive production of hydrochloric acid and the consequent development of **duodenal ulcers.** Sometimes the epithelial lining is atrophic—that is, of poor quality. **Atrophic gastritis** is associated with a low hydrochloric acid concentration in the digestive juice and occasionally there may be no production of acid at all (**total achlorhydria**). The stomach also manufactures in its wall a substance known as the **'intrinsic factor'**. Without the intrinsic factor, vitamin B_{12}, essential for red cell formation, is not absorbed from the bowel. Hydrochloric acid is also needed for the correct use of this intrinsic factor with an extrinsic factor in the food, and for the use of iron contained in food. Lack of acid or lack of stomach wall is therefore commonly associated with severe anaemia of the macrocytic (pernicious) type. Removal of the stomach (gastrectomy) is followed sometimes by the development of a similar condition, or by microcytic (iron deficiency) anaemia.

Acid production in the stomach is set going by the presence of food, acting through the **vagus** nerves which control stomach movement and secretions. In addition, the glands of the pyloric antrum produce a hormone, **gastrin**, which stimulates the cells of the upper part of the stomach to produce more acid. If there is excessive acid production, certain measures can be taken to correct this fault and these are described with the treatment of peptic ulcer (page 523).

The function of the duodenum is to receive the partly digested food and allow it to mix with the alkaline secretions of the duodenum, bile and enzymes from the pancreas.

Upper gastro-intestinal endoscopy

Radiological examination of the intestinal tract gives information on the shape, size and degree of mobility the organs and makes possible an accurate diagnosis in many cases, but a direct view of the inside of the tract is invaluable. Oesophagoscopy and gastrectomy for many years were done with rigid instruments on the same principle as cystoscopy. The development of flexible fibro-optic endoscopes has extended the area of examination and made the operation easier and safer.

Examination of the oesophagus with these modern fibre-optic flexible instruments has already been described on page 509. With instruments of differing lengths and viewing angles of their terminal ends it is now possible to make a complete examination of the stomach and the duodenum as far as the opening of the common bile duct. This opening may be cannulated in order that specimens of bile and pancreatic juice can be obtained and radio-opaque media injected for x-ray examination. The use of these instruments requires special training. Each costs approximately £5,000. The cleaning and maintenance of these pieces of delicate apparatus also needs special training. The stomach may be examined with a rigid metal gastroscope which has a flexible end-piece carrying a lens and light, but the fibre-optic instruments have a channel for irrigation with water and a further channel for passing instruments to enable the operator to take a biopsy specimen or grasp a foreign body. Air is pumped into the stomach to distend it to make possible examination of the fundus and antrum and as the stomach is contractile and moving all the time, the operator has to watch carefully for ulcers which may be hidden in the recesses of the mucous membrane. An attachment is used to enable a second operator to view simultaneously, for instruction and a camera can be attached for photographic records.

Principal surgical centres usually have one side viewing gastroscope for routine examination, but the more specialist investigations with these instruments are usually delegated to someone with a major interest and experience in this particular field. Gastro-duodenoscopy and cannulation of the bile duct is usually carried out under x-ray screening using the image intensifier.

Sometimes gastroscopy is undertaken to determine the site of severe haematemesis and in this case the removal of blood from the stomach may take considerable time before the operator has a clear view. The progress of healing of an ulcer can be checked and information obtained on various types of gastritis.

Preparation for endoscopy. This depends largely on the circumstances and the condition which is suspected. The procedure can be carried out using basal premedication and local anaesthesia. If pyloric obstruction has been present and the patient is known to have retention in the stomach, a preliminary gastric washout is undertaken in the ward.

Post-operative care. There is always a risk of damage to the oesophagus and leakage with subsequent mediastinitis. This is suspected if blood is found on the shaft of the instrument after its withdrawal. Many operators prescribe a small pellet of antiseptic paste (e.g. 3 G sulphathiazole) to be swallowed immediately on return to the ward. Food and drink are withheld for 3 hours after the procedure.

If the patient should complain of severe abdominal pain this must be reported immediately as it may be evidence of perforation of the stomach and x-ray examination of the abdomen is carried out immediately. If there has been a leakage, air will be seen under the diaphragm.

COMMON DISORDERS

Congenital hypertrophic pyloric stenosis

This is quite a common condition in new-born babies and its cause is not known. The thickened pyloric sphincter is spastic and forms a **palpable tumour**. The stomach enlarges and becomes powerful from working against obstruction. Persistent vomiting develops and owing to the force of the stomach this is described as **'projectile vomiting'**. Waves of **peristalsis** may be seen in the child's abdomen and the hard lump of muscle at the pylorus can readily be felt. Occasionally, x-ray examination is used to prove the diagnosis. In severe and neglected cases, gastritis develops. The child becomes extremely ill from dehydration, and constipation is a constant feature, the stools being hard from dehydration and starvation.

Many cases are now treated by Eumydrin (atropine methonitrate) which is an antispasmodic drug given with the feeds. Surgical operation is however very often necessary and in skilled hands is practically without risk; recovery is more rapid and certain after operation, than with medical treatment.

Pre-operative treatment. There is almost certain to be marked dehydration, and subcutaneous saline infusion is usually required. The persistent vomiting results in loss of chloride and the infusion should initially be of normal saline. If operation is contemplated it is better to introduce the infusion into the axilla or into the thighs rather than onto the abdominal wall. Hyalase is used to speed absorption (page 155).

A fine PVC plastic catheter is passed into the stomach and the contents aspirated. The stomach should be washed out several times with normal saline, not more than 20 ml being used at a time. Oral feeding may be completely suspended preceding operation or there may be a preliminary period of observation, during which the child may be allowed small feeds of glucose-saline. Very great care must be taken to see that all feeds are sterilised and all utensils boiled. The catheter, syringe and saline solution used for the stomach wash-out must also be sterile.

Immediately before operation the child is usually attached to a padded wooden cross (page 422).

Operation. This consists of division of the pyloric sphincter muscle (pyloromyotomy) and is **Rammstedt's operation** (Fig. 26.2). It is carried out usually under local anaesthesia

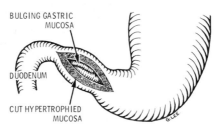

BULGING GASTRIC
MUCOSA

DUODENUM

CUT HYPERTROPHIED
MUCOSA

Fig. 26.2   Rammstedt's operation (pyloromyotomy).

(8–10 ml of 0·5 per cent lignocaine). The operation takes about 15 minutes and when the stage is reached for the surgeon to sew the peritoneal layer there is sometimes a little difficulty if the child cries or strains. This may be overcome by the nurse in charge of the baby inserting into his mouth a teat or a finger covered with a rubber finger cot, either of which should be dipped in glycerine or honey.

The baby relaxes as soon as sucking commences.

Post-operative treatment. There are many schemes of post-operative regime and it is likely that the medical staff will prescribe in detail what is to be administered by mouth.

A satisfactory feeding schedule is shown in Table 42. Feeds traditionally measured in 'drachms' or 'ounces' should now be in metric measure.

Complications. Persistent vomiting may be the result of an established gastritis and feeds will have to be introduced more slowly. Only on very rare occasions is further operative treatment necessary.

Peritonitis can develop if the mucous membrane has been opened accidentally without the surgeon being aware of this.

Pressing on with the feeding schedule too fast results in the intestinal tract being irritated and diarrhoea may develop. This may be a very severe complication and there is no great merit in hurrying with the introduction of food. **Infective gastro-enteritis** can of course also occur by cross-infection from other babies. It is always due to errors of nursing technique. Sometimes the wound becomes infected. If a tiny button of omentum has found its way between the peritoneal stitches, this appears in the incision line and may prolapse, leading to a burst wound (page 469).

Duodenal atresia and stenosis

An error of development of the duodenum may result in a portion of the tube being completely obliterated or very constricted. This obstruction gives rise to persistent

Table 42   Post-operative feeding schedule

Congenital pyloric stenosis

Hours (after operation)	Feed
0– 4	Nil
5– 8	5 ml 5% glucose with normal saline
9–12 —hourly	10 ml 5% glucose with normal saline
13–16	15 ml 5% glucose with normal saline
17–20	20 ml ½ strength milk feed*
22–28	30 ml ½ strength milk feed*
	(i.e. 340 ml of fluid in first 24 hours)
30–36 —2-hourly	60 ml ½ strength milk feed
38–48	60 ml normal milk feed
50–72—3-hourly	90 ml normal milk feed omitting one night feed
	By the fourth day normal breast feeding can be resumed.

Infant fluid requirement is 150 ml per kilo body weight.

---

* The type of milk should be the same as the baby was having before operation. If the baby is very underweight, expressed breast milk is preferable.

vomiting in the neonatal period. The diagnosis is confirmed by x-ray examination and surgical operation is essential. This may be performed under local anaesthesia, as for Rammstedt's operation, but it is more usual to employ general anaesthesia. The pre-operative and post-operative treatment is similar and usually gastro-enterostomy is performed.

Babies with this condition are often premature and almost always in a very bad condition; the operative risk is great.

Foreign bodies

Foreign bodies such as teeth, coins and toys, sometimes have to be removed from the stomach by operation. If an object has reached the stomach safely without becoming jammed in the oesophagus, it is likely that it will pass on by itself, particularly if it is round and no more than 5 cm long. It is traditional to give children who have swallowed sharp objects sandwiches containing a thin teased-out layer of cotton wool so that the spike becomes entangled in the cotton wool and rendered safe. When x-ray examination has confirmed the presence of a foreign body (if indeed it is opaque to x-rays) there is no urgency for operation unless there is evidence that the stomach wall has been perforated. The common practice is to wait for 2 to 3 weeks, because objects such as coins may pass out of the stomach as late as this. Open safety pins or common pins may become arrested anywhere in the intestinal tract. X-ray examination is made every few days and if the pin shows no sign of movement for a week, it is likely that the surgeon will operate.

Gastrotomy involves a simple incision into the front of the stomach with immediate suture after the removal of the foreign body. The wound is closed without drainage and nothing is given by mouth for 6 hours.

Injury

The stomach owing to its size is sometimes injured in gunshot or stab wounds of the upper abdomen. The wound in the stomach is repaired at laparotomy and the post-operative treatment includes the use of an indwelling gastric suction tube, careful observation for the development of peritonitis, and the restriction of oral feeding until peristalsis is resumed.

Gastrostomy

A temporary or permanent gastric fistula is established by means of a catheter introduced through the front wall of the stomach and stitched in place temporarily (Fig. 25.4). The stomach becomes attached to the anterior abdominal wall and the subsequent removal of the tube and its reinsertion is an easy matter.

Gastrostomy is performed as a palliative operation in cases of oesophageal obstruction. It is also necessary as a means of feeding the patient if large operations have been carried out on the pharynx or larynx. Severe fractures of the jaw may necessitate temporary gastrostomy to ensure adequate feeding.

The operation is performed through an upper left vertical or transverse incision and may be carried out under local anaesthesia. At the end of the operation a funnel is connected to the catheter and a feed introduced to make certain that the tube is clear.

Feeding instructions. Whatever the condition for which the operation is performed, there is the immediate post-operative risk of peritonitis and ileus and the resumption of feeding through the tube must therefore be gradual. For the first 12 hours, not more than 60 ml of warm saline or milk should be introduced 2-hourly. If there is any suspicion that ileus is present, the gastrostomy catheter must be used for repeated aspiration. A length of fine polythene tubing may be passed through it.

All feeds must be strained with very great care; hot fluids should not be used. Very soon the patient will learn how much he can tolerate at one feed.

As the conditions for which this operation is performed usually necessitate high calorie diet, special concentrated foods are given. Alcoholic beverages may be administered if desired.

The feeds are administered through a funnel with an additional length of rubber tube connected to the gastrostomy catheter. The funnel should never be held more than 40 cm above the level of the stomach. A spigot is used to close the catheter after feeding.

Various means have been devised for giving semi-solid food to gastrostomy patients and injection guns (modified motor car grease guns) are sometimes used. Such a procedure is dangerous and unnecessary unless the fistula has been established for several weeks.

Care of the skin. However carefully the operation has been performed there will probably be a leak of digestive juice around the catheter. This will lead to excoriation of the skin unless great care is taken. PVA buffer jelly or silicone cream must be smeared on the skin at least twice a day. Various special technical procedures are used from time to time in an attempt to make a valvular opening which will not leak.

Changing the tube. The catheter inserted at the time of operation should be left undisturbed for at least 10 days in order that a firm walled track may develop between the stomach and the skin. After this time there will be no difficulty in changing the catheter which should be as big as the one inserted at the time of operation. If a smaller catheter is used the fistula may close up progressively.

If the gastrostomy is to be permanent or established for any length of time, when the wound has healed a solid rubber plug may be used between feeds instead of the catheter. This keeps the channel open but prevents the escape of fluid.

Closure. If the gastrostomy is no longer required, the fistula will usually close itself without further operation. At first, after removal of the tube, there may be trouble with the skin due to a leak of gastric juice, but by then the patient will usually be ambulant and if he takes care not to overfill the stomach at his normal meal-times there is unlikely to be any significant leak. Very occasionally operation is needed to close the track.

Gastric and duodenal ulcer

Although ulcers in the stomach and in the duodenum produce similar symptoms and have similar complications, the factors which cause gastric ulceration are probably quite different from those which cause duodenal ulcers. Similar 'peptic' ulcers occur in the small intestine around a Meckel's diverticulum which is a congenital abnormality of the ileum. The diverticulum frequently contains gastric mucous membrane which produces acid.

The development of ulcers in the stomach is probably not due to excessive secretion of gastric juice but may be due to reflux of bile into the stomach: this breaks the protective anti-acid film on the surface of the stomach epithelium. On the other hand, duodenal ulceration is undoubtedly connected in some way with excessive production of hydrochloric acid by the stomach (page 513).

Ulcers may occur at any age. They may be very slow-growing and chronic, or an ulcer may develop acutely even to the point of perforating the duodenal wall within a day or so.

There are undoubtedly nervous factors in the production of these ulcers. The very conscientious hard-working individual who is constantly in a state of mental tension is particularly prone to duodenal ulcer. Occupations which incur heavy responsibility or irregular meals are also contributory factors. Excessive smoking, syphilis, and the eating of highly spiced foods have all been claimed as possible causes. In the present state of knowledge all that can be said is that these various factors may be aggravating causes and therefore need to be eliminated in the treatment of ulcer whether this is by medical or surgical means.

Alcoholic drinks, particularly of spirit, and excessive smoking of cigarettes are the most important known aggravating causes. Both these habits are readily acquired by the over-conscientious and anxious individual, who is already predisposed to the development of 'peptic' ulcer.

Acute ulceration may be produced by drugs of which aspirin and potassium chloride are the most common. Even Slow-K tablets used to replace potassium depletion in patients taking diuretics can produce ulceration of oesophagus or stomach.

Complications of peptic ulceration

Perforation. The ulcer erodes the wall of the stomach or duodenum and eventually reaches the peritoneal coat. If this erosive process is gradual, local peritonitis develops and other organs—such as the gall bladder—become adherent to the site of the ulcer. A gastric ulcer may become attached to the undersurface of the liver or may eat its way into the pancreas. If the ulcerative process is more rapid there is insufficient time for adhesion formation, and the ulcer bursts into the peritoneal cavity producing a leak of gastric or duodenal contents.

The occurrence of perforation is usually catastrophic and is followed by the development of peritonitis and collapse. It is one of the most common abdominal emergencies. The sudden onset of violent upper abdominal pain which later spreads to the whole abdomen, associated with a slow pulse (from shock), pallor and low temperature, is quite characteristic. At first the clinical picture resembles that produced by perforation of the appendix or by other grave abdominal emergencies such as acute pancreatitis (page 599). The sudden release of hydrochloric acid or duodenal contents into the peritoneal cavity may at first stimulate peristalsis but very soon leads to complete ileus. The abdomen is therefore silent when a stethoscope is applied. Gas also escapes from the hole in the stomach or duodenum and rises into the upper abdomen. It may be identified between the liver and the diaphragm by x-ray examination, which is diagnostic of a perforation.

Except in very rare instances when perforation has been a gradual process, the condition is treated by urgent operation. The perforation is stitched up and in some cases the peritoneal cavity is drained through a suprapubic stab wound. Pre-operative and postoperative nursing routine is exactly the same as for other forms of acute peritonitis. Continuous gastric aspiration, restriction of oral feeding and attention to chest expansion exercises are the principal features (page 473).

Following perforation, subphrenic or pelvic abscess may develop. The presence of such a localised collection of pus will be shown by the failure of the temperature to return to normal and by persistent toxaemia. If pyrexia develops during the second post-operative week, abscess formation is suspected.

When the peritonitis has subsided and normal bowel action has returned, the course to be adopted will depend on previous history of ulcer symptoms. Operation at a later date may be recommended to prevent a recurrence of the ulcer. Medical treatment will be instituted as soon as possible after operation: this will include diet, antacid medicines and sedatives.

Haemorrhage. If the ulcer erodes an artery in the wall of the stomach, bleeding will occur. In gastric ulceration the haemorrhage may be very great or even fatal. Gastric ulcer is the commonest cause of haematemesis. Large quantities of bright blood may be vomited or the blood may be altered by the presence of hydrochloric acid and appear dark and granular (the so-called coffee-ground vomit). Bleeding from duodenal ulcer may also be devastating and lead to sudden collapse. The blood usually passes down the small bowel and results in the passage of several 'melaena' stools. Blood in the bowel undergoes putrefaction and subsequent distension is sometimes a further complication following this haemorrhage.

A patient admitted to hospital suffering from severe gastro-intestinal haemorrhage of this type is treated for shock. He must be kept absolutely flat, and the foot of the bed may be raised. Blood transfusion must be initiated at once if the systolic blood pressure is under 90 mm. Several pints of blood may be necessary.

Most cases of acute haemorrhage from gastric or duodenal ulcer are treated by medical means with rest and blood transfusion; in the majority of cases the bleeding stops spontaneously within 24 hours. Repeated or persistent bleeding, however, requires surgical treatment and the operation of gastrectomy may be carried out as an emergency. The nursing management of the patient with severe gastric or duodenal bleeding does not differ in any important particular from that of a patient with peritonitis. While the bleeding continues it is probable that a gastric aspiration tube will not be tolerated because of repeated vomiting. The patient is kept under the influence of morphine to reduce the restlessness. Oral feeding is suspended until it is thought that the bleeding has stopped.

Penetration. This is really the same erosive process as perforation, but the ulcer site has become adherent to some other organ and has continued eroding so that the tissues of the liver, pancreas, or perhaps the colon may be subsequently involved. If an ulcer has penetrated into the pancreas it will certainly not heal under medical treatment and surgical operation is called for. The colon becomes attached and eroded, particularly in ulcers which recur after short-circuit operations (gastro-enterostomy) performed for the treatment of duodenal ulcer. A **gastro-colic fistula** forms; faecal material gains entry to the stomach and partially digested food escapes into the colon. Gastro-colic fistula leads to rapid loss of weight and requires radical surgical treatment.

Malignant change. Carcinoma may develop in a gastric ulcer. The change is sometimes indicated by an alteration of the patient's symptoms, especially when he is known to have had an ulcer for many years. On the other hand, a malignant ulcer may develop very rapidly without any previous symptoms or sign of ulceration. X-ray examination may suggest from the character of the ulcer that it is malignant. If there is any suspicion of malignancy in a particular case of gastric ulceration, operative treatment is undertaken. Duodenal ulcer practically never becomes malignant.

Pyloric obstruction. The presence of an active ulcer near the pylorus leads to spasm and oedema. This produces complete obstruction to the passage of food through the pylorus and leads to persistent vomiting, which may subside under strict medical treatment. By a process of repeated ulceration and scarring as the ulcer heals, the pylorus may become permanently obstructed. The gradual narrowing process may take place over many years. The stomach becomes grossly distended.

Pyloric obstruction is shown by repeated vomiting and in severe cases this leads to gross dehydration and malnutrition. Putrefaction of gastric contents reduces the acid-forming property of the stomach so that the patient's digestion is further impaired.

Operation is required for pyloric obstruction. Although the scarring is very unlikely to produce complete obstruction in the lumen of the pylorus, it so narrows the outlet of the stomach that spasm and oedema arising from recurrence of an ulcer will in fact make the obstruction complete. If such a patient is admitted to hospital and the stomach washed out, it is probable that the oedema and spasm may pass off, and normal feeding may be resumed. Nursing treatment therefore involves repeated stomach wash-outs, the administration of small fluid feeds and probably the parenteral infusion of fluid containing electrolytes, glucose and proteins, and vitamins before operation can be undertaken. The pre-operative preparation will include particular attention to oral hygiene and dental sepsis. It is likely that 1 or 2 weeks will be spent in improving the patient's nutrition unless the obstruction is such that vomiting is severe, and nothing is retained.

In addition to the scarring which obstructs the pylorus a similar stricture may appear across the body of the stomach from a large gastric ulcer, producing the **'hour-glass stomach'**. This is also treated by surgical operation.

Diagnosis of peptic ulcer

There are three main channels by which the patient with a peptic ulcer may come to surgical treatment:

(a) By reason of an acute complication such as perforation or haemorrhage. If there has been no previous investigation the diagnosis will rest upon the immediate history and physical signs. In most hospitals, the usual practice is to admit cases of gastro-intestinal haemorrhage initially to medical wards. The surgeon is then called in consultation if the bleeding is not controlled by rest and transfusion.

(b) By transfer from a medical unit or general practitioner owing to the failure of conservative treatment by diet and rest. The majority of cases of peptic ulcer which come for surgical treatment are in this category.

(c) By direct reference to a surgical department on account of abdominal pain, persistent vomiting, or suspicion of malignant disease.

Except in the emergency cases, barium-meal examination is carried out and the diagnosis of gastric or duodenal ulcer is not accepted unless its presence is proved by x-ray examination. Further investigations may be carried out, such as the acid secretion test (page 258), which is of value particularly in cases of duodenal ulceration to assess the degree of hyperacidity. The presence of hyperchlorhydria makes it more likely that further ulcers will develop, and if surgical operation is undertaken steps have to be taken to reduce the acid production of the stomach.

Treatment of gastric and duodenal ulcer

The treatment of these conditions follows the basic principles outlined in Chapter 2. Complete rest is absolutely necessary and this must include freedom from anxiety. Such a period of absolute rest can only be achieved by the patient remaining in bed at home or in hospital, and this is often regarded as essential before resorting to surgical treatment. A duodenal ulcer will usually heal if the patient can be persuaded to stop work and spend several weeks in bed. Septic teeth and tonsils are removed. When anaemia is present it is treated. Sedative medicine such as phenobarbitone is used to allay anxiety. A great deal of attention is paid to diet. The principles of dietetic treatment are that the stomach should never remain empty but the flow of gastric juice should be discouraged.

Medical treatment   Excess acid production can be neutralised by administering alkaline medicines. These are of two types. Powders containing bismuth and magnesium carbonate, and sodium bicarbonate—the so-called stomach powders—combine directly with the acid of the stomach. Pain is relieved and therefore anxiety is allayed. Unfortunately the presence of the compounds formed by the combination of acid and alkalis may upset the digestive processes which normally occur in the intestinal tract. The second group of chemicals neutralise the acid but the compound which results is inert and cannot be absorbed; it does not interfere with intestinal digestion: these are powders or tablets containing **magnesium trisilicate** or **aluminium hydroxide**. Antacid medicines, to be effective, really need to be given at least every two hours.

Gastric acidity can be neutralised readily by the administration of milk or other bland foods which do not excite the appetite. The diet is regulated in such a way that all stimulant foods are excluded; protein of a neutralising type is given every 2 hours, while all meals are small in bulk. The diet also must include essential vitamins, adequate iron, and a total calorie requirement between 2000 and 3000.

One of the most effective ways of treating an ulcer by medical means is by the gastric drip milk feed. A Ryle's tube is inserted in the usual way and connected to a reservoir through a drip chamber. Milk is administered continuously for several days and nights.

Reference has been made on page 258 to the effect of histamine in stimulating gastric secretion. Recently drugs with an action similar to the antihistamines have been found to have a specific effect in suppressing acid and pepsin production. **Metiamide** is one such drug and this may well bring about a really dramatic change in the management of ulcers.

Another group of drugs inhibit the vagus nerve's effect; these are:

propantheline bromide (Probanthine)   **isopropamide iodide** (Tyrimide)
dicyclomine hydrochloride (Merbentyl)   **poldine methylsulphate** (Nacton)
hyoscine butylbromide (Buscopan)

These should never be given if there is a history of difficulty with micturition, or of glaucoma and all may affect visual accommodation. Driving a motor vehicle, fine craft work or even reading may be markedly affected.

Two other drugs are in common use: these are **carbenoxolone** (Biogastrone) for gastric ulcer and a slow release preparation of the same drug (Duogastrone) for duodenal ulcer. Their effect is similar to that of cortisone, probably releasing an anti-inflammatory steroid and the side effects are similar—water and sodium retention and potassium urinary loss. Patients who take these for a long period or in high dose may develop oedema, ascites and heart failure. Hypertension if present may be made much worse.

Economic factors prevent many patients from undergoing extensive courses of medical treatment for ulceration. Financial and domestic considerations have to be taken into account in deciding whether surgical operation is required.

Surgical treatment. Gastric ulcers develop most commonly along the lesser curve of the stomach (the right hand border). Duodenal ulcers almost always occur in the part of the duodenum immediately beyond the pyloric sphincter. The most logical way of treating gastric ulcers is therefore to remove as much as possible of the lesser curvature and the adjacent portion of the stomach, where ulceration is most likely to recur. Similarly, if the first part of the duodenum is removed it might be thought that duodenal ulceration would likewise be prevented. Unfortunately, although removal of part of the stomach is almost always effective for gastric ulceration, removal of the first part of the duodenum is frequently followed by recurrence in those patients who have had duodenal ulcer: ulcers subsequently develop on the stomach or anastomosis to small intestine. An attempt is therefore made to reduce the acid-producing power of the stomach by removing the whole of the pyloric antrum (which produces the hormone gastrin, page 513) and part of the body of the stomach as well. Sometimes the vagus nerves are cut where they travel from the thorax, through the diaphragm, lying against the oesophagus. By these methods the normal physiological process of acid production is intercepted.

In cases of advanced pyloric obstruction from scarring, it is likely that the ulcer has healed and also that the acid-producing power of the stomach has been greatly reduced by long-standing gastritis. Sometimes the simple operation of gastro-enterostomy is performed to by-pass the obstruction at the pylorus.

Fifty years ago gastro-enterostomy had become a safe and short operation and was performed for all types of ulceration of stomach and duodenum. A great many cases of ulcer were relieved by this operation which became extremely popular. Unfortunately, many cases subsequently developed peptic ulcer of the small bowel and jejunum (at the site of anastomosis). Jejunal or **'anastomotic' ulcer** produces more pain and more distress than the original ulceration.

Apart from the treatment of the emergency complications—haemorrhage and perforation—surgical operations performed now for treatment of ulceration are:

1. Partial gastrectomy.
2. Gastro-enterostomy.
3. Partial gastrectomy, vagotomy (division of vagus nerves), with pyloroplasty or gastro-enterostomy.

Partial gastrectomy

This is one of the most common major upper-abdominal operations. It has been made safe by advances in anaesthetic technique, particularly by the introduction of the relaxant drugs.

Two main types of partial gastrectomy are undertaken in the treatment of ulcer— the Billroth I and the Polya or Moynihan type. These operations are named after pioneers in gastric surgery and many modifications of their original methods have been introduced. The essential difference of these two groups is that in the Billroth I operation (Fig. 26.3)

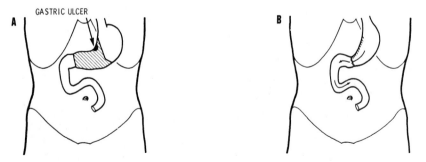

Fig. 26.3   Billroth I type of partial gastrectomy for gastric ulcer: gastro-duodenostomy.

the ulcer-bearing lesser curvature of the stomach is removed, together with the pyloric antrum and the pylorus. The duodenum is joined to the re-fashioned stomach. There is therefore no blind loop and all food passes through the duodenum in the usual way.

The Polya operation (Fig. 26.4) removes a major portion of the stomach together with the pylorus and most of the first part of the duodenum. The duodenum is closed and thus forms a blind loop into which pours bile and pancreatic juice. The jejunum beyond the duodeno-jejunal flexure is taken up in a loop to the divided stomach which is joined to an incision in the side of the jejunum. The gastric contents do not any longer pass through the duodenum but the alkaline duodenal juice and bile passes into the stomach and may help by neutralising the acid. Sometimes the small intestinal loop is brought up to the stomach in front of the colon and sometimes it is taken through the mesentery of the colon. These modifications have no influence on the nursing technique except that in the Polya type it is possible for the aspiration tube to be passed on through the anastomosis into one of the intestinal loops. A false impression will then be obtained from the larger quantities of fluid aspirated (Fig. 26.6).

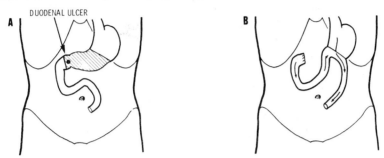

Fig. 26.4 Partial gastrectomy, Polya type for gastric or duodenal ulcer: resection followed by gastrojejunal anastomosis (in the Moynihan operation the intestinal loop is reversed).

Pre-operative preparation. Whatever diet the patient has been having previously will be continued until 24 hours before the operation. No further solid food will be given and nothing at all should be taken by mouth for 12 hours prior to operation. Ascorbic acid (vitamin C) is given by mouth or by injection; probably a total of 2000 mg will be prescribed during the week preceding operation. The patient's blood must be grouped and it is usual for blood to be available for transfusion. If there has been any suggestion of pyloric obstruction, the stomach must be washed out on the evening before operation. Thick residue may require the use of a special pump (Fig. 26.5). A 1 per cent solution of sodium bicarbonate may be used for this purpose as it helps to remove the mucus from the stomach (Fig. 26.5). On the morning of operation a Ryle's tube is passed into the

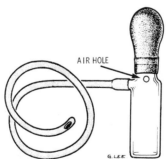

Fig. 26.5 The wide-bore oesophageal or Senoran's tube is passed and the stomach contents aspirated by suction from the bulb. When the pump is connected to the tube the bulb is squeezed and the operator's finger placed over the air-hole each time the bulb is released. If the stomach contents are to be sent for analysis, the glass bottle is stoppered with the various fittings shown. If the stomach is to be washed out, the bottle may be half filled with sodium bicarbonate solution and tilted so that the fluid runs into the stomach by gravity; air is allowed to enter the bottle at this stage: the wash-out fluid is then aspirated by working the suction bulb. Pressure must never be used during the injection phase.

stomach and any residual fluid aspirated. The tube remains in place throughout the operation. According to the routine of the particular unit, intravenous infusion may be set up in the ward before operation or it may be started by the anaesthetist at the beginning of operation. Some surgeons prefer the use of a high colonic infusion through a ureteric catheter inserted after the induction of anaesthesia. The sigmoidoscope is needed for this purpose.

Complications of partial gastrectomy

According to the difficulties which may be encountered and depending on the type of operation which is performed, the operation may vary in length from perhaps 1½ to 3 hours.

Shock, haemorrhage, peritonitis and pulmonary atelectasis are the four principal hazards. The surgeon endeavours to control all bleeding from the cut edges of the stomach and intestine by placing the stitches very close together. Bleeding may however continue or may recur later from infection at the site of anastomosis. Peritonitis may arise from contamination of the peritoneal cavity at the time of operation as the stomach and small bowel are opened in performing the anastomosis. The main fear is that there will be a leak from the site of anastomosis or, after the Polya type of operation, from the stump of the duodenum (Fig. 26.6). It is most likely to occur from back-pressure of fluid which has accumulated in the stomach due to obstruction of the out-going loop, or from distension of the duodenum by kinking of the proximal (afferent) loop. The presence of peritonitis will be suspected if severe abdominal pain persists more than 36 hours after operation, or comes on suddenly (like perforation) after a period of relative comfort.

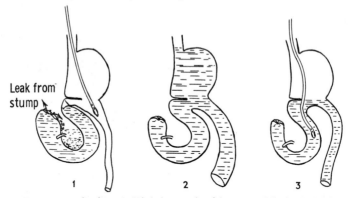

Leak from
stump

1   2   3

Fig. 26.6 Post-gastrectomy aspiration. **1.** Kink in proximal loop: no bile in aspiration: risk of burst from duodenal stump. **2.** Ileus: produces continuous regurgitation. **3.** Excessive aspiration of bile: the tube has been passed too far and has entered the proximal loop.

Drainage. Sometimes a precautionary rubber drainage strip or tube is left in position down to the duodenal stump in case there is leakage from the closed end or from the anastomosis. If the discharge becomes profuse it is tested with litmus paper: a strongly alkaline discharge is coming from the duodenum or small bowel: an acid fluid is coming from the stomach and the tube must remain in position until the discharge ceases. Normally it is withdrawn by repeated daily shortening after the first 3 days.

Similarly, if an ulcer has been firmly adherent to liver or pancreas, a drain is left down to the raw area of the appropriate organ. It is likewise withdrawn by shortening after the 3rd day.

Post-operative routine

The immediate after-care must include:

(a) Maintenance of adequate respiration: If the respiration rate and depth are low, oxygen should be administered without hesitation: consciousness may not be regained for 10 hours or more after an operation of this severity, especially in elderly patients who have had excessive morphine.

(b) Measures to prevent or treat shock: The bed is warmed; pain is relieved by morphine or pethidine as soon as the patient becomes restless, and elevation of the foot of the bed is advisable.

(c) Gastric aspiration by Ryle's tube: This must be repeated at half-hourly intervals at first; bright blood may be withdrawn, as haemorrhage from the inside (mucous membrane) layer of the anastomosis is the most important complication at this time. Some altered (brown) blood and mucus, with regurgitated bile, will be aspirated in most cases, and if there is no bright blood, the intervals can be increased to an hour, after the first 2 hours.

(d) Breathing exercises as soon as consciousness is regained: Failure to encourage this in the first few hours may result in atelectasis.

(e) Parenteral fluid and electrolyte administration: This must be maintained at an intake rate of 2000–3000 ml in the first and subsequent 24-hour periods: oral feeding is normally prohibited until peristalsis has been resumed (as detected by stethoscope), but some surgeons allow fluid by mouth as soon as consciousness is regained. There is very little risk in doing this as any excess amount which accumulates will be withdrawn at the hourly aspiration and the patient is helped by being allowed to sip water or saline. Infusion is rarely necessary after 72 hours.

All fluid administered by mouth or aspirated by the tube is measured and the quantity entered on the fluid balance chart. At the end of each 12-hour period the total fluid administration and fluid loss by urine and gastric aspiration is balanced and the fluid infusion intake adjusted accordingly.

If the amount of fluid aspirated from the stomach exceeds the oral intake by more than 30 ml for each hour it is likely that there is some degree of obstruction to the out-flow from the intestinal loop. Saliva and gastric secretions account for at least an ounce an hour.

If the tube has been passed too far it may have travelled through the anastomosis and the aspiration may be entirely of intestinal or duodenal fluid. The tube should not normally be passed for more than 50 cm from the incisor teeth or it will enter the intestinal loops.

The continued aspiration of large quantities of fluid may arise from:

(*a*) a kink in the outgoing loop of the anastomosis (Fig. 26.6),
(*b*) obstruction at the stoma itself from oedema or haematoma formation,
(*c*) intestinal ileus,
(*d*) mechanical obstruction lower down the intestinal tract, i.e. volvulus or adhesions. The small bowel may be kinked by the presence of a distended loaded colon when pre-operative evacuation of the bowel has not been adequate.

If any of these complications arise, parenteral fluid administration has to be continued, and a second operation may be required. In the majority of cases, the post-operative obstruction is only temporary.

On general lines the post-operative management is the same as for a case of peritonitis. There is gradual resumption of normal light diet towards the end of the first post-operative week.

The patient is usually allowed out of bed within a few days of operation and he is able to leave hospital towards the end of the 2nd week. A further 2 or 3 weeks' convalescence is required.

Late complications of partial gastrectomy

When the immediate post-operative hazards have passed and normal gastro-intestinal rhythm has been established, certain other well-recognised complications may arise. Instructions are given to the patients when they leave hospital in order to reduce the risk of these complications, but it is clearly not wise to suggest to any patient all the things that may arise! Many hospitals institute a follow-up scheme for peptic ulcer patients so that they are reviewed perhaps twice a year, and suitably advised if any complication should have arisen.

Intestinal hurry. Reference has already been made to the risk of increasing the diet too rapidly, and from time to time any patient who has undergone partial gastrectomy may have short attacks of diarrhoea because inadequately prepared food has reached the small intestine. This complication rarely becomes serious, and if the patient realises the cause he can regulate his diet to cure the disability. Tab. codeine co. is often completely effective in patients who find that a meal over-stimulates intestinal activity; two tablets are taken twice a day: this is a convenient form in which to administer codeine which in all normal people has a slight constipating effect.

Post-gastrectomy or 'dumping' syndrome. In this condition the patient experiences a feeling of gross distension after a meal and may not be relieved until he has vomited. This is thought to be due to distension of the duodenal loop from food passing into it instead of being conveyed down the intestinal tract. It may also be due to the accumulation of bile in the rather long proximal loop and most of these patients are completely relieved if they lie down for a few minutes **before** their main meals. This enables the bile to drain from the proximal loop into the stomach whence it passes on down the intestinal tract when the normal position is resumed.

A more severe form of 'dumping' is due to the sudden entry of a large quantity of carbohydrate into the intestinal tract. Its rapid absorption leads to the reflex production of insulin from the pancreas. The insulin secretion is excessive and over-balances the glucose absorption. The patient then experiences the symptoms of hypoglycaemia (insulin overdose) from 1 to 2 hours after a meal. Sickness, pallor, sweating and collapse may occur. The disability may be overcome by reducing the amount of carbohydrate taken at any one meal, or by taking an additional glucose or sugar drink at approximately the time at which the attack usually develops after the main meal.

Anaemia. The great reduction of acid formation which follows partial gastrectomy may result in insufficient absorption of iron from the diet, and so lead to microcytic anaemia (page 513).

Anaemia of a pernicious type (macrocytic) may also develop if a large portion of the stomach has been removed, since the intrinsic factor necessary for red blood formation produced in the stomach wall is now missing.

It is advisable for patients who have undergone radical partial gastrectomy to be given iron-containing medicine and vitamin B preparations for perhaps 1 month in each year.

If a patient complains of lassitude and inability to work, or to concentrate, following his operation, his symptoms may well be due to anaemia and routine blood examinations should be performed every 6 months if possible.

Recurrence of ulceration. A return of the ulcer in a patient who has had a partial gastrectomy for gastric ulceration is uncommon, but a certain number of patients who have a similar operation for duodenal ulceration develop subsequent ulcers in the stomach or at the site of anastomosis— **anastomotic ulcer**. The symptoms are rather similar to the original ones but the pain is mostly on the left side of the abdomen. Treatment by medical means is rarely successful and a further operation is necessary, probably with division of the vagus nerves.

Gastro-enterostomy

This is an operation in which the duodenum is short-circuited by a loop of small intestine being joined directly to the lower border of the stomach. It is performed for three distinct reasons:

(a) Pyloric obstruction or duodenal stenosis due to some congenital deformity.
(b) Pyloric obstruction due to scarring following duodenal or gastric ulceration. (Partial gastrectomy is usually preferable but not always necessary.)
(c) Pyloric obstruction due to carcinoma as a purely palliative measure when the primary tumour cannot be removed (Fig. 26.7).

PYLORIC NEOPLASM

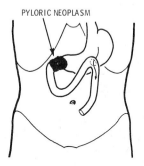

Fig. 26.7   Gastro-enterostomy. Palliative operation for pyloric obstruction.

Pre-operative preparation is exactly as for gastrectomy, but a daily stomach wash-out may be necessary to clean the stomach if obstruction has been prolonged; preparation for at least 3 days is desirable.

Post-operative treatment and nursing is exactly the same as for partial gastrectomy. The risks and complications are, for all practical purposes, the same in nature but less likely to occur.

Vagotomy

Over-secretion of acid is an undoubted factor in the production of duodenal ulcers. Vagus nerve impulses contribute to this acid secretion and reference has already been made to the surgical division of this nerve in the treatment of ulcers (pages 513, 523, 529). If vagotomy is required as the initial surgical treatment for peptic ulceration it is usual to perform the operation through the abdomen and combine it with some further procedure to ensure easy emptying of the stomach. Division of the vagus nerve leads to stasis in the stomach and spasm of the pylorus so the surgeon either does a pyloroplasty or a gastro-enterostomy. The simplest form of pyloroplasty to enlarge the canal is to cut it open in its long axis and sew up the cut at right angles to the axis of the bowel, but whatever operation is performed with vagotomy the possible complications and the management will be the same. If on the other hand vagotomy is being undertaken because ulceration has occurred, perhaps at the site of a former anastomosis, the surgeon may decide to do the operation through the thorax, in which case the post-operative management will be that of a thoracotomy. In either case the operation involves bruising of the diaphragm and there is a tendency for the patient to develop collapse of the left lung. Intensive physiotherapy for chest expansion is desirable soon after operation.

Patients who have had a vagotomy may develop looseness of the bowels which is sometimes very persistent. Intestinal hurry may be controlled completely by the patient having 1 compound codeine tablet a day, but if the looseness continues in spite of codeine and attention to the diet, malnutrition may occur from malabsorption. In 'selective' and 'proximal gastric' vagotomy the main vagus nerve trunks are not divided and no drainage (pyloroplasty) procedure is needed. There is less likely to be bowel function disturbance.

CARCINOMA OF THE STOMACH

There are various forms in which carcinoma may develop in the stomach. Sometimes a large 'cauliflower-like' growth may be present for many months in the upper part of the stomach without producing symptoms. Other patients come first with the symptoms of a gastric ulcer which is subsequently found to be malignant. A third form of carcinoma spreads slowly through the wall of the stomach which becomes hard and leather-like—the so-called 'leather bottle stomach'. The symptoms produced by this last form are due to lack of hydrochloric acid and other secretions of the stomach. Severe anaemia and anorexia arise.

Carcinoma of the stomach is rarely cured by surgical means. Radiotherapy is not effective and it is doubtful whether very large operations are of great value, since they involve the complete removal of stomach and considerable risk to life, with only a very slight chance of genuine cure. By the time carcinoma of the stomach produces symptoms the disease has usually spread to lymph glands and probably to the liver.

A patient may complain only of mild digestive symptoms and yet on examination may be found to have a grossly enlarged liver and ascites.

Operations are undertaken on many occasions to remove the primary growth if it is causing obstruction to the flow of food through the pylorus, although one knows at the time of operation that there is no hope of curing the patient of his disease. Two or three years of useful life may follow before recurrence arises in the liver or elsewhere in the abdomen.

Partial gastrectomy is undertaken whenever it is possible to remove the main growth and the operation is usually one of the Polya type.

Gastro-enterostomy is sometimes performed if the growth is at the pylorus and cannot be removed: the body of the stomach may be free from growth, and it is then a relatively safe procedure to join a loop of small intestine to it so that the patient can eat and enjoy food normally.

When radical excision of the stomach is performed for carcinoma which has not spread elsewhere as far as can be seen, the whole stomach is removed. The duodenal stump is closed and a loop of small intestine joined to the lower end of the oesophagus. Fig. 26.8 shows the resulting anastomosis. Alternatively the transverse colon may be

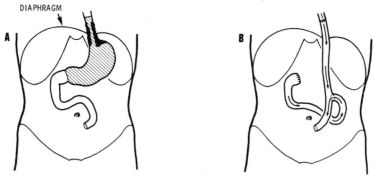

Fig. 26.8   A. Carcinoma of cardiac end of stomach. B. Total gastrectomy, with anastomosis of jejunum to oesophagus, through abdomino-thoracic incision.

separated from the rest of the large bowel and is swung up to replace the stomach. All these procedures carry a high risk, and intestinal obstruction from ileus, peritonitis or mechanical kinking is common. Even if the immediate outcome is successful, the patients often have great discomfort with feeding and suffer from persistent failure to gain weight. The post-operative nursing is similar to that for partial gastrectomy, but it is likely that the thorax will have been opened by the thoraco-abdominal approach (Fig. 26.9) and nursing will involve the general principles in the care of thoracotomy (Chapter 34).

Patients with carcinoma of the stomach are usually suffering from gross malnutrition owing to a prolonged period of loss of appetite or vomiting. Healing after operation is sometimes delayed and particular care is taken to use sutures which will not be digested

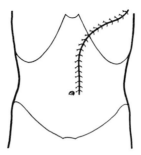

Fig. 26.9   Left paramedian incision with thoracic extension for thoraco-abdominal gastrectomy.

by the tissues. Thread is used instead of catgut for the anastomosis and stainless steel wire or nylon for the abdominal wall.

During the pre- and post-operative periods, large doses of vitamin C will be given as for other gastric cases. Blood transfusion will almost certainly be required, partly to combat the shock of the operation and partly because healing is delayed by the presence of severe anaemia.

The hopeless laparotomy

From time to time the surgeon is faced with a patient with advanced intra-abdominal disease. From barium x-ray investigations and from presence of ascites he may already know that carcinoma of the stomach has become widespread. Exploration of the abdomen may seem a fruitless procedure and yet often we feel it necessary to look and be quite certain that nothing can be done surgically. Releasing the ascites increases the patient's comfort, and chemotherapy may be instituted in the sure knowledge that no alternative procedure will help. After such laparotomy, the patient may be told that nothing further can be done and the aim then is the relief of symptoms. Psychologically the patient has often been considerably helped; it is terrible to be told that operation is not being undertaken because the situation is too bad. With increasing use of anti-cancer drugs even widespread peritoneal secondary deposits may be checked. Metastasis in the liver may be treated by chemotherapy through the hepatic artery (page 435).

Occasionally such hopeless cases improve greatly for a while and the family is given 'breathing space' and time to adjust to the expected outcome.

27

The Small Intestine

In the adult the combined length of the jejunum and ileum is more than 6 metres. The small bowel is completely surrounded by peritoneum and is suspended from the posterior abdominal wall by the mesentery. This is 15 cm long at its base, which curves across the posterior abdominal wall, and resembles a fan. It consists of two layers of peritoneum between which are sandwiched arteries, veins, nerves, lymphatics and lymphatic glands. At the free edge of the mesentery which is 6 metres long, the two layers of peritoneum divide to enclose the small bowel. From the base of the mesentery to the bowel is between 12 and 20 cm. The coils of small intestine pack the inside of the abdomen and are freely movable around the other viscera.

Clinical disorders

Errors of development of the intestine lead, as in the duodenum, to strictures and gaps (atresia). If these conditions are diagnosed soon after birth successful operation is sometimes possible, but the calibre of the baby's intestine is so small that anastomosis frequently fails.

Obstruction. The subject of intestinal obstruction has been discussed in general in Chapter 24.

The most common disorder of the small intestine is obstruction to its lumen. This may arise from:

1. Foreign bodies or large lumps of food, swallowed accidentally.
2. Kinking around adhesions or congenital bands of tissue stretching across the peritoneal cavity.
3. Volvulus (Fig. 24.9). This condition usually affects the sigmoid colon and rarely occurs in the small bowel unless there is a band to cause a loop or twist. A particular type of volvulus affects the whole of the small intestine of a newborn baby. This arises because the bowel develops outside the abdomen. During the later months of pregnancy it is drawn in through the umbilical opening, it takes the wrong path (malrotation) and may then get twisted on an abnormal mesentry. If a diagnosis is made within a few hours of birth the baby can sometimes be saved by surgery.
4. Hernia. A knuckle of small bowel very readily slips into the sac of a hernia and

may become nipped at the entrance. Intestinal contents are trapped in the loop and fermentation increases the distension. The blood vessels then become compressed and the hernia is said to be 'strangulated'. Gangrene of the bowel will develop unless the pressure is relieved by operation or reduction of the hernia by pressure.

5. Involvement by a growth in another organ or by another tumour; the coils of the small intestine become attached to the inflamed area and are subsequently compressed or infiltrated by the growth.

6. Mesenteric thrombosis. This condition affects the veins and sometimes the arteries of the mesentery and sections of the bowel become gangrenous (page 482).

7. Intussusception (page 423, Fig. 27.1). This is a condition which occurs usually in childhood. It is thought to be due primarily to the enlargement of lymphatic tissue in the bowel at a time when the child's digestion is having to deal with a more varied and adult type of diet—towards the end of the first year. The wall of the bowel becomes infolded and carried along so that the peristalsis propels one section of the small bowel into another, often into the caecum and around the transverse colon. Occasionally the 'head' of the intussusception can appear in the rectum. The condition is accompanied by a violent colic and vomiting, and in the intervals between the spasms the child may appear quite well. Quite often, but by no means always, the baby will pass stools described as resembling red currant jelly, from haemorrhage. Immediate operation is required. Usually the bowel can be withdrawn, but sometimes it has become gangrenous and has to be removed. In the adult a similar condition can arise from the presence of a growth which acts as the head of the intussusception, being carried on rather like a bolus of food.

8. Meconium ileus. In the condition muco-viscidosis, sometimes called fibro-cystic disease, there is a congenital enzyme deficiency which leads to the absence of proper mucus production in the lungs, pancreas and the intestinal tract. This in turn produces stasis in the bowel of the baby during its development and the meconium obstructs the intestine, sometimes to the point of perforation before it is born. The baby develops meconium peritonitis and it may then be born prematurely, or even stillborn. After birth the condition shows itself as intestinal obstruction with tremendous distension of the bowel. At operation the whole of the small intestine is blocked by thick putty like meconium which is extremely difficult to remove. If the baby survives the operative relief of the obstruction it is given pancreatin which aids the digestion and may permit normal development.

Meckel's diverticulum. This is a congenital pouch arising from the wall of the ileum. It resembles the appendix and becomes inflamed in the same way. Sometimes its wall contains mucous membrane like the stomach and peptic ulcers develop which subsequently bleed. A diverticulum may become infolded and lead to the development of intussusception.

Wounds. Multiple wounds of the small bowel are produced by the passage of a bullet or bomb splinter through the abdomen. An explosion occasionally bursts the bowel without damaging the abdominal wall. Stab wounds may puncture the bowel even though the abdominal wall shows only a small cut.

Neoplasm. Neoplasms of the small bowel are extremely rare and produce symptoms by obstructing the lumen.

Ileitis. 'Regional ileitis' is a specific chronic inflammatory condition which usually affects the terminal part of the ileum. It produces chronic obstruction but may not be discovered until an abscess forms around the inflamed bowel; the condition is then sometimes mistaken for appendicitis. A similar disease affects parts of the colon. An alternative name is Crohn's disease. Acute ileitis occasionally is due to *Yersinia pseudo-tuberculosis* infection, thought to come from animals, particularly birds. It is a self-limiting infection lasting about 2 months and is usually diagnosed as acute appendicitis.

Both the small and large intestine are affected by typhoid and other forms of acute dysentery and may perforate with resultant peritonitis. The clinical picture is then confused by the severe illness of which peritonitis is the presenting sympton.

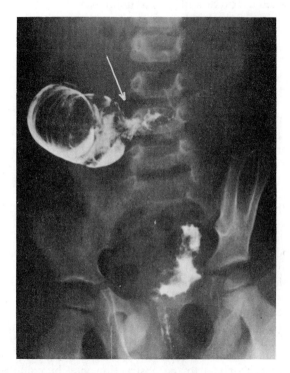

Fig. 27.1 Intussusception. The child has been given a barium enema which was seen to run in as far as the hepatic flexure. The above film taken after evacuation of the enema shows barium adherent to the circular folds of the small intestine, which has travelled up inside the colon to the point shown where it has produced obstruction. Sometimes a barium enema successfully forces the small intestine back out of the colon and reduces the intussusception completely.

Intestinal grafts

Because of its mobility and peritoneal covering the small intestine is sometimes used to replace the stomach or oesophagus in radical operations for cancer (Fig. 26.8): a portion of ileum is used to divert the urinary tract or replace a ureter (page 687).

Diagnosis

Almost every disease of the small intestine requiring surgical treatment produces colic, vomiting, and distension. When obstruction is high up in the small bowel towards the duodenal end, the distension may be very slight and vomiting will come on more quickly. If, on the other hand, the obstruction is at the lower end near the caecum there is a much greater length of bowel to become distended and vomiting will occur later. Chronic obstruction occurs especially where there is a gradual increase of pressure on the wall of the bowel from a growth outside. The majority of patients, however, develop obstruction suddenly or have a series of sharp attacks of colic and vomiting which lead up to a final crisis, when a loop or kink fails to undo itself.

The diagnosis of small bowel obstruction is usually based upon the symptoms. In many cases it is supported by the fact that the patient has had a previous operation and is thus liable to develop adhesions.

X-ray investigation includes plain films which show fluid levels in dilated loops of the bowel. In less acute cases a barium follow-through examination is made.

Surgical treatment

The management of disorders of the small intestine is in fact the management of intestinal obstruction. Severe cases of acute obstruction by bands or volvulus undergo operation as soon as possible after the diagnosis has been made. The abdomen is explored usually through a paramedian or midline incision and the surgeon is frequently able to release the twisted loop without any further operative procedure. Sometimes, however, if there are many adhesions the dissection may be extremely difficult. If the kink or twist has been present for several hours it is likely that the blood supply to part of the bowel will have been interfered with and gangrene may have developed. In such cases, as with severely strangulated hernia, the gangrenous portion is removed, the continuity of the bowel being restored by end-to-end anastomosis.

In cases of gun-shot wound in the abdomen there may be multiple holes or lacerations in the small bowel, which will need either repair or resection.

Pre-operative treatment will naturally depend on the nature of the obstruction. Dehydration, particularly loss of chloride, must be combated by adequate infusion.

Gastro-intestinal aspiration must be established by means of a naso-gastric tube. In some cases the surgeon will wish the patient to have a Miller-Abbott tube passed in order that the intestine proximal to the obstruction may be completely emptied and deflated. Occasionally this 'decompression' is sufficient to relieve the obstruction by altering the position of the intestinal loops. There is no other specific pre-operative treatment except the measures usually taken before laparotomy.

Post-operative treatment

The principal risks are peritonitis and recurrent obstruction from further adhesions or ileus. Oral feeding is therefore restricted or, in most cases, completely suspended until any distension which was present before operation has subsided and peristalsis (audible with a stethoscope) has been resumed. The simple measurement of abdominal girth with a tape measure is a valuable but often forgotten method of assessing distension.

The most important post-operative measure is the maintenance of fluid and electrolyte balance (Chapter 8).

If a portion of a bowel has been resected there is additional risk of abscess formation around the site of anastomosis. Regional ileitis may lead to the formation of abscess before operation: if the abscess is subsequently drained a fistula may develop from the lumen of the bowel—**faecal fistula** (page 539).

Disorders of the mesentery

Cysts sometimes form in the mesentery and may become very large. Lymph glands in the mesentery become infected, especially with tuberculosis. A tuberculous lymph gland occasionally becomes an abscess and bursts into the peritoneal cavity, producing acute tuberculous peritonitis. Usually, however, the gland becomes replaced by chalk—calcification—and symptoms seldom arise. Glands and mesenteric cysts are sometimes removed and as the result of the operation there may be interference with the blood supply to a portion of the small intestine with a subsequent development of ileus or even gangrene.

There is no particular feature in the pre- or post-operative nursing care of these patients. Observations must be maintained for symptoms of obstruction or peritonitis.

Acute inflammation of the mesenteric lymph glands frequently accompanies other infective diseases such as measles, or may follow acute tonsillitis. The abdominal pain which is produced by this condition is sometimes mis-diagnosed as acute appendicitis.

ILEOSTOMY

In the treatment of severe ulcerative colitis, the whole of the large bowel is rested by diverting the faecal stream and subsequently removing colon and rectum. The terminal portion of the ileum is completely divided and the proximal end brought through the skin as an artificial anus. The principle is similar to that of colostomy as a means of draining the colon in cases of lower large bowel intestinal obstruction. There are various methods of forming the ileostomy opening but the aim is to produce a spout of ileum about 4 cm long covered with healthy mucous membrane. A rubber bag is then fitted over its opening and held to the abdominal wall by the pressure of a belt (Fig. 27.2). Some patients prefer to have a square of plaster (adhesive on both surfaces) to stick the flange of the bag to the skin (Fig. 36.7). A plastic disposable type of bag may be used, attached to the skin by special adhesive (Fig. 27.3).

The discharge from an ileostomy is almost continuous and has very active digestive properties which affect the skin. The bag has to be worn continuously but ileal wash-outs are not necessary. The skin may be protected from the effect of digestive juice by a barrier cream (page 469), placed around the stoma after the flange has been applied.

One type of 'continent' ileostomy involves the construction of a large reservoir into which the patient passes a catheter, instead of wearing a bag (Kocks' operation). The presence of an ileostomy does not prevent the patient from following a normal occupation and enjoying good health.

Since the operation is usually performed for ulcerative colitis the patients are frequently in extremely poor condition, emaciated and grossly undernourished. The operation is

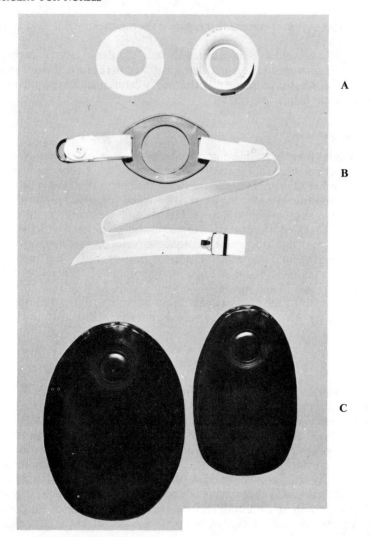

Fig. 27.2   Typical ileostomy appliance pack. **A.** Soft rubber face piece flange with double sided adhesive discs. **B.** Plastic retaining shield and waist belt. **C.** Night and day bags of odour resistant rubber. (J. G. Franklin & Sons Ltd.)

sometimes undertaken as an emergency. The immediate risks after operation for the formation of ileostomy are those of any laparotomy.

In addition to the ordinary risks, aggravated by the patient's poor general condition, the principal local complication is either that the ileum will prolapse through the wound and protrude excessively or be drawn back into the peritoneal cavity, producing peritonitis.

It is essential that the nurse in charge of the patient should see the operation site and the size of the spout at the end of the operation so that she will be able to tell at the first dressing whether or not there has been any change in the length or character. Unless there is constant supervision by the same person, prolapse or retraction may well be missed, with serious consequences.

Attention must be paid to the fluid balance after ileostomy. In the normal individual the main absorption of fluid from the intestinal tract occurs in the colon. When the faecal

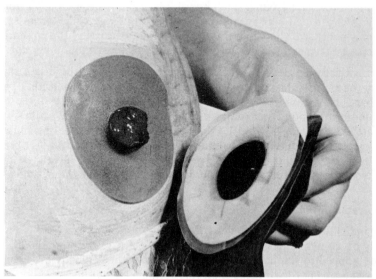

Fig. 27.3   This terminal ileostomy has been surrounded by an adhesive disc of Stomahesive to which the second adhesive disc carrying the bag is applied.

stream is diverted by ileostomy, fluid absorption is greatly diminished and considerable difficulty may be experienced in maintaining correct electrolyte and water balance, especially in the first few days after operation.

Care of the stoma. Patients about to undergo ileostomy or colostomy must have the principle explained carefully so that unnecessary fears may be allayed. After operation detailed and sympathetic instruction in the care of the stoma is so important that some hospitals have a member of the nursing staff concentrating on this subject and supervising a stoma clinic to ensure that patients receive the most appropriate appliances and use them to the best advantage. The management of a faecal ileostomy is easier than that for a urinary ileostomy and the hazard of kidney infection is not present. Similar complications occur. The detailed management of urinary ileostomy is given on page 689 and in general the same rules apply.

Faecal fistula

A communication between the abdominal skin and the bowel leading to faecal discharge is a 'fistula'. This may arise in one of several ways:

(*a*) Abscess formation. A perforated appendix or diverticulum of the colon may lead to the development of an abscess and if this is drained the perforation may stay open (Figs 24.4 and 24.8). The colonic discharge from these large bowel fistulae does not lead to much excoriation of the skin.

(b) Injury to bowel along suture line of laparotomy. A loop of small bowel is caught in the peritoneal closure stitch even without being pricked by the needle. It becomes adherent and ulcerates into the wound, which in consequence breaks down.

(c) Malignant disease eroding small bowel. If the skin surrounding a fistula becomes very inflamed and sore it is likely that the discharge comes from small bowel. Litmus paper will show that it is very alkaline. Because of the presence of strong digestive enzymes a small bowel fistula rarely closes without operation.

As soon as a fistula develops the surrounding skin should be dried, sprayed with Nobecutane or Friar's balsam, and an ileostomy self-adhesive collecting bag applied. If the discharge is profuse a tube may be tied into the bottom corner of the bag; sewing cotton wound firmly round and round will make a leak-proof joint; adhesive strapping is inadequate: bags already fitted with a tape are unsatisfactory as the opening is too small.

Discharge may be reduced by restricting oral intake, but patients with a fistula usually require a high level of nutrition. To sustain nutrition and yet have little or no bowel content, Vivonex is used: it contains essential nutritional elements with virtually no residue.

By-pass operation for obesity

Certain individuals are psychologically unable to stop eating excessively. They become dangerously overweight and ordinary attempts at dietetic restriction fail. Absorption of food can be stopped by joining the upper jejunum with the ileum about 1 metre from its junction with the caecum, leaving the main part of the small intestine as a blind canal closed at its upper end. This by-pass prevents the absorption of food but severe complications can arise from electrolyte imbalance and diarrhoea. Lomotil and codeine phosphate may help in the immediate post-operative period.

It is doubtful if this operation will continue in use as it has been found by biopsy (with a Crosby capsule) that the mucosal villi become enormously hypertrophied in the remaining active piece of intestine thus restoring food absorption and counteracting the effect of the operation.

Small intestine biopsy

In nutritional disorders in which it is thought that there may be defects in the function of the duodenal or intestinal mucosa very small pieces of this tissue can be obtained through a special biopsy tube which is swallowed. A capsule at the end of the tube is moved by peristalsis and observed by radiography. When it is at the appropriate level suction is applied and a sliding cutter inside the capsule slices off the piece of tissue which has been sucked into the eye. The tube is then withdrawn. Occasionally intestinal haemorrhage or perforation may complicate this investigation which is undertaken without anaesthetic. The Crosby biopsy capsule is commonly used. Children require general anaesthesia for the procedure to be undertaken. A period of pre-operative bowel starvation is necessary to ensure that the stomach and bowel are as empty as possible.

28

Appendicitis

The appendix is sometimes referred to as the 'abdominal tonsil' because it is composed largely of lymphoid tissue and is very susceptible to infection. It varies greatly in size, the average length being 7·5 cm. Normally it is a hollow tube lined with mucous membrane, with a muscle wall similar to that of the caecum with which it communicates. Its tip may hang down over the brim of the pelvis to make contact with the bladder, the rectum, or in the female with the ovary, uterine tube or uterus. It may, on the other hand, turn upwards behind the caecum pointing out towards the groin—the retro-caecal position. It may lie on the front of the caecum immediately under the anterior abdominal wall.

Although the cause of acute appendicitis is unknown its occurrence often follows acute infection elsewhere in the body. It can occur at any age and is by far the most common abdominal surgical emergency. It may arise in a patient already in hospital for other reasons.

Table 43 indicates the main types of acute appendicitis, the presenting symptoms, and the conditions with which each type is most commonly confused. The principal complications are also shown.

If acute appendicitis is diagnosed within 24 hours of its onset the risk of post-operative complication is very slight. In children, however, the course may be extremely rapid; perforation and generalised peritonitis may occur within a few hours of the first symptom.

On the other hand, many patients with acute appendicitis recover completely without operation. They may have no further attacks, though this is unlikely. In 'chronic' appendicitis the patient suffers from recurrent symptoms of acute appendicitis as the appendix itself is permanently affected by scarring from previous attacks. This gives rise to dyspepsia and vague abdominal symptoms which disappear when the appendix has been removed.

Appendicitis is mimicked by other conditions such as ileitis (Crohn's disease), Yersinia infection (page 535) and mesenteric adenitis.

Treatment

All but a few cases of acute appendicitis are treated by immediate removal of the appendix. If the patient is not within reach of surgical treatment then his treatment is the same as for acute peritonitis. There must be complete rest in bed, gastro-intestinal suction to rest the alimentary tract, antibiotics or chemotherapy, and parenteral fluid administration (Chapter 24).

Table 43   Acute appendicitis

Type	Common age group	Features	Conditions with similar features	Main complications	Nursing requirement
Catarrhal	Young adults	Short history; loss of appetite; vomit (once or twice); slight pyrexia ($\pm 38\,^{\circ}$C); rising pulse rate; central abdominal pain which is later in the lower quadrant	Salpingitis; pyelitis; enteritis; mesenteric adenitis; cholecystitis	Nil	No drainage
Obstructive	Young adults	Severe colic with sudden onset; vomit; no fever until gangrene develops (several hours)	Biliary, renal or ureteric colic; perforated peptic ulcer; intestinal colic (from inflammation or obstruction); twisted ovarian cyst; ectopic pregnancy	Perforation; peritonitis; pelvic or peri-caecal abscess	No drainage unless perforated; antibiotics (because gangrene is common in this type). As for acute peritonitis if perforation has occurred (see below)
Fulminating	Infants and children mainly	Sudden onset; collapse; rapid pulse; no fever at first until peritonitis advances; ileus; distension	Penumonia; septicaemia (e.g. with meningococcal meningitis); pneumococcal peritonitis; acute infective dysentery; perforated peptic ulcer; acute pancreatitis	Ileus; pelvic or sub-phrenic abscess	Drainage: antibiotics; no oral feeding gastric suction; infusion. As for acute peritonitis
Abscess	Infants and the elderly	Loss of appetite; swinging fever and pallor for several days; palpable mass in abdomen; very high white blood count: pain on attempting to straighten the hip joint (psoas sign)	Carcinoma of caecum with infection; salpingitis; pyonephrosis; perinephric abscess; twisted ovarian cyst	Spreading peritonitis; septicaemia; faecal fistula	(Conservative treatment) drainage; antibiotics; infusion; probably suspension of oral feeding. As for acute peritonitis

If the patient has already formed a palpable inflammatory mass or 'abscess', he will probably not be treated by immediate operation. The same conservative treatment will be established: the abscess may resolve spontaneously or discharge into the bowel (Fig. 24.8). He should, however, always be admitted to hospital for observation, and if the size of the mass remains stationary or even increases, with persistence of fever and high pulse rate, the abscess requires drainage. By this time, the general peritoneal cavity has been walled off: although there is always a risk of spread of infection, rapid resolution usually follows after the insertion of a drainage tube. In the presence of an abscess, the surgeon usually makes no attempt to find or remove the appendix itself. After operation the tube is shortened at regular intervals and removed when the discharge has become very slight. Normally the wound heals spontaneously and the appendix is removed by a planned operation three months later. Sometimes a faecal fistula develops from the abscess and may persist owing to the presence of a hard lump of faeces from the appendix (faecolith) in the bottom of the wound. Operation to locate the site of the fistula and to remove the stump of the appendix is then necessary.

Pre-operative treatment for appendicectomy. Extensive preparation is not necessary in the majority of cases. The administration of anaesthetic premedication (e.g. atropine and morphine) and preparation of the abdominal skin is all that is required. Under certain circumstances however further nursing preparation is needed:

(a) If there has been considerable vomiting or if the patient has had a meal within 4 hours, a gastric tube should be passed and the stomach emptied.
(b) If the appendix is in the pelvic position its presence may irritate the bladder and there may be frequency of micturition. On the other hand, bladder action may be inhibited. It is imperative that the bladder should be empty at the time of operation and catheterisation may be required.
(c) If the patient is thought to have developed peritonitis already, a naso-gastric tube must be left in place and intravenous or subcutaneous fluid administration will be required.

Post-operative care. The majority of cases treated by appendicectomy will have primary wound closure without drainage. A small adhesive dressing is applied, probably sealed with Whitehead's varnish or Nobecutane, is covered with elastoplast and needs no further attention until the clips or stitches are removed on the 5th or 7th day. In the acute emergency, the patient's bowel is not adequately prepared by pre-operative evacuation, and there is frequently discomfort and distension due to constipation after operation. Some surgeons therefore prefer straightforward cases to be given a laxative (e.g. magnesia and paraffin emulsion, Milpar) on the night following operation. When distension causes discomfort an enema should be given without hesitation.

If, at operation, free pus has been found in the peritoneal cavity, this will be removed by suction and swabbing, but the wound may still be closed without drainage. An abscess may develop in the abdominal wall and will be noticed by a rise of temperature towards the end of the 1st week, accompanied by a return of wound pain. It is more likely to occur if a haematoma has formed in the wound from careless surgical technique. The abscess may be evacuated quite easily by the insertion of a probe into the line of the skin incision which has not completely healed.

Similarly, a secondary abscess may develop in the pelvis, when its presence is shown by a gradual rise in temperature towards the end of the 1st week, with the passage of mucus from the rectum and frequency of micturition. Pelvic cellulitis, as the condition is at the beginning, is detected by digital examination of the rectum which reveals a firm tender mass. The temperature chart resembles that shown in Fig. 4.4. If antibiotic treatment has not been given already, it is started. Hot rectal wash-outs night and morning (3 litres each time) aid the resolution of the cellulitis, and if an abscess forms it may discharge into the rectum spontaneously. The condition is in fact the same as the development of a pelvic abscess resulting from diffuse peritonitis (page 472).

Generalised spreading peritonitis can occur without the appendix perforating (or 'bursting') in the ordinary sense of the word. Bacteria escape through the wall of the appendix long before the wall itself undergoes necrosis and bursts. When established peritonitis is present at the time of operation, the surgeon will almost certainly insert a suprapubic drainage tube in the hope of allowing pus to escape from the pelvis, and so preventing pelvic abscess.

Subphrenic abscess is a very rare complication of acute appendicitis of this type. Its possible presence has to be borne in mind if fever persists at the end of the 1st week after an appendicectomy.

Convalescence

If a diagnosis of acute appendicitis is reasonably certain at the time of operation, a transverse muscle-splitting incision will most probably be used. This heals very rapidly and leaves no weakness whatever in the abdominal wall so that the patient is very soon able to return to work. Seven to ten days is an adequate time for the patient to remain in hospital and full manual work can usually be resumed a month after operation.

However, if there has been peritonitis or abscess formation, anaemia and general debility may be considerable and prolonged convalescence will be required.

In straightforward cases, if care at home with medical supervision is possible, patients may leave hospital after 3 or 4 days, stitches being removed by the 'community nurse'. If adhesive strips have been used instead of stitches these can be peeled off by the patient (page 407).

Interval appendicectomy

Sometimes a diagnosis of recurrent appendicitis or appendicular dyspepsia is made and the patient's name is entered on the waiting list for admission at a later date. Unless some unexpected condition is found at operation recovery in such cases is extremely rapid, usually without complication.

Prolonged non-healing

Other conditions may masquerade as acute appendicitis and their presence may not be suspected until days or even weeks after the inflamed appendix has been removed. Infection by amoebic dysentery (amoebiasis) is common in tropical and subtropical countries, but occurs from time to time in persons who have never been to places where the disease is endemic. Treatment by special chemotherapy is prolonged.

Regional ileitis (Crohn's disease), in an acute or chronic form, and tuberculosis sometimes come to light as acute appendicitis.

Thread worms

The common thread worm—*Oxyurus vermicularis*—lives and breeds in the intestine of many children and adults without producing symptoms. Occasionally the worms nest in the appendix, when their presence is responsible for colic and probably adds to the risk of acute appendicitis. Quite frequently children with this infestation develop appendicitis with high fever, perhaps 39 °C, which is otherwise very unusual with acute appendicitis.

The importance of this condition is that the infestation should be treated in the immediate post-operative period and care taken that other patients are not infected by contact. At the end of operation for appendicectomy it is usual for the surgeon to open the appendix and examine its interior: if thread worms are present they will be seen at this time. If their presence is noticed in the first post-operative stool, the fact must be reported to the medical staff.

Carcinoid tumour

This is a little yellow growth which occurs in the appendix particularly but can be found in other parts of the intestine. It is a malignant tumour derived from 'chromaffin' tissue to be found also in the suprarenal gland. A tumour may block the lumen of the appendix and thereby produce symptoms of obstructive appendicitis or it may be found on routine examination of the appendix during laparotomy for some other condition. It rarely spreads to other parts of the body but when it does the metastatic tumours form excessive quantities of a hormone, serotonin (5-hydroxytryptamine). This produces attacks of severe hot flushing of the skin, a purple plethoric appearance, and by its effect on the bowel, chronic diarrhoea and resulting malabsorption of food from the intestines. Sometimes these tumours are multiple, arising in the glandular epithelium of the small intestine, and the 'carcinoid syndrome' is usually associated with these multiple tumours.

Summary

Although very commonplace, acute appendicitis still is sometimes a fatal disease. The patient with severe acute appendicitis requires all possible nursing skill and the post-operative course may be extremely stormy from ileus and other complications. Acute appendicitis may develop in a patient who is undergoing treatment for an entirely distinct condition; the nurse must be familiar with the early symptoms so that they are not ignored.

29

Colon and Rectum

The large intestine extends from the ileocaecal valve to the rectum. From the practical point of view the **colon** is intraperitoneal. The upper third of the **rectum** is covered by peritoneum but the lower two-thirds are below the layer of the peritoneum which covers the pelvic floor. The only very mobile parts of the colon are the transverse colon and the sigmoid loop (pelvic colon), each of which has a mesentery (mesocolon). Before the introduction of chemotherapy it was unsafe to excise and join up portions of the colon

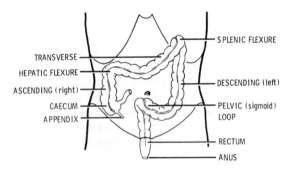

Fig. 29.1 The large bowel—indicating the descriptive terms used in surgery.

which were not completely surrounded by peritoneum, as there was no layer to seal the anastomosis and prevent leakage. Now that the inside of the bowel can be rendered relatively free from organisms, though never actually sterile, these risks are less important. As with other portions of the intestine, the lymph glands which drain the colon lie along the main vessels. If a lymph gland is infected with malignant disease and requires removal, the main vessel alongside also has to be removed. This means that a much larger portion of the colon may have to be removed than would otherwise be necessary, because its blood supply will be cut off in removing the mesentery and affected lymph glands.

When the colon becomes inflamed or affected with growth, especially in its pelvic portion, it becomes stuck to the bladder and other pelvic organs. The rectum is very close to the ureters on either side. They may be involved in growth and are liable to damage in a radical operation on any pelvic organ. The nerve supply to the bladder may also be injured in operations in the pelvis: retention of urine is a common complication.

Diseases which affect the colon can often be diagnosed by direct inspection by sigmoidoscopy and by biopsy (page 573).

Physiology

In contrast to the small bowel, the contents of the large bowel are essentially septic. The main function of the colon is absorption of water. In the caecum and ascending colon the faecal material is very fluid and a large growth may be present without causing obstruction. In the left (descending) colon and sigmoid loop the faeces have become solidified and a much smaller growth will produce obstruction. Caecostomy, an artificial drainage opening from the caecum, is unsatisfactory as a permanent measure because of this fluidity, but in the emergency relief of large-bowel obstruction, the faecal contents of the caecum can be readily drained through a large catheter. The transverse colostomy is also difficult to keep clean because actions are also frequent and usually fluid. If the pelvic colon is brought to the surface as an artificial anus, action is less frequent and the stool more formed. There is an increase of large-bowel activity after a meal and some colostomy patients acquire a habit of evacuation, as with the normal bowel.

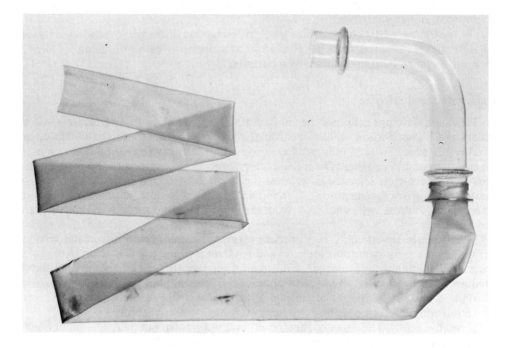

Fig. 29.2   Paul's tube with soft collapsible latex rubber drain. This is sometimes used for caecostomy or colostomy drainage where the content of the bowel is fluid. One end of the glass tube is tied into the lumen of the bowel.

Normal bowel action depends to a large extent on the bacterial fermentation which takes place in the colon. If the organisms become changed, diarrhoea may result with excessive production of mucus. If obstruction is present for a long time, excessive fermentation may suddenly occur with gas production and liquefaction of the stool, so that a bout of constipation is followed by an attack of diarrhoea.

Diseases of colon and rectum

Congenital

Atresia and stricture or congenital volvulus may occur and produce obstruction in the neonatal period. Surgical operation for its relief is essential.

Hirschsprung's disease is a condition in which the nerve supply to the rectum is defective and permanent local 'ileus' is present with subsequent chronic obstruction to the large bowel above. Great enlargement develops and the child's abdomen is enormously distended. In neglected cases colostomy is required until the child's health improves sufficiently for the affected portion of the rectum to be removed. The distal end of the pelvic colon is then joined to the upper end of the anal canal.

Gross neglected constipation or bad training can lead to a similar condition of colon enlargement—megacolon—but this does not require surgical treatment in most cases. A prolonged course of enemas is effective in rehabilitating the bowel, and assisting the development of natural habits.

The use of laxatives such as cascara leads to destruction of the nerve cells in the bowel and thus to an acquired form of Hirschsprung's disease—'cathartic colon'. Chaga's disease is a similar condition caused by a parasite.

Inflammatory and infective

The colon develops little pouches in its walls. This condition of **diverticulosis** affects mainly the pelvic portion. Infection around these pouches leads to the condition of **diverticulitis** which in turn may produce obstruction, abscess formation, adhesions to other organs and peritonitis. The inflammatory process may spread to the bladder and produce a **vesico-colic fistula**. Flatus from the colon is passed with the urine if such a complication arises (**pneumaturia**). Carcinoma of the colon also develops in areas of diverticulitis, and the two conditions, from the point of view of surgery and nursing, are very similar.

Diverticulosis. Diverticulitis may produce vague abdominal symptoms and indigestion, but usually the early symptoms are pain and tenderness in the left iliac fossa. Attacks of acute inflammation with severe pain, constipation and fever require admission to hospital. Frequently such attacks subside with antibiotic treatment, but if obstruction persists proximal colostomy is performed and the obstructed segment is removed later. Abscess formation and perforation require emergency drainage and colostomy.

Ulcerative colitis. The cause of this condition is not known but there are undoubtedly psychological or personality factors. It is a progressive, severe, debilitating and often fatal condition. It frequently starts between the age of twenty and thirty. Very mild cases are treated by medical means and may recover. Ulceration may start in the rectum and spread upwards, involving the whole length of colon, but the rectum is sometimes the last part to be involved. Very severe diarrhoea develops with the passage of large quantities of mucus and a continuous loss of blood from hundreds of ulcers. Almost the entire mucous membrane of the colon may disappear and a very large raw area is then exposed to the faecal stream. The condition has been described as resembling 'a severe burn of an area the size of the leg and thigh on which there is a faecal poultice'. Patients with this condition become grossly emaciated, toxic and anaemic. The bowel itself is very thin and liable to tear or perforate. In recent years radical surgical treatment has been undertaken for this condition and the procedures adopted can be summarised here.

1. Ileostomy (page 537). This may be a temporary measure although it is usually permanent.

2. After ileostomy has been established the whole of the colon may be removed (Fig. 29.3).

3. The rectum also is excised by a combined abdomino-perineal operation (page 552).

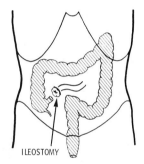

ILEOSTOMY

Fig. 29.3   Terminal ileostomy for ulcerative colitis: with total colectomy and excision of rectum. (The shaded portion is removed.)

The nursing of these patients requires very great skill in the management of nutrition and fluid balance. The complications of operations for ulcerative colitis are those which may follow any intestinal surgery, but the risks are particularly great owing to the poor general condition of the patient and the severe inflammation of the intestinal tract. Prolonged parenteral feeding is necessary and gross malnutrition often requires infusion of protein. A high protein diet is given, with full vitamin supplements. The vitamin reserves of such patients are often very depleted by prolonged diarrhoea and dieting. Ulceration of the large bowel is a complication of typhoid and leads to perforation with faecal peritonitis.

Crohn's disease. This chronic inflammatory condition of the bowel usually affects the ileum (page 534) but may involve the colon as well or alone. If obstruction is present, the affected length is removed: steroid treatment is sometimes given.

Neoplastic

This perhaps constitutes the greatest group of conditions for which surgical treatment is necessary. Innocent growths occur—**adenoma** and **'polyp'**—and one of the features of polyposis in the colon is that it occurs in families with a particular susceptibility. These adenomas are liable to become malignant, and they are usually multiple. In severe cases the whole of the colon and rectum is removed as for ulcerative colitis.

Carcinoma of the colon may occur at any point from the caecum to the anus and the symptoms which it produces depend largely on the position which the growth is occupying. In the caecum the growth becomes very large before it produces any symptoms of obstruction. It may be discovered because the patient complains of vague pain in the area of his appendix, and a large tumour is found on routine examination. In the transverse and left side of the colon, obstruction occurs more readily and the patient becomes constipated and distended. The presence of a growth in the rectum produces an excessive mucous secretion and probably blood. The patient then complains of frequent defaecation with the passage of blood and slime with the motions and sometimes without any faecal matter. This **spurious diarrhoea** is a feature of all inflammatory conditions of the rectum as well (e.g. inflamed haemorrhoids). If this loss of mucus continues the patient becomes short of potassium and magnesium and may develop general muscle weakness (page 109, hypokalaemia).

Carcinoma of the colon is treated by excision of the area involved and as much as possible of the lymphatic field which drains that portion of the bowel. This may involve removal of important blood vessels and consequently the removal also of a longer portion of the bowel. Figs. 29.4 to 29.7 illustrate procedures commonly adopted in the treatment of carcinoma.

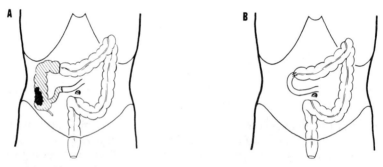

Fig. 29.4 Right hemicolectomy for carcinoma of caecum: ileo-transverse colonic anastomosis.

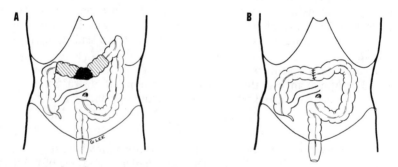

Fig. 29.5 Transverse colectomy for carcinoma: end-to-end anastomosis.

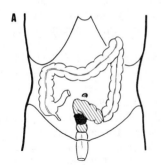

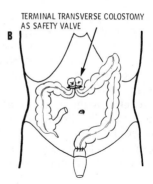

TERMINAL TRANSVERSE COLOSTOMY
AS SAFETY VALVE

A

B

Fig. 29.6   Excision of sigmoid colon and upper rectum for carcinoma; end-to-end anastomosis (restorative resection).

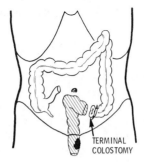

TERMINAL
COLOSTOMY

Fig. 29.7   Abdomino-perineal excision of rectum for carcinoma: terminal iliac colostomy.

Amoebic dysentery due to infection by amoeba histolytica sometimes leads to the development of an inflammatory tumour in the bowel resembling carcinoma. Unless a biopsy is always performed grave errors may occur. It mimics appendicitis (page 544).

Nursing management

Pre-operative treatment

The principles involved in the management of peritonitis and intestinal obstruction (Chapter 24) cover most of the requirements of colonic and rectal surgery. If a patient is admitted for an emergency operation made necessary by the presence of a growth, diverticulitis or ulcerative colitis, there will be little time for pre-operative treatment and the operation will be mainly to establish drainage of the bowel by ileostomy or colostomy.

Fortunately many cases are diagnosed before obstruction has occurred, and in these there is time for adequate preparation. Attention is paid to the patient's nutrition, vitamin requirements and fluid balance. Blood transfusion may be required and preparations must be made for the administration of blood at or after operation in all cases.

The principal special pre-operative measure is the preparation of the intestinal canal throughout its length by low residue diet and antiseptics. Succinyl or phthalyl sulphathiazole, streptomycin or neomycin[1] with metronidazole (Flagyl) by mouth is given for 3 days before operation in non-urgent cases. This reduces the infection in the bowel and by so doing it lessens the fermentation and gas formation in the post-operative period. These drugs are not significantly absorbed from the intestine.

Fashions change in relation to pre-operative bowel preparation. The old-fashioned castor oil is prescribed by some as a safe purgative which really cleans the bowel. Other surgeons require magnesium sulphate (Epsom salts) to be given twice a day until the patient has severe diarrhoea, and is then placed on a fluid only regime.

If a colostomy is present a 'cream' of phthalyl sulphathiazole or neomycin suspension is injected into the distal loop once daily for 3 days before further surgery.

In some cases (particularly in Hirschsprung's disease) large faecal masses accumulate in the rectum. An anaesthetic may be required in order that these lumps may be broken up and extracted from the rectum by the surgeon's fingers. A Veripaque or molasses enema may be used; such preparation may have been given before a barium enema examination but it is important to make sure the barium has been evacuated before operation.

Post-operative nursing

Owing to the severity of operations on the colon and the fact that they usually occupy from one to three hours when a radical excision is performed, shock and haemorrhage are very important complications for which provision has to be made. Intravenous infusion is invariably used during the operation and is continued afterwards in all cases because of the additional risk of peritonitis and ileus. Gastric aspiration is maintained until peristalsis returns. When an anastomosis is performed initially, operations for removal of sections of the colon do not involve any particular post-operative nursing technique except that required for any abdominal operation where peritonitis is a risk. A drainage tube may be left down to the site of anastomosis in case a leak should arise: it is withdrawn gradually by daily shortening on specific instructions from the medical staff. An enema may not be given without the surgeon's consent.

If on the other hand an artificial opening has been made—caecostomy or colostomy—this will involve special nursing procedures which are described later.

Excision of the rectum may be followed by an anastomosis performed through an abdominal incision (Fig. 29.6). If the growth is low down in the rectum the whole of the organ is removed, including the anus (Fig. 29.7). This is usually performed by the combined abdomino-perineal operation. Two surgical teams may work together, one from above and one from below. The upper surgeon frees the sigmoid colon and rectum down to the floor of the pelvis and establishes a colostomy. The lower surgeon closes the anus with a silk stitch to prevent leakage, and excises a large area of skin in the perineum (Fig. 29.9). In the female the posterior wall of the vagina is often removed at the same time. The anal canal and rectum are freed from their surroundings and removed with part of the pelvic colon. The peritoneal floor is then closed by the surgeon working above. The perineal skin wound is also partly stitched and a large cavity is left in front of the sacrum and coccyx (part of which may have been removed to give access to the rectum). Methods

---

[1] In conditions such as ulcerative colitis, neomycin *may* be absorbed and will then produce deafness.

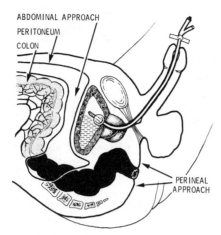

ABDOMINAL APPROACH
PERITONEUM
COLON
PERINEAL
APPROACH

Fig. 29.8 Position and anatomical relations of the rectum. This is partly above the layer of peritoneum across the pelvic floor. The bladder must be kept empty during all pelvic operations.

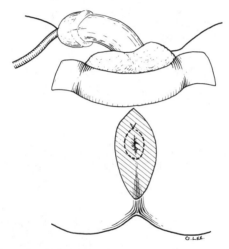

Fig. 29.9 In the synchronous combined abdomino-perineal operation for excision of the rectum (SCAPER), the surgeon operating at the perineal end has the scrotum strapped up out of the way and a urethral catheter in place. He places a stitch around the anus as shown and then the skin is excised over the area indicated.

of drainage of this cavity vary. Some surgeons pack the cavity with a sheet of latex rubber containing a gauze roll. Others merely insert a strip of corrugated rubber (Fig. 29.11).

Post-operative nursing instructions concerning the care of this cavity will be given by the surgeon. Any packing is usually left undisturbed for 3 or 4 days and then withdrawn a little each day. If packing has been used in the perineal wound, anaesthesia may be required for the first dressing and pack removal. The cavity may then be irrigated daily with hypochlorite solution (page 94) and it may take 3 weeks to become completely

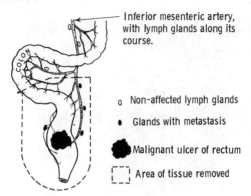

Fig. 29.10   The extent of removal in the abdomino-perineal excision for carcinoma of the rectum.

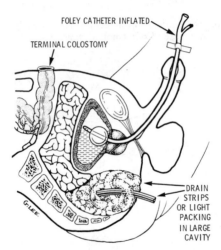

Fig. 29.11   It will be seen that the space previously occupied by the rectum is filled partly by the descent of the perineal floor. The coccyx may be removed to give access for the operation.

healed. It is obliterated by granulation tissue, by the bladder and by the abdominal contents.

The care of the bladder (Chapter 35 for apparatus)

A catheter is passed and left in position before operation. As large retractors are used in all pelvic surgery, unless the bladder is kept empty it may become damaged by pressure. This is particularly important if removal of the rectum is the operation proposed.

After operation, continuous bladder drainage is essential in all cases where the pelvic colon or rectum has been removed. Especially after excision of the rectum the nerve supply to the bladder may be impaired and continuous drainage is usually ordered for the first 2 or 3 days. Alternatively, the patient is catheterised twice a day. After this initial period, tidal drainage may be prescribed in order to maintain the rhythmical filling and emptying of the bladder, which is necessary in order that it shall regain its normal habit (page 664, Cystomat automatic bladder drainage). The exact method of bladder care varies in different surgical units, but occasionally when catheterisation or drainage is stopped, retention persists. It is important then to enquire if the patient feels that his bladder is full, or whether he has in fact no sensation. If he is conscious of his bladder being full and the desire to void, normal function will probably soon return. It may be necessary then to pass a catheter once a day although the patient is voiding some urine spontaneously. The residual urine is measured and its gradual decrease noted. If full bladder recovery is delayed a further period of tidal drainage may be required. It is important to use a *small* catheter—latex Foley not more than 20 F. Charrière gauge—to avoid pressure in the urethra. A tightly fitting catheter prevents the escape of urethral secretion around it and causes severe urethritis.

Particularly in elderly men, the removal of the rectum may precipitate complete urinary retention from enlargement of the prostate. Transurethral resection of the prostate is then necessary, and if this is not practicable, suprapubic cystostomy is performed. Temporary suprapubic drainage by 'intracath' puncture should not be used until the abdominal drainage tubes are out; it is then a satisfactory means of allowing the urethral inflammation to settle and so restore normal voiding.

Post-operative position following excision of the rectum

Owing to the magnitude of such operations as complete removal of the rectum, there is a considerable risk of post-operative haemorrhage. It is important that if bleeding occurs, its presence should be detected as soon as possible. In the first 2 days after operation the patient must be kept in such a position that blood will not accumulate in the perineal wound or track into the peritoneal cavity but will drain outwards. While the immediate treatment of post-operative shock in other cases is to elevate the foot of the bed, this should be avoided after removal of the rectum. Blood transfusion is used liberally and the 'head-down' position can thus be avoided. Some surgeons prefer the head end of the bed to be raised, but the patient should not be lifted into the sitting position owing to the further risk of the sutured peritoneal floor to the pelvis breaking down and allowing small bowel to prolapse.

Caecostomy and colostomy

Caecostomy is performed usually as a temporary measure either in the initial treatment of acute large-bowel obstruction or as a safety valve after an anastomosis has been formed further along in the colon. In either case this method of drainage is temporary. The fluid nature of the small intestinal content as it is discharged into the caecum makes it possible for drainage to be effective through a small rubber tube or large self-retaining catheter. At operation this tube is inserted through a stab wound in the caecal wall which is tied round it with a purse-string stitch. The tube is brought out through the abdominal wall in the right iliac fossa. The caecum becomes adherent to the peritoneum of the anterior abdominal wall: a satisfactory seal is formed very rapidly and prevents leakage into the peritoneal cavity. When the caecostomy is no longer required the catheter is pulled out, and if the normal channel through the distal colon is unobstructed the caecostomy opening will usually close without any further surgical treatment. The Paul's tube method of drainage is sometimes used (Fig. 29.2).

The small intestinal digestive enzymes are apt to damage the skin around the caecostomy opening if there is leakage, and this needs to be protected with a barrier cream. The dressing should not need frequent changing if the tube fits correctly, but a slight leak around the tube is common. The caecostomy drainage tube is connected to a bedside bag.

COLOSTOMY

This procedure is one of the most important in abdominal surgery. It is sometimes necessary as a life-saving measure. It may be temporary or permanent as an artificial anus in the radical treatment of rectal cancer. Because of its appearance, its inconvenience and the very thought of an artificial opening in the abdominal wall a great deal of care is necessary to allay the anxieties of patients and their relatives when colostomy is necessary.

Occasions for use. In some cases of acute intestinal obstruction the surgeon explores the abdomen and finds perhaps a large mass in the region of the pelvic colon or rectum that cannot be removed. An emergency colostomy is then performed in the transverse colon with the immediate purpose of saving life and with the further objective of providing temporary drainage should the growth be removable at a later date. In some such cases, when at first sight the primary cause of the obstruction seems beyond any possibility of surgical removal, after several weeks of colostomy drainage the infection subsides and the affected portion of bowel may then be removed.

Colostomy may be necessary as a preliminary to other operations involving removal of the large bowel. Such an occasion arises if diverticulitis has produced vesico-colic fistula (between the colon and bladder). In some cases of severe incontinence due to abnormality or injury to the anus, a left iliac colostomy enables the patient to be free of the terrible inconvenience of perpetual soiling in the perineum. Injuries or abnormalities of the spinal cord produce paralysis of the anal sphincter mechanism and sometimes colostomy is essential.

Congenital absence of the rectum or anus requires an emergency colostomy within a day or so of birth.

Total excision of the rectum leaves the patient with a permanent colostomy.

Types of colostomy. There are two main forms. First is the **loop colostomy** which has two limbs. The opening is at the apex of the loop and the bowel has not been divided completely across. A variation of the loop colostomy is the double-barrel form in which the two limbs of the loop are separated by a piece of skin after complete division (Fig. 29.13). This is also described as a **defunctioning colostomy** as it prevents the spill of faeces from the proximal to the distal loop. A second variety is the **spur colostomy** and is shown in Fig. 29.14, where a spur is formed by suturing the two ends together for several inches inside the abdomen. This is of particular value if the colostomy is temporary as the spur can be destroyed by a crushing clamp without risk of peritonitis or perforation since the limbs have become sealed together. When the spur breaks down, the artificial opening on the surface shrinks and sinks back below the skin level. The aim is that this should close spontaneously without further operation (page 561). The third type is the **terminal colostomy** in which the distal portion of bowel is removed completely or in the case of excision of rectum the lower end is closed to form a blind end (Fig. 29.12).

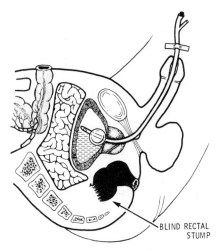

BLIND RECTAL
STUMP

Fig. 29.12 Abdominal excision of recto-sigmoid zone (Hartmann's operation). This operation is performed when total removal of the rectum might be too severe an operation. A terminal colostomy is performed. A self-retaining catheter remains in position after operation: a Foley catheter (as shown) is not inflated until the end of the operation.

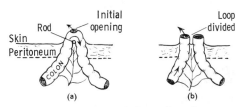

Fig. 29.13 Loop colostomy. This type is used in the formation of a permanent colostomy so that there is complete separation of the two limbs. It is also used as an emergency measure but requires closure by an open operation in order to restore continuity.

In grave emergencies the simplest form of colostomy is performed in which a loop of colon is brought out through the abdominal wall, where it is held by the insertion of a glass rod passed through a small hole in the mesentery. The ends of the glass rod are connected by a loop of rubber tubing which forms a 'bucket handle'. The abdominal wall is closed around the protrusion of the colostomy.

Exteriorisation is another way of performing a colostomy. If a growth is present in a part of the bowel which can be brought readily through the abdominal wall (e.g. transverse or pelvic colon) the affected loop containing the growth is left outside and the peritoneum, muscles and skin are closed around the base of the loop where the two limbs converge. The loop of colon containing the growth is then removed, leaving two open ends of bowel which can later be joined by crushing the spur between them (Fig. 29.15). This operation avoids the handling of growth or unprepared bowel while the peritoneal cavity is open and so diminishes the risk of peritonitis. A formal operation for closure is required if a spur has not been made.

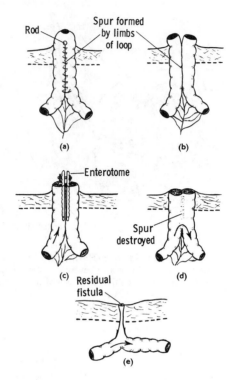

Fig. 29.14 Spur colostomy. The two limbs of the loop are sutured at the original operation so that continuity can be restored without a further operation.

Opening the colostomy. At the end of the operation a small incision is usually made in the apex of the loop to allow the immediate discharge of gas and faecal material which is collected as cleanly as possible before the patient leaves the theatre. A dressing of petroleum jelly gauze or tulle gras is applied on the exposed bowel. The skin incision may be sealed with Whitehead's varnish and a pad of cellulose tissue and wool is bandaged lightly over the opening. The initial opening may be enlarged by the surgeon 2 or 3 days after the colostomy has been raised. The bowel is usually divided (without anaesthetic) by an electric cautery which seals the blood vessels and prevents bleeding from the very vascular mucous membrane and muscle wall of the bowel.

A method of draining the colostomy is by the use of Paul's tube. This is an angled wide glass tube which is inserted through a hole in the colostomy loop: it is tied in position in the same way as the caecostomy catheter and connected to a bedside jar with wide, thin, latex tubing (see Fig. 29.2).

Pre-operative preparation. The surgeon's intention to perform a colostomy should be discussed with the patient. Although this matter is often left to the nursing staff it is really much better that the surgeon himself should discuss with the patient the necessity for colostomy so that any anxiety which arises may be dealt with skilfully, and adequate reassurance given. The idea of a colostomy is so abhorrent to some patients that they refuse consent for operation. The parents of a child who has a colostomy find it very difficult to believe that a well-controlled colostomy is far preferable to an incontinent or unreliable anal sphincter. In emergencies, it is not always possible or wise to broach the possibility of a colostomy, before operation.

No particular nursing measures are required on account of the intention to perform colostomy, but bowel sterilisation will be instituted, as the normal routine before all colon operations.

Post-operative nursing. Certain particular complications may occur.

Bleeding may continue from the opening into the colon. This may require the attention of the surgeon but is usually stopped by a firm dressing, or by a small pad of gauze soaked in adrenaline solution. If arterial bleeding is seen from the cut edge a securing stitch will be necessary and the surgeon must be informed.

The purpose of the glass rod is to avoid the possibility of the loop of colon being drawn back into the peritoneal cavity after the bowel has been opened. If the rod should become dislodged this accident may well occur. Care must be taken to see that the rubber tube on the ends of the rod is firmly attached to prevent the rod slipping out.

A more common complication is that the bowel prolapses through the opening in the abdominal wall and the colostomy loop becomes too long. This is due usually to an error in surgical technique and no nursing measure is required or effective. If the loop appears to have prolapsed the surgeon must be informed.

Strangulation of the bowel may occur if the wound has been closed too tightly. Instead of being bright red the bowel wall will then be purple. In addition to the strangulation the pressure will of course obstruct the lumen to the bowel and it will therefore not be an effective colostomy.

The exposed peritoneal surface of the loop becomes coated with a layer of fibrin and each time the colostomy is dressed it must be covered with tulle gras or some other non-adherent dressing. The patient is nursed in accordance with the surgeon's instruction. Alternatively the surgeon may apply a transparent disposable self-adhesive bag at the end of the operation. This is left undisturbed until the colostomy evacuates. As the formation of the colostomy is usually only part of the more major operation of bowel resection, or has been performed as an emergency measure in peritonitis or obstruction, the post-operative care is mainly determined by the other conditions present. It is wise to suspend oral feeding until audible peristalsis has been detected or until flatus has been passed from the colostomy. If no flatus or faecal material is passed from the colostomy, a finger may be inserted after 24 hours to ensure that the opening is not obstructed. The surgeon may prescribe a small colonic wash-out. Saline may be injected through a soft catheter, but a Higginson syringe should never be used.

The skin stitches can be removed from the colostomy wound after the end of the first week and the glass rod is left in position until specific instructions are given for its removal. This will depend upon the circumstances of the case but it must certainly be left in position until all risk of distension or peritonitis has disappeared. If it should slip out inadvertently during the first 10 days the surgeon must be informed immediately.

If the colostomy has not been completely 'opened' on the operating table a delayed opening will be necessary and this is performed in the ward with the use of a knife or electric cautery.

After a few weeks the mucous membrane from the inside of the colostomy loop spreads through the opening and ultimately grows down over the peritoneal surface and joins with the skin. This protrusion of mucous membrane is essential to prevent a stricture forming where the bowel pierces the skin.

Until the skin becomes accustomed to the presence of faeces it may become excoriated and barrier cream[1] should be used each time the stoma[2] is cleaned. The skin can be further protected by careful placing of the gauze or wool pad which surrounds the stoma.

It may be necessary from time to time to wash out the lower or distal loop of the colostomy. If the operation has been performed as a preliminary to removal of the large bowel at a later date, antiseptic preparation of the intestines before the second operation is achieved by injecting a thin cream of sulphaguanidine into the stoma.

If the bowel actions are too frequent at first the activity of the colon may be slowed down by giving tabs. codeine co. which have a slightly constipating effect. The management of the colostomy and regulation of its habits is described later.

Closure of colostomy. Reference has already been made to the spontaneous closure of a caecostomy after removal of the tube and to colostomy after the crushing of the spur. The instrument used in this latter procedure is an **enterotome** (Fig. 29.15). It consists of two jaws hinged at one end in such a way that the turning of a screw approximates the blades with considerable pressure. The enterotome is applied to the colostomy with one jaw in each limb and the procedure is only safe if the surgeon has sutured the loops of the colon in such a way that the mesentery will not be crushed, when the enterotome is applied. The screwing-up process occupies two or three days, depending on the thickness of the spur. The clamp finally drops off when the spur breaks down after 4 or 5 days.

If no spur has been formed or if the crushing has been incompletely effective, a formal operation to close the opening will be necessary. This operation is sometimes achieved without opening the peritoneal cavity, but the post-operative nursing must assume that the peritoneum has been opened and that there is a risk of peritonitis. Observation, feeding and complications are exactly the same for any operation involving anastomosis of the bowel, or for obstruction. There must be very careful observation for distension, ileus or peritonitis.

Trimming of colostomy. Owing to the risk of distension after large abdominal operations there is the possibility that the colon will be dragged through the abdominal wall. This retraction is prevented in the case of the loop colostomy by the presence of a glass rod. If, however, there is a terminal colostomy, as for instance after excision of the rectum, the risk of retraction is greater. To prevent this a small glass rod is sometimes inserted through the mesentery of the terminal limb of colon, but the usual safeguard is to leave a much longer piece of bowel outside the abdominal wall than is required with the loop colostomy. Subsequently, when all risk of peritonitis and distension has passed, this redundant portion of the bowel is trimmed away. No anaesthetic is required but the procedure is performed in the operating theatre as bleeding may occur. The divided mucous membrane is sometimes stitched over the raw edge of the bowel to encourage its outward growth down to the skin.

[1] Page 469.
[2] Stoma = mouth, opening.

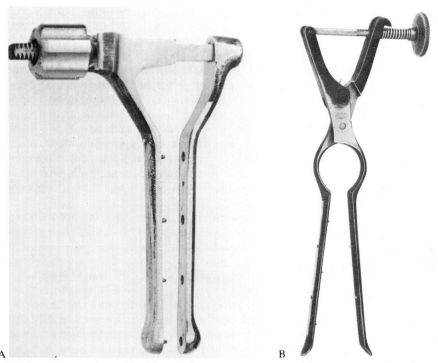

Fig. 29.15 Two types of enterotome used for crushing the spur of a colostomy. **A.** Lloyd Davies' Enterotome and **B.** Mikulicz Enterotome. The pressure is increased by adjustment of the screw daily over a period of 4–5 days: necrosis of the bridge occurs and continuity of the bowel is restored. After the removal of the clamps the redundant mucosa at the stoma gradually shrinks, but a minor surgical excision may be necessary to achieve final closure of the fistula. (Seward Surgical Instruments.)

After-care of colostomy

The patient with a temporary colostomy usually remains in hospital or under nursing supervision continuously. The patient with a permanent colostomy returns home as soon as he is able to manage its care without assistance. The after-care may be considered under five headings:

- (*a*) regularity of evacuation,
- (*b*) management of the blind distal loop (cul de sac) if one is present,
- (*c*) care of the skin,
- (*d*) belts and other appliances,
- (*e*) late complications.

Regularity of evacuation. From the patient's point of view the aim must be to control the colostomy so as to avoid constipation and yet be sure that it does not become soiled by unexpected action of the bowel during his normal daily life. The method by which regular evacuation can be ensured depends rather on the individual. Many patients are able to acquire a regular bowel habit whereby the colon empties itself after breakfast and again perhaps in the evening. In a normal person, the desire to defaecate is brought about by movement of faeces from the sigmoid colon into the rectum. If rectal sensation is impaired (as in paraplegia) severe constipation results. Except for this short time before evacuation the rectum is normally empty. In colostomy, however, the proximal limb of colon has no sensation except that of severe distension and spasm. If the patient can acquire sufficient confidence and lead a regular life, he will be able to develop this regular habit of evacuation. Either he will place a large loose pad over the colostomy before the expected time of movement or he will go to the toilet at the set time and sit with the receptacle beneath the stoma until action is complete. After the bowel movement the stoma and surrounding skin are cleaned with soap and water and a thin square of cotton wool or cellulose tissue applied. Over this is placed the shield and belt and no further leak is expected. Vigorous activity can occur without fear. However, with the free supply of disposable adhesive bags it has become almost routine now for colostomy patients to be introduced to the bag routine. It is convenient and less offensive.

All the world over there are elderly colostomy patients who have acquired regular evacuation habits. Some depend on a regular 'wash-out' and constipation may necessitate this. It is less unpleasant than producing diarrhoea with a laxative.

If a colostomy requires irrigation this is done with a funnel and soft rubber catheter (15 Charrière gauge) using cool water. Warm water will not effectively stimulate peristalsis. Soap is not added as it may irritate the bowel. A rubber appliance is available through which the irrigation catheter can be passed so that there is no risk of leak during irrigation or evacuation. A Higginson's syringe or a rigid nozzle should not be used as there is a serious danger of perforating the colon. Single-use disposable bags are available commercially for colostomy washouts. After an effective morning wash-out there is little likelihood of further action of the bowel under normal conditions. The chief disadvantage of the wash-out method is that it takes time and requires suitable accommodation.

Diet plays a large part in the management of colostomy and the patient learns by experience what articles disturb his colon and what food is safe. Many patients pay no attention whatever to their diet and yet have normal control without limitation of their activity. Green vegetables, particularly sprouts, greens, leeks, and turnip or swede, should be avoided to start with until the patient has discovered how much he will tolerate. Increased action can be brought about by taking fruit or a mild agar laxative. The left iliac colostomy should produce a soft formed stool once, or at the most twice a day. The regularity and consistency of the stool is often helped by the use of **Celevac** granules taken night and morning. Patients should be discouraged from taking a purgative and hoping that a day's diarrhoea will be followed by 2 or 3 days' security!

Management of the blind distal loop. Where there is a double colostomy opening on to the left side the lower orifice normally leads to the distal loop unless a mistake is made in the construction. A distal loop remains if a permanent colostomy has been performed for a congenital abnormality or obstruction by irremovable growth or diverticulitis, or as a 'defunctioning' artificial anus for incontinence. It is a simple matter for the distal loop to be washed through once a week with water or saline. This the patient may undertake himself while on a commode or toilet.

If complete obstruction is present in the distal loop, difficulty may be experienced in emptying it in the process of washing out. A full-length rubber rectal tube should be used instead of a short catheter but should only be passed in one hand's breadth: as the bowel loop is filled the funnel is refilled. While the fluid is still running into the bowel, and the funnel is full, it is quickly lowered into a bucket or w.c. pan. The flow reverses through the wide bore tube and the bowel empties by siphonage.

Care of the skin. When the wound has healed and regular evacuation has been established there is rarely any trouble with the skin surrounding the stoma. It may become excoriated and sore if the patient develops an attack of diarrhoea; a barrier cream should then be used. Any such cream applied to the skin should be made with a silicone base or lanolin rather than with petroleum jelly or paraffin, as grease rots the elastic or rubber belt.

Belts and other appliances. Whatever method of evacuation is used, whether by washout or habit, some form of covering is required over the opening. At night a small pad of cotton wool or cellulose tissue is held in place by a 15 cm crepe bandage taken round the abdomen and iliac crest. A simple and absolutely reliable method of keeping the pad in place is by the 'two-way stretch' abdominal support. If patients prefer a bandage or home-made belt it can be readily washed if it should become soiled. Elasticated cotton net is admirable for retaining dressings in this situation (page 400).

During the daytime, if a bag is not worn, the knuckle of bowel should be covered by a thin layer of absorbent cotton wool over which is placed another layer of non-absorbent cotton or 'draper's' wool. Over this pad may be placed a thick plastic disc which is slightly hollowed and carries on its outer surface four studs which prevent it slipping about under the webbing belt. The belt itself should be made to measure and adjustable. Various forms are available and the type required depends on the shape of the patient and the position of the colostomy. For day use some patients manage very well with the elastic two-way stretch type of corset. It is much cheaper than a colostomy belt, more easily acquired and more readily replaced.

Many patients now rely entirely on the use of a 'stick-on' disposable colostomy bag as is used for terminal ileostomy. The care of the stoma and apparatus is similar to that for urinary ileostomy (page 690).

Late complications

Stenosis or narrowing of the opening may occur and produce gradually increasing obstruction. Dilatation at regular intervals with a finger or metal dilator may be sufficient, but if stenosis becomes troublesome a reconstruction of the colostomy is necessary.

Prolapse of mucous membrane or full thickness of the bowel wall (intussusception) may occur. Surgical treatment is needed.

Bleeding from an established colostomy requires investigation. It may be coming from a recurrence of the growth for which the rectum was removed; it may be from ulceration of the bowel due to impacted faeces. The colostomy can be examined with a sigmoidoscope.

30

Ano-rectal Conditions

A great many people suffer from minor maladies of the anal region. Many of them go untreated because of shyness and an instinctive resort to patent medicines and suppositories.

This region is of particular importance in nursing for two reasons. First, in all general surgical units a considerable number of patients are admitted specifically for operative treatment of ano-rectal lesions; much of the routine surgical out-patient work is concerned with treatment of these disorders. Second, the presence of abnormal conditions in the anal area may only be detected by a nurse during toilet procedures or the administration of enemas. Many patients who are admitted for some entirely different surgical condition are found to be suffering from haemorrhoids or some other anal disorder which requires treatment, or may give trouble in the post-operative period.

Because of the importance of proper bowel management in the prevention and management of these disabilities, the nurse must know the symptoms and be able to recognise the common abnormalities.

Anatomy

The rectum is S-shaped, about 22 cm (9 in) long, and is formed of muscle layers similar to those elsewhere in the intestinal tract. The lower end of the rectum is funnel-shaped and terminates in the anal canal which is lined with a special form of skin. The rectum is 'slung' in the bottom of the pelvis between the **levator ani muscles.** Below this level and around the anal canal is a strong sphincter of voluntary muscle—**the external sphincter. The internal sphincter** is the thickened lower end of the involuntary rectal muscle. Stretching or weakness of the levator ani muscle, or nervous conditions causing paralysis of this or the external sphincter, allow the rectum to drop. The lining mucous membrane is then 'prolapsed'. On either side of the anal canal below the levator ani muscle is a space containing fat—**the ischio-rectal fossa.** This is sometimes the seat of infection and abscess formation.

The anal canal has arteries and veins from the systemic circulation coming from the perineum and buttocks. The arteries join with the branches of the inferior mesenteric artery while the veins join with the tributaries of the portal vein which drain the rectum. If the portal veins are blocked or compressed (as in extreme constipation or in more serious disorders which affect the liver, such as cirrhosis) the haemorrhoidal veins become dilated or 'varicose'. These varicosities around and inside the anal canal immediately underneath the lining membrane are called 'piles' or **haemorrhoids.** Sometimes during strain at stool the veins are temporarily distended and one of them bursts, producing either brisk haemorrhage or a **peri-anal haematoma** (a form of external 'pile', Fig. 30.5*a*).

The rectum is normally empty except immediately before defaecation. The passage of the faecal mass from the colon into the rectum produces the desire to evacuate. If the rectum is insensitive, no such desire occurs, and extreme constipation arises.

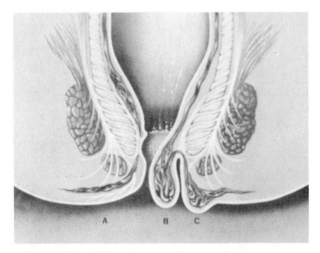

Fig. 30.1   Anatomy of anal canal. **A.** Normal veins with internal and external submucous and subcutaneous plexus. **B.** Prolapsing internal haemorrhoid. **C.** Dilated external haemorrhoidal plexus: if a small vein bursts the haematoma is an external pile.

Pathological conditions

Congenital

During the formation of the rectum and anus certain abnormalities can occur. The anal canal is formed from a pit in the perineal skin and this may fail to break through into the rectum which in turn may not have descended fully into the pelvis. There are several degrees of 'imperforate anus'. The simplest form is one in which there is a very thin membrane across the anal canal: this is readily punctured in the new-born baby and regular dilatations with the finger lead to the development of a perfectly normal channel. If, however, a portion of the rectum is missing it is almost impossible to repair the deficiency surgically and the condition is treated by colostomy. Later the pelvic colon is lengthened and brought down through the perineum, but this is not always possible or successful and colostomy is then permanent. Initially, the colostomy is made in the right part of the transverse colon, but if it is to be permanent the pelvic colon is used.

Sometimes the rectum instead of opening on the perineum turns forward and opens, in the male, into the prostatic urethra: in the female it opens into the posterior wall of the vagina high up towards the cervix, or low down towards the perineum where the opening can be seen. In a male the condition is extremely serious and has to be treated by early surgical operation. It is diagnosed by the absence of a normal functioning anus in the new-born baby: the baby with a recto-urethral fistula passes faecal material with the urine. In the female with a low 'vaginal ectopic anus', stools are passed normally, and the abnormality may not be detected for some days after birth. Occasionally operation is required to enlarge the opening in order to prevent constipation. The child must never be allowed to develop faecal impaction from prolonged untreated constipation.

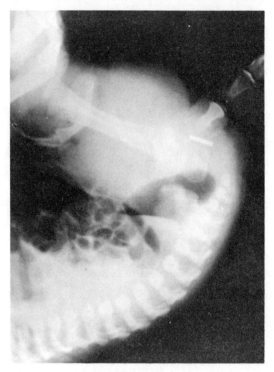

Fig. 30.2 Lateral x-ray of new-born baby with imperforate anus. The baby is upside down and a metal marker is on the anus, held by a nurse's finger. There is a gap between the gas bubble in the rectum and the marker. This baby required urgent colostomy, but construction of a functioning ano-rectal area may be possible.

Prolapse (Fig. 30.3A)

Prolapse of the ano-rectal mucous membrane is very common in young children, especially if they are allowed to sit on a 'pot' for a long time. In infancy the condition very rarely requires treatment, except in the management of the child and the avoidance of constipation. The prolapse may require pushing back after each bowel action. The condition is very likely to occur after an attack of diarrhoea in a child who has lost a great deal of weight and has thus lost also the support of the pads of fat in the ischio-rectal fossa.

Very occasionally, in infants the prolapse is treated by injections of phenol in oil, a method which is used in the treatment of haemorrhoids in adults (page 577).

Prolapse also occurs in old people and often requires surgical treatment. The whole thickness of the bowel is involved, not just the mucosa as in babies. Similar full-thickness prolapse occurs in paraplegic patients. The length of bowel which protrudes may be a

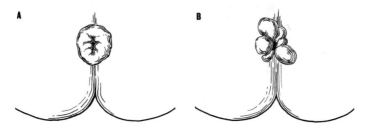

Fig. 30.3   **A.** Rectal prolapse. **B.** Prolapsed (thrombosed) haemorrhoids.

hand's breadth or more. One surgical operation is merely a procedure for amputating this prolapsed portion and stitching the cut ends of all layers together so as to reform the canal. The suture line is then returned through the anal ring. This is **procto-sigmoidectomy.** Minor degrees can be controlled by the insertion of a non-absorbable stitch subcutaneously around the anus within the external sphincter layer. Care has to be taken to ensure that this is not too tight. This is useful in babies, and paraplegic patients, but adults with severe prolapse are best treated by abdominal operation. The end of the sigmoid colon and rectum are surrounded by a sheet of plastic foam (Ivalon sponge) which encourages fibrosis and fixes the rectum but does not stop it contracting.

After this operation there may be great difficulty from retention of urine due to oedema and interference with the nerve supply to the bladder.

Fissure (Fig. 30.4A)

This is one of the most common of all surgical conditions—a simple split of the anal canal. It is almost always produced by the passage of a large constipated stool. The onset is marked by intense pain which recurs each time the bowel acts. The majority of fissures heal as soon as the constipation is rectified, but because of the constant movement, infection, and spasm, healing is sometimes delayed and the fissure is a persistent source of pain and irritation. A skin tag at the outer end of a fissure is a 'sentinel pile'.

In mild cases, the condition is treated by anaesthetic ointments and regular dilatation with a metal bougie dilator which the patient inserts night and morning. Many fissures are cured by this simple method, but some require operation.

At operation, the chronically inflamed skin and the edges of the fissure are excised and the small ring of muscle which lies beneath it is divided to relieve the spasm and allow the fissure to heal as a flat ulcer instead of as a deep crack. After operation the main treatment consists of regular dilatation to prevent the surface bridging across before the depth of the wound has healed.

An additional treatment is the injection of local anaesthetic solution beneath the fissure to relieve the pain and muscle spasm but because of the risk of sepsis and abscess formation this method has fallen into disfavour.

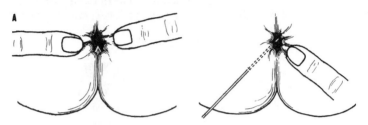

Fig. 30.4 A. Fissure-in-ano. B. Fistula-in-ano.

Fistula (Fig. 30.4B)

A false track develops between the skin and lining of the anal canal or rectum. There may in fact be several tracks communicating with one another and entering the rectum at various levels. Fistula almost always arises from abscess formation, the abscess having burst on to the skin and into the rectum. It must be treated surgically, and will not heal without operation. If it is untreated, persistant discharge and recurrent abscess formation are almost certain to result.

The symptoms are usually continual moisture around the anus and perhaps a faecal discharge and recurrent attacks of inflammation. At operation, the tracks are opened and left to heal by granulation. If the fistula is extensive, operative treatment involves long and deep incisions and painful post-operative dressings. Successful treatment depends largely on meticulous nursing care.

Haemorrhoids

Internal haemorrhoids are due to dilatations of the veins beneath the skin of the anal canal. They fill up during straining and may be so distended that one of the veins bursts. Defaecation is then followed by a variable amount of bleeding. Sometimes these piles prolapse outside the anus and enlarge to such an extent that they are covered partly by mucous membrane, and partly by the external skin (**intero-external or prolapsed piles,** Fig. 30.3B). Thrombosis, infection and gangrene may supervene.

Internal haemorrhoids are frequently treated by injection. Phenol (5 per cent in almond oil) is injected with a special needle (Fig. 16.14) under the mucous membrane above the pile-bearing area. This is done through the proctoscope. If the haemorrhoids prolapse or are large they are treated by surgical operation. This procedure and the nursing requirements are described on page 577.

Under the skin around the anus is a network of small veins which become distended when the patient strains at stool. If one of these bursts, a peri-anal haematoma forms (Fig. 30.5A) just outside the anus. Pain comes on suddenly during bowel action and is very intense. A small purple knob appears which is very tender. If the patient seeks medical advice at this stage, or within 24 hours, a small incision is made into the surface of the lump and the blood clot is released. If no treatment is given the clotted blood may get infected. Infection leads to the formation of a peri-anal abscess. If there is no infection, the surface of the haematoma may ulcerate. The blood is then discharged perhaps ten days after the haematoma has formed and the cavity heals without further trouble. This sequel of events is usually responsible for the so-called 'attacks of piles'. The patient seeks advice from his family doctor, and by the time an appointment has been made for him to see a specialist the haematoma has resolved!

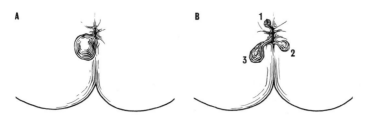

Fig. 30.5   A. Peri-anal haematoma. **B. 1.** skin tag, **2.** inflamed skin tag, **3.** rectal polyp (prolapsed).

The peri-anal haematoma is one form of 'external pile' and sometimes leaves behind a skin-tag (Fig. 30.5**B**). From time to time this tag may get infected and become swollen and oedematous. The tags can be removed with the aid of local anaesthesia.

Polyp

Reference has already been made to benign and malignant adenomas of the colon and rectum (page 550). If these develop a stalk they are called 'polyps'. Polyps of a different type due to congenital malformation of tissue (hamartoma) or inflammation may occur. The rectal polyp of childhood is usually single and harmless except that it bleeds and may prolapse. Polyps are removed from the rectum by diathermy or simple ligature of the stalk. A proctoscope may be needed if the polyp will not prolapse and if it is high in the rectum or in the sigmoid colon it is removed with a wire snare, using diathermy.

Ischio-rectal abscess

The fat-filled space on each side of the anus has already been described. Infection sometimes occurs and spreads to the fat which subsequently undergoes necrosis. A deep abscess forms and has to be drained by surgical operation. The surface skin is excised to prevent the skin healing over too quickly before the cavity has filled up properly with granulation tissue. A small gauze wick or rubber drain is retained in the wound for several days. The development of ischio-rectal abscess is frequently associated with fistula.

Symptoms of anal disorder

The patient's complaint is nearly always one of 'piles'. Common anal symptoms which may occur with any of these conditions are:

pain
pruritus (irritation)
prolapse
passage of blood
passage of mucus
tenesmus (urgent and ineffective desire to pass a motion).

Pruritus is usually associated with infection or with the presence of mucous discharge from inflamed piles or fistula. If something protrudes, it may be 'piles', complete true prolapse or a polyp. Bleeding arises most commonly from fissure or internal haemorrhoids.

Anal or rectal symptoms must never be ignored. The symptom of piles may in fact be due to a carcinoma of the rectum. A fissure may be tuberculous and an indication that there is a tuberculous focus in the lungs. A fistula may also be tuberculous or may be associated with ulcerative colitis or Crohn's Disease. Haemorrhoids by repeated bleeding can lead to the most severe degree of anaemia which requires blood transfusion. Because the amount of blood which is lost each day cannot be estimated by the patient, he does not always appreciate the importance of his anal disorder from which he is becoming exsanguinated. If a patient complains of any of these symptoms whilst in hospital for some entirely different condition, the complaint must be reported to the medical staff as the symptom may have an important bearing on treatment. Piles may be a signal that the patient has cirrhosis of the liver.

The shape of the perineum is very variable. The anus may be very deeply set in some individuals, and there is then a greater liability to constant moisture from sweating and subsequently to infection and pruritus.

Examination of the patient

Any patient who comes to hospital with anal symptoms must be fully undressed for examination by the surgeon. Because of the common association of anal disorders with other more serious abdominal conditions, the *whole* abdomen may be examined. A specimen of urine must be obtained and tested for sugar, as pruritus ani is sometimes due to diabetes.

A red perianal rash and irritation is often the result of infection with candida albicans (monilia) in patients who have recently had treatment with antibiotics, particularly tetracycline. Treatment is with nystatin ointment.

Examination of the anal area must be carried out with a very good light. Finger cots or disposable gloves, lubricant jelly and small squares of cotton wool (page 288) must be available. It is usual for this examination to take place with the patient lying on his left side with hips and knees flexed. Examination is greatly assisted by a large sand-bag placed under the left buttock. An alternative position is the 'knee-elbow position' in which the patient kneels on the examination table with his forearms folded across beneath his forehead and his elbows on the table. This is an impossible position for elderly people and it has no particular merit although some surgeons prefer it.

The nurse should arrange clean, but not sterile, towels so that the patient is adequately covered during an examination which may cause discomfort and will certainly cause embarrassment. In the left lateral position care must be taken that the head is supported comfortably on a pillow and is flexed towards the knees. The legs and feet should be covered with another towel as the surgeon places his head very near the table during the examination with special instruments. The nurse must ensure that the anus has been cleaned and should notice if there is any discharge of pus or blood on the surface. After careful inspection of the anal area, during which he may require a probe, the surgeon carries out a full examination by palpation with the finger inside the rectum. This is followed by endoscopic examination. In the female patient, a digital examination of the vagina precedes the rectal examination. The colloquial abbreviations 'PR' and 'PV' are used for the per rectum and per vaginum examinations.

Proctoscopy

Figure 30.6 shows a standard illuminated proctoscope. It is possible to use a smaller and slightly shorter instrument with direct illumination from a head lamp or from an adjustable spot-light. If the rectum is found full on digital examination, endoscopic examination is postponed until after the next bowel action. This may be induced by suppository so that the patient avoids having to attend an Out-patient clinic on another occasion.

The instrument is lubricated and inserted with the obturator in position. If it is done slowly, it is not painful unless there is a fissure.

After the removal of the obturator the surgeon may need to clean the rectum with small cotton wool balls held in a long pair of non-toothed dissecting forceps.

Injection treatment of haemorrhoids may be carried out at once and the necessary equipment should be available.

A receiving bowl, or paper bag, is used for soiled swabs and the instruments are placed in a separate dish.

After use the proctoscope must be washed thoroughly and boiled, or sterilised chemically. It is not sterilised *before* use. Care must be taken not to boil the lamp. During use, if the surgeon is careful, neither the lamp nor flex will become contaminated. If it should be soiled, it is washed and disinfected in an antiseptic solution. Disposable plastic proctoscopes are used in some clinics, or metal ones are supplied from the CSSD.

Common proctoscope faults

1. The proctoscope has the wrong obturator.
2. The proctoscope has been dropped and the narrow end dented so that the obturator cannot be inserted completely.
3. Light trouble—coiled wire contact is flattened or is short-circuiting on the side of the case.
   the bulb is fused (probably blackened)
   flex faulty
   battery exhausted.

(Fibre-optic lighting for new instruments has eliminated these faults).

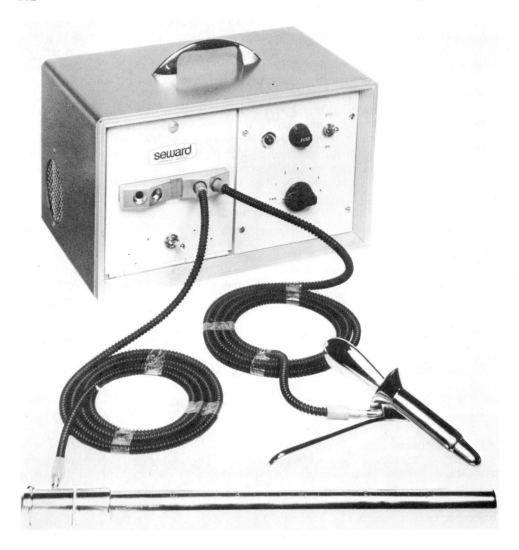

Fig. 30.6 Standard fibre-optic endoscopic unit. This enables four instruments to be lit simultaneously. The illustration shows the standard proctoscope and sigmoidoscope. (Seward Surgical Instruments.)

After the rectal examination is completed the nurse must ensure that the patient's anal area is cleaned, dry, and free from oil and lubricant jelly which would otherwise soil his clothes. This is a most essential point in good nursing technique and one which is very often forgotten; its omission leads to unnecessary embarrassment and inconvenience to the patient.

Sigmoidoscopy

Figure 30.7 illustrates a typical form of sigmoidoscope. Other types of instrument are available with more complicated lighting systems and magnifying lenses, or with fibre-optic illumination. As with the proctoscope, the instrument is not sterilised before use unless supplied from the CSSD, but must be thoroughly cleaned and boiled immediately after use. Spare bulbs must be available. Long swab holders and biopsy forceps are used through the tube and must be at hand.

Preparation. The sigmoidoscope is passed through the rectum to a distance of 25 cm well up into the sigmoid colon. It is inserted blindly through the anal canal. The eyepiece is then fixed in position after withdrawal of the obturator, and the bellows connected. Air is pumped into the rectum continuously and as the pressure rises the air escapes through the anus around the instrument. The surgeon continually 'seeks' the lumen of the bowel and passes the instrument into it under direct vision, inflating the colon as the instrument advances. During this part of the examination he notes the appearance of any faecal matter which is in the rectum and the presence of blood or mucus. In order that no information may be lost, many surgeons prefer that there should be no pre-examination preparation of the patient by means of laxatives or enemas. Under no circumstances should a laxative be given on the night before sigmoidoscopy and no enema or wash-out may be given on the day of examination. The only satisfactory and permissible treatment is that an enema should be given on the previous evening. Further peristalsis may be prevented by giving the patient some codeine compound or morphine derivative after the enema. The rectum then remains absolutely empty and examination on the following morning is rendered more easy.

If there has been no preparation the surgeon may have to spend considerable time removing faecal material with the aid of small cotton wool swabs on a long swab carrier. As described under 'proctoscopy', evacuation may be induced by suppository, and subsequent examination made possible without a second attendance.

Complications. Sigmoidoscopy in unskilled hands can be dangerous and the peritoneum can be perforated if the bowel is torn by a forcible passage of the instrument. This happens most readily if there is growth or diverticulitis and particularly in ulcerative colitis where the bowel wall is extremely thin.

These procedures are normally carried out without anaesthetic, except on small children. There are normally no complications.

If an anaesthetic is required full relaxation is necessary and the patient will need to be retained in hospital on account of the anaesthesia.

Biopsy. Special forceps a little longer than the sigmoidoscope and having a cutting jaw at the distal end are used to snip away a portion of tissue which may be thought to be tumour for microscopic examination. This is an absolute routine to confirm the diagnosis of carcinoma of the rectum. Occasionally bleeding persists from the site where the tissue has been removed.

Sometimes a biopsy of the full thickness of the rectal wall is required for examination particularly by chemical methods to aid in the diagnosis of certain general metabolic disorders and in suspected Hirschsprung's disease. From the nursing point of view such a full thickness rectal biopsy requires the pre- and post-operative care common to all minor anal operations.

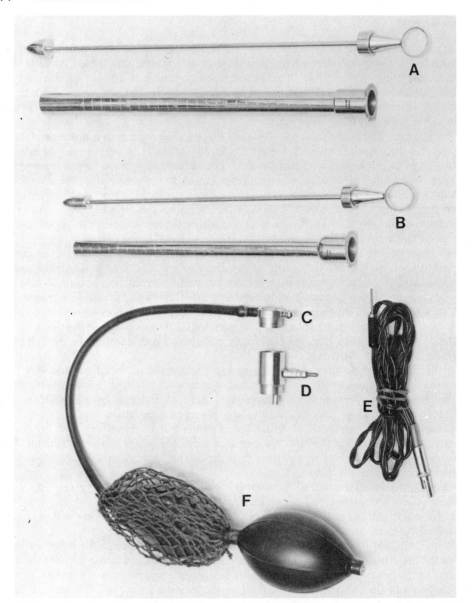

Fig. 30.7 Standard sigmoidoscope. **A.** Wide bore size with obturator; essential when performing a biopsy. **B.** Small bore with obturator for routine examination purposes and for use in children. **C.** Eye piece lens fitting on to bulb carrier. **D.** A light attachment which is inserted into the head of the instrument. **E.** The lighting flex. **F.** Bellows with safety balloon to inflate the rectum for examination.

A tall jar should always be used to receive contaminated sigmoidoscopes; the instrument is easily damaged if it is dropped on the floor and this is unavoidable sooner or later if only a shallow receiver or kidney dish is provided for the dirty instrument.

Operations

General principles

While the operations for these anal conditions are of a relatively minor nature, they are by no means trivial and a great deal of disability has arisen in the past when they have been performed by inexperienced surgeons. The pre-operative preparation and post-operative nursing are equally matters of very great importance.

Infection, spasm of the anal muscle and the development of a painful and persistent fissure are the three important hazards. To deal with these, antiseptic dressings, the avoidance of packing, regular dilatation of the anal canal and regulation of bowel function, all demand special attention.

Pre-operative preparation

The whole of the pubic area and perineum must be thoroughly shaved and cleaned on the evening before operation. An enema should be given to ensure that the lower bowel is empty. No further meal should be taken owing to the risk of stimulating peristalsis. Unless specific instructions are given to the contrary, no wash-out or enema must be given on the day of operation.

Operations on the anus are performed with the patient in the lithotomy position.[1] The legs are held up in the air by being slung in stirrups on the operating table. In this position of hip flexion, the lumbar spine is also flexed. Sometimes patients develop severe back-ache and sciatica following operations performed in this position. If there has been any suggestion of previous sciatica or spinal arthritis the nurse should inform the anaesthetist in order that precautions may be taken to place a pillow or sand-bag under the patient's lumbar spine on the operating table.

Post-operative care

Unless a defunctioning colostomy is present, it is impossible to keep the anal area free from contamination by faeces. All operations are therefore potentially infected but the tissues in this area heal remarkably well in spite of contamination.

After operation, the degree of shock is extremely slight unless there has been great loss of blood.

Haemorrhoids are removed by pulling the individual piles through the anal canal into the prolapsed position. The base of each is then transfixed with a stitch of silk or catgut which is firmly tied. A mass of tissue is cut away, together with a piece of skin around its base. If one of these ligatures should slip profuse haemorrhage occurs. In order that such accidental post-operative haemorrhage should not escape notice by the blood trickling upwards into the colon, a tube is sometimes inserted (Fig. 30.8): the blood then runs outwards on to the dressing where it is observed. With careful surgery this risk is very slight and it is becoming increasingly common for the tube to be omitted.

After most haemorrhoid operations there are three raw areas of skin around the anus with intervening strips which maintain continuity between the rectal mucous membrane and the anal skin. It is an essential part of the operation to leave these strips so that the anus does not become strictured.

[1] Lithotomy position is so named from its use in the stone-cutting operations in which a bladder stone was pressed down towards the perineum and an incision made there for its extraction (Fig. 18.2F).

After excision of a fissure or a fistula a similar raw area remains and the tissues are never stitched together.

At the end of the operation the surgeon places on each raw area a gauze swab moistened with some mild antiseptic such as Savlon or hypochlorite (Milton). Sometimes pieces of tulle gras are used beneath the gauze. Loose gauze packing is added around the tube if one is present. Under no circumstances must the cavity or crater be packed tightly with gauze. A wool pad is held in position by a perineal T-bandage.

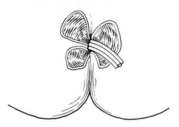

Fig. 30.8 Haemorrhoidectomy. The three raw areas each receive a flat dressing. The corner of each extends into the anal canal. A small drainage tube is left in position for 48 hours.

Whatever the operation has been, the post-operative management of the operation area is for all practical purposes the same. It is left undisturbed for 2–3 days, depending on the surgeon's wishes. The dressing is removed or the patient may be allowed to sit in a salt-bath to soak it off. A moist hypochlorite dressing is applied: no firm padding is used, but care must be taken to ensure that the raw areas are covered and the edges prevented from 'bridging' across.

After an operation for an extensive fistula the raw area may be considerable and an anaesthetic is required for the first dressing. The trilene inhaler (Chapter 18) or intravenous thiopentone is most suitable for ward use. In many cases, on the fourth and subsequent post-operative days the patient is able to take a bath once or twice a day and in this way the healing area is kept clean and fresh.

Considerable trouble occurs sometimes from post-operative constipation. Unless the surgeon has forbidden its use, paraffin emulsion can be given by mouth on the first post-operative day and each evening subsequently. The insertion of a glycerine suppository or the administration of a small olive oil enema may be required to initiate the first bowel movement. Bowel action is discouraged for the first 2 or 3 days, but if constipation is prolonged the faecal mass in the rectum becomes hard and extreme difficulty is then experienced. Digital evacuation of the rectum under anaesthesia is sometimes required, but this necessity should be regarded as a reflection on nursing management.

Another essential in the after-care is regular dilatation of the anal canal until healing is complete. Digital examination is carried out by the surgeon at intervals from the 3rd day onwards. After fissure operation instructions may be given for the patient to insert a metal dilator once or twice a day after his bath. If dilatation is not performed at this stage the anus is likely to become contracted and great difficulty is then experienced in establishing regular bowel action. The patient is instructed to avoid constipation but also to avoid loose bowel actions. The passage of a firm stool daily is the best dilator.

An operation in the anal area may precipitate acute retention of urine in a male patient with an enlarged prostate. This is sometimes an extremely troublesome complication requiring prolonged catheterisation or suprapubic cystostomy, since it is unwise to perform prostatectomy in the presence of an infected anal area.

All patients who have undergone operation for ano-rectal disorders must be nursed for the first day or so on their side. A frequent change of position is necessary and the patient very soon becomes ambulant. It is preferable for patients to remain in hospital until healing is complete owing to the necessity for regular cleansing, dressings and dilatation.

An alternative method of treating haemorrhoids is to 'strangulate' them with a very tight rubber band applied with a special instrument; this is the same procedure as is used to castrate piglets.

A further 'conservative' treatment is full dilatation under anaesthetic; the theory is that by breaking down fibrous bands in the ano-rectal area obstruction to venous return is reduced: the patient has to insert a dilator daily for several weeks. The advantage of both these procedures is that they can be undertaken as 'day admissions'.

Injection treatment of haemorrhoids

In mild cases of internal haemorrhoids, the symptoms can be relieved by injections of phenol (5 per cent) in almond oil into the submucous tissue at the top of the anal canal. Preparation is exactly the same as for proctoscopy and a special syringe is used with a screw-on or bayonet-fitting needle. The needle itself has a shoulder a short distance from its point to prevent it being inserted too deeply into the rectal wall (see Fig. 16.14).

The procedure is usually painless and requires no after-treatment. Sometimes the injected area ulcerates and severe haemorrhage occurs. This usually happens several days after the injection and may be sufficiently severe to require blood transfusion. If bleeding has occurred, proctoscopy is again required and the bleeding area is lightly packed with gauze soaked in 1/1,000 adrenaline solution.

Management of strangulated haemorrhoids

When severe internal piles prolapse they become congested and undergo thrombosis. The term 'strangulation' is often applied to this condition when the prolapsed tissue is virtually 'gangrenous'. The whole of the anal region is extremely painful and the hard purple masses cannot be replaced within the anal canal. The usual treatment is conservative. The patient is kept in bed, lying flat. The foot of the bed is raised on blocks. Cold, 5 per cent saline packs are applied to the anal area in the hope of diminishing the swelling and congestion. Paraffin emulsion is given by mouth to make the bowel action easier. Morphine will be required to relieve pain, but adds to the risk of constipation. Acute distress may continue for several days. In all probability the patient will want 10 to 14 days in bed. In some cases the haemorrhoids are cured by this natural process of thrombosis and no further treatment is required. Frequently excessive skin tags remain and these have to be removed.

To avoid the prolonged disability of conservative treatment in these cases, some surgeons remove the strangulated pile mass as an emergency operation. They consider that the risk is slight and is fully justified by the relief of the patient's distress.

Pilonidal[1] **sinus** (sacro-coccygeal dermoid)

This is not strictly an ano-rectal disorder but is conveniently included in this section owing to its frequent confusion with fistula. The condition is thought to be due to a congenital infolding of skin on the mid-line over the coccyx. It rarely gives rise to trouble in children, but as the body hair develops at puberty the hair-bearing skin lying deeply in this abnormal channel becomes infected. Multiple abscesses form and discharge on the surface as sinuses. There are usually several small holes in the mid-line over the sacrum or coccyx and occasionally these sinuses track out into the buttocks or forward into the perineum around the anus.

The condition is treated by radical surgical operation in which the whole of the infected tissue is excised. A large wound cavity remains and is usually left open, being dressed twice daily in the same manner as anal wounds.

Sometimes the cavity is closed by primary suture, and if this has been done watch must be kept for the development of infection in the depths of the wound. Owing to the risk of persistent sinuses from wound infection, the technique of primary suture is only suitable for certain cases. During healing and for several weeks afterwards the area must be kept shaved. It is thought by some that hair shafts may be driven into the skin and be the initial cause of the condition. Hairdressers occasionally develop a lesion like this in the web between the fingers.

---

[1] pilos = hair; nidus = nest.

31

Diseases of the Liver and Biliary Apparatus

Physiology

The liver has many functions in relation to metabolism; it stores glycogen as an energy reserve; it forms various protein compounds and enzymes, and is the main sorting station for food products absorbed from the intestine. A by-product of its activity is the formation of bile, containing breakdown products of red blood cells, and producing in turn chemicals which are themselves essential for digestion.

Disease affecting the liver may become evident from obstruction of the outflow of bile, by obstruction to the portal venous system or by interference with some metabolic process such as elimination of oestrogens. (Extensive liver disease in the male results in gynaecomastia, page 888.)

Investigation

Various chemical tests are performed on blood to estimate different liver functions. Radio-isotope scanning (page 448) is used to outline areas of the liver which may have become inactive from abscess or malignant deposits. X-ray examination of the bile transport system is carried out by taking dye by mouth or by injection which is secreted in the bile.

The biliary tract

Bile is formed in the liver and transmitted through a network of tiny bile capillaries which join to form the main right and left hepatic ducts. These two again join on the under surface of the liver at the 'hilum' where they form the main or 'common' duct. This in turn runs behind the pylorus and through the head of the pancreas. Here it is joined by the pancreatic duct and the two enter the duodenum by a common orifice, at the papilla of the 'Ampulla of Vater'.

Inflammation of the ducts or a stone within will produce violent contraction of the ducts. The gall bladder, which is a simple muscular pouch placed as a cul-de-sac on the common bile duct, takes part in the spasm.

An additional function of the gall bladder is to store and concentrate bile so that when a fatty meal is taken there is a reserve supply of bile to aid in its digestion. Thus, fat taken by mouth produces a contraction of the gall bladder, and should this be diseased the contraction will produce pain which the patient interprets as indigestion.

Pathology

Interruption of the flow of bile may occur for a number of reasons. There may be defective manufacture of bile due to disease of the liver, perhaps from infection as in infective hepatitis.

The bile capillaries or the main bile ducts may become blocked by pressure from outside or by the presence of a stone or growth inside the duct; if the block continues for more than a few hours the patient becomes jaundiced.

The seriousness of this obstruction to the flow of bile depends on the exact site of the block. If the obstruction is inside or up against the liver, nothing can be done surgically to relieve it. If, however, the duct is blocked below the attachment of the gall bladder, the surgeon may be able to remove the cause of the obstruction or 'short-circuit' the bile. When for instance there is a growth in the pancreas pressing on the bile duct, a relieving operation may be performed, in which the gall bladder is joined to the stomach or to a loop of small bowel (cholecystogastrostomy or cholecystojejunostomy).

In addition to 'mechanical' causes of trouble with the biliary system, the gall bladder and ducts may get inflamed from infection or from deposits of chemicals from the bile. This condition of **cholecystitis** leads to the formation of stones which make their presence known by producing colic or obstruction, or both.

Chronic disease of the biliary system leads to inflammation in the liver around the tiny bile ducts; eventually fibrosis occurs causing biliary cirrhosis (page 588).

Surgical problems

Pain is a marked feature of all forms of gall-bladder disease. It may be located beneath the ribs in the loin, high up between the shoulder blades or in the tip of the right shoulder; this wide distribution of the pain may be a very distressing feature to the patient. If the nurse is aware of this, she may do much to assure the patient that all the symptoms are coming from the one site.

It will be seen that the problems fall broadly into three categories:

(1) Cholecystitis, which shows itself by the presence of a particular form of 'fatty' dyspepsia.
(2) Stones—a condition known as **cholelithiasis**—which produce attacks of colic and jaundice. There may be a single stone or many hundreds of small ones.
(3) Obstructive jaundice. This calls for surgical relief and special measures have to be adopted to lower the risks coming from the presence of jaundice.

Certain operations are therefore undertaken for the relief of these conditions (Table 44). A diseased gall bladder is usually removed whether or not it contains stones. If there has been no history suggesting obstruction of the main duct, the latter is not interfered with. If, however, the patient is or has been jaundiced, the surgeon will open the 'common' duct to make certain there is a clear way for the bile through to the duodenum. Owing to the small calibre of the duct where it enters the duodenum, it is normal practice for the surgeon when he has opened and explored the common duct to leave the special rubber T-tube in the duct to act as a temporary safety valve in case the duct orifice swells and produces further obstruction (page 586). Occasionally, if the patient is too ill for a more extensive operation, the gall bladder is drained to relieve the tension of infected bile within it and to allow the escape of any stones which may have been found there. If there is no remaining block to the duct beyond the gall bladder, this drainage hole will heal up and the bile will go by its normal route when the acute condition has subsided.

Nursing

Patients with gall bladder disease usually come into hospital as emergency cases, either on account of colic or an acute attack of cholecystitis. Otherwise they will be admitted for operation on account of a long-standing history of dyspepsia or recurrent attacks of colic.

In the acute cases, the initial problem will be one of observation and examination until an exact diagnosis is made (pages 452, 462). An appreciation of the nature of the patient's pain, his reaction to it, frequent record of temperature, pulse and respiration rates and the examination of a specimen of urine for bile (page 641), will be routine duties for the nurse. If the patient is severely ill, there may be difficulty in micturition, but the examination is so vital that it is essential to obtain a specimen even if this involves catheterisation.

The common operation for obstruction of the bile duct by a gall stone is choledo-cholithotomy with cholecystectomy (to prevent further stone formation) and temporary drainage of the common bile duct. Though such words seem cumbersome they are useful in practice to indicate exactly what procedure has been adopted.

Sometimes when the gall bladder cannot be removed, part of its wall is cut away and the rest is destroyed by coagulation with the surgical diathermy.

All patients with gall bladder disease suffer from a form of dyspepsia and on account of this there may be a defective flow of saliva, quite apart from the fact that the patient may be febrile and dehydrated. Meticulous attention must therefore be paid to oral hygiene. In addition many patients with gall bladder disease are at the time of life when their teeth are commonly infected and in need of treatment.

Acute cholecystitis

Acute cholecystitis is usually treated without operation, although some surgeons feel that it is better and quite safe to go ahead and remove the acutely inflamed gall bladder. The patient is treated along general lines as for any acute febrile illness, except that this condition is sometimes accompanied by vomiting. Milk drinks and fats must be avoided, and if vomiting is persistent rectal fluid must be given. The patient is usually also given either one of the sulphonamide drugs or antibiotics; penicillin is not excreted in bile and is ineffective in cholecystitis. Magnesium sulphate, which stimulates the flow of bile, is given daily if there is no vomiting or dehydration. Usually the attack subsides without the patient coming to operation. The temperature, which is perhaps running at 38 to 39 °C, falls by lysis over 4 or 5 days. If however the temperature starts to swing and pain persists, this indicates that suppuration has probably occurred within the gall bladder. The condition is then known as **empyema of the gall bladder** and the latter will require draining as any other abscess. At a later date, the gall bladder is removed after the empyema has resolved, just as the appendix is removed after an appendix abscess has settled. Empyema of the gall bladder may burst, producing acute infective peritonitis. During this acute phase of the illness the nurse must be meticulous in her observation of the patient and the patient's stools, since obstructive jaundice may supervene at any time. Constipation will then be a marked feature and the early use of mild laxatives is a great help if magnesium sulphate has not been given already.

Patients with gall bladder disease may be nursed in the acute stage in any position which is comfortable. Some are best sitting up; others are more comfortable lying flat, but normally the sitting-up position relieves the tension on the abdominal muscles, which are usually tender. The patients are very often of a heavy type and the provision of a self-lifting pole ('monkey chain') over the bed helps to relieve the strain of moving when the abdomen is painful.

Colic

In the patient whose presenting symptom is intense pain from colic, shock may be present and the most important thing is to relieve pain. Morphine has for many years been the drug of choice and must be given in doses large enough to relieve the spasm of the muscle in the bile ducts. As morphine is thought to have an adverse effect on the liver, it is probably better to use pethidine (100 mg initially by intramuscular injection in an average size adult, repeated in 4 hours if there is not relief). This drug has a remarkable power of relaxing 'smooth' involuntary muscle. Atropine by injection (gr 1/25–2·5 mg) is also used.

As with acute cholecystitis, fluid intake must be kept high, and the stools watched each day for any change of colour. A paling of the stool indicates that the bile has been dammed back for a while: the pain has most likely been due to a stone producing temporary obstruction. The urine is examined regularly for the presence of bile and no specimen should be thrown away until this has been done. The detection of transient jaundice may be of the utmost help to the surgeon in deciding whether he should explore the bile duct when he operates to remove the gall bladder.

The jaundiced patient

Occasionally a patient will be admitted already in a condition of jaundice. The surgeon has to decide what may be the cause and whether he can do anything to relieve the obstruction. In carcinoma the depth of the jaundice will be usually greater and more persistent. With a stone, it tends to vary from day to day and the stools may not remain as white as in the cases of complete obstruction which are most commonly seen in patients with carcinoma of the pancreas.

A plain x-ray of the abdomen will be arranged at the earliest convenient time in hospital in an attempt to visualise a stone.

There are nursing factors peculiar to jaundiced patients irrespective of whether the jaundice is due to stone or growth.

The patient is depressed and anxious, has lost his appetite and very often his interest in his welfare; he is irritable in mind and body and may have a very troublesome irritation of the skin. He has usually been without food for some days and will almost certainly be dehydrated.

If jaundice has been present for a week or more there may be liver damage. One of the functions of the liver is to build body proteins from amino-acids (products of digestion of protein food), and if this process is impeded the patient will have lost weight from 'starvation'. He is therefore given a high-calorie, high-protein, fat-free diet. He may like a nicely poached egg, but not if the nurse in her kindness spreads butter on the toast. Cane sugar (sucrose) is given liberally. Glucose requires conversion by the liver, and is therefore not utilised if the liver is severely damaged.

If the skin irritation is severe, a soothing lotion may be used (e.g. calamine lotion containing liquor picis carbonis). A sedative will amost certainly be necessary to allow satisfactory sleep, even though the patient may have no real pain. Barbiturates or chlor-promazine must **not** be given.

Fortunately, the patients whose jaundice is due to a stone are readily relieved by operation and the particular nursing care of these patients is dealt with later in this chapter. On the other hand, progressive jaundice is a distressing and constant feature of advanced malignant disease of the liver or pancreas. Where there is complete obstruction to the flow of bile from the bile duct in carcinoma of the pancreas, there is usually also obstruction to the flow of pancreatic enzymes. Though there may be very little pain at this stage, the patient's general condition is distressing and death may not occur for several weeks after the onset of jaundice. If the jaundice is due to secondary deposits from the carcinoma within the liver, it may persist for several months before death ensues.

From the nursing point of view, there is much that can be done to ease the burden of the latter days of such patients. Mention has already been made of the **'pruritus'** or irritation of the skin occurring from the result of jaundice. This may necessitate the repeated administration of drugs, but if the liver is damaged some drugs have a cumulative effect and the patient may become very drowsy after relatively small doses. Morphia is often withheld from patients with jaundice or liver damage for a similar reason. Anorexia is a distressing feature and small amounts of alcohol in the form of white wine or sherry may do a great deal to help the patient to enjoy his food. The severe constipation which occurs in jaundice has already been mentioned and in the cases where there is also an obstruction to the flow of pancreatic juice the patient's bowel function may be further disturbed and distressing distension will occur. Pancreatic extract may be given by mouth to help digestion of such foods as are taken.

Special pre-operative measures in the jaundiced patient. Obstruction to the outflow of bile produces liver damage: protein and glycogen metabolism are disturbed. As the liver forms prothrombin which is vital in the coagulation of blood, a patient who has obstructive jaundice has a reduced amount of prothrombin in the blood (page 59). There is likely to be extensive and persistent oozing of blood at and after operation. Prothrombin is related to vitamin K, and its deficiency can be made good by giving synthetic vitamin K by injection. In severely jaundiced patients 20 mg is given twice daily by intramuscular injection for two days before operation and 10 mg daily after operation for the 1st week. The amount required is determined more accurately by examination of the blood pro-thrombin level.

Jaundiced patients do not heal well and it is particularly important that adequate vitamin C should be given before operation.

Operations upon the biliary apparatus

(Table 44)

Cholecystostomy. Operation for the drainage of the gall bladder and usually the evacuation of stones from it, is performed in patients with acute or chronic cholecystitis who are otherwise unfit for the removal of the gall bladder. An oblique incision is used parallel to the right rib margin. The gall bladder is opened, evacuated and closed around a self-retaining catheter, which is then brought through the abdominal incision. The bile and inflammatory fluid which comes from the gall bladder is drained into a bedside bag. The flow of bile from the tube is measured. If there has been no obstruction to the common bile duct, the nurse will observe that the stools are not pale. If the patient's temperature is normal the tube may be removed at the end of a week and the fistula should close spontaneously by the end of the 2nd week. When the patient's general condition is better, the surgeon may deem it wise to remove the gall bladder by a second operation, but in many cases this is unnecessary.

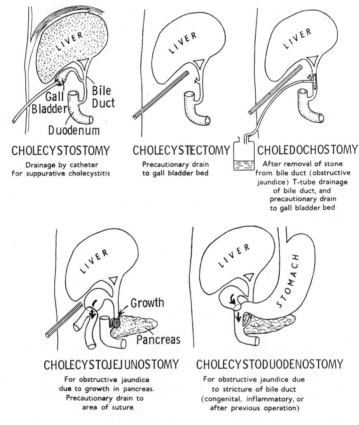

CHOLECYSTOSTOMY

Drainage by catheter
for suppurative cholecystitis

CHOLECYSTECTOMY

Precautionary drain
to gall bladder bed

CHOLEDOCHOSTOMY

After removal of stone
from bile duct (obstructive
jaundice) T-tube drainage
of bile duct, and
precautionary drain
to gall bladder bed

CHOLECYSTOJEJUNOSTOMY

For obstructive jaundice
due to growth in pancreas.
Precautionary drain to
area of suture

CHOLECYSTODUODENOSTOMY

For obstructive jaundice due
to stricture of bile duct
(congenital, inflammatory, or
after previous operation)

Fig. 31.1 Operations on the biliary apparatus showing the method of drainage appropriate to each.

Cholecystectomy and choledochostomy. Removal of the gall bladder and exploration of the bile duct are the most common operations on the biliary system and are usually performed on account of the presence of stones, or chronic cholecystitis without stones. The surgeon may use a mid-line, right paramedian or subcostal incision. Most surgeons, as a routine, perform operative cholangiography before removing the gall bladder. A fine catheter, from which all air has been expelled with saline, is inserted into the cystic duct and radio-opaque dye (e.g. Conray, diodone) injected. A film is taken on the operation

Table 44   Operations on the biliary apparatus (also Fig. 31.1)

Cholecystectomy—Removal of the gall bladder for stones or inflammation or occasionally for growth

Cholecystotomy—Emptying of the gall bladder usually as an emergency measure for stones or infection when removal of gall bladder is considered unsafe

Cholecystostomy—Temporary drainage of the gall bladder for infection; or after cholecystotomy. Cholecystectomy is performed at a later date

Choledocholithotomy—The removal of a stone from the common bile duct

Choledochostomy—Drainage of the common bile duct usually following exploration for stone in the duct

Cholecystogastrostomy—The creation of an anastomosis between the body of the gall bladder and the stomach as a short-circuit for the bile when the common duct is obstructed by growth which cannot be removed

Cholecystojejunostomy—A similar anastomosis between the gall bladder and the jejunum

---

table to show whether the bile ducts are filling completely and whether the opening into the duodenum is clear. This is always done if the patient has been jaundiced. The patients are very often obese and the operation is then difficult. It may require the use of large retractors which, in the upper abdomen, tend to produce a considerable amount of after-pain and a tendency of the patient to avoid using his diaphragm adequately in breathing. These patients are therefore particularly liable to post-operative pulmonary complications: the nurse has an additional responsibility in the prevention of these by encouraging the patient's deep breathing.

After simple cholecystectomy, the main wound is usually closed completely and a separate stab drainage incision is made in the right upper quadrant of the abdominal wall. Through this drainage incision is placed a strip of corrugated rubber which lies snugly in the depression on the under surface of the liver from which the gall bladder has been removed. The purpose of the drain is to allow the escape of a little bile which oozes from the raw surface of the liver and to prevent the accumulation of blood at the operation site. In addition, it acts as a safety measure if the ligature should come off the cystic duct (the point where the gall bladder joined the common bile duct). The drainage tube is usually removed completely at 48 hours and the wound heals up without further discharge.

Cholecystectomy is sometimes combined with choledochostomy (opening of the common bile duct for exploration) if the patient has had attacks of jaundice and it is thought that there may be a stone in the common duct. If **choledochostomy** has been performed in addition, it is usually because there has been some evidence of obstruction to the bile duct. The surgeon explores with special probes up and down the duct and removes any stones that he finds. Owing to the previous inflammation, and the passage of the instrument, the inside of the bile duct may become swollen after operation and produce further temporary obstruction to the flow of bile into the duodenum. A safety valve is necessary in case this should occur, and most surgeons use a specially made rubber T-tube which is placed within the lumen of the bile duct. This T-tube is connected to a bedside bag and the flow of bile is measured each day. The stem of the T-tube is brought out through the abdominal wall, preferably through the upper end of the main incision: when it is removed, this being the highest point, leakage is less likely, and being near the midline it does not drag. It may be brought out through a separate stab incision, connected to a bedside bag and the bile loss measured and recorded daily. This loss of bile reduces the patient's appetite. If the stools are a normal colour, at the end of the 1st week, a cholangiogram is performed to confirm normality of the duct and free flow into the duodenum.[1] The tube is then spigoted and if pain recurs it must be released, but if there is no pain the tube is removed after the 10th day. As long as the T-tube is present and draining into a bag, bile will be continually siphoned off even if the duct system is unobstructed: to eliminate this unnecessary loss, but at the same time avoid risk of obstruction and leakage, some surgeons divide the T-tube after 3–4 days, suspend it by the bedside with a Y-connector allowing an air leak held at a height above the duodenum to prevent siphoning. If pressure should build up, the bile simply flows over the open Y-connector. When there has been severe infection of the bile ducts (cholangitis) and jaundice, siphon drainage is deliberately maintained for longer, sometimes for many weeks. In such cases nutrition is difficult to maintain.

The removal of the T-tube may be momentarily painful; an analgesic should be given an hour before if the patient is apprehensive, so that the nurse is unhurried in the gentle but firm withdrawal which is necessary. If there is difficulty in moving the tube, the nurse must not persist but ask for the surgeon's help. Immediately the tube is out there will be a gush of bile but if the patient is sat up leakage will cease very quickly. If the tube has been brought out low down in the abdominal wall leakage may continue much longer.

Leakage of bile into the peritoneum after operations on the gall bladder or the duct produces the 'biliary peritonitis'. This is a chemical poisoning of the peritoneum and is often fatal. The T-tube is left until its track is firmly walled off.

As the appendix is thought to be a focus of infection, many surgeons remove it as part of the routine when a gall bladder operation is performed for the removal of stones or for chronic cholecystitis. This does not add materially to the nursing problem, except that the additional handling of the intestine may increase the liability to post-operative distension.

Bile short-circuit operations. One of the common sites for the bile duct to be obstructed is where it goes through the head of the pancreas. The cause is usually a carcinoma and during recent years improvements in surgery have made it occasionally possible for such a growth to be removed. If this is done, the bile duct has to be transplanted either into the stomach or the small intestine.

If the extent of the growth, or the condition of the patient, makes an operation for the removal of the growth unwise, then an alternative procedure is to relieve the jaundice by joining the distended gall bladder to the stomach or jejunum. Operations of this type are

[1] Hypaque (acetotrizoate) is injected down the tube and this may produce intestinal colic and diarrhoea for 2 days.

frequently performed on patients whose nutrition is extremely poor and the operative risks are very great.

Post-operative care

Pain and post-operative vomiting are common after operations on the gall bladder and reference has already been made to the risks of pulmonary complications. Mild laxatives are commonly required for a week or so after operation until appetite and digestion return to normal, and in the immediate post-operative periods severe constipation may occur. Vitamin K will be continued by intramuscular injection in cases of jaundice.

The principal post-operative risks are haemorrhage and leakage of bile into the peritoneal cavity. If the bile duct has been explored and a T-tube is in place, there is a considerable risk of peritonitis. Nursing therefore includes the use of a Ryle's tube. Limited oral feeding may be resumed at once but aspiration is repeated 2-hourly so that ileus may be detected early if it should arise. Figure 31.1 indicates the drainage procedures commonly employed.

The 'precautionary' drain to the gall bladder bed is usually removed after 2 days: if bile discharge is sufficient to require daily dressing, the drain should only be shortened by 2 cm daily. The management of the T-tube after exploration of the duct has been described on page 586.

Occasionally, after cholecystectomy, biliary obstruction may occur, and in the post-operative phase careful watch must be kept for paling of the stools, or darkening of the urine, even in patients who have had no previous jaundice or evidence of biliary obstruction. This may arise from accidental damage to the bile duct when the cystic duct is tied and divided; it may be due to a haematoma or abscess forming in the hilum of the liver; or acute infection may spread up the bile ducts—cholangitis. Second and subsequent operations on the biliary apparatus are extremely difficult. The development of obstructive jaundice after cholecystectomy is a constant fear which casts its shadow occasionally over the most skilful surgeons. Further exploration is necessary if obstruction persists. A short length of plastic or metal (vitallium) tube is sometimes used to replace a damaged section of the duct.

It used to be thought that a patient who had his gall bladder removed would require to be careful over his diet for the rest of his life and should avoid fats and pastry. This rigid restriction is entirely without foundation and most patients find that they do not need to restrict their diet in any particular way. The avoidance of a high-fat diet may be wise on the grounds of obesity: gall bladder disease does undoubtedly occur in patients who tend to 'put on fat'. Cooked fats such as fried foods may not be tolerated very well but cold uncooked fat such as butter and milk is a necessary item of diet to stimulate the flow of bile.

Intestinal obstruction by gall stone

The inflamed gall bladder frequently becomes firmly adherent to the duodenum against which it is lying. Occasionally a large gall stone sets up acute inflammation and ulcerates through into the duodenum; the stone is then discharged into the duodenum and sometimes produces acute intestinal obstruction. Laparotomy is performed on account of obstruction and unless the patient is known to have had long-standing gall bladder disease, the association of the two conditions may be unsuspected.

The liver

The liver occupies a major part of the upper abdomen, extending from the right loin to the left side of the epigastric area. Part of it is in direct contact with the diaphragm and the rest of the upper surface is separated from the diaphragm only by a double layer of peritoneum. This forms the subphrenic pouches, being reflected as a ligament by which the liver is held against the diaphragm. When the abdominal cavity is opened at operation, or following perforation of a viscus, air collects above the liver, and allows it to drop away from the diaphragm (pneumoperitoneum, page 460).

Disorders of the liver

The liver becomes involved in many general metabolic disorders, some of which produce the condition of cirrhosis to which reference has already been made in relation to ascites (page 492). Liver disease from any cause adds to the risks of surgery and particularly affects the patient's reaction to drugs.

Liver function tests. A series of chemical tests are used to indicate liver function: these are essentially tests for enzyme function. Jaundice is due to an excess of pigment from the breakdown of red cells. If the liver is working normally this pigment passes through the liver cells and is 'conjugated'; if the outflow of bile is obstructed in the bile capillaries by liver disease such as cirrhosis, or at a lower level in the bile duct, the pigment forced back into the circulation appears in the urine. If on the other hand as in haemolytic jaundice, or in the presence of severe liver damage, the bilirubin has not been processed by the liver cells it is not conjugated and does not appear in the urine, hence the term a-chol-uric jaundice.

Patients with liver disorders requiring operative treatment for unconnected disease need special management.

There are four principal conditions in which the liver is involved and for which surgical treatment is necessary.

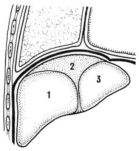

Fig. 31.2   Relations of the liver. Areas **1** and **3** are pockets where the liver protrudes into the peritoneal cavity and area **2** is the 'bare' area against the diaphragm and outside the peritoneum. In general peritonitis (e.g. following perforation of a peptic ulcer), pus may collect in areas **1** or **3**.

Rupture. The liver may be split by injuries in which the abdomen is crushed or in which there is a blow on the right lower ribs. Severe internal haemorrhage occurs and many such cases are fatal before there is time for surgical intervention. Occasionally, however, the tear is only of a minor nature and operative repair is possible. Blood transfusion is essential and post-operative nursing follows the routine for cases of peritonitis. The main risk is one of continued bleeding or of biliary peritonitis, because small bile ducts have been torn and bile may continue to ooze from the repaired area of the liver. The operation site will almost certainly be drained, probably by a stab-drain which may be taken from the right flank.

Abscess. Liver abscess may occur as a complication of some other infective process in the abdomen such as an acute appendicitis. Infection usually travels up the portal vein and multiple abscesses may develop from septic emboli (portal pylephlebitis).

Such abscesses are usually treated by aspiration (with a long needle) and the injection of penicillin or other antibiotic solution. Before the era of chemotherapy, open drainage was undertaken but is now rarely necessary.

One of the most common forms of liver abscess occurs as a complication of amoebic dysentery. Evacuation of the abscess may be necessary and the patient is treated with emetine and bismuth. The abscess forms as part of a general amoebic infection of the

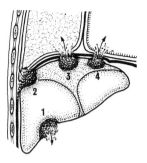

Fig. 31.3   Liver abscess. These may form in any area. According to its position the abscess may: **1.** burst into the peritoneal cavity. **2.** be expelled through the obliterated costophrenic angle (as in Fig. 31.4). **3.** break through into the lung, e.g. amoebic abscess. **4.** break into the pericardium.

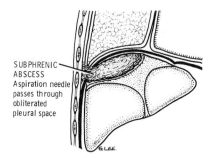

Fig. 31.4   Subphrenic abscess. A subphrenic abscess has formed on the bare area. The diaphragm is raised and the lower edge of the lung compressed. The inflammation spreads and closes the lower part of the pleural space through which the abscess can be aspirated or drained.

liver which is enlarged and tender. The patient at this time is generally very ill and no attempt is made to aspirate or drain the abscess until emetine treatment has been started.

Fig. 31.2 shows the position of the liver in relation to the diaphragm and pleura. If an abscess forms in the liver or in the space between the liver and the diaphragm (subphrenic abscess), there is an inflammatory reaction in the overlying pleura and the narrow space between the chest wall and the diaphragm (costophrenic angle) becomes obliterated. Thus a convenient route is formed through which the surgeon may pass needles for aspiration or through which an open operation may be performed, even with the removal of one or more ribs. The pleural space is not opened and the pleura can be further pushed upwards off the diaphragm at open operation.

If an abscess develops in the upper part of the liver the diaphragm becomes adherent to it; the abscess may then spread and burst into the pleural cavity or into the pericardium. Sometimes the lung also becomes adherent to the abscess site. In cases of amoebic dysentery a liver abscess sometimes tracks into the lung and is coughed up. The sputum is described as being like anchovy sauce because of its brick red colour.

Blood transfusion will probably be required in such patients as there is prolonged malnutrition and may be severe blood loss.

Hydatid cyst. Echinococcus granulosus (the dog tapeworm or taenia) has in its life-cycle a larval stage which normally occurs in the sheep, ox or horse. The dog is infected initially from eating uncooked offal from an infected animal. The adult worm in dogs produces larvae with which man becomes infected. A common site for the formation of hydatid cysts is the liver, where a single cyst may reach the size of a tennis ball without producing significant symptoms. A chalky deposit (calcification) occurs in the wall of the cyst which is then revealed by x-ray examination. Thousands of daughter cysts form inside and the main risk is that the cyst may burst, spreading the daughter cysts all over the peritoneum, where they become established and produce more cysts. The condition is treated surgically by evacuation of the main cyst. At operation, formalin is injected into the cyst to kill off all the parasites immediately before the cyst itself is opened and evacuated.

The main post-operative risks are peritonitis and haemorrhage.

Neoplasm. Primary innocent (adenoma) and malignant (carcinoma) tumours of the liver are rare. Blood-vessel tumours—haemangioma—also occur occasionally. Far the most common neoplasm in the liver is a secondary growth from carcinoma somewhere within the abdomen, and less frequently from other primary sites such as carcinoma of the breast or thyroid. On rare occasions, as part of the treatment of carcinoma of the colon or other abdominal organ, the surgeon may remove a part of the liver containing an obvious metastasis if this appears to be the only one. It is unfortunately extremely rare for there to be a solitary deposit in the liver. Tumours of the liver may be detected by radio-active scanning (page 448).

After partial removal of the liver the risks are the same as those following the repair of a ruptured liver—namely, haemorrhage and biliary peritonitis. The wound is drained.

Liver biopsy

In medical disorders in which the liver is involved a small piece of tissue is sometimes required for microscopic examination. This may be obtained by open operation. A very small fragment of liver is excised from the lower edge. The wound in the liver is closed by sutures and the abdomen closed without drainage. The risk of bleeding or peritonitis is extremely remote.

A more usual method for obtaining a piece of liver for biopsy is by means of a special liver-puncture needle. This special wide-bore needle is inserted into the liver, passing between the lower ribs. It is hoped that the needle will cross the very lowest portion of the pleural space and the angle between the arch of the diaphragm and the chest wall, or that it will miss the pleura altogether. It must of course pierce the diaphragm in any case. As the needle passes through the liver tissue, it cuts a long core of tissue which remains in the barrel of the needle. The operation is performed under local anaesthesia. Careful observation must be kept on the patient's pulse and respiration rate following this procedure. The complications which may arise from liver puncture biopsy are:

(*a*) pneumothorax,
(*b*) haemothorax or pleural effusion,
(*c*) subphrenic abscess or subphrenic haematoma,
(*d*) intra-peritoneal haemorrhage,
(*e*) biliary peritonitis.

This procedure will only be undertaken by someone particularly skilled in the technique. The necessary powerful syringe and special needles will probably be provided by the surgeon, already sterilised by dry heat. Sterile towels, swabs, antiseptic solution, local anaesthetic solution with 10-ml syringe and needle must be provided. Sterile bijou bottles or test tubes must be at hand to receive the specimens of liver tissue which will usually be placed in formol-saline solution, but certain special fixative agents may be used. In the latter case the pathology laboratory will provide the necessary equipment.

Portal vein obstruction—liver failure

Degenerative disease of the liver or secondary deposits from any malignant neoplasm may produce obstruction to the inward flow of blood from the portal vein. In liver disease (cirrhosis) the small intra-hepatic veins are strangled gradually while in malignant disease main vein blockage occurs more rapidly.

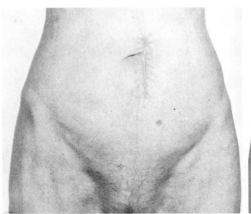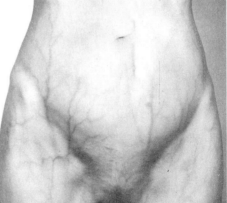

Fig. 31.5 Portal obstruction. *Left*. By plain artificial light. *Right*. By infra-red illumination. Note the great venous dilatation on the abdominal wall, with the vessels converging to the saphenous vein in each groin.

The subsequent venous back-pressure leads to distension of natural communications between portal and systemic venous systems in the abdominal wall, around the lower end of the oesophagus and at the anus. The spleen, whose vein is a tributary of the portal vein, becomes enlarged; oesophageal and anal piles develop and ascites ensues. In certain cases a surgical short-circuit may be made by removing the spleen and joining its vein to the left renal vein (**spleno-renal anastomosis**). Alternatively the portal vein may be joined directly to the vena cava (**porta-caval anastomosis**).

As the liver is severely damaged in most of these cases, there is a grave risk of liver failure, particularly in the post-operative period. The many functions normally performed by the liver are deficient and hepatic coma occurs. It is sometimes preceded by a severe coarse tremor (the 'flapping birdwing') affecting mainly the hands. Severe haemorrhage into the alimentary tract such as occurs from bleeding oesophageal varices, may precipitate hepatic coma. The break-down products formed from the digestion of blood protein are absorbed into the bloodstream but not detoxicated by the liver. Hepatic coma is usually fatal, but with the introduction of the haemodialysis (artificial kidney, page 677 a patient's blood may be cleared of metabolic poisons for a time and this may tide him over the post-operative crisis.

See also:

page 482—phlebitis and thrombosis of the portal vein,
page 492—ascites in portal hypertension,
page 506—oesophageal varicose veins,
page 565—haemorrhoids caused by portal obstruction,
page 595—the spleen in portal-vein obstruction.

32

The Spleen

Anatomy and physiology

The spleen is a solid organ lying between the left wall of the stomach and the diaphragm, protected by the lower ribs and held in position by its capsule which is formed of peritoneum. Its very large artery comes almost directly from the aorta and its vein is one of the main tributaries of the portal system.

The spleen has many functions which are known and probably others which are not known. It contains smooth muscle and is capable of contracting. It has a sponge-like structure in which the sinuses or spaces of the sponge are filled with blood. By its power of contraction it is able to expel into the circulation a large amount of this reserve blood, to meet sudden demands such as may be produced by shock or haemorrhage.

In addition to this reservoir function, the spleen is the 'headquarters' of the reticulo-endothelial system. Cells of this system are found in various parts of the body, the liver, lymph glands and bone marrow. The function of the reticulo-endothelial system with its macrophage[1] cells is to deal with foreign particles which circulate in the blood or gain entrance to the tissues, such as bacteria, viruses and other tissue cells. Red blood cells are being continuously destroyed in the spleen. It is probable that antibodies against disease are also produced by the reticulo-endothelial system and by the masses of lymphatic tissue to be found in the spleen.

Pathology

Trauma. Owing to its position the spleen is very rarely injured. Occasionally, by a blow over the lower ribs the spleen may be split, particularly if it is enlarged. There are two main clinical types of ruptured spleen. In the first, the soft splenic tissue is torn without a corresponding tear in its peritoneal capsule. A large subperitoneal haematoma forms and the patient suffers only from pain in the loin in the region of the spleen, or referred to the left shoulder from irritation of the diaphragm. A common course of such an injury is that after 48 hours the haematoma bursts into the peritoneal cavity with torrential bleeding from the broken surface of the spleen. It is therefore usual to admit to hospital all cases of suspected injury of the spleen until the risk of the delayed haemorrhage has passed.

[1] 'large-eating'.

In the second type, with a more severe injury the patient collapses immediately from profuse internal haemorrhage. The condition is fatal unless operation can be undertaken at once. There is no time for any particular pre-operative treatment. The pre-medication drug is given intravenously and the patient is conveyed straight from the hospital receiving room to the operating theatre, his case taking priority over any other surgical operations.

Blood transfusion is always required. It may be necessary before operation, but is usually deferred until the peritoneum is opened and the surgeon is able to grasp the splenic artery to prevent further loss. No attempt is made to repair the spleen, which has to be removed as rapidly as possible. A rubber drainage strip may be left in the splenic bed and brought through a stab wound in the abdominal wall. It is removed after 48 hours without previous shortening.

Infections. Because of its part in the lymphoid and reticulo-endothelial system, the spleen reacts to generalised infections by becoming enlarged. The spleen is enlarged in glandular fever, malaria, most forms of septicaemia, and in other diseases such as kala-azar, particularly those caused by parasites.

In cases of chronic infection the spleen is only removed if it is so large that its very size is causing embarrassment to the patient by restricting abdominal or diaphragmatic movement. In addition, the peritoneum which covers a large spleen may become inflamed —**perisplenitis**—giving rise to severe attacks of pain. In countries where malaria is endemic and therefore splenomegaly is very common, a noted form of murder was to stab the victim with a small blunt instrument in the upper left part of the abdomen, thus producing rupture of the spleen without any outward evidence of injury.

Reticulosis. This term is applied to diseases of the blood-forming and reticulo-endo-thelial system including leukaemias and lymphadenoma (Hodgkin's disease). Splenectomy is rarely required for these conditions although the spleen is almost always enlarged. When, for instance, neck glands alone are enlarged, it is advisable to know whether the disease is more widespread before starting chemotherapy; the spleen is then removed for histological examination.

Haemolytic jaundice and splenic anaemia. In certain conditions the red blood cells are more fragile than normal and are more rapidly destroyed in the spleen, with resultant severe anaemia. Broken-down blood pigments from which bile is normally formed are released into the blood stream without having passed through the liver. The patient becomes jaundiced. Haemolytic jaundice is sometimes a congenital hereditary condition described as **acholuric family jaundice**[1] and it is treated by splenectomy. The condition may be revealed in a very small baby and there is no age limit to splenectomy. The condition is characterised by haemolytic crises in which there is a series of febrile attacks associated with the development of jaundice and severe anaemia. Splenectomy is not undertaken during these acute attacks but the patient is treated by blood transfusion. At the time of splenectomy the gall bladder is inspected because the condition often gives rise to the formation of pure bile pigment stones from the excessive secretion of blood pigment.

Other forms of anaemia due to over-activity of the blood-destroying function of the spleen are sometimes treated by splenectomy.

Thrombocytopenic purpura. An additional specific function of the spleen is in relation to the destruction of blood platelets. This condition has already been referred to (page 118).

---

[1] '*spherocytosis*' because the red cells swell up into spheres and burst.

The deficiency of platelets which results from this splenic over-action leads to spontaneous haemorrhage or purpura. The spleen is not enlarged in this condition. The only effective treatment is splenectomy.

Following removal of the spleen there is a rapid rise in the number of blood platelets for a short time and it is possible for this to lead to spontaneous thrombosis in important blood vessels. Platelet counts are therefore performed at regular intervals in the first and second post-operative weeks and the surgeon may consider anti-coagulant therapy necessary as a preventive measure if the platelet count rises excessively.

Portal obstruction. This condition has already been described in relation to ascites and cirrhosis of the liver. If the portal vein is blocked the spleen becomes enlarged. Occasionally it is removed.

In the treatment of portal obstruction by operations which short-circuit the portal blood into the vena cava, the spleen is sometimes removed in order that its vein may be joined to the left renal vein. This allows portal blood to run back in the reverse direction through the renal vein, regaining the systemic system in the vena cava without passing through the liver. (See also pages 482, 591.)

Incidental removal. In major upper abdominal operations, such as oesophagogastrectomy or repair of hiatus hernia, the spleen may prevent adequate access and is then removed for convenience.

The operation of splenectomy

There is no particular pre-operative preparation except that the patient's blood should always be grouped and tentative preparations made for transfusion. If the spleen is very enlarged, blood transfusion will almost certainly be required.

The spleen is usually removed through a left paramedian or subcostal abdominal incision (Fig. 24.1) under general anaesthesia. Splenectomy for gross enlargement is more often undertaken in tropical countries than in temperate zones and under these conditions a high standard of anaesthesia may not be available. The operation is then performed under high spinal anaesthesia.

An alternative approach to the spleen is through the thorax, the eighth rib being removed, the pleural space opened and an incision made through the diaphragm from above. This gives very direct access to the splenic vessels which can then readily be compressed to avoid blood loss during removal of the spleen.

Post-operative care depends upon the incision which has been used. In the majority of cases a precautionary drain will be left down to the splenic bed to prevent an accumulation of blood from the oozing surfaces exposed during operation. If the thorax has been opened it is unlikely that there will be any thoracic drainage tube, the lung having been fully inflated by the anaesthetist before the pleura is closed. On the other hand, the thorax may be drained for a short time by means of an indwelling catheter in the pleural space, connected to an under-water seal (Fig. 34.1).

Because of unavoidable bruising to the diaphragm and on account of the position of the incision, the patient may find that respiration is difficult and painful after operation. Collapse of the left lung is then a likely complication.

If persistent discharge comes from the site of wound drainage, it may be pancreatic enzyme; the tail of the pancreas is sometimes injured at operation. Healing is usually spontaneous and the discharge may be lessened by the administration of probanthine by mouth. The surrounding skin requires protection by a barrier cream.

Convalescence should be uneventful and the patient should be ambulant by the end of the first week.

Hiccoughs may be a troublesome immediate post-operative complication owing to irritation of the diaphragm.

Complications of splenectomy are few: the removal of the spleen may reduce resistance to infection and is undesirable in children unless there is a life-saving compelling reason.

33

The Pancreas

Anatomy (Fig. 26.1)

The pancreas is shaped somewhat like a tadpole, having a head, body and tail. The head lies in the curve formed by the duodenum over the front of the bodies of the upper lumbar vertebrae. The mesenteric artery and the portion of the portal vein draining the greater part of the bowel pass through the pancreas at its lower border. The common bile duct enters the upper border of the head, joins with the pancreatic duct and the two enter the vertical part of the duodenum together at the ampulla of Vater. Because of these intimate attachments with vital structures, the pancreas cannot readily be removed without very great risk. The upper part of the pancreas is covered by the stomach and both gastric and duodenal ulcers may penetrate into it. The pancreatic duct has a central trunk and many side branches. It extends into the tail which is in contact with the spleen and may be injured during the operation of splenectomy (page 595).

Physiology

The pancreas, in addition to producing digestive ferments which are secreted into its duct system, is an endocrine gland. Scattered throughout its length are groups of insulin-secreting cells, the islets of Langerhans. A deficiency of insulin produces diabetes mellitus.

The principal digestive ferments which come from the pancreatic juice are **lipase** (fat digesting), **amylase** (starch digesting) and **trypsin** (protein digesting). [The pancreatic cells actually produce **trypsinogen,** which is converted into trypsin by another enzyme in the intestinal secretion.]

In certain conditions the enzymes may escape from the pancreas into the peritoneal cavity. Peritonitis develops with necrosis of portions of the fat in the omentum. Pancreatic juice is very strongly alkaline due to the presence of sodium bicarbonate. It also contains a considerable amount of mucus.

Secretin, a hormone produced in the intestinal mucosa, stimulates the action of the pancreas and is used in tests for pancreatic function.

Disorders of the pancreas

Congenital. Sometimes the pancreas is abnormally placed and actually surrounds and constricts the duodenum (annular pancreas). Obstruction may arise and require surgical treatment.

Congenital fibrocystic disease of the pancreas is associated with other abnormalities, especially in the lungs. It is called 'mucoviscidosis' on account of the stickiness of the secretions and of the intestinal contents. In the new-born infant, the meconium[1] is so thick that peristalsis is impossible and intestinal obstruction occurs. This sometimes requires operative treatment. The abdomen is opened and multiple incisions are made into the intestine, and 'Savlon' is inserted with a catheter to loosen the very sticky contents which are too adherent to be 'milked' along the bowel unless a 'wetting' agent is used. If the obstruction cannot be cleared satisfactorily the terminal portion of the ileum which is the usual site of blockage is brought outside (exteriorisation, Mikulicz operation, see page 557). When the wound has been closed the bowel loop is cut off leaving two ileostomy openings. These are washed out with protein-dissolving enzyme solutions. When the obstruction has been relieved and normal feeding established, the spur between the limbs of the loop is crushed and the opening recedes, as with the spur colostomy (Fig. 29.14).

Infective. Pancreatitis occurs in mumps and in other generalised infections. It may arise also from infections of the biliary tract or duodenum. Chronic pancreatitis may lead to stone formation and the stones may require surgical removal. Pancreatitis may arise from erosion by a gastric or duodenal ulcer or may follow partial gastrectomy when the ulcer has been adherent or if there should be a leak from the duodenal stump (page 526 and Fig. 26.6). The specific condition of acute haemorrhagic pancreatitis is described on page 599.

Traumatic. Injury to the upper abdomen may damage the pancreas and produce a leak of the digestive ferments into the peritoneal cavity. This leak is usually into the lesser sac behind the stomach. It becomes shut off by inflammation of the peritoneum at the opening of the lesser sac. The leak continues and a very large cyst forms. It is called a **pseudocyst** of the pancreas because it is really outside the gland. It may contain several litres of mucous fluid. It is not possible to remove such a cyst entirely and it is usually treated by drainage. If there is reason to suppose that the leak is still open, the drainage tube may have to remain in place for many months. Sometimes the front wall of the cyst is stitched to the anterior abdominal wall to avoid leakage into the peritoneal cavity. This is called 'marsupialisation' as it converts the huge cyst into an abdominal pouch like that of the kangaroo.

Neoplastic. The most common surgical disorder of the pancreas is **carcinoma**. This usually commences in the head of the gland and produces its symptoms by encroaching on the common bile duct and so giving rise to persistent obstructive jaundice. Complete removal of the growth is a formidable procedure but in early cases the risks are justified and operation is sometimes successful. Pancreatectomy for carcinoma (Fig. 33.1) involves:

(a) Removal of the whole of the duodenum and pyloris. The defect is made good by anastomosis between jejunum and stomach.
(b) Removal of the main bile duct. Either the gall bladder or the stump of the bile duct has to be joined to a loop of jejunum.
(c) Excision of the head, body and most of the tail of the pancreas. The duct in the remaining portion of the pancreas is joined to the side of a jejunal loop.

The alternative to pancreatectomy is a palliative operation to short-circuit the bile in order to relieve the obstructive jaundice (Fig. 31.1). Sometimes a seemingly hopeless tumour will respond dramatically to chemotherapy with methotrexate or cyclophosphamide.

[1] Meconium = intestinal contents present at and before birth.

Adenoma of the pancreas is rare but the tumour is usually developed from the islets cells. The tumour produces insulin and the patient suffers from hypoglycaemic attacks resembling insulin overdose. The tumour is removed by operation and the condition is named **spontaneous hypoglycaemia.**

Metabolic. Diabetes mellitus is a medical disorder and patients who suffer from the condition require special precautions to ensure adequate control if they are to undergo surgical operations for other disorders. Diabetes also produces disease of the arteries and diabetic gangrene of the extremities results from this complication. The surgeon has always to be on the look-out for undiscovered diabetes in all cases of chronic ulceration or recurrent sepsis. There is, however, no surgical treatment for the condition. Diabetes can

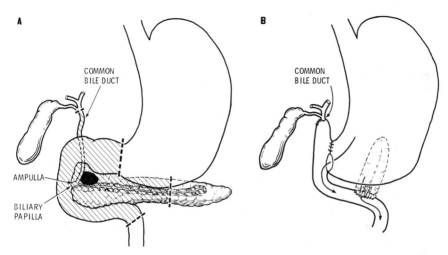

Fig. 33.1   Whipple's operation (pancreatectomy for carcinoma). **A.** Shaded area of organs to be removed. **B.** The re-assembled portions.

arise as a complication of destructive pancreatic disease. In inflammatory lesions of the pancreas the intensity of the diabetes may fluctuate and management is extremely difficult on account of the inconstant insulin requirement.

Acute haemorrhagic pancreatitis. The exact origin of this condition is not known. It was once believed to be due to streptococcal infection. Some have thought that it was due to bile entering the pancreatic ducts by reflux from the ampulla. Whatever may be the cause, it appears that something activates the proteolytic enzyme so that the pancreas begins to digest itself. Its onset is dramatic, with collapse, sweating, high pulse rate and low temperature. The patient sometimes develops a peculiar cyanosed dusky appearance. It resembles perforation of a peptic ulcer and is usually confused with this condition. The treatment is a matter of uncertainty. If the diagnosis is certain operation is not performed. The patient is treated with atropine or propantheline, which are drugs diminishing the vagus nerve stimulation and so reducing the production of gastric and pancreatic secretion. **Fat necrosis** occurs in the omentum and elsewhere in the abdomen. The shock must be treated by infusion probably with additional blood transfusion. In pain relief, theoretically morphine should not be used as it may produce spasm of the biliary ampulla. Pethidine with atropine, as for other forms of severe abdominal pain, is effective in that it relieves the bowel spasm which occurs from peritonitis. Dipipanone and diazepam provide relief similarly.

The enzymes escaping from the surface track up the lymphatics and may cause basal pleurisy with an effusion. Chest pain or shoulder pain (referred from the diaphragm) must be reported.

Chronic relapsing pancreatitis. Recurrent less severe attacks of pancreatitis give rise to minor bouts of peritonitis which subside spontaneously after a few days of pain and distension. Ileus occurs and the patient may develop severe intestinal obstruction. The condition is often associated with infection or stones in the gall bladder. Gradual destruction of the pancreas by repeated attacks reduces the digestive enzyme output and may lead to **steatorrhoea**—the passage of pale bulky stools containing large amounts of undigested fat. This is treated by giving concentrated enzymes by mouth. It is important to note if the stool floats in the w.c. pan as this indicates a high fat content.

By blockage of ducts and auto-digestion, pancreatitis without injury may lead to the formation of a pancreatic cyst or pseudocyst (page 598).

Factors in nursing

Pain from the pancreas is usually experienced in the back, and may pass upwards between the scapulae. This type of pain arising after upper abdominal operations on the biliary system or stomach, indicates that the pancreas may be infected. Back pain should always be reported to the medical staff.

Because of the very close relation of the pancreas to the root of the mesentery and to the main blood supply of the bowel, paralytic ileus is very liable to follow any severe involvement of the pancreas in disease, or any major complication upon it. Peritonitis is the other most likely complication.

There is no particular **pre-operative** preparation or **post-operative** nursing technique other than that required for any major surgical procedure in the abdomen.

Pancreatitis sometimes results in escape of **amylase** into the blood, where it may be estimated by chemical examination. The starch-digesting enzyme appears also in the urine as diastase. Specimens of urine should be saved for examination by the pathological laboratory on each morning following operation upon the pancreas. The specimens must be examined when fresh.

If the pancreas has been involved in any surgical operation, the peritoneal cavity is usually drained for several days and under these circumstances the tube is removed by repeated shortening. A pancreatic fistula may result from injury occurring during the removal of a peptic ulcer which has eroded into the pancreas, and to avoid this the base of the ulcer is usually cauterised with carbolic or diathermy and left adherent to the pancreas. Similarly, a fistula may follow from injury to the tail of the pancreas in splenectomy (page 595).

34

The Principles of Cardio-Thoracic Surgery

This branch of surgery has changed in its scope more than many others in the last two decades. The pioneer surgery in the treatment of pulmonary tuberculosis—thoracoplasty, artificial pneumothorax and other procedures to 'collapse' TB lung cavities is now only of historic interest. Preventive measures and antituberculous drugs in therapy have resulted in a reduction of occurrence and severity of the disease. Carcinoma of the lung, primary in the bronchus, and metastatic from other organs however is very common. Bronchiectasis —infected dilatation of the bronchial tubes—is now also less common. Lung surgery has thus declined but surgery on the heart and great vessels has advanced to take its place. With high speed road travel, severe injuries to the chest are common, and most require surgical intervention as a life-saving emergency.

Major thoracic centres are organised to provide a full service on a regional basis, and not all district hospitals provide experience in nursing these patients.

The nurse in her general training may have little contact with major thoracic surgery, but the 'general surgeon' undertakes surgical procedures which may involve opening the thorax. During difficult operations in the root of the neck, or in the upper abdomen, the pleural cavity may inadvertently be opened. A general surgical unit which deals with injuries may at any time be called upon to operate on the chest: correct post-operative nursing and general management of such injuries is vital. The abdominal surgeon may approach the spleen or the stomach through the chest: he then deliberately opens the pleural cavity, divides the diaphragm and gains wide access to the upper abdominal viscera. The transpleural route is the only approach to the thoracic portion of the oesophagus.

Consequently all nurses must become familiar with the general features and complications of thoracic surgery and the management of the post-operative stage. The more detailed techniques required after lung and heart operations vary from unit to unit and only representative routine and general principles will be described here.

Tables 45 and 46 show some of the operations commonly undertaken outside special thoracic surgical units and in which a knowledge of the principles of special thoracic surgical nursing is required: the pleural cavity may be deliberately or inadvertently opened in these cases. Table 47 gives the operations which are more commonly undertaken in special thoracic surgical centres. There can of course be no strict division and this grouping is only given as a guide to indicate what may be expected in a general surgical unit. Some 'general' surgeons undertake major thoracic surgery while some 'thoracic' surgeons undertake upper abdominal surgery as well. Their respective teams will be specially trained.

Table 45   Operations in which the pleural space may be entered unintentionally

	Operation	Refer to page	Clinical condition for which the operation is required
Operations in the lower part of the neck	Cervical sympathectomy	756	Raynaud's disease, angina pectoris
	Stellate ganglionectomy	943	
	Removal of cervical rib		Pressure neuritis of brachial plexus
	Scalenotomy	762	
	Carotid endarterectomy	944	For atheroma obstruction
	Aneurysm or ligature of subclavian artery	940 914	In arterial injury or prior to forequarter amputation
	Removal of glands in root of neck	760	For biopsy of malignant disease, lymphadenoma, tuberculosis
	Thyroidectomy	773	Goitre, especially if it has extended into the mediastinum
	Thymectomy	608	Myasthenia gravis
Operations in the region of the diaphragm	Nephrectomy or other operation on the kidney	680	Stone, tuberculosis, growth
	Removal of suprarenal gland	701	Tumour or enlargement
	Vagotomy (removal of vagus nerves)	530	Peptic ulcer
Operations on the chest wall	Removal of soft tissue tumour	—	Lipoma, neurofibroma, etc.
	Radical mestectomy	888	Carcinoma of breast

In any of these instances, the puncture of the pleura may not be noticed at the time.

Applied anatomy and physiology of the thorax

To appreciate the principles of thoracic surgical management, it is essential for the nurse to have a thorough grasp of the simple mechanics of the thorax in relation to respiration and blood flow. (See also Chapter 10.)

Lung function

Mechanically, the thorax resembles a syringe; the diaphragm acts as the piston or plunger, being pulled down by its own contracting muscle and recoiling upwards as it relaxes. By an alteration the angles of the ribs, the diameter of the chest and therefore its capacity are also increased: in the healthy adult this chest expansion is from 6 to 10 cm. The pleural membrane lines the thorax and its cavity is completely closed: nothing penetrates it. As the lungs are inflated 'into' the pleural bag, its cavity becomes reduced to a mere slit, lubricated by a little serous fluid. The 'visceral' (lung covering) layer slides against the 'parietal' layer. If the pleural membrane becomes inflamed (for instance, from infection of the underlying lung) the two layers become stuck together: fluid from the inflammation may accumulate as in synovitis of a joint or in peritonitis; it separates the layers widely, preventing lung expansion. This is a **pleural effusion**, and the resultant compression of the lung leads to **compression atelectasis** (Fig. 34.2(4)).

Table 46 'General surgical' operations in which the pleural space is deliberately entered (transthoracic operations)

Operation	Refer to page	Clinical condition for which the operation is required
Abdomino-thoracic gastrectomy	531	Carcinoma of upper end of stomach
Excision of oesophagus and re-	500	Carcinoma or stricture
construction	497	Congenital atresia (performed within a day or so of birth)
Vagotomy	530	Severe peptic ulcer
Nephrectomy or adrenalectomy	680	Large renal neoplasms, especially in infants
	701	adrenal tumour or hyperplasia
Spleno-renal venous anastomosis	591	Portal venous hypertension
('shunt')	595	
Repair of diaphragm	504	Diaphragmatic hernia; 'Hiatus' hernia

In inspiration, the chest wall movement increases the vacuum in the pleural cavity, and since this is closed, the lungs are ballooned out into their respective inspiratory or inflated position. Expiration is produced by the elastic recoil of the lungs as the respiratory muscles relax. If the pleural vacuum space is broken by puncture (deliberate or inadvertent) a state of **pneumothorax** exists. The chest has a right and left pleural space so that when pneumothorax occurs on one side the patient is dependent on greater expansion of the opposite lung. If pneumothorax occurs both sides, the loss of lung expansion may be sufficient to produce asphyxia and death: this can occur from a bullet wound of the chest.

If air enters one pleural cavity, the suction on the opposite side results in the heart and mediastinum moving away from the affected side. This shift is shown by the apex beat, and trachea (which can be felt in the neck). The lung on the affected side collapses.

Methods and physiological aspects of artificial respiration are described in Chapter 10. The effect of inadequate pulmonary ventilation on the blood chemistry is described on page 111.

The under-water seal drain

In order to restore normal lung action after thoracic operations, it is necessary to restore the pleural vacuum or 'negative pressure' and to prevent the accumulation of fluid within the pleura since this would prevent the lung re-expanding. Re-expansion is effected by the anaesthetist inflating the patient's lungs before the pleura is sewn up, or by the surgeon aspirating the air from the pleural space after the wound has been closed. Air is prevented from re-entering by the valvular action of the thoracic wall muscles and skin, but to prevent fluid accumulating a drainage tube is left through the chest wall, the outer

Table 47   Thoracic surgical operations

Region of operation	Operation	Clinical condition for which operation is required
On the chest wall	Rib resection	Bone tumour, infection
	Thoracoplasty	Tuberculosis, especially with cavity
On pleura	Division of adhesions	Tuberculosis; adhesions preventing adequate artificial pneumothorax
	Decortication	Thickened pleura over lung after haemothorax
On lung	Drainage	Empyema
	Pneumonectomy (removal of whole lung)	Carcinoma, bronchiectasis, tuberculosis
	Lobectomy (removal of one lobe)	Carcinoma, bronchiectasis, tuberculosis
	Drainage or excision	Lung abscess
On the heart and great blood vessels (page 625)	Ligature of patent ductus arteriosus	Congenital abnormality
	Arterial anastomosis (Blalock-Taussig operation)	Fallot's tetralogy
	Excision and reconstruction of of aorta	Congenital coarctation (narrowing)
	Mitral valvulotomy	Mitral stenosis (rheumatic heart
	Insertion of valve prosthesis	disease) and similar operations on other valves
	Repair of septal defects	Congenital 'hole in heart'
	Wiring and other procedures	Aortic aneurysm
On other structures in the mediastinum	Excision of cysts and tumours, and operations on the thoracic portion portion of the oesophagus	

end of this being connected to what is known as an 'under-water seal'.[1] As the patient's chest expands, the vacuum created draws water up the tube of the under-water seal, but the weight of the water column prevents it being drawn more than a few centimetres up the tube so that the vacuum is preserved in the pleural cavity, and lung expansion takes place. In fact, when transparent tubing is used, the oscillations of the water are a useful guide to chest movement. Any blood or serum that escapes into the pleural cavity drains off down the tube into the receptacle (Fig. 34.1). Air is absorbed or blown off during coughing or forced expiration.

If air continues to enter the pleural space from a leak in the lung surface (or divided bronchus if part of the lung has been removed), large volumes of air may have to be withdrawn continuously by a special pump connected to the outlet from the under-water seal bottle. In hydropneumothorax—that is fluid with air above it—two drains are used, one intercostal catheter being inserted between the top of the scapular and spine and one at the base. Intrapleural pressure may have to be adjusted using a pressure gauge, but a careful watch for sideways shift of the trachea and early signs of distress or dyspnoea will

[1] The necessary bottles and tubing are available commercially in 1, 2 or 3 bottle sets (Chesebrough-Pond's Ltd.), or may be supplied by the CSSD.

give warning that suction is inadequate: the leak of air from the lung may be too fast for a small pump; if the gauge fails to show a negative pressure its output is inadequate and it will in fact block the escape of air, raising the intrapleural pressure: a larger pump must be used.

If the under-water seal is broken inadvertently, the patient may collapse: sudden introduction of air up the tube allows mediastinal shift and may induce cardiac arrest.

These rules must be very strictly observed in the care of the under-water seal drain:

1. The tube between chest and bottle *must* be clamped before any alteration to bottle stopper, water level, or pump connection is made.
2. The bottle must *never* be lifted to bed level or above as water may siphon into the chest.
3. If the bottle is knocked over the tube must be clamped immediately.
4. The water level in the bottle (or water mixed with drained blood) should not be allowed to rise more than 8 cm above the end of the tube. If the level is higher, air will not be expelled effectively from the chest as too much water has to be displaced from the immersed tube on expiration.
5. Care must be taken to ensure that the tube from the chest does not get kinked or tucked in with the bedclothes.

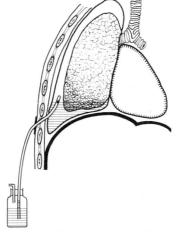

Fig. 34.1 Under-water seal chest drain. Sterile water in the bedside bottle must be sufficient to cover the tube to 8 cm depth: if the drain is immersed to a greater depth the pressure will be too great for the chest movements to expel the air in the pneumothorax. There should be a rise and fall of water in the tube with each respiration: the tube must be clamped when the bottle is changed. Sometimes two bottles in series are used with a low vacuum pump. The purpose of the second bottle is to prevent fluid being sucked over into the pump.

Interference with diaphragm movement impedes lung expansion: this may be brought about by pain and inflammation, especially after upper abdominal operations (page 389). Diaphragm movement may be limited deliberately, in order to rest the lung, by crushing the nerve which supplies one side of the muscle. This **phrenic nerve crush** or the more permanent procedure, **phrenic nerve section** (or 'avulsion'), was part of the planned treatment of pulmonary tuberculosis. The nerve is exposed by a small operation at the root of the neck. The 'crush' has been used also for intractable 'hiccups'.

'Paradoxical' respiration is a complication of thoracic surgery: it sometimes occurs if there is a pneumothorax on one side, open to the air. When the 'healthy' side expands it draws its air partly from the atmosphere through the trachea and partly from the opposite lung around which the pleural cavity has lost its vacuum. During expiration, the sound lung expels its air partly into the atmosphere and partly into the opposite lung. In fact, respiration is taking place from one lung to the other and oxygenation is then inadequate.

The circulation

The heart is enclosed in a fibrous bag which cannot easily expand. This fibrous pericardium is lined by a serous membrane like the pleura which covers the wall and the enclosed heart. If fluid accumulates in this pericardial sac from inflammation (pericarditis) the heart cannot expand (i.e. relax) properly between its beats. It does not fill itself adequately: the output with each beat drops and the pulse rate is increased. A similar constrictive process occurs from inflammation or hardening of the pericardium. Injury to the chest may produce bleeding into the pericardial sac; this certainly occurs with stab wounds or gun shots. The resulting fluid accumulation causes **'cardiac tamponade'**; the pulse volume is lessened during inspiration—**pulsus paradoxicus**. This may be confirmed by taking the blood pressure and setting the pressure just below (say, 10 mm) the point at which the beat is heard—systolic pressure. The sound disappears during inspiration. Cardiac tamponade demands aspiration or drainage. Occasionally infection occurs (suppurative pericarditis) and requires drainage. Constrictive pericarditis is now treated by removing the pericardium to allow normal expansion (diastole) of the heart.

Venous blood is returned from the limbs and abdomen mainly by the suction action of the thorax (page 178), and only partially by the 'vis-a-tergo' or positive pressure in the veins. Inadequate thoracic suction is therefore shown by venous congestion; swelling of the legs and ascites follow. One of the earliest signs of this venous back-pressure is distension of the veins in the neck and this distension also occurs if there is a block or partial obstruction at the entry from the neck to the thoracic cage: such obstruction occurs with mediastinal goitre (page 765) and enlarged malignant glands.

The mediastinum and mediastinoscopy

The space between the two lungs is the mediastinum. The heart and pericardium occupy the lower and front portion while the zone above the heart, the superior mediastinum, is occupied by the great vessels and thymus gland. Behind the heart in the posterior mediastinum are the oesophagus, splanchnic sympathetic nerves and the descending aorta. A considerable number of lymph glands are present in the mediastinum mainly grouped around the hilum of each lung.

The superior mediastinum can be approached surgically from an incision in the neck extended down over the sternum, with division of the sternum. Separation of the two halves carrying the inner ends of the upper ribs outwards gives access to the thymus gland for its removal in myasthenia gravis. The superior mediastinum can be inspected with an endoscope (mediastinoscopy) and a biopsy taken from enlarged glands or tumour: this is done through a small incision in the suprasternal notch below the thyroid gland.

Most operations on structures in the mediastinum are carried out through lateral thoracotomy incisions by rib resection, the appropriate lung being deflated to give access

1.

MEDIASTINAL SHIFT

$+ \longrightarrow -$

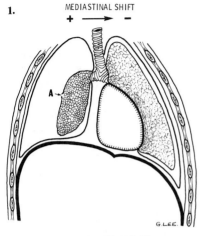

2.

MEDIASTINAL SHIFT

$+ \longrightarrow -$

PNEUMOTHORAX

STAB WOUND

BLOOD

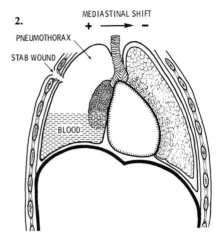

3.

MEDIASTINAL SHIFT

$++ \longrightarrow -$

FLAP
VALVE
OPENING

X

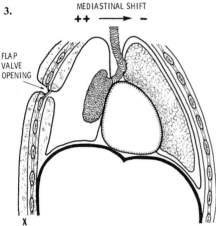

4.

MEDIASTINAL SHIFT

$+ \longrightarrow -$

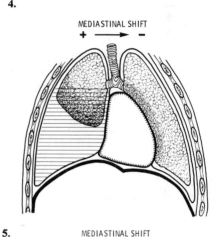

5.

MEDIASTINAL SHIFT

$- \longleftarrow +$

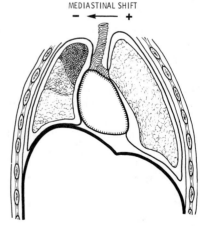

Fig. 34.2 Lesions producing pressure inequality in the pleural cavity. Note the mediastinal shift indicated by tracheal and heart displacement.

1. Pneumothorax—rupture of emphysema cyst on lung (A): can occur from growth or abscess or from stab wound.

2. Haemopneumothorax from penetrating wound.

3. Tension pneumothorax with haemothorax. Progressive mediastinal shift from penetrating wound or leak as in **1**, producing a 'one-way' flap valve. Each inspiration increases the air pressure on the affected side (paradoxical respiration is present). Note surgical emphysema in chest wall X.

4. Collapse of lung by compression: haemothorax or pleural effusion.

5. Collapse of lung from obstructed air entry: bronchus blocked by foreign body, mucus or growth: diaphragm elevated.

across the pleural space. The preparation, risks, and complications are those of any operation which involves an opening into the pleura (page 618).

Myasthenia gravis is a progressive disorder characterised by generalised weakness of muscles including those of respiration. The disease is usually controlled by a specific antidote, neostigmine. It has been found that removal of the thymus produces prolonged remissions and perhaps even cure in some cases. In the nursing management of patients with myasthenia who undergo thymectomy, muscular weakness may be accentuated by the operation and may involve in addition to respiratory paralysis, paralysis of the muscle of swallowing. The post-operative care of such patients is supervised in detail by the medical staff. The disease has an effect very similar to that of curare and the problems which may arise after operation are therefore similar to those which occur when the patient has received a heavy dose of relaxant drugs during the course of anaesthesia (page 220).

Haemoptysis

The lungs are extremely vascular and the capillaries around the alveoli are very fragile. The intercostal spaces are closed by muscle and each contains a major artery and vein. Haemorrhage is therefore a common feature of injury or disease in the thorax. Haemoptysis is the 'coughing-up' of blood; sometimes spitting of blood which has come from a source of bleeding in the mouth or pharynx or nose is confused with true haemoptysis. Injury, infarction (page 392) and infection may produce haemoptysis as an early symptom. Bleeding from the lung may be slight—the sputum being streaked with blood; more severe bleeding, usually from malignant or tuberculous disease, is shown by the coughing of clots of blood: gross bleeding may also occur, the patient being in danger of drowning in his own blood. Haemoptysis is alarming to both patient and relatives and its occurrence in a hospital patient must always be reported, however slight it may appear to be. Pulmonary embolism is the most common cause, in hospital.

Haemothorax

Blood escaping from the lung surface or from the chest wall collects in the pleural sac. This usually follows thoracotomy or injury which may include a rib fracture. The bleeding may be severe, and the accumulation of blood in the pleural space 'compresses' the lung, or, more correctly expressed, prevents its inflation. Dyspnoea is therefore a symptom and the pumping action of the diaphragm tends to encourage the bleeding: the mediastinum is moved towards the uninjured side. Frequently this collection of blood in the thorax (**haemothorax**) is accompanied by some degree of pneumothorax, air having entered either from an open wound or from a puncture of the lung by a rib splinter. This condition is **haemopneumothorax** and its particular danger lies in the risk of infection from the punctured lung reaching the collection of blood.

Conditions which may lead to haemothorax

Any injury of chest wall—stab, gunshot, fractured rib
Pneumothorax.
Operations upon the chest wall or thoracic organs, including paracentesis (needling), or adhesion cutting.
Neoplasms invading the pleura.
Aneurysm of thoracic vessels.

The management of haemothorax. If blood is left in the pleural space it clots: the clot may later liquefy partly and may then be withdrawn with a syringe, but 'organisation' of the fibrin clot into permanent adhesions is the normal outcome. A large clotted haemothorax results in the formation of a thick 'peel' over the lung: the lung is thus prevented from expanding and consequently the pneumothorax (if present) or haemo-pneumothorax cannot be properly obliterated. Though this membrane can be removed (by the operation of decortication) the proper management of haemothorax lies in prevention of clot formation.

As with haemorrhage elsewhere, physical rest, assurance, and sedation are the vital preliminaries to active treatment. Blood transfusion is frequently needed and it must always be remembered that the oxygenating area of the lungs is reduced, so that a small reduction of haemoglobin level is much more serious than a similar reduction from haemorrhage elsewhere in the body. Aspiration may be successful if clotting has not occurred: if it fails or bleeding recurs, an intercostal catheter drain with underwater seal is inserted. If there has been delay and a large amount of clot is present (the extent as seen on an x-ray), the surgeon may open the chest to evacuate the clot. An intercostal drain will be left in place. Probably a pneumothorax apparatus will be required when aspiration is performed, in order that the intrapleural pressure may be correctly adjusted if there has been any degree of leakage into the pleura or if it is desired to maintain collapse of one lung.

The lung surface may ooze blood from a large area: irrigation of the pleural space with a coagulating fluid such as silver nitrate solution or calcium alginate has sometimes been undertaken. If bleeding has followed division of pleural adhesion or is thought to be coming from a well-defined 'bleeding-point' this source of bleeding may be sought through the thoracoscope and cauterised. If through neglect, or perhaps lack of correct diagnosis in the early stage, the haemothorax has become organised into fibrous tissue, an operation becomes necessary. The restricting fibrous coat over the lung has to be peeled off: this procedure is **decortication**.

Pneumothorax

Expansion of the lung in respiration depends upon the fact that the pressure of the atmosphere is constantly greater than the pressure in the pleural space. If air at atmospheric pressure is allowed to enter the thorax, either into the pleural space or between the parietal layer of the pleura and the thoracic wall, the diaphragm and rib movements in inspiration will be ineffective and the lung will remain collapsed. A puncture wound of the thoracic wall which does not actually enter the pleura, may permit the pleura to be pulled off the wall and an **'extra-pleural pneumothorax'** will develop. **'Intrapleural pneumothorax'** may be confined to one zone of the chest by adhesions which have formed between the two pleural layers. It may arise spontaneously or be produced deliberately in treatment.

Spontaneous pneumothorax. This means that air has entered the pleural space accidentally, through rupture of a small cyst on the lung surface or sometimes from the breaking down of a lung abscess or cavity which communicates with the bronchus and erodes onto the surface of the lung. Such cysts may be congenital or may arise with emphysema. This is a state of overdistension of the lungs which follows asthma and chronic bronchitis when there has been longstanding obstruction to expiration. Babies in particular develop spontaneous pneumothorax from the rupture of a tiny lung abscess. Frequently in spontaneous pneumothorax the original connection between the lung tissue and the pleura become sealed off, the air which has escaped into the pleura absorbs in a few days, and no harm results. If on the other hand the opening has resulted from an abscess, it may be too big to seal off immediately and the condition of **'broncho-pleural fistula'** results. Infection is rapidly carried to the pleural space with subsequent development of empyema.

Tension pneumothorax. In this condition, the inspiratory movements of the patient's chest draw air through an open wound in the chest wall or on the surface of the lung, but during expiration the soft tissues close the aperture, forming a 'one-way valve', thus preventing the escape of the air. With each respiratory excursion, air is drawn into the pleural space: not only does the pleural vacuum disappear but the lung is actually compressed by the accumulating air and the mediastinum may be pushed towards the opposite side (Fig. 34.3). Urgent treatment is required—that is, aspiration of the air. The tension may

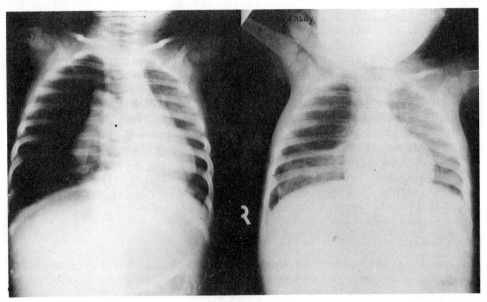

Fig. 34.3 Spontaneous pneumothorax arising from the rupture of a small abscess on the surface of the lung. The baby developed septicaemia from infected eczema. (*Left*) The mediastinum and heart are displaced far over to the left side by 'tension' pneumothorax from broncho-pleural fistula. An intercostal catheter was inserted on the right and air withdrawn. (*Right*) A few days later the fistula became sealed and the lower part of the lung re-expanded. The heart has returned to its normal position. (Author's case.)

rise again within minutes or it may take three or four hours, and repeated or continuous adjustment of the intrapleural pressure is necessary. The detection and management of tension pneumothorax is extremely important in all cases of thoracic wound. If an open communication between bronchial tree and pleura persists, an intercostal catheter is inserted. This is connected to an electric suction pump which is regulated to maintain a constant negative pressure in the hemithorax (pages 604, 284).

Post-operative pneumothorax. After thoracotomy, an attempt is made by the anaesthetist to expand the lung fully, out to the chest wall, before the final closure of the wound.

Some air may remain but will be rapidly absorbed. If the post-operative x-ray photograph shows a persistent pneumothorax, the air is aspirated. Frequently when the chest has been opened an 'under-water seal' type of drainage is used to prevent the re-entry of air which would occur otherwise with open drainage. During respiration any remaining air is blown off through the under-water seal and the weight of water in the tube prevents it being re-aspirated. Pneumothorax may arise some days after operation, from loosening of a bronchial ligature after lung resection. Tension pneumothorax may develop (Fig. 34.3), with surgical emphysema (Figs. 34.2(3), 34.4).

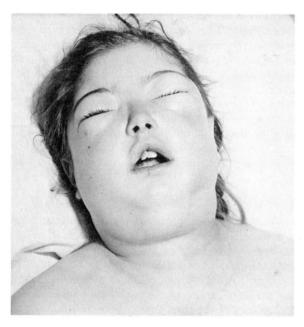

Fig. 34.4 Gross surgical emphysema after lobectomy. In spite of the alarming appearance, the lung was fully expanded and no specific treatment was necessary. The condition subsided completely in four days. Note that the spread of air has extended over the whole face, up to the eyebrows. (d'Abreu, *Practice of Thoracic Surgery*.)

The fate of pneumothorax. Unless the pleura has become thickened by inflammation or is covered by organised blood-clot, air which enters the pleural space is gradually absorbed. Spontaneous pneumothorax or post-operative pneumothorax will normally take care of itself unless the amount of air is very great, or a broncho-pleural fistula develops.

Complications of pneumothorax. Pneumothorax carries with it the risk of other complications. These are:

(a) Excessive displacement of the mediastinum; loss of efficiency of the opposite lung, and subsequent anoxia. The nurse needs to be on the look-out for this complication whatever may have been the cause of the pneumothorax. The trachea is palpated in the suprasternal notch and should normally be in the midline. Its displacement towards the sound side, accompanied by a rise of respiration rate, perhaps a little cyanosis and a rise of pulse rate, indicate most certainly that the pneumothorax is excessive. It will need to be reduced by aspiration of the air.

(b) **Paradoxical respiration** (page 606). It will be difficult for the nurse to detect this complication and its chief evidence will be increasing dyspnoea and cyanosis.

(c) **Haemorrhage.** Reference has already been made to the occurrence of haemothorax and whenever pneumothorax has been produced there is always the risk of bleeding into the space. This may result from the tearing of adhesions as the lung collapses, or from injury to a blood vessel in the thoracic wall when the needle was introduced in the production of artificial pneumothorax: the surface of the lung itself may be injured. Bleeding may be so great as to produce pallor, a rise of pulse rate, and other evidence of internal haemorrhage. On the other hand, the presence of the haemothorax may only be detected radiologically (a fluid level is seen in the pneumothorax), and by subsequent aspiration. If the percussion note over the area of the pneumothorax becomes dull, fluid must be present, either as serum, pus or blood.

(d) **Infection.** Infection arises in pneumothorax, particularly if the lung itself has been damaged or if fluid has been allowed to remain in the pleural space. Any appreciable rise of temperature following the induction of pneumothorax must lead to suspicion that infection has entered. It occurs rarely now in the course of major thoracic surgery or in the management of wounds of the thorax, because of the liberal use of antibiotics.

Surgical emphysema (Fig. 34.4)

If air enters the tissues of the body, particularly in the loose cellular tissue immediately under the skin, its presence is detected by a crackling sensation as the skin surface is palpated. This condition is **'surgical emphysema'** and it develops most commonly in injuries of the thorax because of the continuous pumping action of the thoracic muscles and diaphragm. A puncture of the skin alone may result in air being drawn in with each movement and being unable to escape. Occasionally this condition is present around fractures (for instance, fractures of the tibia where there has been a puncture wound). Air may escape from a pneumothorax into the tissues surrounding the pleura and this happens particularly with fractures of the ribs. It may arise after sigmoidoscopy due to a tear in the bowel which allows the inflated air to escape followed by flatus. The area of surgical emphysema may spread with alarming rapidity beneath the skin over the chest, extending well up into the neck and down onto the abdominal wall. It is sometimes very painful and its presence makes examination of the thorax or the abdomen very misleading.

Surgical emphysema may also be induced by gas-forming organisms—gas gangrene (page 55)—and if the nurse should at any time in the care of *any* surgical case, find an area of skin which presents this crackling sensation, she must report it at once.

Pleural effusion

This term is used to indicate the accumulation of any fluid within the pleural space. An effusion is described as 'clear', 'blood-stained' or 'turbid' according to its appearance when it has been aspirated. It may occur from inflammation of the pleura, especially in tuberculosis; the quantity of fluid may be so great that a lung is completely compressed and the hemi-thorax is filled with fluid right up to the clavicle. Pleural effusion may occur in heart failure or be produced from inflammation below the diaphragm in such conditions as subphrenic abscess, liver abscess, perinephric abscess or cholecystitis. The presence of a pleural effusion is detected by clinical examination of the chest and its extent is demonstrated by x-ray. Apart from thoracic surgery, pleural effusion may occur in surgical patients as the result of post-operative pneumonia or more commonly from the inflammation produced by small infarcts in the lung. These infarcts themselves have arisen from pulmonary embolism. The presence of a pleural effusion is common if there is malignant disease in the thorax, either a primary carcinoma of the lung or secondary deposits from some other organ such as the breast or the stomach. It is not uncommon for such effusions, secondary to malignant disease, to need repeated aspiration, and in a surgical ward this unhappy result of advanced cancer is frequently seen.

Empyema thoracis

This is the condition of pus formation in the pleural space. The pleural effusion which accompanies infective conditions of the lung may itself become infected and form pus. A lung abscess may burst into the pleural space. Haemothorax may become infected.

The symptoms which the condition produces depend on the amount of pus present, and the degree of compression of, or disease in, the underlying lungs. There is some embarrassment of respiration, and 'swinging' fever, typically present whenever pus has accumulated in the body. Fever may sometimes be absent, especially if the patient is being treated with antibiotics. The patient with an empyema is severely toxic, looks ill, loses weight rapidly and becomes severely anaemic. If the pus is sufficiently thin to be removed through a needle, then the treatment is entirely by aspiration. Penicillin or other antibiotic solution may be injected into the pleural space after the withdrawal of the pus. Aspiration needs to be repeated daily until lung expansion is adequate. If the pus becomes too thick for aspiration, the empyema is treated by one of three surgical methods:

- (a) A small intercostal incision is made and a large self-retaining catheter placed into the pleural space to allow the escape of pus. The catheter is connected to an under-water seal. This method of intercostal drainage is rarely used but it is sometimes suitable for children.
- (b) Rib resection and drainage by a wide-bore tube. Part of one rib is removed and the pleural space opened through its periosteum. This tube may be left open at its outer end or may be attached to an under-water seal. One type of tube is the 'Tudor-Edward' empyema tube which has an additional small rubber side tube through which the empyema cavity can be irrigated.
- (c) The empyema membrane which has formed over the surface of the lung is peeled off together with the similar layer lining the chest wall. The procedure is similar to that used for clotted haemothorax (page 609).

Nursing procedures in the care of empyema may be summarised as follows.

- (a) Diet. Because of the fever and toxaemia a high-calorie, vitamin-containing diet is essential.
- (b) Where intercostal or rib resection drainage has been instituted, particular care has to be taken of the drainage tube, to make certain that it never becomes kinked or obstructed and that the wound around the tube is kept scrupulously clean. The

tube is held in place partly by its retaining flange and partly by the intercostal muscles, but for additional safety it is either strapped to the thoracic wall or held in place by a tape passed round the chest.

(c) The posture of the patient has to be such that the drainage tube will be as low as possible in relation to the pleural space. This is made difficult by the fact that the presence of the tube prevents the patient from lying on the affected side. Various methods are adopted to overcome this problem, and perhaps the most satisfactory is to lead the tube out behind the patient between pillows and between the bars of a back rest.

(d) The greatest possible attention is paid to the routine methods for encouraging post-operative lung expansion.

Empyema is a dreaded complication of all operations or injuries involving the thorax because the severe inflammation of the pleura makes it extremely difficult for the lung to expand fully. Apparently trivial errors in the management of empyema, either from the surgical or nursing point of view, may greatly prolong the patient's illness and result in the persistence of a cavity and fistula. An empyema cavity does of course become sealed off from the rest of the pleural space by adhesions between the two layers of the pleura so that the drainage of an empyema does not usually produce pneumothorax of the whole of the one pleural space.

A collection of pus between the two lobes of the lung is an **'interlobar empyema'**.

Lung collapse and atelectasis

The structure of the lung has already been described (Chapter 10). It is held in its expanded state by negative pressure in the pleural space. When this 'suction' on its pleural surface is lost the lung recoils to its contracted state but can be made even smaller by compression. If 'tension pneumothorax' arises or if fluid collects in the pleural space, the lung may be actually *compressed*.

Thus collapse of the lung may be brought about either by pneumothorax or by compression with fluid (effusion or haemothorax).

Collapse may also result from blockage of a bronchus. If a large or small bronchus becomes blocked by growth, foreign body, or more usually by a plug of mucus, the air within the lung beyond the point of blockage becomes absorbed and that area of 'sponge' becomes collapsed. If a whole lobe or a whole lung is thus affected, the condition is **'massive collapse'**. Atelectasis usually occurs in the lower part of the lung and is known as **'basal collapse'**. In the unconscious patient, or in the post-operative period when respiratory movement is embarrassed by drugs or pain (page 390), the presence of minor degrees of infection in the lung leads to the collection of thick bronchial secretion which in turn is apt to block the small bronchial tubes. The cough is not powerful enough to expel this viscid secretion. Thus 'areas of collapse' may occur as a post-operative complication. These areas of collapse or 'consolidation' are in effect areas of pneumonia. Any area of collapse may become a lung abscess.

It will be seen that in the recovery of thoracic cases and in fact in all surgical cases where there may be embarrassment of respiration, the nursing management plays a vital part by eliminating those conditions which lead to pulmonary collapse, and by encouraging conditions which lead to pulmonary re-expansion. Relief of pain, persistent and repeated breathing exercises, and early ambulation all play their part. The trained physiotherapist is responsible for a good deal of this treatment, both in thoracic units and in general surgical units, but the nurse is present most often in the immediate post-operative period and is of course in more constant contact with the patient. It is the nurse who has to encourage and supervise the patient's coughing and the nurse who is responsible for the correct positioning of the patient after operation. The nurse will learn the basic principles involved in the prevention and management of collapse or 'atelectasis', mainly in her contact with abdominal surgery. Methods to encourage pulmonary re-expansion are outlined below.

Most thoracic patients after operation are nursed in the upright sitting position, but sometimes in order to encourage movement of the affected side of the thorax the patient is nursed on the sound side. In other cases it may be necessary to nurse the patient on the affected side, but these are matters which belong to the realm of specialised nursing, and specific instructions will be given by the surgeon in each case. Factors which tend to produce pulmonary atelectasis are described in relation to surgical conditions on page 389. The importance of these 'aggravating' factors is of course increased in all cases where the mechanism of respiration is disturbed by thoracic disease, injury, or operation.

Lung abscess and cavity

An abscess may arise in the lung from various sources and reference to lung abscess is made in other sections.

During the course of any inflammatory disease in the lung, just as with infection in other tissues of the body, pus formation may occur. If the pus is unable to drain away through the bronchus, a local abscess or even several abscesses may occur in the lung. Pneumonia, post-operative atelectasis, and tuberculosis are all conditions in which abscess formation may occur in this way.

A foreign body, such as part of a tooth or a piece of blood clot or something completely extraneous, may be inhaled and pass into the inner recesses of the bronchial tree. Here it sets up an inflammatory reaction and an abscess develops round the foreign body.

A small clot embolus, arising perhaps from a thrombosed vein in the pelvis, may be carried into a small branch of the pulmonary artery which it blocks, producing an infarct (page 62). Infection supervenes and an embolic abscess arises. During the course of any septicaemic process an infected embolus may be caught in the lung tissue and produce an abscess.

The symptoms of lung abscess are those associated with pus formation elsewhere—fever, loss of weight, anaemia. There may in addition be cough.

Sometimes the abscess bursts into a bronchus and pus is discharged by coughing. Healing of the abscess cavity may then occur without any further trouble. Occasionally the thoracic surgeon can break into the abscess by means of a suction tube introduced through the bronchoscope. If the abscess cannot be reached in this way, operation for drainage has to be undertaken by thoracotomy. Inflammation of the overlying pleura during the formation of the abscess may have led to obliteration of the pleural space over the affected area of lung and the abscess may be aspirated, like an empyema, without pus being allowed to escape into the pleural space.

'Cavity' is a term usually applied to lung abscess which is tuberculous in origin. It arises partly by the breakdown of lung tissue and partly by the distension of a small area of the lung from air which is drawn in through the narrow channel of an inflamed bronchus, but which cannot escape owing to the 'check valve' action of the inflamed bronchial lining. As distinct from other lung abscesses, the 'cavity' is air-containing and shows as a clear space on x-ray examination.

Whatever may be the origin of an abscess or cavity in the lung, the purpose of treatment is that the cavity should be drained and then obliterated by re-expansion of the lung tissue around the cavity. Sometimes the abscess or cavity has a wall so rigid that it will not collapse when the contents are removed. It may then need to be cut out by surgical operation. In the case of a tuberculous cavity an attempt is made to collapse the cavity by collapsing the whole lung (page 621) by artificial pneumothorax or thoracoplasty.

Once again it needs to be emphasised that after *all* surgical operations careful nursing, particularly in relation to the prevention of vomiting, the management of vomiting, and conscientious attention to chest expansion, will prevent the occurrence of lung abscess in all but rare cases. When an abscess has occurred, nursing measures will include the following:

(a) High-calorie diet with vitamin supplement and adequate iron intake to counteract the anaemia.
(b) Particular attention to oral hygiene and the collection and disposal of sputum.
(c) Specific measures to encourage lung expansion.
(d) Chemotherapy and antibiotic treatment.
(e) Diagnostic aspiration by needle through the chest wall.
(f) The management of whatever surgical procedure the surgeon adopts.
(g) In many cases, postural drainage (see below).

Postural drainage

Where there is inflammation of the bronchial tree, such as occurs particularly in bronchiectasis, the patient is assisted in his efforts to expel the pus from his bronchi by what is known as postural drainage. The patient is placed in such a position that the part of the lung from which the purulent secretions are to be drained is uppermost. This posturing is achieved by making the patient hang over the side of the bed or by using a special adjustable bed or wedge mattress so that the head and shoulders are lower than the thorax. Continual postural drainage may be maintained by which the patient is kept in this position for long periods, or intermittent drainage may be instituted in which the patient is placed in the specific position for periods of perhaps 10 or 20 minutes, twice or three times a day. Breathing exercises, chest slapping and coughing are all used while the patient is in the 'drainage' position. Fig. 34.5 shows some of the typical positions used to drain particular areas of the lung, but the physician or surgeon in charge of the case will issue specific instructions.

Physiotherapy in thoracic surgery

The trained physiotherapist plays a vital part in the management of thoracic surgery and her personal efforts, no less than skilful nursing by a specially trained team, may eliminate complications and speed recovery, perhaps to a greater degree than in any other branch of surgery. All physiotherapists are trained in routine remedial measures for encouraging lung expansion.

There is no room for 'friction' or 'differences of opinion' between the nurse and the physiotherapist. Each must consider the other's difficulties. The busy physiotherapist may

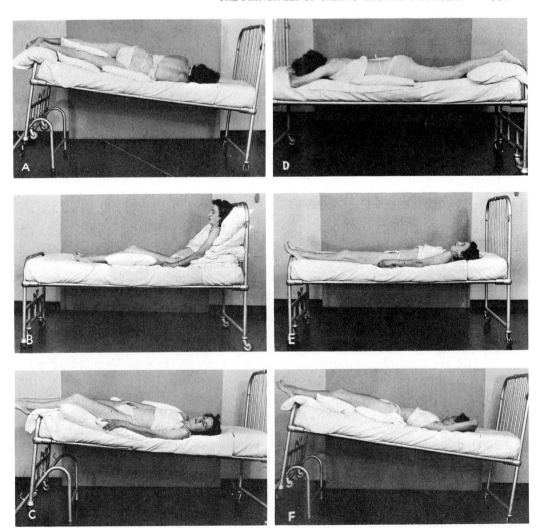

Fig. 34.5 Positions for drainage of individual lung segments. **(a)** Left lateral and posterior basal segments. **(b)** Apical segments of upper lobes. **(c)** Right middle lobe. **(d)** Apical segments of lower lobes. **(e)** Anterior (pectoral) segments of both upper lobes. **(f)** Anterior parts of both lower lobes. (d'Abreu, *Practice of Thoracic Surgery*.)

well appear to interfere with ordinary ward routine and the busy nurse may well miss the opportunities of encouraging a patient's respiratory activity which repeatedly come to her during her routine nursing management. In small hospital units where skilled physiotherapy is not available, the nurse must learn routine expansion exercises and be able to instruct the patient before and after operation. As in other branches of surgery, the patient should, if possible, learn before operation all the exercises which he is expected to perform after operation so that he will have developed the idea and muscle co-ordination required, before pain adds to his difficulty. Physiotherapy required after major thoracic operations such as pneumonectomy and thoracoplasty requires special experience and training.

Pulmonary re-expansion

The main principles of thoracic surgery and the major complications which may arise have now been defined and it may be said that treatment is directed to the ultimate complete expansion of all remaining lung tissue, and to the obliteration of any abnormal cavities either in the lung or in the pleural space. Pulmonary re-expansion is the immediate objective following:

(*a*) Pneumothorax of sudden onset, spontaneous or operative.
(*b*) Consolidation and inflammatory atelectasis.
(*c*) Empyema, haemothorax or effusion.

From consideration of the factors which lead to collapse of the lung, it is clear that in prevention and treatment, the principles may be summarised quite simply. These are:

(*a*) Active movement of the chest wall and diaphragm.
(*b*) Posture, both in relation to drainage and post-operative position.
(*c*) The avoidance of drugs which depress respiration by their action on the brain (the morphine group) and similarly by avoidance of over-deep anaesthesia.
(*d*) By passive inflation of the lungs by the anaesthetist during operation.
(*e*) By the removal of bronchial obstruction, actively by the patient's coughing and passively by the bronchoscopic aspiration.

Active respiratory movement is encouraged by breathing exercises and sometimes by making the patient inflate a rubber balloon or drive water from one glass jar to another by blowing down a rubber tube. Deep respiration may be encouraged by stimulating the respiratory centre in the brain: Nikethamide (Coramine) has been used for years for this purpose. An effective way of stimulating spontaneous deep breathing is by administering a mixture of carbon dioxide and oxygen (carbon dioxide 5 per cent) through a face mask. This effect of carbon dioxide has been described on page 214, but it should not be used if there has been a head injury. Injuries of chest and head are not uncommonly associated.

The nurse will come to recognise that whether in thoracic, abdominal, or other branches of surgery, lung expansion is the aim of a considerable amount of nursing routine. Early ambulation, a strict avoidance of tight binders (for instance after a radical mastectomy) and correct post-anaesthetic management are of paramount importance if chest complications are to be avoided.

Surgical disorders of the lungs

Operations commonly performed for lung disorders are enumerated in Table 47. The thoracic surgeon is mainly concerned with three big groups of case:

(*a*) septic or pyogenic infective conditions of the lung (bronchiectasis, lung abscess and empyema),

(b) tuberculosis,

(c) carcinoma and other neoplasms.

The majority of patients suffering from these conditions are at first a problem of medical diagnosis rather than of surgical management. The necessary investigations are frequently carried out in a medical ward. In tuberculosis, more than in any other group operative surgery is only a small part of the whole management of the patient, who frequently requires prolonged sanatorium treatment.

The surgical treatment of lung disease involves in many cases multi-stage operations on patients whose general condition has been undermined by chronic ill-health.

Diagnostic procedures

The investigation of all cases of pulmonary disease involves repeated examinations of the sputum, for tubercle bacilli, for other infecting organisms, and for malignant cells. Since sputum is swallowed, tubercle bacilli can be recovered from the stomach by means of a saline washout carried out through a naso-gastric tube (page 474). This procedure is frequently necessary in the investigation of cases suspected of pulmonary tuberculosis. The stools are also examined for tubercle bacilli.

Full blood examination, including white cell count, sedimentation rate, and blood group, is carried out on all cases and is frequently repeated during the course of treatment.

Radiological examination

This is in four phases:

(a) Plain x-ray photographs of the chest from various angles. These reveal soft tissue opacities, the collection of fluid in the pleural space, and the degree of aeration of the lung. By tomography different 'layers' of the lung are examined so that the shape and exact position of opacities or cavities can be determined.

(b) Bronchography (Fig. 15.3), in which an iodine-containing contrast medium is injected into the trachea by one of three routes. A soft catheter may be passed through the nose and the contrast medium dripped into the opening to the larynx after the throat has been sprayed with a local anaesthetic. The contrast medium may be inserted over the back of the tongue with a special syringe, carrying a curved metal cannula. Alternatively it may be injected into the trachea through a needle inserted below the larynx (through the crico-thyroid membrane). This last method carries with it a risk of cellulitis of the neck and surgical emphysema, owing to the escape of air and infection from the trachea after the needle has been withdrawn.

The flow of the contrast medium is directed to whichever part of the lung is being examined, and serial x-ray examinations are made.

(c) Screen examination. The movements of the lung, heart and diaphragm are studied by direct vision on the fluorescent screen. This is of particular value if a subphrenic abscess is suspected.

(*d*) Serial follow-up x-ray examination to watch the progress of a lung lesion and particularly to check the re-expansion of the lung after a thoracotomy.

Special radiological techniques are used in studying diseases of the chest, but these are usually inapplicable to patients in the immediate post-operative phase when they are confined to the ward. It is occasionally necessary for a severely ill patient to be moved to the x-ray department in order that adequate examination may be carried out.

Because of the risk of explosion, however slight this may be, all oxygen apparatus must be turned off during x-ray examination in the ward. No x-ray apparatus is completely spark-proof.

Paracentesis thoracis

This is a simple procedure in which the needle is introduced through an intercostal space in order to withdraw pleural fluid for pathological examination or to relieve pressure on the lung. It is carried out under local anaesthesia and, apart from syringes, needles and the anaesthetic solution, no special apparatus is required. Sterile test tubes or bijou bottles (page 256, must be at hand to receive specimens of fluid for laboratory examination. Penicillin or other antiseptic solution may be injected at the end of the aspiration procedure.

Paracentesis for the withdrawal of large pleural effusions requires the addition of a two-way tap or special aspiration apparatus. Short needles are preferable: the two-way tap enables the operator to aspirate with a 20-ml syringe and eject the fluid without detaching the syringe from the needle; to do so would allow air to enter the chest.

Local anaesthetic is injected at the site of aspiration, usually in the mid-axillary line on the appropriate side. The patient is in the sitting position leaning forward with arms folded on a bed table in front of him so he can relax: the pulse is felt frequently during the procedure, and every quarter hour for 1 hour following. Cytotoxic drugs or antibiotics may be injected after withdrawal of the fluid. Unless a two-way tap is being used, the patient breathes out fully and then remains 'expired' while the syringe is changed to lessen the risk of air being drawn in.

Following paracentesis there are three main risks:

(*a*) The development of a haemothorax from inadvertent puncture of the lung surface, with subsequent bleeding,
(*b*) surgical emphysema from an escape of air from the pleural space into the sub-cutaneous tissues,
(*c*) acute pulmonary oedema if a large amount of fluid is removed rapidly: the lung expands and swells.

Bronchoscopy

The general principle of this procedure is the same as oesophagoscopy (page 508) and the instrument is somewhat similar.

Particular care is required with the sterilisation of the bronchoscope as it is frequently used in patients with tuberculosis. It can be boiled but is preferably sterilised in a formalin cabinet or with Cidex, or ethylene oxide gas. Heat sterilisation is usually the most practical method if the instrument is required for a series of cases. Lamps must be removed if the instrument is autoclaved. Modern endoscopes have fibre-optic illumination; the light attachments cannot be heat treated.

Various sizes of bronchoscope are available for different ages of patient. The lighting system and ancillary instruments are similar to those used with the oesophagoscope. Though the instrument is primarily for direct-viewing, a telescope is also used (like that of the cystoscope) to increase the angle of vision. The telescope must *never* be boiled unless it is of a pattern specially designed to withstand boiling.

Bronchoscopy may be performed under local or general anaesthesia. Local anaesthesia is obtained by spraying the mouth and larynx with lignocaine (xylocaine) or other suitable surface anaesthetic. As with other similar procedures, stimulant drugs and resuscitation apparatus must be at hand in case the patient collapses from sensitivity to the local anaesthetic agent. A pre-operative sedative drug is used combined with atropine to limit the secretions in the bronchi.

Bronchoscopy is required not only as a diagnostic procedure but as a means of access to the lower reaches of the trachea and main bronchial tubes for biopsy or for the removal of foreign body. Bronchoscopy is also used for atelectasis to clear a bronchus which has been blocked by viscid secretion. In this case, the procedure may be undertaken with the patient in his bed, if for instance the atelectasis has followed some major abdominal operation (Fig. 34.7).

Complications of bronchoscopy. The surgeon will give instructions concerning the maintenance of the patient's position after bronchoscopy. While the air-passages remain anaesthetic there is a danger of inhalation of secretions from the mouth as the patient is unable to cough. Unless instructions are given to the contrary the patient should be nursed in the 'head-down' position when possible.

When instruments have been passed between the vocal cords there is always a risk of acute oedema of the glottis, and if difficulty is experienced in breathing this fact must be reported to the medical officer *at once*. The oedema may respond to spraying with a vaso-constrictor solution: intubation or tracheotomy might be required (Chapter 10, Asphyxia).

Thoracoscopy

This procedure is commonly used in thoracic units specialising in the treatment of tuberculosis. It is also used in other conditions for diagnostic purposes. Artificial pneumo-thorax is induced to collapse part of the lung in order to produce obliteration of a tuber-culous cavity. Adequate collapse may be prevented by an adhesion between the lung surface and parietal pleura. The introduction of a **thoracoscope** through the chest wall enables the surgeon to see this adhesion and divide it with an electro-cautery.

The thoracoscope is somewhat similar in design to a cystoscope. The lens system and light is introduced through the chest wall by means of a trocar and cannula. The operating instruments are usually inserted through a separate trocar but some instruments combine the two functions (Fig. 34.6).

The procedure is carried out under local infiltration anaesthesia and the principal risk is one of haemorrhage from the divided adhesions or from the chest wall.

Collapse therapy

Since the advent of effective antituberculous drugs, surgical treatment of pulmonary tuberculosis is very rarely needed. In countries where early treatment is lacking and the disease advanced some cases occur which require treatment of cavities (abscesses). This is achieved by encouraging the area of lung involved to collapse to obliterate the cavity. Artificial pneumothorax is induced and maintained by refilling for months till healing occurs. **Thoracoplasty** is a more radical procedure. It involves the removal of several ribs, perhaps as many as eight on one side. This allows the soft tissues of the chest wall to

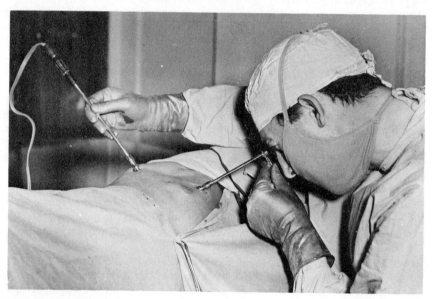

Fig. 34.6 Thoracoscopy by the two-cannula method. The patient is lying on the left side. (d'Abreu, *Practice of Thoracic Surgery*.)

collapse inwards and obliterate a chronic empyema cavity or allow a tuberculous lung to collapse completely (Fig. 34.2). Spinal curvature is very liable to develop after this operation and postural exercises have to be commenced very soon after operation.

A persistent cavity may be resected with the affected lobe, if the disease appears confined to one area. An infected tuberculous effusion (chronic empyema) may lead to fibrosis over the lung and decortication is undertaken as for organised haemothorax.

General nursing considerations

Special beds are used to enable the patient to be postured in such a way that any particular diseased area of the lung is constantly drained by gravity (Fig. 34.5).

Apparatus for administration of oxygen and piped suction is available at every bedside. Electric suction pumps have always to be immediately available to maintain continuous suction. The 'three-bottle method' of suction (page 665) is adequate for babies to maintain pleural drainage. A portable foot-operated suction pump should be available for short term use. Full ECG, pulse and blood pressure monitoring equipment are essential. Many patients are nursed in intensive care units until they are out of danger but, even in the phase of 'intermediate nursing care' emergencies may occur.

Tracheostomy is frequently an added nursing problem, with intermittent positive pressure respiration (IPPR, page 195).

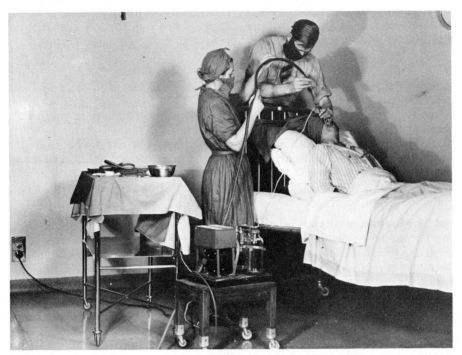

Fig. 34.7 Bronchoscopy and bronchoscopic suction in the ward for post-operative lung collapse. A photograph taken during an emergency bronchoscopy. (d'Abreu, *Practice of Thoracic Surgery*.)

Cross-infection

As the lungs are involved directly in this branch of surgery, airborne infection is a particular hazard. Careless handling of suction catheter, inattention to mouth hygiene, and neglect of ward ventilation are especially dangerous. Collection of sputum, its bacteriological examination and measurement is essential.

Nutrition

All patients undergoing major surgery require a high calorie intake. Parenteral feeding (page 138), quite apart from maintenance of fluid balance, is often required. Patients with heart disease also frequently have poor renal function and dietic restriction may be needed with respect to some items.

Physiotherapy

To ensure pre- and post-operative lung expansion, intensive 'drill' is required. The need is continuous, and the physiotherapist can assist expansion even while the patient is still unconscious. The nature of the surgery focuses attention on the chest and it is easy to overlook the need for leg exercises and forced dorsiflexion of the feet at regular intervals to reduce the risk of thrombosis and embolism.

The student nurse will be very much an observer in the post-operative intensive-care phase of patients who have had cardiothoracic surgery, but her role is nevertheless important in general nursing care, and the discipline learned in relation to observation of cardiac and respiratory function is invaluable in other fields of surgical nursing.

CARDIAC SURGERY

Operations which are performed upon the heart and large arteries occupying the mediastinum are included in Table 47.

Most of the lesions of the heart for which surgery is feasible are either congenital defects in the septa between the atria or ventricles, congenital abnormalities of the valves or great vessels, or scarring of the valves due to rheumatic fever. Any of these conditions demands very extensive investigations before surgery can be contemplated. These tests fall into five main categories:

(a) The electrocardiograph (ECG). This procedure involves measuring the electrical changes produced by each phase of the heart beat. Contact pads are placed on the four limbs and in various positions on the chest wall. An electronic recording device amplifies these minute currents and records them photographically or by direct writing on a strip of paper. During operations upon the heart an electrocardiograph is connected to the patient during the whole procedure and the record can be watched on a small oscillograph (television) screen.

(b) Radiography. In order to watch the flow of blood through the heart, **cardiac catheterisation** is performed. A long plastic catheter is inserted through a vein near the elbow, and passes over the shoulder through the subclavian and innominate veins into the superior vena cava and thence into the right atrium of the heart. It can be directed through any abnormal orifice in the atrium, or through the valves from the right atrium into other cavities of the heart. A contrast medium is injected and the spread of the medium is watched on the x-ray screen, or recorded by cineradiography. During this procedure blood can be sucked back through the catheter and the chemical composition of the blood from various parts of the heart can be determined, especially the concentration of oxygen and carbon dioxide. The great vessels and left side of the heart may similarly be studied by introducing a catheter through an artery.

(c) Blood chemistry. In addition to oxygen and carbon dioxide concentrations in the blood a full analysis is made, because during operation large quantities of blood are given in transfusion, and with artificial circulation and artificial oxygenation it is very easy to disturb the blood chemistry beyond the point of recovery (page 107).

(d) Function tests. The surgeon needs to know the patient's capacity for action and this can be gauged largely from the history—how far he can walk, whether he can climb stairs, or whether he can sleep lying flat. In addition to these simple enquiries, sometimes special tests of function and oxygen consumption are undertaken to assess the patient's recovery.

(e) **Ultra-sound scanning.** This gives additional information on size and shape of major structures.

Patent ductus arteriosus

In **closed** heart surgery the patient's circulation continues through its natural pathways during operation. The chambers of the heart are not opened. The ductus arteriosus (Fig. 34.8) is a congenital shunt between the aorta and pulmonary artery which is normally closed as the child breathes at birth; it may remain open and need tying by operation. If it persists as an open vessel blood escapes from the aorta back into the pulmonary artery and produces lung congestion. Sometimes the shunt is reversed; the heart begins to fail and cyanosis occurs. The most serious complication of this and many other minor heart lesions is the development of infective bacterial endocarditis in later life. This short **patent ductus** can be tied without great difficulty through a left intercostal thoracotomy.

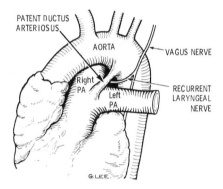

Fig. 34.8   Patent ductus arteriosus between the pulmonary artery **PA** and aorta. Oxygenated blood from the high pressure aorta flows back into the pulmonary circulation where the pressure is lower. Patent ductus is compatible with normal life but may lead to bacterial endocarditis.

Constrictive pericarditis is sometimes treated by excision of the scarred pericardium.

Arterial short circuits came next in the history of cardiac surgery. Sometimes there is congenital narrowing of the great vessels. By clamping the vessels without stopping the heart, cutting out the narrow portion, and joining the ends together again it is possible to overcome this obstruction. Similarly an aneurysm of the aorta (Fig. 48.6) can be excised and the gap made good by inserting a dacron 'prosthesis'.

Fallot's tetralogy is a congenital malformation in which the blood flow from the right ventricle to the pulmonary arteries is inadequate. The left subclavian artery is divided (Blalock's operation) and planted in the wall of the pulmonary artery which is tied off between this join and the heart.

Mitral stenosis was first treated by valvotomy through the auricular appendage. The superior and inferior vena cava were clamped to prevent blood entering the heart. The surgeon made a very small cut into the left auricular appendage. He inserted a finger which carried a special knife blade on a thimble and slit the tight valve between the atrium and ventricle. This whole procedure, apart from opening and closing the chest, could be carried out within the 3-minute period for which the brain can safely be deprived of oxygen. This technique has now been replaced by a closed method using a Brock's or Tubbs' dilator through the ventricle without interrupting the circulation. All this surgery is done through a left thoracotomy across the pleural space.

Pace-makers

In certain forms of heart disease where the beat-conducting mechanism is at fault electronic pace-makers are sown into the heart to maintain a regular beat in case of heart block.

There are two main types. One has an external source of electrical energy and the primary coil is strapped to the skin: the secondary coil which picks up the impulse is implanted beneath the abdominal or chest-wall skin and electrode wires are stitched to the heart (Fig. 34.9). The second type has a built-in battery and is totally enclosed within the body. The latest type is controlled by the natural heart beat and only operates when the heart rate drops to a pre-set level—the 'on-demand' pace-maker. From time to time wires break, batteries require replacement and patients dependent on these pace-makers must live within reach of maintenance centres. Minute nuclear powered batteries have been tried, enclosed in special steel indestructible capsules, able to withstand even the heat of cremation to avoid the danger of nuclear contamination.

Open heart surgery

Open heart surgery involves diversion of the blood and maintenance of the circulation to the brain and vital organs by artificial means. The oxygen requirements of the brain can be reduced with drugs or by cooling. In **hypothermia** the patient's own lungs are left in circulation and perform the oxygenation. With full cardio-pulmonary by-pass a complete shunt is used, replacing heart and lungs.

Open heart surgery includes repair of congenital septal defects and replacement of damaged valves by prosthesis of metal, plastic or graft tissue. Narrowed coronary arteries are by-passed using a length of vein taken from the leg. The range of cardiac surgery is still expanding. Complete heart transplantation requires full cardiopulmonary by-pass. The problem of immunity and graft rejection are discussed on page 38.

Hypothermia. With the advent of positive pressure anaesthesia (page 220), opening the thorax and the pericardium no longer deterred the surgeon. Until some method was found to maintain a flow of oxygenated blood to the brain, no progress could be made towards open heart surgery. It is not possible to deprive the brain of oxygen for more than 3 minutes without risking either permanent damage to the brain, or death. There are two ways in which this difficulty is overcome. The first is to reduce the oxygen requirements of the brain by cooling the patient, thus putting his brain cells in a state of hibernation, aided also by drugs such as chlorpromazine. The oxygen needs can be reduced almost to zero as in an animal that has a natural period of prolonged hibernation without taking food. A safe period of 7–9 minutes can be made available to the

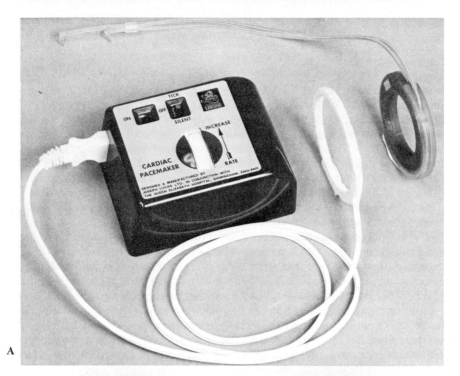

A

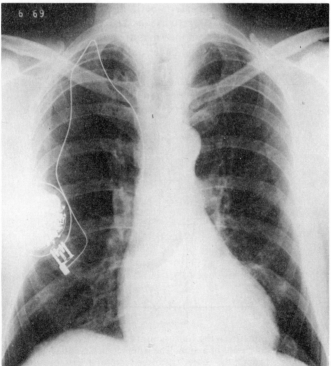

B

Fig. 34.9 Cardiac pace-maker with external source of electric energy. **A**. On the right is the secondary coil which is implanted under the skin of the chest. The two electrodes emerge from this coil and these are stitched to the heart. The white primary coil is strapped to the chest wall over the secondary coil, and energy is transmitted from the pace-maker box which the patient carries. **B**. X-ray showing secondary coil and electrodes in position. (d'Abreu, *Practice of Thoracic Surgery*.)

surgeon in which he can arrest the movement of the heart and perform operations within it. Cooling is achieved by ice packs, baths or special refrigeration apparatus.

Profound hypothermia was a further development of this technique of cooling but is now rarely used. At normal body temperature (37 °C) the brain cannot tolerate anoxia for more than 3 minutes. At 30 °C achieved by 'conventional' hypothermia this time lies between 7 and 9 minutes, but by cooling the brain even further to 15 °C, as long as an hour may be permitted for surgery on the brain or on the heart. This profound drop in temperature is achieved by the use of two pumps which maintain an artificial circulation, but not an artificial oxygenation of the blood. The first pump takes blood from the right atrium and returns it through the right ventricle into the pulmonary artery. The blood is oxygenated in the lungs by positive pressure respiration. The second pump draws the blood from the left atrium, circulates it through a heat exchanger which cools it to the required degree and pumps the blood back through a cannula placed into the thoracic aorta or upwards through the femoral artery, where it is distributed through the aorta to the whole body. When the body has been cooled to the requisite level, pumping may actually cease so that operations may take place on the heart or brain with no bleeding at all. The postoperative care of patients who have been under profound hypothermia is extremely critical as the temperature has to be brought back to normal by a very careful re-warming process. Meticulous observation for evidence of brain damage must be kept continuously; difficulty with speech and twitchings must be reported. Convulsions may occur.

Cardiopulmonary by-pass. An alternative method of maintaining the blood supply to the brain while the heart is operated on is to use 'extra-corporeal' circulation with a pump oxygenator (Fig. 34.10). With this system the lungs are by-passed by withdrawing the blood from both the superior and inferior vena cava, oxygenating it and perhaps cooling it in

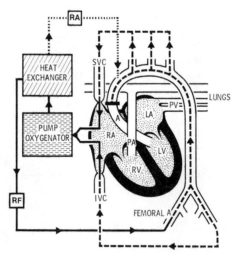

Fig. 34.10 Extra-corporeal circulation—the heart-lung machine. Circulation and oxygenation carried on by pump. Pulmonary circulation out of action. The letters indicate initials of the main blood vessels. Oxygenated blood circulates through the route RF to the femoral artery, or alternatively direct to the thoracic aorta by route RA.

addition before its return to the femoral artery or aorta. This involves the use of very complicated apparatus and a team of between 10 and 15 persons in the operating theatre. The whole pump has to be charged with blood, which is prevented from clotting by the use of heparin (page 59). Great care has to be taken also to prevent bubbles entering the apparatus, or the patient would develop air embolism. At the time of operation when the blood is being taken from the great veins and passed through the pump, artificial lung and delivery tube into another artery, all the vessels which open into the heart have to be clamped to produce what is known as a 'dry heart'. To maintain a supply of oxygenated blood to the heart muscle itself a special cannula may be put into the coronary artery. Unfortunately with this system, in order to keep the tissues adequately oxygenated, there has to be a very large amount of blood circulating and haemolysis (damage to the blood cells) occurs, which limits the time for which this by-pass may be used.

Cardioversion. This term means changing the rhythm of the heart.

Atrial fibrillation is a condition in which the normal rhythmic beat of the atrium is replaced by a fluttering, ineffective movement of the muscle. The impulses passed to the ventricle produce irregular contractions some of which are insufficient to produce a pulse at the wrist. The difference between the apex beat and the wrist pulse rate is the 'pulse deficit' (page 770).

Ventricular fibrillation occurs from coronary or rheumatic disease. This is sometimes deliberately produced in open heart surgery to provide a still heart.

Ventricular fibrillation is fatal unless it can be switched to normal rhythm by defibrillation. The heart which has stopped—cardiac arrest—can be made to fibrillate by injecting adrenaline. Defibrillation is then carried out to restore normal rhythm. This is achieved by giving high-voltage electric shocks to the heart. Figure 34.11 illustrates the apparatus used for this purpose and this equipment should be available in all operation theatres. (See page 191 for external defibrillation). In surgery its most common use is in cases of cardiac arrest, but long-standing cardiac irregularities such as atrial fibrillation or attacks of severe tachycardia may require emergency cardioversion to switch to normal rhythm. The principle is that a direct current shock stops all electrical activity in the heart momentarily and allows the natural pace-maker to start again emitting its regular impulse down the conducting mechanism in the heart. Except in an emergency in an unconscious patient, anaesthesia is required and this is usually achieved with intravenous valium and thiopeptone. In certain conditions the timing of the electrical shock has to be related to the ECG record of the natural electrical discharge already taking place in the heart and the defibrillating apparatus is coupled to an ECG recorder so that the timing of the electrical shock is automatically given at the correct moment in the cycle.

Surgical approach to the heart

The heart may be reached through the left pleural cavity and this is the route used for tying a patent ductus arteriosus, but open heart surgery is performed by splitting the sternum vertically. The heart and great vessels can thus be exposed without deliberately opening either pleural cavity, though there is always a risk the pleura may be inadvertently punctured. As this approach gives good access the return flow of oxygenated blood from the pump in by-pass procedures is directed into the thoracic aorta through a cannula held in with a purse string suture. On withdrawal the hole in the wall of the aorta is stitched.

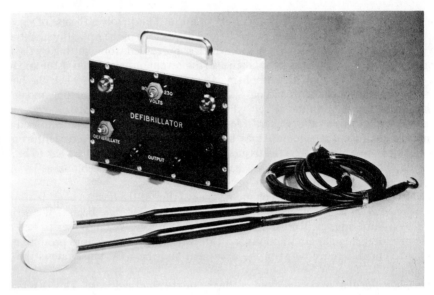

Fig. 34.11 Cardiac defibrillator (internal). The electrodes with insulated handles are placed in contact with the heart. An electric shock arrests the irregular movement of the heart so that normal rhythm can be restored.

Nursing

The post-operative complications which may affect nursing are those associated with other major thoracic surgical procedures. Mitral valvulotomy and ligature of the patent ductus arteriosus often require extremely short convalescence owing to the tremendous improvement in the patient's general condition as soon as a normal blood flow has been established through the heart. After any of the major cardiac operations there has to be minute-by-minute medical supervision for several hours after operation. Usually pulse, blood pressure, temperature and electrocardiograph records are continued on constant monitoring apparatus.

Full resuscitation equipment for dealing with cardiac arrest, asphyxia and bronchial aspiration must be at hand (page 287). In all probability the patient will be on IPPR initially to ensure full lung expansion, and maximal blood oxygenation.

Special problems requiring nursing attention are:

1. (*a*) If the patient is on IPPR, regular suction with full asepsis is required to ensure a clean and clear airway (page 195). (*b*) If the patient is not on IPPR oxygen will be needed through a mask. Physiotherapy to aid respiratory effort is vital.

2. The circulation pressure is monitored through a central venous pressure line and this determines the IV infusion rate (page 148), particularly in relation to blood transfusion. Ventricular fibrillation may occur, calling for external cardiac massage and defibrillation. If ventricular arrest occurs adrenaline may be injected to produce ventricular fibrillation which is then converted by the defibrillator.

3. Fluid balance is critical. Renal function may be defective initially; many cardiac patients are hypertensive and in consequence have kidney damage. Renal function may fall off because blood flow has been inadequate. A self-retaining urethral catheter is used and output recorded very frequently (probably $\frac{1}{4}$-hourly), in order that the intake/output balance can be watched. Overloading the circulation can easily occur. Diuretics (Frusemide) are used freely. Blood electrolyte estimation and blood gas analysis are carried out frequently.

4. Wound drainage. In addition to the under-water seal drain from the pleural cavity if this has been opened, additional suction drains are placed on the pericardial cavity. The outlets from the water bottles are usually connected to a vacuum pump. If the operation has been performed through the sternal split, and neither pleural cavity has been opened there will be no pleural drain. As correct fluid balance is essential, the drainage fluid is intercepted into a separate graduated jar. The connecting tube between the two jars must rise sufficiently high to prevent water being sucked over from the seal bottle (page 603).

5. Temperature observation is required $\frac{1}{4}$-hourly. The rate of return to normal from the hypothermic level which occurs (even if hypothermia is not used deliberately) is regulated by blankets and sometimes an electric blanket is needed.

Conclusion

The nursing of major thoracic surgical cases calls for great devotion to duty. The physical exertion required is heavy and the nurse is called upon to supervise technical procedures which require a thorough understanding of their scientific basis, such as oxygen therapy, repeated blood transfusion and the maintenance of continuous suction. The nurse in a thoracic unit may herself be exposed to tuberculosis and other infection and must maintain her own physical health at the highest possible level. There is no more exacting field of bedside care than that required for major thoracic surgery.

SECTION VII

35

The Principles of Urological Surgery

The function of the kidney is the manufacture of urine. The chemical balance of the body is largely dependent on the ability of the kidney to vary the composition of urine. Any interference with the function of the kidney is reflected in a disturbance of blood chemistry and ultimately in all the chemical processes of the body. Healthy kidneys are essential for the regulation of what is known as 'water balance' in the body (Chapter 8). Disturbances of the **function** of the kidney may perhaps be described as 'medical' rather than surgical diseases, but the management of shock, dehydration, anaemia, and disorders of the urinary tract in particular has to be concerned very intimately with the physiology of the kidney. A great deal of accurate nursing observation is necessary in relation to renal function in all major surgical cases, and the nurse must have a thorough understanding of the chemical and mechanical principles which are involved.

Once formed, the urine is transported automatically through the renal pelvis and ureter on each side, to the bladder. The bladder is emptied through the urethra and this mechanism is under voluntary control. Owing to the long course of the ureter on the posterior abdominal wall and to the close association of the ureters and the bladder with other organs in the pelvis, many tumours and inflammatory diseases outside the urinary tract itself may interfere with the proper conduction of urine. In addition, growths may occur within the kidney or in any part of the urinary tract, and these in turn may obstruct the outflow of urine.

The urinary tract may be injured at any level by accident, in such injuries as fractured pelvis, or in the course of abdominal and pelvic operations. Urine will then leak onto the surface of the body or into the tissues surrounding the tract (**extravasation**).

The urine is of course maintained at body temperature and forms an excellent 'soil' in which germs will thrive. Acute or chronic infection may complicate any other disease of the urinary tract, or may arise for no apparent reason and lead to severe renal destruction.

Stones sometimes form in the urinary tract and it is not clear why this happens. Stagnation of the urine from prolonged partial obstruction and the presence of infection often lead to stone formation. Once a stone has formed it produces pain, probably obstruction to the outflow of urine from the kidney or bladder, and renders the tract liable to further infection, and recurrence of stone.

Table 48 indicates some common causes of urinary retention at various levels.

Table 48   Retention of urine

Site of obstruction	Cause	Result
Kidney	Single calyx by stone	Hydrocalyx
	Pelvi-ureteric junction by stone, adhesions or abnormal renal artery	Hydronephrosis
Ureter	Stone	
	Injury from operation on lower abdominal organs	Hydronephrosis and Megaureter
	Growth in bladder blocking ureteric orifices	(hydroureter)
Bladder	Paralysis (spinal cord disease or injury)	Bilateral hydronephrosis;
	Carcinoma	Megaureter;
	Congenital bladder neck obstruction	Diverticula of bladder
Urethra	Congenital valves	
	Prostatic enlargement senile (benign) or carcinoma	Bilateral hydronephrosis and Megaureter
	Stricture	Diverticula of bladder
	Calculus (impacted during passage from bladder)	

Principles of surgery and nursing

In disorders of the urinary tract, the surgeon is concerned with several major principles.

(a) To ensure complete freedom of evacuation of urine from every part of the urinary tract.

(b) To restore if necessary, and to maintain at the highest possible level, the chemical functions of the kidney.

(c) To protect the urinary tract and kidney from infection or to eliminate infection if it is already present.

(d) To prevent or cure the escape of urine from any abnormal sites—that is from urinary fistula.

(e) To undertake complete removal of any growth arising in the urinary tract or involving it by spread from some other organ such as the rectum or uterus.

The physiological function of the kidney is reduced by interference with its blood supply, by infection, or by back-pressure from obstruction lower down in the urinary tract.

The urinary tract is a muscular tube partly under a very delicately balanced nervous control. This nervous mechanism is easily disturbed by injury or inflammation, and after operation full recovery may be delayed for several weeks. This applies particularly after operations on the bladder and prostate.

After operation, provided the normal way out for urine exists below the point of injury, nature closes up the surgical opening with remarkable rapidity. In the interval between such injury or operation and complete healing, care has to be taken to make sure that any urine leaking from the kidney, ureter or bladder, escapes from the operation wound and does not ooze into other tissues which it will poison. Consequently all operation sites, when the urinary tract has been opened, are 'drained'. The observation and care of the drainage tube is one of the most important duties in nursing urinary cases.

Urinary tract disorders may arise in the course of treatment of any other disease, medical or surgical. The nurse therefore needs to be familiar with the significance of symptoms which are related to micturition or to the function of the kidneys.

The **general symptoms** of urinary tract disorders are either those associated with failure of the kidneys or those associated with infection.

Uraemia—the clinical condition which results from renal failure—may come on very insidiously and be present in a chronic state showing itself as lethargy, headache, loss of appetite, a dirty tongue and constipation. Anaemia is another marked feature of chronic renal failure. With rapid onset, the patient may become suddenly confused, cease to take any interest in his surroundings and become unconscious with irregular 'Cheyne-Stokes' breathing.

Acute infection in the urinary tract is almost always accompanied by a sudden rise in temperature, perhaps up to 40 °C (103° or 104 °F), frequently with rigors.

The more **local symptoms** are referred to the voiding of urine. There may be an increased frequency of micturition, and if this symptom is present, the nurse must take great care to find out if the patient is passing small quantities of urine frequently or if, on the other hand, he is having to empty the bladder frequently owing to the formation of larger quantities of urine. When the outlet of the bladder is partially obstructed, urine may leak past the obstruction owing to the high pressure within the over-distended bladder. The 'overflow' may give adequate warning to allow the patient to avoid incontinence, but if obstruction continues he becomes quite unable to control the flow of urine. He may be able to express a few drops only with great straining. This condition is known as 'overflow incontinence' and has to be distinguished from true incontinence where urine is trickling out of the 'empty' bladder all the time, without any ability on the part of the patient to interrupt the flow.

Pain on micturition is usually due to inflammation of the urethra, and the patient may suffer from 'urgency' or precipitancy—that is the inability to wait until it is convenient to pass urine because the inflamed urethra is oversensitive. Especially in children, this symptom of urgency is often interpreted as incontinence.

'**Anuria**' means that urine is not being formed, while '**retention**' means that the urine is being held up in the urinary tract. The sudden release of retention pressure may produce anuria, or unrelieved retention will so damage the kidneys that anuria follows from back-pressure of the renal cells. **Oliguria** is a reduction in quantity of urine produced and may herald the onset of anuria.

Occasionally, **haematuria,** the passage of blood with the urine, is the only symptom of which the patient may complain. It may come from the kidney or from any part of the urinary tract and must never be ignored (page 679). After operations on the urinary tract, blood is almost always present in the urine for several days. If blood accumulates in the urinary tract it may clot, and the passage of a clot from the kidney down the ureter may produce violent colicky pain, like that produced by the passage of a stone.

The formation of blood clot in the bladder makes the bladder feel full, but the clot obstructs the outlet and the conditioning of 'clot retention' occurs. The patient has an urgent and distressing desire to pass water and the resultant straining makes the bleeding worse. Clot retention has to be dealt with as a serious emergency by washing out the bladder through a catheter. If this is unsuccessful the patient may need a general anaesthetic to allow the passage of a large diameter 'evacuator tube' into the bladder (Fig. 35.1). This apparatus has a rubber bulb attached to it and the bulb, reservoir and urethral tube are filled with sterile water. The bulb is squeezed and released alternately so that the water swirls to and fro into the bladder. Clots which come out sink into the reservoir and are thus prevented from returning to the bladder. Bleeding from small vessels such as those in a papilloma rarely produces clots owing to dilution with urine and the fact that urine contains an active fibrinolytic enzyme **urokinase**: this increases the tendency for 'minor' bleeding to continue.

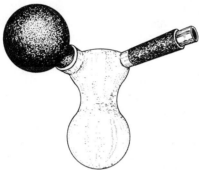

Fig. 35.1   Bladder evacuator (Ellik type). The outlet tube is attached to the cystoscope or special flushing cannula after the apparatus has been completely filled with sterile water. Repeated squeezing of the bulb flushes the bladder and any solid particles sink to the bottom of the glass bulb.

If clots have remained in the bladder for several days without dissolving they become 'rubbery' and a solution of the protein digesting enzyme trypsin (Trypure Novo), or plasmin with another enzyme (Elase) is infused into the bladder, allowed to remain for 2 hours and then washed out. This may be repeated daily.

Haemorrhage is a bugbear of urological operations and the management of the haemorrhage when it occurs is a major problem of nursing. Whatever happens urine must not be allowed to accumulate in the bladder: a catheter must never be clipped or spigoted during the interval between the end of operation and attachment of drainage tubes in the ward: a pad of sterile wool should be placed round the open end to absorb the efflux. Repeated manipulation and change of catheters increases the risk of infection. The steady loss of blood makes the patient anaemic and restless and the subsequent blood transfusion adds to the anxieties of both patient and nurse. Methods used to prevent and to treat clot retention after operation are described later (page 652).

Pain in urinary tract disorders

Pain in urinary tract disorders is sometimes the only symptom. The exact nature and location of pain form the basis of a correct diagnosis. Following operations on the urinary tract, patients frequently experience considerable pain of various types and the nurse must learn to assess from the patient's description what may be the origin of the pain.

Kidney pain arises for three quite distinct reasons. First the kidney may be inflamed from infection or injury, when the pain resembles that of inflammation elsewhere—there is a dull aching pain in the loin on one or both sides. This pain is not relieved when the patient lies down, and is of course frequently accompanied by fever.

Second, there is the pain of renal distension. When there is obstruction to the outflow of urine from the bladder or from a single ureter, or from the pelvis of the kidney into the ureter, the renal pelvis becomes distended. This stretching produces a dull aching pain in the loin rather similar to that of inflammation, but it may be relieved when the patient lies down and it may vary greatly from time to time as urine escapes from the pelvis. If infection supervenes upon the stasis and retention, the pain will become constant and fever will occur. The distension pain follows colic, the third type of pain, if a stone or clot has become impacted in the ureter.

Third, there is the pain of renal colic, or urinary colic. This is the pain of spasm which occurs in any tubular muscular organ which is irritated. The pain is violent, sometimes added to a dull aching 'background' pain of distension or inflammation. The forceful contraction of the muscle of the renal pelvis and ureter provoked by the presence of a stone or the passage of a blood clot comes on in waves, is not relieved in any way by a change in the position of the patient, and is frequently described as travelling round from the loin into the lower abdomen and then into the groin. In the male, pain from the ureter is described as shooting down into the testis and is sometimes misinterpreted by a patient as a sign of testicular inflammation. Because of its intensity, the pain of renal spasm frequently produces reflex vomiting. It is accompanied by shock of varying degree and the temperature is rarely raised. Morphine and atropine (which relieves spasm in the intestinal and urinary tracts) are usually given by injection as soon as it is certain that the pain is really coming from the kidney and is not an early warning of peritonitis. Pethidine is usually very effective in this type of pain, but may precipitate acute retention of urine especially in a patient who has some degree of prostatic enlargement.

Bladder pain is of two types. First there is the pain of distension, which may be accompanied by an urgent but unsuccessful desire to pass water: or there may merely be the discomfort of distension and yet no real desire to empty the bladder. The other type of bladder pain is that which arises from inflammation and is usually accompanied by frequency. It is a 'dull' boring pain which the patient describes as being deep down behind the pubic bone.

'Strangury' means the urgent, intense and yet ineffective desire to void urine when there is in fact no appreciable quantity of urine in the bladder. Injury to the bladder or to the urethra, cystitis, stone or clot all produce strangury.

Pain coming from the bladder outlet (bladder neck), rather than from the whole body of the bladder, is frequently referred to the tip of the urethra. The presence of a suprapubic catheter in the bladder produces the 'bladder outlet' type of pain indicating that the tube is too far in and is pressing on the base of the bladder.

Urethral pain is experienced during the passage of micturition and is often intense: it passes off very soon after micturition is complete. Urethral pain produces a fear of micturition and consciously or unconsciously may lead to retention especially in children.

Extravasation of urine

If during an operation on the urinary tract the kidney, ureter or bladder has been opened at any point, urine is almost certain to leak out for a short time afterwards. A drainage tube will be placed down to the site of incision or injury, but if for any reason this way of escape becomes blocked, urine will seep into the loose tissues round about and will produce the aching pain of inflammation. This condition is known as **'extravasation of urine'** and may involve the whole of the anterior abdominal wall. It may occur also after injury to the bladder. It may arise from injury to the urethra by the passage of sounds or endoscopic instruments. The pain is severe, continuous and distressing, and the skin over the area is tender and bright red.

Urinary tract investigation

Many of the investigation procedures are undertaken in the hospital out-patient department.

Patients whose symptoms suggest that there is some disorder of the urinary tract, invariably undergo a complete series of investigations which seek to determine the following information:

(a) Whether the kidneys are performing their function satisfactorily in controlling the body's chemistry and water balance.

(b) Whether there are in fact two kidneys present and if they are of normal shape and form.

(c) Whether the muscular parts of the urinary tract—the ureter, the bladder and the urethra—are performing their normal functions, and are normal in shape and size. (There are many congenital abnormalities of the urinary tract.)

(d) Whether there is any abnormality in the urinary tract such as stone, growth or infection.

Much information can be obtained from the careful nursing observation of the patient, examination of the urine and measurement of its quantity. The surgeon is absolutely dependent upon conscientious and painstaking nursing for the collection of much of his information. Extensive chemical tests and investigations are carried out in the pathological laboratory and these involve the collection of blood samples and urine specimens at set times. The purpose of acquiring all this information is to confirm the diagnosis already made from the history and the examination of the patient, or to make a more exact diagnosis. In addition, the surgeon discovers how badly affected the urinary tract may be and what complications may be likely to arise from any operation which he plans.

Sometimes patients on arrival in hospital for operations on the urinary tract are already in a very poor state of health and weeks may have to be spent improving their general condition and carrying out the necessary investigations. These patients are apt to become restless, and while not minimising the seriousness of any disease which may be present, the nurse must take care not to alarm the patient in her explanation of the necessity for these prolonged investigations and treatment. Surgical disorder of the urinary tract frequently involves more than one operation and anaesthetic, so that the patient is in hospital for a considerable time. The additional unpleasantness of urinary disorders, and perhaps the leakage of urine through drainage tubes, is a source of embarrassment and discouragement which sometimes produce great despondency.

All patients have their urine examined at the initial out-patient consultation or on admission to the hospital ward. The nurse is expected to examine the urine herself and perhaps the most important test is that of 'naked-eye' inspection. The routine specimen must never be thrown away until the doctor concerned has had an opportunity of seeing it. Normal urine is pale yellow and crystal clear, but from a woman patient it is frequently contaminated with dust and fluff from the receptacle into which the urine has been passed. Urine specimens collected during menstruation other than by catheter are quite useless for examination. The routine specimen must be tested chemically for the presence of albumin and sugar. Its specific gravity must be taken with a hydrometer and its acid-alkali reaction determined by special test paper.

In most cases in a general ward it is not necessary to test every specimen of urine that is passed, but in cases of urinary tract disorder, especially after operation, every specimen without exception must be measured and a sample of it placed in a clear urine glass for inspection for the first 48 hours after operation; once each day subsequently, a specimen must be set aside for inspection. It is only by the examination of successive specimens that the surgeon can obtain adequate information about the progress of healing. The urine specimen must be labelled clearly with the name of the patient and the time at which it was passed, together with the date. It is customary in many hospitals for the consultant in charge of a ward to conduct a full ward round at certain specified times. On such occasions the last urine specimen to be passed must be available at the patient's bedside, or at any rate close by for inspection. The clinician must *see* the specimen. Someone else's description or a simple test report does not give the information which can be obtained by a careful visual inspection.

The hurried emptying of bedpans and urinals must not be allowed to stop the nurse from looking at every specimen of urine, and taking a sample of it if anything untoward is noticed.

Collection of specimens. An 'ordinary' specimen of urine is one collected without any particular aseptic precautions. It is adequate for naked-eye inspection, acidity, and simple tests for albumin, sugar and acetone. It is useless for bacteriology. Contamination with organisms occurs during the collection of such a specimen, and delay in examination which occurs if it is posted to a laboratory or left standing overnight, may well render the chemical tests invalid.

A 'mid-stream' or 'clean catch' specimen may be obtained from both male and female patients without difficulty and such a specimen is usually satisfactory for all laboratory tests. In the male, the patient retracts the foreskin, washes the glans penis with soap and water, and passes a small quantity of urine into a glass jar or urinal. He then interrupts the stream and without touching the inside of the bottlemouth he passes the rest of the specimen into a sterile container. Some laboratories prefer the whole specimen thus collected to be sent for examination; others provide bijou bottles which only contain enough urine for bacteriological examination. The container must be immediately closed with a sterile stopper: cotton wool should not be used to plug the mouth of a specimen container.

The collection of a 'mid-stream' specimen for a female patient is more difficult, but avoids the inconvenience, discomfort, and delay of catheterisation. The vulva is cleansed with soap and water or Savlon, and the labia separated with a dry gauze swab held on each side. The first small quantity, perhaps 10 ml, is passed into the bed pan: this dislodges any mucus or organisms which may be in the urethra. The stream is interrupted voluntarily and then sufficient urine for examination is collected into a wide-mouthed sterile glass jar. This method is infinitely preferable to repeated catheterisation, particularly in children, when specimens may be required at frequent intervals.

Specimens have to be obtained by catheter if the patient is unconscious or unable to co-operate, and sometimes from women patients who are confined to bed. If the specimen is wanted for bacteriology it must also be mid-stream. The first part is therefore rejected as it is contaminated by urethral contents deposited in the catheter eye as it is inserted. The nurse's attention is particularly directed to the advice given in Fig. 35.8 concerning catheterisation. A urine specimen can be collected from infant boys by strapping a test tube or adhesive bag over the penis. A bag over the perineum can be used for baby girls. If bacteriological investigation is needed catheterisation may be used but in babies supra-pubic aspiration of the bladder with a needle is safe and reliable.

Occasionally what is known as the 'three glass' specimen is asked for. Here the patient empties his bladder into three separate urine glasses. The first part of the specimen will contain any pus or debris from the urethra; the second part of the specimen will be ordinary urine from the bladder. He interrupts the flow and prostatic massage is then carried out. The final specimen of urine that is passed washes into the third container the secretions which have been expressed from the prostate into the urethra. This examination is carried out in cases of suspected prostatitis.

'The 24-hour specimen' is collected for certain chemical examinations when it is necessary for the laboratory to have the whole of the urinary output for 24 hours. Some pathologists prefer to have a complete 24-hour specimen when looking for the tubercle bacillus. The output for one day and night is allowed to stand in a large 2-litre container. Microscopic examination of the precipitate is more likely to yield a tubercle bacillus than the examination of an 'ordinary' specimen from one voiding. Pathologists will usually ask for a preservative such as toluol to be added to the container to prevent the growth of other organisms.

Naked-eye examination. Reference has already been made to the great importance attached to the initial inspection of the urine as soon as it has been passed. When the specimen has been placed in a conical glass container, the nurse should notice the presence of any precipitate or cloud. If the urine is absolutely clear, this finding is equally important. Cloudiness developing during the hours which follow the passage of the urine may be due to cooling or crystallisation, or may be due to the growth of organisms from exposure to air. The colour of the urine should be noted, and from the nurse's point of view it is not so much the initial inspection as the observation of succeeding specimens in cases of haematuria and jaundice that is important: this information is a vital clue in estimating the progress of the patient. Particularly is this true of increase or decrease in the amount of blood present in the urine of a patient who has had some operation on kidney or bladder. 'Smokey', mahogany or red urine suggests blood. Nitrofurantoin, ampicillin and certain other drugs make the urine a very dark yellow. Bile produces a more orange tint. The urine may be blue or green if methylene blue has been injected recently for some test.

Specific gravity. Provided the urine is not discoloured by blood or bile its colour is a very fair indication of the concentration. The specific gravity is tested as an essential part of the routine examination; it varies in ordinary individuals from 1010 to 1025. If the specific gravity falls to the region of 1005, either the kidneys are damaged or the patient is receiving too much fluid. If, on the other hand, after operation the specific gravity is over 1020 it is a good indication that the patient is not receiving sufficient fluid.

The special weighted glass float—**the hydrometer**—is placed in the conical glass of urine and a reading taken at a point on the scale where the stem breaks the surface of the urine. If there is not sufficient urine to float the hydrometer then the test must be carried out in a wide-mouthed test-tube.

If the specific gravity is not estimated until the urine is cooled and crystals have settled out into the bottom of the jar, the reading is completely inaccurate.

Acidity. The degree of acidity of the urine is described as its 'pH' and it ranges from 5 to 8·5. Neutral is pH 7 and higher numbers are alkali. The common, but rather unsatisfactory, method of estimating the degree of acidity of the urine is by the use of red and blue litmus papers. A piece of *each* must be placed in the specimen, and a change from red to blue indicates that the urine is alkaline; blue to red indicates that the urine is acid. One usually finds that the little books of litmus paper have been left lying about for a considerable time and both the red and blue books have become rather an unsatisfactory purple. The use of wide range indicator papers[1] (supplied by British Drug Houses Limited) makes the estimation far more valuable. These little strips of yellow paper change to red if the acidity is marked and to varying shade of green with alkaline urine. Similar combined test strips have largely replaced other chemical tests (see below). The exact pH is determined by comparing the colour of the paper with the colour chart on the book.

Chemical tests

The ward staff is called upon to undertake routine chemical tests of the urine of patients admitted for surgical operation. Initial examination for every patient must include a test for the presence of albumin (protein), sugar, bile and blood. Elaborate tests are not necessary and in the majority of hospitals special strips of prepared paper are used for the individual tests. These are supplied in small bottles; they must be kept dry and free from contamination. In addition to strips for testing for individual chemicals there is a combined strip, the Bili-labstix which tests in a few seconds for the presence of blood, protein, glucose, bile and the pH: these are expensive but extremely useful in busy clinics. Where a more accurate assessment of the amount of abnormal chemical present in the urine is required these strips are not of very great value. Certain quick tests are carried out using special tablets.

Albumin. The standard test for protein in the urine depends on the coagulation of the albumin by heat like the boiling of an egg. (If a cloud appears when the urine is heated it may be due to the presence of phosphates which will disappear if acetic acid is added.)

'Strip' test is by **Albustix,** giving a colour range from yellow to green depending on the amount of albumin present. If blood is present the protein test will of course be positive but in inflammatory conditions of the kidney and lower urinary tract albumin may be present without blood.

Sugar. The established ward test for sugar in the urine is by the use of Benedict's solution of copper sulphate, but this is rarely used now.

'Strip' test is by **Clinistix,** but a more sensitive test using **Clinitest** reagent tablets is sometimes used. Clinitest is positive in galactosaemia, but Clinistix is negative. (Galactosaemia is a congenital error of milk-sugar metabolism.)

From the nurse's point of view the presence of sugar in the urine must be regarded as indicating diabetes, although there are certain conditions in which the kidneys allow the excretion of sugar without there being any disease present (**renal glycosuria**).

[1] This wide range indicator paper is also of value in determining the pH of other body fluids such as the discharge from an abdominal sinus: the presence of a strongly acid secretion will indicate a leak of gastric juice.

Acetone (ketone) is a breakdown product of fat and occurs if the body is utilising its fat reserves without sufficient carbohydrate. High fever, cachexia, and diabetes lead to the passage of acetone in the urine. The finding really only indicates the presence of acidosis (ketosis) which will have been suspected from the clinical examination of the patient. In severe fevers, especially in children, the smell of acetone will be detected in the patient's breath. The appropriate quick test is with **Acetest** tablets or **Ketostix** strips.

(Phenistix strips are used to detect phenylketonuria, a congenital metabolic disorder leading to mental deficiency if undiagnosed.)

Bile. Bilirubin, a by-product of red cell breakdown only appears in urine after it has passed through the liver. In jaundice due to obstruction, bilirubin is found in urine: in haemolytic jaundice where the liver is normal, no bile escapes into the urine. Bilirubin is detected by Ictostix test paper or the corresponding section of the combine Bili-labstix.

Blood. Blood is detected in the urine by

(a) an obvious red colour perhaps even with tiny clots,
(b) the finding of red blood cells when the specimen is examined microscopically.

Between these two extremes the presence of blood can only be suspected from a positive albumin test in a urine which is hazy. The standard chemical test for blood in the urine is really a test for blood pigment.

A red blood-coloured urine may be passed by patients, usually children, who have been eating beetroot, or sweets containing red dyes. Occasionally, dissolved haemoglobin is present without there being any red blood cells. This can only be determined in the laboratory.

Occultest tablets are used to detect blood in the urine and **Hematest** strips for blood in the faeces.

Urinary chloride. Complete absence of chlorides in the urine occurs in cases of severe vomiting and alkalosis. The nurse may be called upon to perform a simple test to determine whether chloride is present in the urine, or whether it has returned as a result of intravenous infusion during the treatment of alkalosis. Special reagents are needed and detailed instructions will be available where the test is to be carried out.

A word is necessary concerning the spirit lamp which is used for urine testing. So often these little items are neglected in the maintenance of ward equipment. The wick must be trimmed regularly and must reach to the bottom of the spirit container. Methylated[1] spirit should be used in these lamps. If the lamp is not available or has been broken, a tablet of the urinary antiseptic **hexamine** may be placed on a tin lid and lighted with a match. It will burn long enough for a urine sample to be tested for albumin and sugar. When doing district nursing, the nurse is well advised to carry a packet of such tablets, for the unfortunate emergency which will arise sooner or later, when the lamp has been broken or upset.

Residual urine

This term is used to indicate the amount of urine left in the bladder after normal micturition. In the healthy individual there should of course be no residual urine. However, many disorders of the urinary tract are associated with obstruction to the outlet of the bladder in some form or another and it is extremely common to find several ounces of urine remaining in the bladder after the act of micturition has been completed to the best of the patient's ability. The extreme form of this 'incomplete retention' is that in which the bladder is distended to hold probably 1000 ml while the patient is perhaps passing only

[1] Industrial methylated spirit (purple) is sometimes unsatisfactory in a lamp; a better flame is obtained by using pure SVM (Spiritus vini methylatus). Surgical spirit is no use as it contains castor oil and other ingredients.

a few millimetres every few minutes (page 634). The main clinical conditions in which there is residual urine are:

(a) Congenital conditions such as urethral valves or stenosis of the bladder outlet,
(b) Enlargement of the prostate gland occuring in elderly men, due to hyperplasia or carcinoma,
(c) Certain conditions occurring in women when the muscles forming the pelvic floor have been damaged during child-birth (page 738).
(d) Disorders of the central nervous system, such as injury or congenital defect in the spinal cord (spina bifida), spinal tumour, disseminated sclerosis or tabes dorsalis.
(e) Interference with the nerve supply to the bladder following severe operation in the pelvis such as abdomino-perineal excision of the rectum for cancer.

The amount of residual urine may be measured by passing a catheter immediately after the patient has 'emptied' his bladder. During out-patient investigations when cystoscopy is to be performed under local anaesthesia, the patient empties his bladder immediately before lying on the examination couch. The surgeon then collects the residual urine which comes through the cystoscope. It is usual for this estimation of residual urine to be determined in the ward as one of the earliest tests in urinary cases. The amount of urine remaining in the bladder after micturition can be estimated very approximately by x-rays at the end of the excretion pyelography (page 268).

Surgical operations to relieve the obstruction at the outlet of the bladder are followed by repeated estimations of the residual urine to determine the degree of success of the operation.

Following operations such as abdomino-perineal excision of the rectum or repairs of the perineum and vaginal walls it is usual for a catheter to be left in place for several days because retention is extremely common if this is not done. The catheter is clamped for periods of 2 hours at a time to retain the rhythm of bladder distension and evacuation. If the patient is unable to pass urine naturally when the catheter is removed, then catheterisation has to be repeated until normal bladder control returns. Voluntary micturition, however, usually returns gradually so that the amount of residual urine is perhaps considerable to start with, the bladder taking 2 or 3 weeks to regain normal tone and the power to expel the whole of its contents.

In some cases of urinary obstruction the ureters are also grossly dilated, and when the patient attempts to empty his bladder, urine passes up into the big ureters and kidneys. The bladder also sometimes develops diverticula (Fig. 35.2) or pouches into which urine passes when the bladder itself contracts. In such cases, if a catheter is passed at the end of micturition the urine which flows back into the bladder from the dilated ureters or from a diverticulum will then be drawn off and constitutes 'residual urine'. The presence of more than 60 ml of residual urine is regarded as important since the stagnation frequently leads to infection and stone formation.

When a catheter is passed to measure residual urine, part of the specimen should always be sent to the laboratory for bacteriological examination, and it constitutes the 'catheter specimen' collected under aseptic conditions. If it is known or suspected that there is residual urine, it is unnecessary to collect midstream specimens for laboratory investigation, or to catheterise the patient on separate occasions in order to obtain this clean specimen. The simple precaution of getting the patient to empty the bladder as completely as possible before taking the specimen will enable 'both birds to be killed with one stone'. Even though there is virtually no 'residual' urine, it is extremely unlikely that the amount which comes through the catheter will be insufficient for bacteriological examination: sufficient will have come into the bladder from the kidneys during the few minutes preparation following micturition. 10 ml is quite enough for microscopic examination and the culture of organisms.

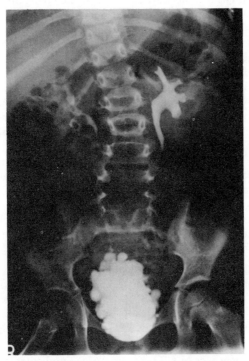

Fig. 35.2 X-ray photograph of the bladder which has been filled with Hypaque through a catheter. There are many pockets (diverticula) in the wall of the bladder and there has been reflux of dye to both kidneys.

Urine concentration and dilution test. The purpose of this test is to determine, by limiting the patient's fluid intake, to what extent the kidney is able to concentrate urine. It is a simple useful test when more sophisticated methods are not available.

The test commences at 8 a.m. and during the normal day period of 12 hours the patient is only given solid food. There must be no drink of any kind, nor soup. All the urine specimens up to 8 p.m. are discarded and all urine to 8 a.m. on the following morning is saved. Each specimen is kept separate and the specific gravity measured with the hydrometer. If the kidney function is normal the specific gravity should rise to between 1026 and 1030. Concentration with a specific gravity below 1020 indicates severe impairment of renal function.

The patient is then encouraged to drink large quantities (at least 3 litres in an adult in the 12-hour period) and the specific gravity of succeeding specimens again measured. The reading should drop to 1010 or lower.

The test is unnecessary if the patient at any time since admission has passed urine with a specific gravity of over 1020. Most urological cases are, however, given increased fluid intake from the time of admission, and ordinary urine specimens consequently give a false idea of the patient's renal function as the specific gravity is low on this account.

Blood urea. In normal health there are between 20 and 40 mg of urea in every 100 ml of blood. The kidneys have an enormous reserve upon which to call if they are damaged by disease, so that it is only in advanced cases of renal disease that the blood urea becomes raised. The blood-urea test is performed in the pathological laboratory and blood samples may have to be collected by the nurse.

If vomiting occurs from any cause, for instance from peritonitis or paralytic ileus, the blood chemistry is so disturbed that, although the kidneys themselves may not have been damaged, uraemia may arise. This blood test is therefore a very common one in cases of severe illness. If the blood urea should rise above 200 mg per cent the patient may become unconscious with uraemic coma: children tolerate a higher level of blood urea without showing signs of coma.

Alkali reserve test. The acid/base balance of the body is maintained by the lungs and the kidneys. Hypercapnia leads to respiratory acidosis (page 129) and reduction in renal function may lead to metabolic acidosis (page 108). The alkali reserve test indicates how much spare chemical corrective capacity is left. It is used in conjunction with other electrolyte estimations. The exact chemical composition of all fluid which is given during the treatment of shock or dehydration is always important but it is even more important if there has been any renal damage (page 133).

The blood for the alkali reserve test must be kept from exposure to air and it is therefore collected in a syringe which will not allow air to leak into the barrel on withdrawal of the piston when the blood is taken from the vein. The specimen is immediately injected into the test tube which contains 2·5 cm of sterile liquid paraffin, the needle being plunged through the paraffin so that the blood does not have any contact with the air. This method of collection is vital to the test, as exposure to the air alters the chemical composition of the blood.

Creatinine and urea clearance test. These are more complicated methods of estimating the function of the kidneys. Specimens of blood and urine are taken at specified times and the pathological laboratory will always provide the necessary instructions. It has only to be emphasised that these instructions must be carried out implicitly with regard to the collection of urine specimens at the correct times.

Dye excretion. Methylene blue (1 ml of 5 per cent solution) or indigo carmine (10 ml of 0·4 per cent solution) is injected slowly into a vein, using a fine hypodermic needle. Care has to be taken in loading the syringe with concentrated dye as it makes a terrible mess if it is spilled. The blue dye is excreted in the kidneys within five or ten minutes of the injection, and if a cytoscope is in place in the bladder the surgeon will see a blue jet of urine come from each ureteric orifice. This gives him some idea of the functional integrity of each kidney. Sometimes there is a delay of excretion, particularly if the patient has been anaesthetised, and the urine may be deeply stained blue or green for 24 hours following injection. In the past, methylene blue has been sold in pill form as a supposed remedy for kidney disease: the blue urine deceived the patient into thinking that the pills were doing good, and 'getting rid of poison'.

Radiology

The x-ray examination of the urinary tract is comprehensive and essential in all but very minor disorders (Chapter 15). Stones which contain calcium salts are shown up on plain films and in many cases the outline of the kidney can also be seen. One of the main problems in x-ray examination is the presence of gas in the intestine, and various measures are adopted to reduce the amount of gas present when the x-ray examination is made.

With children it is almost impossible to have them free from gas, particularly if for some reason, such as paraplegia, the child has been confined to bed for a long time. Instructions for the preparation of the patient are given on page 268.

After the preliminary plain films have been taken an iodine-containing compound is injected intravenously (Table 49). Some patients are sensitive to this drug and on extremely rare occasions severe reactions have occurred and death has followed.

Before the intravenous injection is given, one or two drops of the solution may be injected (with a 1-ml syringe and a fine needle) under the skin: if after 5 minutes there is no wheal it is assumed that the patient is not sensitive to the drug. The rest of the solution is given slowly into a vein. Before the 20-ml syringe is loaded, the ampoule of contrast medium should be warmed by leaving it to stand in a bowl of warm water at 37 °C (100 °F).

Because of the possibility of this untoward sensitivity reaction,[1] an injection of adrenaline hydrochloride must be available, and a 2-ml syringe with hypodermic needle attached. If the adrenaline is needed, it is needed in a hurry, and there is no time to go searching for an ampoule in a far away cupboard. 100 mg of hydrocortisone for injection must also be available.

After the dye injection, x-ray photographs are taken at varying times, occasionally up to two hours. The dye is rapidly excreted by the kidneys and casts shadows which are opaque to the x-rays. Fig. 35.3 shows an excretion pyelogram in which one kidney is normal and one is dilated (hydronephrosis). As the dye passes down the ureters into the bladder the rest of the urinary tract is outlined and any dilatations or defects are shown up.

Excretion urography performed in this way is variously described—intravenous pyelogram, excretion pyelogram or urogram. In most hospitals the investigation becomes known colloquially as the 'IVP'.

Cystogram

Excretion urography may have outlined the bladder in sufficient detail already but certain other information is obtained by injecting a more dilute solution of the dye through a catheter so as to distend the bladder. 10% solution of diodone is used for this purpose. If there is a tumour in the bladder (as for instance when the prostate bulges upwards) the outline of the tumour will be shown as a defect in filling of the bladder. Sufficient dye is introduced to distend the bladder just to the point of discomfort, and the patient

[1] Owing to the unreliability of any single sensitivity test, many clinics have abandoned the tests. The likelihood of reaction is very remote and it may occur even when the tests have not revealed sensitivity.

Table 49.   Radio-opaque dyes used in urography

Diodine (Pyelosil)
  35%   50%   70%
Hypaque (diatrizoate) 25% 45%   ⎱   25% used for retrograde pyelography; dilute
  65% 85%   ⎰   to 10% for cystoscopy, or use diodine which
Diaginol (acetrizoate) 25% 30% 50% is cheaper; up to 300 ml may be needed.
  70%
Conray 280 (meglumine iothalamate injection)
Retro-Conray (for retrograde pyelography) 35%

Note: Meglumine iothalamate solutions are less likely to produce adverse reactions.

is encouraged to resist all tendency to void urine. The x-ray table is tilted so that the head is lower than the pelvis. Dye sometimes runs backwards up the ureters and outlines the kidneys completely. Fig. 35.2 shows a cystogram performed in this way, on a child with congenital obstruction of the outlet of the bladder.

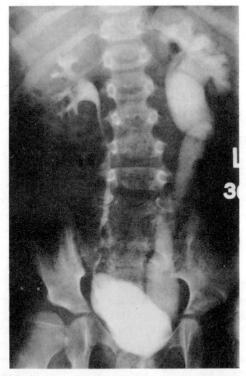

Fig. 35.3   Excretion pyelogram. Film taken 30 minutes after injection of diodone. The right kidney and ureter are normal; the left side shows gross dilatation of the whole urinary tract (hydronephrosis and hydro-ureter).

The urethra is outlined by radio-opaque dye either by taking an x-ray photograph as the dye is being injected through the urethra with a small glass syringe, or by taking a 'snapshot' x-ray as the patient is passing urine into a dish, the bladder having been previously filled with 10 per cent diodone through a catheter.

Where image-intensifier x-ray equipment is available, a visual examination of the voiding is made by the radiologist and recorded with video tape so that it can be 'played back' and studied.

Retrograde pyelography

This is a method of outlining the kidneys on the x-ray film by injecting dye into the pelvis of the kidney through a fine ureteric catheter passed through the cystoscope (page 347).

The solution used for retrograde pyelography is either diodone 10 per cent or iodoxyl 10 per cent. There is a risk of producing pyelitis by this operation, and it is often performed under general anaesthesia.

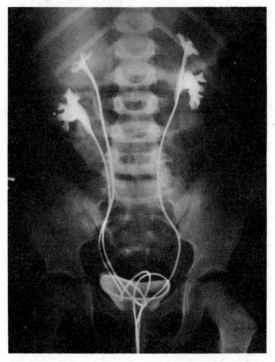

Fig. 35.4 Retrograde pyelogram. Ureteric catheters have been passed by means of a cystoscope. The ureter on the right is double and a catheter has been inserted into each portion of the double right kidney. Ten per cent diodone has been injected to outline the kidneys.

Renal arteriography (Fig. 35.5)

A Seldinger catheter is passed into the femoral artery and threaded up the aorta to the region of the renal arteries, the stylet is removed and the springy tip of the catheter turns down as a crook. By withdrawing the catheter the tip is hooked into the renal artery and contrast medium injected. The vascular supply of the kidney is visualised: a narrow (arterio-sclerotic) artery may be responsible for hypertension. After removal of the catheter from the femoral artery, a haematoma may form unless pressure is maintained for a few minutes.

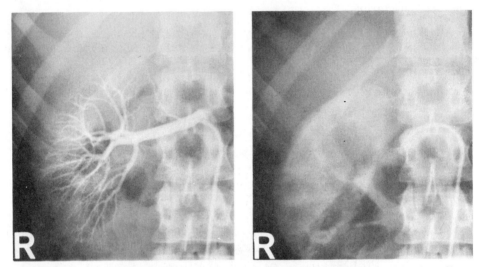

Fig. 35.5 Renal arteriogram. (*Left*) A gap in the arterial tree in the upper part. (*Right*) A later film outlining a cyst. If this had been a growth, it would have been full of arteries.

Ward records

In any general surgical ward there are always a certain number of urological cases. In a special department surgical ward, whether it is neuro-surgical, thoracic, traumatic or orthopaedic, there will always be a certain number of patients whose urinary output has to be watched and carefully recorded. In a special urological unit, the nursing is particularly heavy and in all these cases it is absolutely vital that the information should be accurate and complete.

One of the most essential features of a nurse's training is that she should early acquire the habit of recording her observations in such a way that they are readily available to other people and so that there can be no possible source of error.

Every patient admitted to the ward must have a routine ordinary specimen examined by the tests described on pages 640, 641. If the case is one of urological disorder, an ordinary specimen must be saved for inspection every day of the patient's stay in hospital unless instructions are given that this is no longer required. The results of the routine tests should be recorded on the patient's temperature chart.

All laboratory investigations are usually reported on special forms, and great care must be taken to mount these forms on the patient's notes in serial order so that the most recent one is uppermost.

In all cases of urological disorder, the amount of urine passed at every voiding must be measured and entered either in the ward books or preferably on a special chart of fluid balance (page 251). The time at which the urine is passed must also be noted so that there will be an accurate record of both frequency and output throughout the 24 hours. If the patient is incontinent and the urine is voided into the bed it is usual to guess the amount and record it as +, ++, or +++, though this is obviously a very crude method of estimating the amount which has been lost. Patients are not very co-operative at times, and when an attempt is being made to record their output they will slip out to the toilet and the specimen will be lost.

The normal patient produces more urine during the day than at night—that is more urine is secreted by the kidneys by day. The bladder during sleep is more tolerant of large quantities which accumulate within it. Sometimes, particularly in children, the state of affairs is reversed and the kidneys produce an excessive quantity of urine at night. This is one of the factors which lead to nocturnal incontinence in children and adults, and in the investigation of such cases the day/night urine volume ratio has to be determined by the nursing staff.

If the patient complains of pain on micturition, has difficulty in starting, or is incontinent, such facts must be noted, however trivial they may appear to the nurses at the time.

Blood-pressure recordings are frequently needed in these patients, especially if there has been any suggestion of renal failure. High blood pressure (hypertension) is sometimes the first evidence of renal disease so that repeated observations are necessary before and after operation. The gradual fall of blood pressure following the relief of urinary obstruction is perhaps the best daily indication of improvement.

Provided the nurse understands the underlying principles and the reasons for what may appear to her to be unnecessary tedious measurements, she will find the nursing of urinary cases to be interesting and rewarding and she will not make mistakes. It is because of the patience and skill required in nursing these difficult cases, coupled with the necessity of absolute routine with regard to tests and measurements, that there has been a tendency in recent years to develop special urological units.

Apparatus used in urology

Many of the instruments used in connection with surgery of the urinary tract are used for other purposes as well. Many nurses have great difficulty in understanding the principles of 'plumbing' in connection with the drainage of urine.

Urinary catheters

There are many varieties of urinary catheters with which the nurse needs to be familiar. Broadly speaking, they are divided into two groups, those for use through the urethra, and those for use through artificial openings made into the urinary tract at operation.

Urethral catheters. Many years ago catheters were made of silver or brass with metal plating and curved so as to make introduction through the male urethra more simple. Metal catheters are now practically never used.

Glass catheters are occasionally used for the female urethra, the advantage being that they are cheap, can be sterilised by boiling and are very easy to insert and are painless to the patient.

Flexible catheters were originally made of silk web with a gum compound but today almost all catheters are made of pure latex rubber or some form of plastic such as PVC. Silicone 'rubber' catheters are available: though more expensive they have a wider lumen for the same 'size' and there is no tissue reaction; urethritis is less likely and crusting with phosphate does not occur. A silicone Foley catheter may be left for 6 weeks without being changed. The majority of catheters are now supplied ready sterilised by gamma radiation in individual packs. Such catheters can if necessary be re-sterilised by boiling provided they are not squeezed while hot, but the practice of re-using catheters is unwise as they are very difficult to clean. Catheters in common use are illustrated in Fig. 35.6.

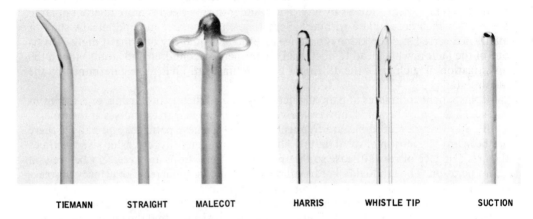

TIEMANN   STRAIGHT   MALECOT   HARRIS   WHISTLE TIP   SUCTION

Fig. 35.6 Catheters in common use. The straight catheter is also described as Nelaton's or Jaques'. The Malecot catheter may have 2 or 4 wings and requires a special stilette introducer to stretch the tip. It is a self-retaining catheter used for suprapubic drainage.

Nelaton's catheter—commonly referred to as Jaques'.[1] This is the most common form of catheter. It is straight and usually has one eye: sometimes there are two eyes and the end of the catheter is solid.

Whistle-tip catheter. This is also a straight rubber or plastic catheter in which the tip is bevelled and open, in addition to there being side eyes. This type is used mainly for post-operative drainage of the bladder following prostatectomy. If the open tip is not bevelled, the catheter is sometimes described as a 'Harris' catheter.

Pasteau's catheter—also known as Tiemann's. This rubber or plastic catheter has a moulded curve at the tip which is both solid and tapered. The shape and stiffness makes it easier to introduce through a male urethra which is obstructed by prostatic enlargement. It is perhaps the most useful catheter for general purposes.

[1] James Archibald Jacques was works manager of the india rubber manufacturing firm, William Warne & Co. He invented and patented the soft rubber catheter about 1885.

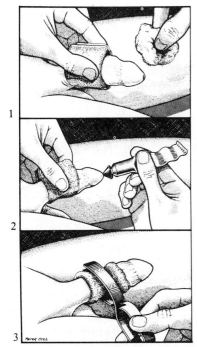
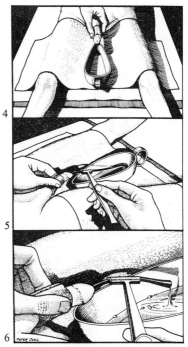

Fig. 35.7 Passing a male catheter. **1.** The penis is held in a gauze swab soaked in cetrimide/hibitane solution and the glans cleansed with the same solution. **2.** Local anaesthetic may be used supplied in single dose tubes with sterile nozzle which is held firmly in the meatus. **3.** A spring penile clamp is applied to retain the anaesthetic jelly or solution for 5 minutes. **4.** The sterile wrapping paper from the catheterising pack is placed across the legs. **5.** The catheter is introduced with a Nash catheter forceps which gives better control than ordinary dressing forceps. **6.** The catheter should slide easily through the urethra and the urine should flow when there is still approximately 10–15 cm of catheter outside.

Dowse's female self-retaining catheter. This type of catheter is straight, made of rubber and has its wall divided into four strips for a short distance from the tip. These 'strips' are moulded to form a soft bulge on the catheter. The catheter is introduced into the female urethra simply by inserting a silver probe through the catheter wall and pressing this into the inside of the tip which is pulled tight on the probe: it is simple and reliable.

Semi-rigid plastic catheters. These are made mainly for use in cases of urethral obstruction in the male, and are only slightly flexible. The principal types are straight with a solid tip with two or three eyes, coudée with a curved tip, bi-coudée with a double curve. There are several other varieties which are less important. The rigidity of these catheters prevents kinking if they are 'tied' into the urethra.

Foley's catheter. This is a straight rubber or polythene catheter with a thin rubber cuff or balloon near the tip behind the eye. This balloon, after introduction of the catheter into the bladder, is distended with sterile water injected through a thin tube incorporated in the wall of the catheter. Most catheters have a 'Luer' fitting plug for the balloon type,

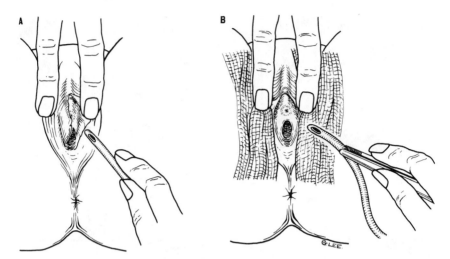

Fig. 35.8 Female catheterisation. After initial cleaning of the vulva with cetrimide/hibitane solution, a cotton-wool or gauze swab is placed on each labium to prevent the finger slipping and to make quite certain that the catheter is not contaminated during insertion. **A** shows the incorrect method with the nurses' fingers on the skin and the catheter held between the fingers. This incorrect method means that the nurse must 'scrub-up' and leave the patient exposed while she does so. **B** shows the correct method. 'Scrubbing-up' is not necessary. After separation of the labia which are held securely with swabs, the inner aspect of the vulva is cleansed with a small wool swab held by forceps. The catheter, in a sterile kidney dish, is then placed on the bed immediately beneath the vulva. The catheter is inserted with catheter or dressing forceps and is untouched by hand. If a Dowse's self-retaining catheter is used, it is stretched on a probe before insertion. The catheter must be lubricated with a *sterile* lubricant.

into which a standard 10–20 ml syringe is inserted. If the syringe is pushed too hard the valve will not operate. Some have a rubber bung through which a needle must be pushed for the injection of sterile water. Over-inflation of the balloon will compress the main catheter lumen and prevent drainage. The capacity of the balloon is marked on the connector end. In addition, a second thin tube is sometimes incorporated and this opens at the end of the catheter within the eye and is used for irrigating the bladder through the catheter (Fig. 35.9).

The Foley catheter is used for two distinct purposes. First with a small balloon holding 5 ml it is a simple form of self-retaining catheter, the balloon merely preventing its withdrawal. Second by using a large balloon with a capacity of 50–150 ml the catheter forms a plug in the cavity left after removal of the prostate. Its presence partly limits bleeding by pressure and prevents the accumulation of clots. There are therefore several types of Foley's catheter depending on the size of the balloon and the presence of an additional irrigating tube. The same principle has been adopted for holding within the bladder radioactive fluids in the treatment of growths of the bladder wall.

A Foley catheter must have its balloon tested before use and it may be necessary to squeeze the distended balloon to make it inflate evenly as a sphere when the catheter being tested is a new one, but this can only be done if the operator has a sterile swab to hold the balloon with, or is wearing gloves.

When the catheter is to be removed the balloon must be deflated: this may be done by cutting the inflation tube. If no water returns and the bag fails to deflate (this occurs sometimes) 2 ml of ether is injected. This vaporises in the bag and bursts it. The bladder is washed out before removing the catheter.

Petroleum lubricants should not be used on these ballooned catheters as the oil tends to rot the rubber: mucilage lubricant jelly should be used instead.

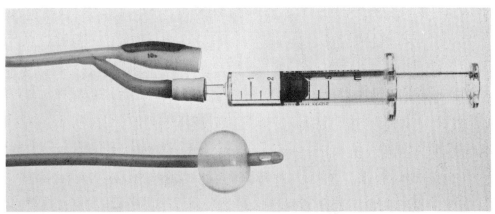

Fig. 35.9 Foley balloon self-retaining catheter. This is now the most commonly used of all catheters. It is made of non-irritant latex or plastic. After insertion the balloon is inflated with water injected through a non-return valve as illustrated. The catheter is supplied with a variety of balloon capacities. Being self-retaining no strapping has to be attached to the penis, thus avoiding pressure on the penis.

Gibbon's catheter. This is a plastic, transparent, semi-rigid catheter 150 cm long, usually supplied in sizes 10, 12 or 14 (Charrière) diameter. This catheter is passed into the bladder to a distance of approximately 25 cm; it curls up in the bladder and does not cause irritation in the urethra. A small plastic strap is sealed to the tube at approximately the right distance from the tip and this is used to attach the catheter to the penis. The remaining long end of the catheter is fitted to a drainage bottle at the bedside without the necessity for any further connectors or tubing. This type of catheter can be tolerated by the bladder and urethra for several weeks without causing inflammation. As the tube is translucent the flow and nature of urine can be observed clearly.

Suprapubic catheters. These are all made of rubber or plastic and have an expanded tip to prevent their accidental withdrawal. They are thus 'self-retaining'. There are various types which differ from one another in the form of the expanded tip. They may be made of red rubber or transparent latex which is less liable to kink but not so durable. Since suprapubic catheters are usually discarded after two weeks' use, this lasting property is immaterial.

For most conditions requiring a self-retaining catheter a Foley latex balloon catheter is used, partly because it is easy to insert and remove. The lumen is relatively small and there is a risk of the balloon deflating so that there is still the occasional need for the more robust type of catheter.

De Pezzer catheter. There is a conical bulb with side eyes and a solid tip.

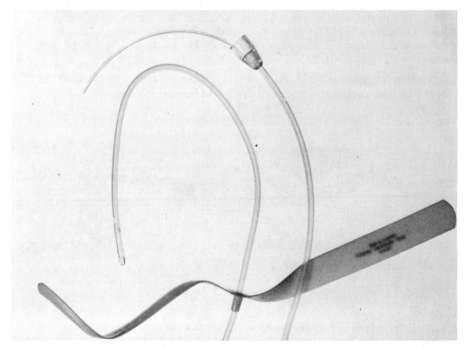

Fig. 35.10   Gibbon's catheter.

Malecot catheter. This is similar in principle but has two or four little rubber wings which prevent it being pulled out accidentally.

These two catheters are inserted by means of an introducer which is a straight metal rod pushed right down to the tip of the catheter to stretch the mushroom-head and thus reduce its diameter (Fig. 35.6). When the introducing stylet is withdrawn the catheter expands inside the bladder. More commonly the self-retaining catheter is put in the bladder before the wound is closed: an introducer is not then needed. Small sizes of this catheter are used in paediatric surgery both in the urinary and alimentary tract where a Foley balloon is too big (e.g. caecostomy in an infant).

Winsbury-White's catheter. This has a wide open circular end which is less likely to become blocked up by clots. A special introducer is needed unless the catheter is placed through an open wound in the bladder. There are two types of shaft to the Winsbury-White catheter, straight and right-angled.

Suprapubic catheters are connected to drainage tubing which leads the urine into a bedside bag.

Sometimes the self-retaining suprapubic catherers are inserted by means of a trocar and cannula (De Pezzer's, Fig. 35.12). This is stabbed into the distended bladder after the introduction of a little local anaesthetic into the abdominal wall, and the catheter or an introducer is passed down the cannula after the withdrawal of the trocar. The cannula is then slipped out of the wound and withdrawn over the shaft of the catheter. This method

of suprapubic drainage is occasionally necessary in an emergency. Other types of introducer are in common use. A Bardic Intracath intravenous cannula may be safely used to
relieve retention.

Catheter sizes

Much confusion arises over the number of catheters, or their 'gauge'. Three systems are
in common use, the English, the French Charrière and the French Beniqué. All three
systems of graduation are based on the outside diameter of the catheter shaft. The difference between the successive sizes varies in the different systems. In 1950 the British Standards Institution published some manufacturing standards to be adopted for flexible
urinary catheters. This system should be used uniformly in hospitals, although catheters
are not consistently marked with the Beniqué scale size (see later).

On the English gauge each size is half a millimetre in diameter greater than the size below. On the French Charrière gauge the increase for each size is one third of a millimetre
and on the Beniqué gauge it is one sixth of a millimetre. Thus a catheter of 5 mm outside
diameter on the Beniqué system will be 5×6, i.e. size 30, or 5×3 diameter, which is size
15 on the Charrière scale. Confusion arises in the English gauge as there is a size 00 and a
size 0. A catheter size 5 mm in diameter is therefore 5×2, that is the tenth size up the scale,
i.e. No. 8 E, because of the additional two sizes at the lower end of the English scale.

The Beniqué scale has been adopted as the international standard, which will make it
very much easier for nursing staff and surgeons to agree upon their requirements. Thus the

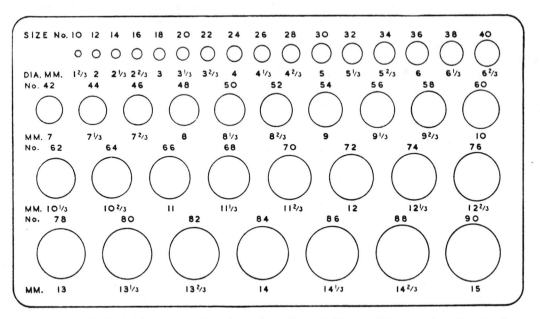

Fig. 35.11 Beniqué catheter gauge. Actual sizes (even sizes only illustrated; 1–8 and above 90 omitted).
(British Standards Institution, 1695–1950, *Catheters.*)

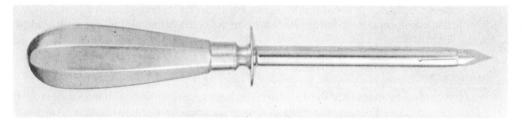

Fig. 35.12. DePezzer's trocar for suprapubic bladder drainage (2/3 size). A 1-cm incision is made half-way between pubis and umbilicus. The trocar and cannula is forced into the distended bladder. The trocar is withdrawn and a finger placed immediately on the opening to prevent a flood in the bed: a self-retaining catheter (De Pezzer or Malecot) is inserted through the cannula, and the latter then slipped out. A Foley catheter cannot be used as the inflation tube will not pass through the cannula. (Seward Surgical Instruments.)

standard is six times the outside diameter of the catheter in millimetres. Under the old system it was usual to use the Charrière scale, although ureteric catheters were frequently described by the Beniqué scale, which added to confusion. The nurse is advised to get accustomed to the Beniqué scale, although she may find many of the catheters numbered according to the old system.

Table 50   Comparison of Beniqué, Charrière and English gauges

Beniqué	Charrière	English	Beniqué	Charrière	English	Beniqué	Charrière	English
1	—	—	25	—	—	49	—	—
2	1	—	26	13	—	50	25	—
3	—	00	27	—	7	51	—	15
4	2	—	28	14	—	52	26	—
5	—	—	29	—	—	53	—	—
6	3	0	30	15	8	54	27	16
7	—	—	31	—	—	55	—	—
8	4	—	32	16	—	56	28	—
9	—	1	33	—	9	57	—	17
10	5	—	34	17	—	58	29	—
11	—	—	35	—	—	59	—	—
12	6	2	36	18	10	60	30	18
13	—	—	37	—	—	61	—	—
14	7	—	38	19	—	62	31	—
15	—	3	39	—	11	63	—	19
16	8	—	40	20	—	64	32	—
17	—	—	41	—	—	65	—	—
18	9	4	42	21	12	66	33	20
19	—	—	43	—	—	67	—	—
20	10	—	44	22	—	68	34	—
21	—	5	45	—	13	69	—	21
22	11	—	46	23	—	70	35	—
23	—	—	47	—	—	71	—	—
24	12	6	48	24	14	72	36	22

Conversion factor: Beniqué = Charrière × 2 = (English × 3) + 6.

Rectal sounds and bougies are graduated in the same way, as are cystoscopes and other endoscopic instruments, but it will be found that the Charrière scale is still the one in common usage for instruments and this is half the Beniqué scale.

Tubing

The urethral catheter may be left in a patient and allowed to drain into the kidney dish or bottle in the bed only while the bedside apparatus is being arranged. Nothing is more messy or unsatisfactory than a badly arranged system for collection or urine. Most hospitals use disposable urine-collecting packs consisting of a length of transparent tubing which is plugged directly into the catheter, and has a plastic graduated bag sealed to the other end, sometimes with a flap valve in the bag inlet to prevent reflux and to help retain the syphon. The bag is suspended from the bed frame. If rubber tubing is used to connect the catheter to the bedside drainage or irrigator, it should be only slightly larger than the catheter and should have a thick wall. Thin tubing becomes easily kinked and compressed even by the weight of the bedclothes. Because of the rigidity of the wall of plastic tubing it holds a column of fluid which therefore acts as a syphon (even though the lower end of the tube is not under water). With rubber tubing under similar circumstances, every time the patient moves the wall of the tubing is compressed a little and urine is ejected from the lower end of the tube only to be replaced by air sucked up from the bottle. The lower end of the drainage tube must not be placed under the surface of the water in the collecting vessel, because the constant drip of urine from the open end of the tube is the only indication that drainage is continuing. **It cannot be over-emphasised that the blockage of bladder drainage even for a short time may have disastrous consequences.**

When collecting jars are used the tubing must be allowed to hang loose in the jar but must be attached to a rigid connector. The use of sterile disposable plastic bags is very hygienic and eliminates a great deal of nursing effort (Fig. 35.13). If the tubing is rubber it should be attached to a connector passing through a cork in the neck of the bottle: the cork must have a second opening in it to allow air to escape. If the tubing is of the more rigid plastic variety it can be passed through one of the holes in the bottle stopper, and no glass connector is necessary.

When a urethral catheter is connected to a bedside drainage bag or bottle, the tubing should not be brought over the front of the thigh for two reasons. First the tube will be raised above the level of the bladder and drainage will not then be effective except by syphonage. Second, if the patient flexes his hips he will make the first fault worse and may well pull the catheter out. The catheter and connector should be strapped to the inner side of the thigh, so that the tubing lies behind the thigh. It will not be compressed by the weight of the leg, if it is the right kind of tubing. The connecting tube must be of sufficient length to allow the patient to move across the bed and care must be taken to prevent kinking. The commonest way in which a soft tube is kinked is by the nurse tucking the bedclothes in as a final gesture when the apparatus has all been fixed up.

If the bladder is being irrigated with antiseptic fluid run in either constantly or intermittently from an overhead flask, a drip chamber should be inserted in the flow tubing so that the rate of flow of the irrigating fluid can be carefully watched. Instructions on irrigation of the bladder are given later.

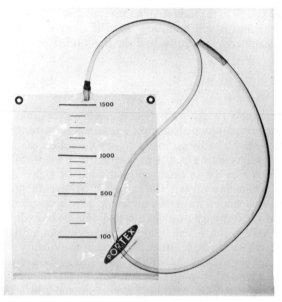

Fig. 35.13   Disposable urine collecting bag. This, slung beneath the bed, eliminates the use of glass jars.[1]

Tubing connectors

These should always be made of some plastic preferably nylon. A large catheter can be attached directly to the plastic tubing. Lengths of plastic tubing are joined by short sections of rubber, or wider-bore plastic. Glass connectors should now never be used: they break easily and this results in nurses cutting their fingers.

Suction apparatus

Drainage of the bladder by gravity is usually satisfactory when it is possible through a urethral catheter and connecting tubing taken underneath the thigh. If, however, drainage has to take place through a suprapubic catheter, it can only do so by overflow unless some form of suction is applied through the tube which connects the catheter to the reservoir There are occasions, particularly after operation for the cure of urinary fistula (that is a leakage from the bladder due to disease or injury), when it is absolutely essential to keep the bladder really empty during the period of healing. In addition, the avoidance of any degree of leakage around a suprapubic catheter makes the patient much more comfortable. Consequently suction is frequently needed and it may be achieved in various ways.

The more luxuriously equipped hospitals have bedside taps connected to a main suction line. The degree of suction with this system is such that it is dangerous to connect it direct to the bladder, and it is interrupted by an interceptor bottle to collect the urine and

[1] With certain types of collecting bag, when there is about 500 ml urine in the bag the walls of the upper part are stretched and held in such close apposition that urine is prevented from draining.

an adjustable air-leak which regulates the amount of suction actually reaching the catheter. Similar suction sockets are provided as part of modern oxygen supply parts.

Urological units are usually equipped with small bedside electric suction pumps (Robert's) which are silent and self-contained.

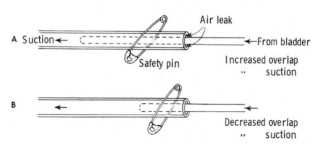

Fig. 35.14   Interruption of suction tube in drainage to provide an air leak. This prevents excessive suction and allows adjustment of the pressure by increasing the overlap of the two rubber tubes which form a loose fit.

If the degree of suction applied to the catheter is excessive, bladder epithelium will be sucked against the open end of the catheter, it will become oedematous and may even bleed and drainage will be unsatisfactory. If mechanical suction apparatus is being used there should be an adjustable air-leak. The Roberts pump has a vacuum gauge and a valve to adjust the degree of suction. A satisfactory simple method is to use a wide-bore rubber tube, with a length of thin tubing inserted for a variable distance inside it to allow an air leak. The two tubes are secured by a safety pin and the degree of suction is varied by altering the length of overlap between the tubes. Should the catheter become blocked by epithelium, the degree of suction will do no harm. When urine accumulates the epithelium will float away again, and allow free drainage.

Another simple and satisfactory way of arranging suction is by the three-bottle method and this is again on the hydraulic principle which the nurse must master. This suction apparatus can be improvised quite simply and is of use in gastric aspiration as well (page 665). A Redivac suction drain jar may be used but the capacity is very small and the 'suction' too strong at first: if a leak occurs the whole suction effect is lost.

Suprapubic drainage apparatus

If the bladder is opened, as it frequently is for operations upon the prostate, the bladder itself or the lower end of a ureter, then it is usual for a drainage tube (suprapubic catheter) to be left protruding from the bladder through the abdominal wall. This is done in order that the suture line on the bladder wall may heal thoroughly without the risk of distension and consequent leakage into the tissues. In the intervening period between the operation and the closure of the suprapubic sinus, all the urine is collected without natural micturition or leakage by using a self-retaining suprapubic catheter. When the time comes to remove the suprapubic catheter, it may be necessary to tie in a urethral catheter to allow the suprapubic hole or fistula to heal.

After the catheter is removed and before healing is complete urine will overflow on to the abdominal wall and can be collected by attaching a self-adhesive ileostomy bag, or if the leak is small, a urine sample collecting bag as used for babies (page 414).

In cases where obstruction to the flow of urine has been prolonged and the kidneys have been damaged, the bladder is sometimes drained through the abdominal wall permanently or perhaps for several months. A rubber catheter of the St Peter's type is held in the bladder by means of a tight-fitting rubber sleeve in the centre of a disc, which itself is kept in position on the abdominal wall by a belt, and the urine is collected into a rubber bag which is slung from the belt and lies against the thigh. The distance which the catheter passes into the bladder can be adjusted by pulling the catheter through the sleeve (Fig. 35.15). Once the fistula has been properly established, the patient can himself change the catheter weekly. Chronic infection of the urine frequently accompanies a permanent suprapubic drainage of this type, although in the majority of cases with modern chemotherapy it is possible to keep the urine sterile. When such an appliance is ordered, it is necessary to make certain that the catheter to be used is of a size sufficient to block the suprapubic opening and to prevent it from contracting down. If too small a catheter is used initially, the hole will become very small and the introduction of the catheter at subsequent changes will become increasingiy difficult.

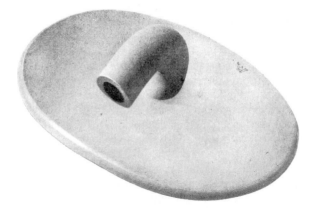

Fig. 35.15 Suprapubic shield with sleeve to retain the indwelling catheter (the Riches pattern has a round shield). (William Warne & Co., Ltd.)

Irrigation of the bladder

On numerous occasions in urological cases, fluid has to be injected through the urethra, through a urethral catheter, or through a suprapubic catheter in order to wash out the bladder. This irrigation may be performed intermittently with syringes or continuously by a gravity irrigation system.

Certain principles have to be observed in bladder irrigation and neglect with any one of these may lead to serious consequences. The rules for safety are:

1. Only very gentle pressure must be used. If the fluid is running by gravity from an overhead flask it should not be necessary to have the flask more than 60 cm above the

patient. Large metal or metal-and-glass syringes of the piston variety should *never* be used by the nursing staff. The surgeon may wish to use a big syringe of this type to inject fluid into the bladder and to withdraw with greater force in order to suck clots out. Small 60 ml (two ounce) glass syringes with a rubber bulb are safe and avoid the risk of too much fluid being injected into the bladder at a time. Plastic disposable syringes of this capacity are available (Fig. 35.16).

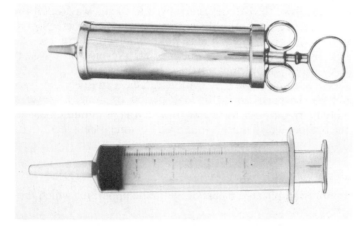

Fig. 35-16   (*Above*) 250-ml all-metal bladder syringe. (*Below*) Disposable 60-ml syringe (Wardill type) for use in wards.

2. Never more than 300 ml should be run into the bladder of an unconscious patient. If the bladder has been injured or opened by operation, never more than 60 ml should be passed in at a time and the injection of 60 ml must not be repeated unless an equal quantity has been returned. There may be a small blood clot on the end of the catheter which does not prevent the injection of fluid but does prevent the return of the fluid down the catheter. If the rubber bulb on the Dakin's irrigating syringe is a good one, the suction may be sufficient to suck the blood clot down the tube. **Under no circumstance must the nurse overlook this rule or she may do irreparable damage by producing leakage from the bladder suture line.**

3. The strictest aseptic precautions must be observed during the irrigation. If the outside end of a catheter is allowed to drop against the side of a thigh or on to a sheet it must be wiped with an antiseptic before the nozzle of the syringe is introduced. So great is the danger of infection from irrigation that surgeons often prefer to run the risk of clot retention rather than have their patients irrigated.

4. Fluids used for irrigation should be mildly antiseptic.[1] Rigid rules about the temperature of the fluid are however ridiculous, as the nurse may test the irrigating fluid in the jug, but by the time it has been drawn up into a glass syringe and injected in the catheter there has been a considerable fall in temperature. For general purposes the irrigating fluid

[1] Bladder irrigating fluids: Sulphacetamide 1 part in 500, Hibitane 1%, Noxytiolin (Noxiflex) 2·5%, or Proflavine 1 part in 1000. Mercury compounds are used very rarely. Silver nitrate (1 part in 10,000) is used to stop bleeding.

should start at 43 °C in the jug. If intermittent or continuous irrigation is being used from an overhead apparatus, then it is usual for the fluid to pass in at room temperature.

5. Great care must be taken not to inject air. When using a rubber-and-glass syringe the nurse must make quite certain that the air is fully expelled from the bulb during the filling or that she keeps the bulb higher than the glass during the injection. Air in the bladder produces discomfort, and airlocks in the irrigation apparatus and tubes prevent satisfactory drainage: the bulb must be kept higher than the outlet.

6. The outflow tube from the bladder is arranged in such a way that if the bladder is being washed through from a urethral catheter to a suprapubic catheter, or vice versa, the end of the outflow tube can be watched: it must not be submerged in a 'receiver'.

7. All irrigating fluid must be measured before and after use, otherwise the patient's fluid balance records will be completely worthless.

8. Repeated and constant bladder irrigation can be extremely exhausting for the patient and should not be persisted in for long periods of time, however enthusiastic the nurse may feel. If an irrigation is not clear of blood in a few minutes then it is likely that there is a clot in the bladder which must be removed by some other means than the nurse's irrigations.

Irrigation apparatus

There are two more complicated pieces of hydraulic apparatus which the nurse must understand.

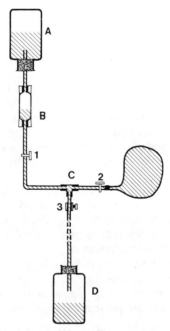

Fig. 35.17 Simple irrigator (Dukes type). **A** reservoir. **B** drip chamber. **C** T-connector. **D** collecting reservoir **1, 2, 3** spring clips.

The first of these is illustrated in Fig. 35.17. It consists of a flask **A** connected through a drip chamber **B** (which is not absolutely essential) to a Y- or T-connector **C**. One limb of the Y- or T-connector is in turn joined by a semi-flexible plastic tubing and connector to the bladder catheter, and the stem of the Y is similarly connected to the reservoir **D** on the floor. Each limb of the Y- or T-connector carries on its adjoining rubber tubing a spring clip.

This apparatus is commonly used when the bladder needs to be irrigated perhaps every two hours and left on open drainage in the interval. Such a procedure is needed in the treatment of severe cystitis or in the post-operative management of the bladder following a major operation in the pelvis such as excision of the rectum.

Suitable apparatus is supplied by the CSSD already autoclaved and assembled. A substitute can be made up using infusion flasks and tubing. Procedure for use:

1. Clips **2** and **3** are closed, and the reservoir filled
2. Clip **2** is opened to expel air and fill the tube: it is then closed.
3. The catheter connection is made.
4. Clip **1** is closed and clips **2** and **3** opened: this allows the bladder to empty.
5. To irrigate, (*a*) clip **3** is closed and **1** is opened to allow approximately 60 ml fluid to flow into the bladder. (*b*) clip **1** is closed and **3** opened, and left open.

If the fluid which has been run in does not return at once it is likely that the catheter is is blocked. Cycle 5 may be repeated once and if there is no return the medical officer must be informed.

Irrigation is carried out 4-hourly or as often as has been ordered.

Tidal drainage apparatus (Fig. 35.18)

In order to imitate the natural rhythmic filling and emptying of the bladder an apparatus is used known as the 'tidal drainage apparatus'. This depends on the principle of siphonage for emptying the bladder at set times. There are various complications and modifications of the apparatus, but in its simplest form it is shown in Fig. 35.18. Sterile antiseptic solution (e.g. noxytiolin) is allowed to drip from a litre flask through a drip chamber to join the catheter which is attached to the stem of a Y-connector. The outlet of this in turn is connected to an inverted U- or Y-tube which provides a small air leak. The size of the air leak is vital and is controlled by a further screw slip. The system depends on the bladder filling gradually from the reservoir and from the kidneys (**A**). When the pressure rises sufficiently to lift the level of the fluid over the inverted U-tube (**B**), flow of urine down to the bedside flask creates a siphon which then reverses the flow of the catheter (**C**). When the bladder is empty (**D**), the siphon is broken by air entry at the leak on the U-tube and the cycle re-starts.

(This system can be made up from standard infusion apparatus and connectors, but is available as a disposable commercial pack, the Cystomat.)

Three-bottle suction apparatus

This simple device can be used for gastric or urine aspiration.

The basic principles are these:

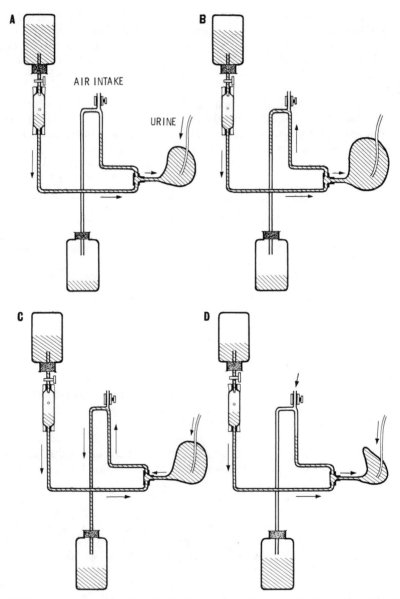

Fig. 35.18   Apparatus required for tidal drainage (automatic intermittent irrigation of bladder).

Water flows from one reservoir to another and it can only do so if it is replaced by more water or air entering the first reservoir. This is very easily illustrated by the ordinary transfusion bottle into which air flows up the long glass tube as the blood runs out under gravity. If this air-inlet tube is connected to another bottle, it will create a vacuum in this last bottle. This third reservoir will in turn be connected to the bladder. The amount of suction provided by a simple apparatus like this is dependent upon the height of the reservoir and the rate of flow from it. The apparatus is illustrated in Fig. 35.19. Blood transfusion bottles can be used for all three reservoirs if no larger bottles are available with suitable stoppers, but the disadvantage is that the lower reservoir bottle has to be changed more frequently. The most suitable are Winchester 'quart' bottles with rubber bungs, pierced with two holes and fitted with glass tubes. A proper bedside stand is ideal but a ward stool inverted on the window-sill or on the bedside locker will in an emergency provide a suitable stand for the top reservoir. Bottle X is filled with tap water and closed with a bung containing a long glass tube reaching to within 1 cm of the bottom of the bottle and the shorter glass outlet tube connected by rubber tubing to a drip chamber and carrying a clip. The drip chamber

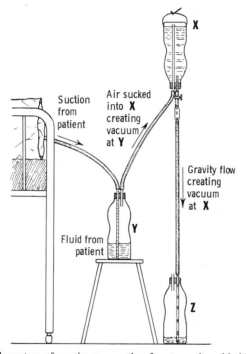

Fig. 35.19   Three-bottle system of continuous suction for stomach or bladder drainage. (See text.)

is connected to a tube through a similar rubber bung in bottle Z which rests on the floor. The long glass tube in bottle X carries a length of rubber tubing with a clip. Bottle X is then inverted in the stand, both the clips on the outgoing tubes being closed. Bottle Y is the collecting reservoir and must have an absolutely air-tight bung through which pass two suitable glass tubes, one of which extends only just through the stopper, on the inside. When the apparatus has been assembled, and the suction tube connected to the catheter, the clip on tube X–Z is released so that the drip rate is about 100 per minute. The clip on the suction tube Y–X should be left closed until the drip rate slows up indicating that all the joints are airtight and a satisfactory vacuum will occur in bottle Y. From now on suction will continue by a rate determined by the clip on tube X–Z until the reservoir X is empty. The nurse *must* then close the clip on tubes X–Z and Y–X and change bottle X for bottle Z. Clearly the frequency of changes necessary will depend on the size of the reservoirs. With a standard 'quart' bottle very adequate suction can be maintained by changing the bottles every three hours. If the suction is being applied to an airtight cavity such as the bladder without a suprapubic fistula the rate of drip need only be quite slow—in fact it need not be greater than the rate of flow of the urine if the apparatus is really airtight: 60 to 100 drops per minute is a safe speed.

If the reservoir Y is always kept lower than the patient and if the reservoirs X and Z are changed over without disconnecting any of the rubber tubes from the bungs, there will be no risk of wrong connections and the apparatus need not be sterilised before use. The author has known an apparatus of this type connected wrongly with the result that the contents of reservoir X has slowly dropped through reservoir Y into a small child's stomach, instead of there being a constant gastric suction. Such a foolish mistake is quite unnecessary and every nurse should be able to improvise a suction apparatus such as this at very short notice.

Urinals for Incontinent patients

If a bedridden patient is incontinent of urine, either a Foley self-retaining catheter must be used, or some form of appliance must be placed in the bed to collect the urine. Unconscious patients who may be incontinent of faeces as well as urine, are sometimes placed on rubber bed-pans to lessen the risk of bed sores. The incontinent male patient may use an ordinary plastic urinal, which must be frequently emptied and sterilised to reduce the risk of infection passing up the urethra. A more satisfactory appliance is the 'Simplic' bed incontinence appliance (Fig. 51.2). The penis should be smeared twice a day with a silicone-containing barrier cream (page 469) to prevent ulceration from constant wetting with urine.

The satisfactory collection of urine from the female incontinent patient—without catheterisation—is extremely difficult. Specially designed rubber urinals are sometimes used.

For ambulant male patients an apparatus is used to collect the urine into a rubber bag strapped to the thigh. A satisfactory pattern is the Stoke Mandeville urinal which has a detachable rubber penile sheath (Fig. 38.3). An apparatus of this type is required for many paraplegic patients. Lighter weight apparatus with disposable plastic reservoirs is being used increasingly with added convenience and reduced risk of infection. The pattern used for paraplegic boys is arranged so that the rubber base presses against the pubis and makes a watertight seal. Such an appliance carefully fitted is absolutely reliable and the wearer can play games without getting wet. Since the introduction of latex and PVC balloon-type (Foley) catheters the management of incontinence in women patients confined to bed is best undertaken by continuous drainage with a catheter. This only needs changing once a week and a maintenance dose of urinary antiseptic prevents infection. After prolonged use, leakage occurs around the catheter.

Women suffering from paraplegia and confined to a wheelchair can sometimes be kept dry with an indwelling Foley catheter, but after prolonged use the urethra tends to enlarge and leakage occurs. Such patients usually require an ileo-cutaneous ureterostomy (page 687). Disseminated sclerosis is another common condition of the nervous system which is associated with urinary incontinence of varying type: some patients have retention with overflow and can be managed with an indwelling catheter: others have precipitate urgent micturition and it is practically impossible for them to retain a catheter in the bladder without considerable pain.

The care of appliances

Apparatus which is used for the collection of urine becomes fouled by deposition of phosphate crystals which collect in the joins and seams of the apparatus. Certain types of rubber absorb the smell of the urine which invariably becomes infected when it has been in the bag for some time. It is quite unnecessary for this apparatus to carry an unpleasant odour, but unremitting care is essential. The patient must have at least 2 sets of apparatus, preferably 3 so there is a spare one if either of the regular sets requires repair or replacement.

The only satisfactory way to prevent encrustation is regular washing with plenty of hot water. This also applies to the webbing or rubber retaining straps. It is not really necessary to clean the appliances with strong antiseptics. Chlorine solutions such as bleach sterilise the apparatus satisfactorily and clean the straps, but constant use tends to rot the material. Other antiseptics such as chloroxylenol may produce irritation of the skin as they tend to be absorbed by the rubber. The best safeguard against infection is routine washing with hot soapy water: the apparatus is then rinsed thoroughly and hung up to dry. Thorough drying of the bag is the best way of guarding against pyocyaneus infections. When the appliance is put on the patient 30 ml of 1% chlorhexidine (Hibitane) solution in water, placed in the reservoir, prevents the rapid multiplication of organisms in the collected urine. If the bag is emptied regularly and a similar quantity of antiseptic solution placed in it the unpleasant smells of putrefying urine will be avoided completely and the life of the apparatus will be prolonged.

Patients wearing external appliances of this type very easily develop skin infections, particularly if there is some leakage. In order to ensure confidence in the appliance patients tend to tighten the straps with increasing vigour which has the effect of chafing the groins and producing areas of pressure necrosis in the perineum. This is particularly likely to happen in paraplegic patients whose sensation is impaired. Once ulceration develops, the appliance must be discarded for the time being and urine collected by an indwelling catheter until the skin has healed. Fungal infections (tinea) develop very readily, producing large scaly red areas in the groins.

Ileostomy and colostomy apparatus requires similar care in maintenance and fitting (page 537) though many patients now are able to use adherent receptacles which are entirely disposable.

In schools, convalescent homes and places of work where there are patients wearing appliances there must be special provision for a patient to attend to hygiene and wash the receptables, without embarrassment.

ENDOSCOPIC AND OTHER INSTRUMENTS USED IN THE URINARY TRACT

Unless she is specialising in theatre work, the nurse will not need to know details of the instruments used for examining various parts of the urinary tract. Tubular illuminated instruments are used to inspect the bladder and the urethra. An examining **cytoscope** consists of an outer sheath carrying a light source at its tip with a removable telescope through which the bladder can be inspected. Before the telescope is inserted, the bladder is distended with water; a valve in the tube prevents the water escaping while the telescope is inserted (Fig. 18.15). Most urologists use an instrument through which water can be run into or removed from the bladder at will so that the bladder wall may be watched as it empties and fills. This ensures that all portions of the bladder are brought within view of the telescope. In addition there are **catheterising cystoscopes** through which the operator can pass catheters into the ureters in order to perform retrograde pyelography.

Larger instruments are used for operating within the bladder, for taking biopsies, or for cutting away pieces of tumour or destroying tumours with a diathermy current. The largest of these instruments used for operating is a **panendoscope.** A **rectoscope** is used for removing strips of prostatic tissue to relieve obstruction.

A **posterior urethroscope** is a similar instrument with a slightly different lens system used for examining the upper part of the urethra again while it is being irrigated with water. An **anterior urethroscope** is used for examining the penile urethra internally, and with this instrument the urethral tube is kept open by inflating with air on the same principle as that used with a sigmoidoscope.

Miniature instruments are used for children, and the smallest cystoscope has an external diameter approximately the same as that of a ball-point pen refill.

With the combination of these instruments, it is possible to examine the whole of the lower urinary tract and to treat small tumours within the bladder and the urethra by destroying them with diathermy.

Cryo-surgery is a procedure for destroying tissue by freezing, and there is a special endoscopic instrument with which this process can be used to destroy the prostate.

Cystoscopy, that is the examination of the bladder, is a routine diagnostic procedure in most urological conditions and when a patient has had a papilloma or malignant tumour of the bladder a life-long follow up of cystoscopy every 6 months is usual routine. There are, therefore, a large number of patients coming through a urological or general surgical unit simply undergoing an examination cystoscopy. This may be performed under a general anaesthetic or by local instillation in the urethra of a lignocaine solution. With a small instrument it is possible to perform a cystoscopy on both men and women without the use of any anaesthetic.

All patients undergoing cystoscopy are given a prophylactic urinary antiseptic for 48 hours covering the operation period to guard against infection being introduced by this procedure, as there are always organisms in the anterior urethra which may be carried into the bladder. 'Catheter fever' from a mild septicaemia can occur and a more severe infection may produce '**bacteraemic shock**' with sudden collapse (page 115).

It is essential that patients going for cystoscopy should empty their bladder if they can immediately before the procedure in order that the residual urine in the bladder may be measured at the time of cystoscopy.

After endoscopic procedures, the patient may have difficulty with passing urine, particularly if there has been some minor degree of obstruction previously. Following operative procedures in the bladder where haemorrhage may occur, a catheter is commonly left in place for 48 hours or longer until bleeding has ceased in order to prevent retention due to clots.

The lighting system on endoscopic instruments was originally by minute electric bulbs at the end of the instruments supplied by a current from the battery or mains transformer source clipped to the end of the instrument. All modern endoscopic instruments are now illiminated through a core of fibre-glass strands built into the sheath of the instrument. The light source is a projector lamp from which the intense light is carried through a flexible fibre-glass cable attached to the head of the instrument. This fibre-optic system has the merit that the light source is always cool, it never fails, and the strength of illumination is very much greater than ordinary electric bulbs.

The care of endoscopic instruments is an extremely important duty for theatre staff. Endoscopic procedures are difficult and the interpretation of what a surgeon sees depend largely on the adequacy of the instrument and the ease with which the procedure is carried out. Badly maintained or faulty instruments are a source of great annoyance and a considerable danger to the patient.

Broad outlines on the care of endoscopic instruments are given on page 350.

Occasionally, cystoscopy becomes an emergency procedure if there is bleeding in order that the source of the bleeding may be located. Very small tumours in the bladder may be difficult to find unless they are actually bleeding at the time of examination, and if the bleeding should be coming from one of the kidneys an emergency cystoscopy during the bleeding may enable the surgeon to discover immediately which side is involved. Often, of course, there is no doubt because the patient has pain in the affected side.

Most surgeons prefer a full radiological examination of the urinary tract to be carried out before examination with endoscopic instruments. The surgeon is then able to plan his endoscopy and be prepared for operative procedures if they should be necessary.

Other Instruments used in urological surgery

Bougies. Following inflammation or injury, the repair processes of the body produce fibrous tissue which gradually contracts. There is therefore a tendency for all tubular structures in the body to develop a narrow area or stricture at the site of damage. Urethral strictures arise following urethritis or urethral abscesses (frequently due to gonorrhoea) or at the site of injury of the urethra. Sometimes the urethra is narrowed by oedema or growth. In order that a normal channel should be restored either for the natural passage of urine or for the introduction of a catheter, instruments are used to dilate the stricture. These are really a series of graduated probes. The finest or filiform bougies may be as small as 1 mm in diameter. They are usually made of plastic material which is flexible. They are graduated in the same way as catheters on the French and English scales. The older bougies were made of silk-web or 'gum elastic', sterilised by insertion in an antiseptic medium or storing in formalin vapour, and they should only be boiled if they are wanted in a hurry; in this case they must be wrapped up and handled with the same care as gum elastic catheters while they are still hot. Plastic bougies which can be autoclaved are now available and will come into general use to replace the gum elastic ones. All these flexible bougies are straight and some have a slightly expanded tip—olive-tipped bougies.

Bougies are also made of stainless steel, in straight and curved patterns, some with olivary tips. The metal bougies are commonly referred to as 'sounds' because they resemble in appearance the original 'bladder sound' which was used for introducing through the urethra to feel round the bladder for the presence of a stone. The term 'sound' was applied to this instrument because it could be heard to click against a large stone within the bladder. Although it is a misnomer, the word is also applied to uterine sounds, graduated instruments for measuring the length of the uterine cavity when passed in through the cervix.

Appropriate urethral and bladder sounds or metal bougies must always be available when endoscopic instruments are being used, as it is frequently necessary to dilate the urethra by the introduction of successive sizes of metal bougies before the large-sized endoscopic instrument can be passed.

The lithotrite (Fig. 35.20). Before the introduction of the aseptic technique of surgery and of more accurate diagnostic methods, the formation of stone in the bladder was more common. By pressure in the suprapubic region, a large bladder stone could be pressed down into the perineum. The patient's legs were held up in the air in what we know as the 'lithotomy position'. An incision was then made down on to the stone in the perineum—a dangerous operation, frequently followed by fistula. To overcome these difficulties, the lithotrite was introduced and this consists of a long metal rod with an outer metal tube. The rod and the tube each carry a jaw. A screw device at the head of the instrument makes it possible to open or close these crocodile jaws while the instrument is in the bladder.

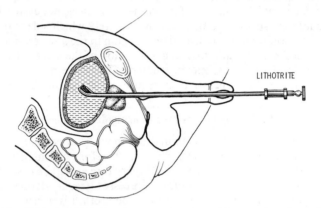

Fig. 35.20   Method of removing a stone in the bladder with a lithortite.

Apart from the cleaning and lubrication, the instrument requires no particular care and is robust. When it is used, a small amount of water (120 ml) is injected into the bladder through a catheter. This ensures that the mucous membrane of the bladder will not get trapped in the jaws of the instrument. The lithotrite is then passed into the bladder and the jaws opened. By manoeuvring the instrument the surgeon may be able to roll the stone between its jaws. By screwing up the wheel on the head of the instrument the stone is then broken in pieces. The particles of stone are then removed from the bladder by washing out through a very wide-bore tube. An evacuator is used for this purpose.

Evacuators. There are various forms of device for removing blood clot or other solid matter from the bladder. The Bigelow or Ellik type is the one in most common use. A straight metal tube (several sizes are provided) is passed through the urethra and a glass receptable (Fig. 35.1) is fitted on to the end of this tube. The receptable carries a large rubber bulb and the whole apparatus is filled with water by immersing it completely in a bowl and squeezing all the air out of the bulb. By alternately squeezing and releasing the large rubber bulb, water is flushed to and fro into the bladder, and as the water rushes out of the bladder back into the receptable, any solid particles that come with it fall to the bottom of the glass bulb and are therefore not squirted back into the bladder with the next squeeze of the bulb.

From the nursing point of view the only real difficulty is the initial filling of the receptacle and bulb to expel all the air. It is essential to have a bowl of water of adequate depth.

Bladder syringes. There are two common types of bladder syringe used for filling the bladder prior to endoscopy or for washing out the bladder on other occasions. The usual sizes contain 250–300 ml. By far the best type is that with a glass barrel and metal piston; although this pattern is more liable to damage, it is less likely to become jammed than the all-metal type. The nozzle of the bladder syringe is detachable in some cases to enable the syringe to be filled rapidly, but others have a specially tapered end which will fit directly into the cannula of the standard cystoscope without the necessity of an intervening piece of rubber tube.

A small glass Dakin's syringe is safe for post-operative bladder wash-out or to un-block tubes. Large bladder syringes should *never* be used by nursing staff (page 661).

50-ml disposable plastic syringes are used for ward 'washouts'. These are already sterilised.

Urethral syringe. For introducing local anaesthetic solution into the urethra or for irrigating the urethra, a small glass syringe with a rubber bulb is used. This is usually known as the Canny-Ryall urethral syringe. The glass syringe and rubber bulb can be sterilised by boiling.

Bladder irrigating stop-cock. This is a metal T-piece with a rotating valve. The inlet is connected to the flow tube of an irrigating apparatus while the other arm of the cross-piece is made to fit the valve opening of the standard cystoscope. With the valve over towards the flow tube, the bladder contents are allowed to escape down the vertical limb of the T into a dish, and with the valve over towards the cystoscope, the irrigating fluid runs straight into the bladder. With the valve vertical all three limbs are closed. The reservoir is graduated so that the surgeon can see the amount of water which has entered the bladder.

Operations upon the urinary tract

Tables 52 and 54 show the operations commonly performed on the various portions of the urinary tract with some of the conditions which are so treated. When, as a result of full investigation, the surgeon is armed with all possible information about the condition of the kidney and urinary tract, he may then be able to plan precisely what operation he is going to perform. On the other hand, he may not be able to decide the nature or extent of the operation beforehand.

Post-operative complications

Many of the complications which follow other surgical operations may occur and there are certain features of urological surgery which must be fully understood so that the complications peculiar to these operations may be watched for and dealt with appropriately.

Haemorrhage

The kidney is a very vascular organ. Removal of a kidney may be followed by fatal haemorrhage if a ligature slips off the renal artery. During the operation for nephrectomy, the surgeon takes particular care over these large vessels owing to their size and the fact that they come direct from the aorta and vena cava respectively. Bleeding may also continue as an ooze from the kidney bed, particularly if the kidney has been inflamed. It is therefore usual for the surgeon to leave a tube or corrugated rubber drain in position through his nephrectomy incision. This tube is rarely left in position more than 48 hours, and its purpose is to prevent the accumulation of serum and blood which might later become infective. Operations upon the kidney or ureter when the kidney is not removed may be followed by bleeding *into* the urinary tract and the formation of small clots. These clots may obstruct the ureter or the urethra and give rise to intense pain and ureteric colic Nothing can be done except to relieve the pain and wait until the clot is finally expelled (page 632).

Operations upon the bladder and prostate may be followed by haemorrhage outside the bladder, and a drainage tube is therefore placed in the wound to prevent this collection of blood, which is even more likely to get infected than a similar collection after nephrectomy, because of the possible associated leakage of urine from a bladder which has been opened. Following such operations, a certain amount of bleeding invariably takes place into the bladder and special methods have to be adopted to prevent the formation of clots and their retention in the bladder. A drainage tube may be left in the bladder so that blood and urine may escape freely. The bladder itself may be closed and a urethral catheter relied upon to drain away such urine and blood as continues to escape. In the management of this complication lies the secret of successful urological nursing. All operations on the bladder and prostate have to be followed by the most careful vigil on the part of the nurse to make quite certain that the outflow from the bladder either through urethral catheter or suprapubic tube continues without ceasing. Once the flow stops, urine and blood collect behind the blockage and clot formation occurs, with dire results (also pages 634, 636).

The bladder and prostatic bed (following removal of the prostate) are particularly liable to infection. Infection leads to the erosion of the small clots in the arteries and veins at their cut ends and secondary haemorrhage is therefore a risk common to most forms of urological surgery. Severe haemorrhage during the second week after removal of the prostate was a very common complication before the advent of chemotherapy and antibiotics. Secondary haemorrhage is now a rare complication though it must still be watched for. Clot formation leads to acute retention of urine and therefore to severe pain. The onset of severe pain at any time following operation on the bladder or prostate, always suggests the possibility of haemorrhage having occurred.

Infection. Operations upon the urinary tract frequently have to be performed in the presence of infection. Infection itself, especially if there is obstruction to the urinary outflow, leads to pyelonephritis (a suppurating condition of the kidneys): severe anaemia develops and ultimately death from renal failure supervenes unless the obstruction is relieved (page 674). In addition, the symptoms of urinary infection are most distressing to the patient—rigors, toxaemia, pain and probably severe frequency of micturition from cystitis.

It is the nurse's duty to observe the urine of every patient and to note any marked change in its appearance. Following operations upon the urinary tract, the urine invariably contains a certain amount of blood, but as the blood lessens each day the urine should soon become crystal clear. If bleeding has ceased and the urine is still cloudy, it is likely that infection is present. The occurrence or persistence of urinary infection may well be due to errors in nursing technique, especially from the imperfect sterilisation and handling of catheters and irrigating tubes or from contaminated irrigating fluid. The more bladder wash-outs, the more instrumentations, and the more dressings the patient undergoes, the more liable he is to acquire a severe urinary infection. On the other hand, when infection is established frequent irrigation may be necessary to clear the pus and mucus from the urinary tract. Particularly is this true if diverticulum formation has occurred in the bladder due to long-standing obstruction. Each case has to be judged on its merits, but the nurse must always bear in mind that she may be the one to introduce the infection into a urinary tract which has hitherto been free from it. The presence of infection already must not be allowed to lead to carelessness, because new and more resistant organisms may be introduced into a urinary tract which is readily tolerating one particular strain. Cross-infection from one patient to another may easily occur if urinals and other apparatus are not adequately sterilised.

Bacteraemic shock (page 115)

The organisms commonly found in the urinary tract are usually 'gram negative'— this means that they do not stain with the gram stain when examined by the bacteriologist as a means of identifying the type. If these germs get released into the blood stream they may produce very rapid septicaemia and collapse. This must be thought of if a sudden fall in blood pressure occurs with perhaps a rigor. Immediate intravenous infusion (dextran) is needed with intravenous antibiotics (gentamycin or carbenicillin). This is a specific condition and may occur without any previous symptoms of urinary tract infection.

Leakage of urine

When a kidney is removed, the cut end of the ureter is usually tied off: leakage due to back flow from bladder is extremely rare. It is, however, particularly liable to occur if the ureter is a dilated one such as is found in tuberculosis or back-pressure dilatation of the ureter and kidney. On account of this risk if the ureter is large and is divided near the bladder, a precautionary drainage tube is inserted through the wound to allow the escape of any urine which may leak. In every operation where the urinary tract has been opened and sutured, whether it is in the pelvis of the kidney, the body of the kidney, the ureter or the bladder, the site of operation is always drained either by corrugated rubber or by tube. In contrast to the drainage tube used to prevent the accumulation of blood (usually removed after 48 hours), the tube in this case is left in position until there is no further urinary escape and is then gradually shortened so that there is no possible risk of urine leaking into the surrounding tissues (**extravasation,** page 636).

If leakage of urine continues for more than two weeks after operation on the urinary tract, it is likely that there is some obstruction below the site of operation or injury. If the natural way out is clear, the unnatural pathway or fistula will always heal up unless there is infection or a foreign body such as a silk or thread suture along the course of the tube track.

Peritonitis

The approach to various portions of the urinary tract involves intentional or accidental opening of the peritoneal cavity. Even if the peritoneum is not itself incised, the retroperitoneal tissues are disturbed and the peritoneum bruised. Peritonitis or paralytic ileus are thus possible complications, and although it is not necessary to withhold oral feeding in the immediate post-operative phase, the occurrence of abdominal distension may be an indication that ileus is present. Fluid intake cannot be limited on account of the additional risk to the renal tract, and parenteral administration is imperative.

Renal failure

Even after fairly straightforward operations such as a simple nephrectomy, complete suppression of urine—anuria—may develop, and it is thought that the mechanism of this is a reflex one, the removal of one kidney producing a temporary cessation of function in the other one. If, however, there has been a long-established infection in the urinary tract, the shock and disturbance of operation may precipitate renal failure. Factors which make failure more likely are inadequate drainage of the urinary tract in the immediate post-operative period (i.e. partial obstruction), the presence of clot within the tract, excessive instrumentation or catheterisation, and shock. The nursing of patients who have shown signs of renal insufficiency (e.g. a raised blood urea before operation) demands particular attention to fluid balance and regulation of salt intake (page 133).

Apart from operations on the urinary tract, severe anoxia from haemorrhage or shock may produce irreparable renal damage even in the absence of previous kidney disease (page 134). Acute kidney failure may arise from poisoning and from mis-matched blood transfusion. Mercury compounds such as mercuric chloride (corrosive sublimate), carbon tetrachloride (used in fire extinguishers) and quite a number of drugs are sometimes taken

Table 51 Causes of acute renal failure for which haemodialysis may be needed

Anoxia of central origin	shock
	haemorrhage
	heart failure
	'crush syndrome' (page 970)
Renal ischaemia	renal artery atherosclerosis
	aortic aneurysm
	compression of artery by malignant glands
	embolus
Renal tubular damage	poisoning: mercury compounds: carbon tetra-chloride: drugs
	mis-matched blood transfusion
'Reflex' (mechanism unknown)	injury or operation on urinary tract
Infection	acute bacterial as in septicaemia
	chronic bacterial pyelonephritis
Renal tissue replacement by	amyloid disease
	lymphadenoma (reticulosis)
	carcinoma, nephroblastoma
	metastatic cancer
Obstetric	renal tubular necrosis
	shock

by accident, or with suicidal intent. There is almost immediate inflammation of kidneys but if the damage is not too severe the patient may survive if he can be sustained over the period required for the kidney to recover.

Management of renal failure. There are four main principles involved here.

1. The bladder must be catheterised to make absolutely certain that there is no obstruction to the outflow of any urine that is formed. If the ureters have been blocked by a growth or injury nephrostomy is required (page 679).

2. Electrolyte balance. Repeated estimations of blood chemistry are required. Intravenous infusion is essential in order that the right quantities of water, sodium, chloride,

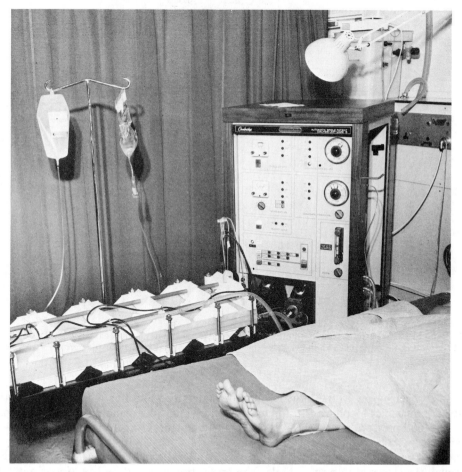

Fig. 35.21 Haemodialysis in progress. The equipment shown is a Cambridge dialyser with disposable dialysing unit. The flow rate, temperature and other controls are monitored by an automatic electronic system as shown.

potassium and other chemicals may be given at the appropriate times. In severe renal insufficiency, the potassium level in the blood rises and cardiac arrest may occur. **Resonium**, a sodium resin compound or **calcium resonium** is given orally or by enema, and its effect is to remove the potassium ions by a natural dialysis in the intestine. These substances are 'ion exchange resins'. If renal fluid output continues, oral diuretics are used to get rid of excess potassium, but if urine flow is greatly reduced they may be ineffective.

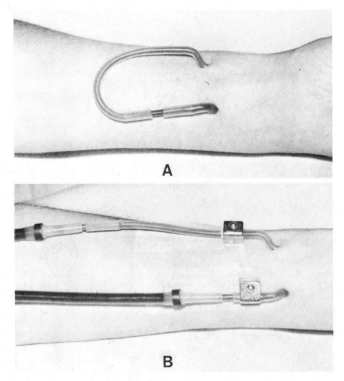

Fig. 35.22   External arterio-venous shunt. **A**. External arterio-venous shunt for repeated haemodialysis. **B**. The shunt is disconnected and the vessels attached to the artificial kidney for the period of treatment.

3. Oxygen supply to the kidneys must be maintained and this is not possible if the patient is anaemic: blood transfusion may therefore be required and repeated estimations of the blood pressure are essential throughout treatment. Oxygen therapy is sometimes a great help.

4. Elimination of urea and other waste products by alternative means. Urea can escape through the skin and into the bowels. The production of excessive sweating is not very helpful and diarrhoea would lead to dehydration. The patient is, however, usually given a laxative such as magnesium sulphate to encourage this elimination.

Artificial kidney

Some patients recover spontaneously if simple nursing methods are carried out along the lines described. In more severe cases, however, the blood can be purified by artificial means. The simplest method is by **peritoneal dialysis** which has already been described (page 494). A more efficient method is to connect an artery and a vein from the patient to a mechanical pump which circulates the blood through a long coiled plastic tube (Fig. 35.21). Substances like urea diffuse through the wall of the tube into the surrounding fluid in the drum in which the coil is immersed. By alterations in the composition of the fluid, any desired changes may be effected in the patient's blood. In fact, the artificial kidney acts in much the same way as the heart-lung machine. The blood has to be treated with heparin to prevent clotting and transfusion is required (to fill the pump initially).

Since the introduction of the artificial kidney many patients whose kidneys are incapable of maintaining health have been kept alive by regular treatment with this apparatus. Methods have been devised for rapid connection of the patient's blood vessels and all that is needed is an overnight stay in hospital. One method is to use an *external* shunt (Fig. 23.22). This is suitable for 'crisis' dialysis when it is expected only to serve for a week or two. For long term dialysis an arterio-venous *internal* fistula is created by sewing an artery in the forearm to a vein. This leads to the enlargement of neighbouring veins which do not thrombose because the blood flow is fast. Thus there is an abundance of sites for venepuncture to withdraw and return the blood.

The artificial kidney is used also in the treatment of drug over-dosage (e.g. by barbiturates, bromides or aspirin) usually arising from attempted suicide.

36

Kidney and Ureter

The right kidney lies mainly behind the liver, but part of its front surface is in contact with the colon. It is possible that this close relationship with the bowel is one reason for common infections of the urinary tract by organisms which are normally found in the large intestine (bacillus coli and streptococcus faecalis). The left kidney is close to the spleen and lies behind the stomach.

Each kidney is surmounted by a small **adrenal gland**. The twelfth and sometimes the eleventh ribs lie immediately behind the kidney on each side and the thick bulk of muscle in the loin is an additional protection against injury. The kidney is surrounded by a layer of fat which is very variable in quantity. This 'perinephric' fat corresponds to the suet found in animals and it is liable to infection which may be blood borne or may spread from the kidney: fat has a very low resistance to the spread of infection and a **'perinephric abscess'** forms.

Table 52 shows the operations most commonly performed upon the kidney and ureter (Fig. 36.1), with complications which may arise.

Common disorders

Congenital

The kidney develops in the bony pelvis immediately in front of the sacrum. The ureter grows as a bud from the vas deferens and joins the primitive mass of kidney tubules where it expands to form the pelvis of the ureter and calyces. The lower end of the ureter ultimately gains a separate opening into the bladder but, because of its origin from the vas or from the corresponding round ligament in the female, the ureter is closely connected with the genital tract at its lower end.

During later development, the foetal kidney travels slowly up the posterior abdominal wall, but this migration may get arrested and result in the adult kidney remaining at the brim of the bony pelvis or low in the loin (**ectopic kidney**). Occasionally the right and left kidneys remain fused together across the mid-line, forming a **horse-shoe kidney.**

Abnormalities of the budding of the developing ureter result in double ureters on one or both sides, each extra tube leading to a well-defined **accessory kidney.**

Sometimes as the result of errors in development, the lower end of the ureter may open into the urethra or, in the female, into the vagina. This condition of **ectopic ureter** gives rise to continuous urinary incontinence which may be overlooked in the young child or regarded merely as a failure of training.

Many of these congenital abnormalities produce no symptoms, but a large proportion of urology at all ages is concerned with complications such as infection, stone formation, and obstruction which have arisen purely on account of the abnormal anatomy of kidney or ureter.

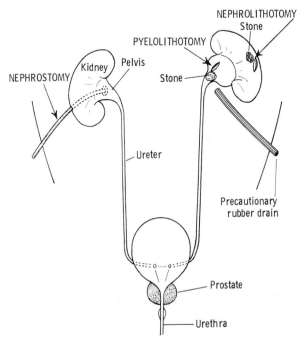

Fig. 36.1   Anatomy of the urinary tract and common operations.

Trauma

Crushing injuries of the trunk or a blow in the loin may bruise or lacerate the kidney. Mild injuries are accompanied by severe pain in the loin which is mostly due to the bruising of muscle. Haematuria is present and the nurse's duty is to save every specimen of urine so that the progress of the bleeding may be watched, each specimen being labelled with the time at which it was passed. If haematuria continues for several days after the injury, open operation may be required to remove or repair the kidney. Renal colic may occur from the passage of clots down the ureter.

The initial injury may be so severe that collapse is sudden from loss of blood into the loose tissues behind the peritoneum. Cases of this type require extremely urgent surgical treatment which almost always involves nephrectomy (page 129). Under such conditions the patient is taken to the operating theatre at the earliest possible moment and there is not time for preliminary investigations to determine whether the other kidney is normal. When

Table 52   Operations on the kidney and ureters

Operation	Description	Disorder	Special complications	Probable Drainage and Management	
Nephrectomy	Removal of kidney	Non-functioning kidney Tuberculosis Growth Stone Congenital abnormality Injury	Primary or reactionary haemorrhage	Precautionary drain (for bleeding) to kidney bed	Tube usually removed at 48 hours
Nephro-ureterectomy	Nephrectomy and removal of the whole ureter	Tuberculosis Megaureter (congenital)	Primary or reactionary haemorrhage	(a) to kidney bed (b) to pelvis in tuberculous cases	If for tuberculosis, re-move by shortening in case any urinary leak develops from ureter stump in bladder wall
Partial nephrectomy	Removal of part of the kidney	Tuberculosis Stone	Reactionary or secondary haemorrhage Urinary fistula	Precautionary drain to kidney bed	Remove by shortening from 4th day, depen-ding on amount of urinary leak (if any)
Nephrolithotomy	Removal of stone from body of kidney	Calculus in small calyx	Haemorrhage (especially secondary) Urinary fistula Recurrence of calculus Anuria	Precautionary (a) to kidney bed (b) sometimes: nephrostomy catheter for irrigation (see below)	Remove by shortening from 4th day
Pyelolithotomy	Removal of stone through wall of renal pelvis	Calculus in pelvis	Urinary fistula	Precautionary drain to kidney	Shortened from 4th day but is not removed until urinary leak has ceased

Operation	Description	Indications	Complications	Drainage	Management
Pyeloplasty	Removal of excessive portion of pelvis after obstruction has been relieved	Hydronephrosis	Urinary fistula	Precautionary drain and nephrostomy catheter	Shortened from 4th day but is not removed until urinary leak has ceased
Uretero-lithotomy	Removal of stone from ureter	Stone	Urinary fistula	Precautionary drain to site of ureteric opening	Shortened from 4th day but is not removed until urinary leak has ceased
Nephrostomy	Catheter drainage through body of kidney	Ureteric obstruction	Haemorrhage Urinary fistula	(a) catheter (b) probably additional precautionary drain	(a) Syphon or straight drainage to bedside bottle. All urine to be measured (b) Remove at 48 hours
Ureteric transplantation	Division of ureters from bladder and implantation into sigmoid colon	For bladder defects Tuberculous cystitis As part of total cystectomy Congenital ectopia vesicae	Peritonitis Urinary fistula Pyelonephritis Anuria	(a) precautionary drain (b) indwelling rectal catheter	(a) Remove by shortening from 4th day (b) Initially to prevent collection of urine in rectum. Usually retained for 1 week

the injured kidney has been exposed the surgeon passes his hand over the opposite side to confirm the presence of a second kidney. Blood transfusion will be required.

Bleeding tissues behind the peritoneum produces severe shock, and by interference with the nerve supply to the mesentery is sometimes responsible for paralytic ileus. The patient with a severely injured kidney is therefore in great danger not only from loss of blood but from shock and ileus.

In the immediate post-operative period the patient should be kept quite flat. A Ryle's tube should be inserted into the stomach and oral feeding not resumed for 48 hours after operation. The blow which has injured the kidney has in all probability bruised or torn the diaphragm. There may be an additional fracture of ribs. The development of basal pleurisy and collapse of the lower part of the lung are very likely complications. If respiratory movements are painful on account of rib or muscle damage, adhesive strapping may be applied around the lower ribs on one side to give support.

Injury to the ureter usually arises from gun-shot wound or surgical operation on some pelvic organ.

Infection

Perinephric abscess has already been mentioned. Early infection of the perinephric fat (cellulitis) may be controlled by antibiotic treatment and operation avoided. If an abscess forms it is almost certain that open drainage will be required. The kidney itself may be undamaged, but its function will be diminished temporarily.

Hydronephrosis (Fig. 36.2) is dilatation of the pelvis, and distension of the kidney due to obstruction in the ureter. Infection may supervene with the formation of pus within the kidney (**pyonephrosis**). This condition requires drainage by open operation. As kidney function recovers urine will escape from the drainage tube and the urinary fistula will persist if the original obstruction to the ureter is still present. Nephrectomy is then necessary.

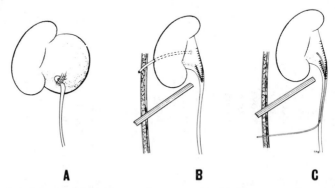

A   **B**   **C**

Fig. 36.2   A large hydronephrosis (**A**) is sometimes treated by nephrectomy or by a plastic operation (**B**) to reduce its size and relieve the obstruction. Oedema of the pelvis will most likely produce temporary obstruction to the opening of the ureter and the pelvis must be drained by a nephrostomy (**B**), or ureterostomy *in situ* (**C**) where a narrow plastic catheter splints the new join.

Occasionally it is possible to aspirate[1] the pus from pyonephrosis, and when the acute stage has passed nephrectomy is performed. Pyonephrosis may be bilateral in cases where there has been prolonged obstruction in the lower urinary tract (bladder and urethra) from prostatic growth or congenital urethral obstruction: the obstruction also requires surgical treatment.

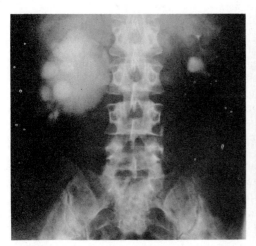 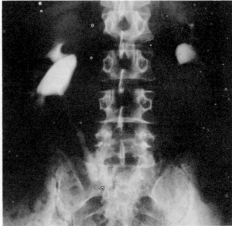

Fig. 36.3   Intravenous pyelogram showing gross right hydronephrosis before and one year after operation. The kidney was drained post-operatively by 'ureterostomy *in situ*' (Fig. 36.2).

Tuberculosis of the urinary tract usually starts in the kidney and spreads to the bladder, prostate, seminal vesicles and epididymis. Full sanatorium treatment is required, but if the tuberculosis process appears to be confined almost entirely to one side, removal of the affected kidney and ureter may be undertaken, but long-term chemotherapy and 'sanatorium' type general treatment is needed. The infection usually comes as a blood-borne spread from a tuberculous lesion in the lung.

Neoplasm

Wilm's tumour (nephroblastoma, embryoma) is an extremely malignant growth which occurs in babies. It is treated by nephrectomy, radiotherapy, and chemotherapy. As it arises in the embryonic tissue it is sometimes bilateral.

Hypernephroma is a carcinoma of the kidney tubules occurring in adults and, like the Wilm's tumour, it is frequently a fatal condition owing to the rich blood supply of the kidney and the ease with which blood-borne metastasis can occur. The condition is treated by nephrectomy.

[1] The procedure requires the same apparatus as for paracentesis abdominis (page 492, Ascites).

Epithelioma (carcinoma) arises from the renal pelvis and rarely produces a large tumour. It is usually discovered by full investigation of a case of haematuria.

Innocent epithelial growths—**papilloma**—are common in the ureter and bladder. They are treated by excision, or by destruction by diathermy (fulguration). They are very liable to recur and become seeded into the rest of the urinary tract. Occasionally an innocent papilloma becomes malignant (epithelioma, squamous cell carcinoma).

Renal hypertension

When kidney tissue is damaged from repeated infection, it is liable to produce a chemical which has an effect on the blood pressure throughout the body. Resultant hypertension produces enlargement of the heart, damage to the eyes and to the arteries.

Many cases of hypertension are therefore submitted to full urological investigation. If one kidney is healthy and the other one diseased, it is likely that the case is one of **renal hypertension** and nephrectomy may result in a permanent lowering of the blood pressure to normal.

Narrowing of a renal artery by atheroma may produce ischaemia and this in turn leads to hypertension. The artery can be shown on x-ray by passing a catheter up the aorta from the femoral artery and injecting hypaque (**renal arteriography**).

Renal calculus

Stones may form at any point in the urinary tract (page 632) and their development is frequently associated with infection. Excessive concentration of the urine is one of the known causes and this accounts for the frequent occurrence of renal calculus in tropical countries. Certain metabolic disorders result in the production of stones.

A renal calculus produces its symptoms by obstructing part of the renal tract—a calyx, the renal pelvis, or the ureter. Severe renal colic is usually due to the presence of a stone and if this becomes impacted in the junction of the ureter and pelvis, hydronephrosis results. A stone can be removed by opening the renal pelvis, but sometimes it is necessary to split the kidney if the stone is growing in the solid portion (Fig. 36.1). If the stone passes down the ureter, it may be extruded into the bladder and subsequently voided with the urine. On the other hand, it may become jammed in the lower end of the ureter (Fig. 36.4). It is then removed by incision into the dilated part of the ureter, which is usually approached through a muscle-splitting incision in the iliac fossa.

A precautionary rubber drain is always left in position after the urinary tract has been opened for the removal of a stone.

Unfortunately small portions of calculus may break off and act as seedlings upon which a subsequent stone forms. Nephrectomy is sometimes necessary if the kidney is filled with stone (Fig. 36.5).

If, following a pelvic operation, or indeed following any abdominal operation, suspicion arises (from the smell) that urine is escaping from the wound, the attention of the medical staff must be drawn to the matter immediately. If there is any doubt about the nature of the escaping fluid, some of it may be collected and sent to the laboratory to be tested for urea. Alternatively an intravenous injection of methylene blue may be given (page 644). The dye will be excreted by the kidney, and if the escaping fluid contains urine the blue dye will be seen at the same time as it appears in urine which is passed naturally.

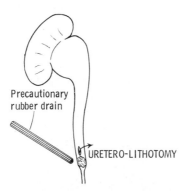

Fig. 36.4   Obstruction of the ureter has been produced by the impaction of the stone formed in the kidney. The stone is extracted through an incision into the ureter. The ureter is carefully repaired and a tube left in position in case of leakage. The tube is subsequently withdrawn by repeated shortening.

Ureteric transplantation

The ureter may be injured during operations in the lower abdomen, particularly in those for cancer of the uterus, vagina or rectum. If the injury is discovered at the time of operation, the ureter is completely divided and re-implanted into the wall of the bladder. A drainage tube is always inserted down to the site of implantation to guard against extravasation of urine following the operation.

Urinary diversion

(a) **Uretero-colic anastomosis.** For certain congenital abnormalities and for cancer, the bladder is completely removed. This involves transplantation of the ureters into the rectum or sigmoid colon. The operation is sometimes undertaken in stages to lessen the risk of renal failure, which is very considerable if both ureters are transplanted on the same occasion.

Patients who have ureters transplanted into the colon are able to lead perfectly normal lives although they are liable to recurrent renal infection.

Pre-operative treatment must include a full course of sulpha drugs or streptomycin for bowel sterilisation (page 551). For 24 hours before operation, a urinary antiseptic drug will be administered in addition.

Post-operatively, very careful observation must be kept for the passage of urine through the rectum. Oedema of the ureter at the point of anastomosis frequently produces complete obstruction for 24 to 48 hours so that no urine is passed in this period. As soon as the urine begins to flow freely, inflammation of the rectal mucosa may occur and become quite troublesome. The frequent desire to pass the urine from the inflamed rectum may be very distressing and at the same time an indwelling rectal tube may not be tolerated. In the majority of cases the rectum becomes acclimatised to its new function in about 2 weeks. The patient is instructed to empty the bowel at set times and at gradually increasing intervals, but should not attempt to wait until he experiences a desire to void urine.

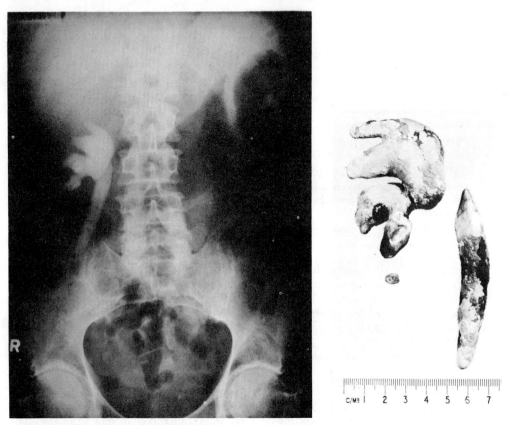

Fig. 36.5   Massive renal calculus forming a 'cast' of the pelvis and ureter. (*Left*) Plain radiograph. (*Right*) Stone removed at operation.

Because of the initial inflammation, the rectum becomes irritable, and if *routine* regular emptying is not instituted at the beginning, incontinence occurs and the patient will be greatly discouraged. A mildly antiseptic barrier cream should be smeared on the peri-anal skin and a pad of absorbent cotton wool retained in position with a T-bandage or diaper until the patient has gained complete confidence in his control.

Many surgeons recommend the continuous use of small doses of urinary antiseptic following transplantations. 0·5 G sulphadimidine taken at bedtime and in the morning is sufficient to prevent recurrence of pyelitis in the majority of cases. If, in spite of this, acute pyelitis occurs, the patient must be kept in bed and a rectal catheter left in place for 2 or 3 days to ensure continuous drainage.

(b) Urinary ileostomy. Ileo-cutaneous ureterostomy The large bowel, when used as a urinary reservoir, tends to permit absorption back into the blood of certain excretory products. If the anal sphincter mechanism is faulty as in paraplegia, clearly uretero-colic anastomosis would be useless. In such cases a loop of ileum about 25 cm long is isolated with its own section of mesentery. The divided bowel is rejoined to establish intestinal continuity; one end of the isolated loop is closed and the other end brought through the abdominal wall as an ileostomy. The ureters are severed from the bladder and implanted into this conduit (Fig. 36.6). The kidneys are thus protected from back-pressure and infection and the patient is absolutely 'dry'. An ileostomy bag with a tap is worn as a receptable. The patient usually takes a small daily dose of urinary antiseptic. This operation is of particular value for children with congenital spinal paralysis (page 869).

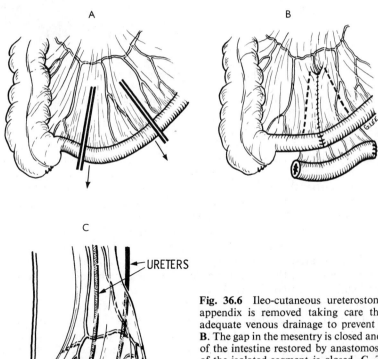

Fig. 36.6 Ileo-cutaneous ureterostomy. **A.** The appendix is removed taking care that there is adequate venous drainage to prevent congestion. **B.** The gap in the mesentry is closed and continuity of the intestine restored by anastomosis; one end of the isolated segment is closed. **C.** The divided ureters may be included in the closure of the end of the bowel segment or implanted separately. The free end of the 'loop' is brought through the abdominal wall and everted to form a mucosa-covered spout.

As the operation is performed most commonly on paraplegic patients who have no rectal sensation, there is usually severe chronic constipation. At least a week of intensive bowel preparation with enemas, laxatives and neostigmine is required. If at operation the surgeon finds the colon full of faecal masses the operation is made extremely difficult. Finally, the bowel is sterilised before operation by oral chemotherapy (Streptomycin and Neomycin). A self-retaining catheter is left in the bladder for the operation, and a rectal tube is strapped in position to allow full deflation of the lower bowel.

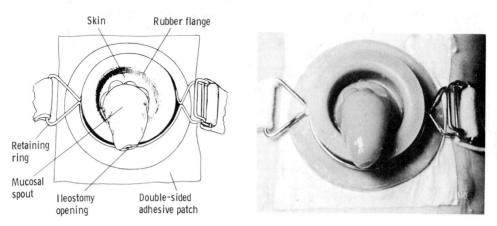

Fig. 36.7   Typical ileostomy spout. In this case it has been constructed to drain the ureters. A rubber or plastic bag is fitted over the flange.

Post-operative care involves all those observations required after a major abdominal operation. There is a risk of ileus and peritonitis, and of renal complications. Initial collection of urine from the ileostomy spout is by adhesive transparent bag so that the condition of the spout can be inspected readily. If the protruding bowel is purple (cyanosed), or if it sinks back into the abdomen, this must be reported immediately.

A latex catheter (Foley without inflation of balloon) may be left in the ileal conduit to ensure free drainage. Sometimes ureteric catheters are left in the ureters and threaded down through the ileal segment cut into the bag. Such catheters may be expelled by spontaneous movement of the loop. Urine should drain freely soon after operation and may be blood-stained for two to three days.

A stab drain is usually placed in the left iliac fossa to prevent collection of urine in the peritoneum if there is leakage from the junction of ureters to ileum. This may discharge urine for the first few days and is removed by shortening when the flow ceases.

Abdominal distension is common and an enema may be needed early, since the patient is often chronically constipated. Sometimes.the stoma becomes oedematous but this subsides provided the flange is not too tight. Care must be taken to avoid the weight of bed clothes on the stoma, and a bed cradle is advisable.

The natural bladder will not have been removed in paraplegics, but may have been if the operation is for bladder cancer. A residual bladder may accumulate infected mucus and inflammatory exudate for a while. A catheter should be passed and the bladder washed out gently on the third day and this is repeated if there is a urethral discharge.

The patient will now have to be taught the care of stoma and detailed routine for ensuring a satisfactory control with her appliance (see below).

Urinary diversion may be achieved by using a segment of the sigmoid colon instead of ileum. The same principles apply and after-care is similar.

The operation has involved considerable re-arrangement of structures within the abdomen and certain specific considerations may arise apart from those at risk with all abdominal surgery.

These are:

1. Intestinal obstruction from internal herniation, adhesions or volvulus.
2. Prolapse of stoma.
3. Retraction of stoma.
4. Strangulation of stoma (purple).
5. Retention of urine in stoma.
6. Intra-peritoneal leakage of urine.
7. Peritonitis from intestinal leakage.
8. Haemorrhage from intestinal loop or ureters.
9. Acute pyelitis.

Long-term management of urinary ileostomy

This is similar to the care of a colostomy or ileostomy performed for ulcerative colitis, but there are important differences. The greatest problems arise when this operation has to be performed on patients with severe spine and chest deformity from paralysis, as the abdominal wall provides little space for the appliance.

Perhaps the first requirement is for the patient to realise that this operation is not at all uncommon, and there are literally thousands of people with an ileostomy, either bringing the water to the surface or, in certain diseases of the bowel, bringing the bowel contents to the surface similarly. With adequate routine care and meticulous attention to detail an individual can lead a normal life as far as toilet management is concerned. There are many variations in the design of applicances used to collect the urine. The majority of these are held in place by an adhesive or special form of glue. Some adults manage without any adhesive, but the majority of children with spina bifida also have a disability of the legs which gives them excessive rocking movements of the trunk when they walk. This makes it difficult to keep the appliance in place. A rubber cap to replace the bag is provided for bathing or swimming.

We can consider the management under four headings:

1. The care of the spout and the surrounding skin.
2. Types of appliance.
3. The method of applying the apparatus and holding it in place.
4. The care of equipment.

The care of the stoma

Immediately after operation the spout is somewhat swollen, but it shrinks and should normally be a bright red colour with a slightly rough moist surface. Sometimes it is an active contracting spout moving and ejecting a stream of urine every few seconds. This is the ideal. Occasionally it may 'prolapse'. That means it will lengthen and become too big and cumbersome. The size and movement and variation in length of the stoma is to some extent dependent on the amount of abdominal muscle that is active. Some paraplegics have weak abdominal muscles and the stoma tends to prolapse. Others have very powerful tight abdominal muscles which are inclined to obstruct the outlet and when the surgeon makes the hole in the abdominal wall he has to make quite certain that it is big enough to prevent the muscle nipping the stoma. If the protruding piece of intestine becomes damaged it will develop raw patches which bleed or have a white patch rather like a scab on the skin. This can occur from infection, or from rubbing on the rubber bag. The management of this condition is to put a little antiseptic ointment (framycetin, soframycin) around the stoma inside the flange. The doctor may prescribe an antibiotic or chemical which will be passed in the urine and act as a constant sterilising agent. If the skin around the stoma becomes very sore or ulcerated it may be necessary to abandon the apparatus for a few days and for pads to be worn, but this very rarely occurs once the skin has become accustomed to the sticky patches.

Appliances

These are supplied through a hospital supplies department or on prescription from the family doctor. There are various recognised manufacturers and each produces a 'set'. A typical lightweight appliance is shown in Fig. 36.8. A patient must have at least two complete sets of apparatus so that one may be 'in the wash' and one in use. The essential parts of the appliance are:

1. The bag, which may be rubber, nylon or PVC with a turn-tap or a screw stopper at the end. More recent models have a sliding 'tap' which is unhygienic as it remains wet externally.

2. A flange. The bag is applied to the abdominal wall either directly or by being attached to the rubber or plastic flange. The flange has the merit of protecting the stoma from friction or injury from pressure.

3. An adhesive patch which is sticky on both sides and joins either the flange to the abdominal skin or, in the case of a bag used without a flange, the surface of the bag to the skin.

4. A retaining belt which may be made of webbing with a buckle to attach it to the bag, or to the flange; sometimes, particularly if the abdomen is a difficult shape, a two-way stretch miniature girdle is used with a buttonhole to fit over the flange before the bag is attached.

There is no such thing as a standard appliance suitable for everyone and often the most satisfactory compromise is achieved by using some parts from one manufacturer and others of a different make.

The bags. Some patients prefer opaque rubber bags and find these entirely satisfactory. The standard bag is stretched over the rubber or plastic but with a new bag this might be a difficult manoeuvre. Disposable plastic bags are intended for use without a flange by direct application with a double-sided patch, but they may also be used with a flange instead of a rubber bag. The advantage of course is that they are less likely to become infected, and smell is avoided. Some patients whose skin is allergic to rubber cannot tolerate the rubber bag or flange: the plastic bags produce less reaction. Unfortunately, they are not as robust as rubber bags and often leak. Some disposable bags have a Karaya gum seal washer at the neck which helps to prevent leakage.

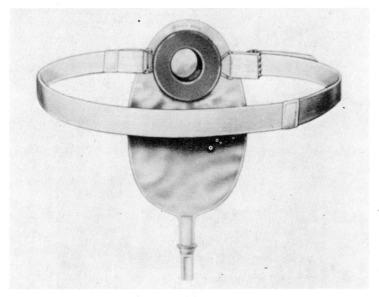

Fig. 36.8   Mitcham urinary ileostomy appliance with disposable bag. (Down Bros.)

Lightweight-black rubber bags are also available for use without a flange, the bag carrying its own flexible and self-adhesive base.

Various sizes of bags are available and for patients who have a high night output a large bag is preferable, or an outlet spout may be connected by a tube to a bedside bottle.

Disposable plastic bags and some of the latex type of rubber bags have an internal sheath in the form of a funnel which is meant to prevent splash-back from the main container.

There is no need for the spout to be covered when the patient is in the bath, but for swimming, or if the patient prefers for a normal bath, a thin latex cap can be provided to fit over the flange for a short period.

Patients who are confined to a wheelchair sometimes find that the bag folds up in the groin and such patients manage best with a double-chambered bag similar to a male urinal, the upper chamber being smaller and draining through the neck of variable length into the main bag which is on the thigh or at the side of the wheelchair.

It is recommended that a teaspoonful of 1 per cent chlorohexidine (hibitane) solution be placed in the bag when it is applied to the flange as this amount of antispetic discourages the rapid growth of germs in the urine that has been passed.

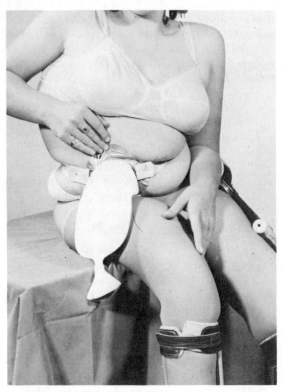

Fig. 36.9   Urinary ileostomy in a paraplegic patient. This illustrates the difficulty in retaining a leak proof attachment of the appliance, particularly in obese patients. With care and instruction, however, this can be made completely reliable. The principal problem is that the patient finds it difficult without a mirror to see what she is doing when applying the flange.

When a **flange** is used this may be made of rubber with a soft backing which is flexible, or it may be rigid or semi-rigid plastic. The latter is less liable to lift at the edges but requires a very flat area of skin for satisfactory application. For patients who have weakness of their hands and have difficulty in stretching the bag over the flange when the latter is already attached to the abdomen, the Russell screw flange is used. In this the flange itself is threaded and the bag is stretched over the separate threaded holder: thus an individual can have several bags already attached to screw fittings which she can change as necessary without having to seek assistance.

Adhesives. The less expensive and most commonly used is the double-sided zinc oxide patch. These very rarely produce skin irritation but the adhesive on these varies from batch to batch and old stock becomes dry. *Stomaseals* and similar plastic transparent adhesive patches produce less skin reaction and are preferred by some patients. There are also small kidney-shaped patches used to reinforce the initial patch by being applied over the edge of the flange, creating a sort of adhesive sandwich: these are waterproof and adhere on one side only. Alternatively waterproof *Elastoplast* from a reel can be used. Some patients find waterproof adhesive strapping useful in addition when trouble is experienced with keeping the flange in place. The Chiron Seal single-sided patches are particularly easy to use for this purpose. *Stomahesive* is a soft plastic material supplied in squares to use sandwiched between the skin and the standard patch: it adheres to moist or perspiring surfaces (Fig. 36.7).

Belts. Reference has already been made to the variety of belt which may be tried. Under no circumstances must the belt be too tight or it may produce pressure sores over the iliac crest or lumbar spine. If a narrow webbing belt is used it may help to place under it a 6 cm (3 inches) wide strip of thin plastic foam which will discourage the webbing from slipping and also prevent it causing friction sores. Additional security may be given by the provision of a small two-way stretch girdle, or specially constructed belt which is placed over the flange before the bag is attached. Belts are now supplied with *Velcro* fastenings to allow any amount of adjustment in tension.

Technique of application

Well illustrated booklets are supplied by the manufacturers on how to apply the particular apparatus. Each patient finds personal points which help in the application and reliability of the appliance. With the type which has a flange independent from the bag, the flange itself should remain unchanged for up to a week if the method of application is satisfactory. Each morning and evening the bag will be removed and the alternate bag applied after cleansing the stoma and the area within the flange with wet cotton wool. No antiseptic should be used unless this has been specifically prescribed by the doctor. Those patients who use a Karaya gum washer will replace it at this point. Care must be taken to ensure that when the bag is stretched over the flange it is attached in such a position as to hang vertically during the day, and over towards the right side at night if the patient habitually sleeps flat or on her right side.

The bag which has been removed should be washed thoroughly with warm soapy water, rinsed and then hung up to dry with one teaspoonful of 1 per cent Hibitane solution in it. The tap must of course be open for the washing-out process and closed when the bag is hung with the Hibitane in it. It is a mistake to use a strong antiseptic, which not only injures the material from which the bag is made, but impregnates it and eventually irritates the patient's skin.

The most difficult operation is the changing of the flange weekly or as often as it becomes necessary. If a one-piece disposable apparatus is used without a flange some of the following remarks cannot apply.

When the used bag and flange have been removed the skin must be cleaned thoroughly and all trace of adhesive removed with a solvent—acetone or a substitute for it.

To keep the skin dry and to prevent urine flowing on it during the process of attaching the adhesive patches, and depending on the size of the spout, an inverted egg-cup or small table-napkin ring may be found useful, or a small piece of cotton wool placed on the stoma may be adequate to absorb any urine that emerges, and it does not matter if this small piece of cotton wool goes into the bag as it is applied. It might, of course, block the outlet, but can be displaced by tipping the end of the bag.

If a spray or liquid adhesive is used this must be allowed to dry fairly well before the first double-sided patch is applied. When a one-piece apparatus is used without an independent adhesive or patch the stoma is inserted into the hole in the bag, which is then pressed firmly onto the skin avoiding air bubbles or wrinkles.

If the patient is paraplegic the apparatus is best applied with the patient lying flat and the abdominal wall relaxed. This means that the patient must arrange the pillows to support her head so that she can see without actively raising the head and shoulders and thus displacing the abdominal wall. Those who have adequate balance either by leaning against a table, or a wall, in front of a mirror often find it more satisfactory to apply the apparatus this way (Fig. 36.9).

Having worked out an exact technique each patient should have the steps of the procedure clearly written down. It is particularly important that the patient should learn to assemble every item required before starting to change and to have everything within easy reach.

Causes of leakage

After operation the skin beneath the patch continues to perspire and it may be some weeks before the sweat glands under the patch cease to function. Apart from this initial problem, leakage may arise from inflammation or excoriation of the skin, and under these circumstances it may be necessary for pads and nappies to be worn until the skin has healed. Very often, spraying the skin with Nobecutane or Octaflex will exclude the air and allow the patch to adhere whilst the skin heals beneath the patch.

Otherwise leakage is usually due to one of the following causes:

1. Failure to dry the skin before application of the first patch.
2. Allowing mucus or urine to wet the surface of the patch before the flange or second patch is attached.
3. Wrinkles in the patches.
4. Careless application of the bag to the flange causing a displacement of the flange and the patches, or a failure of the seal between the bag and the flange due to over-stretching of the rubber or inadequate application of the plastic bag.
5. Insufficient care being taken to press the air out of the bag, after it has been applied to the flange, with the tap open—not forgetting to shut the tap again. If a disposable no-tap bag is used the air must be expelled before the bag is applied.
6. Repeatedly allowing the bag to overfill so that the flange is constantly immersed in urine. The additional weight of the bag tends to cause separation.
7. Leakage of the bag, which again may be caused by allowing it to be overstretched, by pinpricks, or because it is too old. Plastic bags tend to break at the seams.

If the skin round the stoma becomes sore a period without the use of the appliance is essential. Under direction by the doctor or nurse, a Foley catheter may be passed into the stoma with the bag inflated to less than 5 ml; sometimes effective drainage into the bag through a catheter will enable the patient to remain in bed and keep completely dry.

Watching for complications

A spout whose layers have not become firmly stuck together may vary greatly in length from day to day and may in fact retract completely and a little later, after coughing or straining, may protrude to a finger's length. This does not matter provided the stoma remains sufficiently short to prevent it getting damaged. At least it means that there is no obstruction in the abdominal wall. If the spout becomes purple this is a sign of interference with its blood supply and medical assistance must be sought. The blood vessels to the stoma may be twisted inside the abdomen so that this complication can arise without there being an obstruction to the outflow of water. If it is noted that there are long periods of say half an hour or more when no urine is ejected from the spout it is likely that there is obstruction in the abdominal wall; this is one of the complications which occur particularly in an active child with good abdominal muscles. The surgeon will determine the tightness of the opening by inserting a finger through the mouth of the stoma. It should be possible for an index finger to pass right through the abdominal wall. Alternatively he may insert a large catheter which also enables him to find out if there is any appreciable amount of urine retained in the loop.

A dusky coloration or pallor of the spout, associated with abdominal pain and sometimes distension, is an indication for immediate surgical advice as it is likely that something has become twisted inside the abdomen. Such an event is occasionally produced by constipation and this must be avoided. Straining to evacuate the bowels is bad for the ileostomy as it encourages the development of prolapse.

Bleeding is usually from the surface of the stoma due to injury but it can occur from severe infection, the blood coming either from the kidney or a piece of bowel. If it continues for more than a day, or if it is accompanied by pain in the loin, medical advice should be sought.

Pyelitis or infection of the kidneys can occur in any of these patients just as it can in a normal individual. Those whose kidneys have already been damaged and dilated by previous urinary obstruction and infection are naturally more prone to further infection after diversion than those whose urinary tract has always been healthy. On the other hand, once the obstruction has been removed by a diversion operation, patients who were previously liable to recurrent obstructions may now remain free from them and x-ray examination will show a remarkable degree of recovery in their kidneys, in their shape and function.

The risk of infection cannot, however, be ignored, and unless a really adequate flow of urine comes through the conduit all the time, bacteria will multiply in the piece of bowel and sooner or later affect the kidney. Times of particular danger from this point of view are:

1. During any febrile illness such as measles, mumps or gastritis.
2. During or after a long journey when insufficient fluid has been taken.
3. During holidays at the seaside or under conditions of excessive exposure to the sun.
4. In hospital admissions for orthopaedic or other operations in the immediate post-operative period, particularly if there is vomiting.

The Bladder. If the operation of urinary diversion has been carried out on an adult in the treatment of bladder disease, then the natural bladder may be removed altogether. In children with paraplegia, however, the bladder is usually left behind and occasionally an accummulation of fluid occurs within it when the urine is no longer passing through. The natural bladder has no normal secretion but mucus from the urethra, and in the male from the prostatic glands, may accummulate and become infected. After operation the latter is washed out several times by means of a catheter, but if subsequently there is apparently a discharge from the urethra, medical advice must be sought. Accummulation of fluid within the natural bladder will not occur if the urinary obstruction that was present before the diversion has been adequately dealt with.

Summary

In surgical cases involving the kidney or ureter, there is inevitably, for many, a long period of investigation. Otherwise the pre-operative nursing includes the procedures adopted for all abdominal surgery. In the post-operative phase the risks and complications are those common to other types of abdominal surgery with the additional hazard of renal failure or urinary fistula. Post-operative nursing observation is of supreme importance in the management of catheters and drainage tubes. Incompetent observation may mislead the surgeon and result in prolonged disability or death from renal failure.

A descriptive booklet, 'The Management of Urinary Ileostomy', explaining the purpose and care of the urinary stoma for patients and parents of child patients is available from the Ileostomy Association.

37

Adrenal Glands

These two flat yellow glands are attached to the upper poles of the kidneys lying up against the diaphragm. The right gland is behind the liver and the left one is behind the stomach. The adrenal glands produce several hormones.

Physiology

The central portion of the glands, the **medulla** produces two principal hormones, the catechol amines **adrenaline** and **noradrenaline**. These have different effects. Broadly they simulate the activity of the sympathetic nervous system. 'Adrenergic receptors' are the sites responding to these chemicals and are of two types. **Alpha** receptors respond to noradrenaline mainly and **beta** receptors respond to both adrenaline and noradrenaline. The combined effect of both noradrenaline and adrenaline may therefore be mainly **beta** stimulation. The general vascular bed responds to adrenergic drugs; alpha receptors constrict and beta receptors dilate. Excessive beta stimulation therefore may produce peripheral vasodilatation and a state of shock without pallor. **Isoprenaline** is a synthetic drug with pure beta response.

Alpha **blockers** are thus drugs which prevent the effect of noradrenaline and to some extent adrenaline. Beta blockers inhibit adrenaline effects principally. Phenoxybenzamine (long acting) (Dibenyline) and phentolamine (short acting) (Rogitine) are alpha blockers. Propranolol (Inderal) and practolol (Eraldin) are beta blockers. Hormone-producing medullary tumours may produce adrenaline or noradrenaline.

These details of adrenal physiology are included because the use of alpha and beta blocking drugs in management of shock and other conditions is increasing greatly (page 111).

The **cortex** or outer portion of the gland produces steroid hormones which control the metabolism of carbohydrate, nitrogen and electrolyte balance. Cortisone is the predominant hormone but there are androgen and oestrogen substances as well. The development of the adrenal gland is under the control of the pituitary. Adrenocorticotrophic hormone (ACTH) from the pituitary circulating in the blood determines the output of cortisone. In times of stress from injury or infection the body requires more cortisone and if for any reason the adrenal glands are not functioning properly collapse may occur (page 92). In very young children who suffer from acute septicaemic conditions such as meningogoccal meningitis, haemorrhage occurs into the adrenal glands and death ensue (Friderichsen-Waterhouse syndrome). Adrenal insufficiency is therefore a very real problem in modern surgery. This is why cortisone is sometimes a life-saving drug in grave states of collapse. Cortisone has to be given by mouth if the pituitary has been removed, as for instance for the treatment of advanced malignant disease of the breast.

The nitrogen-retaining 'body-building' effect of certain steroids allied to testosterone (the natural adrenal product) is used to speed up weight-gain in convalescence, to stimulate growth and to overcome osteoporosis (decalcification of bone) in the elderly.

The relationship of the adrenals to the sex glands is confusing. Androgen and oestrogen are antagonistic, but the normal balance of production is disturbed by disease, surgery or hormone medication. Testosterone is produced in the adrenal and testes. If the testes are removed (castration), as for instance in the treatment of carcinoma of the prostate, oestrogen from the adrenal predominates and the male develops breast enlargement and a loss of body hair—effects similar to those produced by administration of stilboestrol.

If the ovaries are removed, adrenal androgens predominate but there is still oestrogen production in the adrenals, hence the need for adrenalectomy or suppression by prednisolone if oestrogen production is to be stopped.

Aldosterone is the mineralo-corticosteroid produced in these glands and is responsible for the control of sodium, potassium and water balance. Excessive production leads to sodium retention and oedema. In Addison's disease, the resultant electrolyte balance is often fatal due to salt depletion.

Sometimes the adrenal glands grow too big—adrenal hyperplasia—and if this occurs in a boy it produces the premature development of adult sex features—the so-called infant Hercules—and similarly premature puberty and virilism in a girl. If the condition arises in a female foetus early the baby may be born with 'male' external genitalia—pseudo-hermaphroditism.

Adrenal overactivity produces Cushing's syndrome—excessive hair growth on the face and body—obesity and hypertension (Fig. 37.1). This in a woman leads to virilism or masculination.

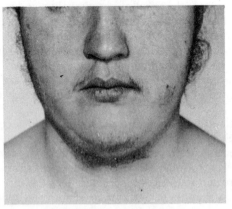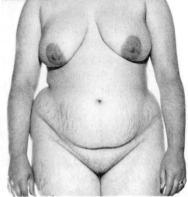

Fig. 37.1 Cushing's syndrome. Virilism in a female patient who has developed an adrenal tumour. Note the great increase in body and facial hair and heavy striae on the abdomen.

Tuberculosis of the adrenal gland or other lesions destroying their function leads to Addison's disease—skin pigmentation, hypotension and renal failure. There is gross salt depletion (lack of aldosterone). The pigmentation may be due to failure of the glands to manufacture adrenaline of which the pigment melanin is a chemical precursor.

Tumours of medulla

Because the medullary tissue stains in microscopical sections with particular chemicals it is known as **chromaffin** tissue. Ectopic 'seeds' of adrenal tissue are sometimes found along the course of the ovarian or testicular blood vessels, in the inguinal canal or even in the wall of the bladder. A tumour of medullary tissue is called **phaeochromocytoma**. Adrenaline and noradrenaline and their presence is usually detected by the occurrence of a very high blood pressure coming in attacks with shivering and a high pulse rate. Such attacks have been associated with bladder voiding in the case of ectopic tumours. Extensive chemical tests are carried out on the urine before the diagnosis can be made. As a result of long-term overproduction of vasoconstrictive hormone the peripheral circulatory pool has an artificially low capacity. When the tumour is removed, sudden withdrawal of this hormone may result in hypovolaemic shock—that is, a sudden reduction in the rate of venous return to the heart. During operation a continuous intravenous infusion is maintained so that appropriate amounts of alpha and beta blocker, or conversely of noradrenaline, may be given to maintain a correct blood pressure. This infusion has to be continued with drugs 'at the ready' in the immediate post-operative period.

Tumours arising within the adrenal gland produce mainly adrenaline because cortisol from the cortex is needed for the final stage in producing *adrenaline*. Tumours arising from ectopic adrenal tissue produce mainly *noradrenaline*. In the local adrenal gland tumour, the patient has paroxysmal tachycardia, sweating and pallor: in the ectopic tumour the symptoms are due to hypertension with a slow pounding heart—the subtle difference between **fast palpitation** and **slow palpitation**.

Operative removal is needed but sometimes malignant tumours cannot be removed completely. At operation the handling of the tumour squeezes hormones into the blood stream, with resultant great changes in blood pressure. To reduce the risk of fatal hypertension, the patient is prepared for several days with adrenergic blocking drugs, mainly alpha blockers (phenoxybenzamine). Practolol (beta blocker) is used to control the heart rate. The management in the post-operative phase is very difficult.

Tumours of the cortex

An adenoma may produce aldosterone which leads to the body retaining sodium and losing potassium. Extreme muscular weakness results, with other chemical disturbance— Conn's syndrome.

Most tumours, benign or malignant, lead to virilism—the development of male characteristics—as occurs with cortical hyperplasia.

In certain cases of cancer of the breast when metastasis has occurred, both adrenal glands are removed in an endeavour to reduce the amount of oestrogen circulating in the blood and this is usually undertaken when oophorectomy—removal of the ovaries—has failed to control the growth. The patient has to be given cortisone continuously to replace gland function. Large doses of prednisolone (a cortisone-like chemical) switch off the pituitary stimulus and treatment has an effect similar to extirpation of both adrenal glands.

Investigations

Reference has already been made to the chemical tests required to verify the diagnosis of a medullary tumour and similarly intricate investigations have to be undertaken where there is a hormone disturbance. This involves analysis of the urine for ketosteroids, the group of chemicals which include the sex hormones. '17-ketosteroid' output will be estimated. These are breakdown products of the hormones and the total gives an estimate of the androgen-oestrogen activity of the glands.

X-ray investigation of the adrenal glands is achieved by injecting air or oxygen into the loose connective tissue spaces behind the peritoneum. The air acts as a contrast medium

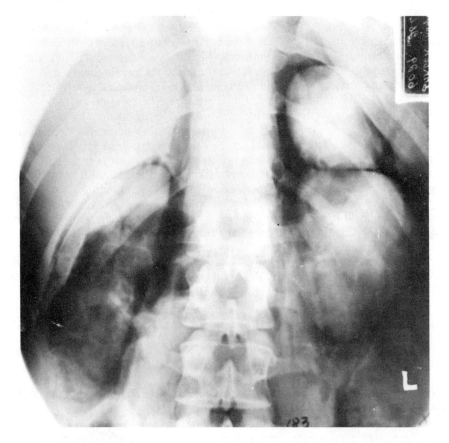

Fig. 37.2 Radiograph showing a normal right kidney and the left kidney surmounted by an adrenal tumour outlined by air injected into the retro-peritoneal tissues through the abdominal wall.

and outlines the kidneys and the suprarenal gland, revealing any enlargement of the glands.

It will be apparent from Table 53 that many metabolic changes occur with adrenal gland dysfunction. The pituitary controls the glands and thus pituitary disorder can produce all these adrenal changes as a secondary effect.

Table 53   Adrenal hormones

	Physiological effect	Excess production	Deficiency
Medulla			
Adrenaline Noradrenaline	Vaso-constrictor maintains vascular tone. Functioning tumour is phaeo-chromocytoma	Hypertensive attacks	Collapse
Cortex (Cortical Steroids)			
Cortisone	Inhibits nitrogen metabo-lism (protein). Maintains carbohydrate (diabeto-genic)	Delays wound healing Glycosuria	Collapse Hypoglycaemia Addisonian crisis
Androgens—Testosterone (also produced in the testes)	Increases nitrogen metabo-lism and skeletal growth Functioning tumour is a carcinoma	In the embryo, pseudo-hermaphroditism* In boys, precocious puberty In girls, precocious puberty and virilism In women, virilism In men and women, Cushing's syndrome	Hypogeni-talism Feminism
Oestrogen (also produced in the ovaries)	Female sex hormone (small fraction of total)	In men, feminisation In women, maintains oestrogen effect after re-moval of ovaries	
Aldosterone—mineralo-corticosteroid	Maintains electrolyte balance	Sodium and water retention leading to hypertension. Potassium depletion leading to myasthenia (weakness)	Addisonian crisis. Salt loss and collapse
	Functioning adenoma produces Conn's syndrome		

* True hermaphroditism or **Intersex** is a chromosome abnormality and is quite different.

Adrenalectomy

The operation may be performed by one of three routes. If the surgeon is removing one gland which is already known to contain a tumour the operation may be similar to a nephrectomy through an incision in the loin.

If both adrenals are to be removed for hyperplasia or in the treatment of breast cancer this may be done with the patient lying on her face, through an incision on each side over the 11th rib which is removed to gain access to the adrenal from above. The pleural space may be entered when this approach is used and then special attention has to be paid to the chest condition post-operatively.

Occasionally both adrenal glands are removed through a midline incision in the abdomen particularly when the operation is being undertaken for breast cancer.

Whichever route is chosen the operation is a severe one and special attention has to be paid to electrolyte balance and to hormone replacement. Frequent blood pressure readings are required; intensive physiotherapy to ensure that there is no collapse of the bases of the lungs is needed early as the diaphragm is in the operation area and the patient will be reluctant to use the muscle fully.

The amount of cortisone, additional salts and other chemicals to be given will be scheduled by the surgeon and the programme must be carried out meticulously.

38

Bladder, Prostate and Urethra

The general principles of surgery in treatment of disorders of the lower urinary tract have already been described. The management of these cases involves the procedures necessary for complete investigation of the urinary tract, while post-operative nursing is largely the management of catheters and drainage tubes. Table 54 indicates the operations most commonly performed on the bladder. Many of these operations are to provide a temporary diversion of the urinary stream to relieve obstruction due to lesions in the urethra, or while plastic operations are being carried out for congenital abnormalities or injuries to the urethra or penis.

The principal symptoms which arise from bladder disorders are described in Chapter 35. Table 48, page 633, indicates the common causes of retention of urine at various levels in the urinary tract. Suprapubic cystostomy is required for many of these in which the obstruction has produced dilatation of the ureters and kidneys (Fig. 38.1).

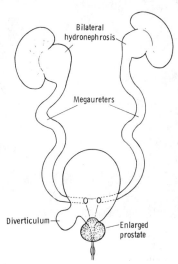

Fig. 38.1 The effect of obstruction at the bladder outlet. The ureters become wide and tortuous. Diverticula form in the wall of the bladder.

Bladder

Congenital abnormality

A gross abnormality sometimes occurs in which the bladder is open on the abdominal wall, owing to a deficiency of the skin and muscle. This condition of **ectopia vesicae** is usually associated with a bony abnormality of the pelvis. The iliac bones are divided at the back in infancy and the open pubic symphysis brought together in an attempt to close

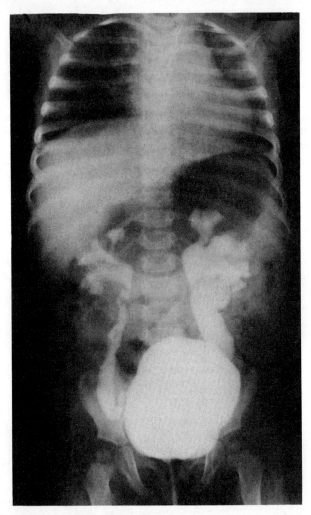

Fig. 38.2 Cystogram of child one year old showing the effects of obstruction to the outlet of the bladder. Both kidneys are grossly dilated and have been filled by reflux of diodone from the bladder. The obstructing muscle bar was excised at 1 year old and the child is very well 6 years later. This x-ray photograph also shows clearly the relation of the gas-filled stomach to the diaphragm and heart. It will be seen that the lung area is relatively small in a child. Breathing is mainly abdominal by diaphragm movement.

Table 54 Operations on the bladder

Operation	Description	Disorder	Special complications	Drainage and Management
Cystostomy	Opening and tube drainage of bladder	Temporary—as preliminary to prostatectomy Permanent—for incurable urethral obstruction	Extravasation of urine	Indwelling catheter to bladder —connection to bedside bottle Precautionary drain to retropubic area —remove at 48 hours
Cystotomy	Opening of bladder for removal of growth, foreign body or stone		Leakage and extravasation	(a) temporary catheter drainage (i.e. cystostomy) (b) urethral catheter and precautionary drain to retropubic area
Cystectomy *Partial* *Total*	Partial removal of bladder Complete removal of bladder	Carcinoma or diverticulum	Haemorrhage and extravasation	If partial cystectomy, as for cystotomy—temporary drainage of bladder and precautionary retropubic drain If total cystectomy—ureteric transplantation will have been performed (page 685)

the bladder. Very rarely is it possible to make the bladder outlet continent and the ureters may be transplanted to the colon or an isolated ileal segment.

There is sometimes a congenital obstruction to the bladder outlet which requires surgical excision. Figure 38.2 shows the effect of such obstruction on the kidneys and ureters, which are damaged in the same way as those of the elderly patient with prostatic enlargement.

Trauma

The bladder may be ruptured by crushing injuries, usually in association with fractures of the pelvic bones. Extravasation of urine occurs into the tissues of the pelvis and abdominal wall; if the tear involves the intraperitoneal portion of the bladder peritonitis ensues. Immediate operation is essential and temporary suprapubic catheter drainage is used to prevent the possibility of distension rupturing the suture line (page 659).

Infection

Infection of the urine may produce only mild and symptomless inflammation of the bladder. In severe infections, there is pain, dysuria and subsequent spread of infection to the kidneys. There is often haematuria.

Severe cystitis sometimes requires repeated irrigations or tidal drainage.

Vesical[1] calculus. Persistent infection may lead to the formation of stone. A small calculus can be removed by means of the lithotrite (page 670), which crushes it. If this is not possible suprapubic cystotomy is performed. Bladder stones are almost always due to chronic urinary obstruction. Stones from the kidney may pass into the bladder and increase greatly in size.

Neoplasm

The lining epithelium of the urinary tract—the renal pelvis, ureters and bladder—is called **urothelium.** It has a peculiar characteristic of producing wart-like growths which 'seed' down the tract. The whole urothelial surface is liable to this change; recurrence is common and 'benign' tumours progress to become malignant.

Papillomas are fern-like structures growing from the bladder wall. They produce haematuria and are diagnosed by cystoscopy. They are destroyed by diathermy applied by a cystoscopic electrode. This is a simple procedure and apart from a slight risk of haemorrhage there is usually no complication. The patient is not detained in hospital for more than 24 hours. Widespread or large but superficial tumours can be treated by inflating the bladder with a special balloon catheter to maintain a pressure of 20 cm water above the diastolic blood pressure for 6 hours. This kills the tumours by producing ischaemia.

Carcinoma may affect the bladder by malignant change occurring in a papilloma or by the development of a malignant ulcer. Small malignant growths are treated by diathermy coagulation. Growths involving the full thickness of the bladder wall require excision or radiation. If the growth is in an area away from the bladder base, **partial cystectomy** is performed. The bladder is repaired: a suprapubic drain is left in place to guard against leakage

[1] Vesical = relating to the bladder, e.g. vesico-colic fistula.

and a urethral catheter is retained for a week. Excision of part of the bladder may involve transplantation of one ureter if the growth is near the ureteric orifice. **Total cystectomy** is necessary if the base is involved and this requires the transplantation of both ureters into the colon or a urinary ileostomy; nursing aspects of these procedures are described on page 685.

Radiotherapy may be used after surgery, or alone. Sometimes cystectomy is performed if growth recurs following radiotherapy. Radon seeds may be planted into the area of the growth in the bladder wall, but the usual form of radiation is with an external source, cobalt or linear accelerator. All forms of radiotherapy produce an intense cystitis which may be extremely troublesome. There is the additional risk that oedema in the wall of the bladder following radiotherapy may lead to blockage of one or both ureters. A complaint of pain in the loin may indicate that this complication has arisen (page 446). Radiotherapy for the bladder almost always produces proctitis (inflammation of the rectum), and diarrhoea may be troublesome. Prednisolone retention enemas are used to relieve the symptoms.

Patients who have had growth in the bladder require regular follow-up examination. This may be done by 'cytological' examination of the urine and by cystoscopy. 'Screening' by cytology is used as a routine method of examination of workers exposed to toxic chemicals known to induce carcinoma of the bladder.

Paralysis

Any disorder which affects the spinal cord, either from congenital abnormality, injury or growth, may result in bladder paralysis. The outlet of the bladder is normally controlled by a sphincter mechanism whose nerve supply is balanced with the nerve supply to the bladder muscle itself. Any interference with this co-ordination results in complete incontinence or in retention. Patients with paraplegia, arising for instance with spina bifida, may suffer from true incontinence or from retention with overflow. In the latter case a small wedge of tissue may be removed from the outlet of the bladder to make it possible for the organ to be emptied by manual pressure applied to the suprapubic region. There is sufficient spasm in the muscle at the bladder outlet to prevent incontinence between the routine manual expression times. Tidal drainage may be needed (page 663).

Paralysis may occur in the course of other nervous disorders and lead to retention or incontinence. A permanent suprapubic cystostomy by catheter drainage was the common method of dealing with this but is not satisfactory. Transplantation of the ureters into the rectum may relieve obstruction and deal with the incontinence, but this is not possible if the nervous control of the anal sphincters is also defective. Incontinence in the male is usually managed by a penile appliance with the type of flange and bag shown in Fig. 38.3. Incontinence in the female is best dealt with by a urinary ileostomy (Fig. 36.8).

Foreign bodies in the bladder

Children, usually from curiosity, and adults suffering from perversions occasionally insert foreign bodies into the urethra. From time to time such objects slip into the bladder inadvertently and have to be removed, usually by suprapubic cystotomy. Their presence may not be discovered until a stone has formed around the object. The patient's guilt may lead to concealment. The hair-clip of the Kirbigrip type is said to be the most common foreign body, and as it is longer than the length of a small girl's urethra it may become lodged in the bladder wall. Unexplained haematuria occurring in children leads to a suspicion of injury having been caused in this way.

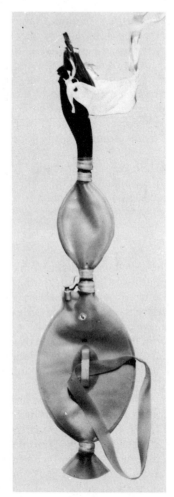

Fig. 38.3 Adult male incontinence appliance with double bag to prevent reflux. (J. G. Franklin & Sons Ltd.)

Post-operative care (also page 671)

Operative procedures on the bladder are always followed by drainage either through a transurethral catheter or suprapubic tube. There is the constant fear of leakage until healing is complete and the drainage must be such that there is no possibility whatever that the pressure rises within the bladder. Similarly care must be taken in the post-operative period to prevent the accumulation of clot within the bladder. If haemorrhage has occurred it is usual for the surgeon to order regular irrigation by means of a simple apparatus of the Riches-Dukes type (Fig. 35.17), or automatic tidal drainage using the 'Cystomat' (page 663). Not more than 60 ml (2 ounces) of irrigating fluid are run in at any one time and the outlet tube must be watched to make quite certain that the fluid escapes (page 664).

Warning has already been given that the large type of metal bladder syringe should never be used by nursing staff (page 661).

Care of suprapubic cystostomy

In the immediate post-operative period, a corrugated rubber drain in the retropubic space may be employed to prevent accumulation of any fluid which may have leaked from the bladder. There may, however, be no such precautionary drainage, the surgeon depending on careful suturing and a tight closure of bladder around the suprapubic catheter. Watch must be kept for signs of spreading cellulitis in the lower abdomen after operation, as this will indicate that extravasation has occurred. The incision usually heals without any trouble and the initial catheter is not changed for at least 10 days after operation.

If the cystostomy has been a temporary measure as a safety valve, the next step is to re-establish normal micturition provided the obstruction has been removed (e.g. hypertrophy of the prostate).

Two methods are employed. The first is to use an indwelling urethral catheter after removal of the suprapubic tube. The abdominal wall is firmly strapped to obliterate, as far as possible, the sinus at the site of catheter. As soon as the abdominal wound is soundly healed the urethral catheter is removed and it is hoped that normal micturition will be resumed. If the obstruction has not been adequately removed the suprapubic fistula will reopen.

An alternative method is to clamp the suprapubic tube for increasing periods from 1 to 4 hours, encouraging natural micturition at the end of this period. Once the normal channel is open and the patient has obtained the necessary control of the sphincter mechanism, the suprapubic tube can be withdrawn. It is likely that the wound in the bladder will be closed by muscle contraction and will heal soundly within a few days. If a urinary fistula persists it is due to infection or persistent obstruction to the outflow through the urethra. The inconvenience of suprapubic leakage from this persistent fistula can be dealt with by the application of an adhesive bag or the reinsertion of a small suprapubic catheter.

When the cystostomy has been performed as a permanent measure in cases of malignant disease of the prostate or in nervous disorders, it is hoped that the fistula between the bladder and the abdominal wall will become lined with epithelium which prevents its natural tendency to close, but a permanent cystostomy is rarely satisfactory.

The suprapubic catheter (usually St Peter's or Harris open-end pattern) is changed weekly and during normal activities it is held in place by a rubber disc with a central sleeve through which the catheter slides to the requisite length within the bladder (Fig. 35.15). A Foley catheter may be used instead but leakage may occur around it. Silicone catheters require less frequent changing.

A patient with a suprapubic cystostomy *must* be instructed in its care, and essential training must be given concerning asepsis and the handling of the catheter and the care of the skin surrounding the fistula. If urinary obstruction has been present for any length of time before the operation it is likely that there will be many diverticula in the walls of the bladder and infection will be well established, with production of mucus and pus. In such cases regular bladder irrigation is necessary when the catheter is changed. This may be performed by the patient with a glass or plastic syringe of the Wardill or Dakin type (sterilised by boiling)—(Fig. 35.16). A weak antiseptic solution (sulphacetamide 1/500 or noxytiolin) is injected very gently down the suprapubic catheter and withdrawn by the suction action of the bulb. This process is repeated several times until the returning fluid is clear. Care must be taken not to inject more than 60 ml (2 ounces) owing to the risk of causing reflux up the ureters and subsequent kidney infection.

If restoration of normal voiding is impossible and the patient is fit for operation, some form of urinary diversion is preferable.

The catheter must never be left out for more than a few hours at a time as its track very soon becomes narrow by the contraction of fibrous tissue around it. When ordering replacement catheters it is essential that one of the correct size should be obtained. If it is too big, insertion will be difficult and pain will be produced with subsequent infection from pressure. If it is too small leakage will occur around it.

There are many types of collection apparatus (urinal) for attachment to the suprapubic catheter. The majority of the receptacle bags are made of rubber with canvas reinforcement and must be kept clean by thorough daily washing with hot soapy water. Polythene disposable bags are available and their use avoids the necessity for the thorough cleansing process which is required with the other types of bag. A teaspoonful of 1 per cent Hibitane placed in the bag after it has been emptied and washed helps to stop decomposition and smell.

Prostate

The prostate gland develops at puberty and surrounds the neck of the male bladder. It is composed of muscle and glandular tissue and the urethra passes through its centre. This prostatic portion of the urethra becomes obstructed by enlargement of the prostate which occurs with the formation of adenomas in the latter years of life. Sometimes the bladder outlet becomes obstructed by a small knob of prostatic tissue protruding inwards underneath the mucous membrane at the base of the bladder. A small 'middle lobe' enlargement is dealt with simply by transurethral resection with diathermy (see Fig. 38.6). The majority of cases of prostatic enlargement require removal of the prostate gland. Removal is only possible because the development of the adenoma has produced a false capsule which enables the surgeon to shell out the offending mass without damaging other surrounding tissues. The prostate is so firmly attached to fascia in the pelvis and has such a rich blood supply that the removal of its true capsule is impossible without the simultaneous removal of the bladder to which it is closely attached. Carcinoma of the prostate is not amenable to surgical treatment for this very reason, though a carcinoma is often found within an enlarged prostate that has been enucleated.

Prostatic hypertrophy

This is the term applied to senile enlargement of the prostate which is by far the most common urological disorder in the adult male. The symptoms are many and varied. There are three clinical types for which the surgical nursing procedures are distinctive.

(1) The irritable bladder type. The presence of a large tumour in the region of the neck of the bladder leads to occasional involuntary leakage of the urine through the sphincter into the prostatic urethra. This initiates the desire to pass water, and the patient's main symptom is frequency. The upward projection of the enlarged gland also prevents complete emptying of the bladder and there is an increasing amount of residual urine (page 641). This adds to the frequency and discomfort. The obstruction in these early cases has been insufficient to produce permanent changes in the bladder, and when the diagnosis has been confirmed by cystoscopic examination the patient is ready to undergo prostatectomy without any period of preliminary treatment.

(2) Acute painful retention. Perhaps following a cold or some other apparently unrelated incident such as operation for hernia, the patient develops acute retention of urine which is painful. On being questioned, such a patient almost invariably gives a history of increasing frequency of micturition and perhaps difficulty in passing his water, but he has regarded the symptoms as 'normal for a man of his age' and has not sought advice until this attack of acute retention. The main problem here is the relief of the acute condition and the majority of surgeons treat such a case by catheterisation. The catheter is left in position for 2 or 3 days. If its removal is followed by persistent retention the prostate is removed by a one-stage operation.

(3) Chronic painless retention with overflow incontinence. Prolonged and increasing back-pressure on the bladder has led to gross distension. The over-distended bladder loses the normal sensation of desire to void: the patient is conscious only of constant dribbling of urine from the urethra and the inability to pass any appreciable quantity of urine except by straining. This patient is usually in great danger from the effect of prolonged retention upon his kidney function. He may in fact seek advice first because of loss of appetite and a general feeling of lassitude, these being the first signs of uraemia.

The condition requires prolonged treatment on account of the renal damage, and removal of the prostate is not undertaken until opportunity has been given for the renal function to improve. If the blood urea is found to be raised there may be an initial period of 2 or 3 weeks urethral catheter drainage or the surgeon may perform an initial suprapubic cystostomy. Prostatectomy is then undertaken as a 'second-stage' operation several weeks later. Very occasionally such patients do not become fit to undergo the second stage and the cystostomy remains permanent.

Complications. Whatever the features of any particular case, the greatest risk is that of infection. This may occur spontaneously or is most likely to follow the passage of catheters or cystoscopes. Some surgeons believe so fervently that catheterisation is impossible without infecting the bladder that they advise emergency prostatectomy in all cases of acute retention due to prostatic enlargement. To those accustomed to more conservative methods, the 'midnight prostatectomy' may seem somewhat unorthodox, but if the patient's condition is in other respects good the emergency prostatectomy eliminates a great deal of wasted time and certainly avoids the risk of infection which is otherwise considerable when urinary obstruction occurs.

If there has been chronic retention there is always the possibility of renal damage. The sudden release of urine from the bladder lowers the pressure in the ureters and pelves of the kidneys so rapidly that bleeding may occur and aggravate the kidney damage. It is however considered wiser to drain the tract completely, as infection is then less likely. A urinary antiseptic is given and great care taken to prevent infection gaining entry along-side the catheter. It is tied in a dressing soaked in Hibitane and placed around the penis to discourage infection.

Pre-operative preparation. Estimation of renal function is determined and other abnormalities in the urinary tract are discovered by excretion pyelography and cystoscopy. Preparations are made for blood transfusion. The genital area must be shaved and thoroughly cleansed. It is usual for the patient to be given chemotherapy for 24 hours preceding operation to reduce the risk of acute urinary infection. The rectum must be empty.

Operation for prostatectomy

The various surgical methods of prostatectomy are illustrated in Figs. 38.4–38.7. There are many modifications of technique and most urologists have their own particular method of after-treatment, but fundamentally the principles are the same in all methods.

1. Suprapubic prostatectomy (Fig. 38.4). A transverse suprapubic incision is usual, the bladder having been distended previously by an injection of sterile water through a urethral catheter or cystoscope used in the initial examination. The bladder is opened and emptied. The surgeon inserts his index finger into the bladder outlet between the lobes of the prostate. By working his finger around the prostatic bed he forces the adenomatous mass away from its false capsule. The urethra is divided with scissors or torn across with the finger at the lower border of the prostate: the gland is then extracted. A wedge of tissue is cut away from the bladder neck to prevent the formation of a shelf, which can cause subsequent retention. During this procedure there is usually severe bleeding from the prostatic bed. This is controlled temporarily by packs and the use of diathermy.

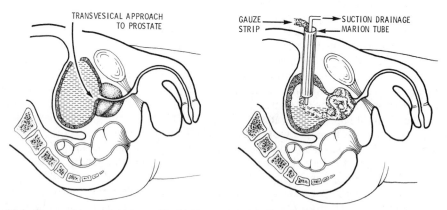

Fig. 38.4 Suprapubic prostatectomy. (*Left.*) The approach is through the bladder which is exposed below the level of the peritoneum. (*Right.*) Post-operative drainage by Marion tube. The bladder is drained through a wide bore rubber tube and the prostatic cavity may be packed with ribbon gauze.

In the Harris prostatectomy the bed of the prostate is repaired by sewing the bladder base into the floor of the cavity previously occupied by the gland. A urethral catheter is passed and left in position and the bladder is closed completely, a small corrugated rubber drain being left in the retropubic space in case of leakage.

A simpler and more common technique after the removal of the gland, is to leave a loose pack in the prostatic cavity, the main bleeding points having been tied or coagulated with diathermy. The ribbon gauze which is used for this packing is pulled out through the opening in the bladder into which has been inserted a wide-bore rubber tube. Marion's tube is sometimes used for this purpose. A metal connector is inserted into its outer end, attached to the continuous suction apparatus which keeps the bladder empty. Alternatively the tube may be left open and covered with absorbent dressings. The packing is removed 3 or 4 days later by pulling it through the wide-bore Marion's tube. The tube is withdrawn during the 2nd week after operation and is replaced by an adhesive stoma bag (page 691). A urethral catheter may then be inserted and encourages the rapid closure of the suprapubic fistula.

2. Retropubic prostatectomy (Millin) (Fig. 38.5). This is now the most common method of prostatectomy and eliminates a good deal of the distress and inconvenience of a suprapubic fistula. The bladder is not opened in this operation except at its outlet, a direct approach being made to the prostate by incising its capsule. After removal of the gland the capsule is repaired and a urethral catheter left in position for several days. A precautionary corrugated rubber drain is left in the retropubic space, but if there is no urinary leakage it is removed at 48 hours. The urethral catheter can usually be withdrawn on the 5th day and normal micturition is resumed immediately in the majority of cases as the bladder neck mechanism has not been stretched or disturbed (page 715).

3. Transurethral resection (Fig. 38.6). (*a*) An instrument similar to a cystoscope is passed through the urethra and carries a diathermy cutting loop with which the surgeon scoops pieces out of the prostate. A stream of water is used to irrigate the bladder during this procedure as the field of vision becomes obscured by bleeding. A catheter is left in

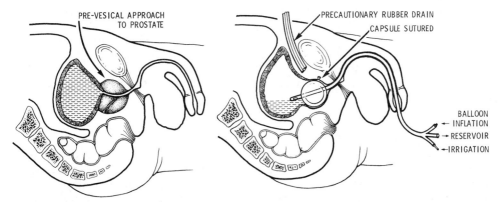

Fig. 38.5 Retropubic prostatectomy. *Left.* The bladder is pushed upwards and the false capsule of the prostate opened to expose the adenomatous mass. The capsule is repaired and post-operative drainage is by indwelling urethral catheter. A precautionary retropubic drainage strip is left in position for 3 or 4 days. *Right.* Post-operative drainage by self-retaining Foley balloon catheter (with irrigation tube).

position after operation and can usually be removed after 2 or 3 days. This operation is eminently suitable for obstruction due to carcinoma and may have to be repeated after an interval of several weeks or months. It is used in some cases of retention precipitated by operations on the rectum or anus, a formal removal being performed at a later date.

(*b*) 'Cold punch'. The prostate is sliced away similarly by a transurethral instrument with a sliding tube with a cutting end, within a sheath with a large side eye, into which the gland is pressed for each cutting movement. Haemorrhage is considerable.

(*c*) By **cryosurgery.** This is used for the very frail, or 'bad risk' cases. A 'freezing' probe cooled by liquid nitrogen is positioned in the prostatic urethra: a temperature probe is inserted into the prostate through the perineum and another recorder is placed in the rectum. The prostate is 'frozen' to death and is passed as necrotic tissue during the next week or so.

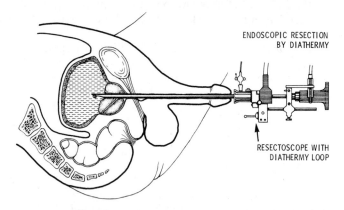

ENDOSCOPIC RESECTION
BY DIATHERMY

RESECTOSCOPE WITH
DIATHERMY LOOP

Fig. 38.6   Transurethral prostatectomy.

4. Perineal prostatectomy (Fig. 38.7). This is hardly ever performed now but was popular at one time as it did not involve abdominal operation. The only occasions on which the prostate is approached by this route are for the drainage of an abscess or for the insertion of radium needles.

As part of prostatectomy, the vas deferens on each side is exposed and divided to prevent the spread of infection to the epididymis. A small incision is made in the top of the scrotum on each side.

Complications of prostatectomy

Primary, reactionary or secondary **haemorrhage** are common following prostatectomy, and considerable difficulty may be experienced in keeping the bladder free from clots in the immediate post-operative period. Continuous irrigation is sometimes employed using a solution of sodium citrate as the irrigating fluid. **Clot retention** is the most serious complication and produces severe shock from distension of the bladder. Management of clot retention is essentially a matter for the surgeon, but good nursing can prevent its occurrence. Reference has already been made to the danger of using spigots or clips on any catheter drainage even for the short period between the patient leaving the operating theatre and being placed in bed in the ward. If drainage is interrupted for a few minutes by inadvertent compression of the outlet tube, this may be sufficient for a clot to form in the catheter, with very serious consequences (see also pages 634, 671).

Renal failure may occur from reflex anuria. Its onset will be shown by a diminished urinary output. It is of course imperative that all irrigating fluid should be measured and recorded on the fluid balance chart.

Urinary infection is common in cases of prostatic obstruction, but with modern anti-septic treatment it rarely gives rise to serious complications. When normal micturition has been re-established there is no longer any residual urine. The infecting organism may be identified by the pathologist and the appropriate antibiotic or chemotherapy instituted to sterilise the urinary tract.

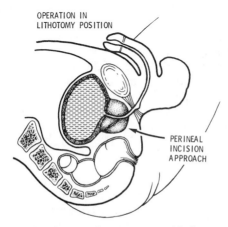

OPERATION IN
LITHOTOMY POSITION

PERINEAL
INCISION
APPROACH

Fig. 38.7   Perineal approach to prostate and bulbous urethra.

Acute **epididymo-orchitis** may occur in the 2nd week after operation and constitutes a serious set-back in an otherwise straightforward case. It is unlikely to occur if the vasa deferentia have been tied (**vasectomy**) (page 728 for treatment).

Post-operative incontinence. Considerable difficulty may be experienced in regaining complete control of the outflow of urine, especially if the bladder has been distended by chronic obstruction. The sphincter mechanism is sometimes interfered with by the opera-tion. If after removal of the urethral catheter there is any suggestion of incontinence, the patient should make an attempt to void urine at hourly intervals while awake and be allowed the use of a urinal at night. The interval between acts of micturition can be grad-ually extended over succeeding days. The patient cannot be expected to hold his urine for several hours but he must not be encouraged to have the 'bottle' constantly at hand or he will develop a 'habit incontinence'.

Recurrent retention. Sometimes as the result of sepsis in the prostatic bed, or from errors of technique, scar tissue forms at the outlet of the bladder and produces a recurrence of the prostatic symptoms from retention. Dilatation of the urethra under anaesthetic or subsequent transurethral resection of the fibrous bar may be required.

Carcinoma of prostate

This condition produces symptoms similar to that of benign senile hypertrophy described above. If the growth is advanced it may be suspected from the hardness of the gland on rectal examination, but often secondary deposits have formed before there are prostatic symptoms. This form of growth spreads readily by the blood stream and hardly ever by lymphatic vessels. The metastases have the peculiar property of encouraging the formation of dense bone wherever the malignant cells lodge in the skeleton. Fortunately the growth of these metastases is almost entirely controlled by the administration of female sex hormones (oestrogen), although these have very little effect on the primary growth. The majority of patients are therefore treated by hormone administration, though surgical operation (transurethral resection) may be necessary if the obstruction becomes severe. The one great disadvantage of hormone treatment is that it is apt to produce retention of sodium in the body and thus to produce oedema. This may become severe and affect the patient's heart. Treatment should therefore be started when the patient is still in hospital and if there is any untoward reaction over the first 2 weeks of treatment this is continued, but the patient is instructed to weigh himself weekly and report any weight gain to his doctor. Only by careful observation of the weight can oedema be detected in its early stages. Treatment may have to be intermittent and combined with one of the diuretic drugs.

Frequently, the carcinomatous nature of the growth is only discovered by microscopic examination of what was thought to be senile benign enlargement.

Prostatitis

Chronic inflammation may result from past gonorrhoea infection, but often the infection is non-specific especially in paraplegic involvement of the bladder (page 707). The gland becomes hard and stones form within it. Transurethral resection is needed to relieve obstruction.

Prostatic biopsy

To establish a diagnosis when the prostate is found to be hard and carcinoma is suspected, a needle biopsy is performed through the rectum. A special Franzen needle is used attached to the surgeon's finger by a ring so that he can guide it accurately.

Urethra

Disorders of the urethra are important because of their interference with the normal flow of urine, and the consequent added risk of infection. Pain and distress is considerable.

The **female urethra** is very short and apart from rare congenital abnormalities, the only common abnormal condition is the **urethral caruncle** (Fig. 40.3), a mass of vascular tissue like a pile at the urethral orifice. The caruncle is extremely painful and is treated by simple surgical excision or diathermy. **Prolapse** (Fig. 40.3) of the urethral mucous membrane also occurs in women and sometimes requires surgical excision of the cuff of prolapsed mucosa. If the nurse observes either of these abnormalities during procedures such as catheterisation or vaginal douch the medical staff must be informed.

The **male urethra** is a long channel which has important anatomical relations. The prostatic portion of the urethra is the innermost section and becomes obstructed by enlargement of the prostate. Into this portion open the ducts which carry the seminal fluid from the vesicles and prostate. The next portion of the urethra—the membranous portion —is surrounded by a sphincter muscle and is supported in a ligament which crosses the pubic arch. In severe fractures of the pelvis where the pubic bones are separated the membranous urethra may be torn across. The urethral injury is indicated by haematuria following an accident. The bulbous portion lies behind the scrotum in the perineum. The longest section of the urethra is the penile portion and is the part most commonly affected by congenital abnormalities.

Common disorders

Congenital abnormality

The development of the urethra is a complicated process and many forms of abnormality occur. Little flaps of mucous membrane may be present in the prostatic portion of the urethra. These act as valves, allowing the easy passage of a catheter but preventing the free escape of urine. The condition is usually discovered because a child fails to thrive owing to the back-pressure effects of retention of urine with subsequent uraemia. The valves may be removed by means of a miniature resectoscope.

The urethral tube may be incompletely formed and instead of being incorporated in the whole length of the penis may terminate to open in the perineum or somewhere along the undersurface of the penis. This condition is **hypospadias** (Fig. 38.8). In the severe forms

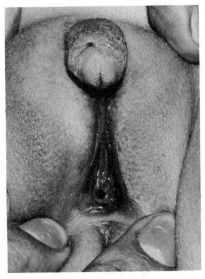

Fig. 38.8.   Severe degree of hypospadias in a boy with primitive vagina and uterus (pseudohermaphrodyte).

where the urethral opening is far back towards the perineum the right and left halves of the scrotum are separated. In the new-born baby this appearance, with a very small penis and central urethral opening, very strongly resembles the anatomy of the female baby and the sex is mistaken. Minor degrees of this deformity result in the urethral meatus being only slightly displaced from the normal position: it is then sometimes very small and requires enlarging by **meatotomy**.

Severe cases of hypospadias are treated by a two-stage operation, the first stage consisting of a plastic operation on the undersurface of the penis to increase its length as this area is usually contracted. When the second stage of the operation is performed to fashion a new tube on the undersurface of the penis, the urinary stream is diverted temporarily by perineal urethrostomy. An opening is made into the urethra immediately behind the scrotum and an indwelling catheter passed into the bladder from this point.

Occasionally the urethra is formed on the upper surface of the penis and does not become closed into a tube. It remains as a gutter running beneath the pubic arch directly into the bladder. The sphincter mechanism is sometimes defective and incontinence occurs. This condition of **epispadias** is also found in baby girls, the abnormal cleft resulting in the urethra opening above the clitoris. Plastic operations are performed for the repair of this condition. The nurse may observe this condition in female patients who are unaware that there is an abnormality.

Infection

Acute urethritis occurs in gonorrhoea and there are other infections which have a special affinity for the urethral mucous membrane. Urethritis produces intense pain on micturition and sometimes leads to retention. Abscess formation along the course of the urethra leads to subsequent stricture (page 719). The presence of urethritis is shown by the development of a urethral discharge. Urethritis from irritation of the mucous membrane lining the urethra follows the use of an indwelling catheter, and if the catheter is too large necrosis of the mucous membrane may be produced: infection is inevitable but the urethritis can be diminished by using the smallest adequate size of catheter and by the use of urinary antiseptics. Stricture formation sometimes follows the prolonged use of a catheter.

Trauma

Rupture of the urethra has already been described as a complication of fractured pelvis. The urethra is sometimes damaged by the passage of bladder sounds or endoscopic instruments.

The repair of the ruptured urethra requires highly skilled surgery and suprapubic cystostomy is almost always used to divert the urinary stream during the healing process.

Neoplasm

Carcinoma occurs in the urethra but is extremely rare. It affects the penile portion of the urethra and is treated by amputation of the penis.

Urethral stricture

In civilised communities where the treatment of venereal disease is carried out effectively, urethral stricture following gonorrhoea is now extremely rare. Narrowing of the urethral channel is produced by any inflammatory lesion in the urethra. It may follow prostatectomy or injury. The symptoms are those of increasing difficulty with micturition and sometimes retention with overflow. Acute retention may occur and require suprapubic cystostomy. The initial treatment of retention due to stricture consists of the passage of bougies of gradually increasing size. The dilatation is carried out at regular intervals and may be required for many years. Operation is sometimes required to divide the stricture, and reconstruct the urethra, using a buried strip of scrotal skin.

Circumcision

The removal of the foreskin (prepuce) is carried out in Jewish and certain other races as a religious rite. It is sometimes necessary on medical grounds if the foreskin cannot be drawn back over the glans penis. In babies the prepuce is normally adherent to the sensitive bright red mucous membrane at the end of the penis and the separation is not completed for several months after birth. Unfortunately it has become a custom to anticipate the natural separation of these layers of skin by forcing the prepuce back over the glans. If it is too tight for this to be done, circumcision is then frequently undertaken, for tradition, rather than for medical necessity. If the prepuce is removed, ammonia dermatitis, which is so common in small babies, produces burns of the glans and the urethral meatus frequently becomes ulcerated. As the result of this ulceration the child has pain on micturition and sometimes passes blood. Subsequent scarring produces stenosis (stricture) of the meatus.

Circumcision of the new-born baby, when required, is usually undertaken without anaesthetic and the penis is surrounded by a strip of ribbon gauze smeared with a mild antiseptic cream or moistened with friar's balsam (tinct. benzoin co.). The principal risk of circumcision is haemorrhage and a very careful watch must be kept, as a tiny baby cannot stand a severe loss of blood. Healing occurs very rapidly, and in spite of its situation, infection of the cut edges of the skin (which are sewn together) is very rare. The baby is bathed normally a week after operation and no special after-treatment is required except cleanliness and the use of a mild antiseptic powder. Catgut sutures are used to stitch the divided skin edges. These come away naturally in the bath and no stitch removal is necessary.

Circumcision is required in the older child and in the adult if there has been recurrent infection beneath the prepuce (**balanitis**). In the adult there is a considerable amount of pain from congestion and hyoscine hydrobromide is usually administered to reduce the post-operative discomfort.

Phimosis is a condition in which the prepuce is abnormally tight and cannot be drawn back over the glans.

Paraphimosis is present when the tight prepuce has been withdrawn behind the glans but cannot be returned to its normal position. The end of the penis then swells enormously and the condition requires emergency operation to divide the constricting ring of skin.

Paraphimosis sometimes occurs in babies when the mother has been advised to force the prepuce back to 'stretch' it.

In the elderly the prepuce is less elastic and when an uncircumcised patient is catheterised, particularly if the catheter is to remain in, care must be taken to ensure that the prepuce is drawn forward. If this is ignored and the patient complains of pain only to be told, 'it's just the catheter', serious trouble arises and surgical relief is needed.

Genital oedema

Owing to the looseness of the skin of the penis and scrotum, and of the labial skin in the female, oedema develops very easily from injury or infection. Operations in this area sometimes result in the development of a degree of swelling which becomes alarming to the patient but which is usually painless.

Generalised oedema occurring in the course of a severe illness such as peritonitis or nephritis can very often be detected first in this loose genital skin.

Tight bandages or dressings are not necessary in this area, and after operation for conditions such as hypospadias, the risk of oedema and infection is actually reduced by eliminating dressings completely and leaving the repaired tissue exposed to the air. Antibiotic powder is applied frequently by an insufflator.

Fungus infections

Tinea, monilia and other 'fungus' type infections become established readily in the skin of the genital area and in the vagina. Sometimes chronic fungus infection of the finger nails originates from vaginal infection, and reinfection of the finger occurs unless the genital infection is cleared. **Nystatin** or **candicidin** is used as a local application in ointment form or solution. **Griseofulvin** taken by mouth for several months may be needed to get rid of chronic lesions. Overgrowth with secondary bacterial infection sometimes prevents discovery of the underlying fungus (page 739).

Cross-infection

Certain troublesome organisms are commonly introduced into the urinary tract by careless catheterisation, through baths or improperly sterilised equipment, especially bedpans and urinals. *Pseudomonas pyocyaneus* thrives in moist surroundings and is easily conveyed from patient to patient. A green discharge indicates its presence and any suggestion of this must be reported. A spread of this infection to other patients is a reflection on ward hygiene and nursing management. Patients with urinary disorders should have special marked bedpans and urinals and these should be sterilised. Chlorine solutions are satisfactory for this purpose if heat methods are not available.

39

Hernia and Testis

Hernia

The term 'rupture' signifies that something has burst. In the majority of cases of hernia, a protrusion of peritoneum has occurred at some point of anatomical weakness in the abdominal wall as a result of abnormal strain (Fig. 39.1). This protrusion is the hernial sac. The most common site for a hernia of 'congenital' origin is in the **inguinal** region. The protrusion accompanies the spermatic cord in the inguinal canal of the male or the round ligament in the inguinal canal of the female. Though inguinal hernias of this type are seen in new-born babies, frequently the sac does not manifest itself until later life when, as the result of some strain or muscular weakness, a piece of omentum or bowel is forced into it. The congenital inguinal hernia is usually referred to as 'indirect' and the acquired hernia as 'direct', the terms describing the course which the hernia pursues through the inguinal canal.

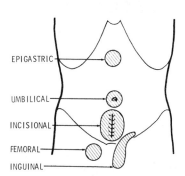

EPIGASTRIC

UMBILICAL

INCISIONAL

FEMORAL

INGUINAL

Fig. 39.1 Common sites of abdominal hernia.

A similar protrusion occurs behind the inguinal ligament into the upper part of the thigh, medial to the femoral artery and vein. This **femoral** type of hernia is more common in women and is more liable to the complication of strangulation which will be described later. **Umbilical** hernia also occurs and is common in children (Fig. 39.3).

Following abdominal operation weakness may develop at the site of the incision. A very large peritoneal protrusion follows, forming an incisional or **ventral hernia** (Fig. 39.4). This may reach enormous proportions so that the major part of the intestinal tract lies within the sac.

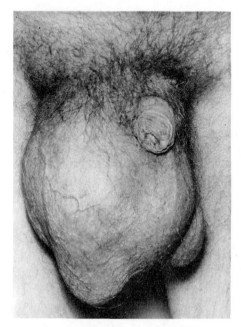

Fig. 39.2   A large right-sided 'scrotal' inguinal hernia containing intestine. The outline of the left testis can be seen at the side of the enormous scrotum.

The majority of hernias require surgical operation, because they are not self-curing, and cannot be treated satisfactorily by any other means. In certain exceptional cases, where operation is considered unnecessary or unwise, a special supporting 'truss' is fitted, but this is only effective if the contents of the hernia can be pushed into the abdomen. The truss then presses on the opening and prevents refilling of the sac.

Apart from congenital weaknesses, and operation scars, hernias develop in the inguinal region as a result of excessive strain or prolonged muscular effort. Chronic constipation and straining at stool, difficulty in micturition from an enlarged prostate, or the violent effort of lifting heavy weights are all factors which lead to the production of hernia. They are also factors which need to be eliminated after operative cure, to lessen the chance of recurrence. Chronic cough, due to bronchitis, is a major factor in causing enlargement of the hernia, and perhaps the greatest post-operative strain placed on the repair is the development of bronchitis following operation.

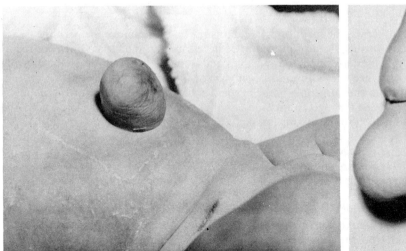

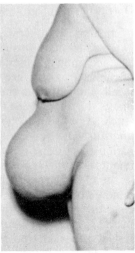

Fig. 39.3 A large umbilical hernia in an infant three weeks old. This was cured by reduction and strapping of the abdominal wall. Operation is not required in the majority of cases.

Fig. 39.4 Incisional hernia following abdominal operation many years previously. The hernia contained the transverse colon and most of the small intestine. It was repaired completely by the use of fascial strips from the thigh (Gallie's operation).

Complications of hernia

The peritoneal sac may become inflamed and its contents, which includes omentum or bowel, become adherent. A hernia is described as **reducible** if the 'lump' of omentum or bowel can be pushed inside the peritoneal cavity. As the result of inflammation the hernia may become **irreducible.** If the sac contains a coil of small intestine or colon this may become **obstructed.** By compression of the veins and later of the arteries at the point of entrance to the sac, the bowel may be deprived of an adequate blood supply and it is then **strangulated** (Fig. 39.5). A strangulated hernia requires immediate operation if it cannot be reduced by skilful manipulation.

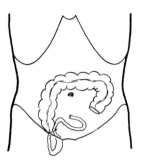

Fig. 39.5 Strangulated inguinal hernia. The proximal loop of bowel is distended by the obstruction.

Operative treatment

In all types of hernia, the main principle in operation is to remove the peritoneal sac.

In children no further surgical procedure is necessary and the hernia does not recur. The operation may be performed in tiny babies and is infinitely preferable to the wearing of rubber trusses which are both unsatisfactory and unhygienic. The operation is technically difficult from the surgeon's point of view owing to the delicacy of the patient's tissues. It is performed through an incision less than 3 cm long which is closed with one stitch. Admission to hospital is unnecessary for more than 24 hours and the baby is undisturbed. The wound is covered with a sealed dressing which prevents any contamination from urine or faeces. This applies to inguinal hernia: umbilical hernia in tiny infants is strapped or disregarded.

In adults where there is marked weakness in the abdominal wall, not only is the sac removed but the weakness is repaired usually by a darning operation. The material used to close the gap may be thick silk, nylon, or stainless steel wire. Both nylon net and wire mesh has also been used to patch the gap in the muscle wall. Many surgeons use a graft of fascial strip taken from the external oblique muscle in the abdominal wall. If the deficiency is very large, as in incisional hernia, long strips of fascia are taken from the side of the thigh. This procedure is 'Gallie's operation'. The strips are obtained by making a long incision down the side of the thigh or through a very small incision just above the knee, using a fasciotome or stripper. This consists of a long rod carrying a ring at the end. It is pushed up the thigh underneath the skin. The strips of fascia are threaded on to special needles and used as laces to darn the deficiency in the abdominal wall.

Pre-operative treatment

The elimination of upper respiratory infection, especially if it is associated with chronic cough, is the most important preliminary to hernia operation. The post-operative course is more comfortable if heavy cigarette smoking is curtailed for 1 or 2 weeks before operation. The abdomen and pubic area must be thoroughly cleaned and shaved. If a fascial strip has to be taken from the leg one side must be prepared and shaved from the iliac crest to a point 8 cm below the knee.

Abdominal and breathing exercises should be taught before operation.

There is no other special pre-operative measure.

Post-operative care

In the simple forms of operation where the sac has been removed (**herniotomy**) and no further procedure carried out, there is very little after-pain or interference with mobility. If a repair operation has been performed (**hernioplasty, herniorrhaphy**) there is more pain and the patient is very unwilling to use his abdominal wall for respiration or coughing. There is then a likelihood of post-operative pulmonary complications and particular care must be taken over breathing exercises.

Abdominal exercises are started usually 3 or 4 days after operation. Routine methods of wound care are employed and the patient is allowed up on the day following operation unless otherwise ordered. The surgeon may wish to defer ambulation if a large incisional hernia has been repaired.

Haematoma formation in the wound sometimes delays discharge from hospital.

Post-operative retention of urine is a common complication but usually responds to an injection of carbachol (page 388) which is a drug having a specific bladder-stimulating action.

If haematuria occurs, it must be reported instantly: it signifies that a stitch may have penetrated the bladder wall. A catheter is inserted to maintain constant bladder drainage to prevent extravasation.

Convalescence. Sedentary workers may return to their duties 2 weeks after operation, while manual workers are not permitted to resume for at least 6 weeks any employment which might involve the lifting of heavy weights.

Special management of strangulated hernia

Strangulated hernia is an acute emergency condition. It is not always possible for the surgeon to tell whether the hernia is simply irreducible or whether strangulation has occurred. When this condition arises in babies the child is admitted to hospital and his legs are suspended from a bar across the sides of the cot. A clove-hitch knot of flannel bandage is passed round each ankle to hold the legs sufficiently high for the buttocks to be clear of the bed. A sedative is given and in the majority of cases the hernia reduces itself or can be reduced manually by the surgeon within an hour. If this method fails operation is necessary.

In the adult, strangulated or 'irreducible' hernia may also be reduced by the surgeon's manipulation. The foot of the bed is raised on blocks as high as possible, and application of an ice pack to the 'lump' may be prescribed in the hope of reducing the oedema and making reduction more likely.

The pre-operative treatment is the same as for intestinal obstruction. A Ryle's tube is inserted into the stomach and the contents aspirated. If there has been severe vomiting due to pain or obstruction, an intravenous infusion will probably be required.

At operation the bowel may be found to be in such a condition that it will recover. It is then duly replaced into the abdominal cavity and the hernia treated in the usual way. If, however, the bowel is gangrenous a portion of it will require resection.

Whether or not there has been resection, the post-operative treatment must provide for the risk of peritonitis. Gastric suction is maintained until peristalsis is resumed. Antibiotic therapy will most probably be ordered. Once the risk of peritonitis has passed the convalescence will be uneventful (pages 485 *et seq.*).

Testis

The testis is suspended in the scrotum by the vas deferens and spermatic blood vessels (Fig. 39.6). The vas is a small muscular tube which conveys the spermatozoa (male sex cells) from the testis to the seminal vesicle which lies at the base of the bladder. The epididymis is a comma-shaped structure closely attached to the back of the testis and composed of a very long and closely coiled tube. It connects the outlet ducts at the top of the testis with the vas deferens at the lower end of the epididymis. The proximity of the testis and epididymis means that many conditions which involve one structure, inevitably involve the other.

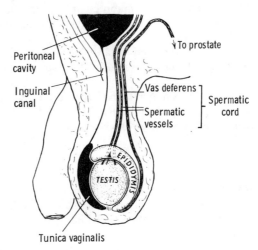

Peritoneal
cavity

Inguinal
canal

To prostate

Vas deferens

Spermatic
vessels

Spermatic
cord

EPIDIDYMIS

TESTIS

Tunica vaginalis

Fig. 39.6   The anatomy of the testis and associated structures showing the relation of the peritoneum and its attachment to the tunica vaginalis.

In the development of the foetus, the testis is formed behind the peritoneum of the posterior abdominal wall. During development it migrates towards the inguinal region and emerges by passing through the inguinal canal into the scrotum. Its progress may be interrupted at any point leading to the pathological condition of **undescended testicle.** In some cases the testis traverses the inguinal canal and becomes attached in the wrong position instead of passing into the scrotum. This is referred to as **ectopic testis.** Although in some boys the descent of the testis is completed by puberty without surgical interference, many cases require operation to free the testis from its surroundings and place it correctly in the scrotum **(orchidopexy).**

The condition of undescended testis is frequently associated with the presence of inguinal hernia. The hernial sac is removed at the same time as the operation for fixing the testis in the scrotum.

Hydrocele. The testis is contained in a cavity formed originally from peritoneum—the **tunica vaginalis.** The membrane which lines this cavity can produce fluid in the same way as the peritoneum; such an effusion is a **hydrocele.**

Figs. 39.7 and 39.8 illustrate the conditions which can arise from abnormalities of this peritoneal process. Obliteration may occur at each end, leaving a centre portion in the inguinal canal.

Hydrocele can also arise from injury to the testis or from inflammation due to infection. In many cases there is no known cause and the cavity may become enormously distended containing perhaps half a litre of fluid.

Bilateral hydrocele is often seen in small babies. The fluid is absorbed during the first few months of life and no treatment is necessary. In older boys and in adults, if the swelling is causing inconvenience the hydrocele is 'tapped'. The fluid is withdrawn by means of a trocar and cannula (Fig. 24.10) inserted through the scrotal wall under local anaesthesia. A solution of procaine, a fine hypodermic needle and a 2-ml syringe are required. Instead of a trocar and cannula a 20-ml syringe and serum needle may be used to aspirate the fluid. Many hydroceles refill after this procedure and repeated tapping is necessary. Operation

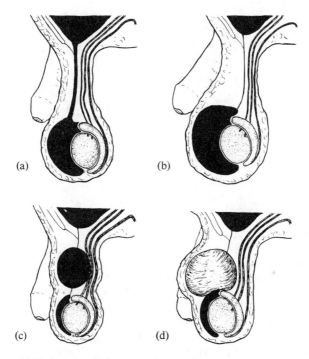

(a)   (b)

(c)   (d)

Fig. 39.7 Hydrocele. **(a)** Hydrocele which communicates with the peritoneal cavity and varies in size. The operation is the same as for inguinal hernia. **(b)** Simple hydrocele treated by repeated tapping (aspiration) or by excision of the sac. **(c)** Hydrocele of the cord. Excision is required as for hernia. **(d)** Spermatocele (cyst of epididymis). Excision is required.

is undertaken to remove the hydrocele sac through an incision in the groin or on the front of the scrotum. Pre- and post-operative nursing is exactly as for hernia, but there may be considerably more swelling of the scrotum which needs support by a wool pad and T-bandage. Sometimes a drainage tube is inserted through the scrotal wall to prevent the collection of blood: it is removed after 48 hours.

Hydrocele may also be treated by injection of sclerosing fluids. Aspiration of the fluid is carried out in the usual way and a small quantity of Ethamolin or other irritant fluid may be injected. A further effusion usually occurs and requires subsequent aspiration and the method of treatment is not always successful. A suspensory bandage[1] should be provided after aspiration.

In the female the round ligament follows exactly the same course as the vas deferens which it resembles. It is accompanied by vessels forming a rope-like structure in the inguinal canal. A peritoneal process accompanies this ligament, and if it is not completely obliterated, hydrocele and hernia can occur as in the male. The condition is treated by simple surgical excision.

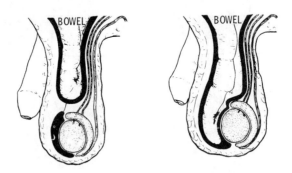

Fig. 39.8   Inguinal hernia. (*Left*) Incomplete but containing bowel. (*Right*) Complete communicating with tunica vaginalis.

Epididymo-orchitis

Infection may reach the testis by passing from the urethra via the vas deferens, or it may be carried direct to the testis by the blood stream. If the infection originates in the urethra the primary lesion is epididymitis: thus tuberculosis produces lesions in the epididymis without involving the testis: this infection is usually a complication of renal tuberculosis. Syphilis, on the other hand, appears as a gumma of the testis without involvement of the epididymis since the infection is carried in the blood stream.

Most infections, however, involve both structures. Epididymo-orchitis occurs as a complication of mumps. It can also arise from infection in the urethra following prostatectomy, in which the lower ends of the vasa deferentia are necessarily cut across. To prevent this complication the vasa are exposed at the neck of the scrotum and divided at the end of a prostatectomy operation.

Acute epididymo-orchitis is liable to arise after the passage of instruments (bougie, sound, cystoscope) through the urethra. It may also occur for no obvious reason and is frequently unconnected with other disease. It may be a manifestation of gonorrhoea.

It is characterised by high temperature, great pain and sometimes by vomiting and rigors. There is great swelling of the scrotum and the skin becomes oedematous.

The patient is treated in bed: antibiotic cover or sulphonamide therapy is usual even

---

[1] A suspensory bandage is a cotton net bag attached to a waist-band. It is used in the convalescent stage of cases of epididymo-orchitis and is sometimes worn to relieve discomfort from the weight of a hydrocele.

though the infecting organism is not known. Mumps orchitis requires no specific treatment except rest and local applications to decrease the inflammation.

To diminish the risk of the condition arising from instrumentation, routine chemotherapy (e.g. 2 G of sulphadimidine or 100 mg nitrofurantoin) is given after endoscopic examination, and repeated in 6 hours, if the urine was previously sterile.

The scrotum must be supported and the simplest method is to place a large piece of cotton wool underneath the scrotum and hold it in place with a T-bandage. Adhesive strapping attached to both thighs and acting as a shelf is sometimes used for bed patients, but is extremely uncomfortable since it limits movement of the legs. Loosely applied hypertonic saline packs are helpful in reducing inflammation of the scrotum, but no local application can affect the inflamed testis or epididymis. A suspensory bandage should be worn when the patient gets up.

Tuberculosis of the epididymis frequently results in attachment of the scrotal skin, ulceration and sinus formation. It is treated by removal of the epididymis, and sometimes of the testis as well.

Orchitis occurs following injury to the testis. It is treated by support and bed-rest.

Torsion of the testis is due to the organ becoming twisted on the spermatic cord, the vessels become obstructed and the symptoms resemble those of inflammation. Operation is required.

Neoplasm

Malignant disease of the testis is rare. There are two main forms, **seminoma** and **teratoma.** The former is a malignant growth (carcinoma) of the germ-forming cells and spreads in a similar manner to other forms of carcinoma. The lymphatics in the testis pass to glands on either side of the aorta in the renal region. Excision of these glands is not a practical method of treating a patient who has a carcinoma of the testis but radiotherapy is given to the gland fields to diminish the risk of metastasis. Teratoma of the testis is a form of growth in which the germ cell produces various kinds of foetal tissue. The teratoma may also be malignant and the treatment is the same as with carcinoma (seminoma). Some testicular tumours produce hormones which affect the patient's general physiology.

Pre- and post-operative treatment

Table 55 indicates the operations performed on structures within the scrotum. There is no particular pre-operative treatment except skin shaving and preparation. Sometimes the scrotum is drained for 48 hours following operation. It should always be supported by a bandage after operation.

Orchidectomy and other operations on the testis or epididymis are usually performed through an incision in the inguinal region. It is unlikely that the patient will need to remain in bed for more than 2 or 3 days.

If the incision is made through the scrotal skin instead of in the inguinal region, it is usually sutured with catgut to avoid the difficulty of removing fine stitches from the thick wrinkled skin of the scrotum.

Table 55   Operations on testis, epididymis and penis

Orchidectomy	removal of testis for infection, maldescent, torsion or growth.
Orchidopexy	fixation of testis in scrotum for ectopic or undescended testis.
Epididymectomy	excision of epididymis, usually for tuberculous infection.
Excision of hydrocele	
Excision of spermatocele	
Operation for varicocele	ligature of dilated veins in spermatic cord.
Ligature of vas deferens	after prostatectomy to prevent infection (page 714). For sterilisation of male.
Amputation of penis	for carcinoma.
Circumcision	for phimosis.
'Dorsal slit'	division of tight prepuce, in paraphimosis.
Meatotomy	enlargement of urethral meatus for stenosis (congenital; with hypospadias; due to repeated ulceration).
Reconstruction of urethra	for hypospadias.
Reconstruction of urethra	for epispadias.
Excision of urethral structure and reconstruction.	

Spermatocele

Figure 39.7 shows this condition. A very large cyst develops in the upper part of the epididymis and contains spermatozoa. The cyst may vary in size from perhaps 1 cm to 10 cm in diameter. If it is large, the cyst is removed.

Varicocele

In this condition the veins from the testis are dilated and cause enlargement of the spermatic cord in the upper part of the scrotum and groin. The condition is sometimes responsible for aching pain. Operative treatment is not usually necessary but sometimes portions of the veins are excised. This is a minor operation and can be performed under local anaesthesia.

Castration

This means the removal of both testes. In animals the operation is a routine veterinary procedure partly to sterilise the male animal but mainly to remove the hormone-secreting interstitial tissue of the testis, which is responsible for the development of male characteristics. The reduction of the male hormone permits the full physiological action of oestrogen which is present to a small extent in the male as well as in the female: the animal gains weight.

In man, castration may be the inevitable treatment of bilateral tuberculosis. It is sometimes performed in a patient with carcinoma of the prostate since it is known that this condition is more easily controlled if the male hormone is removed. The majority of patients with carcinoma of the prostate can be treated satisfactorily by the administration of artificial female hormone (stilboestrol) in tablet form, but some elderly patients are unable to tolerate stilboestrol treatment and castration is essential.

Vasectomy

Excision of a short length (1 cm) of each vas deferens at the top of the scrotum is performed under local anaesthesia as a means of producing male sterility. It is widely practised as an outpatient procedure as a safe and economic method of population control. Consent has to be obtained from the man *and* his wife. Vasectomy does not produce impotence. It is also performed to prevent infection travelling through the vas after prostatectomy (page 714).

An incision is made at the neck of the scrotum on each side: the vas is isolated, divided, a segment removed and the ends turned back and stitched to reduce the possibility of their joining up. The wound is closed with Dexon catgut substitute. The testes may be painful for a few days and a scrotal support is advised. If the procedure is being done to secure sterility, semen examination is essential one month and three months after operation to ensure that no live spermatozoa remain, stored in the seminal vesicles. The patient must be warned that until there is a negative test other methods of contraception must be continued. The semen specimen is secured by masturbation or by natural intercourse with a latex sheath (condom).

Although restoration of continuity of the vas to restore continuity is possible no guarantee of success can be given, so for practical purposes a man has to accept that the effect of vasectomy is irreversible.

40

Gynaecological Surgery

Medicine, surgery, and obstetrics with gynaecology form the great triad upon which medical education has been built. Each of these great specialities has a separate section in the qualifying examinations for medical students, and the interests of each speciality are represented by a Royal College. The special study of gynaecology is widely separated from general surgery, but there are numerous occasions in which the general surgeon has to undertake gynaecological operations in the treatment of abdominal disease. Abdominal emergencies of gynaecological origin may be indistinguishable from intestinal or other lesions. The general unit thus overlaps with the special department in this branch of surgery.

It is not intended here to cover the whole field of gynaecological nursing but to introduce the terms commonly used in this speciality, and to outline main methods of treatment and special nursing procedures which may be required. Much of the technique and care is that required for other forms of abdominal and urological surgery.

The development and constant physiological changes in the female reproductive organs are under hormonal control and disorders which arise are in many cases medical rather than surgical.

Common gynaecological disorders

Gynaecological disorders may be divided into five groups:
1. Congenital abnormalities.
2. Disorders of menstruation.
3. Disorders connected with pregnancy and childbirth.
4. Infections.
5. Tumours.

In describing the conditions which affect various organs the terms commonly used are derived from the Greek:

Ovaries—oophorectomy.

Uterine tubes—salpingectomy, salpingitis.

Uterus—hysterectomy (from Greek 'husteros', ὑστηρος).

Vagina—colporrhaphy, haematocolpos (from Greek 'colpos', κολπος).

Traditionally the womb is the seat of the emotions, and the term hysteria has the same root.

Anatomy

The **uterus** is a thick muscular organ about 8 cm long in the adult and placed between the bladder in front and the rectum behind (Fig. 40.1). It is surrounded entirely by peritoneum except for the narrow lower portion, the **cervix** or neck, which protrudes

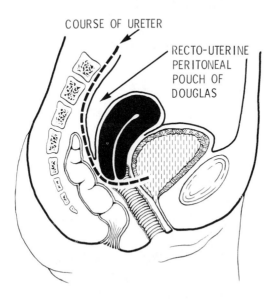

COURSE OF URETER

RECTO-UTERINE PERITONEAL POUCH OF DOUGLAS

Fig. 40.1 Section through pelvis showing the relations of uterus and vagina to peritoneum, bladder and rectum.

into the vault of the vagina. The cavity of the virgin uterus is reduced to a mere slit and opens into the vagina through the cervical canal. It also communicates with the peritoneal cavity through the uterine tubes which are held in the upper free border of a double fold of peritoneum, the **broad ligament**, on each side of the uterus. The **ovary** is attached to the outer end of this ligament. The **vagina**, at its upper end, is in contact with the peritoneum between the back of the uterus and the front of the rectum. In front it lies against the bladder and the urethra which opens at its lower end. The ureters lie against the side of the vagina towards its upper end as they pass forward to the bladder. They may thus be easily injured during operations on the uterus or vagina.

On either side of the vaginal orifice is Bartholin's gland which occasionally develops a cyst or abscess (Fig. 40.3).

The pelvic floor is formed by a sling of muscle—the levator ani—passing from the pubis to the sacrum on either side. This forms an active support for all the pelvic organs. It becomes greatly stretched during childbirth and the muscle and surrounding ligaments are so severely damaged that the pelvic organs sag. The central body of the perineum, between rectum and vagina, may be torn in childbirth: if it is not repaired at once, prolapse is very likely to occur. Prolapse of the uterus, bladder and rectum are among the disorders most commonly requiring surgical treatment in middle-aged and older women (Fig. 40.7).

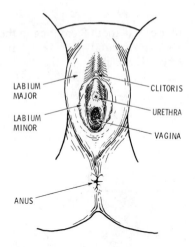

Fig. 40.2   Normal anatomy of vulva.

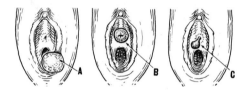

Fig. 40.3   Disorders apparent on examination of the vulva. **A.** Bartholin's cyst, or abscess. **B.** Prolapse of urethral mucosa. **C.** Protruding urethral polyp, or caruncle.

Congenital abnormalities

There are many congenital abnormalities which affect both uterus and vagina. The uterus may be divided into right and left halves, and the vagina may be a double tube. Either structure may be absent. Occasionally the rectum opens into the posterior wall of the vagina forming a **rectovaginal fistula**[1] which is associated with imperforate anus (page 565). Sometimes the anus lies immediately adjacent to the vaginal orifice (ectopic anus) and the opening is then frequently inadequate and requires dilatation or operative treatment.

The vaginal opening in the virgin is restricted by a circular membrane, the **hymen**. Sometimes, as a congenital abnormality, this is a sheet of tissue closing the lower end of the vagina completely. Secretions which are dammed up behind an imperforate hymen may become infected forming **pyocolpos.** If the condition is not discovered until the girl has her first menstrual period, **haematocolpos** develops. An incision through the imperforate hymen is then necessary.

---

[1] Rectovaginal fistula arises also from injury to the vagina in childbirth or by operation of the rectum or vagina; a colostomy is required to allow healing. A vesico-vaginal fistula arises between bladder and vagina as a complication of carcinoma of the cervix, or of childbirth.

Another congenital abnormality, which is sometimes noticed for the first time during catheterisation of a child, is the congenital fusion of the labia minora (Fig. 40.4). In this condition the vaginal orifice is completely covered by an abnormal membrane which may extend forward over the urethra with the result that urine accumulates in the vagina each time the bladder is emptied. The two labia are easily separated by passing a probe between their adherent edges. Antiseptic ointment, applied daily for a few days, prevents re-fusion.

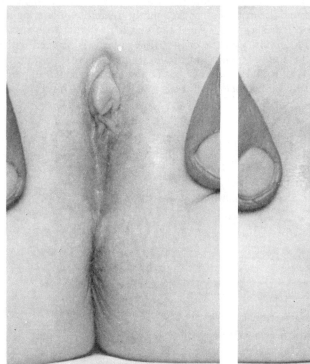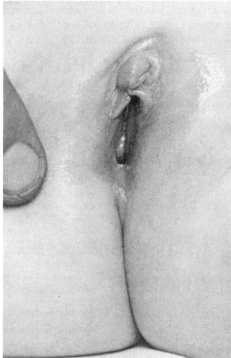

Fig. 40.4   Congenital adhesions of labia minora. (*Left*) Closure obscures urethral orifice. (*Right*) After splitting apart with probe, a normal hymen and vestibule is revealed.

Disorders of menstruation

The frequency and duration of the periods is affected by the patient's general health. An abnormality in the cycle may be the first symptom of some otherwise symptomless anaemia, or endocrine disorder such as thyrotoxicosis, or it may be due to local disease of the reproductive organs.

When menstruation does not start at puberty the condition is **primary amenorrhoea.** If the periods cease the condition is one of **secondary amenorrhoea**, the commonest cause of which is pregnancy.

Dysmenorrhoea is pain associated with the periods, and although in many cases there is no organic disease, the pain may be an important symptom of infective or other disorders.

Epimenorrhoea is an increased frequency of the periods.

Menorrhagia indicates an excessive loss in quantity or duration.

Many of these disorders are associated with an unhealthy condition of the lining epithelium of the uterus, the surface layer of which, in healthy individuals, separates completely and is discharged with each monthly period. If the separation is incomplete or the replacement is inadequate these abnormal conditions arise. Although in many cases the irregularity is due to endocrine disturbance, it is frequently treated by **dilatation and curettage**. Under full general anaesthesia the cervix of the uterus is dilated with special metal bougies (Hegar dilators, Fig. 40.5) and the cavity of the uterus is scraped with a curette, Fig. 40.6. Pieces of the lining membrane are examined microscopically for malignant or other disease. This procedure is known as 'D and C'. It is thus sometimes undertaken for therapeutic reasons and sometimes for diagnostic purposes only.

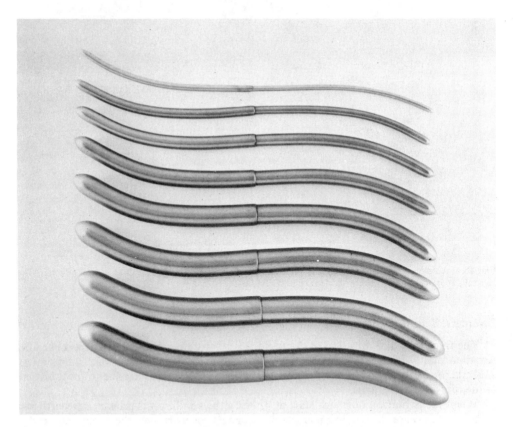

Fig. 40.5 Double-ended dilators (Hegar type) used for dilating the uterine cervix, and canal, and stomal (colostomy or ileostomy) strictures ($\frac{1}{2}$ size).

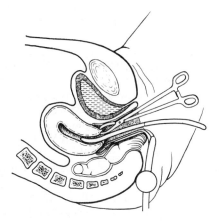 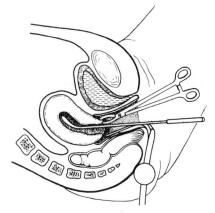

Fig. 40.6 (*Left*) With the patient in the lithotomy position the Auvard's speculum is kept in position by its own weight; the cervix is held firmly with tissue (vulsellum) forceps. (*Right*) Hegar's dilators enlarge the canal of the cervix to allow the passage of the curette with which the endometrial lining is removed.

Disorders connected with pregnancy

The ovum is shed from the ovary into the peritoneal cavity and enters the open end of the uterine tube. If it is not fertilised, it passes into the uterus and is discharged with the normal secretions. Abnormalities of the uterine tube resulting perhaps from pelvic peritonitis prevent the passage of the ovum and lead to sterility (page 751).

If fertilisation takes place, this occurs usually in the uterine tube. The ovum then passes into the uterus. It becomes adherent to the lining membrane, into which it grows, with the subsequent formation of the placenta.

Ectopic gestation (Fig. 40.8). Sometimes the fertilised ovum is held up in the uterine tube and continues its development there as an **ectopic gestation** (tubal pregnancy). After a few weeks of normal growth the wall of the uterine tube is eroded. Grave and sometimes fatal haemorrhage occurs into the peritoneal cavity if the condition is not detected and treated by immediate surgical operation. This condition produces low abdominal pain. The patient may not be aware that she is pregnant since a period may have occurred after fertilisation, as the ovum is not actually in the uterus. If the gestation has occurred on the right side the condition may be misdiagnosed as acute appendicitis. At operation the uterine tube is removed. Blood transfusion is frequently required owing to the severity of the haemorrhage. Ectopic pregnancy is one of the main causes of internal bleeding (Chapter 8).

Abortion (miscarriage) is the termination of a pregnancy before the 28th week which is the earliest age at which a fetus is regarded as capable of separate existence. Abortion may occur as the result of some endocrine disturbance, injury or other disease. If it is **incomplete** (that is if the placenta or membranes remain within the uterus) there is a very heavy loss of blood; dilatation and currettage may be required as an emergency procedure.

Criminal abortion is usually attempted by the introduction of a knitting needle or similar object into the vagina in the hope that it will pass into the uterus. Owing to the angle between the uterus and the vault of the vagina (Fig. 40.1) the instrument commonly perforates the vault of the vagina, entering the peritoneal cavity and producing peritonitis.

Pregnancy may legally be terminated on medical grounds if the mother's physical or mental health is expected to be adversely affected by the continuation of the pregnancy. The 1967 Abortion Act in Great Britain led to a wide demand for termination. Even in skilled hands there is a risk of haemorrhage, peritonitis and perforation of the uterus. In the early months abortion may be produced by dilatation of the cervix. Later in pregnancy the uterus is stimulated to expel the fetus naturally; prostaglandin (page 94), an intravenous infusion of oxytocin induces this action; hypertonic saline injected through the cervix has a similar effect. In the past the fetus was removed by **hysterotomy**, a surgical operation like Caesarean section. If it is desired to prevent further pregnancy, sterilisation is produced at the same time by dividing the uterine tubes (page 753).

If the baby is born after the 28th week and before full term the term 'abortion' is not used, but the birth is described as premature.

Chorion-epithelioma. This is a rapidly growing malignant tumour which arises from the placenta-forming membranes which surround the fetus. It is treated usually with chemotherapy using methotrexate, by mouth or intravenously. Arterial perfusion may be needed.

Carneous mole. If the fetus dies but is not expelled it becomes mummified in the uterus or tube: surgical removal is required.

Prolapse. After childbirth the most common disorder is one of prolapse which increases with successive pregnancies. The function of the bladder and urethra is affected and urinary incontinence adds to the disability. Various operations are undertaken for the repair of the prolapse, and these may involve removal of the uterus (Fig. 40.7).

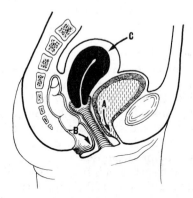

Fig. 40.7 Section through pelvis showing the effects of damage to the pelvic floor. The central part of the perineum has been torn in childbirth: the bulky uterus has stretched its ligamentous supports. Similar prolapse occurs in paraplegia owing to paralysis of the pelvic supporting muscles. A. Cystocele—bladder prolapse. B. Rectocele—rectal prolapse. C. Enlarged heavy uterus.

If operative treatment for prolapse is not advisable, artificial support is provided by the use of a **pessary**.[1] There are various types of this appliance but the most commonly

[1] The supportive pessary is to be distinguished from medicated pessaries which are large oval tablets containing penicillin or other chemical in a soluble base, and used in the vagina for the treatment of infection or for contraception.

used is a rubber ring containing a metal spring to give it rigidity. The pessary is inserted into the vagina and it bridges the gap between the separated levator ani muscles and strengthens the pelvic floor. A pessary has to be of the correct size; it is inserted initially by the doctor or nurse. It is changed at regular intervals.

Infections

Acute infection of the uterine tube (**salpingitis**) may affect either side, but on the right side it may be confused with acute appendicitis. An abscess may form in the tube— **pyosalpinx**. The condition is usually treated as one of peritonitis; antibiotics are given and operation is rarely required. Salpingitis is frequently a complication of gonorrhoea. Inflammation of the ovary is **oophoritis** and it occurs in association with salpinigitis. It may be a complication of mumps.

Chronic salpingitis may be **tuberculous**; operation is sometimes required to remove the tube. Tuberculous salpingitis is a common cause of sterility.

Endometritis is inflammation of the uterine epithelium. **Parametritis** is cellulitis of the broad ligament and adjacent pelvic connective tissue.

Cervical erosion is a condition of the cervix of the uterus. It is associated with **cervicitis** in which the lining epithelium from the inside of the cervix spreads out to replace the normal skin-type covering. It is treated by local applications and cauterisation.

Leucorrhoea[1] or vaginal discharge is due to a variety of infections and is a common cause of symptoms. If a nurse discovers that a patient has leucorrhoea this must be reported in order that the necessary investigations may be made. It occurs in small girls, and is sometimes gonococcal in origin (**vulvovaginitis**), or due to diphtheria infections or foreign bodies. Swabs are taken for bacteriological examinations (page 745). Severe discharge may be the first indication that carcinoma of the cervix is present.

Pruritus vulvae (intense irritation) may result from leucorrhoea or may be due to some primary skin infection such as tinea (ringworm). It is also frequently associated with diabetes and particular attention should be paid to urine testing in a patient who complains of this symptom.

Following antibiotic treatment of some general infections, monilial and trichomonas infections are common causes of vaginal discharge and vulvitis. For many years such infections were treated by vaginal washout ('douche') but modern chemotherapy eliminated the need for such treatment. **Erythrasma** is a particularly troublesome condition in this area and responds specifically to treatment with erythromycin. It is characterised by the skin being bright red and simulates infection with tinea. Other causes of vulvitis are virus infections, which may cause soft pink papillomata (**condylomata** —viral warts), or crops of vesicles (Herpes genitalis). Sexually transmitted virus infections produce ulcers on the labia with inguinal gland enlargement (lymphogranuloma venereum or granuloma inguinale). Treatment is with tetracycline, sometimes excision, and the lesions may become malignant. A syphilitic granuloma (chancre) is a raised warty lump which is painless. It is, therefore, very important that any abnormality seen on the vulva of a patient who is being catheterised should be reported to the medical staff.

---

[1] Leucorrhoea, literally 'white discharge' (cf. *leuco*cyte = *white* cell), but it is applied to any vaginal discharge that is not blood.

Local application of drugs to the vagina is achieved by the use of a pessary. This is a pellet the size of a large rectal suppository. The waxy base which dissolves at body temperature contains an antiseptic or hormone which is thus dispersed over the vaginal epithelium. Alternatively the substance to be used is made up in a cream and inserted with a tubular applicator. Substances commonly used in this way include Flagyl (metronidazole), antibiotics and povidone iodine.

Urinary infection. Cystitis and pyelitis are complications of gynaecological disorders owing to the shortness of the female urethra and the ease with which infection can enter the bladder. Prolapse produces retention and residual urine (page 641); this in turn favours the development of infection.

Low-grade chronic infection of the glands in the wall of the urethra causes dysuria and frequency. It is treated sometimes by repeated urethral dilatation.

Ovarian tumours

Ovaries develop cysts which may be innocent or malignant.

Follicular cysts are due to retention around an ovum. Lutein and endometrial cysts are also found in the ovary and are small and nonmalignant; they may cause pain and haemorrhage. Endometrial ('chocolate') cysts are part of endometriosis (page 743).

Benign tumours can form huge cysts occupying almost the whole abdominal cavity; one type is a dermoid cyst and contains hair, and sometimes teeth.

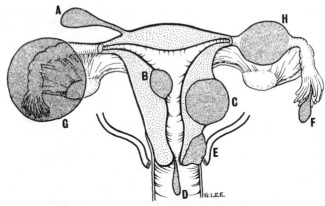

Fig. 40.8   Common disorders of the female reproductive organs. **A.** Pendunculated fibroid. **B.** Submucous fibroid. **C.** Intra-mural fibroid. **D.** Fibroid polyp protruding from the cervix. **E.** Carcinoma of the cervix, eroding ureter and vagina. **F.** Fimbrial cyst. **G.** Ovarian cyst. **H.** Distension of uterine tube—pyosalpinx or ectopic gestation.

Malignant ovarian cysts are also common and may be very large. They often produce ascites and spread widely in the peritoneum: cytotoxic drugs are used in the treatment of the peritoneal spread.

Ovarian tumours produce symptoms by their size and pressure on other organs. They may twist (torsion) and cause intense pain and shock.

Secondary neoplasms from the breast, stomach and colon grow in the ovaries. From the breast, the melantoin is blood born and grows in the ovary because of its oestrogen content: from other sources the malignant cells are implanted across the peritoneum.

Rarely endocrine-producing tumours arise from the ovary and may produce masculinisation. Such a tumour is the **arrhenoblastoma** and it has a virilising effect like an adrenal cortical tumour.

Uterine fibroids

'Leiomyoma' is a tumour of involuntary muscle and the uterus produces many varieties of fibromyoma, commonly referred to as 'fibroids'. These may develop near the peritoneal surface (subserous) of the uterus, beneath the lining membrane (submucous), or in the cervix (cervical). Symptoms may be bleeding (submucous), torsion (subserous, or apedicle), sterility (cervical) or abdominal distension from the very large type. Treatment if symptoms warrant it is hysterectomy, but small fibroids can be excised from the wall of the uterus (myomectomy).

In pregnancy, a fibroid may degenerate and have internal haemorrhage, causing great pain.

Many women have symptomless fibroids and these may calcify as they get older (Fig. 40.8).

Carcinoma of the uterus

This occurs in two distinct sites—the cervix and the corpus (body) of the uterus.

Cervical carcinoma occurs in the younger age group, particularly in women who have borne children. Changes occur in the cervical epithelium before invasive growth is present and this is the basis of the 'cervical smear' test. A scraping of the cervix taken with a wood 'spatula' is spread on a microscope slide and stained: an expert cytologist can detect the pre-cancer cells. If the test is positive, a 'cone biopsy' is performed and if more serious disease is present surgery or radiotherapy is used.

More advanced growth produces vaginal discharge or bleeding, and as the growth extends it invades the ureters and bladder, producing hydronephrosis.

Carcinoma of the corpus (that is, of the endometrium as opposed to the cervical epithelium) occurs in an older age group, and the usual symptom is post menopausal bleeding.

Treatment

Total hysterectomy, with removal of ovaries and tubes, is the usual method of treating carcinoma of the endometrium, the lining of the body of the uterus. Radiation may be used in those unfit for surgery.

In carcinoma of the cervix, pelvic lymph glands are often involved. Extensive surgery—total hysterectomy and gland excision—is necessary.

Alternatively radiotherapy is used, and this is one of the principal areas in which caesium (previously radium) is now used. A tube containing the radioactive needles is placed in the uterine cavity, and 'ovoid' rubber-covered applicators or silver tubes containing the radioactive material are placed in the vault of the vagina with a spacer to keep them in position (Fig. 40.9). The cervix and body and adjacent tissues are irradiated for several days. The vagina is packed with gauze to keep the rectal and bladder walls as far away as possible, and a Foley self-retaining catheter is kept in the bladder during treatment.

Special nursing instructions are always given for patients having radiation treatment. A card showing that radiation is taking place is attached to the foot of the bed. The patient

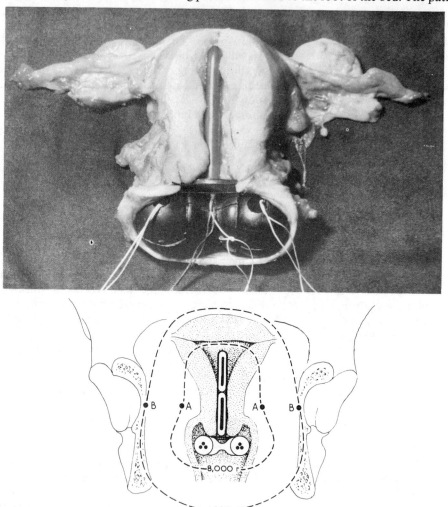

Fig. 40.9 (*Above*) Specimen of uterus and vagina to show how radium applicators are positioned in the vault of the vagina and in the uterine cavity (Manchester technique). (*Below*) Diagram to show section across pelvis indicating the zones of radiation achieved by the use of applicators. (*Gynaecology*, Ten Teachers, Arnold.)

is x-rayed to check the position of the radiation tubes and applicators immediately after insertion. Each tube or ovoid has a tape which is strapped to the thigh.

At the conclusion of treatment, under sedation with pethidine or valium, the catheter is deflated and removed; the tapes are used to extract the applicators: these are quickly rinsed and placed in the lead protective box which is kept by the bedside throughout treatment in case any tube is extruded.

Radiation produces cystitis and proctitis and may cause blockage of the ureters by oedema. Necrosis of the irradiated tissue may lead to a urinary fistula.

Epithelioma affects the vagina and vulva and is usually treated by radiotherapy, or wide excision. It spreads to inguinal glands and these are treated by excision or radio-therapy.

Endometriosis. This is a condition in which tumours are formed within the abdomen from tissue resembling the lining of the uterus. This tissue responds to the hormone stimulation of the menstrual cycle. The tumours become engorged before each period

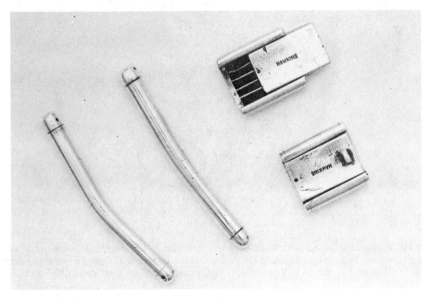

Fig. 40.10 Silver vaginal boxes and intra-uterine tubes containing radium. (*Gynaecology*, Ten Teachers, Arnold.)

and then bleed; thus they produce regular rhythmic pain and other symptoms. If this tissue grows in the ovary it produces 'chocolate cysts'; sometimes the disease affects the bowel and results in bleeding from the bowel at the same time as the periods. Endo-metriosis develops in those who have never borne children. In others a similar condition, 'adenomyosis', spreads out from the uterus, or grows within the uterus. Both these conditions subside spontaneously after the menopause, though surgery is often required because of pain or bleeding.

An **endometrioma** may be found anywhere in the abdominal cavity or groin. Sometimes a deposit is in the wall of the colon. Cyclical swelling and haemorrhage produces pain and rectal bleeding, related to the menstrual cycle (Fig. 40.11).

Gynaecological aspects of general surgery

Nurses and doctors are very familiar with the type of patient who makes the most of every symptom. There are, however, a great many patients who conceal important symptoms, not deliberately, but because they do not realise that these may be significant. A woman may state quite casually that her periods are normal when in fact they occur every 3 weeks and each period lasts perhaps 10 days. Similarly a woman who has passed the menopause may pay little attention to a small loss of blood from the vagina when in fact it is an indication that she has carcinoma of the cervix. Such facts as these may come to light during a period of hospital admission for a condition quite unconnected with the gynaecological disorder, and nursing staff must report any such abnormalities in amount or duration of a patient's menstruation.

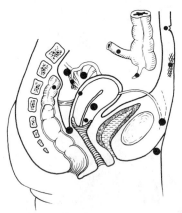

Fig. 40.11 Endometriosis—sites at which deposits are found. Haemorrhage is the usual presenting symptom, preceded by pain at the time of the periods. It can be seen that these deposits may be found in the bowel wall, at hernial sites as well as in the immediate vicinity of the uterus and its adnexa.

Gynaecological symptoms sometimes arise from conditions which really come within the sphere of general surgery. Any inflammatory condition of the pelvis—diverticulitis, appendicitis, Meckel's diverticulum—can aggravate **dyspareunia** (pain during intercourse). Conversely, uterine disorders, vaginitis or intercourse may be precipitating causes of urinary infection. Haematuria and minor vaginal bleeding are sometimes confused by the patient. Varicose veins may be due to pressure from a uterus enlarged by 'fibroids'.

It used to be considered unwise to undertake surgical operations on women patients during their menstruation. A decision in each case must depend on the distress which the patient normally suffers with each period and clearly if the loss of blood is excessive any operation which will add to the anaemia should be postponed. Patients are frequently very concerned that they will be called for admission to hospital when a period is due and the nurse may well be asked for a decision. In all urological cases, menstruation holds up investigations and prohibits operative surgery owing to increased risk of infection and the inability to watch the progress of postoperative haematuria. Other operations in the pelvis are also postponed until after menstruation, partly on account of the congestion of the pelvic organs which occurs at this time. The patient who has started her period should never be allowed to go to the operating theatre unless the surgeon has been informed and has stated clearly that he is able to proceed with the operation. This must be an absolute rule but is a matter which can be easily overlooked in a busy ward where the preparation of patients for an operating list is divided between several nurses.

Operations have to be undertaken during pregnancy for emergency conditions, but it is usual to postpone non-urgent operations until after the 4th month owing to the risk of producing abortion by the disturbance of the anaesthetic or operation. By the 4th month the fetus is more firmly secured in the uterus.

Examination

Care must be taken to ensure that the patient has emptied her bladder immediately before the examination takes place. A full bladder or loaded rectum may make pelvic examination difficult, if not impossible.

The full examination of gynaecological patients begins with a general physical examination, including the record of blood pressure, heart and lungs. The patient should accordingly be properly prepared by the nurse, and nothing is more embarrassing for the surgeon and the patient than unsuccessful attempts at examination because insufficient clothing has been removed.

After routine abdominal examination the patient is prepared for internal pelvic examination. This is usually undertaken with the patient on her left side, with the hips and spine flexed and the lower buttock at the extreme edge of the examination couch or bed. Sometimes the examination is carried out with the patient lying on her back and her legs supported in special stirrups. After the examination of the vulva, the surgeon, using a gloved hand, examines by palpation the vagina and cervix. Bimanual examination is used to assess the condition of the uterus, broad ligaments and ovaries, the surgeon's left hand being placed in the suprapubic region in order to press the pelvic organs down towards the vagina.

After digital examination, a speculum is used in order that the cervix can be seen directly. There are three commonly used types of speculum. The double-ended Sims's pattern is the smallest. The hinged, Cusco (duckbill) speculum has the advantage that its blades can be separated after the insertion of the instrument (Fig. 40.12). When the vaginal walls are prolapsed a double-bladed or tubular speculum is needed to expose the cervix.

Adequate examination of the vagina is not possible in a virgin owing to the discomfort produced when the hymen is stretched. General anaesthesia may be required for full examination.

Swabs for taking specimens for bacteriological examination must always be available and the technique used may require the use of a Pasteur pipette (page 260) to aspirate the vaginal secretion. Smears of the epithelial cells of the vagina are also taken for microscopic examination and clean glass microscope slides must also be at hand. The slides are examined for the presence of malignant cells and cytological examination is being used

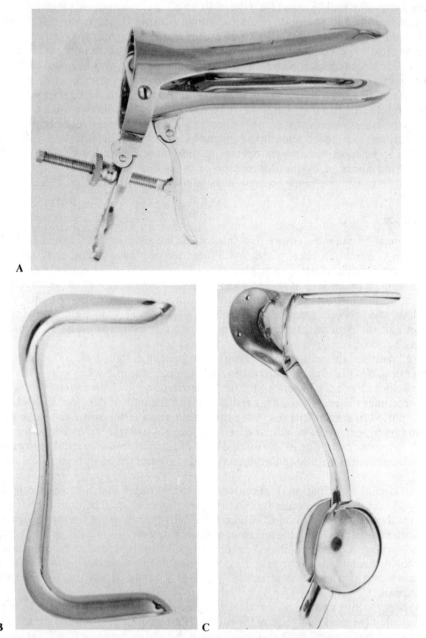

Fig. 40.12 Specula used for vaginal examination. **A.** Cusco's stainless steel vaginal speculum. This instrument is also available in disposable plastic form thus avoiding repeated sterilisation in busy clinics. **B.** Sim's vaginal speculum. **C.** Auvard's vaginal speculum. (Seward Surgical Instruments.)

increasingly in the early detection of carcinoma of the cervix in otherwise healthy women. Rectal examination and proctoscopy form part of the routine pelvic examination.

Consent forms

A patient who is to undergo a pelvic examination must always be asked for her verbal consent and in some centres written consent is demanded from the patient, just as for operation or anaesthetic.

Before any operation is undertaken which may result in sterilisation of the patient, she must have this explained to her, and if she is married the consent of her husband is also obtained in writing, the reason for the operation being explained to the husband by the medical officer. Circumstances may arise when the husband will not give his consent.

If a pregnancy is to be terminated on medical grounds it is usual for the surgeon to obtain a second opinion, perhaps from a physician or psychiatrist, according to the underlying medical disease. The consent of the patient and her husband are obtained in writing. These steps are necessary in Great Britain because the artificial termination of pregnancy is a crime (criminal abortion) unless it can be shown that the action was necessary to save the mother's life or on other general medical or psychological grounds, or in the interests of the rest of the family under certain circumstances.

Treatment

The treatment of gynaecological conditions may be medical, with hormones or other drugs administered by mouth, by injection, or applied locally to the affected areas. Drugs may be applied to the vagina in the form of pessaries or tampon (a gauze or cotton wool pack), or very occasionally in solution as an irrigation.

Surgical treatment of gynaecological disorders falls clearly into two categories, abdominal operation, or operation from below through the perineum or vagina.

Abdominal operations. Pre-operative and post-operative care for those conditions requiring abdominal operation is the same as that for other abdominal conditions (Chapter 19). If there is, however, a likelihood that the vagina will be opened, as in total hysterectomy, the surgeon may wish the vagina to be washed out with an antiseptic on the morning of operation. If there is any suspicion that the colon or rectum is involved in growth or inflammation, bowel preparation with enemas and oral anti-bacterial drugs (phthalyl-sulphathiazole or neomycin) is essential.

In order that the bladder is protected from injury during operation, it must be emptied by catheter immediately before the operation commences, and this is usually done in the theatre.

Haemorrhage, paralytic ileus, retention of urine and peritonitis are all complications for which special post-operative nursing observation is essential. The bladder may have been bruised, and micturition is often difficult and painful. Tidal drainage may be needed.

Perineal and vaginal operations (Table 57). Apart from relatively minor operations on the vulva or for Bartholin's cyst, the most common operations are those for the repair of prolapse and the procedure of dilatation and curettage.

Pre-operative treatment varies with different clinics and the surgeon will give instructions concerning the technique he wishes employed. The vulva must be shaved. The vagina may be irrigated with antiseptic and it may be necessary to pack the vagina with ribbon gauze. This latter procedure will be undertaken by a medical officer. The rectum must be emptied and this is best ensured by the use of a laxative 2 nights before and an enema or suppositories the evening preceding the operation. The bladder must be emptied and the natural voiding of urine is not sufficient to guarantee an empty bladder in a case of

Table 56   Abdominal operations

Name	Description	Reason
Oophorectomy or removal of ovarian cyst	Removal of ovary	Cyst formation on account of size, malignancy or torsion
Bilateral oophorectomy	Removal of both ovaries	To produce artificial menopause or in treatment of carcinoma of breast to reduce oestrogen formation (page 885)
		Infection (probably tuberculous)
Salpingectomy	Removal of uterine tube	Tubal pregnancy (ectopic gestation)
Sterilisation	Division of uterine tubes	General physical or mental unfitness for pregnancy (pulmonary tubercle, heart disease)
Total hysterectomy (Fig. 40.13)	Removal of uterus (including cervix)	Uterine disease; fibroids; prolapse. (Sometimes in radical removal of malignant disease of bladder or rectum)
Subtotal hysterectomy (Fig. 40.14)	Removal of uterus and tubes, leaving cervix (less severe operation than total hysterectomy, but cervix may become malignant)	Uterine disease; fibroids; prolapse
Wertheim's hysterectomy	Removal of uterus, ovaries and all lymphatic drainage areas	Carcinoma of body (endometrium) or cervix
Ventrisuspension operations	To attach uterus to abdominal wall	Treatment of uterine prolapse
Myomectomy	Removal of fibromyoma from uterus	
Hysterotomy	Opening uterus to remove fetus	To terminate pregnancy on account of disease in mother
Caesarean section	Delivery of baby by open operation	Natural labour unsafe or impossible
Emergency operations		
Oophorectomy, or removal of cyst	For twisting (torsion)	
Salpingectomy	For ruptured (bleeding) ectopic gestation (tubal pregnancy)	
Peritonitis—drainage	From salpingitis or criminal abortion	

prolapse. A catheter is therefore passed either before the patient goes to the operating theatre or by the surgeon at the start of the operation. He may leave the catheter in position or withdraw it.

After operation the routine care must be the same as for abdominal procedures. Even if the peritoneum has not been opened, infection may gain entry into the peritoneal cavity through the uterus. Usually, however, normal feeding can be resumed at once, but it must always be borne in mind that the risk of intraperitoneal complications (e.g. ileus) is present in all pelvic operations performed by the vaginal route. Naturally the risks are greater when the peritoneum has been deliberately opened as in the operation of vaginal hysterectomy.

Table 57   Perineal operations

Name	Description	Disorder
Dilatation and Curettage ('D and C')	Dilatation of cervix Scraping of uterine cavity	For treatment of disorder of endometrium
Amputation of cervix		Chronic erosion (ulcers) or laceration of cervix
Cone biopsy	Coring out of the cervix	Carcinoma in situ of the cervix
Vaginal hysterectomy	Removal of uterus through vault of vagina	In treatment of prolapse
Vulvectomy	Excision of labia and reconstruction of urethra and vaginal outlet	Epithelioma of vulva
Anterior colporrhaphy	Repair of tissue in anterior wall of vagina	Treatment of prolapse where bladder is sagging: (cystocele). Stress incontinence
Posterior colporrhaphy	Repair of posterior vaginal wall	Treatment of prolapse where rectum is mainly affected (rectocele)
Colpoperineorrhaphy	Complete repair of pelvic outlet and perineum	Severe prolapse and perineal injury from childbirth
Insertion of radium	Application of radium in a special container, or in needles (page 741)	Treatment of carcinoma or cervix or vagina: production of menopause by irradiation of ovaries
Salpingography	Injection of contrast medium into uterus to detect obstruction in uterine tube	Investigation of sterility

The vaginal tissues are almost always repaired with catgut to avoid the difficult procedure of stitch removal. Sometimes the vagina is packed at the end of the operation. In all cases the external skin requires cleansing after the use of a bed pan and vulval swabbing is always performed from in front backwards to avoid conveying organisms from the anal region towards the urethra. A mild antiseptic solution such as Savlon may be used.

Alternatively, vulval toilet is performed by sitting the patient on a bedpan and pouring warm water, containing a teaspoonful of sodium bicarbonate to 500 ml sterile water over the vulva. The patient is then dried by using sterile swabs if it is after a vaginal operation. For patients having radiotherapy (x-ray or radium) the skin is very delicate and to avoid abrasion, drying is done preferably with an electric hair drier. Occasionally, as for instance in the repair of vesico-vaginal fistula, non-absorbable stitches of nylon or stainless steel wire may be used and these will require removal, probably under anaesthesia.

The post-operative care of the bladder depends on particular circumstances. Sometimes instructions are given for a self-retaining catheter to be left in place with simple gravity or syphon drainage. Post-operative catheterisation may not be required unless retention occurs from the tightness of the vaginal repair in the region of the urethra and from post-operative oedema. If natural micturition is not resumed within 12–18 hours, catheterisation is necessary, and the catheter is left on open drainage for 2 days: if voiding still fails after 8 hours and the bladder is full, catheterisation is repeated; alternatively, the surgeon may wish the catheter to remain undisturbed for 6–7 days. If difficulty presents, carbachol may be tried (page 388). The patient endeavours to void urine before the catheter is passed on each occasion, and the residual urine is measured and recorded. Considerable quantities of residual urine are found for some weeks after certain repair operations and the recovery of bladder function is considerably delayed. During this recovery period urinary antiseptics are administered to prevent the development of cystitis.

If prolonged catheterisation is necessary the surgeon may order tidal drainage (page 663) to maintain the normal rhythmical relaxation and contraction of the bladder.

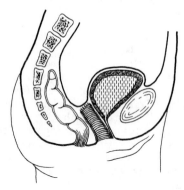

Fig. 40.13 Total hysterectomy. The vagina is shortened and closed after removal of the cervix. The ureter may be injured during this operation.

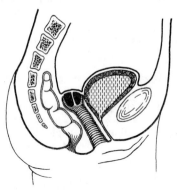

Fig. 40.14 Subtotal hysterectomy. The cervix is not removed in this operation and remains as a possible source of infection and carcinoma in the vault of the vagina.

Post-operative activity

Thrombosis of iliac veins and the veins of the legs is particularly liable to occur after gynaecological operations. This is probably because of the presence of very large veins in association with the uterus. Post-operative abdominal and leg exercises are essential in the prevention of this complication and most patients are able to get out of bed within the first 48 hours. After operations for the repair of prolapse the avoidance of strain is essential but patients are mobilised early to discourage venous thrombosis, common after pelvic surgery. A strain much greater than that produced by walking will result if the patient is allowed to become constipated or to develop retention of urine. Prevention and management of these conditions has been described in Chapter 20.

Infertility

Clinical investigation into the cause of a childless marriage is undertaken in a gynaecological department or special 'fertility' clinic.

There are many causes of sterility in both the male and the female. In the woman, the presence of abnormalities of the vagina or uterus which may prevent intercourse are discovered on clinical examination. Other minor structural changes in the uterus, tubes or ovaries, may prevent the spermatozoa reaching the ovum. Salpingitis, endometritis and fibroids are frequent causes of sterility.

The husband is also examined and the seminal fluid is subjected to laboratory examination.

If there is then no apparent reason for the patient's inability to conceive, x-ray investigation is undertaken. Radio-opaque contrast medium is injected through a special catheter introduced into the cervix. Photographs reveal the outline of the uterine cavity and indicate whether the tubes are open.

Similarly, air may be injected into the uterus, a special apparatus being used so that the pressure can be recorded and over-distension avoided. As the air escapes through each tube into the peritoneal cavity, there is a drop in pressure. 'Tubal insufflation' may also unblock a tube which has been obstructed by mild inflammation. This may be combined with laparoscopy (peritoneoscopy); methylene blue dye injected through the cervix may then be seen to escape from the uterine tubes if they are open (Fig. 40.15).

These two procedures, **salpingography** and **tubal insufflation,** are sometimes carried out under general anaesthesia but are commonly performed now with the patient admitted just for a day, and having sedation with ketamine, valium or oral medication. A further method of investigating pelvic disorders is the injection of carbon dioxide gas into the peritoneum. The patient is tilted into the head down position and x-ray examination outlines the pelvic viscera; cystic conditions of the ovary can be detected by this method.

During the course of investigation for sterility, the patient is asked to keep a 'basal temperature chart'. A daily vaginal temperature record is made on waking. The purpose of this is to note whether there is a fall of perhaps half a degree below the normal morning temperature for the individual, when ovulation occurs. This is usually about the tenth day of the menstrual cycle. A subsequent rise to perhaps one degree above normal is maintained during the second half of the cycle and indicates that the normal physiological process has occurred.

Changes in the lining membrane (endometrium) of the uterus which occur following ovulation can be verified by biopsy performed through the cervix with a curette (page 736).

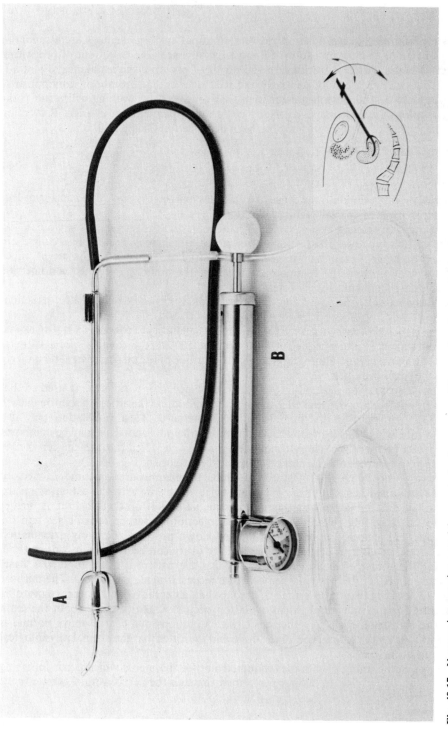

Fig. 40.15 Vacuum intra-uterine sound for use during laparoscopy. The cup **A** makes an airtight seal over the cervix; the pressure produced by the pump **B** is recorded on the dial. The diagram illustrates how the uterus can be manipulated to bring the various parts into view at laparoscopy. (**Rocket of London.**)

Sterilisation and contraception

If on medical or sociological grounds it is deemed necessary for conception to be permanently prevented, the only absolutely reliable method is division of the uterine tubes or removal of the ovaries. Frequently the condition on account of which pregnancy is contra-indicated may warrant removal of the uterus in any case—for instance, severe prolapse. Removal of ovaries is undesirable simply to prevent contraception. The tubes may be divided by open operation or through an endoscope at 'laparoscopy'. The closed method carries risks of haemorrhage, damage to the bowel and peritonitis, the tubes having been divided with diathermy.

Oral administration of hormone tablets—'the pill'—is most commonly used for women who have not yet borne children. Whatever the composition of these preparations they suppress ovulation. They are administered on a date cycle: cessation produces an artificial period, but they are only effective if taken regularly. Patients need to be warned that they should not rely on this method until they have been taking it for 2 weeks and that if they should miss taking a pill for more than 36 hours they should use an alternative method. Most packets state clearly how many days should lapse before taking the next cycle and this must be adhered to even if menstruation has not finished.

Women who have borne children are often advised to have an intra-uterine contraceptive device fitted. This consists of a little plastic coil or loop (Fig. 40.16) inserted into the cavity of the uterus; it remains embedded there, and sets up a mild inflammatory reaction

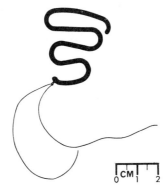

Fig. 40.16   Lippe Loop—one form of intra-uterine device, left in the cavity of the uterus unless pregnancy is desired.

which prevents a fertilised ovum from becoming attached. The loop may come out accidentally, or it may in fact perforate the uterus and produce peritonitis. The most popular device now is the Copper '7' which can be fitted for nulliparous women as well as those who have borne children.

Both these methods have superseded the use of the Dutch cap, a rubber diaphragm mounted in a small spiral spring, which is inserted in the vagina by the patient when required. For complete security it is usually used with a chemical spermicidal jelly. The diaphragm has to be fitted initially by a doctor to ensure that it is of the correct size.

Permanent prevention of conception in cases of severe or chronic ill-health (e.g. psychosis, heart disease) is achieved by tubal ligation. This necessarily involves abdominal operation though it is often done at the time of Caesarean section for the delivery of the first child.

Before major surgery, patients are usually advised to stop taking the contraceptive pill. They do, however, need reminding that they should use an alternative contraceptive during the waiting period before the operation.

41

Surgery of the Neck

A great many surgical conditions arise in the neck because of the numerous vital structures which are packed into so small a space. From a nursing point of view many of these conditions require no particular description. On the other hand, conditions affecting the larynx, thyroid gland or structures at the root of the neck, in the area above the clavicle, all involve operations and after-care of a more specialised nature. The surgery of the thyroid gland perhaps best illustrates the details of pre-operative preparation and post-operative care; the nurse who is familiar with the management of the thyroid case will find little difficulty in the care of patients with other surgical lesions in the neck. The surgery of the larynx is somewhat different and is described separately (Chapter 43).

Common disorders of the neck

From faulty development there may remain in the neck cysts and small openings connecting the skin with the pharynx. Though these **congenital branchial cysts** and **fistulae** are present from birth, they may not be noticed until later years when they become infected. **Infective** conditions arise in the lymph glands of the neck, particularly in those below the angle of the jaw which are connected with the tonsils; these infected glands may give rise to abscesses and they are frequently affected with tuberculosis. The salivary glands, of which there are two principal ones on either side of the neck, also become inflamed and sometimes need to be removed if they develop tumours. The neck is sometimes the site of **injury** of which the suicidal 'cut-throat' is a well-known example.

Neoplastic disease affecting the lymphoglandular system (e.g. lymphadenoma) is a common cause of enlarged glands in the neck. The lymph glands in the neck drain lymph from the tongue and the floor of the mouth. In cases of cancer in the mouth, these glands may require complete removal (block dissection) or radiotherapy to deal with possible secondary growth.

A further group of surgical conditions arises in the part of the neck immediately above the clavicle. Some of these are associated with the important bundle of nerves (**brachial plexus**) and large blood vessels which pass from the neck down into the arm, behind the clavicle. It is not uncommon for there to be an extra little rib (**cervical rib**) in this area, and overcrowding due to its presence results in pressure on the nerves, with

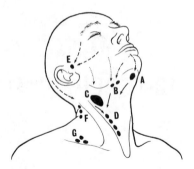

Fig. 41.1 Lymph glands in the neck. **A.** *Submental,* from chin and front of tongue. **B.** *Submandibular,* from side of tongue and cheek. **C.** *Tonsillar,* from back of tongue and pharynx. **D.** *Deep cervical,* draining all these previous groups. **E.** *Pre-auricular,* from face, forehead and ear. **F.** *Occipital,* from scalp. **G.** *Supraclavicular,* from shoulder and skin of upper chest.

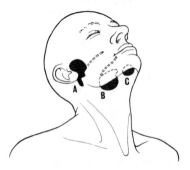

Fig. 41.2 The salivary glands. **A.** *Parotid:* the duct traverses the cheek to open opposite the upper molar teeth. **B.** *Submandibular:* the duct lies in the floor of the mouth and opens beneath the tip of the tongue. **C.** *Sublingual:* several openings in the floor of the mouth.

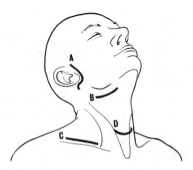

Fig. 41.3 Common incisions. **A.** For parotid gland and temporo-mandibular joint. **B.** For tuberculous lymph glands or submandibular salivary glands. **C.** For operations at the root of the neck—brachial plexus, subclavian vessels, cervical rib or sympathectomy.

consequent neuritis. Here also are found the sympathetic ganglion (**stellate ganglion**) and nerves which control the blood supply to the arm, and **'cervical sympathectomy'** is performed through an incision above the clavicle (Fig. 41.3).

Pre-operative treatment

Dental sepsis is treated before operation in order to lessen the risk of wound infection (cellulitis) and adenitis. Apart from cases of thyrotoxicosis, no specific treatment is required. If the operation is in the upper part of the neck, the lower part of the scalp should be shaved (i.e. below and behind the mastoid process).

Post-operative nursing

Apart from the removal of lymph glands for microscopic examination, most surgical operations on the neck are performed under general anaesthesia, given through an intra-tracheal tube. The general post-operative care is usually straightforward but particular attention has to be paid to the following points:

1. While the patient is still unconscious, care must be taken not to move the neck excessively or to let the head fall back unsupported. A sudden jerk of the head may well tear some of the stitches or pull off some ligatures which have been placed on arteries or veins.

2. If haemorrhage should occur into a wound in the neck it may produce pressure on the trachea, with difficulty in breathing and swallowing. If this pressure is great asphyxia may result (page 774 for emergency action).

3. As the result of handling, retraction, and interference with the tissues of the neck, there may be some inflammation of the lining of the trachea and larynx—tracheitis and laryngitis. This results in a weakness and huskiness of the voice and the production of a cough. Any movement of the larynx (necessary, of course, in swallowing) is also painful, so that feeding and drinking are difficult. Inhalations for the tracheitis and a completely fluid diet may be required for several days.

4. The pleural cavity extends up into the root of the neck and may be damaged during an operation low in the neck. If this has occurred it will usually be known to the surgeon and special instructions will have been given to ensure the adequate expansion of the affected lung (page 603). Should air escape into the tissues of the neck, a crackling sensation will be present when the skin is pressed. This is **surgical emphysema** (page 612), and if the nurse suspects this complication to be present, she must report it at once.

5. The tissues of the neck heal very rapidly and therefore it is possible to lessen the risk of stitch marks by early removal of the stitches or clips (probably on the 2nd day).

6. Because of the constant movement of the tissues of the neck, collections of blood may occur and it is usual for the operation wounds to be drained for perhaps 24 hours; if in spite of drainage, a haematoma develops, it is aspirated through a serum needle. Major procedures such as block dissection usually require two (Redivac) suction drainage tubes.

7. If the original condition is due to infection or if an infection should complicate the operation, there is an additional risk of spread of this infection down into the mediastinum between the two lungs, as there is no natural barrier of connective tissue. **Mediastinitis** is extremely grave unless it can be controlled by antibiotics (page 511).

Thyroglossal cyst and fistula (Fig. 41.4)

In the embryo the thyroid gland is formed at the base of the tongue, and during subsequent growth of the baby it takes up its normal position in the lower part of the neck. Very occasionally this migration is arrested and the whole thyroid gland remains in the base of the tongue. This condition is very rare and cannot be treated surgically. Between the normal thyroid gland and the base of the tongue there are sometimes remnants of the original connection. These may be present either as a cyst or a narrow sinus which passes from the base of the tongue behind the central part of the hyoid bone down towards the top of the thyroid gland. The importance of these conditions lies in the fact that the remnants frequently become infected and give rise to a discharge. They are difficult to remove and, unless the operation is carried out with great care, the fistula will recur.

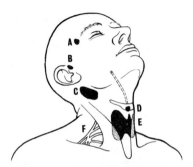

Fig. 41.4   Surgical conditions in the neck. **A.** *External angular dermoid cyst.* **B.** *Pre-auricular dermoid cyst and fistula.* **C.** *Branchial cyst,* connecting with pharynx in the region of the tonsil. **D.** *Thyroglossal cyst* with tract opening at the back of the tongue. **E.** *The thyroid gland* surrounding the lower part of larynx and upper end of trachea. **F.** *The brachial plexus* lying between the muscles of the neck and the first rib.

When a surgeon removes a thyroglossal fistula, he tries to trace it right up to the base of the tongue; he usually removes the centre part of the hyoid bone. (Small bone-cutting forceps and nibblers must be available at this operation.)

In nursing such cases there is no particular pre-operative treatment. Occasionally diodone or other iodine-containing compound opaque to x-rays is injected into the sinus to determine the length of the track. At the time of operation, in order to help him to find the upper part of the fistula, the surgeon may inject methylene blue (1 per cent) with a blunt-ended needle on a 2-ml syringe. A warning is needed in connection with the methylene blue because if the fistula communicates with the back of the tongue, the dye may be squirted through into the mouth and stain the mouth, or even find its way down into the lungs. It must always be realised that though the fistula may appear to be small, the operation is far from simple and, as removal of part of the hyoid bone is usually necessary, there may be considerable discomfort in the post-operative stage: a fluid diet is usually essential for several days.

Branchial cyst and fistula

These congenital remnants are similar to thyroglossal cysts and fistulae, but arise from the 'gill cleft'[1] development in the embryo, and are situated at the side of the neck usually just in front of the sternomastoid muscle. Frequently they communicate with the pharynx through a long sinus which threads its way among the large blood vessels and other structures deep in the neck. The operation from the nursing point of view is similar to thyroidectomy, and a syringe with methylene blue should be available for injecting into the sinus so that it can be identified at operation.

In the case of a long fistula reaching to the lower part of the neck, the surgeon may make two separate incisions in the neck at different levels in order to trace the track up to its origin.

There is a risk of wound infection, on account of the pharyngeal connection of the cyst or fistula.

Acute cervical adenitis

The glands of the neck are commonly affected by pyogenic (pus forming) organisms from the throat. The infection may be so severe that an abscess forms. Swelling occurs in the region beneath the jaw; diffuse cellulitis may spread from the gland and cause difficulty in swallowing and breathing. With chemotherapy and antibiotics these serious conditions now rarely arise. Cellulitis of the neck[2] is a grave condition as the infection may spread downwards around the larynx and produce oedema of the glottis, leading to asphyxia; it may descend into the mediastinum, setting up mediastinitis.

Because of the risks of spread of infection, patients (usually children) with acute cervical abscesses are usually admitted to hospital. As well as general measures to combat infection, kaolin poultices are used to relieve pain, and cold hypertonic saline packs may equally relieve oedema and give comfort. Abscesses may be incised and a piece of 'glove' drainage or corrugated rubber left in for 2 to 3 days. Alternatively the abscess may be aspirated and penicillin solution injected into it. Great care has to be taken over oral hygiene, as the patient has pain on swallowing and is usually very loath to move the jaw adequately for mouthwashes to be effective.

Tuberculous adenitis

The glands of the neck may be unhealthy from chronic tonsillar infection, and fall an easy prey to tuberculosis bacilli gaining entry through the tonsil or adenoid.

Sometimes the tuberculous glands heal themselves by calcification; sometimes they form 'cold' abscesses (so called because they do not exhibit the heat of acute inflammation). The glands are usually removed surgically and sanatorium treatment is advisable. An abscess may be spirated and para-amino salicylic acid (PAS) injected into it as an anti-

[1] The human neck in development resembles a fish head, with gill (branchial) arches and clefts. Each arch has a special nerve; the clefts become buried by fusion of adjacent arches.

[2] Sometimes described as Ludwig's angina.

septic. Streptomycin or isoniazid (isonicotinic acid hydrazide) is given in many cases. The infection may spread to the overlying skin and ulcerate, leaving a tuberculous sinus.

If the tonsils have not already been removed this forms part of the routine. Particular attention is paid to the patient's nutrition. Extra vitamin D (e.g. 50,000 units calciferol) is given daily. Anti-tuberculous chemotherapy or an appropriate antibiotic may have to be continued for many months (page 89).

Secondary infection with germs such as staphylococcus aureus may complicate tuberculous adenitis, and other antibiotics are then used.

At any stage, and especially if there is secondary infection, the surgeon may order complete rest by 'splinting' the neck. This may be achieved in two ways:

1. If the patient is to be in bed, he is kept quite flat without a pillow: a sandbag is placed on either side of the head, which is held by a folded hand towel passing across the forehead and under the sandbags.

2. A Plastazote collar may be used.

Block dissection of glands of the neck

This operation, as its name implies, involves the removal of a block of tissue including all the upper deep lymphatic glands of the neck, the internal jugular vein and the sternomastoid muscle. It is performed in cases of cancer of the tongue to remove all lymph glands in which there may be metastasis. It is a severe operation and is sometimes performed on both sides of the neck. In post-operative care particular attention is paid to oral hygiene and diet; the nursing difficulties are increased by the previous removal of the tongue or impairment of its function by disease. The patients are elderly and especially liable to chest complications. Feeding by means of a nasal tube may well be necessary in order to maintain adequate fluid intake and eliminate the discomfort of swallowing.

Malignant disease originating in the lung, stomach, oesophagus or pharynx may not be discovered until secondary deposits of growth cause enlargement of cervical glands. Lymphadenoma and other generalised glandular disorders frequently give rise to large masses of glands in the neck. These may be removed for diagnostic purposes or, occasionally, as the only possible treatment really as a palliative measure. Tight bandaging is not possible and usually two suction drainage tubes are used to prevent haematoma formation.

Salivary glands (Fig. 41.2)

The parotid gland in front of the ear is sometimes the site of a growth. The typical **parotid tumour** is usually not malignant at first but may become so if left or if only partly removed. If the tumour is malignant the facial nerve is usually involved; the whole gland has to be removed and facial paralysis results.

The parotid gland and the submandibular salivary gland beneath the mandible may become infected, especially if the mouth or teeth are unhealthy. The parotid is particularly liable to infection after any severe operation (e.g. gastrectomy) if oral hygiene has been neglected. Such infection is treated with chemotherapy and occasionally incision of an abscess in the gland is needed.

Salivary calculus

Stones form in the ducts of the salivary glands, often with infection. A stone may be removed by operation upon the appropriate duct inside the mouth, usually under general intratracheal anaesthesia. A stone may block the duct and cause painful swelling of the gland when salivation is stimulated by eating. Pus may be seen exuding from the duct by the frenum of the tongue (Fig. 41.5).

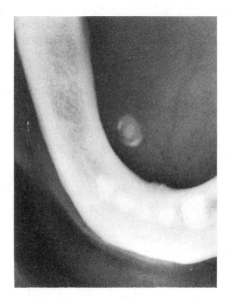

Fig. 41.5   X-ray of floor of mouth showing a stone in the submandibular duct under the tongue.

Sometimes the whole affected submandibular gland is removed if chronic infection persists. The nursing management is the same as for excision of thyroglossal cyst. Infection in the wound may occur from the connection with the mouth.

Pharyngotomy

A congenital pouch sometimes springs from the pharynx or upper end of the oesophagus behind the larynx and trachea, giving rise to symptoms of choking and regurgitation of food.

Cancer of the pharynx or of the oesophagus, or the impaction of foreign bodies, may require open operation. Infection of the loose tissues of the neck is the main risk and the wound is always drained for several days. Feeding has to be by naso-gastric tube initially to diminish the risk of leakage from the pharyngeal wound. (Also Larynx, page 811, and Oesophagus, page 500.)

Parathyroid tumour

A non-malignant tumour may arise in one of the parathyroid glands. The cells of the tumour produce in excess the normal parathyroid hormone—**parathormone**—which alters the use of calcium in the body. The bones become weak and develop cysts; stones form in the kidneys. There are normally four parathyroid glands placed on the back of the thyroid gland, but frequently one or more of these are displaced into the mediastinum. When a tumour is known to be present, the surgeon first searches in the region of the thyroid gland, but if he is unsuccessful the sternum has to be split and separated to search in the space around the great vessels and thymus (page 606). To assist in identifying parathyroid tissue at operation methylene blue (5 mg per kilo body weight) is given in 500 ml dextrose-saline 1 hour before operation. The glands concentrate the dye.

In order to determine which of the four glands has developed a tumour, blood samples taken from different positions in the internal jugular veins are assayed for parathormone levels. The blood is obtained through a cardiac-type catheter passed up the femoral vein and venae cavae, under x-ray control; a spot of radio-opaque dye is injected to confirm the exact position of the tip. This is a time-consuming investigation. Recently, isotopic scanning with ^{75}Se selenomethionine has been used with success.

To confirm that hypercalcaemia is in fact due to hyperparathyroidism and not to some other cause such as sarcoidosis, a **steroid suppression test** is used: hydrocortisone given at 40 mg three times daily for 10 days depresses blood calcium *except* in parathyroid over-activity.

The blood calcium level may fall too low after the tumour has been removed and tetany may develop (page 775), and require calcium gluconate injection.

The post-operative nursing management is identical to that for thyroidectomy.

Operations at the root of the neck

In the small space (Fig. 41.4) immediately behind and above the clavicle, bounded by the curve of the first rib, lie the subclavian artery and vein, the brachial nerve plexus and the sympathetic nerves which control the circulation of the arm and of the same side of the head and face. The anterior scalene muscle lies in here and an extra 'cervical' rib is sometimes to be found. The phrenic nerve, responsible for diaphragm movement on that side, crosses the scalene muscle. The apex of the lung, in a cone of pleura, protrudes upwards into the area. Each of these structures is of surgical importance.

1. The subclavian artery and vein may be operated on for aneurysm, embolus or injury.
2. A cervical rib or the scalene muscle may be removed if there has been compression of the brachial plexus and neuritis.

3. The phrenic nerve is frequently exposed and crushed to rest the lung on that side in the treatment of pulmonary tuberculosis (page 622). The operation is performed under local anaesthesia.
4. The 'stellate' sympathetic ganglion or sympathetic chain may be removed for vascular disorders of the arm, such as Raynaud's disease. A diagnostic injection of procaine may be made to determine the likely response of the circulation to sympathectomy (page 943).
5. Minor strokes or syncopal attacks may be due to compression of a thickened vertebral artery where it enters the cervical spine at the root of the neck. Vein patch grafts have been used with success to enlarge the narrowed vertebral artery at this point. Similarly, blockage of the subclavian artery may lead to a reversed flow down the vertebral artery, producing syncope when the arm is used vigorously (subclavian 'steal' syndrome).

Nursing, after any of these procedures, does not usually involve any difficulty; patients are very soon ambulant. Wounds are sometimes drained for 24 hours. Occasionally the pleural cavity is opened accidentally at operation and in such a case the nurse will watch particularly for surgical emphysema (page 612), difficulty with breathing or cyanosis. Owing to bruising and inflammation of the nerves, patients may be troubled with pain in the arm and may need analgesics (such as codeine or aspirin). Bruising of the phrenic nerve from pressure or retraction may produce severe hiccough: if this occurs and does not respond to simple measures, the surgeon may inject a little local analgesic (such as procaine 1 per cent) around the nerve.

Post-operative dressings in this area need only be small and are better held in place by adhesive elastic strapping than with bandages.

Torticollis

'Wry-neck' is a condition in which the head is held to one side by spasm or shortening of the muscles.

Fibrositis, an acute inflammation of the trapezius muscle, produces severe torticollis and is often very sudden in onset. It may occur in a patient already in hospital, and relief is usually obtained with warmth from a radiant heat lamp or kaolin poultice and occasionally an injection of procaine is given into the muscle.

There is a 'congenital' form of torticollis in which the sternomastoid muscle on one side is shortened, from birth. Usually there is an associated asymmetry of the baby's skull. If the muscle tightness is not corrected in infancy, operation is undertaken later. This consists of dividing either the upper attachment of the muscle to the mastoid process or the lower attachment to the clavicle and sternum, by open operation. Sometimes the tight lower tendon above the clavicle is divided by 'closed' tenotomy; a very small tenotomy knife is inserted through the skin and the tendon cut by 'feel'. Haemorrhage and haematoma formation may follow this 'closed' procedure.

After tenotomy, the muscle has to be stretched by vigorous physiotherapy: the surgeon may 'strap' the head into an over-corrected position or he may wish the head held towards the opposite side with sandbags in the immediate post-operative stage.

The thyroid gland

The thyroid gland consists of a right lobe and a left lobe joined together by a narrow bridge of tissue in the mid-line. The gland lies in the lower part of the neck between the two sternomastoid muscles. It is folded round the front and sides of the trachea and larynx and is one of the most important structures in the body. Its function is to produce a hormone, **thyroxin**, which controls general body activity. The thyroid itself is controlled by the pituitary gland, and all the endocrine glands are to some extent linked up, so that a disorder of one is reflected in disorder of the others. Persons may be born without a thyroid gland or with the gland displaced from the normal position.

At certain times in a person's life when there is an increase of physiological activity, the thyroid gland becomes enlarged. This is sometimes referred to as **physiological goitre** and such enlargement may occur during adolescence, during pregnancy and to a lesser extent, with each menstrual period. The physiological enlargement of pregnancy is carried on through the period of lactation. After each of these spells of physiological enlargement, the increase in cellular activity and enlargement of the gland should recede, but this does not always occur. Sometimes the whole gland or only small portions of it remain in a more active state. Consequently, when the next need for increased activity comes along, there is an unequal subsequent enlargement of the gland which we believe leads to a process of nodule formation in the gland. At the menopause there may also be an increase in hormonal activity, and perhaps a production of thyroid overactivity.

The normal activity of the thyroid gland is dependent on the presence of iodine in the diet. If there is a shortage of iodine in the food or in the water (and in certain areas of the world there is a natural iodine deficiency in the drinking water), then in its effort to produce normal thyroxin with poor material the thyroid gland produces a large amount of jelly-like substance called 'colloid'. In some cases the gland becomes enormous. With the passage of years this uniformly enlarged thyroid gland gets too big for its blood supply and undergoes a process of degeneration with partial shrinkage, which again leads to a form of nodular or irregular goitre,

With any of these physiological or 'colloid' goitre patients, symptoms of thyrotoxicosis may develop. The classic picture of 'Graves' disease, with severe weight loss, exophthalmos, a very rapid pulse and great nervousness is now rare. Uncommon forms in which thyrotoxicosis appears include recurrent diarrhoea, or atrial fibrillation (usually in the elderly) with no other obvious symptoms. The onset of the toxic condition may be very gradual and insidious. It may go unnoticed for years until eventually the patient's heart is affected before a diagnosis is made. On the other hand, the onset may be acute and the general symptoms very severe.

Pressure symptoms. The thyroid gland, by its enlargement and subsequent degeneration, may produce symptoms by reason of its very size. These symptoms arise from pressure on the trachea, which is displaced (Fig. 41.6). and may be reduced to a narrow slit. There may be increasing difficulty in swallowing from pressure on the oesophagus. Pressure on the nerves to the larynx produces a husky and weak voice. Inability to reach the high notes in singing may be the first symptom. Haemorrhage may occur into the nodules of a nodular goitre from 'rotting' of the tissues: this accounts for the sudden appearance of the lump in the neck, of which some patients complain. Patients with 'non-toxic' goitres have with them the constant hazard of becoming thyrotoxic, as well as the risk of pressure symptoms.

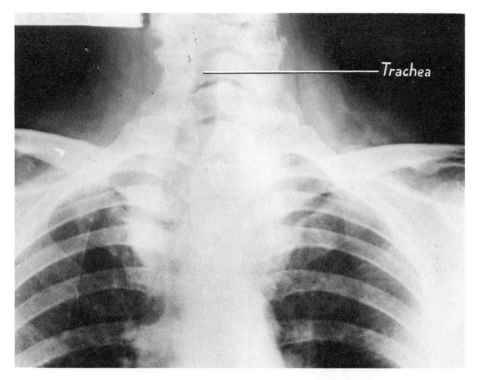

Trachea

Fig. 41.6 Radiograph of root of neck. The trachea is pushed away from the mid-line by a large goitre which is causing a shadow in the mediastinum.

Primary thyrotoxicosis or 'Graves' disease'. This is a condition in which thyrotoxic symptoms arise in a patient whose thyroid gland has previously been normal in size. With the onset of the condition the gland enlarges, although sometimes this increase is only very slight.

Mediastinal or intrathoracic goitre. Sometimes the thyroid gland enlarges downwards into the superior mediastinum behind the sternum. It is then known as a 'plunging' goitre (Fig. 41.8). In some cases the whole of the thyroid gland may be in the mediastinum. Now that mass radiography is applied to many thousands of persons, quite a number who have never suspected that they had any thyroid enlargement are found with a goitre in the upper part of the chest, displacing the windpipe to one side or actually enveloping it. These patients are usually advised to have the abnormal thyroid gland removed because of the possibility of pressure symptoms or malignancy arising at a later date.

Lymphadenoid goitre and neoplasms. Lymphadenoid goitre (Hashimoto's disease) is a condition in which the thyroid gland becomes replaced by lymphoid tissue. The cause is unknown. The gland enlarges symmetrically and loses its ability to produce thyroxin; consequently the patient shows, in advanced cases, myxoedema, although the thyroid gland is enlarged. Another similar condition occurs, known as Reidel's thyroiditis, in which the gland shrivels and usually produces its symptoms by strangling the trachea. In the first of these two the thyroid gland is usually removed, and in the second, sometimes the isthmus is divided in order to release the pressure on the trachea.

A true benign neoplasm (adenoma) occurs usually as a single nodule in the thyroid gland and may, by enlargement and a change in its character, produce symptoms of thyrotoxicosis. At operation what may have been thought to be a single nodule is often found to be part of a multinodular goitre. Malignancy in a nodule cannot be excluded without biopsy and so advice is usually given to remove nodules. Carcinoma is not uncommon and any rapidly enlarging goitre is regarded as malignant. The management of thyroid cancer is described on page 777.

The influence of pathology on nursing

The thyroid gland is removed for simple enlargements because it is known that these goitres may give rise to symptoms later. Prevention is better than cure and in order to avoid sudden increase in size from haemorrhage and the damaging effects of thyrotoxicosis,

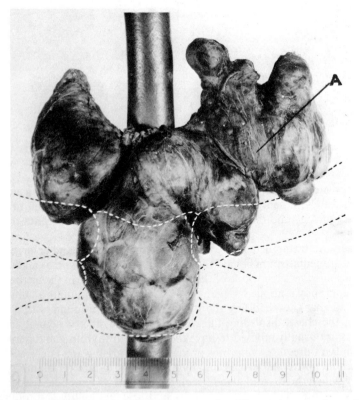

Fig. 41.7 Photograph of nodular goitre removed at operation. The specimen has been placed across a length of rubber tubing which represents the trachea. The portion A was folded behind the larynx. The dotted line shows the position of the clavicles and sternum. Downward projection of the gland into the thorax impeded respiration and swallowing.

the patient is usually advised to undergo operation. The surgeon is also called upon to remove the thyroid gland because of thyrotoxicosis which has already developed as a primary condition or in a patient who has had a 'nodular' goitre for some years. Consequently from the nursing point of view there are two major aspects of thyroid surgery. The first is the technical aspect of the removal of the gland, the after-care and complications of the operation; the second aspect covers the specific factors which arise from thyrotoxicosis which is a disease affecting the whole body, and in particular the function of the heart.

Operation for the removal of part or the whole of the thyroid gland is performed for a variety of reasons. Broadly speaking these patients may be divided into two categories:

(*a*) those with established or suspected thyrotoxicosis,
(*b*) those who have a tumour of the thyroid gland without any general metabolic disturbance; there may be symptoms from pressure.

The assessment of the severity of thyrotoxicosis is made usually only after the patient's admission to hospital and is dependent largely upon nursing observations. Some patients who previously have had no evidence of thyrotoxicosis develop symptoms and signs while under observation, before or after operation for the removal of an enlarged gland, and in practice the nurse must regard all goitre patients as potentially 'toxic'.

Nursing routine will therefore be discussed particularly in relation to the care of the thyrotoxic patient. The lesser considerations of the non-toxic patient are naturally included in the greater considerations.

Period of observation and preliminary medical treatment

As there is very little risk in operation for patients with non-toxic goitre, an initial period of rest is not vital, although it is ideal to have such patients under observation for several days before operation. On the other hand, all patients with recognised thyro-

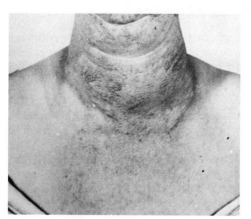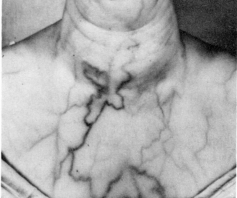

Fig. 41.8 'Plunging goitre' causing venous obstruction and consequent dilation of veins on the chest. (*Left*) Normal photograph showing very little enlargement of the thyroid in the neck. (*Right*) Photograph taken with infra-red illumination, which reveals the enormously dilated veins. There is very little enlargement of the thyroid in the neck although the gland extends down into the mediastinum (Fig. 41.7).

toxicosis will have undergone a period of preliminary medical treatment. Sometimes it is possible to complete this period of rest aided by barbiturate sedatives while the patient is still in his or her own home.

In mild cases, immediately prior to operation the patient receives a daily dose of iodine, usually in the form of Lugol's iodine solution, for a period of 2, or at the most 3 weeks. If it has not been thought advisable to complete this period of iodine treatment before admission to hospital it will be necessary for the patient to spend at least 2 weeks having a maximum amount of bed rest in hospital. In the more severe cases the commencement of iodine therapy will be delayed and during this initial period of rest, very careful observations of the patient's pulse and rhythm rate will be necessary. Electrocardiography will be undertaken if there is any doubt about the heart's action. Until the introduction of **thiouracil** in 1943, long periods of rest and sedation were necessary before the most severe cases were deemed fit for operation. Nurses today would find it difficult to appreciate how gravely ill were some of the cases of thyrotoxicosis which had to be treated surgically before the introduction of the anti-thyroid drugs.

Carbimazole is now used almost exclusively. It is possible to render nearly all toxic patients virtually non-toxic—and in fact quite a number become myxoedematous. Unfortunately, the drug does not control the gland disorder indefinitely. Sometimes the gland enlarges as a result of treatment. Partial thyroidectomy still remains the final treatment of choice.

Severely ill patients are usually treated in a medical ward until they are considered fit for operation. Carbimazole is stopped and replaced by iodine for the last 2 weeks of the pre-operative treatment. If iodine is not given after carbimazole, the operation is made extremely difficult by the great increase in vascularity of the gland.

In mild cases with very little thyroid enlargement, radioactive iodine may be used as the chosen treatment.

If the portion of gland remaining after thyroidectomy grows and produces a recurrence of thyrotoxicosis, ^{131}I is used to reduce the gland activity in preference to a second operation (page 447).

The nurse has a very important role throughout this preliminary phase. Although sedatives, antithyroid drugs and iodine all play a very large part in preparing the patient for operation, a restful and yet cheerful atmosphere, where the patient is free from anxiety and physical exertion, goes a long way to reduce the risks of a surgical operation on the patient whose nervous system and heart have been affected.

The voice. In advanced cases of thyroid enlargement—and usually with those due to neoplasm—the voice is appreciably affected by pressure on the nerves to the larynx. The nurse, however, in conversation with the patient may learn that the patient is no longer able to sing well or to reach high notes: she may have an irritant cough at night, about which she has not complained: such information should always be passed on to the surgeon as it may give an indication that the recurrent laryngeal nerves are already affected. It is usual for the larynx to be examined with a mirror in order to determine the degree of mobility of the vocal cords, before operation.

The pulse. There are certain well-recognised and easily detected disturbances of the heart which result from excessive thyroid activity. The nurse must be familiar with their main features and significance (Fig. 41.9).

(a) Simple tachycardia. Because of the over-secretion of thyroid substances the body tissues are working faster, and consequently there is a rise in pulse rate. This represents the normal

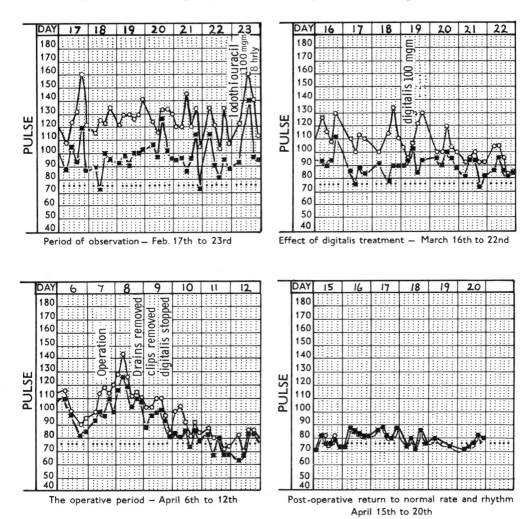

Period of observation — Feb. 17th to 23rd

Effect of digitalis treatment — March 16th to 22nd

The operative period — April 6th to 12th

Post-operative return to normal rate and rhythm
April 15th to 20th

Fig. 41.9 Severe toxic goitre. Extracts from pulse chart of patient with atrial fibrillation who was prepared for operation by anti-thyroid drugs and digitalis. The upper line indicates the apex beat; the lower line indicates the radial pulse counted at the same time.

(a) A pulse deficit of between 20 and 30 beats per minute.

(b) Although there has been a fall in both the apex and radial pulse with iodothiouracil treatment, there is still a pulse deficit between 10 and 20. The apex rate was further reduced with digitalis.

(c) Very small pulse deficit before operation, the heart being controlled completely by digitalis. Following thyroidectomy there is a continuous fall of heart rate.

(d) Normal rhythm was restored spontaneously on the 8th post-operative day.

heart acceleration occurring from increased demands by the body for oxygen. It is analogous to the rise in pulse rate due to exertion. Usually this diminishes during sleep but even in mild degrees of thyrotoxicosis it may be running at 90 to 100 beats a minute during the first few days in hospital. This 'basal' pulse rate is one of the most important factors in assessing thyrotoxicosis. The pulse may increase appreciably with any small amount of exertion or during conversation, particularly if the patient is discussing the possibilities of operation. The nurse will note these temporary accelerations and report them as 'an irritable pulse'. A 4-hourly record must be charted and sleeping pulse rates specially marked.

(b) **Paroxysmal tachycardia.** Here, owing to the sensitivity of the cardiac muscle, although the basal pulse rate may be only slightly raised, the patient has attacks of tremendous pulse acceleration during which the heart may be going so fast as to be uncountable. Such attacks are alarming both to the patient and to the nurse if she happens to be counting the pulse during one of the attacks. As the 'paroxysms' are frequently short-lived (seconds, minutes or rarely an hour or so), it may well be that the nurse is the only observer on the spot. The patient's description of these attacks is often adequate to make an accurate diagnosis possible, even if no attack has been observed by doctor or nurse. In itself, paroxysmal tachycardia is not a very serious condition but it is an indication to the doctor that the heart muscle is in a very irritable state. This condition may merely be a precursor of other more serious disturbances of rhythm.

(c) **Paroxysmal atrial fibrillation.** For short periods of minutes or perhaps hours, the heart rhythm becomes irregular. The patient will describe her pulse as being 'all over the place'. Such attacks are usually unrelated to exercise, and again, as with paroxysmal tachycardia, the nurse may be the only observer to detect this irregularity and she must not be depressed if, when she finds in her routine pulse recording that the pulse rate is irregular, her ward sister fails to confirm this! A regular rhythm may have been restored but the warning will have been given. If the nurse suspects that the pulse is irregular she should at once obtain a colleague to count the apex beat with a stethoscope independently while she herself counts the radial pulse. The observation will not only confirm the presence of the irregularity but will give the number of heart beats which failed to produce a pulse sufficiently strong to be felt at the wrist. This difference is known as **pulse deficit**. One has on many occasions heard both doctors and nurses talking of patients 'fibrillating less today' or 'not fibrillating very much' or even 'fibrillating badly'. Such expressions are very misleading. If a heart is fibrillating, it is *indeed* fibrillating and degrees of fibrillation do not exist. The pulse deficit is the important observation.

Atrial fibrillation is a condition in which the normal 'wave' or sinus rhythm of the heart does not spread over the auricles and ventricles regularly; each part of the heart develops a beat rate of its own. Consequently, the ventricles often contract when they are incompletely filled, and such a contraction results in the output being low and the pulses not reaching the wrist. If the cardiac muscle is badly damaged by thyrotoxicosis it becomes very irritable, and consequently the rate of the irregular beat of the ventricles becomes very high. The pulse deficit is therefore large and the irritability of the ventricle has to be damped down by the use of digitalis. Even in the pre-operative phase, where there is paroxysmal atrial fibrillation it may be thought wise by the physician or surgeon in charge to 'digitalise' the patient, to diminish the risk of the heart 'running away with itself' during or immediately after operation. If the ventricular rate is too high in spite of digitalis, **propanalol**[1] is given. Digoxin is given by mouth or in extreme emergency may be ordered by injection.

(d) **Established atrial fibrillation.** This condition is rather different from the paroxysmal

---

[1] This is a drug known as a β-blocker because it blocks the stimulation of heart by adrenaline-like substances. Muscle fibres have trigger mechanisms responding to different chemicals, alpha and beta receptors—Greek letter α, β.

fibrillation. It indicates a greater degree of damage to the heart muscle and is usually found in older patients, often without symptoms. The heart has become enlarged as a result of over-activity for a number of years, and having now become irregular, the ventricular beat may well be slow. On the other hand, the patient may have developed atrial fibrillation fairly rapidly and may seek advice first because of symptoms of heart failure; it is not immediately apparent that thyroid disease is the cause of the heart failure. Such patients may be saved from their attacks of cardiac failure and greatly improved in their general condition by partial thyroidectomy. Frequently the regular rhythm becomes restored after operation but long-standing cases may never regain a normal rhythm. They continue with their fibrillation, apparently without discomfort.

Clear understanding of these cardiac disturbances is vital to any nurse who is going to look after thyroid patients, and although the incidence of these abnormalities is more common in the immediate post-operative period it is equally important at this stage of observation.

Embolism. In cases where the rhythm of the heart has become irregular and the beat of the auricle reduced by fibrillation to a mere flicker, thrombosis occurs on the walls of the auricular appendages of the heart. Clots remain attached to the wall of the heart until a normal rhythm is restored. When, as a result of treatment, the thyrotoxicosis abates and the patient's cardiac irregularity suddenly switches to normal rhythm, these little clots may be shot off and passed into the circulation as emboli. They may occur in the right side of the heart and therefore appear as pulmonary emboli causing infarction of the lung, pain in the chest, a rise of temperature, and haemoptysis. There may be showers of such emboli. If clots are dislodged from the left side of the heart they pass into the main arterial circulation, sometimes producing embolism of a major artery such as the femoral. In this event, the patient will complain of sudden pain at the site of embolism and the limb distal to the clot will become blanched. Embolectomy may be needed (page 68). An embolus may lodge in the vessels of the brain and produce a sudden loss of consciousness or paralysis. It is essential for the nurse to be acquainted with these possibilities and to report any occurrence which suggests that embolism may have taken place (e.g. haemoptysis; pain in chest, legs or arms; incoherent speech or strange conversation).

Weight and appetite. The patient will normally have been weighed on admission or transfer from the medical ward and it is essential that weekly weight records should be kept and entered on the temperature chart. In some cases where the basal pulse rate is not raised, the increase of weight under initial medical treatment is the best sign of progress. Most thyroid patients have a very good appetite and normal digestion, but there are certain cases of thyrotoxicosis in which intermittent dyspepsia and diarrhoea is a feature. Excessive looseness and frequency of stools should be reported, and sigmoidoscopy will usually be undertaken to exclude ulcerative colitis, the many manifestations of which somewhat resemble thyrotoxicosis.

Mental state. During this phase of observation the nurse has an excellent opportunity of observing the general mental condition of the patient. The change in demeanour when a thyrotoxic patient undergoes preliminary medical treatment is often very striking and these patients are among the most cheerful and the most grateful. There are, however, certain cases in which depression is a marked feature, and these have to be treated very carefully as they do not respond so readily to surgical treatment as far as their mental condition is concerned. Such features of the case may escape the notice of the doctor, since his interviews with the patient take place under rather abnormal conditions.

The eyes. Exophthalmos, or protrusion of the eyes, is a marked feature of certain cases of thyrotoxicosis (Fig. 41.10). The degree of protrusion may be so severe that the lids provide incomplete protection against injury and drying; the patient then develops a soreness of the eyes and **ulceration of the cornea**. Paralysis of certain eye muscles may also occur, the so-called **exophthalmic ophthalmoplegia**. This produces **diplopia** (double vision) which may be a passing symptom, mentioned quite casually by the patient when she first notices it. It may be necessary to cover and protect the eye: the greatest risk is the possibility of damage to the exposed eyes during operation. Liquid paraffin is best avoided as 'eye drops' since it tends to produce inflammation of the lids: mild antiseptic 'drops' such as Soframycin may be prescribed (page 838).

Glycosuria. There is sometimes a disturbance of sugar metabolism in thyrotoxicosis and it is not uncommon for patients to suffer from glycosuria, although they have not true diabetes. The urine should, of course, be tested weekly, and if sugar is present, then blood examination will be performed to determine the importance of the glycosuria.

Sedation. The selection of an appropriate sedative is a matter for the doctor in charge. Most commonly an adult patient of average size will be given 30–60 mg of phenobarbitone night and morning; some patients become very depressed when taking phenobarbitone and an effective and suitable sedative is diazepam.

These, then, are the main aspects of thyrotoxicosis. It cannot be emphasised too strongly that the nursing in its broadest sense plays a very big part in the restoration to normal health of these patients. These manifestations of thyrotoxicosis may appear for the first time in the immediate post-operative phase in the milder cases, so that the nurse must carry in her mind the possibility of these complications, such as cardiac irregularities, occurring at any stage during observation or convalescence. Mild symptoms which have

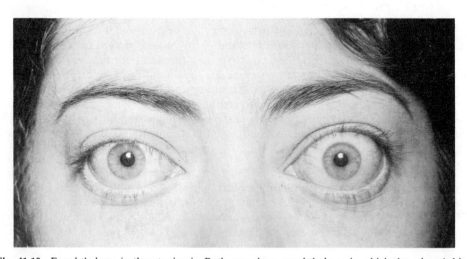

Fig. 41.10 Exophthalmos in thyrotoxicosis. Both eyes show exophthalmos in which the sclera (white) is exposed above the iris. In the normal eye the upper lid overlaps the margin of the iris.

been present before operation may be made more obvious or even become severe after operation, due to the general upheaval of the patient's metabolism which interference with the thyroid gland produces. Fortunately nowadays, the pre-operative preparation is so satisfactory that we rarely see these gross reactions to the operation.

Immediate pre-operative treatment

As thyrotoxicosis can be controlled in most cases by antithyroid drugs, the majority of patients have been made temporarily 'non-toxic' by the time of operation. Except in those less severe cases which have had no antithyroid drug in preparation, there is little risk of cardiac crises at or after operation.

The pre-operative routine is straightforward and differs very little from that for any major operation. Adequate sedation (valium or butobarbitone) is required for the night before operation. The patient's neck is prepared in accordance with the wishes of the surgeon, usually with a detergent solution such as Savlon (2 per cent), and the skin should be cleaned from the chin down to the nipple line including the front of both shoulders; the area should then be covered with a sterile towel fixed in place by a loosely applied bandage. **Adhesive strapping should not be used to fix sterile towels, since traces of the strapping are left on the skin.** Preferably a head cap made from a length of tube gauze or stockinette is applied: this must retain all the hairs which tend to stray into the field of operation when the surgeon applies the double head towel! It is helpful to grease the hair margins in the neck as an added precaution against contamination of the hair with blood. If the back rim of the head cap is lined with a 'gamgee' pad this further prevents blood seeping up into the hair and considerably lessens the discomfort of the patient after the operation. This may seem a small detail but it is nevertheless a very important point.

In all cases of large goitre or where an extension into the mediastinum is suspected, the patient will have had an x-ray photograph of the neck to show if there is any displacement of the trachea at the thoracic inlet. This x-ray must accompany the patient to the operating theatre. It may to some extent guide the anaesthetist and the surgeon.

Post-operative nursing

The most convenient method of securing the dressing is by a stoll of elastic adhesive strapping. The wound is usually drained at each end by rubber strips or vacuum drain, and when the anaesthetic tube is removed a pillow must be immediately available to place under the head so that at no time shall the head drop back into the extended position. If, while the patient is recovering from the anaesthetic, it becomes necessary to turn her head or swab out the mouth, great care must again be taken not to extend the neck. A folded towel should be placed under the chin as soon as the ward nurse takes the patient over, in case any vomitus should find its way down on to the dressing. On being returned to bed the patient is placed with two pillows under the head and quarter-hourly pulse readings recorded by the nurse, who must not leave her until consciousness is regained. Owing to the difficulty which thyroid patients experience in taking fluids by mouth for the first few hours, it is usual for the patient to receive intravenous fluid for 12 hours.

Shock is not a common feature of thyroidectomy but the nurse must be very vigilant for haemorrhage. It is not uncommon for the dressings to become deeply stained with blood, but should a main ligature become displaced blood may collect very rapidly in the wound and produce pressure on the trachea. The patient exhibits distress in breathing and will be asphyxiated unless the pressure is rapidly relieved. Such a complication becomes a dire emergency and, if the doctor is not available within seconds, the dressing must be removed and the skin stitches or slips taken out quickly in order that the wound may burst open and allow the escape of blood. A firm sterile pack is then applied until medical assistance arrives. Any nurse who has the post-operative care of thyroid patients will be warned about this possibility. Apart from this, the nurse's most important duty is to observe any change in the pulse rate or rhythm.

A description of the cardiac irregularities which occur in thyrotoxicosis has already been given (page 768). Paroxysmal atrial fibrillation is the most common post-operative cardiac disturbance, and may in fact, be quite alarming. Again, before the days of anti-thyroid drugs, the so-called **thyroid crisis** was one of the terrors of thyroid surgery. There is probably an overspill of thyroxin into the circulation by handling of the gland at operation: there is a sudden increase in tissue activity, hyperpyrexia, sweating, tremor and rapid rise of pulse. Hot weather and humid conditions make post-operative trouble more likely in thyrotoxicosis and operation is sometimes postponed if the temperature is too high. The patient's metabolism rises extremely rapidly, the temperature may go up to 40·5 °C, the pulse is uncountable and the patient becomes delirious. The treatment calls for urgent medical care, and the nurse's primary duty lies in dealing with the hyperpyrexia and in administering oxygen. The doctor in charge may prescribe drugs for controlling the rate of the heart, as in other cases in which, short of a true thyroid crisis, auricular fibrillation is accompanied by a large pulse deficit. In all probability, this complication will have been anticipated from the severity of the patient's previous degree of toxicity, even though it may have been controlled. Such a patient will already be having propanolol or be digitalised.

A thyroid crisis is treated by:

(a) tepid sponging, and fans,
(b) morphine by injection, or chlorpromazine,
(c) oxygen (preferably in a tent, page 283, if adequate cooling is available), as a mask will not be tolerated.

The average patient after thyroidectomy, quite apart from cardiac disturbances, will require fairly heavy sedation, and in the first 24 hours this is usually achieved by the use of morphine 20 mg (owing to the high rate of metabolism of thyrotoxic patients they tolerate fairly large doses of drugs). It is debatable whether iodine treatment should be continued after operation and whether it serves any useful purpose, but it may be prescribed as a precautionary measure. Owing to interference with the muscles of the neck, swallowing is difficult and the patient may be unable to swallow solids for 2 days; the difficulty may be overcome by giving an aspirin mucilage mixture to relieve the pharyngeal discomfort. Unless very great care has been taken to prevent straining of the neck on the operating table, the patient may have severe pain down the back of the neck; this is usually relieved by an aspirin mixture, but may be very troublesome: the patient also benefits from the temperature-lowering effect of the aspirin. This should never in such cases be given as a tablet owing to the swallowing difficulty, but a mucilage mixture should be used.

As soon as the patient is fully conscious, additional pillows should be given in order to bring the head forward as far as is comfortable. The drainage tubes are removed 24 hours after operation and the skin clips usually 48 hours after operation. Thereafter, bandages are unnecessary and a gauze dressing is kept in place by a 'bib' for 2 or 3 days.

Sometimes a haematoma develops in the wound. It may be immediately under the skin from the start, or it may track forwards from the deeper tissues during the 2nd week. The skin becomes red and shiny at one point of the scar and usually the haematoma can be emptied very easily by the insertion of a silver probe through the incision line at perhaps a week or even 10 days after the operation. If induration (hardening) persists in the scar, short-wave diathermy for a few days helps to resolve it.

The patient must be rested until the pulse rate has returned to the normal base line. Unless the patient has been rendered non-toxic before operation, exercise is limited post-operatively for at least 2 weeks, but it is not necessary for patients to be confined to bed strictly. The rapid recovery of patients after thyroidectomy is one of the most gratifying events in surgery, but in toxic cases the patients must be made to realise that the operation has only started them off on their recovery and a further period of rest for 3 or 4 weeks may be necessary before they are restored to normal physical activity.

The voice is often affected during the first few days after operation by tracheitis. This is due to interference with the trachea and larynx and by the difficulty which the patient experiences in coughing. The persistence of a weak and husky voice at the end of the first week suggests that the nerves to the muscles of the vocal cords have perhaps been damaged, and in such cases a special laryngeal examination is usually called for. Post-operative tracheitis is greatly relieved by pine or tinct. benz. co. inhalations. There is a modern tendency to despise such simple remedies but the fact remains that the patient feels greatly comforted and eased, mainly by the inhalation of the steam. Menthol should not be used as this tends to provoke coughing, which is again very painful, and the vapour may affect the protruding eyes of the exophthalmic patient.

A 'red eye' must be regarded as serious and may be due to corneal ulceration from exposure (page 394). A pad and bandage should be applied to the eye immediately for protection.

Parathyroid tetany. On very rare occasions all the parathyroid tissue may be removed or bruised. In such cases the patient exhibits, perhaps 2 or 3 days after operation, irritability of the muscles, shown by twitching of the face and spasm of the hands and feet. She may complain of a feeling of tightness in the hands. This parathyroid deficiency is usually only temporary and is overcome by intramuscular injection of 10 per cent calcium gluconate (10 ml). This injection may be repeated for a day or so, or large doses of calcium lactate (10 G per day) may be prescribed. It is usual for the parathyroid deficiency to be only a passing phase where some of the glands have been removed and the remaining ones damaged; recovery of the remaining tissue occurs and there is only very rarely any permanent damage. Occasionally the deficiency does not become apparent for several months.

Post-operative mental disturbance. Reference has already been made to psychological changes which may occur in thyrotoxic patients; in those in whom such changes were noted before operation there may be an accentuation of the symptoms in the post-operative phase. The moody and very excitable patient may occasionally become quite uncontrolled and the operation may have precipitated a major psychotic disturbance. Cases in whom the mental changes are most prominent usually do not recover so well after thyroidectomy simply because they have a bad psychological make-up beforehand. The nurse must, therefore, be on the lookout for any strange behaviour which may show itself by irrational conversation.

Cardiac complications. If cardiac complications have occurred, these will take pre-eminence in the recovery phase. When auricular fibrillation persists after operation, normal rhythm may be restored suddenly and spontaneously, usually about the 10th post-operative day; if after 2 weeks the irregularity persists, medical treatment with quinidine is usually instituted to attempt to 'switch' the rhythm to normal. If this fails the patient, under general anaesthesia, is given an electric shock with a special direct-current external defibrillator (page 191).

Embolus. This is discussed on page 771. Thyrotoxic patients who have had persistent auricular fibrillation are particularly liable to atrial embolism when the heart regains its normal rhythm after operation, dislodging clots from the atrial wall.

Late complications. These include persistent voice changes, an excessive gain in weight, and other symptoms of lack of thyroid gland. Fibrosis, the gradual formation of scar tissue, continues in the area of operation for several months and in this process the parathyroid glands and recurrent laryngeal nerves may become damaged by 'strangulation'. Voice changes and cramps in the muscles are the respective warning signs.

Myxoedema. Hypothyroidism is always present after total thyroidectomy for neoplasm or lymphadenoid goitre and sometimes follows thyroidectomy for other forms of goitre unless it is prevented by thyroxin taken by mouth. The dose is regulated in accordance with the patient's weight changes. It is therefore essential that thyroidectomy patients should be weighed immediately before discharge from hospital, and at intervals in follow-up examinations for at least a year.

The onset of myxoedema is marked by the patient complaining of stiffness of the face, or a feeling of swelling of the cheeks and hands. The skin becomes dry and coarse, hair is shed, and the whole surface of the body seems to be padded with rather inelastic fat. Weight gain is excessive, the patient becomes lethargic and depressed, and the blood choles-terol test shows a very high figure. The voice is lower in pitch and rough. Myxoedematous thickening of the vocal cords is sometimes the result of prolonged medical treatment with anti-thyroid drugs *before* the patient comes to the surgeon. Hypothyroidism may take from 6 to 12 weeks to develop after total thyroidectomy, and similarly response to treatment is slow. The patient will feel no immediate benefit from taking thyroid tablets.

Sometimes an individual can develop antibodies against his own thyroid secretion. This strange process of 'auto-immunisation' produces a condition in the gland resembling inflammation. This process results in the development of lymphadenoid goitre (Hashimoto disease), or self-destruction of the thyroid which in turn leads to myxoedema. Certain virus diseases affect the thyroid gland in a similar way.

The management of thyroid cancer

Cancer may arise from the thyroid-secreting alveolar (follicular) cells, from the para-follicular 'C' cells which produce calcitonin, or from the lymphatic tissue which predominates in lymphadenoid goitre. Arising from the alveolar tissue there may be a *papillary* carcinoma which is often a solitary nodule. If such a nodule has been excised widely and no other nodules have been found in the gland, probably there will be no further treatment. A more aggressive *follicular* type carcinoma arising from the alveolar cells spreads more rapidly to the blood stream and it is treated more vigorously. The growth arising from the 'C' cells is *medullary* carcinoma and is even more malignant.

Scanning with radio-active iodine, or technetium will reveal whether a nodule is active ('hot'), or inactive ('cold'). A malignant nodule is usually cold even though the tissue may be functioning since the isotope is taken up by the much more active normal part of the gland. A cold nodule is therefore suspect of being malignant, or of being a cyst. The generally accepted method of treating thyroid cancer of the follicular type is by total thyroidectomy, preserving at least one parathyroid gland and both recurrent laryngeal nerves. As it is difficult to be certain of removing every trace of functioning thyroid tissue without doing damage to these structures, a tracer dose of radio-active iodine is given post-operatively to locate any residual tissue. This is then destroyed by a further 'therapeutic' dose, and the patient is subsequently treated with thyroxin to meet the normal metabolic requirements. If it is thought that secondary deposits are present in the glands or have been traced at any other site, thyroxin is withheld until the radioactive iodine treatment is complete: this allows the thyroid stimulating pituitary hormone (TSH) to activate the metastasis and make it 'iodine-hungry' so it will then take up the radio-active iodine.

At routine reviews, usually at 3 month intervals, the patient is given a further tracer dose of radio-active iodine in a search for metastasis, or if metastases are known to be present, a therapeutic radio-active dose is given which will be taken up by the deposit, thus destroying itself. Before isotope treatment is given the patient's thyroxin maintenance dose must be stopped for 4 weeks, or if maintenance has been with L-tri-iodothyronine, only a 2 week suspension of treatment is necessary.

Cytotoxic drugs have not been shown to be very effective in the management of carcinoma of the thyroid though they are used if there are extensive bone metastases. X-ray therapy is used on some patients.

Prognosis for many of these cases is good, but growths arising from the calcitonin-producing cells—medullary carcinoma—or from the lymphoid tissue are much more highly malignant.

Exposure of the neck to radio-activity is known to be one causative factor in the production of thyroid cancer. A number of people now in middle age have in childhood had x-ray treatment for an enlarged thymus gland, or for tuberculous infection of glands in the neck, or possibly for thyrotoxicosis occurring in childhood. The incidence of cancer of the thyroid in such patients is much higher than in the normal population.

42

Oral Surgery

Disorders affecting the mouth and tongue are treated in various special departments of surgery which necessarily overlap in their interests. The general surgeon is called upon to deal with cancer of the lips, tongue and floor of mouth. The nose and throat surgeon is usually asked to treat growths of the palate because of the involvement of the adjacent maxilla and maxillary antrum. Surgery of the lower jaw is undertaken by a general surgeon or dental surgeon, and in the management of injuries to the facial bones the co-operation of all three departments is essential. Congenital cleft palate is more commonly treated by the plastic surgeon because it is frequently associated with cleft (hare) lip.

Whatever the disease or disorder the general principles of surgical nursing care are the same.

Anatomy

The red surfaces of the lips, gums, palate and tongue are covered with squamous epithelium similar to the skin, but studded with mucus-secreting glands which keep the surfaces moist. The lips, tongue and cheeks have a very rich blood supply. Injury or operation produces profuse bleeding, but healing is rapid and the tissues have a high resistance to infection.

The sensory nerve supply of the mouth and teeth comes mainly from the trigeminal (fifth cranial) nerve and the troublesome intractable condition of trigeminal. neuralgia frequently has its origin in some localised disease within the mouth. Unfortunately the neuralgia may persist long after the disease itself (for instance an infected tooth) has been treated. Part of the palate and tongue is supplied by the ninth (glossopharyngeal) and part by the tenth (vagus) cranial nerves.

Saliva is poured into the mouth from the ducts of the **parotid glands**, which pierce the inner surfaces of the cheeks opposite the upper molar teeth. The **submandibular**[1] salivary glands discharge their secretion into the mouth through a tiny orifice on each side of the frenum of the tongue behind the incisor teeth. The **sublingual glands** open through additional ducts beneath the tongue (Fig. 41.2).

[1] Many years ago the mandible was called the inferior maxilla and surgeons who were accustomed to the old name still speak of the **submaxillary** salivary gland.

The **lymphatic drainage** from the inside of the mouth and tongue passes almost entirely through the floor of the mouth into groups of glands situated beneath the mandible (Fig. 41.1). The **submental** lymph glands under the chin drain the lower lip, front of the tongue and floor of the mouth; the **submandibular** group beneath the body of the mandible drain the side of the tongue and floor of the mouth and both the inner and outer surfaces of the cheek. The **tonsillar** gland which lies against the jugular vein behind the angle of the jaw drains the tonsil and pharynx. Lymph from all these groups passes downwards and backwards to the **deep cervical** chain of glands situated along the internal jugular vein and carotid artery at the side of the neck deep to the sterno-mastoid muscle.

Enlargement of any of these glands leads immediately to a search for a possible focus of infection or growth in the area drained by the affected group.

Common disorders of the mouth

Congenital. During the development of the face two prong-like processes of tissue grow from each side to form the jaws and underlying soft tissues. A central process grows from the region of the forehead to join with the upper prongs on each side, forming the nose, palate and lip. When these processes fail to fuse various forms of cleft face, cleft lip and cleft palate arise. In these conditions, no tissue is actually lost and the surgeon's task is to weld the tissues together in such a way that both natural shape and movement are given to the lip and palate.

Congenital tumours of the tongue may produce obstruction to the infant's feeding or breathing (haemangioma, lymphangioma, sublingual dermoid cyst).

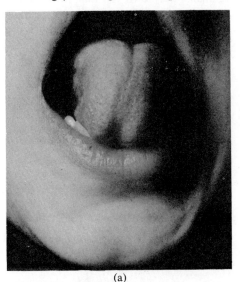

(a)

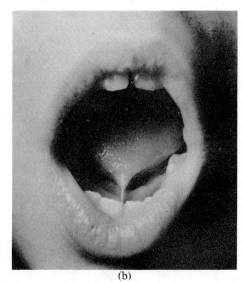

(b)

Fig. 42.1 Tongue-tie.
(a) Forking of the tongue on protrusion.
(b) The short tight frenum extending to the tip of the tongue. This interferes with speech development, particularly with the pronunciation of the letter *R*. This child should have been treated in infancy.

Errors of development of the teeth may be discovered in infancy. The baby may be born with some teeth already erupted, or the milk teeth may be displaced.

The later development of the maxilla and mandible depends to a large extent on the normal function of the tongue. **Tongue-tie** is a condition in which the tongue is tethered to the floor of the mouth and cannot be protruded: if severe, the tethering may interfere with sucking and subsequently affects speech (Fig. 42.1). Tongue-tie is treated by dividing the band underneath the tip of the tongue. In tiny babies this frenum is torn by the surgeon's finger; the child is kept under observation for an hour to make sure that bleeding does not continue; there is no after-treatment. If the condition has been neglected a set operation under general anaesthesia is required.

Thumb sucking or the constant use of 'dummies' leads to protrusion of the upper jaw. Mouth breathing from nasal obstruction by adenoids also leads to impaired development of the palate and upper jaw. All these conditions result in an imperfect fit between the upper and lower jaws. Not only is the child's appearance disfigured but the function of the jaws is impaired and the teeth deteriorate because of the imbalance. The science of the correction of jaw deformities is **orthodontics.** Special orthodontic clinics are held in the large general hospitals and in school centres so that corrective appliances may be fitted to the teeth when the second dentition erupts.

Mucus retention cysts, usually the size of a small pea and translucent, occur on the inner surface of lips or cheeks, or on the tongue. The treatment is to cut off the protuberant mucosa and cauterise the base under local anaesthesia, but if the cyst recurs excision is required. Children often effect a self cure by biting the cyst cap away.

Infections. The mouth is normally teeming with bacteria which play a part in maintaining its healthy condition. Some of these organisms are destroyed and the bacterial 'balance' is disturbed by sucking penicillin tablets or pastilles. Abnormal disease-producing germs are then able to thrive and fungus infections in particular arise. **Thrush** is a fungus infection which produces extensive ulceration.

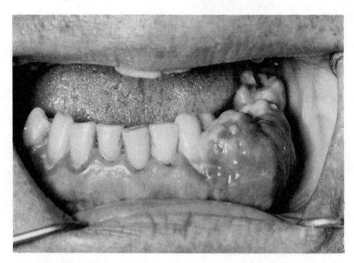

Fig. 42.2   An epulis growing from the gum in the region of the left lower pre-molars.

Abscesses occurring in association with the teeth are **gum boils** if they are on the surface of the jaw. An **apical abscess** is a pocket of pus within the bone at the root of the tooth. **Dental caries** or decay is really a degenerative condition with subsequent infection which destroys the body of the tooth. **Pyorrhoea** ('running pus') is a suppurative condition around the necks of the teeth. **Gingivitis,** inflammation of the gums, may arise from dental infection but it occurs also in vitamin deficiencies and in various forms of poisoning.

Chronic infection around a tooth produces a tumour of granulation and fibrous tissue which can reach a large size. This is an **epulis** (Fig. 42.2).

Glossitis, inflammation of the tongue, arises in vitamin B deficiency (page 85). It may be caused by thrush or any infection which thrives when the normal organisms in the mouth have been destroyed by antibiotic therapy. Oral hygiene is therefore very important when prolonged chemotherapy or antibiotic treatment is being given. Syphilis produces glossitis in the 'secondary' stage.

Chronic superficial glossitis is sometimes associated with syphilis but frequently occurs without this infection. Areas of the tongue become white (leucoplakia) and subsequently smooth and sore. The condition is very prone to become malignant if the affected areas are untreated.

Osteomyelitis of the mandible is a serious destructive infection which may follow a compound fracture or may arise from sepsis around the root of a tooth.

Infection of the salivary glands arises usually from the presence of infection in the mouth. Acute inflammation **(sialo-adenitis, parotitis)** is treated by chemotherapy. Chronic infection may lead to calculus formation in the ducts (page 761).

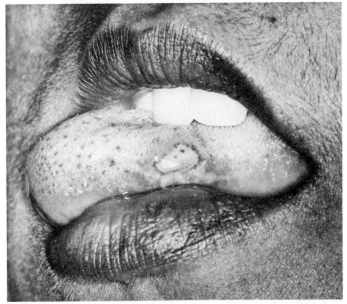

Fig. 42.3   A dental (traumatic) ulcer on the side of the tongue caused by constant abrasion on a broken tooth. Note the overcrowding of the upper teeth which prevents cleansing by the normal flow of saliva.

Traumatic conditions. Minor injuries to the lip and tongue are very common. They bleed freely at first but because the tongue and the lips are both muscular, bleeding soon ceases. In all but the smallest cuts, stitching is required to hold together the cut ends of the muscle fibres and prevent gaping of the wound. The stitches may be inserted under local anaesthesia. The tongue after injury may swell excessively and cause difficulty with feeding and swallowing.

Fractures of the jaws are almost always compound because of the tight attachment of the gum to the bone. Teeth may be broken and fragments swallowed or inhaled. Lacerations of the palate occur especially in children who fall while they are sucking sharp objects such as pencils, toffee apples, or lollipops.

Ulcers develop on the tongue from constant friction with a broken tooth or ill-fitting dental plate (**dental ulcer,** Fig. 42.3).

Neoplasms. Many different types of 'tumour' arise in the jaws in association with the developing teeth or as true neoplasms. They require surgical excision, sometimes of a very radical nature. Half the mandible may have to be removed; it is usually replaced by a bone graft.

The most common form of neoplasm in the mouth is cancer of the tongue. It usually appears as a small ulcer and arises frequently at the back of the tongue where it cannot be seen by the patient. It is a relentless condition which spreads on to the floor of the mouth and into the surrounding soft tissues and bone. It is treated by excision of the affected portion of the tongue, sometimes of half of the tongue (hemiglossectomy) and occasionally by removal of the whole tongue. It may be treated by radium needles, cobalt bomb or x-rays (Fig. 23.4 and page 445). The glands which drain the tongue are also treated either with radiotherapy or by radical surgical excision (block dissection). In this latter procedure all the tissues in the area between the undersurface of the tongue and the sterno-mastoid muscle on the affected side are taken as one 'block' of tissue. This includes the submandibular salivary gland, submental and submandibular lymph glands, muscles, external carotid artery, deep cervical lymph glands and internal jugular vein. Block dissection operation may be required on both sides of the neck. The operation wound is drained for 2 days, and there may be considerable difficulty in swallowing owing to oedema of the pharynx (page 760).

If carcinoma of the tongue or floor of the mouth has already invaded the mandible it is extremely difficult to treat because radiation further destroys bone. Apart from mutilating operations to remove the mandible there is very little effective treatment. The condition is extremely painful and the patient's distress from infection, inability to eat and severe pain is one of the most difficult problems of surgical care.

Factors in treatment

Surgical operations involving the inside of the mouth are inevitably exposed to infection both during and after operation. It is not practicable to sterilise the inside of the mouth although mild antiseptic mouth washes limit the infection to some extent; in normal life the constant movement of cheeks and tongue ensure continuous cleansing with the aid of the saliva. If the arrangement of teeth is perfect the constant movement of the cheeks washes the crevices between the teeth, but if the teeth are overcrowded, pocketing of food debris occurs and leads to infection. Inexpert filling of decayed teeth similarly leads to pocketing if insufficient gap is left between adjacent tooth surfaces.

Any interference with this movement of cheeks or tongue, from disease or operation, results in stagnation and sepsis. Even facial paralysis on one side leads to the accumulation of food in the trough between the jaws and cheek and particular care must be paid by the patient to ensure thorough cleansing after each meal. Swelling of the tongue, which is inevitable after operations or the insertion of radium, limits its movement and prevents the natural cleansing of the palate or inner surfaces of the teeth.

A reduction in the flow of saliva very rapidly leads to food decomposition and infection in the mouth. This occurs after radiotherapy has been used in the treatment of carcinoma of the mouth. Dryness of the mouth accompanies severe dehydration.

The presence of infection in the mouth, either as a primary condition or complicating some other disease or injury, is very liable to lead to lung infection, particularly after general anaesthesia.

Oral disease interferes with mastication and swallowing. It is difficult to maintain sufficient food intake to meet the patient's calorie requirements and other nutritional needs.

Because of the constant natural movement which is very difficult to avoid unless the jaws are fixed together by splints, pain is a troublesome feature of oral conditions. Particularly is this true when the root of the tongue and pharynx are involved. In addition, impairment of swallowing and tongue movement may result in the dribbling of saliva which adds to the patient's distress and discomfort.

Nursing considerations

In all medical and surgical nursing, oral hygiene is of paramount importance, but in surgery of the mouth the success or failure of an operative procedure depends largely on the after-care in relation to cleanliness. Nursing technique has already been discussed (Chapter 2). The patient may be able to use mouth washes if the cheeks are uninjured and if the mandible is free to move. After dental operations or when splints are in position on the teeth the only satisfactory way of ensuring thorough cleansing is with a pressure spray. In the presence of special splints and appliances, it is usual for this procedure of cleansing to be undertaken by a dental or medical officer, or by a member of the nursing staff with special training.

Adequate nutrition is ensured by planning a high-calorie diet with added vitamin supplement. In all probability appetite will be poor owing to interference with taste. The preparation and presentation of the food is important. It must be tasty, unless there is inflammation of the salivary glands, which produces pain when the appetite is excited. Purées and fruit juices such as tomato juice, should be strained, to avoid the presence of pips or seeds in the mouth. Hot food should be avoided. Fluid is sometimes taken readily by 'straw' when the use of a feeding cup is difficult. If, on account of other injuries, the patient is unable to sit up, he can be provided with a length of rubber or plastic tube with which to suck fluid from a jug or from a transfusion type bottle on his bedside table. This is much more satisfactory than attempts to manage a feeding cup.

Tube feeding may be required. If the condition in the mouth is sufficient to interfere with swallowing, it is unlikely that a wide-bore oesophageal type of tube can be passed and a nasal Ryle's tube is then necessary. Before an attempt is made to insert the tube the patient should be allowed to suck an anaesthetic lozenge to diminish the pain of swallowing. The feeds must be very carefully strained to avoid blocking the narrow tube.

In some cases where oral feeding is not possible owing to severe injury to the jaw, a temporary gastrostomy is the most satisfactory way of maintaining the patient's nutrition.

Chronic infection in the mouth from dental sepsis or carcinoma of the tongue is often accompanied by infection of the respiratory tract, even before any operative procedure is undertaken. Except in acute cases, all steps possible are taken to eliminate dental sepsis before the treatment of the primary condition. Complete clearance of infected teeth may be necessary before radium treatment can be commenced for carcinoma of the tongue.

A further major problem is the relief of pain. Interference with swallowing, the presence of foreign particles or splints in the mouth, and unquenched thirst make the patient miserable and therefore much more sensitive to pain. Analgesic drugs are essential: methadone (physeptone) and codeine-phenacetin mixtures are effective in many cases, but if the patient is particularly anxious and restless, barbiturate sedatives may be required. Very severe mental distress may arise in nervous patients who develop a feeling of suffocation and choking. An acute anxiety state may develop and demand the use of heavy sedation such as diazepam. When such a situation arises, it is usually in the course of treating a severe fracture or a serious condition such as carcinoma, and the treatment cannot be interrupted in spite of the patient's distress.

Pain and discomfort will be increased if there is the slightest relaxation in measures to safeguard oral hygiene. A cough may become very troublesome as it is difficult to cough effectively when the movements of tongue or jaw are limited. Inhalations and sedative cough mixtures are required in such cases.

Great sympathy and tolerance is required in nursing patients with disease in the mouth. A writing pad and pencil should always be at hand if the patient is having difficulty with speech.

It is advisable for a patient to be warned, before operation, concerning any appliance which is going to be placed in his mouth, so that as he regains consciousness, he is not tempted to pull it out or to think that he is being choked. This is particularly important before the insertion of radium needles.

In the immediate post-operative period, the patient must be nursed on his side with the head lower than the shoulders to prevent the entry of blood into the larynx. Mouth gags and anaesthetic airways must be used with great caution. To diminish the need for these, the surgeon frequently leaves in place on the upper surface of the tongue, a silk or nylon stitch, the long ends of which are held in an artery pressure forceps, to enable the nurse to pull the tongue forwards. The stitch is not removed until the patient is fully conscious. During this post-anaesthetic recovery period, or later, vomiting may occur and under such circumstances aspiration of vomited material into the lungs is inevitable if nursing help is not at hand. A suction pump should be kept in the ward in order that the pharynx may be cleared if vomiting occurs, because the patient will be unable to swallow naturally in order to clear his throat.

When there has been a period of restricted feeding in which only fluid has been given, and that probably by tube, care must be taken to restore normal diet gradually in order to avoid gastro-intestinal disturbance. Vitamin supplement is essential.

Dental surgery

The work of the dental surgeon is, like medicine, divided into general dental practice and specialist dental surgery, although there is in Great Britain more overlap between these two fields than there is between general medical practice and hospital practice. Many dental surgeons are also fully qualified doctors.

The general dental practitioner is concerned mainly with 'conservative' dentistry. His object is to preserve and repair teeth. If this work of conservation fails, then he extracts diseased teeth and supplies dentures. Most of his work is done with the patient in the dental chair. The dental surgeon is assisted by a dental orderly who is sometimes a trained nurse and has had a special training as a dental assistant.

A specialist dental practitioner, in addition to general work, undertakes orthodontic treatment, major surgery of the jaws and, in collaboration with the general or plastic surgeon, he undertakes the treatment of jaw fractures. **Maxillo-facial surgery** is a term used to describe the work undertaken by a team of general and dental surgeons especially in the treatment of fractures. Hospital organisation in Great Britain has encouraged the development of maxillofacial and plastic surgical centres side by side because the plastic surgeon is so often required to undertake repair of the soft tissues of the face and nose after facial injuries which have resulted also in jaw fracture.

Dental mechanics are technicians especially trained in the manufacture of dental splints, false teeth and other appliances. They carry out their work in the dental laboratory attached to a hospital dental department.

Anaesthesia in dental surgery

The majority of 'chair' work—conservative dental surgery and minor extractions—is carried out under local anaesthesia. The nerves to the upper and lower jaw are sufficiently close to the surface, inside the mouth, to enable the surgeon to produce regional anaesthesia by an injection of procaine or lignocaine solutions. For convenience and economy multi-dose containers are used for the anaesthetic solution and self-sterilising preparations are commonly employed; these contain a mild antiseptic which does not damage the tissue into which the solution is injected.

In a hospital dental department or in private practice the nurse will be required to supervise the storage of these solutions and to ensure that the containers are not muddled. Serious accidents have occurred through injection of the wrong solution. All bottles must be very clearly labelled and those containing anaesthetic solutions should be of a type which cannot be confused with those containing any other substance.

Many dental surgeons use the cartridge type of syringe (Fig. 16.18) in which a small quantity of the necessary anaesthetic solution is supplied in a sterile sealed glass tube. The syringe frame and needle is readily sterilised by boiling and the risk of infection is very greatly reduced. Needles used for dental injections are very thin and flexible (Fig. 16.17) and because of their narrow calibre it is virtually impossible to fill the syringe through the needle. Hence, the cartridge type of syringe saves a great deal of time.

Nitrous oxide is employed for chair work as a general anaesthetic and is administered either by the dental surgeon or by a doctor. It is not possible to obtain relaxation of the muscles with nitrous oxide and a prop is therefore placed between the jaws before the induction of anaesthesia (Fig. 12.10). A sponge, to which is attached a long tape, is inserted into the pharynx before dental extractions commence to ensure that no tooth or blood is inhaled or swallowed. The extracted teeth must not be thrown away until they have been inspected and counted by the dental surgeon. If one has been lost, in spite of all precautions, it is likely that a chest x-ray will be required to make certain that the missing tooth has not been inhaled. Sponge packs must never be used without a tape attached because if the gag or prop slips the dental surgeon may be unable to retrieve the sponge before the patient has been asphyxiated. The sponges are washed in plain water, immediately after use, and sterilised by boiling.

Recovery from nitrous oxide anaesthesia occurs rapidly while the patient is still in the chair, but he should not be allowed to leave hospital until it is certain that bleeding has ceased and he is steady on his feet. No patient who has undergone nitrous oxide anaesthesia should be allowed to drive a motor-car for several hours. After dental extraction or minor operation the patient should be provided with a bowl into which he may spit, and with swabs of gauze to wipe his mouth. He should not be returned to the waiting room and expected to use his handkerchief. Neglect of this simple procedure is a mark of inefficiency and lack of sympathy.

Sensitivity to procaine and allied drugs sometimes occurs after the injection of a very small quantity: unexpected collapse requires urgent measures for resuscitation (page 285). Adrenaline solution or injection must be at hand. Oxygen must be given.

The dental formula

The first set of teeth, the **milk dentition,** consists of twenty teeth and begins to erupt towards the end of the normal period of breast feeding when the baby is 6 to 9 months old. The milk dentition is complete by the end of the third year. The **second dentition** begins to appear from 6 years onwards and there are normally thirty-two permanent teeth. The

DENTAL FORMULA

Child by the age of 4

E D C B A | A B C D E
———————————
E D C B A | A B C D E

A, central incisors
B, lateral incisors
C, canines
D and E, milk molars

Adult

8 7 6 5 4 3 2 1| 1 2 3 4 5 6 7 8
———————————
7 6 5 4 3 2 1| 1 2 3 4 5 6 7

(Note lower wisdom teeth are unerupted)
1, central incisors
2, lateral incisors
3, canines
4 and 5, premolars
6, 7 and 8, molars

Example of a child about 9—partial milk and partial adult dentition.
The first lower left molar has not yet erupted to replace the lost milk molar.

6 E 4 3 2 1| 1 2 3 D E 6
———————————
6 E 4 C 2 1| 1 2 C   E 6

third molars sometimes remain unerupted, or grow at such an angle that they impinge on the second molars and are unable to break through the surface of the jaw completely. They are then described as **impacted molars.** The term 'wisdom teeth' arose because the eruption of these last four is frequently delayed until after adolescence and in a considerable number of people never occurs! All the molar teeth of the permanent dentition arise in an area of the jaw which has not previously borne teeth, whereas the premolar, canine and incisor teeth displace the milk dentition as they grow.

If a tooth is incompletely erupted the bone around it or the cavity in which it is fixed may become infected, and it is this infection which necessitates the removal of many imperfectly erupted third molars.

The teeth of the milk dentition are lettered for descriptive purposes A to E on each side of the upper and lower jaw. The permanent teeth are numbered 1 to 8. On hospital notes and dental records the letters and numbers are used to describe the patient's dental state. In clinics where extractions are taking place it is essential that each patient has a separate card indicating which teeth are to be extracted, so that confusion and error is avoided.

A nurse may be called upon during the examination of school children, to know and record the dental formula in each case.

Complications of dental extractions

During extraction under general anaesthesia the jaw may be dislocated or fractured and severe pain on movement, particularly in the region of the temporo-mandibular joint, should be regarded as an indication that the jaw has been damaged.

Considerable swelling of the cheek frequently follows dental extraction due to interference with the lymphatic drainage which adds to inflammatory oedema.

Lung abscess and other pulmonary complications which arise from the inhalation of blood or tooth fragments can all be prevented by careful packing of the throat before extraction commences.

If the removal of teeth is carried out under local anaesthesia the two main complications are persistent infection in the tooth socket and haemorrhage. Infection may spread to surrounding bone and if it persists the cavity fails to heal. Haemorrhage under normal circumstances ceases very rapidly as the socket becomes filled with clot. If there is a disturbance of the clotting mechanism or the gum has been badly torn, bleeding may be extremely troublesome. Hot mouth washes are used initially. If this is ineffective the patient may be made to bite on a pad of folded gauze. Persistent bleeding usually requires surgical attention and plugging of the socket with wool soaked in adrenaline. Suture of the gums may occasionally be necessary. (Page 799—Antro-baccal fistula.)

Fractures of the jaws

The bones of the face and jaws are fractured most frequently by 'high velocity injuries'. Minor fractures occur from blows on the face received in sport, falls or personal fights. For descriptive purposes in relation to fractures, the face is divided into thirds. Fractures of the upper third are really fractures of the frontal bone and skull; these may involve the frontal sinus and lead to meningitis.

Fractures of the middle third are subdivided into those affecting the lateral portion and those affecting the centre section. In the lateral middle third the prominence of the cheeks is formed by the zygomatic or malar bone which may be driven in towards the orbit or into the maxillary antrum. An open operation is sometimes required to lever the prominence of the cheek bone back into position or to push it out by making an opening into the maxillary antrum, from inside the mouth (Fig. 43.6, antrostomy).

Fractures of the central middle third of the face may be very minor. For instance, a simple fracture of the nasal bones is reduced by moulding the nose with forceps under general anaesthesia. In a severe injury, the impact drives both maxillae and the whole

Table 58   Common oral operations

Site	Disorder	Operation
Lips	Congenital cleft (hare lip)	Repair
	Carcinoma	Excision and repair probably with skin graft
		Insertion of radium needles
Palate	Congenital cleft	Reconstruction, probably in two stages, including removal of tonsils, and repair of cleft lip
	Carcinoma or other neoplasm	Excision; insertion of radon seeds
Tongue	Tongue-tie	Division of frenum (frenoplasty)
	Leucoplakia	Excision of affected area
	Carcinoma	Partial glossectomy
		Hemi-glossectomy (right or left half of tongue)
		Total glossectomy
		Insertion of radium needles
Floor of mouth	Cysts—congenital dermoid cyst, mucus retention cyst, salivary cyst (ranula)	Excision (wall of cyst may be cauterised)
	Salivary calculus (submandibular duct)	Extraction of stone
	Carcinoma	Excision
		Destruction with diathermy
		Insertion of radium needles
Teeth	Injury, displacement, overcrowding, decay	Extraction
	Impaction of 'wisdom' teeth	Extraction
	Apical abscess	Apicectomy (removal of part of root) without disturbing the tooth
Gums	Gingivitis, pyorrhoea	Gingivectomy (excision of gum around the necks of all the teeth)
	Tumours (epulis)	Excision of tumour
Maxilla and mandible	Fractures	Wiring, manipulation and splintage: extraction of teeth in fracture line
	Cysts and neoplasms	Excision
	Osteitis	Drainage of abscesses
Temporomandibular joint	Dislocation	Manipulation
	Derangement; 'clicking'; recurrent dislocation	Excision of fibrous joint disc (as in knee injury)
	Arthritis	Condylectomy

centre portion of the face back towards the base of the skull. The air sinuses on the inner side of each orbit are damaged and the roof of the nose may be splintered with the result that there is a communication with the inside of the skull: cerebrospinal fluid escapes through the nose (**cerebrospinal rhinorrhoea**). The most severe fracture of this type is frequently associated with cerebral injury, and the patient is probably unconscious. Because of the associated head injury, the jaw condition is sometimes overlooked. As soon as it is possible the maxilla, which carries the teeth, has to be drawn forwards into its normal position where it is splinted to the mandible until healing has taken place.

Fractures of the lower third of the face involve the mandible. They may affect the tooth-bearing segment or the vertical portion to which are attached the muscles of mastication.

Fractures of the jaws are almost always compound, the fracture site communicating with the mouth, nose or maxillary antrum. Infection is likely and union is then delayed. Unless the fracture is correctly reduced the position of the teeth will be abnormal and the bite distorted. The jaws are splinted by the application of specially cast metal **cap splints** to the teeth. The splint on the upper jaw is fixed to that on the lower jaw so that the mouth cannot be opened during the period of healing.

The cleansing of the mouth when splints of this type are used can only be achieved effectively by the use of high-pressure spraying, and watch has to be kept for ulceration of the cheeks or lips by pressure from any prominent portion of the splint. The gap will be noticed between the jaws behind the position of the last teeth. Food can usually be introduced at this point if there is no opening further forward.

In fractures of the mandible, pins are sometimes placed into the bone through the cheek, the protruding outer ends being joined together by a metal bar which holds the fragments in position during healing (Fig. 42.4).

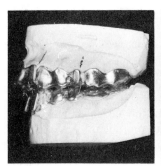 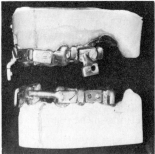 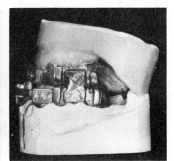

Fig. 42.4 Cap splints. The cast metal splints are made to fit plaster models which in turn have been made from the wax impressions of the patient's jaws. The splints are subsequently cemented to the teeth in the treatment of fractures of the mandible or maxilla. The correct bite is obtained by adjustments on the models. (*Left*) Simple cap splints with lugs to which are attached wires fixing upper and lower jaws together. (*Centre*) Cap splints with screwed fish plates which are used to lock the upper and lower jaws. (*Right*) The splints shown in centre, locked into position.

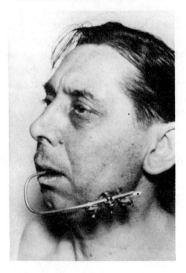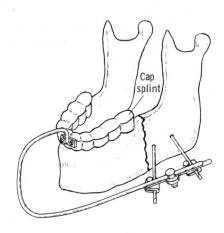

Fig. 42.5 Oblique fracture of the body of the mandible treated by a cap splint attached to the main fragment, coupled to pins inserted into the posterior fragment. Adjustment of the locking bar maintains the fragments in firm apposition.

Nursing management

In the initial treatment of patients with facial injuries the nurse will be concerned with the following problems:

(*a*) The management of any associated cerebral injury.

If the patient is unconscious continuous supervision is essential. Observation must be kept for cerebrospinal rhinorrhoea (page 789).

(*b*) The maintenance of a free airway. Tracheostomy may be made.

Reference has already been made (page 173) to the risk of asphyxia in jaw injuries when the patient is unable to protrude his tongue voluntarily. Patients with fractured jaws are therefore nursed during the 'first-aid period' in the prone position with the forehead propped on a cushion. This is essential in order that the tongue may fall forward: the accumulation of blood and secretions in the pharynx is thus prevented.

(*c*) The dressing and protection of lacerations of the face.

(*d*) The care of any associated eye injury.

(*e*) The administration of fluid.

Surgical treatment for the reduction and immobilisation of the fracture is undertaken as soon as possible and the associated injuries are dealt with at the same time.

When operative treatment is undertaken the nursing care must follow the lines described above for oral surgery in general.

43

Ear, Nose and Throat Surgery

The prevalence of infections of the upper respiratory tract in densely populated industrial communities has been largely responsible for the development of this special department of surgery. The association of the ear, the nose and the throat, as communicating parts of the upper respiratory tract, means that all three parts are commonly involved in the same disease processes. Many of the surgical procedures are highly specialised. Diseases of the ear are sometimes dealt with in a separate aural department.[1]

The investigation and treatment of deafness requires special apparatus and special rooms with sound-proof walls. In large hospital departments in Great Britain there is also the **hearing-aid centre** responsible for the provision of electric deaf-aids.

Speech therapy is an auxiliary method of treatment of defects of speech which may be either primary, such as stammering, or may be secondary to operations on the larynx. The primary defects may be associated with deafness. Speech therapists have a special technical training and usually work under the supervision of the surgeon in charge of the throat and ear department.

As in some other special departments the basic principles of nursing are simple, but advanced experience in the surgery of the department enables a trained staff nurse or sister to perform duties of a much more technical nature.

Clinical examination of the ear, nose and throat

Full examination can only be carried out adequately with special lighting and equipment. For simple routine ward examination of the ear, an electric battery-lighted auriscope is used. Illumination in the special department examination is provided by a 'bulls eye' lamp. This stands behind the patient and projects a beam of light on to the surgeon's head mirror, which has a central hole through which he can examine the patient who is seated on a chair in front of him. By this means, he can direct the reflected beam down the narrow channel of a speculum or on to the laryngeal mirror.

The nose is examined with a Thudichum-type speculum (Fig. 43.1) which resembles a pair of spring sugar tongs. Various sizes are provided.

The larynx is examined by means of a small circular mirror held above the epiglottis.

[1] **Otorhinolaryngology** is the technical term used to describe the work of the combined department.

To prevent it being steamed-up by the patient's breath, the mirror is warmed first in the flame of a spirit lamp, the temperature being tested on the back of the surgeon's hand.

Full examination of the ear requires not only an auriscope speculum but apparatus for removing wax (probes and wax-hooks) and for mopping away any discharge which obstructs the drum. Wire swab carriers are used covered with a small twisted swab of special wool. These are inserted through the speculum. Tuning forks of different frequency and other special appliances are used for testing hearing and the function of the semi-circular canals.

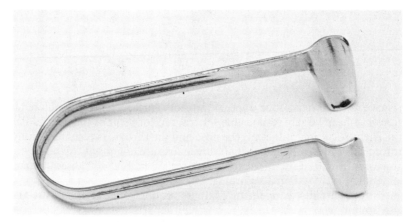

Fig. 43.1   Thudichum nasal speculum.

In addition to the specula, lamp and mirror the minimum equipment necessary for the examination of the ear, nose and throat includes also:

wool-carrying probes for local anaesthesia in the nose,
swabs for bacteriological culture of pus and nasal secretion,
Eustachian catheters,
an atomising spray for local anaesthetic solution,
a spirit lamp,
matches,
tongue cloths and spatulas,
special bellows used for inflating the nose in an attempt to overcome blockage of the Eustachian tube (page 818).

With this last appliance is a rubber tube with an ear-piece (like those on a stethoscope) at each end. This connects the patient's ear to the surgeon's and a click is heard if the surgeon is successful in inflating the Eustachian tube.

Apparatus which needs to be sterilised is boiled. The instruments are always placed in a constant position on the trolley beside the surgeon so that he may pick up the ones he wants without moving his head and losing sight of the particular area under inspection. Used instruments are placed in a special receptacle. Some of them are small and may accidentally be thrown away.

Most surgeons wear a gown and face mask during the examination as the patient is apt to cough. An apron is used around the patient to protect his clothing.

When they are healthy, the frontal and maxillary sinuses are translucent. A small lamp is placed in the patient's mouth to test the maxillary sinus and the light should be visible as a glow on the face over the antrum. The frontal sinus is tested by pressing the lamp into the orbit beneath the eyebrow. This transillumination test has to be carried out in a dark room and most special departments have a special cubicle for this purpose.

Radiology

Routine x-ray films are taken in the examination of the paranasal sinuses and, if antral infection is present, the films are repeated at intervals to watch progress under treatment.

Infection of the mastoid air cells is also shown by x-ray examination.

Examination of the teeth is frequently required as dental sepsis is often associated with sinus infection.

DISORDERS OF NOSE AND SINUSES

Obstruction and infection

In the healthy state there is a free airway on either side of the nasal septum. Into this airway open the ducts of the many **paranasal air sinuses** which are an integral part of the bones forming the face. These sinuses are lined by ciliated epithelium in which minute tufts protruding from the surface cells maintain a constant drift of the mucous secretion out of the sinuses into the nose, **Rhinitis** or inflammation of the nose produces swelling of the mucous membrane and blockage of these tiny ducts from the sinuses. Infection of the sinuses supervenes (**sinusitis**) (Fig. 43.2).

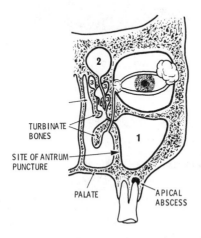

Fig. 43.2   Section through front of skull showing paranasal air sinuses and orbit. **1,** maxillary antrum. **2,** frontal sinus. **3,** ethmoid air cells. The lacrimal gland and naso-lacrimal duct are also shown. Note the site of intranasal antrostomy and the proximity of the roots of molar teeth to the antrum.

Obstruction to the free airway of the nose may be produced by swelling of the mucous membrane or by deviation of the septum from disease or injury. **Nasal polyps** form in the upper recesses of the nose and protrude like grapes into the airway producing further obstruction. They are removed under local anaesthesia.

Obstruction to the nose or to the orifice of a sinus leads to retention of secretions and to infection. A vicious circle develops in which infection, swelling with obstruction and retention follow in relentless succession.

Sinusitis may be chronic or acute. An acute infection is accompanied by severe pain and fever and is a regular occurrence during the course of the common cold. If the obstruction persists and the sinuses cannot drain, surgical intervention is sometimes necessary.

Chronic sinusitis leads to great thickening of the mucous membrane lining the sinuses and radical operations for the removal of necrotic bone and this diseased epithelium are sometimes necessary.

The treatment of nasal obstruction and sinusitis is directed to restoring free drainage

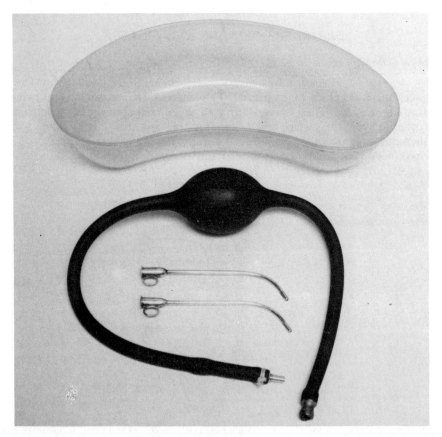

Fig. 43.3   Antral washout set. Higginson syringe and metal antral cannula which is introduced through the nose.

and a free airway, and thus to breaking the vicious circle. Various procedures are employed for this purpose.

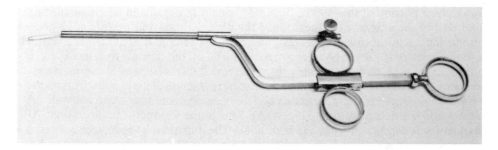

Fig. 43.4 Nasal snare. The sliding wire loop is placed over a polyp and closed.

(a) Nasal wash-outs or douching

The patient is made to sniff normal saline solution through each nostril into the pharynx. He spits out the solution and the mucopurulent material which it has carried from the nose. Douching of the nose with a pressure syringe is dangerous since infection may be carried up the Eustachian tube into the middle ear.

(b) Sinus drainage

Antrostomy (Fig. 43.5). The natural opening from the maxillary sinus to the nose is in such a position as to make the introduction of a cannula through it almost impossible.

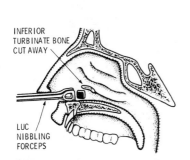
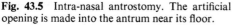

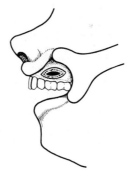

Fig. 43.5 Intra-nasal antrostomy. The artificial opening is made into the antrum near its floor.

Fig. 43.6 Caldwell-Luc operation. Antrostomy through the side wall of the maxilla above the teeth.

Also, the opening is very near the top of the antrum, since the natural drainage is by the action of the ciliated epithelium. If the epithelium is damaged by infection, gravity drainage is essential and an artificial opening is made below the inferior turbinate bone. This may be by 'antral puncture', a trocar and cannula being used under local anaesthesia. The sinus is washed out with a Higginson syringe. Sometimes, in chronic infection, a small polythene tube is left in place for several days and penicillin solution introduced daily.

A permanent nasal antrostomy is sometimes made to provide better drainage. In this procedure, a portion of the inferior turbinate bone is removed and a hole nibbled in the nasal wall of the antrum near the floor of the nose. Regular wash-outs can be given by introducing an antral catheter through this enlarged opening without further anaesthetic.

Sometimes it is necessary to explore the inside of the antrum to remove polypoid mucous membrane, to deal with growths, to remove a displaced root of a tooth which has been broken off during extraction, or to treat a severe fracture of the maxilla. This operation is performed under general anaesthesia and an opening made into the front wall of the antrum above the canine tooth (Fig. 43.6). This is the Caldwell-Luc operation. After-treatment will depend on what has been done. The antrum may have been packed with antiseptic ribbon gauze, or it may require washing out daily. Attention must be paid at very frequent intervals to oral cleansing, but mouth washes are avoided.

The bone of the maxilla is thin in front of the antrum and oedema of the overlying cheek is very marked if the antrum is acutely infected. Facial swelling follows the Caldwell-Luc operation but subsides without any special treatment.

Frontal sinus. Acute infection of the frontal sinus may require open operation for drainage (Fig. 43.7). An incision is made above the inner end of the eyebrow and a pathway is opened into the nose to re-establish free drainage. Temporary external drainage with a small rubber tube may be necessary.

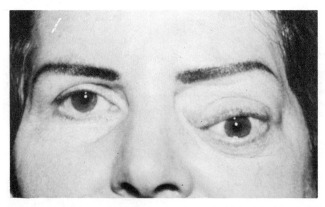

Fig. 43.7 Mucocele of the left frontal sinus arising from sinusitis. The eye is displaced downwards (page 398). Infection of the ethmoid sinuses may cause orbital cellulitis, producing a similar protrusion and inflammation of the eye (page 827).

(c) *Management of allergy*

Allergy is a major cause of sinusitis. Sensitivity to house dust, tobacco smoke or pollen causes chronic oedema of the nasal epithelium: this in turn leads to infection. Antihistamine drugs are taken systematically and may be applied locally with a nebuliser (e.g. Antistin-Privine of Otrivine (xylometazoline).

Injury

Reference has already been made to fractures of the central middle third of the face (page 787). A blow on the end of the nose may fracture the septum or the bridge of the nose. Not only is there disfigurement by loss of the normal contour but the septum becomes deviated and may obstruct one nostril. Fractures of the nasal bones are treated by manipulation under anaesthesia. A two-bladed Walsham forceps is used, one blade passing into the nostril. The instrument grips the septum or nasal wall and enables the surgeon to mould the front of the nose into position. Various forms of plastic splint are applied to maintain the position of the nose during healing.

The nasal septum consists of a cartilage and bony central plate with lining epithelium on each side. If it is badly deviated and causing obstruction to the airway part of it is removed. An incision is made on one side through the epithelial mucous membrane and the central portion of the septum which is causing obstruction is resected, care being taken not to puncture the mucous membrane of the opposite side. The operation can be performed under local anaesthesia, but as it is combined with other operations on the sinuses general endotracheal anaesthesia is frequently used. The operation is described as **submucous resection** (SMR).

Occasionally as the result of a blow, a haematoma develops in the septum. If this becomes infected necrosis of the septal bone and cartilage leads to collapse of the nose and loss of contour. A large haematoma of the septum is therefore drained by simple incision to prevent this risk of infection and necrosis.

A foreign body may become impacted in the nose accidentally. Food particles may enter the nose from the nasopharynx during vomiting or coughing. A child may put beads or seeds or other tiny objects into the nostril. A profuse discharge from one nostril should lead to a search for such a foreign body. No attempt should be made to dislodge a foreign body by syringing or douching the nose. By syringing, the object may be made less accessible and in douching it may become inhaled into the larynx. Removal under direct vision is necessary.

Neoplasm

Rodent ulcers, a special form of skin carcinoma, may affect the nose. This type of growth does not spread to lymph glands and is usually cured by radium or x-ray treatment. A portion of the nose which has been destroyed by the ulcerative process may require replacement by skin grafting (page 799, rhinoplasty). Carcinoma of the antrum of the maxilla may be treated by radiotherapy or by complete removal of the maxilla.

Anaesthesia

A major portion of the out-patient treatment undertaken by the Ear, Nose and Throat Department comprises operations on the nose and sinuses performed under local anaesthesia. This is applied by means of a nebuliser[1] or by pads of wool soaked in cocaine or other solution.

Long metal probes are covered for a distance of about 3–4 cm (1½ inches) with a special high-quality cotton wool which does not disintegrate. This material is sometimes described as 'ear' wool because it is used for covering probes for mopping the external meatus. It is also described sometimes as ophthalmic wool because it is equally important that there should be no fluff on wool pads used to cover the eyes. The wool must be twisted on the probe so that there is no fear of it becoming detached and remaining in the nose. The wool-covered probes are soaked in a local anaesthetic solution and inserted in the floor of the nose. The whole of the inside lining of the nasal cavity is rendered insensitive after a few minutes of this application. Antrum puncture or the removal of polyps can be undertaken with the patient sitting in the chair.

When general anaesthesia is used for nasal operations the pharynx is packed by the anaesthetist to prevent the risk of blood entering the larynx. Particular care must be taken in the checking of swabs used in the theatre to make certain that no small pack is left behind in the nasopharynx. Fatal accidents have occurred because a swab has been overlooked and during the recovery period has become displaced and has dropped down into the glottis, producing asphyxia.

Epistaxis

Nose bleeding may follow injury or may occur spontaneously in patients with very high blood pressure. The most common injury is damage to the very vascular septum by 'nose-picking'. A particularly prominent vessel which is the source of recurrent bleeding may be destroyed by use of the electric cautery (page 354).

Nose bleeding occurring as a complication of severe injury of the face must be treated by nursing the patient in the face-down position so that the blood runs forward out of the nostrils rather than into the pharynx, from which it will be swallowed or inhaled. If the patient is conscious, he should sit up, leaning slightly forward so that the blood escapes from the nose. Sometimes packing may be required (see below).

Nasal packing and post-operative care

After certain operations on the nose the nostrils are packed with ribbon gauze, and if bleeding is occurring in the posterior part of the nose post-nasal packing has to be inserted. This is a procedure for the medical officer or specially trained nurse. Packing which is inserted by the surgeon at the time of operation is usually removed three or four days later. A loose end is left protruding from the nostril and is attached to the cheek with adhesive strapping to prevent it becoming pushed back into the nose out of reach. Removal is sometimes quite painful and light anaesthesia may be required with gas or trilene. Dry gauze is used on most occasions for packing the nose, nasopharynx or antrum,

[1] Nebula (Latin) = mist, cloud.

but if the packing is to remain in place for several days, an antiseptic gauze is preferred to prevent foul decomposition of blood. BIPP gauze (ribbon impregnated with 'bismuth-iodoform-paraffin-paste') is commonly used for this purpose.[1]

If the nasopharynx is to be packed, a pad of gauze may be used with two tapes attached. The nose is sprayed with anaesthetic solution and a rubber catheter inserted. The end which emerges beyond the palate is pulled forward through the mouth and one tape of the gauze tied to it. As the catheter is then withdrawn through the nose the pack is pulled into the nasopharynx. The second tape comes out of the mouth and is used for removing the pack in due course. This method may be necessary for severe bleeding from the raw area after removal of adenoids.

Nasal discharge which occurs following operation has to be mopped frequently from the nose and the patient is provided with gauze swabs in a bowl on his bedside table. No attempt must be made to plug the anterior opening of the nostril. Douching and inhalations may be prescribed to cleanse the airway and relieve congestion.

Rhinoplasty

Reconstruction of the nose is sometimes necessary after injury or when part of it has been destroyed by growth or lupus vulgaris (a tuberculous condition of the skin). A pedicle skin graft is used (page 952).

Antro-buccal fistula

Following the removal of an upper molar tooth whose root has protruded into the floor of the antrum a communication may develop between the mouth and the maxillary sinus. This fistula requires closure by open operation, usually under full general anaesthesia.

DISORDERS OF THE PHARYNX

The pharynx is the area bounded below by the epiglottis and the opening of the oesophagus, and in front by the anterior pillar of the fauces, and at a higher level by the posterior choanae (the posterior opening of the nasal air passages). The roof is formed by the base of the skull in which is the sphenoid sinus and the pituitary fossa. There is a ring of lymphoid tissue around the pharynx with the adenoids posteriorly and the tonsils further forward on either side. In practice the principal clinical conditions which arise are those due to infection and neoplasm.

Tonsils and adenoids

Each tonsil is a soft pad of lymphoid tissue lying between the base of the tongue and the edge of the soft palate. It becomes infected by organisms which gain entry through the nose so that chronic tonsillitis is frequently present with chronic nasal infection. Tonsillar infection gives rise to enlargement of glands in the neck. Acute tonsillitis is sometimes accompanied by the development of an abscess in the tonsillar bed. Great swelling is seen

---

[1] Iodoform is also used in Whitehead's varnish, for sealed dressings, for its prolonged antiseptic effect (page 398).

at the back of the mouth and the tonsil may protrude almost as far as the midline. An abscess in this situation is a **quinsy**. The spread of infection around the tonsil can now usually be controlled by antibiotic treatment, but if an abscess forms, an incision is made through the front wall and the pus discharged into the mouth. Anaesthesia is not necessary, as the abscess is opened by a sudden stab with a small scalpel, the blade of which has been protected with adhesive strapping except for the point. If a quinsy is not treated effectively the cellulitis may spread down the neck and produce oedema of the glottis. After the drainage of a quinsy the patient should be given gargles and mouth washes, more for the cleansing effect than with any intent to destroy organisms.

The removal of tonsils and adenoids constitutes one of the major problems of in-patient organisation in this department. Two principal methods are in common use in Great Britain, the **dissection tonsillectomy** and **guillotine enucleation.** In the dissection operation the patient is admitted to hospital the day before operation. Full pre-operative sedation with barbiturate or other drugs is essential to remove fear in these patients, most of whom are children. The operation is carried out under full general anaesthesia. This is administered through a tube incorporated in a special Boyle-Davis mouth gag, or by means of an endotracheal nasal tube. Bleeding from the tonsillar bed usually stops spontaneously but occasionally blood vessels are tied with thread or catgut. If bleeding is particularly troublesome the surgeon may stitch the pillars of the tonsillar fossa together with catgut stitches; these will absorb and do not require subsequent removal. After both tonsils have been removed and bleeding has been controlled satisfactorily the adenoids are removed with a curette. This produces profuse bleeding and the patient is immediately turned on his side so that the mouth is lower than the throat. Small blocks of ice are often used to apply to the bridge of the nose and face, as this produces a reflex constriction of blood vessels and helps to stop the bleeding from the raw area at the back of the nose. The patient is nursed on his side in the semi-face-down position until consciousness is regained and the cough reflex has returned. Great care has to be taken to prevent inhalation of blood.

Many years ago tonsils were guillotined. In this procedure the protruding portion of the tonsil was cut off without the removal of the deep portion. This procedure has been abandoned but a blunt bladed guillotine is still used in many centres for enucleating the tonsil. The guillotine is passed into the mouth and pressed against the tonsil which is pushed towards it by the surgeon's finger placed in the neck below the angle of the jaw. When the guillotine is closed it grips the tonsil which is then wrenched from its bed by rotation of the instrument. The guillotine-enucleation method is extremely rapid in skilled hands but the blood loss is greater than with dissection and even greater care has to be taken to prevent the possible inhalation of blood.

Haemorrhage is the most feared complication of tonsillectomy and this may occur within the first 48 hours or from infection (secondary haemorrhage) several days later. If post-operative haemorrhage is severe transfusion may be required, but it is usually controlled, after removal of the clots in the tonsillar bed, by the application of an adrenaline soaked pack. This procedure is undertaken by a medical officer. The pulse rate is recorded every quarter of an hour for the first 2 hours after tonsillectomy and very close supervision is maintained during the first 12 hours. If bleeding continues the blood may be swallowed without anyone being aware of what is happening. The partly digested blood is subsequently vomited.

In the healing process the tonsillar bed is covered with slough which is naturally infected. Infection may spread to the middle ear so that acute otitis media, indicated by rise of temperature and earache, is a complication which must be watched for. The ears are inspected daily by the medical officer, following tonsillectomy, as reddening of the drum may be the first sign of this complication. Many patients, particularly children, are able to consume a normal diet the day after tonsillectomy. It is usual to restrict food to soft items and fluid for the first 48 hours. In the adult and older child, pain is relieved by aspirin gargle, at frequent intervals. Also, pain may increase after the first 48 hours, owing to infection in the tonsillar bed.

Retropharyngeal abscess

Behind the pharynx, at the level of the soft palate, there is a pad of lymph gland tissue which may become infected in the same way as the tonsil. Occasionally an abscess forms here. Its presence is detected by pain, fever and a visible bulge in the wall of the pharynx. An incision is made into the abscess through the mouth.

In tuberculous disease of the spine a much deeper form of retropharyngeal abscess develops on the front of the cervical vertebrae. That type is not opened into the pharynx.

Neoplasm of the pharynx

The lining epithelium of this area is squamous and carcinomas which arise from it may be called therefore epitheliomas. Rapidly growing tumours also arise in the lymphoid tissue—lymphosarcoma, adenolymphoma—both in children and the elderly.

The first clinical sign of any neoplasm in the pharynx may be the appearance of enlarged glands in the neck. The primary growth in the naso-pharynx or at the back of the tongue may only be discovered by the surgeon during full examination under general anaesthesia.

The majority of neoplasms of the pharynx are treated by radiotherapy and these growths respond very well. Extensive or infiltrating growths may, however, be treated by radical surgery, particularly if they have arisen in the lower part of the pharynx and involve in addition the wall of the larynx. Surgical excision necessitates the patient having a tracheostomy and possibly gastrostomy as well at least as a temporary measure. Reference is made again to this in relation to carcinoma of the larynx.

Owing to the proximity of the glottis both inflammatory and neoplastic conditions of the pharynx render the patient liable to glottic obstruction and the need for emergency tracheostomy. Occasionally acute glottic oedema arises during a course of radiotherapy.

DISORDERS OF THE LARYNX

The larynx is formed by the **hyoid bone**, the **thyroid cartilage** and the **cricoid cartilage**. It is held in position in the neck by a lower group of muscles which extend between the larynx and the clavicle, and an upper group between the larynx and the base of the skull, while the muscles of the tongue are also attached to the hyoid bone. The vocal cords are formed by two folds of mucous membrane stretched between the front and the back of the larynx. In the normal resting position the space between the cords, **the glottis**, is less than half a centimetre. The position of the cords is varied by muscle action so that the gap between them can be opened and the tension of the cords varied also. The muscles controlling the cords derive their nerve supply from the recurrent branch of the vagus which comes up from the thorax on each side of the neck behind the thyroid gland.

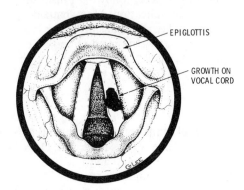

Fig. 43.8   View of the glottis (entrance to larynx) by indirect laryngoscopy, seen in a laryngeal mirror held behind the soft palate. A carcinoma is present on the left vocal cord. By use of a laryngoscope, a direct view is obtained.

If the **recurrent laryngeal nerves** are damaged by operation in the neck, or by growth in the chest or neck, the voice is affected. There may be obstruction to respiration if both cords are completely paralysed: tracheostomy is then necessary, followed by some operation to separate the vocal cords.[1]

The mucous epithelium which lines the larynx swells very easily from allergy or infection. This oedema produces alteration in the voice and occasionally complete respiratory obstruction which itself may require tracheostomy.

The larynx is closely attached to the front of the oesophagus and pharynx and may be involved from growth in that region.

The treatment of laryngeal obstruction

Irritation of the larynx from the presence of foreign bodies, such as crumbs, produces violent spasms of coughing. The spasm may at the same time close the vocal cords together and produce asphyxia. This happens during anaesthesia if mucus from the pharynx or vomitus is inhaled into the larynx. Under hospital conditions, acute obstruction of the glottis is treated initially by intubation—that is a laryngoscope is inserted into the mouth and an endotracheal tube passed through the glottis. Babies develop acute tracheobronchitis and laryngeal obstruction very easily. Intubation in the casualty department may be urgent and life-saving. Even in hospital, if intubation equipment is not available or the procedure proves to be very difficult, emergency tracheotomy or laryngotomy has to be performed.

In **laryngotomy** (Fig. 43.9) an opening is made between the cricoid cartilage and the

---

[1] **Tracheotomy** = making an opening into the trachea. *Tracheostomy* is the established opening. *Tracheostomy* is now used almost universally in describing the operation whether temporary or permanent. Cf. cystotomy and cystostomy.

lower edge of the thyroid cartilage. It is quicker and easier than the operation of tracheostomy but may result in damage to the vocal cords. A laryngotomy tube is oval in section.

In **tracheostomy** (Fig. 43.9), an opening is made usually in the second or third ring of the trachea which is exposed by dividing the isthmus of the thyroid gland.

Tracheostomy implies more than a short-term opening into the trachea as an emergency. A stoma or mouth is made into the windpipe and this term is in more general use today.

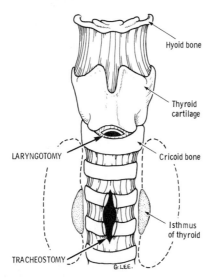

Hyoid bone

Thyroid cartilage

LARYNGOTOMY

Cricoid bone

Isthmus of thyroid

TRACHEOSTOMY

G.LEE.

Fig. 43.9   The larynx and trachea showing the position of artificial openings in laryngotomy and tracheostomy. Owing to the spring of the cartilage rings in the trachea, a dilator is necessary to hold the edges of the opening apart during the introduction of a tracheostomy tube.

The most frequent need for tracheostomy is in the intensive care of patients with respiratory disease. This may have occurred as a complication of major surgery, or from accident, or be associated with unconsciousness and head injury. Any condition which produces paralysis of the respiratory muscles such as myasthenia gravis, poliomyelitis or a high fracture of the spine may lead to the need for artificial respiration by a mechanical ventilator (page 186). Intermittent positive pressure respiration can be performed through an indwelling endotracheal tube passed through the mouth for short periods but for anything more than 48 hours a tracheostomy is preferable.

Tracheostomy tubes and technique

In the real emergency tracheostomy, a rigid metal tube made from silver is used; this is easy to handle (Fig. 43.10). All casualty departments have a tracheostomy set at hand. The procedure is performed under local anaesthetic, or if the patient is unconscious without anaesthesia, through a small incision in the midline of the neck across the thyroid region, the patient's head being extended over a pilllow. The tissues over the trachea are separated and an incision made vertically over the second, third and fourth rings of the trachea. Violent coughing is produced when the trachea is incised and to prevent this, if there is time, a small quantity of local anaesthetic is injected into the trachea between

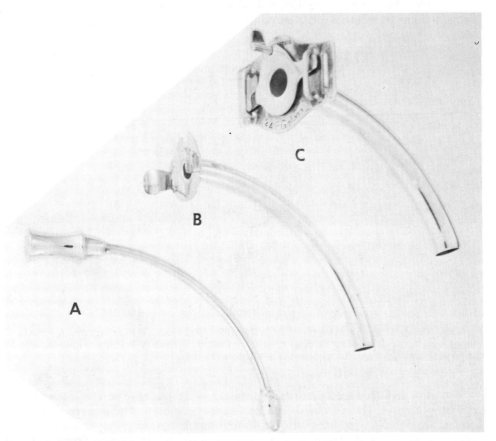

Fig. 43.10 Silver tracheostomy tube (Chevalier Jackson). **A.** Introducer. **B.** Removable inner tube. **C.** Outer tube which carries a loose fitting flange to which the tape is attached. A turn catch is seen at the top and this anchors the inner tube which can be quickly removed if any degree of blockage occurs with mucus. (Seward Surgical Instruments.)

the rings. The edges of the tracheal opening are held apart with the special dilator provided and the silver metal tube is inserted with its curve downwards. The edges of the wound are sutured and a thin gauze dressing placed under the flanges of the tracheostomy tube, which is held in place by a tape around the neck.

When, however, the operation is being performed in order to institute intermittent positive pressure respiration with a mechanical ventilator, a rubber or plastic tracheostomy tube is used with an inflatable cuff. Even if artificial respiration is not going to be used, but the patient has weakness of the pharyngeal muscles or excessive secretion and is unable to swallow, a cuffed tube is used to prevent pharyngeal secretion or blood from trickling into the trachea. This is a 'planned' operation and often done under general anaesthesia.

When tracheostomy has been performed to improve respiratory function rather than simply to relieve laryngeal obstruction, one of the most important advantages is that bronchial secretions can be removed regularly by suction catheter. All forms of tracheostomy require meticulous attention to asepsis and regular suction through a sterile catheter (see below).

Oxygen may be administered through a tracheostomy tube; a small catheter and humidifier are used, until an oxygen tent is available.

If the patient is to receive radiotherapy to the neck, the tracheostomy tube must be a rubber or plastic one.

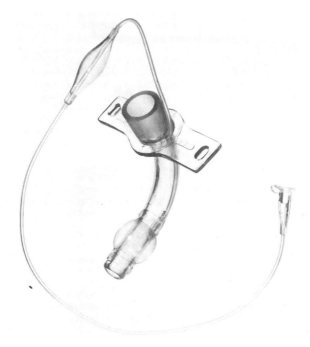

Fig. 43.11   Portex PVC cuffed tracheostomy tube. (Feldman and Crawley, *Tracheostomy and Artificial Ventilation*, Edward Arnold.)

On rare occasions when no surgical appliance has been available and laryngeal obstruction has occurred, life has been saved by rapid incision into the trachea with a penknife and the introduction of the stem of a smoker's pipe. The onset of oedema of the glottis after burns or scalds from flame or steam may be so rapid as to require urgent desperate action such as this.

Nursing management

Apart from the extreme life-saving emergency, as for instance when a child has a foreign body impacted in the pharynx, it is likely that the tracheostomy is going to be needed for a considerable time.

The tube is fixed in position to prevent its ejection by coughing, by paired tapes tied around the neck, with the reef knots placed on the *side* of the neck so they can be seen: the correct tightness of the tape is important, and it should be secured with the head bent forward slightly: 'night gowns' or bed jackets with neck tapes must not be worn: loose tapes become confused with the tracheostomy tapes or may even be sucked into the stoma. Assuming the patient is breathing naturally through the tracheostomy and does not require artificial respiration, the tracheostomy tube is covered with a small square of loose gauze but must never be bandaged. The loose gauze acts as a protection against the inhalation of foreign particles and absorbs the secretions which are coughed from the tube. The gauze should be changed every hour for the first day or so. If this pad is allowed to become sodden it may be drawn over the tracheostomy tube and obstruct it.

A writing pad and pencil must be at hand as soon as the patient recovers consciousness.

Metal tracheostomy tubes consist of an outer sheath and an inner flanged tube which is removable (Fig. 43.10). The inner tube is taken out and washed several times a day and whenever there appears to be irritation or obstruction. The outer tube also requires removal and sterilisation from time to time, but the nurse should never remove this unless specific instructions are given, as its replacement may be extremely difficult in the first few days after operation. The first tube is left at least 5 days so that a track is established. A special curved introducing forceps is used to maintain the airway through the opening while the outer tube is changed.

In paralytic conditions such as poliomyelitis or a high cervical spine fracture or myasthenia gravis, the purpose of a tracheostomy is twofold. The first is in order to reduce the resistance to respiration so that any natural breathing that the patient is able to perform will be more effective, or alternatively it is in order that intermittent positive pressure respiration with a mechanical ventilator can be performed. The second purpose is to prevent the patient drowning in pharyngeal secretions.

The nurse in training may come in contact with tracheostomy patients in the Ear, Nose and Throat Department, but the majority of tracheostomies are performed for patients having intensive care, either as a result of injury or in the post-operative phase. In these special units, very clear rules for procedure are laid down in order that the routine treatments for the cardio-respiratory problems and other aspects of nursing are carried out to a strict schedule (page 195).

Suction

The trachea or tube may be blocked by mucus: this is prevented by regular aseptic suction with a sterile catheter.[1] The suction tube has a Y-connector to produce an air leak. The catheter is inserted with special holding forceps (Fig. 35.7), or with the fingers of the nurse's right hand wearing a sterile glove. The catheter is inserted gently for 12–20 cm if tolerated, the air leak closed with a finger, and suction thus applied as the catheter is

---

[1] The catheter must be less than half the diameter of the tracheostomy tube. This is vital in children, to avoid the risk of excessive suction on the lung tissue.

withdrawn. If the patient is being ventilated suction must be done through a T-piece in the connector; the suction 'act' should not take more than 10 seconds as the patient is not being oxygenated while this is taking place.

In the unconscious patient suction is needed regularly and whenever respiration becomes 'rattley'.

Humidification

Various attachments are available for keeping the air passages moist—a function normally performed by the healthy nose and pharynx. Fig. 10.20 shows a plastic box attachment which acts similarly to the partial re-breathing oxygen mask. Mechanical ventilators usually have a built-in vaporizer, e.g. Bird respirator (page 190).

Inflatable cuffs

When a cuffed tube is being used with IPPR, the cuff is inflated just sufficiently to prevent an air leak. Very little pressure is required. Over-inflation quickly produces ulceration of the tracheal lining. In some units it is routine practice to deflate the cuff for 2 minutes every hour, but this has the disadvantage of repeated manipulation and the possibility of secretions running past the tube. A tube with a floppy redundant cuff is ideal to avoid ischaemia of the lining mucosa.

Complications of tracheostomy

Clearly complications are more likely when the operation has been undertaken as an emergency, under difficult circumstances, than when it has been a planned procedure. The successful outcome of tracheostomy depends very largely on skilled nursing with meticulous attention to detail.

Obstruction. (*a*) A metal tube or a rubber cuffed tube may become blocked by a plug of mucus coughed from lower down the respiratory tree.

(*b*) A cuffed tube may break and part of the cuff become dislodged below the inlet of the tube, the lumen of which it will then obstruct.

(*c*) If the cuff breaks, the tube may be partially rejected or a metal tube may become loose due to slackening of the tapes; it may slip out of the trachea and yet appear to remain in the neck.

Surgical emphysema. This means the escape of air either from the ventilator or from the trachea by natural expiration into the tissues of the neck. This may occur if the tube becomes dislodged or if it does not make a firm fit in the opening of the trachea. The emphysema may spread with alarming rapidity and the swelling of the neck tissues surrounding the stoma may make it very difficult to replace the tube that has become dislodged.

Haemorrhage. Assuming that the bleeding has been stopped adequately at the construction of the tracheostomy, subsequent bleeding may come from the edges of the wound due to friction from the tube or may come from the trachea. Bleeding may be started by the

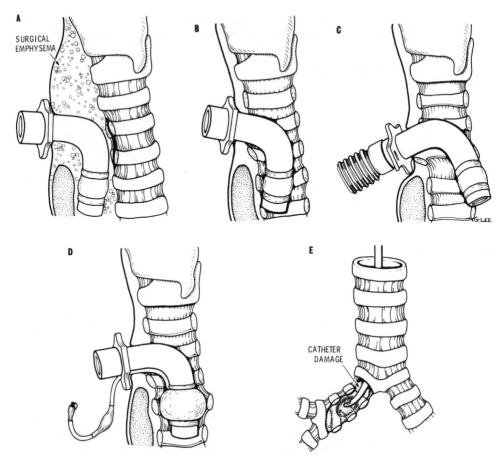

Fig. 43.12 Tracheostomy. 'Cut-away' views of cuffed tube showing complications which may arise. **A.** Short tube has slipped out—surgical emphysema. **B.** Anterior ulceration—tube too short and elevated. **C.** Tube dragged by respirator tube—posterior ulceration. **D.** Over-inflation of cuff—pressure necrosis. **E.** Careless suction with hard catheter causing bronchial ulceration.

aspiration catheter if it is used rather roughly. Torrential bleeding can occur from ulceration of the trachea wall by pressure from the tube. Such pressure can be produced by over-inflation of the cuff or by angulation of the tube where it is a metal one or a rubber one.

The lining membrane of the trachea becomes inflamed and is, therefore, very ready to bleed if it is damaged in any way by tubes or catheters. Severe bleeding must be managed at once by putting the patient into the head down position and repeating aspiration sufficiently frequently to keep the airway clear.

Dysphagia. The conscious patient may have difficulty in swallowing after a tracheostomy because of the discomfort produced by movement of the tube. The cuffed tube may cause compression of the oesophagus. If the patient is having difficulty in swallowing or clearing his pharynx, even greater than normal care must be taken to ensure that there is no accumulation of saliva which may get inhaled.

Pulmonary infection and collapse. A pre-existing inflammatory condition of the lung may spread, particularly if there is poor humidity and inadequate suction. Because of the moist conditions which exist, infection with the pyocyaneus organism can easily occur and this may be resistant to all antibiotic treatment.

Closure of tracheostomy

After a short term tracheostomy, when the normal airway has been restored through the larynx the tracheostomy tube is removed and the sinus closes naturally within a few days. If the resultant scar is ugly, or spontaneous closure is slow, excision of the scar and surgical closure may be required. If the operation has been performed as a preliminary to complete removal of the larynx, or in a case in which obstruction is permanent from growth or scarring, the tracheostomy opening becomes lined with skin.

Long-term tracheostomy

In certain cases tracheostomy is permanent even if the larynx has not been removed; for instance if there has been injury to both recurrent laryngeal nerves perhaps from thyroidectomy for cancer, or if there has been scarring of the larynx from injury. In order to enable the patient to talk, an inner tube is fitted with a flap valve. The patient is then able to breathe in freely through the tube and can talk while breathing out through the narrow larynx (Fig. 43.13).

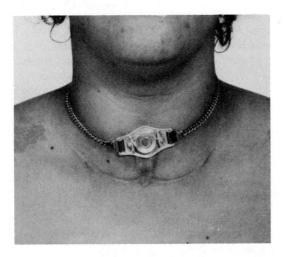

Fig. 43.13 Permanent tracheostomy. The metal inner tube has a flap valve. This closes during expiration and thus enables the patient to speak.

Foreign bodies in the larynx

The inhalation of foreign bodies accidentally by the conscious patient results in coughing and spontaneous expulsion of the particle. More often than lodging in the larynx, the foreign body enters the trachea and falls into the lung. If the object remains impacted in the larynx and is not expelled by coughing it sets up acute inflammation and laryngeal oedema which may later produce obstruction. The foreign body is removed with angled laryngeal forceps. Local anaesthesia is used since the induction of general anaesthesia would probably produce asphyxia from spasm of the larynx. The first and urgent measure if a foreign body lodges in the larynx is to spray the throat and air-passages with anaesthetic solution and prevent spasm and coughing. Large foreign bodies do not enter the larynx but produce spasm from their presence in the pharynx. Usually such an object can be hooked out by a finger introduced over the back of the tongue.

Infection

Laryngitis occurs most commonly as part of a general infection of the upper respiratory tract. It may also be part of an acute specific infection of the trachea in small children, in whom it is rapidly fatal if untreated. Diphtheria also affects the larynx and occasionally produces complete obstruction requiring the introduction of a tube between the cords (**intubation**) or tracheostomy.

Injury

If the larynx is fractured or bruised, the resulting oedema may produce respiratory obstruction requiring tracheostomy. Suicidal cut-throat wounds, or bullets, may open the larynx and respiratory obstruction then occurs from the entry of blood and from spasm. Tracheostomy with suction is required. Cellulitis of the neck and surgical emphysema are likely complications.

In severe injuries of the larynx when the air-passage has been opened the principal first-aid measure is to control haemorrhage by pressure and to separate the edges of the wound in the larynx so that air may enter freely. If much blood has entered the lungs, artificial respiration will be necessary with posturing, to drain the trachea and bronchi.

The initial hospital treatment may involve tracheostomy and insertion of a cuffed tube through which the lower respiratory tract is cleared of blood by suction. Surgical repair may be very complicated, particularly if the pharynx has been opened in addition to injury of the larynx itself. If the larynx has been crushed or lacerated it is usual for the surgeon to leave a large-bore soft tube between the vocal cords to act as a former during the healing process. A nasal tube is used down the oesophagus to maintain the patient's nutrition and vacuum drainage tubes are left in the wounds (Fig. 43.14).

Neoplasm

A type of innocent tumour (**papilloma**) occurs on the vocal cords, as a wart. It is removed or cauterised under direct vision. Occasionally tracheostomy is required as a preliminary measure.

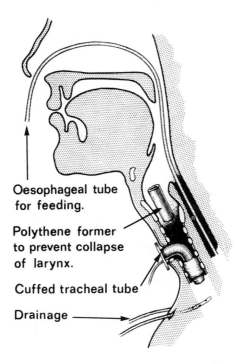

Oesophageal tube
for feeding.

Polythene former
to prevent collapse
of larynx.

Cuffed tracheal tube

Drainage

Fig. 43.14   After laryngeal injury—crush or laceration in 'cut-throat' wound, tubes are placed as shown.
Similar intubation is needed after extensive throat and neck operation (except for the polythene 'former').

Carcinoma (epithelioma) of the larynx is a common form of cancer. The first symptom
is an alteration in the voice, and persistent hoarseness in persons of the cancer age-group
(over 40 years of age) always leads to a suspicion of carcinoma.

Early cases are treated by excision of the affected portion of the larynx or by the implantation of radium. Access is gained by the operation of **laryngofissure** (Fig. 43.16) in
which a window is cut in the side of the thyroid cartilage after preliminary tracheostomy.
For more advanced cases the whole larynx is excised, by **laryngectomy**. Tracheostomy in
this case is permanent.

The post-operative care is mainly that of a patient with tracheostomy, particular
attention being paid to the prevention of pulmonary complications from inhalation of
blood and secretions into the air passages.

Temporary tube feeding is necessary after laryngectomy unless a gastrostomy has been
performed, as the swallowing movements have been impaired.

Surgical emphysema, cellulitis of the neck and lung infections are the most likely
complications. Preventive antibiotic treatment is usual after such operations.

The voice is not necessarily lost after removal of the vocal cords. In the immediate
post-operative phase great sympathy and tact is required in the management of these
patients, since they are unable to speak. As with oral cases a pencil and writing pad must

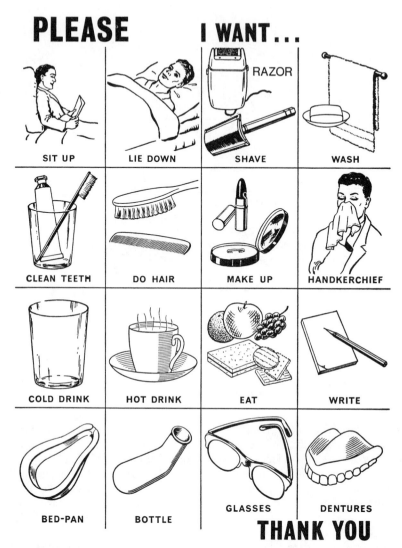

Fig. 43.15 Aid to communication for patient unable to speak, as for instance after laryngectomy, or patients with tracheostomy, or on ventilation with endotracheal tube. (Reproduced from *Word and Picture Chart* by permission of The Chest and Heart Association.)

always be at hand. Inability to communicate with the nursing staff in the immediate post-operative period can be alleviated by the use of a chart such as that devised by the Chest and Heart Association, one side of which is reproduced in Fig. 43.15. Speech therapy is required in the convalescent stage, and the patient learns to talk with the aid of oesophagus and pharyngeal muscle.

In advanced carcinoma of the larynx, excision of the adjoining pharynx and oesophagus may also be necessary. Either as a one-stage or two-stage procedure, repair is effected by swinging the transverse colon beneath the skin of the chest and joining it to the lower end of the pharynx as a replacement. A normal oesophagus cannot be mobilised and stretched as it has a very poor blood supply, and the only way of making good a deficiency is by using an intestinal graft (page 501).

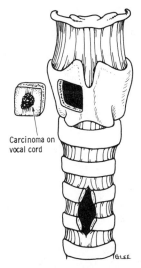

Carcinoma on
vocal cord

Fig. 43.16 Laryngo-fissure. A window is made into the side of the larynx through the thyroid cartilage: note temporary tracheostomy.

DISORDERS OF THE EAR

Pain and deafness are the principal symptoms of aural disease. In acute conditions, pain is outstanding and hearing is only slightly affected, whilst in chronic conditions, deafness is the main symptom. Discharge from the ear is the third important indication of disease.

The external ear

This consists of the **pinna** and the **external auditory meatus** which is just over 2·5 cm (one inch) long. The pinna consists of a sheet of cartilage covered on both sides by thin vascular skin. If the skin becomes separated from the cartilage by abscess or haematoma the cartilage may die since it derives its blood supply entirely from the attached skin. The **pinna** grows from a series of small lumps of tissue which join together: extra pieces containing cartilage are sometimes left in front of the ear, or dermoid cysts form at the points of fusion of the component elements (Fig. 43.17). These are harmless but are removed for cosmetic reasons. There may be a dimple marking the opening of a sinus or fistula which goes through to the meatus: this is often a site of infection (Fig. 43.18).

Congenital protuberance of the ear away from the sides of the head, **'bat ear'**, requires surgical treatment if the deformity is marked.

It is not necessary to shave a wide area around the pinna: the hair is kept out of the operation area by being smeared with soft paraffin: a surgifix or netalast or stockinette cap is fitted with slots for the ears.

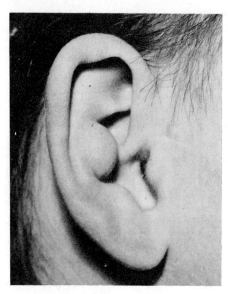

Fig. 43.17   Dermoid cyst of pinna: note dimple and small scar in front of meatus on site of removal of 'accessory pinna'.

The defect is in the cartilage ridge in the upper portion: this is restored by folding the cartilage with stitches inserted through an incision on the back of the pinna. Some skin is also removed and sometimes the cartilage is cut. A pressure bandage after carefully moulded packing in the pinna maintains pressure for 10 days after operation. The principal complication is a haematoma in the pinna. Skin stitches are removed at 10 days and the child continues to wear a bandage at night for a further 3 weeks.

Injury to the ear may produce a haematoma which must be opened: a compression bandage is applied to prevent it refilling. Lacerations of the ear occur accidentally, but if the injury is repaired without delay, healing is very satisfactory.

The external auditory meatus passes forwards towards the middle ear and is closed at the inner end by the **tympanic membrane** (ear drum). The lining skin produces **wax** which may accumulate, blocking the meatus completely. It has to be removed by means of a wax hook or, more commonly, by a jet of water from a syringe.

Infection of the skin occurs with pyogenic organisms (most commonly staphylococcus) or it may be excoriated as part of a more generalised skin disease such as seborrhoea or eczema. As the skin in the meatus is hair bearing, boils frequently develop (**furunculosis**).

These usually discharge spontaneously after several days' intense pain which is sometimes relieved by placing in the meatus a strip of ribbon gauze with magnesium sulphate paste to reduce the swelling.

In all forms of **otitis externa,**[1] the meatus requires regular cleaning and this is best achieved by the use of a wood or metal probe upon the end of which has been twisted a piece of special non-fluffing cotton wool. Care must be taken not to enter the probe far enough to produce pain, for fear of damaging the drum. The probe should always be held lightly so that if the patient moves his head the handle of the probe will slide through the nurse's fingers.

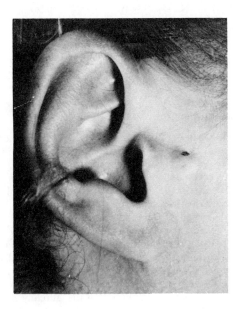

Fig. 43.18 Pre-auricular dermoid fistula.

Aural conditions are frequently treated by the instillation of 'drops'. In cases of eczema of the meatus, zinc cream or zinc paste is commonly applied. The meatus must never be plugged firmly; if required, a small piece of well-loosened wool should be placed very lightly in the outer part of the meatus only.

Various antiseptic solutions are used in the ear, including combinations of sulpha drugs and antibiotics. Spirit is frequently used to harden the skin of the meatus and dry up infection in the middle ear in cases of chronic otitis media.

Aural discharge is usually swabbed for bacteriological culture. When taking such a swab, care must be taken not to contaminate the swab also with any antiseptic solution which has been used in the ear.

[1] 'Otorrhoea' (running ear) may arise from otitis externa or otitis media.

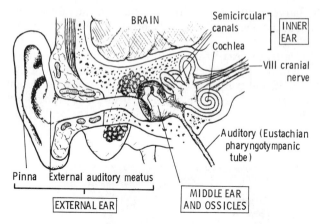

Fig. 43.19   The ear.

Aural syringing and the instillation of drops

A Higginson's syringe with a rubber nozzle may be used, drawing the water from a basin held by the patient or by an assistant, or placed on the table. Alternatively a metal ear syringe can be used, but care must be taken that this is working smoothly and that the piston has not been damaged by being dropped. Warm water should be used for the irrigation; cold water may produce giddiness and hot water will damage the drum. The temperature should not exceed 38 °C.

The patient should be seated with a towel over the shoulders and he should hold a kidney dish against the side of his cheek beneath the ear.

Whatever type of syringe is used, the operator must at all times hold the pinna firmly between the index and middle finger, using the thumb as a guard against the end of the syringe. This ensures that if the patient moves his head the nozzle will not be accidentally forced into the meatus. As the meatus passes forwards and inwards, when an attempt is being made to dislodge wax by means of syringing, the jet of water is directed towards the roof of the meatus and forwards (Fig. 43.20). The nozzle must be placed correctly so that the jet really enters the meatus and does not impinge on the pinna. The first 'jet' must be very gentle, as the element of surprise may make the patient jerk suddenly.

Considerable pressure is needed to dislodge pellets of wax, and after each syringeful has been injected, the meatus should be inspected and any visible pellet removed with forceps.

When it is thought that the meatus is clear, the drum is inspected with an auriscope, and the meatus dried with wool-covered probe or with a pledget of wool on angled aural forceps (Fig. 43.21).

The ear should never be syringed in the presence of a perforation of the drum. If there has been the slightest suspicion of otitis media, or any discharge of pus from the ear, the nurse must never undertake this procedure without medical advice.

Occasionally aural wax is so hard that it cannot be dislodged by syringing or by means of a wax hook, and it is softened by the instillation of olive oil drops for several days prior to syringing.

If drops are to be inserted, the patient must lie down with the affected ear uppermost and the nose pointing towards the pillow. Three or four drops of the necessary solution are placed directly into the meatus and a loose piece of wool placed over the opening. The patient must remain lying down for at least a minute in order that the solution may reach the drum.

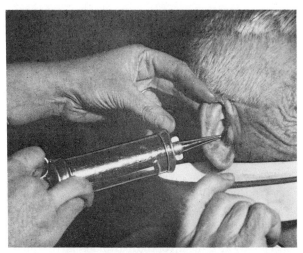

Fig. 43.20 Syringing the ear. The pinna is pulled upwards and backwards: the thumb and ring finger are used to steady the syringe, to prevent its accidental insertion, should the patient move.

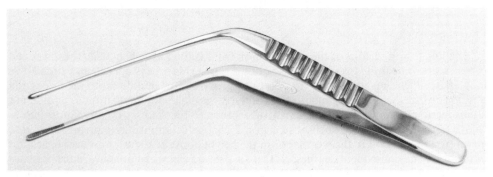

Fig. 43.21 Keene's aural forceps for use in cleaning the external auditory meatus and removing wool or debris.

Foreign bodies in the ear

Beads and other small particles are sometimes inserted into the ear by children, and insects occasionally enter the meatus. Foreign bodies are best removed by aural forceps under direct vision, but if this is not possible, the ear may be syringed. If an insect has entered the meatus and cannot be withdrawn, it is killed by the insertion of a few drops of cocaine, procaine or spirit, and then removed by syringing.

Patients sometimes force plugs of wool into the ear and forget to remove the entire piece. A foul plug of wool is then found as a cause of continued irritation and discharge.

The middle ear

The **drum** or **tympanum** is a cavity in the temporal bone. The **drum membrane** lies at the inner end of the meatus. The cavity communicates behind with the mastoid antrum and

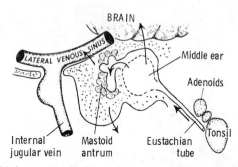

Fig. 43.22   The spread of infection in middle ear disease. The germs enter from the pharynx, producing acute otitis media. In the absence of effective treatment, the infection may spread upwards to the brain, backwards to produce mastoiditis and lateral sinus thrombosis. Infection may spread through the bone to form an abscess in the neck below the ear.

mastoid air cells which lead towards the tip of the mastoid bone behind the pinna. Immediately above the middle ear, separated only by a thin layer of bone, are the dura mater and brain.

Eustachian block

Leading from the floor of the middle ear in front is the **Eustachian tube,** the lower end of which opens near the tonsil at the back of the nose. This tube is opened and closed by a muscle. Its function is to allow air to pass to and fro from the middle ear to the throat and thus to equalise the pressure on both sides of the ear drum at different altitudes or different atmospheric pressures. The Eustachian tube becomes blocked by inflammation due to catarrh. In the presence of such obstruction a change of atmospheric pressure brought about by an alteration in the weather or in the height above sea-level, produces deflection of the drum and consequent deafness. If there is a severe change of pressure in the presence of a Eustachian block, the ear drum may burst. This condition is referred to as **barotrauma** and is one of the complications of air travel. By repeated swallowing or by chewing when climbing or descending in an aeroplane the Eustachian tube is opened frequently and the pressures become equalized. Eustachian catarrh frequently accompanies a common cold and persists in the presence of nasopharyngeal infection. In treatment, a Eustachian catheter is passed through the nose and guided into the Eustachian tube. Air is injected into the catheter and the Eustachian tube opened by force.

Otitis media

The Eustachian tube also acts as a channel for infection of the middle ear from the throat and consequently **otitis media** is a very common condition. It is usually produced by a streptococcal infection and in the acute stage the patient has intense earache and fever. The drum membrane becomes inflamed and oedematous. The majority of cases subside with ordinary anti-infective treatment including probably antibiotics. If pus forms in the middle ear, the drum membrane bulges and a tiny incision is made into it by the surgeon, through an aural speculum (**myringotomy**). General anaesthesia, probably nitrous oxide, is used. Following this procedure the meatus is swabbed daily and discharge will continue until the healing is complete. In many cases this is only for 2 or 3 days and there is no subsequent loss of hearing.

The infection is usually by a streptococcus which produces streptokinase, a fibrinolytic agent (page 60): the pus is thin and watery and escapes readily through a small perforation or drum incision. However, with the widespread use of antibiotics a troublesome complication sometimes arises known colloquially as **'glue ear'**. This occurs when the antibiotic treatment has been sufficient to limit the infection, but insufficient to eliminate it: the inflammatory exudate in the middle ear becomes extremely thick. The infection lingers on and the ossicles become glued together by this sticky secretion. Its presence is indicated by deafness. Although pain and temperature may have subsided myringotomy has to be performed and a special high-powered suction cannula used to draw out this exudate. In order to ensure complete drainage so that the ossicles can move freely a teflon **'grommet'** —a minute double-flanged button with a central hole—is placed in the drum as a temporary measure. When this is removed the drum heals. If a child is particularly susceptible to recurrent infections he may be given prolonged antibiotic chemotherapy in a maintenance dose for perhaps a month after the acute infection has subsided. 'Glue ear' may occur when there is no known history of infection and the cause is uncertain.

In all cases of otitis media, the temperature must be recorded 4-hourly and observation kept for the development of swelling or tenderness behind the ear as this indicates infection of the mastoid air cells.

Mastoid infection

If the spread of infection is not controlled by chemotherapy, pain and aural discharge persist, with increasing swelling behind the ear, and the patient develops **mastoiditis**. This is usually regarded as an acute surgical emergency. The patient is admitted to hospital and under general anaesthesia a curved incision is made behind the ear and the bone chiselled away to expose the mastoid air cells, remove dead bone and release the pus. This is the **Schwartze operation.**

Pre-operative preparation. Since the introduction of penicillin and sulpha drugs there is less urgency for operation and it is usual for the patient to be given antibiotic treatment for at least 24 hours before operation. The scalp must be shaved for an area 5 cm above the pinna and 5 cm behind the tip of the mastoid process. The hair at the edges of this shaved area should be smeared with soft paraffin (petroleum jelly). This fixes stray hairs and to some extent prevents blood contamination from the operation wound.

Post-operative care. The wound is usually drained with a strip of rubber. The auditory meatus is not plugged. A firm pad of wool behind and over the pinna is kept in place by means of a crepe bandage. Antibiotic treatment continues after operation and it is usually not necessary to re-dress the wound until the third or fourth day. The tube, and probably the stitches, are then removed. Any subsequent cavity is treated according to the surgeon's instructions either by irrigation, instillation of antibiotic solution, or by light packing with BIPP gauze.

The temperature should subside to normal within 48 hours of the operation. Any subsequent rise indicates insufficient drainage or a spread of infection.

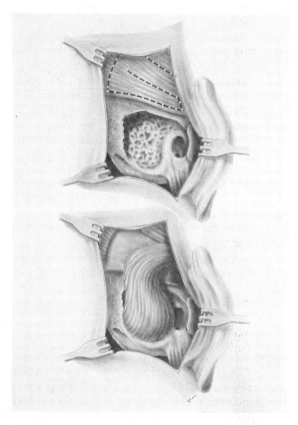

Fig. 43.23   Right radical mastoidectomy showing exposure of the bone and application of a muscle graft to fill the gap.

Complications of otitis media and mastoiditis. If infection of the middle ear spreads upwards it may produce **meningitis** or **brain abscess**. If the patient after operation complains of pain in the neck or intense headache, these symptoms must be reported, as they may be serious.

Sometimes the infection spreads beyond the mastoid air cells into the lateral venous sinus on the inner aspect of the skull. Thrombosis occurs here (**lateral sinus thrombosis**) and septic emboli may travel down the jugular vein producing **septicaemia**. The development of rigors is an indication that this process is occurring but it is a very infrequent complication of otitis media since the introduction of sulpha drugs.

Drainage of the middle ear may be insufficient and persistent infection of middle ear or bone may be kept going by continuous re-infection from the pharynx in the presence of infected tonsils and adenoids. As the result of the bone infection, pieces of bone may die and the infection becomes chronic. Sometimes acute otitis media is a very short-lived condition which may not be diagnosed and the patient, usually a child, is brought for treatment first on account of a chronic discharge from the ear. **Chronic suppurative otitis media** (CSOM) is an extremely common condition, particularly in areas of dense population and low resistance to infection.

Chronic suppurative otitis media. In the treatment of this condition the external meatus is mopped out daily and drops instilled. If healing does not take place it may be necessary to remove tonsils and adenoids or to operate to secure better drainage of the middle ear. Sometimes infected bone in the mastoid area has to be removed by the operation of **radical mastoidectomy**. A muscle graft may be used to fill the hole left by bone removal (Fig. 43.23). The pre- and post-operative treatment is similar to that for the Schwartze operation. Occasionally skin grafts are used and in such cases the initial post-operative dressing will be undertaken by the surgeon.

The inner ear

The inner ear has two main functions. It is embedded in the dense part of the temporal bone on the inner side of the middle ear. The **semicircular canals** are so arranged that no matter in what direction the head is moved, the fluid in one of these canals travels from end to end setting up currents which stimulate the vestibular part of the eighth cranial nerve. By this means the brain is able to maintain a constant record of the position of the head. Further information about position is received from the eyes and the two receiving stations are very closely related in the special brain centres. Disease of the inner ear, by alterations in the semicircular canals (**vestibule**), may produce **nystagmus** (jerky, swinging movements of the eyes).

The second function of the inner ear is the detection of sound by means of the **cochlea**. This consists of millions of tiny fibrils which vibrate in harmony with sounds of different rates·of vibration (frequency). Certain forms of deafness are simply due to disease of small portions of the cochlea. This cuts down the range of frequency which the patient can perceive. Thus a person may suffer from 'high tone deafness'. The volume of sound (loudness) is not the only factor in hearing. In the examination of a person who is suffering from deafness, appliances are used to determine the range of pitch which he can perceive at different intensities of volume. The simple methods used in this assessment include the tuning fork, a loudly ticking watch, the whispered sounds of different types such as low-pitched words like 'Birmingham' and high-pitched words like 'pip squeak'. The nurse working in a special department may be called upon to perform certain routine hearing tests carried out with standard apparatus.

Thus, in addition to disease of the middle ear which subsequently affects the inner ear, deafness may be due to a primary defect of the auditory nerve.

Surgery of deafness

Middle-ear disease produces deafness without involving the inner ear, by damping down the vibrations of the ossicles (malleus, incus and stapes) which transmit the vibrations from the drum membrane across the middle ear to the cochlea. Injury or infection of the drum membrane has a similar effect. In 'middle ear deafness' the patient's hearing is better if the sound is transmitted through the mastoid bone than if it is transmitted through the air in the auditory meatus. The vibration of the mastoid bone is conveyed direct to the inner ear. Bone conduction is tested by placing the tuning fork on the mastoid bone and opposite the meatus, comparing the intensity of sound in the two positions.

There have been great advances in the surgical treatment of deafness. Conditions of the middle ear arising from injury, infection or a constitutional disease of the bone interfere with the conduction of vibrations from the tympanic membrane to the oval window of the cochlea, a tiny opening closed by the foot of the stapes (Fig. 43.24). The tympanic

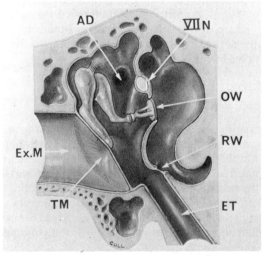

Fig. 43.24   The ear: a vertical section across the plane of the skull. **Ex.M**—external meatus. **TM**—tympanic membrane. **AD**—aditus, the opening into the mastoid antrum from the middle ear. **VII N**—the facial nerve. **OW**—oval window to which the stapes bone is attached. **RW**—round window connected also with the cochlea; these windows together act as a microphone picking up the sound vibrations. **ET**—Eustachian tube opening into the naso-pharynx.

membrane may be destroyed by infection; the ossicles themselves may be diseased and immobile and in otosclerosis the foot of the stapes becomes 'arthritic' and ceases to vibrate. The transmission of sound vibrations depends on the integrity of the tympanic membrane and chain of ossicles causing vibration of the fluid within the cochlea at the oval window. These vibrations can only be transmitted properly through the cochlea if there is a second 'round' window which is not subjected to the same external vibrations. The air space in the middle ear is essential therefore for hearing and this is kept at the correct pressure by the repeated opening of the Eustachian tube. If the tube becomes blocked fluid accumulates in the middle ear and the effect of the sound vibrations transmitted by the ossicles is lost.

Surgery therefore is designed to ensure adequate transmission of sound vibrations to the oval window and the provision of adequate protection of the round window. These operations in the middle ear are performed through an operating microscope.

Figure 43.25 indicates some common causes of middle-ear deafness. Otosclerosis is treated by excision of the stapes and is replaced by a small plastic prosthesis. Eustachian block is treated by attention to naso-pharyngeal sepsis. See Fig. 43.24 for detailed anatomy.

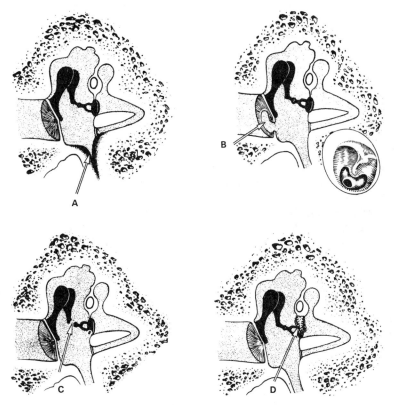

Fig. 43.25 Causes of deafness. **A.** Middle ear deafness due to Eustachian catarrh blocking the tube and preventing correction of air pressure. **B.** Perforation of ear drum by sepsis (inset as seen through auriscope). **C.** Break of continuity of 'ossicles' by sepsis or injury. **D.** Otosclerosis in which the stapes is fixed and cannot vibrate effectively.

Vertigo (giddiness)

Ear disease is sometimes accompanied by giddiness from interference with the vestibular apparatus and in such cases the **caloric test** may give valuable information. Menière's disease is one such condition where the patient suffers from severe attacks of giddiness, vomiting and headache.

The prolonged use of streptomycin for tuberculosis sometimes poisons the eighth nerve, producing deafness and blocking the pathways from the vestibular apparatus. This unfortunate side-effect of treatment has, however, been used in the treatment of Menière's disease to damp down the effects of the abnormal action in the vestibule.

Caloric test. The function of the vestibular apparatus (semicircular canals) may be tested by this means. Everyone is familiar with the fact that cold water is heavier than hot, and if a vessel containing water is warmed, the water circulates by the constant rising of the hot water. In this test, with the patient lying down, the ear is syringed with water above or below the normal body temperature. (Warning has already been given in the instructions for ear syringing that cold water should not be used because it produces giddiness.) As the warmth or cold is transmitted from the middle ear to the semicircular canals the endolymph fluid within these canals circulates, setting up the same nerve impulses as if the patient were spinning in space. This has the effect of making the eyes flicker (nystagmus) if the normal nerve pathways are intact. If the drum is perforated a jet of cooled or warmed air is used instead of water.

Earache

There are many causes of earache. In addition to that from otitis externa or otitis media, pain may arise from the temporomandibular joint following strain or loss of balance in biting. It may also be referred from the molar teeth in the upper or lower jaw or from the tongue in carcinoma. The skin of the pinna derives some of its sensory nerve supply from nerves which arise from the middle of the neck. Malignant glands in the neck may thus also produce severe pain in the ear.

44

Surgery of the Eye

Ophthalmology is the study of disease of the eye. From the nursing point of view the subject falls into two main sections, medical and surgical. Vision is affected in medical disease either from interference with the structure of the eye or by interruption of the visual nerve pathways and of the visual centres in the brain. Such conditions require no special treatment as far as the eye is concerned, but the ophthalmic department is involved in the assessment of visual defect and the treatment of secondary effects on the eyes.

This chapter is concerned with the surgical aspect of eye disease and with the diagnostic procedures which comprise a great deal of the eye department's routine work.

In the organisation of ophthalmology, there are two classes of doctors. **The ophthalmic surgeon** with special qualifications has been trained as a surgeon and has specialised in operative surgery of the eye. He is also an expert in the diagnosis and management of the medical lesions of the eye. The second type of doctor has little or no operating experience and is concerned mainly with diagnostic work, and special eye examinations for the prescription of spectacles (refraction). He is sometimes referred to as a 'refractionist' or ophthalmic optician.

An **optician** is one who supplies spectacles and may in fact prescribe the necessary corrective lenses without previous examination by a qualified doctor.[1]

Orthoptic treatment is an ancillary service which provides for special exercises and training of the eye muscles in cases of squint, particularly in children. This treatment is given by a specially trained technician (**orthoptist**).

Organisation

Many of the operations carried out on the eye and surrounding structures are of a relatively minor nature, although they call for a high degree of technical skill. A very large out-patient department is necessary, though there may be only a few in-patient beds.

In the out-patient department, the work falls into two categories, diagnostic and therapeutic. The nurse may be called upon to help with the diagnostic work by carrying out simple tests for visual acuity and helping the ophthalmic surgeon with other examinations. In therapeutic procedures, irrigation of the eye, instillation of drops and the application

---

[1] 'Oculist' is used loosely and incorrectly to denote either a refractionist (doctor) or an optician.

of ointment are routine treatments undertaken by the nurse. Preparations for and assistance at minor operations such as the removal of foreign bodies is a further part of her routine duty.

In distinction from other departments of surgery, the eye ward is usually arranged so as to have a fully equipped treatment room or operating theatre attached, where post-operative dressings and routine daily treatment can be performed under ideal aseptic conditions with adequate illumination. The sister in charge of the eye ward is then also the theatre sister and assists with the major operations so that she is completely conversant with the details of pre- and post-operative care.

Anatomy and physiology

Ophthalmology is concerned with:

(a) the eyeball (globe),
(b) the muscles in the orbit attached to the eyeball and responsible for its movements, and the other orbital contents,
(c) the eyelids and conjunctiva,
(d) the naso-lacrimal apparatus which manufactures and transports the tear fluid from the lacrimal gland to the nose.

The eye ball. This is a 'cyst' with a fibrous capsule (Fig. 44.1). The translucent aperture at the front is the **cornea** which is very easily damaged by abrasion or by drying, particularly if it is insensitive from local or general anaesthesia. It is kept moist by the lacrimal fluid,

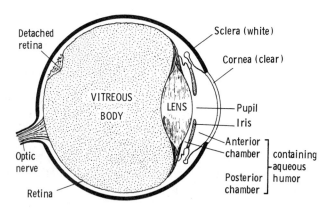

Fig. 44.1 The anatomy of the eye. Retinal detachment may be produced by haemorrhage from injury or hypertension.

and if it is exposed to the air without the constant movement of the lids **corneal ulceration** occurs. Healing of the cornea may leave a scar which interferes with the transmission of light. Similarly the cornea may be scarred by inflammation (**keratitis**). The amount of light which passes to the back of the eye is regulated by the coloured **iris** which is a disc of muscle in the centre of which is a hole, the **pupil**. The size of the pupil is varied by movements of the muscular iris. Immediately behind the iris is the **lens**, slung from an elastic ligament which tends to keep the lens capsule tight, thus flattening it and focusing it for long distance vision. This ligament can be stretched by the ciliary muscle which relaxes the lens capsule, allowing it to become more spherical and to bring in focus objects nearer the eye. This ability of the eye to vary the shape and focus of the lens is '**accommodation**'. When the eye accommodates, it also varies the amount of light passing through the lens by a corresponding alteration in the size of the pupil. In bright lights, the pupil is also constricted to reduce dazzle, whereas in the dark the pupil dilates. The pupil is therefore said to 'react to light and accommodation' in normal individuals. When the reaction to light or accommodation is diminished or absent it is an indication that there is partial or complete blindness or disease of the nerve which works these muscles. Reactions of the pupil are important in the observation of patients with head injury (page 857).

Lining the back part of the eyeball is the sensitive **retina** which receives the light rays and converts the impression into nerve impulses transmitted to the brain through the **optic nerve**.

By means of an ophthalmoscope placed immediately in front of the eye all these structures can be inspected in detail, including the retina or **fundus.**

The cavity between the front of the lens and the cornea is filled with a fluid, **aqueous humor**. This circulates freely through the pupil and escapes from the anterior chamber of the eye (in front of the iris) through a minute canal at the outer edge of the iris (Fig. 44.2A). In certain diseases this channel becomes blocked and the **intra-ocular pressure** rises in the anterior chamber due to accumulation of the aqueous humor. This condition is **glaucoma**. As the result of inflammation, the iris may become adherent to the front of the lens (**posterior synechia**) so that it cannot contract and relax adequately and the communication between the anterior and posterior chambers in front of the eye becomes obstructed. The iris may become adherent to the cornea (**anterior synechia**) (Fig. 44.3).

If the iris muscle is relaxed so that the pupil enlarges, the bulk of the muscle obstructs the canal of Schlemm (Fig. 44.2B) and may precipitate an attack of glaucoma with subsequent blindness. This effect may be produced by atropine given as a pre-operative drug in the course of treatment in other surgical conditions or put in the eye as drops in order to dilate the pupil for adequate ophthalmological examination. A drug with the reverse effect, eserine or pilocarpine, is used to contract the pupil in the treatment of some types of glaucoma.

Owing to the normal intra-ocular pressure from the secretion of aqueous humor, any perforation of the eye, whether by accident or during surgical operation, leads to escape of the fluid and in cases of accidents to collapse of the eyeball, which is thus destroyed.

It is very difficult to immobilise the eye in disease and therefore almost impossible to achieve the first great principle of treatment, rest. The eye is covered to minimise the movements of the globe which accompany vision. This also eliminates the entry of light which can cause pain if the eye is inflamed. Further rest is obtained by paralysing the intra-ocular muscles by the use of a **cycloplegic** drug (e.g. atropine), which paralyses the ciliary muscle and sphincter pupillae.

Ocular muscles and orbit. The eyeball is held in the orbit by a group of flat muscles attached to the back of the bony wall. By synchronised action of these muscles, the two eyes are moved together to follow a moving object, to alter the field of vision or to converge in order to inspect close objects. Any imbalance of the action of muscles in the two eyes results in inco-ordinated movement, and produces double vision (**diplopia**). Most

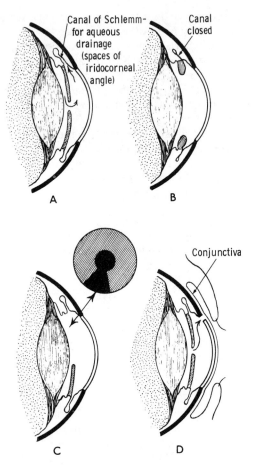

Fig. 44.2   Section through front part of the eye. **A**. The aqueous humor circulates through the iris and into the canal of Schlemm. **B**. Full dilatation of the pupil (produced by atropine) allows the canal to be blocked by the retracted iris. The sphincter pupillae muscle is paralysed. **C**. Iridectomy performed in the relief of glaucoma. **D**. The trephine operation which permits the aqueous humor to percolate beneath the conjunctiva.

commonly, an error in the focusing and lens system (**refractive error, astigmatism**) leads to an excessive strain on these muscles, and a squint (**strabismus**) occurs. The affected eye may diverge (swing outward) or converge (swing inward). Squint arises usually in childhood and may be precipitated by some unconnected severe illness or strain. It may occur from paralysis of the eye muscles (ophthalmoplegia) by damage to their special nerves (cranial nerves III, IV and VI) in skull fractures or paralytic diseases such as poliomyelitis.

If diplopia occurs, the brain for convenience suppresses the image from one eye. After several months of severe squinting, a child may develop **amblyopia**, that is blindness in one eye as a result of this suppression. In the initial treatment of squint the good eye is covered with an Elastoplast patch, an eyeshade, or dark spectacle lens to force the bad eye back into normal activity and restore the brain function in respect of its images, by eliminating confusion from visual impressions in the normal eye.

Refractive errors are corrected by spectacles and orthoptic exercises are used to attempt to build up co-ordinated ocular muscle tone and movement. In severe cases, operation is required. Individual muscles are detached from the globe and re-attached further forward or further back to change their range of action (**advancement** or **recession** operation).

The globe is surrounded by fat, which becomes infected (**orbital cellulitis**) from ethmoid sinusitis or by the spread of infection from the face. The eye protrudes and the conjunctiva becomes oedematous (**chemosis**). The swelling of the conjunctiva may be so great that the lids cannot close.

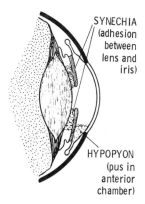

SYNECHIA (adhesion between lens and iris)

HYPOPYON (pus in anterior chamber)

Fig. 44.3   Infection producing iritis leads to adhesion formation.

Thrombosis of the plexus of veins behind the eye produces similar chemosis.

Frontal and ethmoid sinus lesions may protrude into the orbit and push the eye forward (**exophthalmos**). In thyrotoxicosis the similar protrusion is due partly to increased muscle tone and partly to excessive orbital fat. The protrusion may be so great as to prevent co-ordinated movements of the eyes: the exposure and inadequate lubrication by the eyelids leads to corneal ulceration. After surgery for thyrotoxicosis the eye condition usually improves (page 772) but may be exacerbated due to pituitary overaction when the excessive thyroxin is withdrawn.

Primary and secondary malignant growths may occur in the orbit and produce exophthalmos.

Eyelids and conjunctiva. The upper and lower lids each have a stiffening plate of cartilage (**tarsal plate**) covered on the outside by thin loose skin, and on the inside by firmly attached conjunctiva. The lashes are set in special hair follicles, which may become infected, and develop a boil or stye (**hordeolum**). In the tarsal plates the lids are special tarsal glands (Meibomian) which may be infected or may develop cysts. Sometimes a lash grows inwards and sets up irritation, necessitating its removal. Inflammation of the lids is **blepharitis**, frequently associated with **conjunctivitis**.

The lids are closed by a circular muscle surrounding the orbit in front, **orbicularis oculi muscle,** under control of the facial nerve.

Ptosis is the drooping of an upper eyelid, and may be congenital or due to paralysis of the lid-elevating muscle. This muscle (levator palpebrae) may be shortened by operation, if ptosis is severe.

The conjunctiva covers the globe in front as far as the edge of the cornea as well as lining the lids. It is translucent and very vascular. This pocket between the globe and the lids is the **conjunctival sac,** with an upper and lower **fornix**.

Any operation on the eye necessitates an incision through the conjunctiva, which swells rapidly from irritation by infection or injury. It heals easily. The cornea is covered by a specially thin and firmly attached epithelium in continuity with the surrounding conjunctiva.

Naso-lacrimal apparatus.[1] The lacrimal fluid is formed in a gland which is like those producing saliva, at the outer margin of the orbit above the globe. This antiseptic fluid lubricates the cornea and protects it from ulceration which may occur if the cornea becomes dry. The lacrimal fluid normally enters two tiny ducts at the medial end of the conjunctival sac (Fig. 44.4). Below this point, on the inner wall of the orbit is the **lacrimal sac**, with a communication into the nose by the **naso-lacrimal duct.**

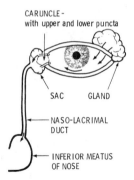

CARUNCLE –
with upper and lower puncta

SAC   GLAND

NASO-LACRIMAL
DUCT

INFERIOR MEATUS
OF NOSE

Fig. 44.4   The course of the lacrimal fluid. (Compare with Fig. 43.2). The ducts sometimes require probing.

The duct system may be blocked from congenital disease, inflammation or injury, and an operation may be performed (dacryocystorhinostomy)[1] to restore the normal channel and so prevent the constant trickle of tears.

Special **lacrimal probes** (Bowman) are used to unblock the duct, and specially designed syringes are used for irrigation of the sac.

In Sjögren's syndrome the lacrimal and salivary glands dry-up. Corneal irritation and ulceration can be alleviated by the use of methyl cellulose (1 per cent) drops as a lubricant and this substance is a constituent of many other eye drops.

[1] *Lacrimal* is derived from *lacrima*, a tear (Latin). A corrupt mediaeval spelling was *lachryma*, from which have arisen the alternative spellings *lachrymal* and *lacrymal*. The Greek *dakruon* (δακρυον), a tear, gives the term *dacryocystorhinostomy*.

Table 59 Operations on the eye

Site	Lesion	Description	Treatment
EYEBALL Retina	Elevation of part from its base by injury or haemorrhage	Retinal detachment	Operation for **retinal re-attachment** by diathermy or cryotherapy silicone 'plomb' or strap
	Neoplasm	Glioma Retinoblastoma	**Enucleation** of eyeball: irradiation
Lens	Opacity [congenital: in diabetes: 'senile' following injury (traumatic)]	Cataract	**Cataract extraction or discission** Removal of opaque lens in suitable cases (A specially powerful spectacle lens is used to restore vision.)
Iris	Iritis	Inflammation and adhesion (synechia)	**Iridodialysis.** Division of synechia
Anterior chamber	Blockage to circulation of aqueous humor	Glaucoma (acute or chronic)	**Iridectomy** (excision of part of iris) **Trephining** (artificial fistula from anterior chamber through sclera to subconjunctival space) Cyclodialysis
Cornea	Inflammation (sometimes syphilitic)	Keratitis	Medical: **corneal grafting**
	Ulceration (exposure, injury, infection)	Corneal ulcer	Medical: cauterisation; **grafting**
	Foreign body	Impaction of foreign body	Removal
OCULAR MUSCLES	Squint	Strabismus	**Advancement** and **recession** of muscle attachments
EYELIDS AND CONJUNCTIVA	Infection (stye)	Hordeolum	Hot bathing: sometimes puncture
	Meibomian cyst		Incision and curettage
	Meibomian abscess		Puncture
	Ptosis	Drooping of lid	Muscle shortening
	Paralysis of orbicularis oculi or exophthalmos	Suture of lids together, to protect insensitive cornea from ulceration (e.g. after operation or after trigeminal nerve block)	**Tarsorrhaphy**
	Infection	Conjunctivitis Blepharitis	Irrigation: instillation: protection from injury and ulceration
NASO-LACRIMAL APPARATUS	Blockage to ducts or sac		Probing: **dacryocystorhinostomy**

(Operative treatment is shown in bold type)

Common disorders of the eye

In relation to diagnosis and treatment it is convenient to describe pathological conditions of the eye under the categories described in the foregoing section.

Table 59 indicates the principal disorders set out in this way with the main features of treatment.

Ophthalmic conditions may also be described in relation to the causes and age groups in which they occur.

Congenital disorders

If a woman contracts rubella (German measles) during the early months of pregnancy at a stage when the eye and heart are developing very rapidly in the embryo, either or both of these structures may be severely and permanently damaged. The baby is born blind, or may have congenital heart disease, or both. There is no preventive treatment. Other congenital disorders are a form of cataract, errors of refraction, squints and forms of visual defect associated with structural abnormalities in the eyeball. At birth the baby may contract infection from the maternal birth canal, such as gonococcal conjunctivitis (**ophthalmia neonatorum**); because of the seriousness of this condition, in many centres, antiseptic drops are instilled into every baby's eyes immediately after birth. Congenital syphilis affects the eye, producing keratitis and other lesions. There are familial disorders which also affect the eye and produce, in addition, changes in the central nervous system further impairing vision. **Retinoblastoma** (Fig. 44.5) may be present at birth.

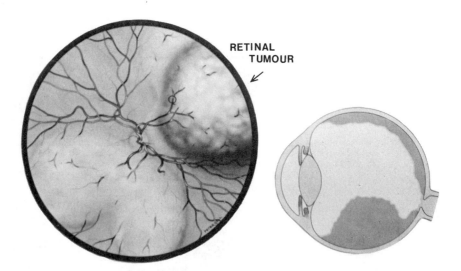

RETINAL
TUMOUR

Fig. 44.5 Tumour of retina. (*Left*) Ophthalmoscopic appearance: the vessels radiate from the optic 'disc': the bulge on the right is a retinoblastoma. (*Right*) Diagram shows how the retina is raised and vision grossly disturbed: radioactive 'seeds' or plaques can be attached to the outside of the eyeball over the tumour.

Retrolental fibroplasia is a condition of blindness arising at or soon after birth, especially in premature babies. It is thought that the use of very high concentrations of oxygen in the incubators in which premature babies are kept, may be a cause of this condition.

Infection

Almost any organism can infect the eye. Resistance to infection is low if the structures of the globe are involved and infection may spread through the optic nerve to the opposite eye.

Conjunctivitis may arise from direct infection from the air, contamination from fingers, or from surrounding infected tissue.

Conjunctivitis (inflammation as distinct from infection) may arise from the presence of foreign body, allergy or injury: the irritation leads to rubbing of the eye by the patient, and secondary infection supervenes.

Keratitis (cornea), iritis, cyclitis (ciliary body) and retinitis may occur individually due to specific infections, or together as a total infection of the eyeball (**ophthalmia**).

Inflammation can lead to a rise of intra-ocular pressure, **glaucoma**, which in turn produces blindness and even loss of the eye. The chain of events can be very rapid and eye treatment is therefore urgently needed in all acute cases.

Infection with the organism *Pseudomonas pyocyanea* (producing a green discharge) is very dangerous and can be made more intense by penicillin. Culture of organisms from the conjunctiva is very important. A swab must be taken *before* antiseptic or antibiotic drops are used.

Trauma

The most common injury is the entry of a foreign body. Particles of dust enter the conjunctival sac and may be rapidly washed away by the flow of lacrimal fluid which is increased by the irritation. If a foreign body cannot be located, the eye should be covered lightly to prevent injury and handling, until skilled assistance is available. Sharp foreign bodies such as glass and metal splinters from grinding machines may be impacted in the cornea. Removal is urgent; it is performed under local anaesthesia, using a Bowman's needle which is a very tiny spade for lifting the particle with minimum damage to the cornea. Normally the resulting ulcer heals in a few days. Irritant dust such as lime or cement is washed out by irrigation, and **sodium calcium edetate** (EDTA) 0·4 per cent is used as a specific solvent for lime.

Irritation from allergy (hay fever) may lead to rubbing which aggravates the inflammation by self-inflicted injury. The local condition can be relieved harmlessly by instillation of Antistine-Privine or weak steroid solution, or if not available adrenalin solution 2 drops (1 : 1000).

Penetrating injuries of the globe require immediate surgical attention. From a blow on the eye, haemorrhage may occur within the globe or the retina may be detached in part, leading to distortion or loss of vision. The iris may prolapse through the cornea.

Metallic foreign bodies are sometimes extracted with the aid of a very powerful magnet.

Infection readily gains entry after injury and when a foreign body has been removed from the conjunctiva; antiseptic drops (chloramphenicol, neomycin or framycetin) are instilled as a routine, or ointment applied in the conjunctival sac.

After injury special watch must always be kept on the opposite eye for the development of iritis (**sympathetic ophthalmia**) which may occur at any time, even 20 years later. Appearance of this is an indication for removal of the damaged eye and intensive treatment of the 'good' eye with local steroids and atropine. Sympathetic ophthalmia is a blinding condition requiring constant vigilance on the part of nurse and doctor alike.

The so-called 'black eye' is due to haemorrhage in the loose tissues of the eyelids. Following a direct blow, compression of the orbital contents may burst the thin bony wall, usually down into the antrum, producing a 'blow-out' fracture. The patient will have double vision due to the eye muscles being trapped in the fracture (page 787).

Neoplasm

Growths occur in the globe, especially from the nerve tissue (**glioma**). **Retinoblastoma** arising from the retina is hereditary and often affects both eyes. Secondary (metastatic) deposits from malignant disease elsewhere arise in the orbit and compress the globe. Primary growth in the maxilla or parotid gland may invade the eye by direct spread. Rodent ulcer and epithelioma of the face also sometimes encroach on the orbit. Malignant disease in the eye is treated by radiotherapy or excision of the eye. Light coagulation is sometimes used for small tumours at the posterior pole.

Radiotherapy is rarely used to treat disease near the eye as the rays may damage the eye, leading to the production of cataract years later. If the eye is already involved in growth, the risk of cataract is irrelevant.

Metabolic disorders

The eye is frequently involved in diseases affecting metabolism. Diabetes leads to cataract and to retinal changes (**diabetic retinopathy**) and may cause blindness. Retinopathy is treated by photocoagulation (Fig. 44.6 and page 845) and sometimes by the removal of the pituitary gland (hypophysectomy). Deficiency of vitamin A produces blindness. Other nutritional disorders affect the eye. Thyrotoxicosis produces exophthalmos and ophthalmoplegia.

Degeneration

Cataract occurs in old age owing to degenerative changes in the lens. Optic nerve atrophy may occur from various causes, including infection. Hypertension, nephritis, and arterial disease lead to changes in the retina which may produce blindness. Ophthalmoscopic examination of the fundus reveals these conditions.

Diagnostic procedures

Full ophthalmic examination requires the use of special apparatus and some of the routine procedures may be carried out by the nurse.

Visual acuity. This is a measure of accuracy of vision, theoretically, at different distances, but the examination is standardised to use one distance only (6 metres) by means of Snellen test types. The test card bears letters of different sizes to correspond in appearance

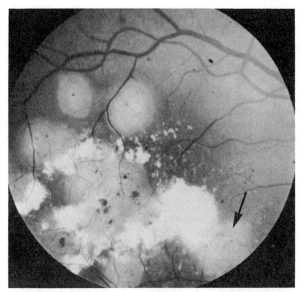

Fig. 44.6 From a colour photograph of the right retina 24 hours after light coagulation of the abnormal vascular patches and exudate in a patient with diabetic retinopathy. (From Keen and Jarrett, 1975, *Complications of Diabetes*. Arnold, London.)

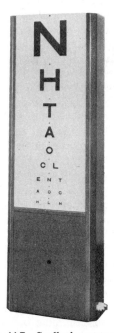

Fig. 44.7 Snellen's test types.

to the largest letter as it would appear at varying distances up to 60 metres. Several cards are used with a different arrangement of letters so that the patient cannot memorise the different lines. Fig. 44.6 shows a sample card. With normal vision the lowest line but one (6/6) should be visible clearly at 6 metres. If the examination room is less than 6 metres in length a mirror system may be used to give the same effect.

The patient stands or sits (according to the height of the type) 6 metres from the test type which has even illumination. His left eye is covered with a card and he reads the letters from above downwards. The lowest line which he can read clearly and accurately, using distance spectacles if he wears these normally, is recorded as his VAR (Visual acuity, right). This procedure is repeated with the other eye. If he is unable to read any letters his VA is less than 6/60 and is recorded as 'counting fingers' (CF) or 'hand movements' (HM) at whatever distance this can be appreciated. In refraction examination by the doctor or optician, this procedure is repeated using different lenses in the spectacle test frame.

Visual field. By means of the **perimeter** a plan is made indicating the width of visual field in each eye. There are sometimes defects in the visual field from lesions of the retina or nerve pathways. Any blind area is a **scotoma.**

Ophthalmoscopy. The examination of the fundus of the eye is part of the normal clinical examination of all patients. If no ophthalmic disease is suspected, the examination is carried out by the patient's medical officer without any previous special treatment of the eye. If the findings are in doubt or there is any reason to suppose that retinal disease is present, the pupil is dilated by paralysing the iris muscle with homatropine or cyclopentolate drops. In children this is achieved by instillation of atropine drops for the two days preceding the examination. Atropine also paralyses the ciliary muscles which work the lens, so that the patient is unable to accommodate for near vision. This is of particular value in children as the refractive power of the lens can be determined accurately by avoiding any action on the part of the child's muscles. No patient who has had atropine or homatropine in the eye should be allowed to drive a motor vehicle and warning must be given that care is needed in using stairs owing to paralysis of the focusing mechanism. Full recovery after atropine does not occur for several days.

Examination of conjunctival sac. If a foreign body has entered the 'eye'—i.e. is in the conjunctival sac—a search is made by holding the upper eyelid away from the globe and asking the patient to look in those directions at the limits of his eye movements. Very commonly a particle lodges in the deep surface of the upper lid and in this examination the lid is everted. In order to achieve this the lashes are held while a probe or match is placed lengthwise against the upper edge of the tarsal plate on the outer surface of the lid. When the lid is flicked over, it will remain everted while the inspection is carried out.

The lower fornix of the conjunctival sac is examined by pressing the lid with the tip of the finger immediately beneath it.

A drop of **fluorescin stain** is put in the lower fornix and the patient told to blink. The dye makes any abrasion or ulcer of the cornea clearly visible.

Refraction. This may be determined in one of two ways. A surgeon may use a special mirror with a central hole. He examines the fundus from a distance by reflected light, interposing lenses of different strengths. Alternatively, the refraction might be determined by using Snellen test types with various combinations of the lens before each eye.

Special examination of minute structures. The cornea and other parts of the eye may be further examined with a special hand lens (**loupe**) or a type of microscope built for this particular purpose (**slit-lamp**).

Symptoms

Pain arising from inflammatory lesions in the globe is intense, continuous, and accentuated by light. It is due partly to a rise of intra-ocular pressure, as in glaucoma. Pain may be 'felt' in the eye when referred from disease elsewhere, through the trigeminal nerve (trigeminal neuralgia). Frontal, maxillary or ethmoidal sinusitis, or dental infection may produce pain referred to the eye. The pain of conjunctivitis is an intense 'soreness' or 'grittiness' accompanied by restlessness and inability to keep the eye still. It is aggravated by exposure to draught or light. 'Watering' of the eye is a most troublesome symptom.

The cornea is normally extremely sensitive and ulceration from infection or injury can cause great pain. Sometimes, however, the cornea is insensitive and it then becomes ulcerated or injured because the protective reflex movement of the lids is lost and the patient is unaware of the injury. Pain from corneal or conjunctival lesions can be alleviated by local analgesic solutions.

Headache is a common symptom of eye disease, usually from a refractive error.

Visual disturbances. Diplopia (double vision) may be continuous or intermittent. The patient may not mention the symptom if it is intermittent but the occurrence of diplopia must always be reported as it may be the first symptom of serious neurological disease.

Defects of vision such as blurring, short-sight (**myopia**) or long-sight (**hypermetropia**) are common complaints, and occasionally more specific defects such as **hemianopia** (ability to see to one side only) are noticed.

Transient **amblyopia** (blindness) or the appearance of images such as bright lights or patterns of light occur in migraine.

The presence of **colour blindness** in varying degrees is frequently unknown to the patient until it is detected by some routine examination such as that required for military service. **Word blindness** is a peculiar form of defect in the brain centres: the visual pathway is intact.

Watering of the eyes may occur in conjunctivitis or from blocking of the naso-lacrimal duct. **Squint** is noticed by parents in their children, but is rarely observed by the patient. **Exophthalmos** similarly is usually first noticed by the patient's relatives.

Drugs

Apart from the use of antibiotics, the relief of pain and other general medical treatments, certain drugs are used specifically in ophthalmic work, in the form of 'drops' (**guttae**) for instillation into the conjunctival sac. The drop diffuses through the conjunctiva and cornea into the anterior chamber and thus reaches the inside of the globe. 'Drops' are washed away rapidly by lacrimal fluid and drugs are used in special ointment for more prolonged effect. The choice of antibiotic is influenced by its ability to diffuse into the eye. Drops should be instilled 2–3 hourly and ointment 6–8 hourly. A tiny soluble disk of drug (**lamella**) is sometimes placed in the conjunctival sac where it dissolves slowly and releases the drug in constant concentration.

Drops (guttae pro oculis). Many drugs are used for instillation in the eye and they are grouped according to the purpose of use.

    (a) **Antiseptic and antibacterial**
        Neomycin 0·5%
        Soframycin (framycetin) 0·5%
        Chloramphenicol 0·5%
        Sulphacetamide 10%
    (b) **Anaesthetic** to relieve pain following an abrasion or to produce complete anaesthesia of the eye for operation.
        Amethocaine (Anethaine) 1% or 2%
        Cocaine 2%
        Note. Procaine is *not* used in the eye.
    (c) **For dilating the pupil (mydriatic, cycloplegic)**
        Atropine sulphate 1%   Phenylephrine 1:10,000
        Homatropine 2%   Cyclopentolate 0·5% (short action, reversible with pilocarpine)
        The effect of homatropine is shorter than that of atropine: there is consequently less visual defect after its use.
    (d) **To constrict the pupil**
        Eserine (physostigmine) 0·5% or 1%
        Pilocarpine 1%, 2%, 4%
        Adrenaline drops 1/1000 or 1/100 (the only purpose for which adrenaline of this concentration is used in the whole of surgery) to prevent bleeding by constricting the blood vessels during operations on the eye.
        Fluorescin drops are also required for bathing the cornea to detect ulcer.
        Hydrocortisone 1% drops for chronic inflammatory conditions often combined with an antibiotic to prevent infection. Betnesol or Betnesol-N with neomycin.

Instillation of drops

This must be done with great care to prevent unnecessary discomfort. The drops should not be allowed to fall direct on to the exposed cornea which is much more sensitive than the conjunctiva beneath the lids. The patient must be seated or lying down. The nurse stands behind the patient and asks him to look upwards. The left index finger is placed upon the cheek immediately below the eye so that light pressure draws the lower lid away from the globe. A glass pipette should be held 5 cm above the eye (Fig. 44.8), and one drop is allowed to fall into the lower fornix. The pipette must not be allowed to come into contact with the skin or with the eye lashes which are of course infected. If this precaution is not taken when the pipette is returned to the bottle the solution will be contaminated. Single-application pipettes are preferable, but if bottles are used, a separate pipette and bottle, clearly labelled, is used for each eye.

Ointments. Certain drugs, some of which are also used as drops, may be incorporated in special ointment from which the chemical is absorbed to give a more prolonged effect. These ointments (**oculenta**) are usually supplied in a collapsible tube with a very fine opening so that the patient can apply the ointment direct to the eye without the use of any appliance or the risk of contaminating it with his finger. Antibiotics, yellow oxide of mercury (golden eye ointment) and atropine are those most commonly used. Antibiotics may cause severe sensitivity conjunctivitis. Neomycin 0·5 per cent, framycetin 0·5 per cent and chloramphenicol 0·5 per cent are the least harmful and most effective ointments.

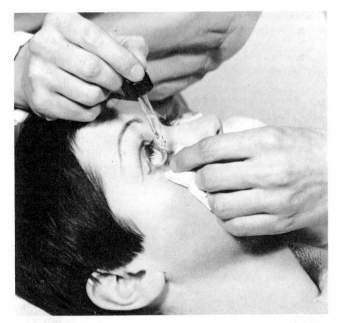

Fig. 44.8 Instillation of eye drops. The lower lid is depressed with a finger on the cheek and the drop falls into the lower conjunctiva fornix. The pipette is held well above the eye to avoid possible contact and the nurse's hand is steadied on the patient's forehead.

If the ointment is provided in a small tube, the lower lid is depressed and the ointment squeezed direct into the lower fornix as a thin thread. Alternatively, a small pellet of ointment is taken on a glass rod or probe and placed carefully in the lower fornix of the conjunctiva, the rod being kept parallel to the lid so that there is no risk of poking the eye with the point. Single application packs are now available containing various drugs. The use of these disposable capsules and tubes removes all risk of cross infection. (Fig. 44.9.) Certain drops and ointments affect vision and care must be taken that they are not applied to both eyes unless this is necessary. Patients who are given either drops or ointment to take home must be instructed in the correct method of application and warned against the risk of infection being introduced by careless handling.

Heat. The pain of eye disease is frequently relieved by the application of heat. In hospital, this may be supplied by a small electrically heated pad which is bandaged very lightly over the eye. It must be properly earthed and be of the correct voltage for the appropriate electricity supply to avoid any risk of over-heating.

Short-wave diathermy is also used with special applicators in the treatment of intra-ocular disease or conditions of the lid and orbit.

The simpler methods of hot bathing or steaming may be used in clinic, ward, or home.

A wooden spatula or wooden spoon is used with a pad of cotton wool tied to the end with thread. The bigger the pad the more effective will be the heating. A basin full of boiling water is used for steaming but this should never be allowed if the patient is in bed owing to the risk of spilling the boiling water. The padded spoon is dipped into the water, the excess being removed by pressing it against the side of the basin. The steaming pad is held as close to the eye as the patient will tolerate, the eye being kept closed to avoid contact. It is safer and probably more effective to use water which has been cooled to a safe temperature and allow the patient to place the wet pad against the eye as warm as he can stand it. As with hot fomentation, the effectiveness of these simple measures depends on the frequency with which the procedure is used and the length of time on each occasion. Fifteen minutes every 2 hours should be attempted.

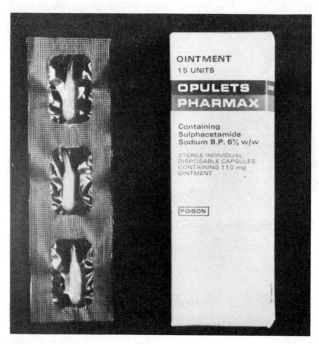

Fig. 44.9   Single dose ointment capsules. Drops are also supplied in single application tubes.

Irrigation of the conjunctival sac

The eye frequently has to be washed out to remove foreign bodies such as lime, cement, sand or chemicals. It is also necessary to remove the pus in severe conjunctivitis. Normal saline is used as the irrigating fluid but 10 per cent solution of ammonium tartrate should be kept at hand if it is likely that patients may be seen with plaster or cement dust from lime in the eye. EDTA drops are inserted.[1]

A small glass flask (**undine**) is used. There are various patterns of undine. The main feature is a fine glass spout. The aperture through which the undine is filled can be closed by the finger to regulate the flow of fluid. A Canny-Ryall urethral syringe is a very good substitute and is less likely to be broken in routine use.

The saline must be warm and its temperature tested on the back of the hand before one starts the irigation. The patient is seated comfortably on a chair with the head resting on a cushion, or

[1] Ethylene-diamine-tetra-acetic acid (sodium calcium edetate).

he may be on a couch. A waterproof apron is placed round his neck and he should hold a kidney dish to rest against the side of his face below the eye.

The lower fornix is exposed as for the introduction of drops and the stream of lotion is directed first on to the patient's cheek so that he will appreciate the temperature and be less startled when the solution is run into the eye. The upper and lower fornices are washed out by everting the appropriate lid.

Sometimes it is necessary to anaesthetise the eye by placing in it one drop of amethocaine before the irrigation commences. If the eyelids are greatly swollen so that they cannot be opened voluntarily, irrigation will be necessary at frequent intervals and the lids may need separation with wire retractors in order that the lavage may be effective.

Surgical operations

Many minor operations are performed on the eyelids in the out-patient clinic, using local anaesthesia. There is no particular preparation and post-operative treatment consists of the application of drops or ointment. Such procedures include the removal of foreign bodies, Meibomian cysts, and the opening of a Meibomian abscess. A pad and bandage are applied and the patient is detained for perhaps an hour to ensure that bleeding has ceased.

For in-patient surgery, operations upon the lids, muscles and other orbital contents are described as **extra-ocular** and are mainly undertaken in children. This group includes operations for squint, ptosis, and obstruction to the lacrimal duct.

Operations on the globe and the structures inside it are described as **intra-ocular**.

Special nursing considerations. The majority of patients admitted to hospital for ophthalmic operations are in other respects well and ambulant. The enforced temporary blindness may easily lead to boredom and great sympathy and understanding is necessary in the care of these patients who are unable to pursue their usual pastimes of reading or sewing. Smoking may also be impossible and in any case is dangerous owing to the risk of fire. Only rarely are both eyes covered after operation, but if the only 'seeing' eye has been operated on, the patient is temporarily blind for perhaps 2 or 3 days and must therefore be accompanied to the bathroom or on exercise walking around the ward. Patients are rarely now confined to bed for more than 24 hours after surgery except in some cases of corneal graft or retinal detachment.

Particularly after intra-ocular operations, post-operative pain though not severe may be persistent, and patients may find this and the immobilisation intolerable; heavy sedation is, however, seldom necessary; these patients are often elderly and drugs produce confusion.

The eye is very subject to infection and great care must be taken to avoid cross infection when dressings are performed. The post-operative treatment of the eye, including the removal of stitches when necessary, is usually undertaken by a specially trained member of the nursing staff or by the medical officer.

Irreparable damage may be done in the globe by haemorrhage from the tiny vessels within it. Complete rest of the head is ensured with pillows. Straining from constipation or coughing may produce bleeding. The patient must be told not to press or squeeze his eye.

Young children need to be fed and helped with every drink. Toddlers and some older children may require arm splints (Fig. 22.9) to prevent them rubbing the eyes or displacing dressings, but often the eye is now left uncovered.

Many intra-ocular operations are of necessity performed on old patients, especially those for cataract. Such patients may be infirm and the added disability of poor vision makes the first few days out of bed after operation particularly hazardous.

Anaesthesia. The majority of extra-ocular operations are performed under general anaesthesia mainly because the patients are young and there is no merit in using a local anaesthetic. The usual pre-medication is required as for any other operation performed under general anaesthesia.

Intra-ocular operations may be performed under local anaesthesia which is achieved by the instillation of cocaine 2 per cent drops several minutes before the operation is begun. Its vaso-constrictive effect reduces bleeding. Structures deep to cornea and conjunctiva are anaesthetised by an injection of 5–10 ml of local anaesthetic around the optic nerve behind the eye, 'retro bulbar injection'.

Procaine or other local anaesthetic is sometimes injected beneath the skin at the side of the eye to 'block' the branch of the facial nerve which supplies the orbicularis oculi muscle. This prevents the patient moving the eyelids during the operation, and squeezing the eye immediately afterwards.

Pre-operative preparation. Specific instructions are given in each case concerning the instillation of penicillin and other drops on the day preceding operation. The detailed drug treatment depends on the operation to be performed and no drops should ever be inserted in the eye unless they are prescribed by a medical officer.

Reference has already been made to the necessity for avoiding strain after operation and attention is therefore necessary to bowel action. The use of a magnesia and paraffin emulsion regularly, even though the patient has not been accustomed to taking a laxative, will diminish the risk of post-operative strain due to constipation. Neglect of such details as this may materially influence the result of the operation.

Most ophthalmic surgeons require the eyelashes to be cut, but in small children this should be left until the child is anaesthetised. A pair of blunt-pointed scissors is used, the blades being smeared first with soft paraffin (petroleum jelly). The cut lashes then adhere to the scissors and do not fall into the eye.

A pre-operative bacteriological swab of each conjunctival sac is taken as part of the routine investigation and is essential before all intra-ocular operations.

Immediately before operation, even if local anaesthesia is being used, dentures, ear-rings, hair clips and other jewellery must be removed and the patient otherwise prepared as for other surgical operations.

Before intra-ocular operations antibiotic drops (chloramphenicol or framycetin) and a mydriatic to dilate the pupil (e.g. 1 per cent cyclopentolate) are instilled probably 4 times in the hour preceding operation; the forehead facial skin is cleaned with Savlon.

The nurse should take particular care to see that the patient is familiar with his surroundings before operation, that he knows the position of the bell switch and that any necessary 'last-minute letters' are written the night before operation.

Post-operative care. During the operation sutures may have been used to hold the upper lid away from the globe. These stitches may be left in position, pulled down and attached to the cheek with strapping to prevent the patient opening the eye before healing has taken place: a square of tulle gras is placed over each closed eye and a pad, eye-shield and bandage may then be used.

The patient must make no effort to lift himself from the operating table, and care must be taken to avoid jarring when moving him. To reduce this risk the patient is usually transferred direct to his bed from the operating table, the bed being brought into the theatre.

After general anaesthesia the patient must not be left until consciousness has returned. He will then require reassurance as he will be unable to see.

After squint operations the eye is covered until the child is conscious and able to co-operate.

Special care after cataract extraction and other intra-ocular operations

The regime to be followed after the removal of cataract is that most commonly employed for all intra-ocular operations, with very little modification. The patient is placed in bed in a semi-sitting position with pillows suitably arranged to limit head movement and effort. The necessity for avoiding head movement must be explained to the patient.

The majority of cataract extractions are performed under general anaesthetic as this allows greater speed to the surgeon. Local anaesthetic is used if some medical condition such as ischaemic heart disease makes general anaesthetic unwise. After general anaesthesia, straining during the recovery period may produce haemorrhage and sedation is vital.

The effect of local anaesthesia lasts 2 to 4 hours and as it wears off the patient may complain of pain and the feeling of dizziness. Pethidine or compound codeine tablets are given to relieve the pain but morphia should be avoided owing to its effects on the eye.

Pain is not usually severe and the occurrence of severe, acute pain suggests that some complication such as prolapse of the iris may have occurred and the medical officer should be informed without delay.

The patient must be warned to avoid if possible coughing, sneezing and any sudden movement. Vomiting may do considerable damage and if a patient is nauseated post-operatively an anti-emetic such as intra-muscular metoclopramide monohydrochlor (Maxolon) 10 mg 6 hourly should be given. Care should be taken during the giving of feeds, as choking may well be produced by trying to feed the blind patient too rapidly. Care should be taken never to surprise a patient who cannot see following operation as it may cause him to jump and the eye will be damaged. Noise should be avoided: particularly the banging of doors or the dropping of enamel ware which may also startle the patient.

If the patient is restless the arms should be lightly bandaged to the side of the bed so that they are restrained sufficiently to prevent them reaching his eyes when he is not fully conscious. The bandage can be adjusted to allow enough movement for him to reach his nose and mouth.

Two major problems occur after intra-ocular surgery. The fluid escaping from the eye may lead to collapse of the bulb: reduction of intra-ocular pressure encourages bleeding and blood may accumulate in the anterior chamber (hyphaema). Prolapse of a portion of the iris through the incision is serious and requires reporting.

The first dressing is done by the Sister-in-charge on the day after operation; the patient is then allowed to sit out in a chair 1 hour twice a day if the eye is all right and there is no hyphaema. The patient may use a commode, which is less of a strain than using a bed-pan. He is allowed out of bed for increasing periods of time and may walk to the toilet accompanied by a nurse on the second day and have a bath on the sixth day. He usually leaves hospital during the second week.

Post-operative bowel action is not encouraged for the first 2 days but if a lubricant type of laxative has been given there should be no straining. Enemas should be avoided but it must be remembered that severe constipation, which often follows operation and the use of sedatives, may be followed by the passage of a large hard stool. The patient may then leave hospital with a troublesome anal fissure which has not been brought to the notice of the ophthalmic surgeon.

After full-thickness corneal grafts a more prolonged period of immobilisation is necessary and the patient is usually kept quite flat.

After retinal detachment operations the position of the patient will depend on the site of the detachment and the nature of the operation which has been performed. Specific instructions will be given by the surgeon, and immobilisation is only rarely needed but may in certain cases be prolonged.

The care of a patient after removal of an eye is similar but specific instructions will be given concerning the socket. There is a post-operative risk of severe haemorrhage and a further risk of infection spreading to the opposite eye.

Corneal grafts

Scars in the cornea from ulceration, keratitis or injury, obscure vision. It is possible to replace the damaged cornea by living tissue from another person. The graft is cut from eyes which have to be enucleated for injury, or may be taken from the eye of a person who has been dead only a few hours. In Great Britain it is very difficult to obtain sufficient eyes from dead persons owing to the very strict regulations which prevent any operation whatever being undertaken on a corpse without permission of relatives or, in cases of accidental death, permission of the Coroner. There is therefore a great shortage, and corneal surgery is limited. Grafts may be preserved by refrigeration for several days, and in certain centres 'eye banks' have been established for the collection and supply of corneae.

The graft may replace the whole thickness of cornea and the anterior chamber is opened in removing the scarred tissue. A less dangerous operation removes only the anterior part of the cornea (lamellar graft), and if this operation is not successful, it can be repeated.

Cryotherapy[1]

This is becoming widely used, particularly for cataract extraction and in operation for retinal detachment. When used for lens extraction, a fine point is super-cooled using liquid nitrogen, and when the lens is touched a firm bond of ice crystals is formed enabling the lens to be worked free from its ligamentous attachments.

In operation for retinal detachment where the object is to 'stick' the retina to the sclera, the super-cooled point causes a retinoscleral reaction. Freezing in this way only injures the sclera temporarily whereas diathermy causes a burn.

[1] Greek Kruos ($\kappa\rho\upsilon os$) cold.

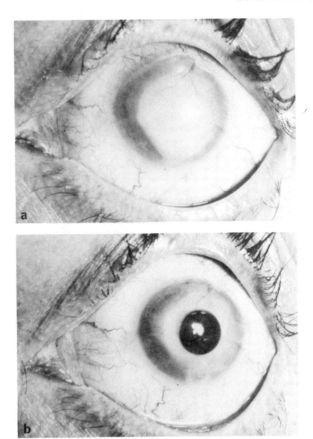

Fig. 44.10 Corneal graft. **a**. Complete opacity of the cornea treated by the insertion of a free corneal graft in the centre. **b**. The sight has been restored to normal through the clear graft. (*Institute of Ophtholmology*).

Photocoagulation (light and laser beam) therapy

A xenon arc produces a beam of white light which is focused through a special appliance to produce a burn on the retina. The diameter of the burn and the intensity of the burn can be varied. An infra-red beam from an **argon laser** is used for the same purpose: the beam is applied for a fraction of a second: local or general anaesthetic is used, depending on the likely reaction of the patient and his ability to co-operate. The technique is used for three main conditions:

(*a*) to coagulate bleeding or leaking capillaries as found in diabetic retinopathy, or central serous retinopathy. The affected blood vessels are shown up by injecting a 5 per cent fluorescein solution intravenously, photographing the retina through a blue filter at intervals.

(*b*) For sealing the retina in place as in retinal detachment when there is no fluid between the retina and choroid.

(*c*) To destroy very small malignant tumours at the posterior pole of the eye.

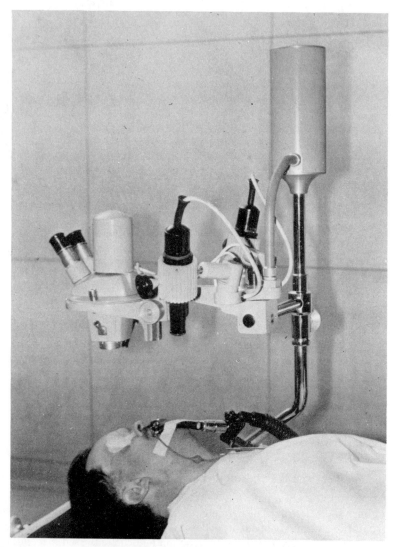

Fig. 44.11   Binocular operating microscope for corneal grafting or intra-ocular surgery.

Plastic and silicone prosthesis

Plastic implants are used after enucleation for injury or other non-malignant conditions. The extra ocular muscles are sutured to the rounded implant and the conjunctiva closed over it. The advantage of such an implant is to hold the artificial eye forward in the socket and to enable some movement of the eye as the socket implant is moved. Some retinal detachment operations utilise plastic rods of different sizes and types to produce a ridge inside the eye in order to plug the retinal hole (one of the commonest causes of detachment). These rods may be made of silicone rubber. Severe retinal detachment may require the application of a strap of silicone rubber to produce a ridge right round the inside of the eye.

Non-operative treatment and general post-operative management

Cases of deep-seated inflammation of the eye, such as iritis and iridocyclitis, may require prolonged hospital treatment during which the patient's activity is considerably curtailed. Enforced blindness, though rare in ophthalmic nursing today, demands skilful handling and encouragement where it is prolonged. The patient is in constant fear of losing his vision, and this fear is aggravated by boredom. Post-operatively a patient's sight is often diminished due to the drops used and to the fact that glasses may not be prescribed for several days. The boredom can be slightly overcome by the radio and by the use of 'talking books'. The latter are tape machines that are easily turned on and off by the patient although any other operation needs to be done by the nurse. If the patient is in a small ward and does not wish to disturb other patients, then the 'pillow phone' is used. This is rather like a large earpiece enclosed in foam with a washable cover and the patient can lie in bed with his pillow phone beside his ear and can hear the tapes. The tapes are usually well-known books read by very articulate people and can give hours of pleasure.

The hours can also be occupied by reading large print books which are often easier for elderly people. Permission must be obtained from the doctor first before a patient is allowed to use one of these.

The care of the blind

The special needs of the blind are provided for in Great Britain partly by voluntary organisations and partly by the State. The St Dunstan's Welfare Hospital was founded in 1915 to care for men who had been blinded during the first World War. This has continued as one of the most important charities, extending its activities to provide training for blind persons and special factories where they can earn a living.

The Sunshine Homes for Blind Babies care for those who are born blind or who lose their sight before education has commenced. Local education authorities are compelled by law to provide special schools for those who are blind and for partially sighted children. The latter group is particularly important since impairment of vision can soon lead to backwardness, and a child who is physically handicapped needs intellectual training more than the physically fit child.

Blindness as a result of injury or disease in the adult can soon lead to poverty, and dependence upon charity makes the patient even more conscious of his disability.

Re-education and social adjustment is an absolutely vital part of the management of serious eye conditions. Psychiatric help may be needed in some cases during this period of re-adjustment. Persons who are otherwise able-bodied and have become blind may be provided with a guide dog in order that they may be mobile. This provision is all part of the convalescence.

45

Neurosurgery

The development of specialist neurosurgical centres has to a large extent removed 'head cases' from the general surgical ward. Probably the only ones which may be seen in the course of general nursing training are those of mild cerebral concussion.

Neurosurgery is concerned with three main subjects, each of which overlaps with other special departments.

(a) Cranial surgery: head injury, cerebral tumour, cerebral abscess and the surgical treatment of mental disease and nervous disorders such as Parkinsonism.

(b) Surgery of the spinal cord: the relief of compression by prolapsed intervertebral discs, by tumours of the spinal cord or by abscess in tuberculous disease of the vertebrae.

(c) Surgery of peripheral nerve injuries: complicated wounds of the limbs involving injury or division of such nerves as the radial and median.

In the surgical management of brain conditions there is a very close liaison with the neurologist. Surgery of the spinal cord and peripheral nerve injuries is also undertaken by some orthopaedic surgeons.

Anatomy and physiology

The brain is enclosed in three distinct membranes. The **pia mater** is adherent to the brain surface and follows its crevices and divisions. The **dura mater** is the tough outer layer which lines the skull and spinal column. It is attached to the bone. The **arachnoid mater** is intermediate and is loosely attached to the inside of the dura. It forms the outer boundary of the **subarachnoid space** which is filled with **cerebrospinal fluid**. Within the brain are cavities, the **ventricles** which intercommunicate and into which is poured the cerebrospinal fluid from the very vascular **choroid plexus**. The cerebrospinal fluid escapes from the hindmost ventricle into the space surrounding the brain and spinal cord. Any interference with the circulation of the cerebrospinal fluid leads to compression and distension of the ventricles (**internal hydrocephalus**, Fig. 45.2), or if it escapes to the outer surface of the brain but is not properly absorbed back into the blood circulation, **external hydrocephalus** develops, and the brain is compressed. The normal passage-way is clear between the ventricles and the subarachnoid space surrounding the spinal cord, and there is free communication between the **spinal theca** (the expansion of the subarachnoid space in the lumbar region) and the ventricles.

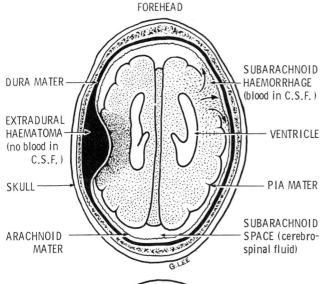

FOREHEAD

DURA MATER

EXTRADURAL
HAEMATOMA
(no blood in
C.S.F.)

SKULL

ARACHNOID
MATER

SUBARACHNOID
HAEMORRHAGE
(blood in C.S.F.)

VENTRICLE

PIA MATER

SUBARACHNOID
SPACE (cerebro-
spinal fluid)

G.LEE

Fig. 45.1 Horizontal section through the brain showing the relation of the meningeal membranes. **Subdural** haematoma produces symptoms by compression of the brain. It may spread over a large area. **Extradural** haemorrhage strips the meninges from the skull and also produces compression. **Subarachnoid** haemorrhage produces symptoms by meningeal irritation from the presence of blood in the cerebrospinal fluid.

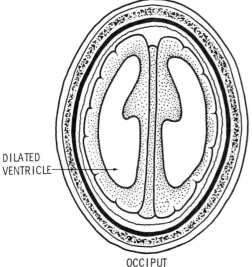

DILATED
VENTRICLE

OCCIPUT

Fig. 45.2 Internal hydrocephalus. Great expansion of the ventricles leads to thinning of the cerebral cortex and the constantly high intracranial pressure produces expansion of the skull in the young patient.

In the first few years of life abnormal increase of cerebrospinal fluid leading to hydrocephalus results in expansion of the skull and the development of grotesque features. If, however, there is an interference with the cerebrospinal fluid when the skull bones have fused, compression of the brain occurs. Similarly if the brain is infected or injured, the inflammatory oedema which follows (as it does in all other tissues) leads to a rise of intracranial pressure. The brain can only expand at the expense of the subarachnoid space and the ventricles. Any further increase of pressure is shown by changes in the function of the brain, described collectively as the effects of **cerebral compression**.

Cerebral tumour, whether neoplasm, abscess or haematoma, is described as a **space-occupying lesion** and it shows its presence in two principal ways. First it produces cerebral compression resulting in headache and, from pressure on the vital centres in the medulla, slowing of the pulse and respiration rate. Second, by interference with some particular region of the brain there is a disturbance of function. Thus if the lesion is in the frontal area there may be mental derangement such as hallucinations, and if the lesion is in the temporal lobe the patient may complain of abnormal sensations of smell or he may suddenly be unable to write. Similarly lesions at the back of the brain produce disturbances of vision.

By **concussion** is meant the condition of the brain in which its functions are disturbed as a result of the brain being shaken. The whole organ becomes slightly oedematous and there may be many tiny haemorrhages.

Certain arteries of the brain are liable to undergo thrombosis and the evidence that this has occurred will be somewhat similar to that produced by a space-occupying lesion: that is, there is a disturbance of a particular function such as writing or reading, but in the case of thrombosis there is no evidence of cerebral compression.

On the other hand, if a cerebral artery bursts, the haemorrhage both destroys brain tissue, which is very soft, and produces compression by haematoma formation.

Nursing considerations

The care of the head case, whether one of accidental injury or one requiring a planned surgical operation, has to take account of certain features which may develop at any time and which can, to a large extent, be prevented by skilful nursing. In cranial surgery, the nurse is the chief observer upon whose records the surgeon will depend in planning treatment.

The principal complications which may arise are: infection (meningitis), cerebral swelling (oedema), loss of consciousness, paralysis and loss of sensation (anaesthesia).

Infection. Meningitis may arise from compound injuries of the skull or infection may gain entry at operation. Infection may reach the subarachnoid space from the bursting of a brain abscess or by direct spread from the middle ear or nose. The symptoms and signs of meningitis are intense headache, pain in the neck, and fever with photophobia (dislike of the light). Lumbar puncture is performed in cases of suspected meningitis, and if infection is present the cerebrospinal fluid is hazy. As the condition increases in severity signs of cerebral compression develop.

Oedema. Increase in cerebral oedema leads to a fall in the pulse rate and slowing of respiration. This is most clearly seen from the chart of a patient with mild concussion following a road accident (Fig. 45.3). As the oedema develops, the depth of unconsciousness increases, and if the respiration is severely disturbed, cyanosis occurs. There is then an associated loss of normal swallowing reflex and secretions accumulate in the back of the throat, leading to 'drowning'. The management of this aspect of the condition is discussed in Chapter 10.

Specific measures are taken to reduce cerebral oedema. The patient is kept flat with the bed horizontal and only one small pillow. If the depth of unconsciousness is such that secretions are accumulating in the throat, there must be repeated aspiration with a soft catheter, and the foot of the bed is raised on small blocks. Sometimes hypertonic solutions of glucose (50 per cent) or magnesium sulphate are given intravenously. Magnesium sulphate may be given rectally: it withdraws water into the bowel, whereas intravenous solutions withdraw the fluid from the tissues, including the brain, and hold it in circulation for only a short time. The purpose of both these procedures is to dehydrate the brain, but the effect is only temporary. In cases of head injury, there are very often associated injuries of the limbs or abdomen and intravenous infusions of blood and haemorrhage. Unless very great care is taken to limit the quantities used there is an added risk of increasing the cerebral oedema from the head injury, by over-infusion. Dexamethasone (a steroid preparation) is used similarly to reduce cerebral oedema and a diuretic such as bendrofluazide or frusemide may be given.

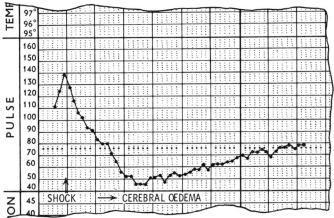

Fig. 45.3   Pulse record showing the daily change due to the onset of cerebral oedema which has produced an abnormally slow pulse. The pulse rate returns to normal as the oedema subsides.

The features of compression due to haemorrhage are described later (page 858).

Gravity increases oedema and this is why the foot of the bed should not be raised unless it is necessary on other grounds.

Paralysed and unconscious patients are turned from side to side at frequent intervals to avoid the development of pressure sores, but this turning also diminishes the risk of oedema developing in the dependent part of the brain. Sometimes, on account of spinal or limb injuries repeated change in position is not possible, but the head can be turned from side to side and so the same object is achieved as far as the brain is concerned.

Other causes of oedema such as heart failure and renal failure may contribute to the development of cerebral oedema, and a complete examination of the heart and renal system is essential before operation.

Loss of consciousness. The care of the unconscious patient has been described in Chapter 11. Reference has been made to the features of the varying depths of unconsciousness. Loss of consciousness may be accompanied by excitability and the stages resemble those seen in the patient recovering from general anaesthesia. After operations on the brain, the nature of unconsciousness is not easy to determine, and continued and careful observation for changes in temperature, pulse and respiration is essential in order that incipient cerebral oedema and compression can be detected and its progress arrested.

Paralysis and anaesthesia. Lesions involving 'motor' areas of the brain produce paralysis. This may involve one limb, both limbs on one side, or the effect may be scattered. The right side of the brain supplies movement to the left side of the body, and vice versa. The paralysed limbs are 'spastic' or 'flaccid', depending on muscle tone. In spinal or peripheral nerve injury there is always flaccid paralysis. If the spinal pathways are intact, automatic contraction of the muscles occurs, producing spasm but absence of co-ordinated voluntary movement when the higher motor centres in the brain have been destroyed. In brain injuries, therefore, there is usually spasticity of the limbs. Spastic hemiplegia is also common after birth injuries (page 862). The spasticity may be only slight leading to impairment of fine movements which prevent the growing child walking properly or using his hand correctly.

Very severe injuries of the brain produce a condition called 'decerebrate rigidity' in which the whole body is in spasm and its functions entirely automatic, the depth of unconsciousness being extreme.

Sensation in a paralysed limb may be quite normal. There may in fact be increased sensitivity, but owing to associated unconsciousness the extent of sensory loss cannot always be determined. Different types of sensation are tested, light touch (with cotton wool), pin prick, deep pain and temperature.

Whatever form of paralysis has occurred the nurse has seven primary duties.

(a) To protect the paralysed limb from injury by faulty position, or by burns from hot-water bottles, since the patient is unable to withdraw his limb although he may be aware of pain sensation.

(b) To protect insensitive areas against ulceration from pressure or injury.

(c) To prevent over-stretching of paralysed muscles by splints, sand-bags or pillows. For instance, if the anterior tibial muscles are paralysed foot drop must be prevented.

(d) To prevent relaxed ligaments or muscles from becoming short by contracture. Exercises and passive movements are required regularly and splints may be needed. If foot drop is not prevented the tendo-Achilles becomes shortened and prevents the heel being put to the ground when the patient walks.

(e) To prevent joint stiffness by encouraging active movement and performing passive movement of all limb joints at least twice a day, including those of the toes and fingers.

(f) To prevent retention of urine and consequent infection of the bladder which has in the past been a common cause of death in these cases.

(g) To guard against faecal incontinence or severe constipation if rectal control and sensation have been impaired. Incontinence is common in head injuries but retention of faeces and gross constipation leading to faecal impaction is a more common sequel of injuries to the spinal cord.

Other complications of brain disorder. Following injury or operation, cerebral oedema may interfere with the vital centres controlling respiration and heart action. The slightest obstruction to respiration leads to rapid rise of the intercranial pressure and further deterioration of the patient's condition. The maintenance of a very clear airway and the use of oxygen have already been discussed in this connection (page 172).

If the oedema spreads to the brain stem, it affects the heat control centre and **hyperthermia** may result. This is sometimes fatal. A rise in temperature is therefore a danger signal after head injury or operation. Measures are taken to reduce the cerebral oedema, and produce artificial cooling by removing bedclothes and by the use of tepid sponging.

Convulsions ('fits') are due to the sudden release of energy in the brain. The brain tissue may have been stimulated by alterations in the blood supply, by pressure or by toxins. The presence of a tumour is sometimes shown by the occurrence of fits before any other symptoms develop. At any stage in the management of head cases, local cerebral irritation may be indicated by twitching of the face or one arm or leg, before the development of a major fit. 'Jacksonian epilepsy' or 'Jacksonian fit' describes a particular type of fit in which there is a constant pattern of movement indicating involvement of some specific site in the brain (e.g. left-sided fit beginning in the arm and spreading to face and leg). Such fits are distinguished from fits of ordinary epilepsy by the persistence of this particular pattern on each occasion. The onset of fits following an injury to the brain is often delayed for many years, since it may arise from scarring or inflammation in a brain cyst or old subdural haematoma.

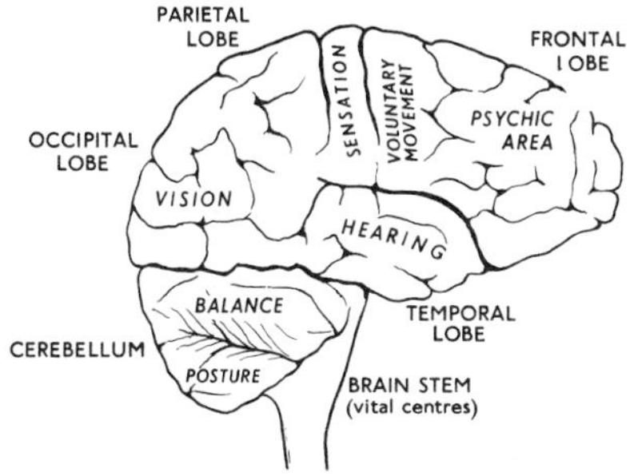

CEREBRAL HEMISPHERE

PARIETAL
LOBE

FRONTAL
LOBE

SENSATION

VOLUNTARY
MOVEMENT

PSYCHIC
AREA

OCCIPITAL
LOBE

VISION

HEARING

BALANCE

TEMPORAL
LOBE

CEREBELLUM

POSTURE

BRAIN STEM
(vital centres)

Fig. 45.4   The right side of the brain showing the areas in which the principal functions are located.

Amnesia. When a patient who has had a head injury or operation recovers from his delirium, there is often an impairment of memory for events immediately preceding the accident or operation. This is **retrograde** or **post-traumatic amnesia**. The duration of the period for which memory has been lost is a very good indication of the severity of the injury. This period of retrograde amnesia is used to assess the time of convalescence necessary after concussion which has been uncomplicated by other injuries.

Common disorders of the brain and their treatment

Congenital abnormalities

Part of the brain may be absent at birth (agenesis). Sometimes large areas of the brain are honeycombed with cysts (**porencephaly**). Interference with the cerebrospinal fluid circulation produces **hydrocephalus**. A common abnormality in the formation of the spinal column leads to herniation of the meninges, usually in the lumbar region. The resultant tumour is a **meningocele** and a similar herniation of the meninges may occur through openings in the skull. In severe deformities of this type, part of the spinal cord is spread out into the dura mater sac and there is always associated paralysis, because the spinal nerves in the region are defective. This more severe variety is a **meningomyelocele**. With a large defect in the skull, brain may be herniated into the meningeal sac forming an **encephalocele** (Fig. 2.1). Many of the gross deformities of the brain and spinal cord are incompatible with survival and the babies are either born dead or die in the first few weeks of life. Those with spina bifida and meningocele frequently survive, with varying degrees of paralysis of the legs and sphincters (page 869).

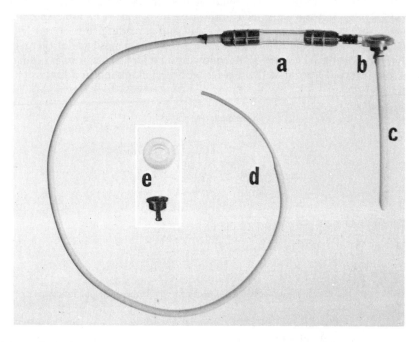

Fig. 45.5   Holter valve assembly. The valve **a** has a centre plastic section which acts as a pump with a non-return valve at each end. It is connected at **b** to the catheter **c** which goes through the skull into the ventricle. The right-angled catheter may be used or, as shown in the diagram, a Rickham reservoir which has a plastic cap to enable cerebrospinal fluid to be withdrawn through the skin by a fine needle. The other end of the valve is connected to a long silastic catheter **d**, passed through the jugular vein into the right atrium. If the cerebrospinal fluid is infected the catheter **c** is inserted initially and attached to the Rickham reservoir **e** with no side tube. Daily aspiration of c.s.f. and injection of antibiotics can take place. When infection has been controlled the cap **e** is replaced by one with a side tube and the valve then inserted.

The basilar artery at the base of the brain is sometimes affected by congenital aneurysm. Spontaneous haemorrhage occurs from this weak vessel (subarachnoid haemorrhage) and leads to sudden death. In most cases **basilar aneurysm** goes unnoticed for many years before the first haemorrhage, and if a diagnosis can be made before any major attack of haemorrhage, operative treatment is possible.

Hydrocephalus. In the normal brain cerebrospinal fluid (c.s.f.) is formed in the lateral ventricles (Fig. 45.11), passes through the central 3rd ventricle, through a tiny canal, the **aqueduct**, to the 4th ventricle and then out through two small openings into the **cisterna**, a pool in the subarachnoid space. The fluid circulates over the brain and spinal cord and is absorbed into the blood through veins in the skull.

If the communication between the ventricles becomes blocked by congenital defect, inflammation or tumour, **internal hydrocephalus** occurs. If meningitis or other lesion blocks the openings into the cisterna there is again internal hydrocephalus. External hydrocephalus can occur with compression of the brain instead of distension. In the congenital forms, often associated with spina bifida, the brain distension stretches the skull in which bones have not fused, and the appearance may be grotesque. Now it is possible to relieve

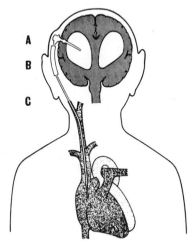

Fig. 45.6   Holter valve with Rickham cap. **A.** Ventricular catheter through burr hole in skull, and mounted on Rickham cap. **B.** Holter valve with plastic centre 'pump'. **C.** Atrial catheter inserted through jugular vein into right atrium.

hydrocephalus by inserting a plastic tube into the brain cavity. This is connected to a 'non-return' valve placed between the scalp and the skull. The outflow tube passes down the neck into the internal jugular vein as far as the heart. It is made of silicone rubber to which blood will not adhere (thus eliminating clots). The valve can be felt under the skin, and pumped by pressure to test it; normally it releases c.s.f. into the blood stream when the brain pressure rises above normal. Various types of valve are used. The Holter valve is shown in Fig. 45.5. The Pudenz valve has a silicone rubber reservoir at the upper end under the scalp: this also can be used as a pump. The operation preserves life and saves the brain from damage which might otherwise produce blindness and insanity. As the baby grows the cardiac catheter becomes too short and revision operations are undertaken at about 6 months old and perhaps again at about the age of 2. Sometimes the brain catheter becomes blocked and has to be replaced. Drowsiness, vomiting or fits may indicate that the valve system is not working. Some children with hydrocephalus which has been treated in this way lose the need of the valve as they grow. Occasionally blood-borne infection settles in the valve or tube, maintaining chronic septicaemia. This is shown by poor health, repeated attacks of fever, anaemia and weight loss. The valve is removed and if still needed a new one is placed in the opposite side of the brain and neck after an interval of 2 weeks treatment with antibiotics. As an alternative to placing the outlet tube in the jugular vein and heart, it may be led under the skin of the chest wall and fixed into the peritoneal cavity:

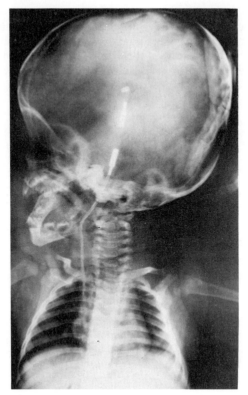

Fig. 45.7 Spıtz Holter valve in place.

fluid is readily absorbed through the peritoneum; special 'peritoneal' catheters may be used to lessen the risk of omentum adhering to the tube.

Infection

Brain abscess may develop from septic embolus arising in the course of some other infective condition, or in a general septicaemia. Infection may spread from paranasal sinuses or otitis media. Treatment is by evacuation of the abscess through a burr hole in the skull. Drainage tubes are used but alteration in the position and the removal of the tube is always undertaken by the surgeon himself.

An extradural abscess may arise from infection of a haematoma or from the spread of infection following a compound fracture, otitis media or sinusitis. It is drained by a burr hole in the skull.

Osteomyelitis of the skull sometimes follows injury or infective conditions of the scalp such as a boil or carbuncle. Between the skin and skull is a dense aponeurotic layer of fascia which connects the muscle of the forehead and that of the occipital region. Infection may spread beneath this layer following puncture wounds of the scalp.

Surgical intervention is sometimes called for in the treatment of tuberculous meningitis. Burr holes are made through the skull in order that fine polythene tubing may be inserted into the lateral ventricles for the repeated injection of streptomycin. An alternative method of treatment is by daily ventricular puncture, using a fine brain needle through the burr holes. Very great care is necessary to prevent infection.

Injury

Head injury may be **open** or **closed**. An open injury is one in which the cranial cavity communicates with the air through a scalp wound and fracture of the skull. A closed injury is one in which there is no such communication though there may be lacerations of the scalp or face. The brain may be damaged slightly or severely in either case. Because of the gelatinous nature of the brain, when, for instance, the head strikes the ground in a fall, the brain injury is frequently on the side (*contre à coup*) opposite to the point of impact of the skull. Fractures of the base of the skull are sometimes associated with damage to the cranial nerves which cross it. Fractures of the frontal bone may enter the paranasal sinuses and result in cerebrospinal rhinorrhoea (page 789). Skull fractures are not always accompanied by loss of consciousness, and conversely very serious brain damage may be present with little external evidence of injury.

Depressed fracture is one in which a portion of the skull has been driven inwards. Fragments may not be completely free but merely form a bulge on the inside of the skull. Sometimes, however, the bits of bone are driven into the brain. Depressed fractures require surgical treatment in order that the fragment may be elevated and any loose pieces removed. The dura mater is repaired to prevent adhesion of brain to the inner surface of the skull.

A baby's skull bones are soft and springy and may be dented by a fall. The 'pond fracture' which results is like a dent in a table-tennis ball. It is elevated by using a lever through a small burr hole by the side of the fracture

Severity of brain injury

Injuries to the brain, with or without associated skull injury, have three degrees of severity.

(a) Concussion. This has already been described (page 850). It is a general injury of the whole brain produced by a jar. Oedema follows, without any physical signs developing to indicate injury to a particular area of the brain. In a mild case for the first 2 or 3 days of observation, the pulse rate falls gradually to a subnormal level (perhaps 40 to 50), and as the oedema subsides the pulse rate climbs gradually back to normal during the 2nd week (Fig. 45.3). There is a varied period of unconsciousness but the depth is usually not great except for the few minutes immediately after the accident. A blow on the head from accident or assault stuns the victim and for a brief time there may be cessation of breathing, giving the impression that the patient is dead. Asphyxia may occur during this short interval before the patient's swallowing and respiration reflexes recover.

(b) Compression. In this condition the brain substance is compressed by a haematoma forming between the dura mater and the skull (**extradural haematoma**). This arises from the rupture of an artery or vein which is in the line of skull fracture, and the vessel most commonly involved is the middle meningeal artery or its accompanying vein. The principal feature of this condition is that after the initial stunning, the patient recovers consciousness partially or completely. There is then a return of unconsciousness after this lucid interval.

Physical signs develop indicating a localised lesion and the pulse rate falls progressively. There is soon interference with the rhythm of respiration and unless surgical operation is undertaken immediately, death ensues. At operation the blood clot is evacuated through a skull burr hole and the bleeding vessel secured.

The development of this condition is one of the very few occasions on which really urgent surgical treatment is required for head injury.

(c) **Laceration.** The brain may be torn by the jar or by the entry of pieces of bone, or by the passage of a bullet. Laceration of the brain produces haemorrhage into the sub-arachnoid space. There is usually deep coma. Lumbar puncture reveals the presence of blood in the cerebrospinal fluid. Surgery is of no avail except for the removal of foreign bodies.

The nursing management of these conditions is essentially the management of the unconscious patient with particular attention to temperature, pulse and respiration records, so that compression can be detected early (page 202).

Evidence of compression

One of the early signs of irritation of the brain by pressure is constriction of the pupil on the affected side. As the pressure is further increased the pupil dilates, but at the same time the mild degree of pressure exerted on the opposite side produces contraction of the opposite pupil. Finally both pupils dilate. Note must therefore be taken of the size of the pupils at frequent intervals following head injury and any change or inequality must be reported at once. Morphine is avoided in the treatment of head cases for two reasons. First it depresses respiration and second it has a constricting effect on the pupil which may mask these physical signs.

Late effects of cerebral injury

Mental and personality changes, post-traumatic headache, 'dizziness' and fits are complications which follow brain injury. In children only a very short period of convalescence is required after concussion but it is usual for an adult if he has been unconscious for more than 3 minutes to be confined to bed for at least 3 weeks. Manual workers are able to return to duty sooner than those whose work involves strenuous mental activity. Inability to concentrate on work is frequently a serious difficulty after head injury, and when associated with headache leads to the development of 'traumatic neurasthenia'. This term is applied to the state of ineffectiveness into which some of these patients drift. Special facilities for rehabilitation, both mental and physical, are provided in a few convalescent homes set aside for this purpose.

After severe brain injury, consciousness may take months to return.

Illustrative case report: E.Y., a student aged 24, injured in a road accident was admitted deeply unconscious with the following injuries:
Fractured skull (base).
Fractured facial bone (zygoma).
Three fractures of the mandible.
The blood from these facial injuries was causing respiratory obstruction and the broken jaw had dropped back. There was cerebrospinal rhinorrhea (cerebrospinal fluid running from the nose, escaping through the fractured skull base).

Severe chest contusion with several fractured ribs.

Compound fracture of right tibia and fibula.

The deep coma and pharyngeal obstruction from blood demanded immediate tracheostomy. The breathing rate and depth were inadequate and intermittent positive pressure (IPP) automatic respiration was instituted using a mechanical ventilator.

The leg wound was cleansed and sutured under local anaesthetic and the fractures temporarily reduced with the application of a full-length leg plaster which was split to allow for swelling.

The urethra was catheterised with a Gibbon plastic catheter.

A naso-gastric tube was passed.

Blood transfusion was set up immediately and this was followed by the maintenance of fluid balance by intravenous infusion controlled by daily analysis of the blood.

Nursing measures, apart from ¼-hourly observation of pulse, respiration and blood pressure, included hourly aspiration of the stomach, hourly tracheal suction using a sterile catheter on each occasion.

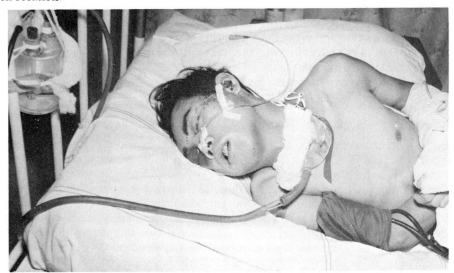

Fig. 45.8 The patient whose condition is described above, with a tracheostomy tube and humidifier. Note the naso-gastric tube, the blood pressure cuff and intravenous infusion. His extreme restlessness required very firm splinting of the infusion arm. He was sedated with large doses of intra-muscular phenobarbitone and paraldehyde from time to time. At the time of the photograph he was not 'on the respirator' but was breathing naturally through the tracheostomy which was being supplied with a trickle of humidified oxygen.

There was little change in the patient's condition for the first 6 days, fluid then seemed to be passing normally through the pylorus and the intravenous infusion was stopped and gastric tube feeding continued with a high-protein, high-calorie intake supplemented with Complan.

The urethral catheter was removed and replaced by a length of Paul's tubing strapped over the penis. Undoubtedly this measure greatly reduced the nursing hazard from incontinence.

On the 5th day cap splints were manufactured for the sections of the jaw. These were applied and elastic bands connected the various sections, exerting gradual traction on the fractures. On the 15th day the jaw fractures seemed to have been reduced satisfactorily by the elastic traction and locking plates were applied to the cap splints (page 789).

The patient remained irresponsive and very restless for 2 weeks after his injury and there was mild spasticity of the right arm and leg indicating severe injury to the left side of the brain.

At 4 weeks the level of consciousness began to rise.

As it appeared that the patient was going to recover, during the 3rd week the tibial fracture was treated by open operation with plate and screws. This wound became infected and the plate had to be removed at 9 weeks.

At 6 weeks he was beginning to talk as much as the jaw splints would allow him to. The talk was meaningless as he was not orientated to his surroundings and had complete amnesia for the previous 6 weeks' events. At 8 weeks the jaw splints were removed and the fractures had united satisfactorily leaving fairly good bite position. At 12 weeks he was able to be out of bed and began to walk and at 16 weeks he was discharged to a rehabilitation centre. By then he had recovered his sense of humour and, as far as could be told, his intellectual capacity.

In the middle of his period in hospital he contracted chicken pox from a visitor and had to be isolated.

This case history illustrates the tremendous burden of nursing involved with patients suffering from multiple injuries, particularly if they are unconscious. This man owes his survival to nursing skill and meticulous attention to detail. Perhaps the most important single measure in his management was the tracheostomy followed by immobilisation of the jaw fractures. Up to the time the splints were applied the nursing staff found it extremely difficult and upsetting to perform the routine oral hygiene as the various pieces of the jaw were very movable.

Neoplasm

Both innocent and malignant tumours arise in the skull as primary growths. Secondary malignant disease affects the brain, particularly if the primary growth is in a very vascular organ such as the lung, kidney or thyroid.

The symptoms of brain neoplasm are those of the space-occupying lesion (page 850). Physical signs develop indicating the involvement of some particular part of the brain such as the visual cortex. If the tumour develops in the 'silent' areas (mainly with psychological function) headache from cerebral compression occurs without any localising signs (Fig. 45.4). The rise of intracranial pressure produces papilloedema (swelling in the fundus of the eye at the point of entry of the optic nerve) which is seen with an ophthalmoscope.

Certain types of brain tumour develop from the meninges and can be removed without damage to the underlying brain. Others arise in and infiltrate the brain tissue and their removal is often impossible. Radiotherapy is sometimes used. Tumours also develop in the skull from bone, or from the nerve trunks on the base of the brain, particularly from the route of the 8th (acoustic) nerve.

The **pituitary gland** is an extension of the brain and tumours arising in it produce two sets of symptoms. It lies between the two optic nerves and a tumour may cause early blindness or symptoms of raised intracranial pressure, i.e. headaches and behaviour changes. Some of the neoplasms produce an excess of hormone and the secondary body changes draw attention to the presence of the growth. Treatment is by removal or radiation.

The pituitary is also removed in the treatment of advanced breast carcinoma (page 885) and sometimes for diabetic retinopathy (page 832).

Anterior craniotomy, the brain being lifted up from the base of the skull, is the normal approach for tumours. The gland can be removed or destroyed by radioactive gold seeds implanted through the nose and the sinus in the sphenoid bone. Hormone replacement is always required—cortisone and thyroxine—as the secretions which normally activate the other endocrine glands are no longer produced.

Vascular disorders

From degeneration in the wall of the arteries in atheroma (arteriosclerosis), blood vessels of the brain may burst, the resultant haematoma ploughing up the brain tissue and producing the same effects as an injury with brain laceration. If haemorrhage is severe, signs of compression develop rapidly, with stertorous breathing and increasing loss of consciousness.

Atheromatous vessels are also liable to undergo thrombosis. Part of the brain is rendered ischaemic; it loses its function, again producing paralysis, anaesthesia, blindness or loss of some other function which may be quite specific, such as inability to write words. The particular features of a patient's disability make it possible to locate the site of thrombosis. There is no treatment for the initial disease but full recovery depends to a large extent on skilful nursing in the weeks immediately following the vascular accident. So often, stiff joints, contractures and stretched ligaments, all of which could have been prevented, prohibit the patient from making a full recovery, or from once again becoming mobile though perhaps weak in one arm and leg.

Cerebral embolus occurs by the displacement of clots from the heart. Air, malignant and septic emboli also affect the brain. Fat embolism is usually diffuse and produces loss of consciousness and delirium rather like a mild concussion. There is no specific treatment for cerebral embolus. General nursing care of the patient must be of the highest possible order. Septic embolus may produce a cerebral abscess or meningitis.

Mental disease

Certain forms of severe mental disturbance are treated by surgical operation. These procedures are not in any way cures but may remove particular symptoms of the disease such as depression. In **frontal leucotomy**, which was historically the earliest of these operations, part of the frontal lobe on each side of the brain was cut, through a small burr hole in the skull. Recent advances have led to more selective operations in which only specified nerve pathways are cut. In all these operations, there is a risk of altering the patient's personality adversely and there are grave ethical problems raised by any such procedure. The effect, while curing worry and depression, may produce irresponsibility and foolhardiness.

A very common method of treating severe mental disorder is by **electro-convulsive therapy.** Artificial fits are produced by special high-frequency electric apparatus which delivers a shock-current to the brain. The violence of the convulsion may result in fractures of the spine or long bones, and sometimes relaxant (paralysing) drugs are given to prevent this side effect of the brain stimulation. A gag is placed in the patient's mouth to maintain an airway. Oxygen and other resuscitation apparatus must always be available. No pre-medication is used but the patient must be kept under observation for several hours after the treatment. The immediate after-care is the same as that of a patient who has had a general anaesthetic.

Special note on cerebral palsy. The term 'cerebral palsy' is used to denote those cases of partial paralysis in which the primary disorder is in the brain, as a result of congenital abnormality or birth injury. The condition leads to delayed progress in walking, and is often associated with fits and mental retardation. The affected limbs are spastic, usually an arm and leg on the same side or both legs. Treatment is directed to overcoming spasticity by special relaxing exercises, developing speech and the maximum use of the bad limbs. In 'athetoid' forms, the child is constantly moving his head, limbs, eyes and tongue in an entirely purposeless fashion, but may be mentally bright. By the operation **topectomy** areas of the brain are removed to prevent the unnatural and embarrassing movement.

Operations are undertaken frequently for lengthening tight tendons, dividing some tendons which cannot be lengthened, and for cutting the nerve supply to muscles which

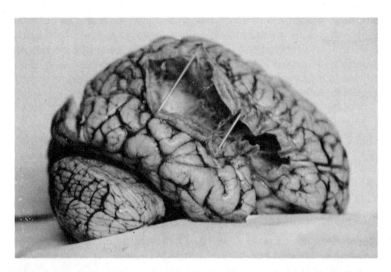

Fig. 45.9   The brain of a child of seven years who died suddenly under anaesthesia during an abdominal operation. She had hemiplegia from birth and a large cyst was found to occupy the centre of the right cerebral hemisphere. Death is produced in such cases by any minor strain which may lead to a rise of intracranial pressure.

are so spastic that they interfere with the function of the opposing group. The calf muscles are treated in this way, by nerve section, and sometimes the adductor muscles of the thigh are denervated by division of the obturator nerve (**obturator neurectomy**).

Special x-ray examinations are carried out (ventriculography, etc.) to assess the condition of the brain. Apart from these diagnostic procedures, the management of the condition is mainly an orthopaedic one. In nursing these children, much patience is required because if they are hurried or frightened, they are apt to lose control over their muscles completely, and emotionally they are unstable.

As the disease is usually one affecting a special part of the brain involved in 'voluntary' muscle control, there is no anaesthesia or loss of bladder or bowel sphincter control.

Parkinson's disease (paralysis agitans)

In this condition there is a coarse slow tremor of muscles usually in the arms, but eventually affecting gait and speech. In severe degrees of the condition, selected areas of the brain in which the abnormal nerve cell activity is taking place are destroyed by chemical or physical means or nerve tracts cut. The part of the brain involved is the **globus pallidus**, and where chemical injection is used the procedure is **chemo-pallidectomy**.

Diagnostic procedures

Several special methods of investigation are used to determine the nature of lesions inside the skull.

Lumbar puncture

Apparatus required for this routine investigation is usually supplied to the ward in a complete pack (Fig. 45.10). The surgeon may require sterile gloves but the procedure can be done with the 'no touch technique'. With the patient lying on his side, knees drawn up to chin, a special needle is inserted through the ligaments which join the neural arches of

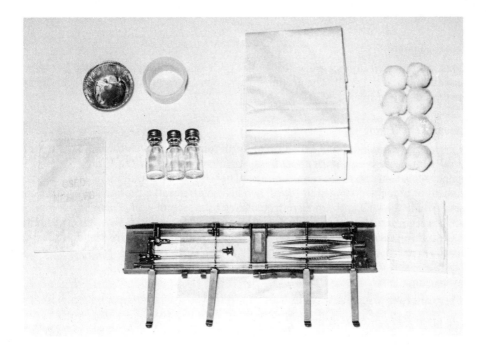

Fig. 45.10 Sterile lumbar puncture pack. These needles are non-disposable. The tray holds a glass manometer and rubber connecting tube: disposable needles and manometers are also available.

the lumbar vertebrae. Local anaesthesia is sometimes used for this procedure if the patient is conscious. The needle enters the spinal theca and fluid is withdrawn from the subarachnoid space. The fluid is normally crystal clear; turbidity indicates infection; a specimen is sent to the laboratory for microscopic and chemical examination. By means of a glass manometer attached to the lumbar puncture needle the cerebrospinal fluid pressure is taken. This varies according to circumstances. It is measured in centimetres of cerebrospinal fluid in the manometer. In the normal adult the pressure is about 12 cm. While the manometer is still connected to the puncture needle, both jugular veins are compressed in the neck by an assistant. This prevents venous return from the brain and temporarily raises the intracranial pressure. The rise of pressure is reflected in a corresponding rise of pressure in the spinal theca if there is the normal free communication between the cranial and spinal subarachnoid space. This is **Quickenstedt's test**. The nurse is usually required to press the jugular veins while the medical officer reads the cerebrospinal pressures.

Certain precautions have to be taken with lumbar puncture and these are only in reality a very rigid enforcement of those precautions which should be taken whenever hypodermic equipment is used. The needles must be sterilised by dry heat or autoclaving. Before insertion care must be taken to make certain that there is no block in the shaft of the needle. Most lumbar puncture needles have a fitted stilette which ensures that the tube is clear and that the point is undamaged. The surgeon will give instructions concerning the position of the patient for the first few hours after this procedure. Severe headache may occur after lumbar puncture. Pain in the neck, back or legs must be reported to the medical officer: it may arise from bleeding into the theca or from infection.

Cisternal puncture

This is similar to lumbar puncture but is performed through the space between the upper vertebra and the skull. The needle is inserted into a cavity of the subarachnoid space at the base of the brain.

Ultrasonic echo testing

This is used as an aid to the detection of brain tumours and in estimating the size of the cerebral ventricles. It depends upon the transmission through the head of a very high frequency vibration above the range of normal hearing. This 'sound wave' is reflected back at changes of tissue density just as sound is reflected off a wall although some of the sound passes through the wall and can be reflected back off a second wall. The rebounding sound waves are recorded, amplified and shown on an oscilloscope like an electrocardiograph. This procedure, **echo encephalography,** has the merit of carrying no risk and producing no discomfort (page 943).

X-ray investigations

There are four principal ways in which radiology is used to assist in diagnosis:

(*a*) plain x-ray photographs,
(*b*) air contrast photographs,
(*c*) opaque contrast media,
(*d*) angiography.

Plain x-rays. In order to obtain satisfactory photographs a powerful x-ray plant is needed. Considerable difficulty is experienced in obtaining adequate x-ray photographs of patients with head injury as it is not always possible for them to attend in the x-ray department. Consequently many of the examinations have to be carried out with a mobile x-ray set in the ward. The radiographer, being unfamiliar with a patient's condition, will be very loath to move the head to obtain correct positions, but movement, provided it is slow and gentle, rarely does any harm. It is extremely important that proper x-ray photographs shall be obtained and the nursing staff need to co-operate to the full in this procedure. If there is a scalp or facial injury the x-ray casette (film holder with screen) should be wrapped in a towel to protect it from contamination with blood.

Air contrast photographs. Air or oxygen is injected through a lumbar puncture needle into the spinal theca. It rises through the subarachnoid space if there is a free communication, and enters the ventricles. This procedure is **encephalography** and the injection of air is performed with the patient sitting up. Severe headache may follow due to a reactionary increase of intracranial pressure.

By **ventriculography** similar pictures are obtained outlining the ventricles to demonstrate indentations from tumour, or displacements; it is an operating theatre procedure. The

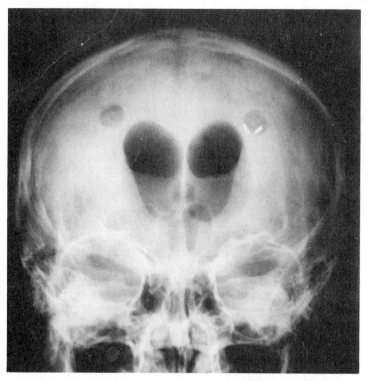

Fig. 45.11 Ventriculography. The lateral ventricles have been filled with air through two burr holes which can be seen clearly above and behind the shadow of the ventricles. Note the two silver clips which have been used to stop bleeding from meningeal vessels near the burr holes.

scalp has to be shaved completely and a full skin preparation with cetrimide or other antiseptic is essential. Pre-operative sedative is given and local anaesthesia is produced by injection into and beneath the scalp. A small burr hole is made in the skull on either side of the midline and a brain needle introduced into the ventricle. Cerebrospinal fluid is withdrawn, the intraventricular pressure is measured and the air is then injected. X-ray photographs are taken in various positions. The ventricle is outlined as a translucent area on the skull pictures.

Certain particular dangers arise, as these investigations are usually performed on patients with a brain tumour or other disease which has already produced a rise of intracranial pressure. There may be sudden collapse from interference with the vital centres. Hyperthermia may occur; coma or convulsions may be precipitated by stimulation of the brain, or by bleeding into the ventricles following the injection.

Severe headache almost always follows the injection of air and may require heavy sedation for its relief. The patient must be kept absolutely flat and quiet in a darkened room if the headache is persistent.

Opaque contrast media are injected into the spinal theca to outline the space around the spinal cord (**myelography**) in the search for protrusions of the intervertebral discs or spinal tumours. The procedure is as for lumbar puncture and the after-treatment similar.

Angiography is the demonstration of the vessels of the brain by injecting diodone solutions into the carotid artery or vertebral artery. The injection is performed under local or general anaesthesia by direct puncture or in some cases through an operative incision in the neck. While the dye is injected into the artery, rapid serial photographs are taken of the brain in order to demonstrate aneurysm or the presence of thrombosis. It will also indicate the location of haemorrhage or tumour and is one of the most useful emergency x-ray examinations. (Fig. 45.12).

The complications of angiography are similar to those of other investigations. Thrombosis may occur, cerebral oedema may be precipitated or an epileptiform attack may take place. In addition, haemorrhage may occur in the neck from the site of arterial puncture.

Electro-encephalography

Brain activity is accompanied by the discharge of electrical impulses. By placing suitable electrodes at various points in contact with the scalp the electrical impulses can be picked up and magnified by a powerful and complicated valve amplifier. The current is used to trace a graph on a moving strip of paper. Six or more leads are taken at the same time and by comparison of the electrical waves it is possible to locate a tumour in the brain with considerable accuracy.

Anaesthesia in head surgery

Some major operations on the brain are performed under local anaesthesia in order to avoid the risk of increasing intracranial pressure by general anaesthesia. If a general anaesthetic is used it is sometimes combined with the 'hypotensive technique' in order to reduce bleeding from the brain (page 243). Hypothermia is also used (page 626). The anaesthetic is given through an endotracheal tube and great care must be taken not to

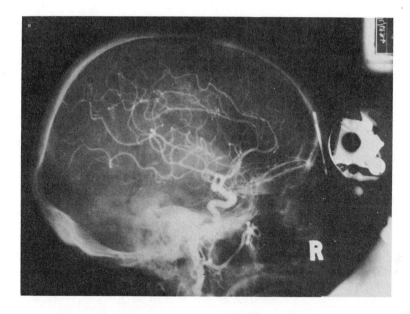

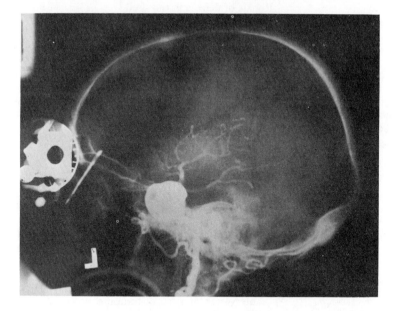

Fig. 45.12   Carotid angiography.
(a) Contrast medium injected through the right carotid artery shows a normal distribution.
(b) Injection on the left shows a pool of dye in a carotid aneurysm in the middle cranial fossa with relatively little blood being distributed to the left side of the brain.

obstruct the veins in the neck by any form of gown or towel as this by itself would raise the intracranial pressure dangerously.

Pre-operative preparation

Except in emergency admissions due to head injury or some other acute cerebral condition, there is bound to be a considerable period of observation before operation is undertaken.

In the immediate pre-operative period the scalp is shaved completely and the skin prepared with antiseptic. Care must be taken to prevent any of the solution entering the eyes. The crevices and meatus of the ear must be thoroughly cleansed.

Blood loss may be considerable during operation partly owing to the vascularity of the scalp and skull and partly due to the length of the operation. It is likely therefore that

Table 60   Common operations on the nervous system

Name of operation	Procedure
Craniotomy	Exploration of skull (as for instance for removal of tumour)
Decompression	Removal of part of skull to relieve abnormal intracranial pressure
Cranioplasty	Repair of defects in the skull
Ventricular puncture	For ventriculography (x-ray examination)
	For measurement of CSF pressure
	For repeated or continuous drainage and instillation of antibiotic (e.g. in tuberculous meningitis)
Excision of gasserian ganglion	Interruption of Vth cranial nerve in trigeminal neuralgia [the cornea is made anaesthetic and may be protected from ulceration by tarsorrhaphy—see page 831]
Section of sensory root of trigeminal nerve	
Injection of trigeminal ganglion	
Elevation of depressed fracture	For fractures of skull, usually compound
Operation for middle meningeal haemorrhage	Relief of pressure from extradural haematoma: the middle meningeal artery is torn in certain fractures of the skull
Leucotomy*	Cutting of certain areas of the brain in mental disease to destroy abnormal function
Chordotomy	Division of certain nerve pathways in the spinal cord in cases of intense pain (such as that from advanced malignant disease)
Laminectomy	Excision of part of neural arch of vertebra, for exploration of decompression of spinal cord, in removal of prolapsed intervertebral discs, or tumours.
Neurectomy	Excision of a nerve, to relieve muscle spasm or pain (e.g. obturator nerve in spastic paraplegia)

* *leucos*—white, i.e. cutting of 'white matter'. White matter is nerve fibres. Grey matter is nerve cells.

intravenous infusion will be set going before the operation and cross-matched blood must be available. Chemotherapy and antibiotic treatment is used prophylactically in many instances.

At operation it is essential that the brain is as 'slack' as possible. Intracranial pressure may easily be raised from a little venous congestion during induction or from oedema, and to lessen this hazard it is usual for patients to be given in the immediate pre-operative period something which has a powerful diuretic effect to shrink the brain, such as an intravenous infusion of urea or 20 per cent mannitol (1 g/kg).

Post-operative care

This is essentially the care of the unconscious patient, but restlessness and respiratory obstruction of a degree which would produce no permanent harm in the other types of patient may prove fatal after cerebral operation. Morphine must be used with great care; paraldehyde, chloral and bromide are frequently used as sedatives in preference to morphine derivatives. Before feeding, even if the patient is conscious, the swallowing reflexes must be tested by a very small trial drink and if there is any doubt about the patient's ability to swallow naturally, tube feeding must be used. Post-operative coma may persist for several days, during which nursing attention must be unremitting to prevent sores or lung infection (Chapter 11).

In order to relieve post-operative intracranial pressure, repeated lumbar puncture may be necessary. Hypertonic glucose or magnesium sulphate may be used as described in the treatment of cerebral oedema. Hyperthermia is a particularly important risk in operations in the region of the base of the brain.

Convalescence is slow and account has to be taken of the mental rehabilitation of patients as well as physical recovery. The general principles of nursing care have already been described and these must be followed rigorously in all cases.

Operations on the spinal cord

Exploration of the spinal canal for the removal of tumours, parts of prolapsed intervertebral discs or division of certain nerve pathways in the relief of pain, are all performed through a **laminectomy** incision. This involves cutting through the very thick spinal muscles in order to remove one or more laminae or neural arches. The post-operative nursing care is similar to that required after head cases as the same complications may arise from interference with the cerebrospinal fluid system.

The rate of convalescence depends on the condition for which operation has been undertaken. Many patients who have spinal operations need to wear a support for some months after the operation to prevent back strain.

Spina bifida (page 853)

This condition is caused by a failure of the spinal column to close over the spinal cord. This in turn may be due to an overgrowth of the spinal cord in the very first month of foetal life. There is a tendency for the condition to run in families and there are many varieties ranging from a fatty lump—a lipoma over the buttocks—to a large cystic swelling containing spinal cord with complete paralysis of the lower part of the body. Between these two extremes there are two main groups. The first includes **meningoceles** which are completely covered with skin and do not require immediate surgery although there may be involvement of roots and subsequent paralysis (Fig. 45.13A). In the second type the skin

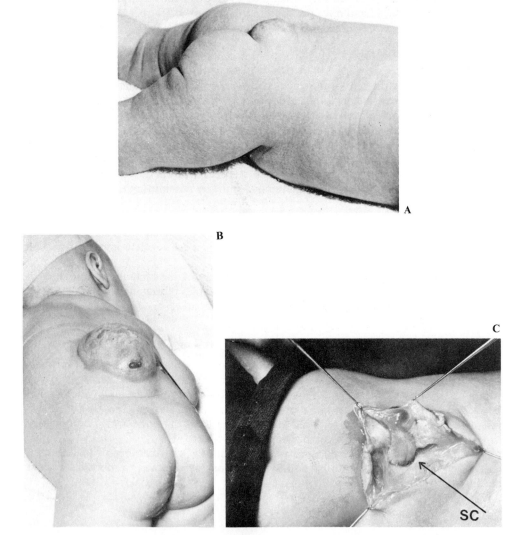

Fig. 45.13 Spina bifida. **A.** A skin-covered meningocele: no paralysis. **B.** Myelocele protruding through defect in spine: the irregular dark zone is exposed nerve tissue. **C.** A meningomyelocele at operation showing the spinal cord **SC** emerging from a small bony deficit and fanning out onto the roof of the sac. This end piece of spinal cord is often overgrowth of tissue and can be removed without causing paralysis.

overlying the cyst is deficient and there is a raw area of nervous tissue exposed (Fig. 45.13**B**): the condition is referred to as a **meningomyelocele**, or simply **myelocele**. There is then always some degree of paralysis and cerebrospinal fluid may be escaping through a puncture in the thin membrane. There is always a risk of infection and subsequent meningitis. Immediately after birth the raw area on the back is covered with a sterile non-adherent dressing such as Melonin: under no circumstances must the greasy tulle gras be applied. The baby is nursed on its face or side to prevent pressure being applied on the area of the myelocele. A paralysed baby loses heat very quickly and special care has to be taken to maintain the baby's body temperature by wrapping it up in some insulating protective sheet such as polythene. Most obstetric units have special aluminium foil sheets in which to wrap up newborn premature babies whose heat loss may be very rapid.

Many years ago the majority of these children died from infection and there are still doctors and midwives who think nothing should be done to preserve the life of a baby who is going to be paralysed. It is indeed a problem when parents are faced with the possibility of having to care for a child who is severely handicapped, but the surgeon has no alternative but to advise and perform any operation which he knows from experience will diminish the degree of paralysis or improve the quality of life should the baby survive. Any nurse who has to care for a child in this particular condition will undoubtedly be concerned about the rights and wrongs of operation and there are very occasional cases in which the baby is so badly deformed and perhaps has a congenital disorder of the heart and severe hydrocephalus, that there is little prospect of saving its life. Only the surgeon can, from his experience, judge when it is right to operate and when it is better to refrain. With early surgery, skilful nursing and really intensive follow-up treatment, well over half these babies that are born alive grow up to lead independent lives.

Operation. As soon as possible after birth, certainly within 24 hours, the spinal cord, spread out as a plate in the raw area, is released from skin, reconstructed as the cord and covered with dura mater taken from the lining of the sac. The skin defect may require rotation flaps if the edges will not come together by direct suture. Fig. 45.13**C** shows the open sac with the abnormally large end of the spinal cord protruding through the gap in the bone and then opening out like a flower on the surface of the sac, from which it is dissected free.

Hydrocephalus may occur in association with this condition and regular measurements of the skull circumference at weekly intervals during the first few weeks of life should be recorded on the patient's weight chart. A normal skull circumference at birth is about 35 cm. Operation for the relief of hydrocephalus is now safe and essential (page 854).

The paralysis which accompanies the condition is very variable (Fig. 45.14). In mild cases the child's only obvious disability may be claw feet. He is then able to walk reasonably well, but many of these mild cases have an area of anaesthesia in the feet and in the saddle area (buttocks and perineum). Trophic ulcers may develop on the feet, and because of the lack of pain they go unnoticed and untreated. The infection penetrates bone and the resultant osteitis sometimes necessitates amputation of the foot or leg. In the more severe cases of paralysis, gross deformities occur in the lower limb, and amputation may be necessary because of the deformity. In the care of these infants, the legs and hips must be extended regularly to prevent deformities and the joints must be moved daily to prevent stiffness.

Complications. Interference with the bladder muscle and sphincters leads to complete incontinence or to retention of urine with dribbling overflow and severe back-pressure changes in the kidneys. Regular examination of the urine for infection is necessary and the medical staff are really dependent on the nurse's observation for accurate information on the function of the bladder. Waterproofing barrier creams (e.g. cetrimide with silicone) must be used liberally to prevent ammonia dermatitis and subsequent infection. Deep pressure sores may develop in the older children over the ischial tuberosities, from sitting

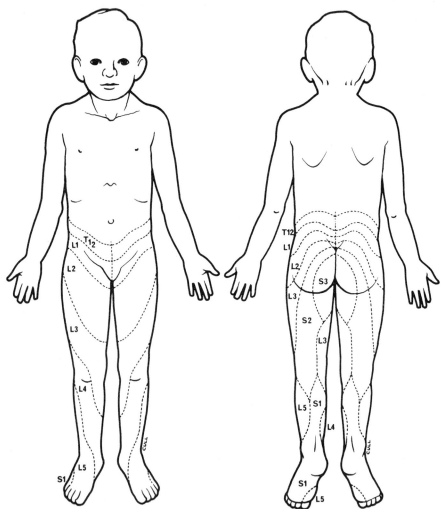

Fig. 45.14 The segments of the body develop with individual nerve roots known as dermatomes. By mapping the area of loss of sensation the surgeon can determine the level of the spinal cord involvement. In injury or congenital malformation involving the lower part of the spine below the end of the spinal cord where the lumbar sacral nerves form the cauda equina, these nerves are damaged; it will be seen from the illustration that the 'saddle area' also involves the nerve supply to the sphincters of the bladder and the anus: on the sacral nerve roots the nerve may be picked off while those above and below may be normal. Anaesthetic areas are prone to injury and particularly to trophic ulceration.

on hard chairs. In severe cases there is a constant danger of osteomyelitis from penetrating ulcers of the legs, sacral area or buttocks, of urinary infection, and of meningitis or hydrocephalus.

Faecal incontinence is common in the mismanaged case from constipation with overflow. It is an unnecessary complication and a regular enema two or three times a week will completely eliminate soiling except in an attack of diarrhoea. With habit-training and mild laxatives it is frequently possible to avoid the necessity for enemas. Urinary incontinence is managed by the use of appliances or the urine is diverted into an ileostomy (page 687).

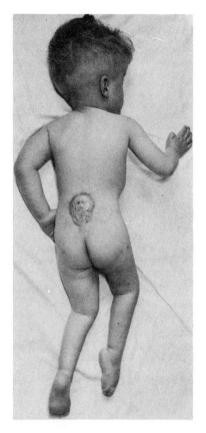

Fig. 45.15 Spina bifida. This boy, born with spina bifida and meningomyelocele survived without operation on his back. His head enlarged from hydrocephalus, he was almost completely paralysed from below the waist: the pelvis and legs were relatively small from lack of use. To avoid pressure on his back, as an infant he was nursed on his side and in consequence his hips, knees and feet became fixed in the position shown. These deformities from long association with chronic sickness are known as 'infirmary legs'. Corrective and other operations were needed on the hips and other joints. The boy became entirely independent over toilet matters with the aid of a penile urinal. He walked with calipers but spent most of his time in a wheel chair. He drove an invalid car and earned his living in factory work but died at the age of 24 from meningitis, infection having gained entry through the original cyst. The quality of his life from early operation would have been very much better.

Children with spina bifida who survive the first few months of life and have paraplegia usually attend special schools for the physically handicapped child; some of these are boarding schools. Some children are able to attend normal schools, and take a full part in school activity. Because of paralysis and inability to crawl around and explore their environment mental development is very slow. For this reason every effort is made to encourage a baby to move around on a trolley and to stand as soon as possible in a frame.

On average in Great Britain one baby in 800 born alive suffers from spina bifida.

Many cases have an associated mental defect due to hydrocephalus.

Spinal injuries

The spinal cord may be injured as a complication of vertebral fractures. These most commonly occur as the result of crushing injuries or by accidental falls in which the patient drops from a considerable height on to his feet or buttocks. Gunshot wounds through the spine may produce complete division of the spinal cord. Lesser injuries which result in herniation of the central part of the intervertebral discs lead to compression of one or more roots and the exact site of injury is determined by the location of sensory change in the skin and of motor weakness.

As with the brain, the initial shock may produce spinal concussion and apparent immediate paralysis and loss of sensation which to a great extent will recover. Any such recovery will usually occur within a week of the injury and the outlook is extremely grave if paralysis persists beyond this time.

The principal complications which may arise are:

(a) Increasing paralysis from the spread of oedema or haemorrhage up the spinal cord during the days succeeding the injury.

(b) Pressure sores in the sacral area and on the heels unless a very rigid nursing discipline is maintained in which the patient is changed in position at least every hour except for permitted periods of sleep. From this point of view the care of such patients is the same as that of the unconscious patient but the skin which has lost its sensation is much more liable to ulcerate after spinal injury than when the anaesthesia is due to cerebral injury. In a thin or heavy patient a large area of sacral necrosis may develop within a few hours of a spinal injury. There is a particular risk that such a patient when admitted to hospital in a state of shock is treated on a hard stretcher or bed, and during this critical period of low blood pressure and poor oxygenation is not turned repeatedly. Irretrievable damage occurs by what may appear to be a trivial oversight. These patients should be nursed on an open foam mattress or, if one is available, an automatic ripple mattress (Fig. 45.16). An alternative is a floatation water-bed (page 276).

(c) Retention of urine. Acute and complete urinary retention almost always follows spinal injuries but automatic bladder action may return after a few days. The normal procedure is to catheterise the patient twice a day with very strict aseptic precautions. The patient is given prophylactic chemotherapy. If automatic bladder action does not return tidal drainage may be instituted (page 663). There is an ever-present danger of acute ascending urinary infection with fatal pyelitis, and chemotherapy should be continuous.

(d) Intestinal ileus is extremely common following spinal injury even in the absence of any obvious paraplegia. The resultant distension is so great that it is unwise to put patients with spinal fractures involving the thoracic or lumbar region into a plaster jacket until several days have elapsed and bowel function has returned. If paraplegia is present with definite damage to the spinal cord, faecal incontinence results from paralysis of the anal sphincters, but the loss of rectal sensation very soon leads to constipation. This in turn, if not dealt with by enemas, may lead to faecal impaction and overflow faecal incontinence. Severe constipation may predispose the patient to urinary infection.

(e) Paralysed limbs require protection from injury by heat, infection or pressure. They also require regular passive movements of joints and splintage to prevent contractures. General oedema commonly occurs in limbs which have been completely paralysed by spinal cord injury since there is stagnation of venous blood and lymph by the absence of muscle movement. This oedema cannot be treated by pressure bandaging for fear of skin necrosis and the only effective measure is to elevate the limbs with the knees very slightly flexed on a soft pad; special frames may be used. When the patient is turned on to his side a

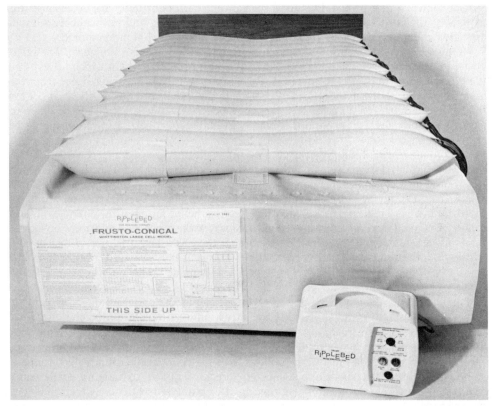

Fig. 45.16 Ripple bed. The air cells inflate and deflate alternately, producing an ever-changing pattern of pressure areas. Only a thin blanket and sheet must be placed over the mattress. These mattresses can be hired and save an enormous amount of effort and time in the care of unconscious or paralysed patients. Cushions activated in the same way are also available for paraplegic wheelchair-bound patients (Fig. 51.12). (Talley Surgical Instruments Ltd.)

pad must be placed between the knees to prevent firm contact which might lead to necrosis of the skin on the inner side of the knees (Fig. 11.2).

The spinal cord does not heal after injury and a patient with traumatic paraplegia is permanently disabled. He is liable to all the complications of spina bifida except hydrocephalus. He requires intensive treatment to prevent gross deformity and necrosis.

After the initial period of urinary retention and when the immobilisation which has been required for the treatment of fractures has been completed, the patient is usually able to manage his bladder by pressing it empty with his fist placed above the pubis at regular intervals of perhaps 2 or 3 hours. Occasionally a suprapubic cystostomy is required with permanent catheter drainage, but this is not always satisfactory as a persistent urinary leak through the penis may occur. The management of urinary incontinence in a woman is even more difficult. Various appliances are used to collect the urine and prevent continual soreness from soiling of the clothing. In Great Britain there are special centres for the management and rehabilitation of patients with spinal injuries and it is clearly in the patient's interest that he should enter a special centre if opportunity arises, because it is extremely difficult to maintain the full programme of nursing and medical care without special facilities and staff who are familiar with the various techniques required.

In high cervical spine injuries, there may be quadraplegia (arms and legs). The intercostal muscles are paralysed and the phrenic nerve to the diaphragm which arises from the cervical spine may also be involved. Respiratory paralysis may thus occur from the moment of injury or from the spread of oedema in the spinal cord during the 2 or 3 days following the injury. In all cases of injury to the cervical spine steps should be taken to ensure that some form of respirator is readily available if artificial respiration should be required (Chapter 10).

A common form of injury to the neck occurs in motor-car accidents. If a car runs into another vehicle or a fixed obstacle the passengers' heads are jerked forwards and a flexion injury of the neck occurs. This may crush one of the cervical vertebral bodies. If a car is struck from behind by another vehicle the passengers' heads are jerked backwards. In each case there is a rebound in the opposite direction, hence the descriptive term, whiplash injury. The sudden to-and-fro movement dislocates the vertebrae and may break the odontoid process of the 2nd cervical vertebra. If there is a high fracture or dislocation, traction has to be applied to the cervical spine. This is usually achieved by applying some form of 'ice-tong' calipers (Fig. 45.17). A drill hole is made in the outer layer of the skull in the temporal region and the blade of the caliper is hooked into this opening so that its prong slides up between the two bony layers into the soft more-spongy bone between them. The necessary weight is then applied to exert traction over a pulley at the end of the bed against the weight of the body. As soon as the patient is able to swallow, oral feeding may commence but drinks will have to be given through a long plastic tube: the cup from which the fluid is being sucked must be kept *lower* than the head or the drink will continue to siphon after the patient has stopped sucking and this will lead to choking. Little points like this are terribly important when looking after paralysed patients as their ability to cough 'if something goes the wrong way', is very limited and great distress may be produced.

If a cervical spine injury is unstable the surgeon may decide that a bone graft is necessary. Open operation will be required if the spine is dislocated and cannot be reduced by simple traction.

Whether the spinal cord has been involved or not, fractures of the vertebrae may require prolonged immobilisation. If there is no paralysis, this is achieved usually by a plastic jacket for the thoracic or cervical spine, but if bed rest is required the use of a turning frame greatly reduces the nursing load and improves the patient's morale and circulation (Fig. 47.3).

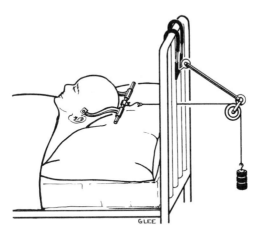

Fig. 45.17   Blackburn skull traction. Traction caliper hooks inserted in outer table of skull, for fracture dislocation of cervical spine.

Surgery of the peripheral nerves

Spinal nerves may be damaged near their origins from the spinal cord or at any point along their course. The resulting amount of paralysis or anaesthesia clearly depends on the level and degree of injury. If a nerve is bruised (**neuropraxis**) it ceases to conduct impulses for a varying time from minutes to several days. The function of the nerve recovers completely. A slightly more severe injury (**axonotmesis**) breaks the continuity of the insulating material round the nerve fibres and function is lost for several months. The nerve fibre to the point of injury degenerates and fails to respond even to electrical stimulation; its recovery is likely in due course as the nerve fibre grows along the path of the old one. The third and most severe degree of injury (**neuronotmesis**) is when the nerve with its sheath is actually severed. In this case when the nerve is repaired immediately, the minute fibres cannot possibly be opposite the distal ends from which they were severed and the degree of recovery is therefore less satisfactory, but nevertheless takes place in many cases.

If a nerve is injured in a dirty wound such as a lacerated wrist, the surgeon may decide not to repair the nerve at the time but to wait until the wound is healed and is completely free from infection. In other sites when a nerve such as the facial is injured during the removal of the parotid gland, another active nerve (for instance the hypoglossal from one side of the tongue) can be grafted on to the distal end of the facial nerve to take the place of the nerve trunk. Nerve grafting is, however, a very uncommon procedure.

Nerve tissue heals very slowly, and operations for the repair of peripheral nerve injuries or for nerve grafting have to be followed by prolonged periods of immobilisation in a plaster cast and many months' physiotherapy. Any area in which the sensation has been impaired must be protected from injury—the hand must be protected from burns, perhaps inadvertently acquired by holding a lighted cigarette between anaesthetic fingers; the foot must be prevented from developing ulcers on the weight-bearing areas. Electrical stimulation of paralysed muscles is continued until the new nerve fibres grow into the muscle.

New techniques using an operating microscope have led to greatly improved recovery rates after nerve injuries. Great accuracy of repair is possible and regeneration is thereby speeded up.

There are no particular features in relation to nursing in this section of neurosurgery. The same post-operative risks are present in all forms of limb surgery, namely ischaemia, oedema and anaesthesia (page 896; care of the injured limb).

46

Surgery of the Breast

The mammary gland develops from skin by the inward growth of tiny ducts which invade the fatty tissue by repeated branching. In the walls of these ducts develop the special cells which ultimately produce milk.

At birth the amount of breast tissue beneath the nipple is very slight and it remains as a small button of firm gland until puberty, unless some abnormal irritation or infection leads to its premature growth. The subsequent development of the breast is largely an expression of general body maturity in the female and in the male the true breast tissue remains as a small plaque very little bigger than the dark area (**areola**) surrounding the nipple. The activity and development of the breast is controlled by hormones from the pituitary, ovary and adrenal glands. Its function and growth is stimulated also by any abnormal increase in blood supply, such as occurs in inflammation.

It is not uncommon, even in male babies, to find during the first week or so of life that the baby is producing milk which may be squeezed from the breast with quite a forceful jet. This phenomenon, **neonatal mastitis**, is spoken of as 'witch's milk' and is due to the entry of breast-stimulating hormones into the baby's blood from the mother before the baby was born. Later in life, as the result of an injury or more particularly from constant pressure or rubbing, as for instance by trouser braces passing over the nipple, the male breast may become enlarged and painful, although it does not produce secretion.

In the young girl the breast may undergo a similar increase in size on one side or both sides as the result of minor injury followed perhaps by rubbing which has been intended to relieve the pain. The further development of the breasts occurs with the onset of menstruation at puberty. Thereafter, it is common for the breasts to become uncomfortable at the time of menstruation and this association is due entirely to the influence of female hormones. Sometimes this physiological recurrent activity is sufficiently troublesome to require treatment. This condition will be referred to later.

The 'normal' breast varies very greatly in size and occasionally the enlargement is disproportionate to the patient's normal body size. A clear or slightly turbid secretion can frequently be expressed from the breasts of women who have never been pregnant and the presence of secretion is not therefore a reliable sign of pregnancy.

During pregnancy the blood supply to the breasts increases very greatly and there is full development of all its tissues. Towards the end of pregnancy, if the pale yellow secretion is expressed regularly, lactation may commence before the baby is born. It used to be thought that this yellow **colostrum** fluid which precedes the flow of milk might be the natural food for the new-born baby whose sucking stimulated the breast to produce complete milk. The present view is that it is better for the breast to be rid of the colostrum before the baby is born so that the ducts are completely free and the dead epithelial cells and stale secretion have been discharged.

Occasionally a milk duct becomes blocked and leads to the development of a large milk cyst within the breast (**galactocele**). This is aspirated with a serum needle and 20-ml syringe, but if infection occurs, either open drainage or aspiration with the instillation of penicillin is necessary.

There is considerable variation in the prominence of the nipple. Flattened or depressed nipples give rise to difficulty in breast feeding and the presence of a depressed nipple on one side only may lead to confusion in the diagnosis of breast tumours.

Investigation

Mammography. This is a special x-ray examination of each breast. Malignant tumours often have tiny areas of calcification and when there is doubt about diagnosis this examination can be very helpful. Occasionally mammography reveals suspicious areas which have not been felt on clinical examination and which then turn out to be carcinoma.

In 'well-women' clinics where cervical cytology is performed, mammography is frequently used as an additional screening procedure.

Radio-opaque dye may be injected into individual ducts to detect duct growth or dilatation. It is painful and is rarely useful.

Thermography. This is a further diagnostic test dependent on the detection of infra-red (heat) emission from the tumour tissue—a form of photography.

Xeroradiography (xerography). This is a special technique of x-ray examination of the breast, using the same process as 'Xerox' document copying apparatus. A selenium x-ray-sensitive film is used and the contrast between dark and light is increased greatly, thus revealing differences in density of soft tissue.

Cytology. Discharge from the nipple is collected in a small tube or spread on a glass slide if the quantity is very small. Microscopic examination may reveal cancer cells if there is growth in one of the ducts, even though no tumour can be felt.

Clinical disorders

Congenital disorders

Supernumerary nipples are quite common. It is unusual for any of these extra nipples to develop an appreciable amount of breast tissue beneath it. They are always found on a line running from the normal nipple to the pubis. Their development is a reversion to the multiple mammary glands of the lower mammals. Sometimes such a nipple may be mistaken for a wart. If one of these accessory nipples becomes sore and in any way causes inconvenience it can be excised.

Inflammation and infection

Neonatal mastitis has already been mentioned. This is a hormonal engorgement but may become infected and form an abscess. Pyogenic infection of the breast can occur quite apart from lactation, although this is unusual. **Acute infective mastitis** usually results from a crack in the nipple and the entry of infection down one of the ducts. Cysts may also become infected.

Special care is taken in antenatal clinics to instruct the expectant mother in the care of the nipple to prevent such cracks and subsequent infection.

The symptoms of the condition are pain, swelling and tenderness localised to an area of the breast which becomes hard. There is a rise of temperature and the condition of cellulitis spreads through the surrounding breast tissue. If suppuration occurs it may go undetected for some time if the affected area of the breast is deep in the gland. The onset of pus formation is shown by the development of a swinging temperature (Fig. 4.4). Before the introduction of chemotherapy, in order to follow the basic principle of rest for the diseased or inflamed organ, it was always considered wise to stop lactation. This was achieved by administering oestrogen (stilboestrol, hexoestrol), by bandaging the breasts firmly, and by allowing the patient to become dehydrated. Because of the risk to the baby from pyogenic infection in the milk, breast feeding was discontinued. With the advent of antibiotics and chemotherapy, it became possible to avoid extensive drainage incisions into abscesses of the breast, and more often than not the condition can now be aborted by penicillin or other antibiotics alone. If an abscess develops, instead of open drainage it can be aspirated and a solution of antibiotic introduced through the aspiration needle. The surgeon may wish breast feeding to continue if the infection has occurred in a nursing mother.

In the management of acute infective mastitis during lactation, it is essential that engorgement of the breast should be avoided. If the child is removed from the breast, milk must be evacuated by means of a breast pump. Various types of pump are used. No attempt should be made to squeeze the milk out as this only spreads the infection and increases the engorgement of the breast. If it is thought unwise to allow the baby to suck during this stage of acute infection, the flow of milk may be maintained by use of a breast pump and the baby subsequently returns to breast feeding when the infection has subsided.

An inflamed breast requires support to relieve pain. A firmly applied many-tailed bandage is preferable, but a suitable brassière in which is placed a pad of sterile wool is sometimes adequate. The nursing treatment of acute mastitis may be summarised as:

(a) General anti-infective measures—rest, nutrition, hygiene, attention to the bowel and the relief of pain. If instructions have been given to stop breast feeding and interrupt lactation then the usual anti-infective measure of increasing the fluid intake is not possible and, in fact, the fluid intake has to be reduced below the normal three pints every 24 hours.

(b) Systemic antibiotic treatment, usually with penicillin.

(c) Local measures to combat infection; drainage of abscess or aspiration, instillation of penicillin solutions, withdrawal of milk by breast pump. Kaolin poultices are sometimes prescribed on the basis that heat relieves pain. Unfortunately the heat increases the engorgement of the breast and thus increases its activity in the production of milk. Cold hypertonic saline packs are just as effective in relieving pain and act by relieving congestion.

Short-wave diathermy is sometimes used in cases which have not formed an abscess but which are not resolving with usual measures.

Chronic infections of the breast may be due to tuberculosis or actinomycosis. **Tubercu-**

lous mastitis is very rare in the human but the special form of **bovine** tuberculous bacillus which affects mainly the udders of cows has led to the development of modern dairy practice which centres round the elimination of tuberculous infection in milk.

Fungus infections sometimes attack the nipple, leading to ulceration and excoriation. Scabies may produce deceptive lesions resembling Paget's disease of the nipple which is a form of carcinoma. Occasionally a syphilitic chancre (primary sore) arises in the nipple.

Any abnormal condition of the patient's nipple which is noticed by the nurse should be reported to the medical officer in case it has escaped his attention.

Injury

Occasionally a large haematoma forms in the breast from direct injury. Bleeding may take place into a cyst, leading to its sudden enlargement. Blood-stained discharge from the nipple may also be the result of an injury, though it more often indicates the presence of a growth (duct papilloma or carcinoma).

Fat necrosis is a term used to describe the development of a hard lump resembling a carcinoma, but arising from degeneration of fat which has been injured. Very often in the diagnosis of breast tumours the patient states that she discovered the lump by feeling the breast after she had sustained some minor injury. The history of such an incident increases the difficulty of diagnosis of carcinoma as it misleads the patient and the doctor.

The effect of repeated or chronic injury has already been described. It produces increase in the size of the breast, associated with discomfort.

The injured breast requires support by a bandage, brassière or strapping.

Metabolic disorders

Fibro-adenosis: Chronic cystic mastitis: Fibro-adenoma

Confusion arises over the use of the term mastitis which is literally 'inflammation' as has already been described in relation to hormonal stimulation in the neonate, and from trauma.

With the cyclical hormone activity associated with ovulation, the breast undergoes hyperplasia and resolution back to normal with the same rhythm. As in the thyroid gland, sometimes the physiological changes are excessive or disordered and lead to nodularity. The local response in the breast tissue is variable and sometimes irregular, leading to blockage of ducts by epithelial debris and to the formation of cysts and of solid innocent tumours referred to sometimes as **fibro-adenomas**; very rarely are these solid tumours true benign neoplasms. **Fibrosis** occurring in the breast as a result of this chronic inflammatory process leads to areas becoming hard. The importance of this condition lies in the fact that the cysts or areas of mastitis may be confused with carcinoma, or a carcinoma may be wrongly regarded as a cyst and left untreated.

The condition of chronic cystic mastitis is incurable but only causes symptoms by virtue of the fact that lumps appear and lead to confusion in diagnosis. The areas affected are tender, particularly the axillary tail of the breast, and it is for that reason alone that this portion of the breast may have to be removed to relieve pain. Single or multiple benign rubbery tumours—the fibroadenomas—are removed as and when they are found. This is done to dispel doubt and anxiety about the diagnosis. If a surgeon is fairly certain from his examination of a patient that her 'lump' is a cyst he may aspirate this with a fine needle and 20-ml syringe. The fluid is sent for cytological examination in case malignant cells are present: occasionally carcinoma is found within a cyst. The mental relief for the patient when a breast lump disappears in this way is enormous and far outweighs the very slight risk of misdiagnosis. If a lump can still be felt after aspiration of the swelling, the surgeon will probably excise it.

The contraceptive pill sometimes induces the formation of areas of fibroadenosis in the breasts of young women. Chronic cystic mastitis and chronic hypertrophic mastitis sometimes produce pain which is accentuated by menstruation. The most important factor in the treatment of this condition is reassurance, when this is possible, that the condition is not in any way serious. 'Mastalgia' (painful breasts) is frequently associated with anxiety and other nervous disorders.

A retention cyst occurring during lactation is a **galactocele**. It is aspirated and if it becomes infected excision and drainage may be needed.

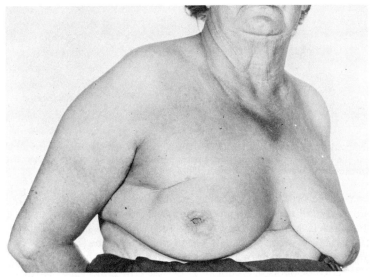

Fig. 46.1 Carcinoma of the breast. The crease above the nipple is the site of a deep tumour which had gone unnoticed for many months. Puckering of the skin is frequently the first indication of carcinoma.

Carcinoma

Malignant disease of the breast is one of the most common forms of cancer. In educated communities every lump in the breast is regarded by a woman as cancer until her fears can be allayed. So intense is this fear and so ingrained is the idea that treatment is of no avail that many women still conceal their disease until it is widespread and hopeless.

Carcinoma of the breast is usually painless. At one time it was thought that chronic mastitis (described below) led to cancer, but this is not so. The surgeon, in his management of patients with lumps in the breast, is necessarily cautious and in many cases it is not possible to make an accurate diagnosis by clinical examination.

Carcinoma is very variable in its rate of growth. In pregnancy it is extremely malignant. Generally speaking, the younger the patient the more virulent the neoplasm. In the very old the rate of growth is extremely slow and metastasis is less likely. The development of carcinoma is to some extent governed by hormones, and this is important in management of the condition.

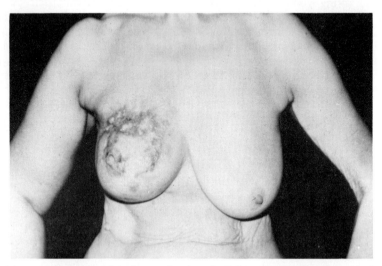

Fig. 46.2   Advanced carcinoma of the breast showing ulceration and elevation of the nipple. The lower outer portion of the breast skin shows an orange peel appearance (*peau d'orange*). Note also the swelling of the arm (lymphoedema due to blockage of axillary lymphatics with growth).

Carcinoma of the breast may remain confined within the breast capsule for several years but ultimately infiltrates the underlying muscle of the chest wall or breaks through to ulcerate the skin. It spreads to the lymph glands of the axilla and to those behind the front ends of the ribs. By blood spread, metastasis arises in bone (Fig. 46.4). Sometimes the patient, though quite unaware of the presence of a growth in one of her breasts, first complains of sciatica or pains in a bone. It may reach the lungs through the blood stream or by direct spread through the chest wall. Metastasis may remain dormant for more than 10 years, the patient being apparently 'cured' during this time.

Figure 46.5 indicates the lymphatic drainage of the breast upon which is based the surgical treatment of carcinoma. There are two main methods of treatment, surgical excision or radiotherapy. In the majority of cases both methods are combined, a surgical operation being used for the removal of the breast, sometimes with the axillary lymph glands; radiotherapy is then used to treat the whole area of chest wall, axilla and intercostal spaces.

In cases where the diagnosis is uncertain, a primary tumour may be removed by simple excision of a portion of the breast, the specimen being sent for immediate microscopic examination by the 'frozen section method'. Examination takes about twenty minutes and if the laboratory reports that carcinoma is present the surgeon proceeds to the major operation for removal of the whole breast.

Occasionally radium is used for irradiation (Chapter 23).

In advanced cases, radiotherapy may be used before excision of the lump, or there may be no operation at all, treatment being confined to x-ray therapy.

In patients who have reached the menopause, owing to the importance of oestrogen activity, smears of the vaginal epithelium are examined microscopically and, if the type of cell which is present indicates that the patient is producing an appreciable quantity of oestrogen hormone, removal of both ovaries by laparotomy is now considered advisable.

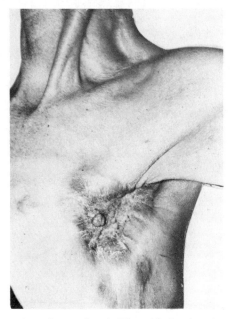

Fig. 46.3 Even more advanced carcinoma than in Fig. 46.2 showing that the breast has been almost completely destroyed.

Removal of the ovaries before the menopause is sometimes undertaken in a case in which the outlook seems otherwise grave. Male hormone (methyltestosterone) is also used and in some cases appears to control widespread secondary deposits of growth. The drug is given by mouth, by injection or by means of very slowly dissolving pellets introduced into the muscle of the abdominal wall by implantation. (A special trocar is used.) Bilateral adrenalectomy is performed in some advanced cases (page 701). The pituitary gland may be removed or destroyed by implanting radio-active seeds into it, thereby cutting off the supply of adrenocorticotrophic hormone. Alternatively large doses of corticosteroid drugs such as betamethasone may be used to achieve by medical means an adrenal gland 'cut off' secretion (page 434).

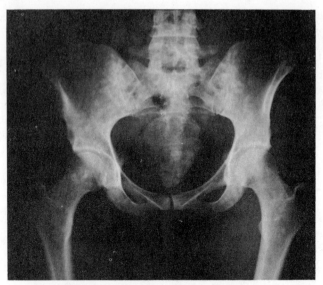

Fig. 46.4 Pelvic bone metastasis from carcinoma of the breast. The patient was unaware of her breast tumour: the white spots on the bones of the spine, pelvis and thighs were seen during the course of x-ray examination for cholecystitis and a thorough search for a primary malignant tumour from which these growths might have come led to discovery of the breast lump.

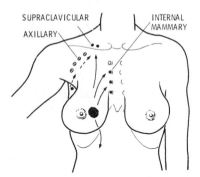

Fig. 46.5 Carcinoma of the breast showing spread to intercostal, axillary and supraclavicular glands. Such a case is beyond treatment by radical mastectomy and the lymph gland areas are dealt with by radiotherapy.

Recurrence of carcinoma

Unfortunately breast carcinoma cells may be dormant in the body for years and suddenly spring to life again. Metastasis to bone is very common and often comes to light as back-ache or sciatica. X-ray may not at first reveal any lesion and radiotherapy may be given to a painful area on the assumption that there is a deposit. Bony secondaries are treated successfully by radiotherapy if not very widespread. The pelvic bones or femur may be involved, or a vertebra may collapse.

Similarly a single rib metastasis may lead to a spontaneous fracture of the rib and will heal with radiotherapy. Even widespread bony metastasis may be controlled for many months by cyclophosphamide and radiation. When secondary deposits are too numerous to deal with individually, hormonal control and chemotherapy are used as described already for the advanced primary growth.

Occasionally the disease spreads widely in the skin infiltrating over the shoulders and down the back. The skin becomes hard and inelastic and on account of the shape of spread this is referred to as carcinoma 'en cuirasse' (Fig. 46.6).

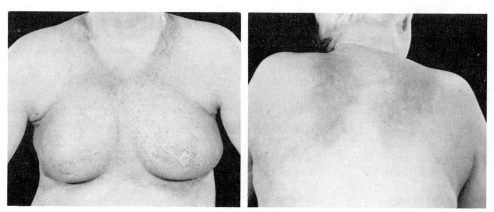

Fig. 46.6   Carcinoma 'en cuirasse' cutaneous spread over the chest and shoulders.

Severe anaemia may require blood transfusion and this contributes very greatly to the patient's sense of well being.

Dyspnoea arises from radiation pneumonitis. 'Lymphangitis carcinomatosa' is a term used to describe the condition in which the lung fields become extensively involved and produce pneumonia. Large pleural effusions occur, and are relieved by paracentesis. Nitrogen mustard or radioactive gold may be instilled into the pleural cavity to discourage the refilling with fluid.

Cerebral metastasis occurs late in the disease but is the explanation very often of a change in personality or the onset of confusion.

The nursing management of patients in the terminal stages of carcinoma of the breast, which has usually run a long course, calls for much wisdom and sympathy.

Male breast

Reference has already been made to the enlargement of the infant breast at birth in neonatal mastitis and the later enlargement of the breast from irritation. Bi-lateral hard enlargement of the breast in men is more often due to liver disease in which the liver has failed to destroy the normal amount of oestrogen found in the male. Similar enlargement occurs during stilboestrol treatment of carcinoma of the prostate.

Carcinoma occurs rarely in the male breast and usually responds to castration and hormone treatment. Even widespread metastasis may disappear (Fig. 23.3).

Occasionally, a male breast grows excessively and resembles that of a woman: the cause of this condition, **gynaecomastia**, is unknown. It is usually treated by amputation if the enlargement is embarrassing; the nipple is left intact.

Operations

Table 62 indicates the operations which may be performed on the breasts. Apart from the radical mastectomy these procedures are straightforward and rarely have complications. There is, however, associated with the thought of operation upon the breast the fear of mutilation, and it is very easy for those accustomed to dealing with surgical cases to overlook the degree of anxiety occasioned by what may seem to be a trivial operation. Carcinoma of the breast is one of the most common types of malignant disease with which the nurse will meet, and in no condition is more care needed in avoiding unnecessary mental suffering by contradictory statements on the part of those who have care of the patient. The ethical aspects of dealing with malignant disease have been discussed in Chapter 23.

Table 61 Operations on the Breast

Radical mastectomy*	Removal of breast, pectoral muscle, axillary glands and fat
Mastectomy with axillary clearance	Same as 'radical' but pectoral muscles not removed
Simple mastectomy For benign tumours or cysts, and advanced carcinoma	Removal of breast
Partial Mastectomy For benign tumours or cysts	Removal of part of breast; the nipple is usually left intact
Mammoplasty	Plastic operation to reduce the size of abnormally large pendulous breasts

* The standard operation now in use is known as the modified Halsted's operation. The original operation included removal of part of the clavicle to gain access to the glands which lie behind it. Halsted (1852–1922), an American surgeon, introduced the use of rubber gloves in aseptic surgery.

Pre-operative preparation

Skin preparation is most essential and must include careful shaving of the axilla. The skin must be cleansed above the clavicle, well up into the neck and down as far as the elbow for the whole circumference of the arm and shoulder. Preparation must also extend across the midline to the nipple on the opposite side and below the costal margin to the level of the umbilicus. The incision for the 'radical mastectomy' operation may extend from the upper arm to the epigastrium, and unless instructions are given to the contrary the nurse must always prepare this complete area *in all breast* cases. In a particularly apprehensive patient on whom it is known that only a minor operation is necessary, the nurse should enquire from the surgeon whether the full area should be prepared or not.

An x-ray picture of the chest must always be obtained and the film should be available in the operating theatre.

These measures are not of course required before the drainage of a breast abscess or such minor procedures as aspiration of a cyst or galactocele.

The patient may be anxious about the deformity produced by removal of one breast and she should be told that if it is necessary, an appliance will be provided to wear under her brassière to restore the normal contour.

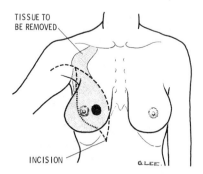

Fig. 46.7   Modified radical mastectomy.

Post-operative care

Operations involving the removal of a complete breast are sometimes complicated by the fact that a large area of skin has been removed. If the skin flaps have been pulled together too tightly, necrosis may occur at their edges, with delayed healing or the development of gangrene of one flap.

Usually if the flaps cannot be approximated without tension an immediate skin graft is used to fill up the gap.

Breast tissue is very vascular and haematoma formation is common if portions of the breast have been removed and no drainage tube has been introduced. After removal of a complete breast with dissection of the axilla, a large space remains beneath the skin flaps in the armpit. Blood which oozes from the raw surfaces may accumulate there and various steps are taken to prevent the development of a haematoma. A simple corrugated rubber drain through a stab wound in the posterior flap may be used. After the closure of the wound the skin flaps are bowed across this gap and the withdrawal of the air by a needle and syringe is sometimes sufficient to suck the skin into the axilla, rendering open drainage unnecessary, but Redivac or similar continuous suction drainage is now most commonly used. The amount of serum which exudes is variable. The drainage is usually discontinued when there has been no further leakage for 24 hours.

Instructions will be given by the surgeon as to whether the arm should be moved early in order to prevent stiffening of the shoulder, but some surgeons prefer the arm to be kept bandaged to the side to diminish the risk of axillary haematoma with its subsequent complication of fibrosis.

Pneumothorax occurs occasionally from injury to the thin membrane between the ribs when the breast and underlying muscles are removed. X-ray examination of the chest may therefore be required after radical mastectomy to exclude this complication. Any alteration in respiration rate, the occurrence of haemoptysis, or any pain which suggests pleurisy must be reported immediately. The development of surgical emphysema beneath the skin flaps may indicate a pleural leakage.

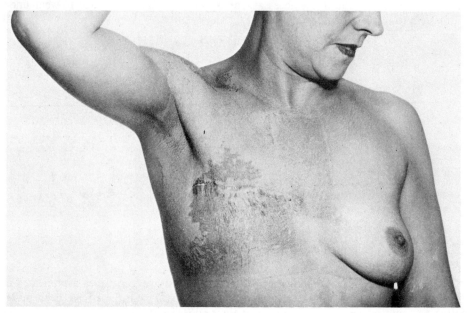

Fig. 46.8   Mastectomy and clearance of the axillary glands has been performed without removal of the pectoral muscles. Radiotherapy has been completed, and the fields of radiation are outlined by pigmentation and desquamation of the skin.

If a skin graft has been used, pressure dressings must be maintained until an adequate time has elapsed for the graft to take. It is not necessary for dressings to be done daily provided the bandage is correctly applied with adequate protective gauze beneath it. Even if a sealed dressing has been used with the overlying gauze held in place by adhesive strapping, a well-padded bandage is an advantage, especially when only part of the breast has been removed.

Radiotherapy

Post-operative therapy with x-rays or cobalt cannot be commenced until the wound has healed firmly. The care of the skin and of the·patient's general condition has been described in Chapter 23.

Convalescence

Even apparently trivial operations on the breast may be followed by considerable bruising. Every time the arm is moved the breast also is moved and as the majority of women who return to household duties use their arms vigorously, convalescence must be adequate to allow complete healing. When only part of the breast has been removed, it should be explained to the patient that the area of the breast adjoining the incision will remain hard for several weeks. If this is not done she may fear that a further tumour has developed.

Prosthesis after amputation of the breast[1]

Arrangements must be made for the patient to be fitted with a specially padded brassière if she so desires. Several types are available. Some are made of plastic foam, others are inflatable to any desired size and the patient may like to choose a particular type and weight. Various models are available.

Camp **Trulife** is a very satisfactory type with a fluid compartment in front of a plastic foam mould, giving a consistency similar to that of the normal breast.

Spencer **Confidante** has a fluid centre with an outer air-filled pocket which can be varied in size by inflation. It is eliptical in shape and unsuitable on this account for some patients.

The **Malpro** is filled with small polystyrene particles which 'flow' like fluid and take up the shape of the brassière cup. It is very light.

In ordering a breast prosthesis, the side (right or left) must be stated, and a suitable brassière with a pocket for the mould can usually be obtained from the same suppliers. Two or three units are needed to allow for washing. If worn for swimming, the prosthesis can be protected from sea water simply by a polythene bag.

---

[1] A *prosthesis* is an appliance used to simulate part of the body—e.g. dentures, artificial leg, glass eye.

SECTION IX

47

Orthopaedic Surgery

The purpose of this chapter is to serve as an introduction to orthopaedic[1] surgery and give sufficient information to cover the requirements of the nurse in training. The wide range of appliances and methods used in orthopaedic surgery makes it impossible to include in the compass of a single chapter more than a brief reference to method and general principles.

The scope of orthopaedic surgery is wide and may include virtually all surgery of the limbs and spine. In practice, surgery of the blood vessels in the limbs is usually undertaken by general surgeons, through whose research the scope of vascular surgery has been greatly extended during recent years. Orthopaedic surgeons dealing with major trauma undertake the necessary vascular surgery themselves. The growth of surgical techniques in which the very tiny blood vessels and nerves such as those supplying the finger are rejoined after injury has extended the field of reconstructive surgery and repair. There is a great overlap between the work of neuro-surgeons and orthopaedic surgeons, and in spinal surgery procedures involving peripheral nerves. Minor surgery and septic conditions of the soft tissues are also dealt with by the general surgical team, though in some centres 'hand' clinics have been established to ensure specialist treatment for all conditions of the hand, to lessen the risk of prolonged incapacity.

First, in many large surgical centres the traumatic (accident) cases are segregated into special units equipped and staffed for the specific purpose of dealing with fractures and associated injuries. In other hospitals the initial treatment of fractures is undertaken by the general surgical staff and the cases admitted to general wards. Every nurse must be familiar with the care of these patients with limb injuries. If in addition to limb damage there are associated abdominal or thoracic injuries these take priority over procedures involving the limbs.

The second great group of orthopaedic cases includes patients with bone tumours,

---

[1] 'Orthopaedic' is derived from two Greek words: *orthos*, meaning straight, correct or right (e.g. orthodox), and *paideia*, meaning childhood. The English spelling is usually '-paedic', while the American contraction is '-pedic', both in this speciality and in 'pediatrics'. There is a common misconception that the -pedic part of the word refers to the foot (*pedis*, Latin for foot). The Greek word *paedeia* is also used generally for 'discipline' and 'training', and it is interesting to note that much of the technique of orthopaedic practice is the long 'training' of bones during their period of growth or healing, much as one trains a plant or tree to the desired shape. It is a slow process extending over months or even years, in many cases of bone deformity.

acute infections, and arthritis. Lesser disorders, tears of the semilunar cartilages in the knees, bunions, hammer toes and other foot deformities form the largest section of orthopaedic cases. The development of surgical techniques for the treatment of both osteo- and rheumatoid arthritis has led to a very great increase in procedures for the reconstruction of both major joints such as the hip and of those of the fingers.

Third, there are congenital defects of the skeleton such as dislocation of the hip (CDH), club feet and spina bifida, and deformities arising from neuromuscular disorders such as cerebral palsy and poliomyelitis. Bone and joint tuberculosis is now very rare in Great Britain. Whereas 30 years ago it frequently involved long hospitalisation, modern drugs and surgical techniques have virtually eliminated these cases from long-stay hospital care.

These conditions affect children principally, and their admission to special hospitals makes it possible to provide education side by side with active treatment. Especially is this necessary if several operations are required during the course of treatment.

If the child lives in an urban area and can attend hospital easily, long-term admission is avoided. Day special schools for the older child provide physiotherapy in the school.

Permanent disability in a child interferes with every aspect of development and parents need constant help and sympathy.

Some congenital conditions though severe are treated very successfully and leave no marked disability. CDH is one such lesion. If detected in early infancy (and inspection specifically for this condition is routine in examination of the newborn), the legs are splinted to keep the head of the femur in the ill-formed acetabulum. The cup gradually deepens as growth proceeds (Fig. 47.1).

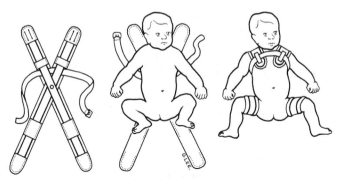

Fig. 47.1   Barlow cruciform splint for congenital dislocation of hip. The four limbs are held in the pliable padded struts to maintain the hip continuously in the abducted position.

In her general training the nurse will have experience in the care of patients with fractures. She must always remember that after an injury a patient is apt to be resentful—someone may have been the cause of the injury. Patience and encouragement are essential.

Major planned orthopaedic surgery has also a prolonged convalescent period in which the patient must co-operate with exercise: both occupational therapist and physiotherapist are involved.

Some nurses in general training have already spent a period in a long-stay orthopaedic hospital and will have had experience of the third group of patients. A nurse who has had special orthopaedic training is capable of making and finishing plaster-of-Paris casts, assembling extension apparatus for traction, and of supervising the recovery stage of patients who have had major orthopaedic operations.

Out-patient departments. Owing to the prolonged supervision required in the treatment of orthopaedic conditions the out-patient section is usually a very large and busy clinic. Plaster casts have to be changed; many minor operations and manipulations under anaesthesia are undertaken; splints and special appliances have to be fitted and maintained. Many of the patients attending the orthopaedic department are also receiving physiotherapy.

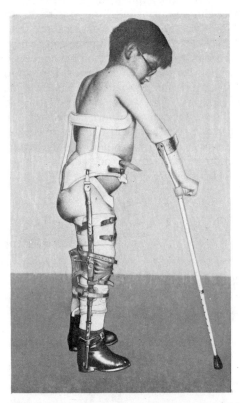

Fig. 47.2   A typical orthopaedic appliance. This boy has complete paralysis of the leg muscles and buttocks. The spinal brace is hinged to the full length calipers. In addition there is a hinge at the knee and the side irons fit into sockets in the heels. The boy unlocks the hips and the knees by hand when he sits down.

PRINCIPLES OF ORTHOPAEDIC SURGERY

Bone is a living tissue which is constantly growing and being moulded by the periosteum which is firmly attached to its surface. Most long bones consist of a **diaphysis** (shaft) and **epiphysis** at each end. At birth the ends of the bones are made of cartilage which gradually becomes converted into bone as growth proceeds. A special plate of cartilage between the epiphysis and the shaft of the bone (**epiphyseal plate**) is the site of continuous growth by which the bone gains its adult length. Between the ages of 15 and 20, the epiphyseal plate stops producing new bone and the epiphysis fuses to the shaft.

During the growing years, the normal strains and stresses of weight-bearing may lead to unequal growth and subsequent deformity, especially if the health of the bone is impaired. Such bone softening is produced by deficiency of vitamin D in rickets. By the use of splints and exercises abnormal strains may be placed deliberately on these epiphyseal lines to alter the growth of the bone artificially, and thus to correct deformity. Once puberty has been reached, deformity can only be corrected by open operation in which the bone is divided and 'set' in a corrected position (**osteotomy**).

When bone is injured accidentally or by operation, the surrounding periosteum is capable of producing new bone which repairs the gap and eventually moulds it to the correct shape. During this period of repair the divided bone has to be maintained in correct position and alignment, with contact between the bone ends, which must be prevented from moving.

If muscles are paralysed as in poliomyelitis, or their function is impaired by injury or alteration in the nerve supply as in cerebral palsy, the affected limb is not used normally and its growth may lag behind its fellow.

Muscles that are not used become smaller ('waste'). Opposing groups become short and the resulting contracture limits the movement of joints, which themselves become stiff from disuse.

Mild inflammation, involving the synovial membrane which lines the joint, produces an effusion of fluid which temporarily limits the use of the joint by pain and swelling (**synovitis**). Inflammation of the smooth articular cartilage surfaces of joints (**arthritis**) leads to a roughening process and sometimes to the complete loss of movement in a joint (**ankylosis**): the joint is like a rusty hinge.

Although bone has a rich blood supply from its periosteum and marrow cavity, it has very little resistance to any infection introduced by accident, by operation or by the blood stream. Tendons and joints are similarly susceptible to infection to a much greater extent than skin or muscle. The effect of infection on bone and joints may produce permanent crippling and constitutes a grave risk to life (page 925). Every conceivable aseptic precaution is taken to diminish this risk of infection during orthopaedic operations and in the pre- and post-operative care.

In the majority of orthopaedic cases there are three stages of treatment. First, there is reduction of deformity or other treatment of the primary condition such as excision of a tumour or drainage of infection. Second, there is the prolonged period of rest for the disordered part, usually in a plaster cast or extension, while healing of bone takes place. Third, when the bone, joint or tendon has regained its normal strength there is a period of intensive exercise and re-education in order to restore normal function. One of the main aims of treatment is to maintain as much of the patient's general activity as possible by regular exercises of all muscles and by movements of all joints, except those which need to be immobilised to achieve healing. Great emphasis is therefore placed on the part played by the physiotherapist in the orthopaedic team. Tolerance and co-operation are necessary and the nurse can always contribute to the success of treatment by encouraging the patient in his exercises and activity.

Nursing care

In many cases an injured limb or one upon which an operation has been performed is encased in plaster-of-Paris cast. The nurse has no access to the site of operation. Plaster-of-Paris (POP) may be used to make a gutter splint, a complete case for a limb, a plaster jacket or a plaster bed. When fractures of long bones have been fixed by plates or internal nails external splintage is not always required.

Nursing practice includes four main subjects:

1. The care of the injured limb.
2. The preparation, use and care of plaster-of-Paris splints and cases.
3. The erection and care of limb traction (extension) apparatus.
4. The care of amputation stumps.
5. General attention to the patient's welfare and disability in order that he may be well adapted to the restricted life which is necessary for the recovery period. This includes the correct placing of his locker and easy access to his personal belongings in order that the patient may be as independent as possible.

Where necessary the nursing staff must enlist the help of the occupational therapist so that the patient may be provided with any special aids which may be needed when he returns home.

The injured limb

The deep tissues of both the upper and lower limb are divided into compartments by the attachments of the deep fascia along the length of the bones. Each compartment contains a group of muscles, its appropriate main nerve and blood vessels. The fascial barriers between these compartments tend to limit swelling so that oedema due to infection or injury leads to greatly increased tension. The skin is only slightly elastic and it therefore further restricts expansion of the deep tissues from oedema. Thus in the injured or infected limb there is a rapid and sometimes very great increase of internal pressure. The small veins and lymphatics are compressed and the back pressure in the small veins adds to the engorgement of the limb. The continued rise of tension compresses the arteries, leading to **ischaemia**. Gangrene of tissues is sometimes the ultimate result of unrelieved swelling. Tissue tension is responsible for pain. Oedema, particularly of the skin, prevents healing.

In the management of an injured or infected limb certain principles follow from these considerations of anatomy and physiology. Engorgement should be prevented if possible and all steps taken to relieve oedema which has already occurred. Tight bandages, especially on the thigh or upper arm, are particularly dangerous. It may seem contradictory to condemn tight bandaging and later to describe the use of pressure bandaging. However, if the swelling, particularly in the leg, is chronic, such as that arising from varicose veins, tissue tension will never be great and it is safe to bandage the limb firmly from below upwards: this will reduce the swelling and, if pressure is maintained, it will prevent recurrence. In many cases of gravitational oedema the swelling disappears during the night's rest; if crepe bandages are applied in the morning, the swelling can be kept under control. Similarly after the removal of a plaster cast from the leg, oedema is very common, due to the impaired vascular and lymphatic circulation which accompanies disuse of the limb. A crepe bandage or other form of support is used for a week or so. Whether the injury is limited

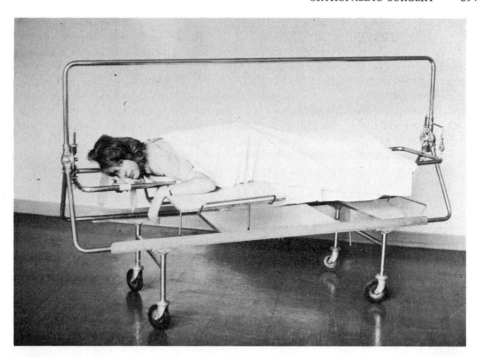

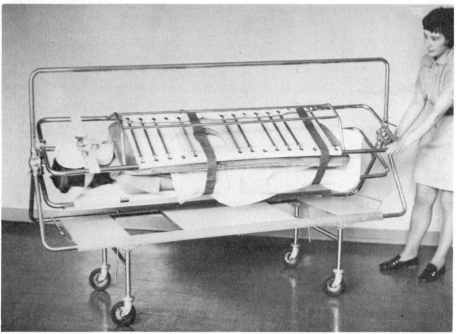

or whether there is an accompanying fracture or a joint injury, the basic principles of treatment are not affected—namely, rest and elevation of the limb to increase the venous and lymphatic return and diminish oedema. Reference has already been made to methods of elevating the arm and leg (Fig. 4.5). In inflammatory conditions of joints (arthritis), whether the condition is due to infection or injury, the joint is immobilised during the acute stage, usually by means of a complete plaster cast or a back splint, sometimes with traction. Similarly when a patient has had a plaster cast applied and is being sent home he must be warned to keep the injured part elevated as much as possible in order to diminish the risk of oedema and the plaster becoming tight.

Gravitational oedema is entirely different from that following injury such as fracture and particularly from the gross oedema which follows burns. After injury, pressure bandaging must *never* be used in the 1st week.

Damaged muscle is very fertile ground for gas gangrene organisms. The development of anaerobic infection of this type leads to rapid spread of muscle necrosis and increased oedema.

If a plaster cast is used after injury, it is applied over a layer of wool to allow some room for post-traumatic swelling, and it is usually split to guard against restriction. Sometimes a slit is made in a plaster cast for almost the whole of its length. The cast cannot expand at once but if its removal becomes necessary owing to evidence of increasing pressure from oedema, it is a simple measure to cut the remaining ends of the plaster and separate the edges (see later).

The arteries of limbs are very susceptible to irritation and if an artery is injured it may go into spasm to such an extent as to restrict the blood flow through the limb to a dangerous level.

Impaired circulation to the distal part of the limb following injury may then be due to:

(a) vascular spasm
(b) compression of the vessels due to oedema,
(c) restriction of the venous return by tight dressings or plaster.

One of the main peripheral nerves may be involved in the limb injury. A nerve may be cut, bruised or nipped between the fragments of a fracture. Nerve damage is indicated by loss of sensation in the distal part of the limb and in loss of movement. Anaesthesia and paralysis may also be due to ischaemia and if a patient complains of numbness or tingling in the toes or fingers, this must be taken as a danger signal.

In the treatment of limb injuries the surgeon is concerned not only with the treatment of the site of injury but that the general condition of the limb, the tone and power of the muscles, and the position of the other joints should be kept as normal as possible during the period of healing. Great attention is therefore paid to exercises. For instance, following an operation on the knee for the removal of a torn cartilage, ankle and hip movements are practised every day. Knee movement is not encouraged at first but the patient is taught to perform sustained contractions of the quadriceps (thigh) muscles for periods of perhaps

Fig. 47.3 Stryker turning bed. *Upper*. The patient is in the prone position, with head rest and arm tables. A tray (at the foot of the bed in the illustration) is placed on the sub-frame for meals or reading. *Lower*. The turning movement to the supine position is nearly complete. Note the central opening in the mattress for toilet purposes. As the canvas is translucent and the springs are made of rubber x-rays can be taken without disturbing the patient.

5 minutes every hour throughout the day. By the time knee movement is allowed, the muscles are then in sufficiently good condition to protect the ligaments of the knee from abnormal strain and walking is resumed with the minimum risk of joint strain.

Plaster of Paris

This, in its prepared form, is a fine white powder derived from calcium sulphate (gypsum) by the removal of its water content. When the dry powder is mixed with water, a chemical reaction takes place and the powder sets into a solid cake. This takes place in 5 to 10 minutes and final hardening occurs by the drying off of excessive quantities of water. In clinical use the powder is applied on a bandage. The manufacture of plaster-of-Paris bandages by hospital nursing staffs has largely been abandoned, since commercially prepared bandages are more convenient to handle and less liable to deteriorate with storage.

Prepared bandages must be kept absolutely dry, being stored in damp-proof containers. If exposed to the moisture of an operating theatre annexe they will become useless in 2 or 3 days. If the bandage is found to be hard on removal from its wrapping it is likely to be useless and a sample from each batch may be tested. If it has been damp at any stage it will become lumpy when soaked and will not set correctly. The incorporation of one faulty bandage in a cast may weaken it and render it quite useless.

Preparation for the application of plaster. A plaster cast may be applied directly to the skin surface to which it adheres, thus preventing movement and friction. In cases of recent fracture where swelling may occur, a light wrapping of special draper's wool may be used, or a strip of stockinette of appropriate diameter is rolled over the limb like a stocking. Areas which may be splashed with plaster during the application, but which are not to be included in the cast, must be protected by the application of soft paraffin or a barrier cream. It is particularly important to protect the pubic area as it is difficult to remove the plaster from the hair-bearing regions. Orthopaedic felt may be applied to the skin to protect various bony prominences but the majority of surgeons rely on even and careful moulding to the contours of the body to prevent the development of pressure and friction ulcers: a minimum of padding is used.

The application of plaster may be required after the reduction of a fracture, after the surgical treatment of a soft tissue wound, or to retain the position of the limb or spine following a major operation on a bone or joint. The equipment is usually assembled on a special table or trolley and includes the following items:

Rubber mackintosh sheets.
Two deep bowls or buckets.
An adequate supply of fresh plaster bandages of various widths; the waterproof wrappings must not be removed until the bandages are required.
Rolled, thin strips of draper's wool of various widths (Orthoban).
Stockinette in at least three widths for the limbs and two sizes for applying to the trunk as a vest beneath a plaster jacket.
Orthopaedic felt. This must be fresh. If it has become dry from being stored in a hot place the linen backing will be difficult to remove and the adhesive surface will not stick.
Adhesive strapping of various widths, including waterproof strapping.
Large plaster shears and small plaster cutters (Fig. 47.4).
Strong scissors and plaster knife. The latter should be a small cobbler's knife with a short

blade and stout handle. A scalpel can be used but it is a dangerous and unsatisfactory tool which is not designed for cutting plaster.

Tape measure (for measuring the length of stockinette and plaster slabs).

Skin pencil.

Any special appliance to be incorporated in the plaster such as a wooden rocking heel or Böhler leg iron.

A selection of cotton bandages and Viscopaste (zinc oxide paste) bandages should be readily available if required.

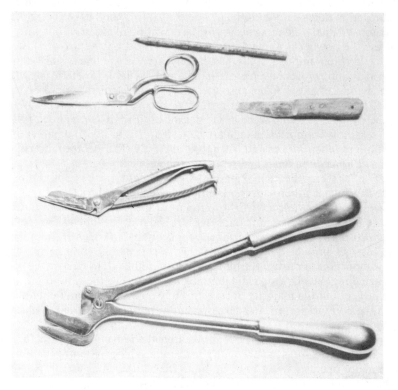

Fig. 47.4 Instruments for the preparation of plaster casts and for their removal. From above down—skin pencil; dressing scissors; plaster (cobbler's) knife; small plaster cutters; Stille pattern plaster shears.

Construction of the cast. The patient, bedding and floor must be protected with sheets or mackintoshes, leaving exposed only the part to be plastered. If a jacket or bed is to be made, the patient must wear a head cap and the hair edges must be greased. Underclothes must be removed if there is any possibility that the leg or arm of the garment is too small to pass over the finished limb cast.

The majority of splints or casts are made by the skilful and even application of a series of wet plaster bandages. Care is taken to produce a regular covering of the limb, each layer being smoothed down to fuse with the preceding layer, the whole field being kept wet. It is essential that the layers are welded together by the plaster cream which exudes from the bandage. Care is taken to avoid rough edges or lumps. 'Slabs' are made by measuring the required length and unrolling a bandage to and fro to make a flat slab of five or six thicknesses. Special shapes may be cut from the dry plaster sheets which are provided commercially: these wide sheets are of use in the construction of plaster beds. Slabs may be made dry and then simply drawn through the water, compressed lightly to remove excess water, and applied. They may be made with a wet bandage instead.

When a surgeon is ready to use a plaster bandage, it should be immersed *carefully* in cool water, for approximately 10 seconds or until air bubbles cease to rise from it: it should never be squeezed while under water as this expels much of the useful plaster. The bandage is lifted carefully from the bowl or bucket and excessive water removed by squeezing gently from the ends towards the middle. This avoids loss of plaster. If a spindle is provided inside the rolled bandage this is left in place: care must be taken not to allow it to fall out as it simplifies the handling of the bandage. The plaster begins to set very quickly and if bandages are not used immediately or even if they are left in the bowl of water they become hard and caked. No attempt must be made to incorporate them in the cast once the setting process has started. Hot water should not be used for plaster bandages as setting will probably occur before the layers have been moulded adequately together.

The 'cream' that remains at the bottom of the bowl after the bandages have been soaked can be used, provided it has not partially set, to fill the surface crevices of the cast and produce a smooth finish. A well-finished and polished (with French chalk) plaster does not get dirty as soon as a rough plaster, and is more durable.

The cast becomes hot as it dries owing to the chemical reaction, but unless bandages have been used in a particularly wet condition, artificial heat is not required during the drying process. The splint must be exposed to a free current of air, and for the leg an open-ended bed cradle is used. A spinal jacket, or a thick cast for a leg or shoulder may take 24 hours to dry completely and weightbearing should not be permitted until the plaster is crisp and has a resonant note when tapped.

After care

Circulation. The importance of elevation of an injured limb after treatment has been stressed already. The most important immediate risk from the application of a plaster splint is restriction of venous return. The fingers or toes are always left uncovered and the circulation must be inspected repeatedly during the first few hours.[1] If at any time there is swelling or blueness of the exposed part beyond the plaster the matter must be reported. Sometimes after a severe injury or fracture, it is very difficult for the surgeon to determine whether the plaster has become too tight owing to post-operative swelling. In recent injuries or in major operation cases, a slit is made into the plaster cast from top to bottom so that it can be expanded if pressure within becomes excessive. Sometimes two such splits are made converting the complete case into a 'divided plaster'. The two halves are bandaged together lightly. Either may be removed for wound examination or removal of stitches.

One of the earliest indications that the circulation is impaired is loss of touch sensation

---

[1] If a coloured antiseptic is used in pre-operative skin preparation the toes should be left unpainted and treated with a *colourless* antiseptic so that post-operative circulation can be observed.

in the toes or fingers. This can be tested very easily by the nurse with a piece of cotton wool. Pallor of the nail beds and failure to flush again when squeezed indicates that the circulation is severely impaired; this may be due to vascular spasm (page 898).

The skin at the edges of a plaster cast must be watched very carefully for the development of pressure sores. Pieces of cotton wool must never be stuffed in at the ends for protection. If pressure is occurring and causing discomfort by chafing of the skin, the plaster must be cut or remoulded: this is a matter for the medical staff. A very loose plaster is dangerous for two reasons. First, it fails to produce adequate immobilisation, and secondly, the movement leads to the development of friction sores over bony prominences.

Pressure ulcers may also develop inside plaster casts where there is a bump on the inner surface or where excessive pressure is applied to the skin, as for instance over the subcutaneous surface of the tibia. Careless handling of a wet splint may leave indentations made by the nurse's fingers.

Plaster casts are not waterproof and the patient must be warned not to wet the cast during toilet operations. In children, a pelvic or leg plaster may be protected from contamination with urine by binding the edges of the exposed areas with Elastoplast adhesive waterproof strapping. Ordinary non-waterproof strapping is useless.

Immediately after the application of a plaster cast, particularly of a pelvic plaster or jacket, the patient may develop a state of acute anxiety and agitation with the feeling of being totally enclosed. The use of sedatives is sometimes necessary until the patient becomes accustomed to this restriction. Children adapt themselves to life in a plaster cast very much more readily than adults, but particular care is necessary to make certain that the child does not become twisted in his plaster and produce areas of pressure necrosis. The child on whom a plaster splint has been applied must be seen at frequent intervals owing to the very obvious risk of damage from excessive activity.

All plaster casts should be inspected daily for cracks, and patients who are sent home in plaster must be told to watch for the development of cracks and report them if there appear to be any. Cracks in plaster casts can be reinforced by the addition of further bandages but these do not adhere firmly and the repaired splint is rarely a satisfactory one. The addition of further plaster makes the removal more difficult and the extra weight adds to the patient's burden.

Removal of cast. The nurse must obtain practical experience in the removal of plaster-of-Paris cases. Considerable physical effort is required and care must be taken to keep the point of the plaster shears, which is inside the cast, away from the skin surface. Small bites must be taken and the shears moved repeatedly from the slot which has been cut in order to clear the blades. Damp plaster is extremely difficult to cut and thick casts may require the use of a plaster saw. Various devices are used to facilitate the removal of plaster by incorporating a tape, wire or metal strip during the application of the cast.

The skin beneath a plaster is soft and sensitive if the cast has been on for more than a few days. After removal of the splint, the skin should be cleaned gently and powdered with a simple dusting powder. If pressure sores have developed, it is best to cover the affected area with a disc of adhesive strapping beneath which healing will usually occur rapidly.

The leg tends to become oedematous after removal of a plaster, and for 1 or 2 weeks a compression bandage of elastic strapping or crepe is applied. **Tubigrip**, a form of elasticated stockinette is often used for this purpose. Ordinary Elastoplast applied as an overlapping spiral over stretched stockinette can also be used. If oedema is allowed to develop, it may be extremely difficult to obviate later unless the patient is confined to bed with the leg elevated.

When a patient has been in a plaster cast for several weeks the muscles become weak and are unable to guard the joints against abnormal strain. After the removal of the cast the patient is therefore encouraged to regain joint movement by intensive exercises without bearing weight at all on the limbs. This means that in the case of leg fractures the patient will either have to remain in bed or in a wheelchair with the leg elevated on an extension board. Once full control is adequate the patient then begins weight-bearing aided by elbow crutches or a walking frame. If care is not taken at this stage joint strain and effusion of fluid (synovitis) may occur.

Plastic splinting

Special materials are now available for making lightweight more-permanent splints to fit individual patients. Perforated polyethylene foam sheets (Plastazote) are supplied in different thicknesses. The material is cut to pattern and heated to make it malleable. It is moulded on the patient over stockinette while it is still hot. Splints and in fact many instruments and calipers are held in place by velcro straps which have a surface composed of thousands of tiny nylon hooks (Fig. 47.5).

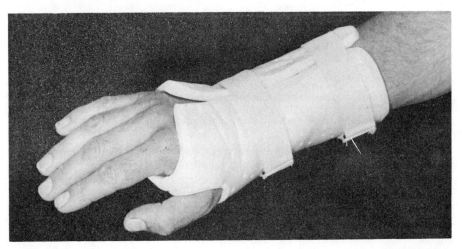

Fig. 47.5 Moulded polyethylene splint, detachable and fixed with Velcro straps. It is used to rest an arthritic wrist. (Smith & Nephew.)

Limb traction

A simple illustration of the principles of limb traction can be drawn from its use in fracture of the shaft of the femur. The broken ends of the bone damage the surrounding muscle. The intense pain of the fracture produces spasm of the muscles which is a reflex action to prevent abnormal movement. If the distal end of the limb is pulled slowly and constantly, muscle spasm is gradually overcome. As the strap-like muscles are straightened by the pull, they act as splints around the fractured bone. Traction has the additional effect of preventing abnormal movement at the fracture site during healing. The degree of pull is varied according to the requirements. Only a very light pull (5 to 10 lb—2 to 4 kilos—on the leg) is necessary to overcome muscle spasm and relieve pain, but a much heavier weight may be needed in order to reduce the fracture by 'over pulling' the overlapping bone ends. If excessive traction is used and the fracture fragments are kept apart for 2 or 3 days, union is greatly delayed by the formation of fibrous tissue between the bone ends.

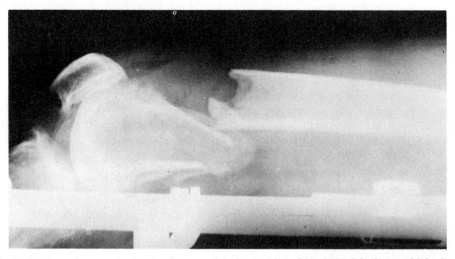

Fig. 47.6   X-ray photograph, showing fracture of the lower third of the shaft of the femur with backward displacement of the lower fragment. The popliteal artery is in danger from pressure by the projecting fragment. The bars of the Thomas splint and the splint clip are shown in the x-ray photograph.

Even if a fracture is correctly reduced under anaesthesia and splinted, when consciousness returns muscle spasm returns, and the bone fragments may slip. Certain types of fracture are particularly unstable in this respect and in such cases traction has to be maintained after reduction until the healing process is well established, unless internal fixation of the fracture by plates, screws or nails is undertaken.

As a temporary measure traction may be obtained by tying a folded triangular bandage or a piece of rope with a non-slip clove hitch knot around the ankle. As a first-aid measure the traction is applied over the patient's boot. In the hospital treatment of fractures and other bone and joint conditions such as arthritis, traction is applied to the limbs in one of two ways, **skin traction** or **skeletal traction**.

Special non-stretch adhesive strapping is applied to the sides of the thigh or leg and a bandage wound firmly over the two strips between the ankle and the knee. The distal ends of the strapping are attached to a spreader to avoid pressure over the malleolar bony prominences. Commercially prepared extension strapping sets are available with the spreader mounted in the centre and plastic foam padding at the sides of the ankle (Fig. 47.7). The traction weight is then applied to the spreader (Fig. 47.12). Skin traction is useful

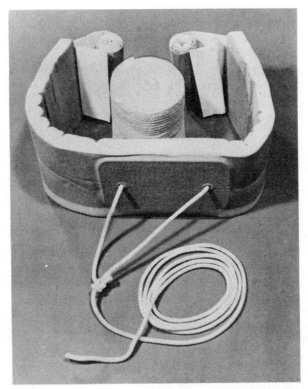

Fig. 47.7 Elastic skin traction pack: spreader and foam ankle-protecting insert: crepe bandage. (Seton Products Ltd.)

in children to suspend the legs from an overhead gallows in the treatment of arthritis of knees or hips, or in the management of fractured femur (Fig. 47.8). In adults skin traction is adequate for some fractures of the femur and to correct deformities arising from disease of the hip or knee.

In fractures of the lower leg and very often of the femur, skeletal traction[1] is used. A steel pin or wire is passed through the upper or lower end of the tibia, sometimes through the lower end of the femur or through the os calcis. A steel stirrup is applied to the ends of the pin and traction obtained by a cord attached to the stirrup (Fig. 47.10).

The pins can be inserted under local anaesthesia if necessary. Sometimes the surgeon uses a sealed dressing on the point of entry and exit from the skin but many prefer to leave the skin punctures dry with an occasional dusting with antibiotic powder (bacitracin). When traction is no longer required, one protruding end of this pin is cleaned with a strong antiseptic and the pin easily withdrawn through the bone without anaesthesia, since it becomes loosened in its track from atrophy of the surrounding bone.

[1] Skeletal traction is also used on the skull by means of 'ice-tong calipers' in the treatment of cervical spinal fractures. One prong is inserted in a small burr hole on each side of the skull (page 877).

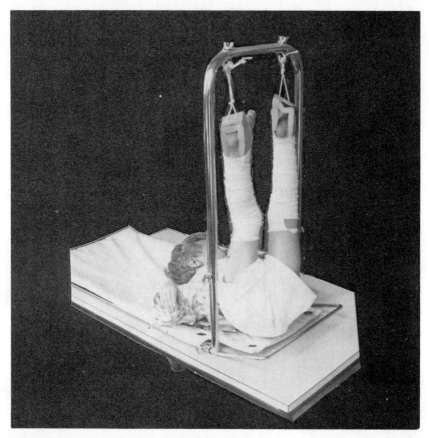

Fig. 47.8 Gallows traction for femur fractures of hip: the sacrum must be clear of the mattress. The traction splint with its own canvas base and frame is completely transportable for x-ray purposes and use in the home.

When skin traction is in use, very careful watch is necessary on the circulation of the toes as the drag of the strapping and bandages may restrict venous return and lead to oedema.

Whatever form of traction is employed, the weight of the limb is supported on some type of additional splint. For the lower limb, most commonly the Thomas[1] **knee** splint is used extending from the groin to beyond the foot, but for fractures of the tibia and lower end of the femur, the Böhler-Braun frame (Fig. 4.5) is sometimes substituted. The limb is slung between the bars of the splint on strips of flannel (domette) bandage which can be adjusted individually to distribute the weight of the limb evenly. It is important that the

[1] Hugh Owen Thomas, pioneer orthopaedic surgeon designed a double hip splint for fractures of the neck of the femur, and a knee splint for acute infections of hip and ankle. The Thomas knee splint is one of the most frequently used splints 100 years later, mainly for fractured shafts of femur.

knee should be very slightly flexed otherwise the posterior capsule becomes stretched and the joint is subsequently unstable. Foot-drop and contracture of the tendo-achilles is prevented by a footpiece which keeps the ankle at a right angle.

Two different principles are used in the application of the Thomas splint with traction. **Fixed traction** is obtained by tying the traction strapping or pin to the end of the Thomas splint **A** (Figs. 47.9 and 47.10), the ring of which is pushed firmly into the groin and up against the ischial tuberosity. The pull is then exerted by the tension of the cord between the

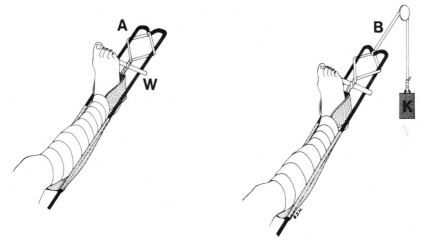

Fig. 47.9 (*Left*). Extension with skin strapping, spreader and cord tied over the end of the Thomas splint, the windlass **W** tightening the cords to produce fixed extension **A** with the top ring of the splint against the grain and ischial tuberosity. (*Right*). Floating extension is applied over a pulley and this draws the ring away from the groin: the **effective** traction **B** is now the floating weight **K**.

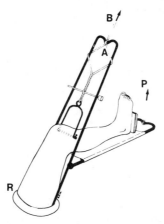

Fig. 47.10 A Steimann pin inserted behind the tibial tubercle provides attachment for a stirrup to which fixed traction **A** is applied; when the splint is suspended from the frame floating traction is applied at **B**. A Pearson bent-knee attachment allows flexion of the knee, to prevent stiffness.

pin (or strapping) and the end of the splint, counter pressure being exerted on the ischial tuberosity through the ring **R** in the groin. Two cords taken from the spreader or pin passing over the sides of the splint are tied together over the end of the splint: a piece of wood or metal—for instance two wooden tongue spatulae—can be inserted and used as a windlass **W** to twist the cords together, thus tightening up the tension to any desired degree of pull. The splint is then slung from an overhead beam and an additional cord and weight attached to the end of the splint at **B** (Fig. 47.9); this further floating traction is added to the original fixed pull. Any elongation in the limb such as occurs when a fracture is pulled out from its overlap position, is shown by the upper ring of the splint being pulled away from the ischial tuberosity, by the floating traction.

If the weight extension is attached direct to the skin-traction straps or skeletal-traction pin without the use of fixed extension, the splint may tend to ride down the limb. Fixed extension with added weight traction is regarded by most surgeons as being preferable as it maintains a more satisfactory position of the splint. Also the surgeon is able to apply fixed traction in the operating theatre, knowing that a fracture, for instance, of the shaft of the femur, is unlikely to be displaced on the journey back to the ward, where the additional floating traction can be attached.

If a Thomas knee splint is used the upper and lower ends of the splint are themselves supported by cord which passes over pulleys on the suspension frame. Appropriate weights are attached to each of these cords so that the leg is balanced at the correct height from the bed (Fig. 47.11). It is best to have two cords from each end of the splints and variation in the weights on the outer and inner cords is used to adjust the degree of rotation of the limb inwards or outwards. If the patient moves up or down the bed, the splinted limb 'floats' with him.

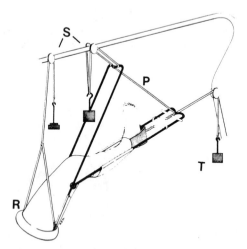

Fig. 47.11   The limb is suspended from a beam with adjustable pulleys (Fig. 47.15). Two cords at each end of the splint are attached to the suspension weights S, about 2 kilograms each. These cords slope towards one another from the two ends and are not vertical. Here the bent-knee attachment is shown carrying the traction and kept at the correct angle with the cord **P**. Subsequently a further cord may be attached and carried over pulleys to the head of the bed, to enable the patient to exercise the leg, by pulling the cord.

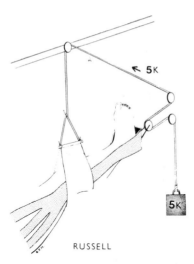

Fig. 47.12 Russell traction. This has no splint but a sling at the knee: it is useful for lower femur fractures and makes use of three pulleys to double the effect of a weight: the cords are arranged as shown: 5-kilogram weight is applied in two directions and the knee in suspension provides the weight.

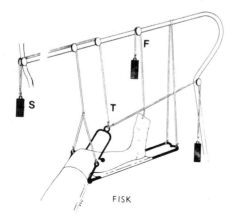

Fig. 47.13 Fisk traction. This uses a modified Thomas splint which has no lower half, but a hinged 'knee' attachment. It has a leather thigh cuff. Note traction is divided into an upward pull and a pull toward the foot of the bed, an effect similar to that of Russell traction. The foot-drop-preventing weight also provides a resistance against which to exercise the foot.

For fractures of the femur immediately above the knee a Böhler-Braun splint may be used with skeletal traction as shown in Fig. 47.14. This splint may also be used when traction is required for fractures of the tibia.

Whatever form of traction is used, the apparatus requires daily attention to adjustment of cords and weights to ensure that the limb is maintained in exactly the correct position in the splint.

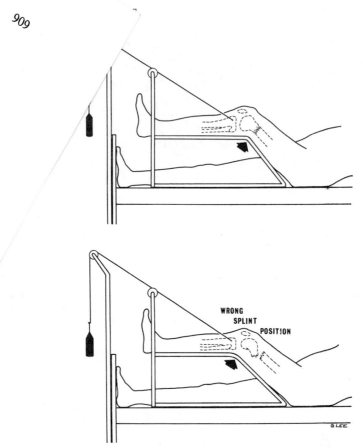

Fig. 47.14 The Böhler-Braun splint (page 906) with pulley attachments is used in the treatment of fractures of the lower third of the femur as shown. The essential nursing point is that the splint must be high to maintain the angle at the point of fracture; if this position is not retained the fracture will re-dislocate.

The salient features of a limb extension apparatus and its management provide that:

(*a*) It should be effective in providing the right amount of pull.

(*b*) The limb is kept in position on the splint, and the splint is kept in the correct position on the bed. With all lower limb traction, the foot of the bed is raised to prevent the patient being pulled down the bed. The weight of the body acts as counter traction.

(*c*) As far as possible the patient is able to move his other limbs and lift himself clear of the bed by a monkey chain.

(*d*) The whole apparatus looks tidy. Loose ends of cord are rolled up and tied. Weight bags or shot cans are adjusted to the correct height so that they swing clear of the bed. The foot-piece is kept in correct position and a cover of gamgee tissue is cut to go over the exposed upper surface of the limb, as a 'blanket'.

(*e*) Care is taken to check the position of splints, cords, and weights after attention to the patient's toilet or the use of bedpans.

(*f*) Toe (or finger) movement and circulation must be checked repeatedly during the day and during the night. Any complaint of pain or of pressure on some point on the limb must be investigated immediately. Inability to move the toes or fingers is a danger signal.

There are many methods of suspending and applying traction to an injured leg. The particular method chosen depends to a large extent on the apparatus available. Commonly used methods are described in Figs. 47.9–47.14.

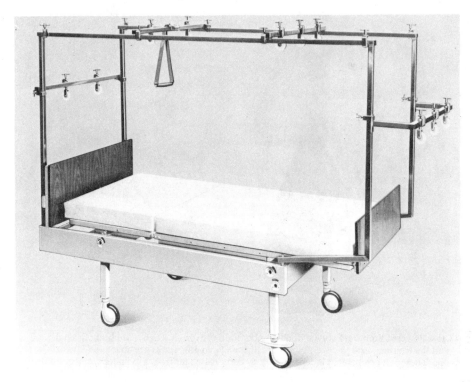

Fig. 47.15 Ellison Manulift bed with complete orthopaedic frame for extensions. This bed provides variable height and tilt. (George Ellison Ltd.)

Traction is rarely required for the upper limb. If it should be necessary, skin traction is used from the forearm. Occasionally extension is applied by means of special 'pulp pins' inserted through the pulp of the finger or through the terminal phalanx. Traction on the thumb or an individual finger for metacarpal fractures is obtained by incorporating the Böhler finger splint in a plaster cast, and using skin strapping.

Amputation

A child may be born with 'congenital amputation' of one or more limbs: the arm, forearm or leg resembles a surgical amputation stump covered with skin, sometimes with a primitive toe or finger in the tip. There is nothing to do for such cases except to provide an artificial limb as the child grows. Absence of a limb is **amelia**. Thalidomide, a tranquilliser drug given to relieve the vomiting and distress of early pregnancy, interfered with limb growth and resulted in the birth of thousands of babies with one, two, three or even four limbs absent or grossly deformed (Fig. 7.1). This accentuation of an age-long problem has stimulated interest in the provision of power-operated prostheses (Fig. 47.16).

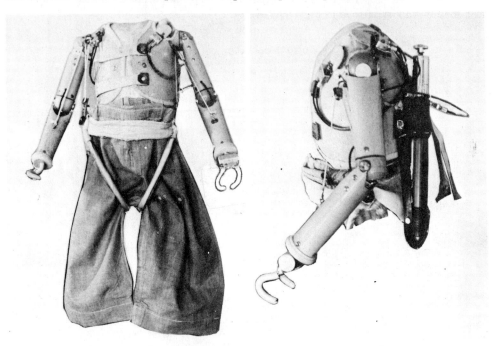

Fig. 47.16   Powered limb. Jacket type double upper limb prosthesis. (*Left*). Method of attachment to the trunk, and the trousers used to cover 2 limb prostheses when all 4 limbs are affected. (*Right*). The 2 arms and hooks. These can be operated independently by compressed air from a cylinder attached to the jacket. The valves may be worked by shoulder movement, or the primitive digits sometimes found in the shoulder region.

In young children, amputation may be required for injury or in cases of paraplegia (from spina bifida, page 869) when a paralysed limb is severely deformed or infected. In the active older age groups, amputation may be called for after crushing injuries or gunshot wounds. In patients in the upper age groups, arterial disease produces gangrene which frequently necessitates amputation of the leg below the knee or in the mid-thigh.

Emergency amputation, performed because a limb is too severely damaged for repair to be reasonable, may be performed by the 'guillotine' method. The skin, muscle and bone are all divided at the same level. No skin flaps are formed to cover the exposed end of the limb. Skin traction is usually attached to the skin on the stump to prevent it retracting. Subsequently when the risk of infection has passed and the patient's general condition has improved re-amputation takes place with the fashioning of a skin-covered stump of correct length for the fitting of an artificial limb.

In other cases, amputation is planned and performed in such a way that the bone end is adequately covered with skin, and the muscle and fascia is closed to prevent bone becoming adherent to the scar.

Amputations are performed usually under general anaesthesia and with the use of a tourniquet applied over a pad at the highest convenient point on the limb.

Levels of amputation

When deciding at what point to divide the bone the surgeon takes into account the likely function of the remaining portion of the limb. In general every little bit of finger or thumb that can be left is useful. For instance if the index finger is removed the head of the first metacarpal with its ugly protuberance gets in the way of useful hand movement, so this is removed. In the upper limb where there is no weight-bearing, the surgeon endeavours to leave as much length as possible as a short stump of forearm or upper arm is useful to work the prosthesis (artificial limb).

On the lower limb weight-bearing is a major consideration. Amputation stumps can be either end weight-bearing or non-weight-bearing. In the latter the weight has to be taken on the ischial tuberosity as with a caliper, or through a gaiter around the limb well above the end of the amputation stump.

In addition to considering the useful length of a limb and the weight-bearing possibility, the surgeon has to take into account the blood supply of the skin. In arterial disease for which many lower limbs have to be amputated, the skin nutrition is poor and the level of the amputation has to be sufficiently high to ensure good nutrition to the stump. In children whose limbs continue to grow after an amputation re-amputation may be necessary as the bone may grow faster than the skin overlying the stump. Sometimes infection occurs in the bone end and this requires re-amputation at a higher level.

In the upper limb, if the hand has to be removed completely or has already been removed in the accident and the forearm stump has healed, operation may be performed to separate the radius and ulna so that it forms a fork-like grip. In the lower limb the common levels of amputation are:

1. Immediately above the ankle—a **Syme's amputation**—in which the thick skin at the back of the heel is used on the end of the stump as a weight-bearing pad. With this amputation the patient is able to walk about without an artificial limb for short distances, in the bedroom and bathroom for instance. This is a useful amputation if the foot has been badly deformed and the patient can then wear a lightweight artificial foot with suitable looking shoes.

2. The most common form of lower limb amputation is the '**below knee**' where 15–20 cm of the tibia are left below the knee joint. The weight is taken then on the tibial tuberosities and the artificial limb grips the thigh so that no shoulder straps are necessary. For instance, patients with double below-knee amputations do extremely well and have very good function.

3. If it is not possible to do a below-knee amputation because of inadequate blood supply or injury, the operation may be performed **through the knee joint** and a large anterior skin flap taken back over the end of the femur. The patella becomes attached to the end of the bone and this again is a weight-bearing stump.

4. Above the knee the common site of amputation is the '**mid thigh**'. The patient then

wears an artificial limb with a hinged knee which he can lock at will. Shoulder straps are usually necessary.

5. If there is a growth in the femur, operation is performed through the hip joint— 'disarticulation'. The patient then has a flat sloping side to the pelvis which, as it were, sits in the artificial limb on that side.

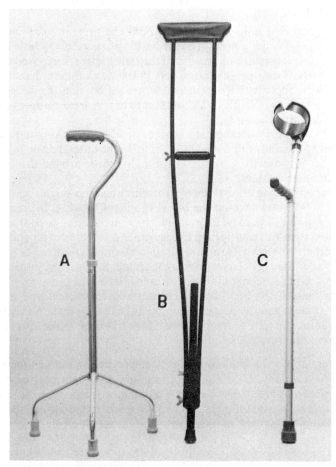

Fig. 47.17 Walking aids. **A. Quadruped crutch** to assist balance (e.g. stroke patients). **B. Axillary crutch** for leg amputees or patients unable to use forearms for weight bearing. **C. Elbow crutch**—weight taken on hand with arm steadied in ring.

Occasionally, due to the presence of malignant disease in the arm, **'fore-quarter' amputation** is called for. The whole upper limb including the scapula and part of the clavicle is removed together with the shoulder girdle muscles. The subclavian artery is tied at the beginning of the operation as clearly no tourniquet can be used. Blood transfusion is a necessity.

Similarly for extensive malignant disease in the thigh or in the region of the hip joint, **'hind-quarter' amputation** is necessary and this includes removal of half the pelvis. The common iliac artery is exposed by abdominal operation and tied or compressed to control blood loss.

Except in grave emergencies, it is usual for surgeons to obtain the opinion of a colleague before deciding upon an amputation.

Nursing care

The patient is usually informed of the surgeon's intention but he may withhold this knowledge from elderly people who are very ill with gangrene and require a life-saving

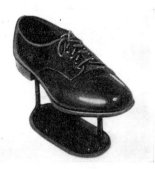

Fig. 47.18 Patten fitted to shoe to compensate for loss of leg length, or more often to lengthen the good leg so that an injured leg, in splint or plaster, clears the ground when the patient walks with crutches. (Pryor and Howard.)

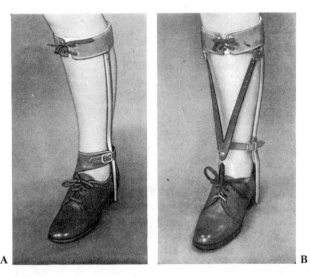

Fig. 47.19 (A) Outside iron and T-strap for ankle weakness. (B) The same with a 'toe-raising' spring to prevent the foot dropping after poliomyelitis affecting the anterior leg muscles. (Pryor and Howard.)

amputation. Care must be taken in such cases, as in those following injury, that the patient is not made aware of his loss by some careless reference by the nurse. Following amputation, the patient still feels the limb and frequently complains of pain in the toes or fingers which have been removed. The severed nerve stumps send impulses of pain and other sensation which the brain interprets as coming from the tissues which have gone. After amputation of the lower limb, bedclothes may be arranged in such a way that the patient cannot see the amputation stump.

The care of the stump

When sepsis was common following injury or operation, secondary haemorrhage was also common and two rules followed as tradition. The first was that a tourniquet must be kept immediately available, usually fixed to the foot of the bed where it can be seen by all the staff, and placed in such a position that it is not constantly visible to the patient as a warning of what might happen. This practice has largely been abandoned and is not routine, but may be requested particularly by a surgeon if there is a special risk. The second tradition is that the bandaged stump must never be covered by bedclothes; any staining of the dressing with blood is then at once visible to the nursing staff. A bed cradle is used with envelope-end type of bedclothing so that the limb can be seen from the end of the bed.

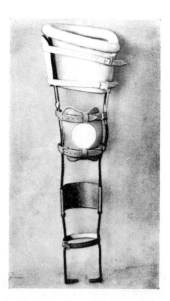

Fig. 47.20 A weight-bearing caliper. The patient 'sits' on the ring: the lower end pegs into sockets in the heel of the boot. The length is adjusted so that the ischial tuberosity takes the weight on the top ring, thus relieving the knee, a healing femur fracture or diseased hip joint. (Pryor and Howard.)

Although secondary haemorrhage is now extremely rare, these precautions are wise and serve as a constant reminder that fatal haemorrhage may occur from any amputation stump.

In the guillotine type of amputation a non-adherent dressing is placed over the raw surface with a light pad and crepe bandage. Where skin flaps have been sutured in the ordinary amputation method, the wound is usually drained for 48 hours by a strip of corrugated rubber or latex tube which allows the escape of serum and blood coming chiefly from the cut muscle surface.

After removal of the drainage tube, to prevent oedema of the skin flaps and to produce a correctly tapered stump which is most suitable for the fitting of an artificial limb, a pressure bandage is used to exert even compression, particularly over the lowest few inches of the stump.

For a few days following operation a leg stump is supported on a pillow. As soon as the pain has passed off the pillow must be removed in order to prevent flexion contracture of the hip and ensure maximum possible activity to restore function and prevent muscles from wasting. Occasionally there are spontaneous spasmodic movements of the limbs. This disturbs the patient. In such circumstances the thigh may be controlled to some extent by placing a roller towel or folded pillowcase over it, anchored at the side by sandbags.

When the wound has healed soundly, intensive stump exercises begin in order to develop the remaining muscles on which the patient is dependent for the satisfactory manipulation of the prosthesis.

An interval of 3 months is usually required before the stump is ready for the fitting of an artificial limb.

Complications of amputation. Apart from haemorrhage and infection, certain delayed complications may arise which may add to the patient's disability and prevent the use of an artificial limb.

The skin may become adherent to bone. It is then thin and unstable and may break down under pressure from the artificial limb. Re-amputation at a slightly higher level is sometimes required.

Severe pain may be experienced from the development of buds at the ends of the nerves in the stump (**neuroma**). Excision of the nerve ends does not always cure the pain. The term 'phantom limb' is used to describe abnormal sensations which the patient suffers, giving him the impression that the limb is still present, and producing pain.

These complications apply equally to the amputation of a finger as to the amputation of the thigh.

The artificial limb

With planned amputations where the patient is aware of what is necessary, the usual arrangement is for the patient to be seen at the limb-fitting centre before operation in order that measurements can be taken and a limb of the correct design planned. This is not always possible and frequently a lower limb amputee is allowed a pylon artificial limb—a wooden stalk with a 'bucket' on the top—until the fully formed prosthesis is available.

Fractures

Orthodox definitions of fractures are used to describe the type, severity and complications.

Closed (simple) fracture. There are two bone fragments. No other structures are involved except the bone and surrounding muscle. This is the most common form of fracture.

Open (compound) fracture. This is similar to a simple closed fracture but the site of bone injury communicates with the surface of the body through a skin wound or opening into a body cavity such as the thorax. Most fractures of the jaw are compound. The significance of this communication is that the fracture site is potentially infected by the entry of organisms from the skin, or by contamination carried in on such foreign bodies as bullets or bits of bomb splinter. A fracture may be compound from 'within-out'—that is, one of the bone ends has pierced the skin. This type of fracture is less likely to be infected than one which is compound from 'without-in' by the penetration of some missile or sharp instrument.

Comminuted fracture. There are more than two bone fragments. Such a fracture is more difficult to reduce and to keep in correct position as there is unlikely to be an accurate fit between the broken ends of the bone.

Complicated fracture. This term indicates that some other important structure has been damaged. This may be a peripheral nerve or indeed the spinal cord in a fracture of the vertebral column. A main vessel may be damaged or the fracture may extend into a joint. Most fractures of the skull are complicated (page 857).

Greenstick fracture. This describes accurately the nature of the injury. The bone is partly fractured and partly bent. A greenstick fracture only affects the bones of the young and there is no complete separation of the two fragments. Greenstick fractures heal rapidly and rarely require an anaesthetic for their reduction.

Impacted fracture. The bone fragments are jammed into one another and traction may be necessary to disimpact the fracture before setting it in the correct position. A **crush** fracture of a vertebra is one form of impaction, in which the body of the vertebra is compressed.

Fissure fracture. This term is used to indicate a crack without any displacement of the bone. A fissure fracture occurs in the patella, in the skull, and sometimes in the long bones, particularly in elderly people whose bones are more frail. This type of fracture occurring in the limb bones is sometimes referred to as a **stress fracture.**

Pathological fracture. If a bone is weakened by disease or previous injury, it may break as the result of a trivial accident or from a strain which would quite easily be borne by a healthy bone. The most common cause of pathological fracture is a bone cyst or secondary malignant tumour from carcinoma of the breast, liver or alimentary tract. The development of a pathological fracture may be the first symptom of such malignant disease.

In patients whose limbs are paralysed, the muscle wasting results in osteoporosis—or failure of the bones to become really hard; fractures occur with trivial strain. In such patients, though there may be no pain and therefore no spasm or deformity, the fracture may go unnoticed until a hard lump is found due to callus formation which fortunately in these conditions is abnormally rapid (Fig. 47.22).

Repair of fractures

Healing of fractures takes place by the formation of a temporary callus on the outside of the bone followed by subsequent internal callus in the marrow cavity. Finally there is

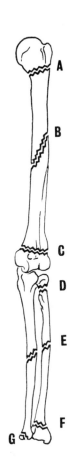

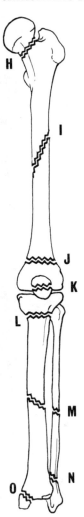

Fig. 47.21

(*Left*) Upper limb fractures. **A.** Neck of humerus—impacted. **B.** Shaft of humerus—spiral; radial nerve in danger. **C** Supracondylar humerus (common in children); median and ulnar nerves and brachial artery in danger. **D.** Neck or head of radius—usually excised. **E.** Ulna and radius—forearm; danger of cross union between the two bones. **F, G.** Colles' fracture.

(*Right*) Lower limb fractures. **H.** Neck of femur —impacted; treated with pin or excision of head and total hip joint replacement. **I.** Shaft of femur—traction; frequently Kuntscher nail (Fig. 47.23). **J.** Supracondylar—skeletal traction and Böhler frame (Fig. 47.14). Popliteal artery in danger. **K.** Patella—if transverse, usually wired; if comminuted, excised. **L.** 'Bumper' fracture of tibia—knee joint often involved. **M.** Tibia and fibula—often screwed or plated. **O, N.** Pott's fracture—dislocation of ankle.

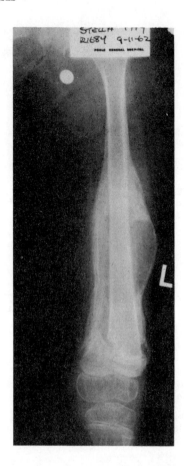

Fig. 47.22   Pathological fracture of femur in paraplegia. Note the massive formation of callus.

complete fusion of the bone ends. Normal **union** is dependent on the patient's general health, age, site of the fracture and the efficiency with which it has been treated. Certain factors delay union: these are infection, imperfect reduction, inadequate immobilisation, malnutrition, anaemia and intercurrent infection such as tuberculosis or syphilis. **Delayed union** indicates that the fracture has not united after the period which is regarded as the usual healing time for that particular site of fracture.

Mal-union indicates that union has occurred in a faulty position.

Non-union or **fibrous union** indicates that there is still movement between the fragments. Movement produces pain in some cases. The factors which produce non-union are the same as those leading to delayed union. Non-union is frequently treated by excision of the fibrous tissue between the bone ends and by bone grafting.

Minimum times for healing in healthy adults are:

	Weeks
Phalanx, metacarpal and metatarsal	2
Forearm	4
Humerus	6
Tibia and fibula	8
Femur	12

In children the time of immobilisation in plaster is frequently less than this period and in elderly people it is considerably greater. Many other factors which are known to be present and which may delay union must be taken into account when assessing the total period of disability of the patient.

It is natural that the patient admitted to hospital with a fracture is anxious to have an approximate estimate of his period of disability, and in most cases with manual workers it can be assumed that at least twice the above period is necessary before work can be resumed.

Treatment of fractures

The stages in the management of a case of fracture are:

(a) first aid,

(b) reduction of the deformity,

(c) maintenance of the corrected position during the period of healing, by external splint or internal splint (bone nail or plate),

(d) restoration of function.

Throughout the whole duration of treatment, attention has to be paid to the patient's general condition.

First aid. The most important general principle is the prevention of unnecessary movement, since movement at the fracture site causes further damage, produces pain and aggravates shock. There is no doubt that the handling of casualties by trained first-aid teams greatly diminishes the complications which arise, in comparison with those occurring in patients who are incorrectly handled immediately after an accident. Fractures of the upper limb are immobilised by tying the arm to the patient's trunk. Fractures of the lower limb are fixed by tying the legs together above and below the knees. The use of the Thomas knee splint for fractures of the femur is only recommended if those responsible for its application are really familiar with the principles involved and are able to put traction on the leg by means of a clove hitch bandage round the ankle. Unless the first-aid crew is really familiar with the handling of injured persons much unnecessary movement and suffering may be produced by attempts to use this splint.

No attempt should be made to manipulate the limb in order that projecting bone ends may be drawn back inside. A tourniquet should not be applied merely because a fracture is compound, since the bleeding can nearly always be controlled by a pad and bandage firmly applied over the wound.

If a fracture of the spine is suspected in the cervical region, the patient should remain flat on his back with a pillow in the hollow of the neck so that the head is extended. Fracture of the spine in other regions is best managed with the patient lying on his face, with pillows placed under the upper chest. Fractures of the spine are often associated with head injuries and if a patient is unconscious he should be placed on his face with his head turned to one side with a small support under the forehead.

Reduction of the fracture. If there is only slight displacement at the site of fracture, no formal reduction is necessary.

The majority of fractures require manipulation under anaesthetic or gradual correction of the deformity by limb traction. During the manipulation by the surgeon, traction in the long axis of the limb is applied by an assistant or by the surgeon himself, the position being checked from time to time by x-ray screening or photographs.

Fractures of the femur and lower leg are sometimes treated immediately by traction, no manipulation being required. Methods of applying traction have already been described.

The initial reduction may be performed under local anaesthesia, procaine or some allied substance being injected into the fracture haematoma. Alternatively brachial plexus block for the upper limb, or general anaesthesia for the lower limb, may be preferred.

After a patient has been admitted suffering from injury of any type, no food or drink should be given until specific permission has been obtained from the medical officer in charge. If it is likely that a general anaesthetic may be required within 4 hours, then nothing will be allowed by mouth. If the patient is known to have had a recent meal and general anaesthesia is required, the stomach should be washed out by means of a tube unless the operation can be deferred beyond this 4-hour period.

In preparation for the reduction, as much of the patient's clothing as possible should be removed without disturbing the fracture site. This may necessitate cutting certain articles of apparel, and whenever possible, seams should be opened so that the garments can be repaired. It is unlikely that any degree of skin preparation will be demanded until the patient has been anaesthetised.

During the 'undressing' stage the nurse must inspect the patient thoroughly for bruises and any signs of injury other than those which have been noted initially by the medical staff. It is particularly important to look for evidence of bruising over the spine or in the loins. The development of bruising on subsequent days must also be reported.

During the period of waiting, observation must be kept for any change in circulation in the fingers or toes due to the development of swelling and haematoma at the site of fracture. The injured limb should be elevated immediately after admission and this simple measure may contribute greatly to the patient's recovery.

It is said that every fracture of a major bone results in loss into the tissues of 300–500 ml of blood. A patient with several fractures has therefore suffered a severe loss of blood from the circulation and blood transfusion will be required, though he may have no external wounds.

Maintenance of corrected position. Once the fracture has been reduced, in the majority of cases a limb is treated in a plaster-of-Paris cast. If there has been a compound fracture and the injured tissues have been excised and the wound sutured, the plaster cast is *always* split, and anti-tetanus serum and gas gangrene serum is given routinely.

X-ray photographs are again taken after the plaster is complete.

Steel pins may be incorporated in the plaster, these passing through the bone to fix it in position. Traction may be used in addition to plaster.

Fractures at certain sites are known to be particularly unstable and are treated initially by open operation. This is not necessarily performed on the day of admission if the fracture is not compound; time is allowed for skin preparation. At operation, any tissue, such as muscle, which has become entangled between the fragments of the fractured bone, is excised and the bone ends placed in complete and accurate apposition. Some form of internal splintage is then used. In the case of the patella the fragments may be wired together. Bones of the forearm may be splinted by screwing **vitallium metal plates** across the fracture site, and other bones such as the femur and humerus are sometimes splinted by a large spike (**intramedullary nail**) inserted into the marrow cavity through a hole in the cortex (Fig. 47.23). Fractures of the neck of the femur are frequently treated by a special nail passed through the great trochanter, or the head and neck of the femur may be removed and replaced by a new socket and prosthesis (page 930).

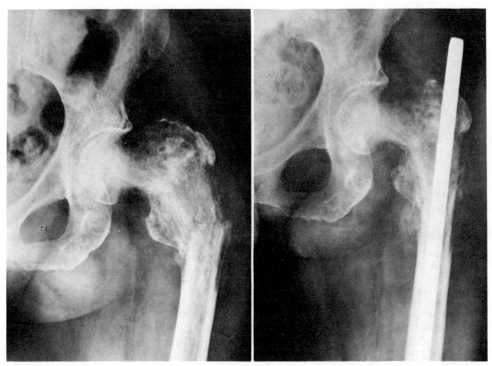

Fig. 47.23 (*Left*) Pathological fracture (due to growth) of the upper end of the femur. (*Right*) The fracture has been reduced and splinted internally with an intramedullary (Kuntscher) nail.

In all these cases, the nursing principles are identical. The limb still requires immobilisation and the metallic splint cannot be relied on to produce complete protection of the fracture during healing. It does however prevent re-displacement of the fragments, and permits much earlier mobility.

After operation, watch must be kept for the development of infection, for haemorrhage from the wound, or for increasing swelling adding to impairment of the limb circulation (page 896).

After reduction of a fracture, particular care must be taken while the patient is recovering from general anaesthesia. In the semiconscious state he may attempt to get free from his traction apparatus or plaster.

Restoration of function. The word 'rehabilitation' is used to describe the continuous process whereby a patient is restored to his normal state of health and activity during a period of illness. It is correctly said that rehabilitation starts from the moment of injury. By this is meant that every effort must be made, right from the beginning to maintain the patient's general fitness. He must be made to use all those parts of his body that are not injured, and even in an injured limb muscles must be kept as active as possible in readiness for the time when the splints are discarded and joint movement begins. The general principles have already been discussed. Particular attention must be paid to respiratory movement to prevent the development of chest complications. Patients are encouraged to help themselves as much as possible.

One of the principal difficulties of rehabilitation is with the patient who is discharged from hospital still wearing a plaster cast, or who is treated purely as an out-patient. The difficulty of getting to and from hospital frequently outweighs the advantage of attending for supervised exercises. Before such patients leave hospital, really adequate instructions must be given concerning the activity which they are expected to undertake while at home. Immediately before discharge the plaster must be inspected for cracks or soft places and specific instructions must be given to report back to hospital if severe pain develops under the plaster or if there is any swelling, blueness, or loss of sensation of the fingers or toes.

Most large hospitals run a specially organised out-patient clinic—**the fracture clinic**—so that all patients wearing plasters are seen at regular intervals of 2, 3 or 4 weeks depending on the stage of their disability. The majority of plaster-changes are undertaken in the out-patient department but occasionally patients have to be admitted for 48 hours. Change of a plaster jacket necessitates detention in hospital for at least 2 days to make certain that the plaster is dry, hard and comfortable.

Complications of fractures

Many of the late complications of fractures are due to inefficient treatment. At the time of injury, however, major nerves may be damaged, main arteries may be bruised or severed, and tendons torn. If a fracture enters a joint there is almost always subsequent limitation of movement and perhaps later chronic arthritis—post-traumatic osteoarthritis. Nerves may also become involved in callus or by being stretched around a deformity. Severe fractures complicated by nerve injuries sometimes result in a useless and painful limb and amputation is required.

When a bone is broken accidentally or by operation droplets of fat from the marrow may pass into the circulation producing **'fat embolism'**. This is sometimes fatal.

Occasionally if union is delayed, open operation and bone grafting is required. Compound fractures of the tibia and fibula are sometimes complicated by the development of a chronic ulcer over the subcutaneous surface of the tibia, and skin grafting is required. This is usually achieved by the cross-leg flap, a pedicle graft being used from the opposite calf (page 952).

The particular problems of spinal fractures

Involvement of the spinal cord in fractures of the vertebral column has been described on page 872. Major fractures of the spine usually occur from forced flexion injuries which crush the vertebral bodies. Falling on the feet from a considerable height or 'run over' injuries in road accidents cause this type of lesion. Widespread complications arise from involvement of the nervous system (page 874): these may be transient and in a matter of days there may be no residual weakness or interference of vital functions. In such cases, involving the thoracic spine, the patient is mobilized, wearing a plaster jacket. If the lumbar spine or pelvis are fractured, more prolonged bed rest may be needed. Fractures of the cervical spine may require traction, operation and bone grafting.

The nursing problems may be those of the paraplegic patient. The complications or involvement of the nervous system and other injuries such as spleen or kidney damage usually determine the line of management.

Infection of bone

Infection arising from sepsis elsewhere in the body (e.g. boil, pneumonia) may enter a bone from the blood stream. It settles usually at the growing end of a bone in the marrow spaces, setting up **osteomyelitis**. Bone infection may also occur from a compound fracture or from an open wound which exposes bone. **Acute osteomyelitis** is accompanied by severe pain and toxaemia and is in fact usually part of a septicaemic condition. The inflammatory reaction in the rigid bone leads to its death from pressure and thrombosis of its blood vessels. Dead bone (**sequestrum**) has to be removed by surgical operation, or in chronic cases may be extruded through a sinus. Infection may spread to, or arise in, the periosteal layer, stripping away the membrane and forming a **subperiosteal abscess**. The raised periosteum produces a 'shell' of new bone around the old which is thus increased in girth. If the inner bone is dead, the new shell is described as the **involucrum**.

The most common acute infections are by pyogenic organisms, especially staphylococcus aureus.

Chronic osteomyelitis sometimes ensues if treatment has been inadequate. Sinuses develop between the bone and the skin. Chronic sepsis leads to general toxaemia, anaemia and amyloid disease.

Tuberculosis affects both synovial membrane and bone, starting usually in the end of the bone; in countries where treatment is insufficient sinuses develop between bone and skin and secondary infection with pyogenic organisms ensues.

Septic arthritis. A joint may become infected in the same way as bone, by blood stream infection, direct spread from disease in neighbouring bone, or from open wound penetrating into the joint. Mild infection (**synovitis**) produces a joint effusion, pain and diminished movement. If infection proceeds, pus forms within the joint (**suppurative arthritis**): the joint surfaces may then be destroyed, leading to fixation of the joint (**ankylosis**) by adhesion between the adjacent bone surfaces.

The treatment of acute bone or joint infection follows the basic principles of treatment in all infective lesions. There are four major considerations, in order of urgency:

(a) antibiotic and sulphonamide therapy,
(b) general anti-infective measures—fluid balance, nutrition, relief of pain,

(c) local treatment—splintage, elevation of a limb, aspiration for drainage of abscesses, or open operation on the bone,

(d) management of complications—anaemia, septicaemia, or chronic osteitis.

Intensive antibiotic treatment is usually effective and, if the condition is detected soon after its onset, no surgical measures are required. If aspiration of abscess or open operation on the bone is needed, there may be insufficient time for more than one skin preparation. Splintage is usually by plaster cast. Post-operative dressings are required if the wound has been left unsutured. Drainage tubes and packing are removed by gradual withdrawal, allowing the abscess cavity to heal by filling with granulation tissue. If a wound has been packed, the first dressing and change of plaster is usually carried out under anaesthesia, by the surgeon. Subsequent dressings are done at infrequent intervals, the limb being totally enclosed in plaster on each occasion, until the wound has healed. In cases where an open operation has been performed and the wound left open, a second operation may be undertaken when the critical period of acute infection has passed, and the wound is then sutured to accelerate healing (**delayed primary suture**).

During the acute recovery periods, the urine must be tested weekly for albumin. Four-hourly temperature records must be maintained. A high-calorie diet is needed on account of infection.

Occasionally amputation is required for chronic osteomyelitis.

Chronic arthritis

There are two forms of chronic arthritis. The first—**rheumatoid**—is a generalised disease usually affecting the small joints, especially of the hands and feet. This condition is accompanied by considerable constitutional disturbance, periarticular thickening and pain. It is a slowly progressive disease which may arise in childhood in an acute form. In adults it is commoner in women than in men. In the acute phases, splints, heat and cortisone are used with drugs to relieve pain. In the 'quiet' chronic phase various surgical procedures are used to fix joints which are painful, or to increase the mobility of other joints. Rheumatoid arthritis is a very crippling disease and accounts for a great many of the home-bound elderly disabled persons for whom supportive welfare services are required. Great strides have been made in surgical treatment. In the knee, the whole affected synovial membrane may be removed and excellent pain-free movement restored. Stiffened crippled fingers may now be treated by cutting out the joints and inserting an elastic 'springy' joint, covered with silicone rubber which produces no reaction in the surrounding tissues.

Osteoarthritis is quite a different condition and is degenerative in nature, affecting usually the large weight-bearing joints and the spine. It is essentially a 'wear and tear' disease which develops particularly in joints that have been injured, or are the subject of particularly heavy strain. Sometimes only one joint such as a hip is affected; the bone becomes roughened and the synovial membrane thick. Sometimes infection plays a part in the development of osteoarthritis but frequently no trace of infection, either locally in the joint, or elsewhere in the body can be found. Fibrous tissues and new bone form around the weight-bearing surfaces of the joint and gradually movement becomes limited. Pain leads to further disuse and the wasting of the muscles which in turn increases the strain on the joint. If the condition progresses the joint surfaces become so destroyed that they fuse and bony ankylosis occurs.

Treatment is directed to maintaining mobility, building up the muscles and relieving pain. The condition is almost universal in the spines of old people and is extremely common in the knees, particularly in patients who are overweight. When the condition occurs in the hip it leads to adduction and flexion deformity and difficulty in walking. Surgical procedures are undertaken to remove the arthritic bone surfaces and create a new joint, or to improve the angle of the joint for weight-bearing (page 929).

It is important for nurses to realise that many patients admitted for the treatment of other conditions, suffer from arthritis which may be aggravated by acute illness, inconsiderate handling, or unsuitable hospital beds and fireside chairs. Deterioration of this arthritic condition may well prolong convalescence.

Miscellaneous orthopaedic procedures

Muscle and tendon repair. Tendons, particularly those of the wrist and fingers, are severed by incised wounds. Violent force sometimes avulses a tendon, such as the patellar tendon or Achilles tendon, from its bony attachment. The larger tendons are repaired by direct suture of the torn ends. For the finger tendons special techniques are employed to guard against adhesions between the tendons and the sheaths through which they slide.

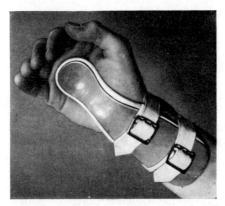

Fig. 47.24 Simple cock-up wrist splint. (Pryor and Howard.)

Stainless steel sutures are used, inserted in such a way that they can be pulled out through the skin when the tendons have united. Occasionally **tendon grafts** are necessary to replace lengths of important tendon which have been injured. Less important tendons, such as that of palmaris longus on the front of the wrist, are used to provide the graft.

From the nursing point of view, tendon injuries are treated in the same way as fractures. The limb is immobilised usually in plaster, and the limb elevated, only such movements being encouraged as are specifically ordered by the surgeon (page 901).

Tendon transplantation is also used in the treatment of paralysis, especially of the foot. After poliomyelitis, if there is severe foot-drop and the peroneal muscles are active, the lower attachment of the peroneal tendons may be transferred to the attachment of the anterior tibial muscles on the inner side of the foot. Similarly in hands crippled by leprosy tendon grafts are used to connect the muscles of the forearm to the bones of the fingers in order to restore the grip when the lumbrical muscles have wasted. Again, as with tendon injuries, a period of immobilisation is required followed by a period of rehabilitation.

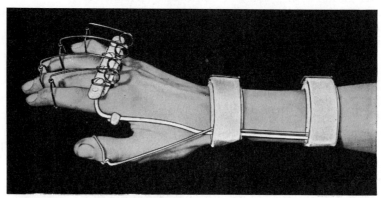

Fig. 47.25   An example of a special splint for wrist and fingers to prevent flexion contractures, 'clawing' in arthritis or paralysis. (Pryor and Howard.)

Bone grafting. Pieces of bone are used as internal splints for un-united fractures, in the treatment of recurrent dislocations of joints or to produce **arthrodesis** (artificial stiffness) of joints. The graft is usually taken from the tibia by means of a twin-blade motor saw and blocks of bone several centimetres long are inlaid into the length of a fractured femur or other bone which has not united. Similarly bone-graft blocks are employed to fuse several vertebrae together in the late treatment of tuberculous disease or chronic strain of the back. Smaller pieces of bone, **bone chips**, are occasionally used to fill cavities which have been left after the removal of bone tumours or cysts. Grafts of this type are normally taken from the iliac crest.

The pre- and post-operative nursing care involves attention to the donor site as well as to the grafted area. Full skin preparation is required for both areas and the donor limb is treated post-operatively as any other injured limb. The grafted site is immobilised in plaster for several weeks in order that the implanted bone may be completely incorporated in the surrounding structures. Cut bone bleeds very profusely and a haematoma may arise from the donor site unless a firm pressure dressing is maintained after operation. The principal risk in bone grafting is infection, but this has been almost entirely eliminated since the introduction of antibiotics. More massive grafting is therefore possible with very little risk of failure. When the iliac crest is the donor site, watch must be kept for abdominal distension and ileus due to haemorrhage spreading behind the peritoneum from the area of the donor site.

Meniscectomy. The semilunar cartilages in the knee are frequently torn by a twisting type of injury while the limb is weight-bearing. A damaged cartilage usually requires removal because it leads to sudden and unexpected locking of joint movement which prevents the patient walking and which is accompanied by severe synovitis and effusion into the joint. Opening a joint is *arthrotomy*.

Operation is preceded by a 2-day skin preparation with a chosen antiseptic. Quadriceps exercises are given before operation and are resumed immediately the patient regains consciousness. The patient is usually allowed out of bed in a wheelchair or on crutches after 4 or 5 days and commences weight-bearing when the effusion in the joint has subsided. The nursing care is again that of an injured limb, particular attention being paid to circulation, toe movements and quadriceps exercises.

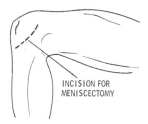

INCISION FOR
MENISCECTOMY

Fig. 47.26 Arthrotomy by oblique incision over medial side of knee joint commonly used for operations on the knee cartilage (meniscus).

Synovectomy. In certain types of rheumatoid arthritis the inflamed synovial membrane lining the joint is completely removed. This restores function to joints which have lost their movement due to the thickening of these tissues.

Osteotomy is the division of a bone by open operation, thus creating a surgical fracture. It is used in the correction of severe deformities, particularly in the management of the osteoarthritic hip where the femur has become severely adducted. The bone is divided below the great trochanter and allowed to unite in the abducted position in which the deformity is far less of a disability to the patient. The hip requires immobilisation in plaster for 3 months following such an operation. Osteotomy is sometimes combined with the insertion of a bone graft. Arthroplasty (see below) is more commonly chosen as the best treatment for the arthritic hip.

Arthrodesis. A joint which is stiff from arthritis is frequently painful. If the range of movement is not sufficient to be really useful, pain is eliminated by fixing the joint completely. What remains of the articular surface of each bone is removed and the two bones fixed together by metal pins, plates or bone grafts. Immobilisation as for fractures is required after operation.

Arthroplasty. This is a refashioning procedure most commonly applied to the hip, in the treatment of osteoarthritis. In certain selected cases, the hip joint is opened by operation, the head of the femur removed, the acetabulum reamed out into a smooth hollow once more, and a metal or plastic artificial head fitted to the femur. Various methods have been used and sometimes a metal cup is placed between the head of the femur and the acetabulum (**cup arthroplasty**).

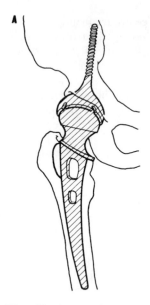

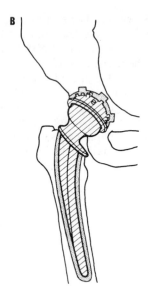

A. Ring. Metal to metal; no cement; short neck; lag screw up into ilium taking vertical stress.

B. McKee-Farrer. Metal to metal; cup carries studs which lock it into the reamed-out acetabulum; bone cement to shaft.

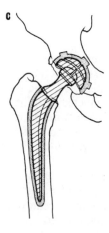

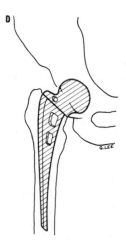

C. Charnley. Metal to plastic; small head with low friction polypropylene cup.

D. Austin Moore. Metal to bone; the acetabulum is reamed out to take a large head.

Fig. 47.27   Total hip replacement.

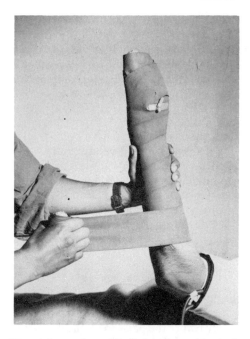

Fig. 47.28 Application of Esmarch tourniquet. The limb is elevated for 1 minute: the sphygmomanometer cuff is then fixed over a cloth pad: the elastic rubber bandage is applied from finger tips to just below the elbow, giving two pulls for each turn and overlapping the bandage: the cuff is inflated to 200 mm mercury and a pressure forceps clipped on the inflation tube at the cuff to avoid accidental deflation. The rubber bandage is unwound, and the time recorded on the swab board. In the illustration, a Gordh needle is seen in position: through it regional intravenous local anaesthesia has been produced.

Total hip replacement is now the most frequent technique. Fig. 47.27 shows the various combinations of ball and socket which may be used. The blood supply of the head of the femur is not good and consequently after an operation such as cup arthroplasty the head of the femur may degenerate even more. It has been found that it is best therefore to remove the head and the neck of the femur and put in a complete prosthesis which is fixed into the hollow shaft of the femur with special bone cement. Similarly after fractures of the neck of the femur the result of total hip replacement with removal of the fractured neck and head gives a better result than the simple use of a nail to hold the fragments together.

The immediate post-operative complications are those of any severe operation which is accompanied by considerable blood loss. Transfusion is sometimes required and there is a risk of phlebitis, thrombosis, and embolus, increased by immobilisation of the limb in the immediate post-operative period.

To lessen the risk of dislocation of the hip in the immediate post-operative period the thighs must be prevented from going into adduction. This is usually achieved by placing a large pillow between the knees. Similarly when the patient's buttocks are raised to be placed on a bed-pan, hips are pushed forwards and for this reason again to lessen the risk of dislocation, a slipper type bed-pan is preferable. After the first 2 or 3 days the patient is usually moving about freely, but must not roll from side to side. Muscle exercises are very important.

After total hip replacement the patient can move around freely and muscle exercises start almost at once. The patient is very soon moving around on crutches or in a wheelchair. This early mobilisation has greatly reduced the complications from prolonged rest in bed with resultant embolus.

Other joint replacements

Satisfactory hinged metal knees and elbows have been developed and are being used increasingly to restore the function to stiff and painful limbs.

The nursing management of these patients involves particularly vigilance over the circulation of the bandaged limb as swelling and haematoma formation are major complications. Bruising of the nerves at operation may lead to temporary loss of sensation.

In major procedures on long bones where a metal implant is placed in the marrow cavity two particular complications may arise. There may be a reaction to the acrylic cement that is used to keep the metal in place and an unexpected fall in blood pressure. The second hazard is fat embolus (page 924).

Tourniquet

Many operations on the limbs are performed in a 'bloodless field'. In the upper limb a sphygmomanometer cuff or pneumatic tourniquet is used to compress the main arteries in the upper arm. Immediately before the pressure in the cuff is raised, a rubber Esmarch bandage is applied firmly to the limb from the fingers upwards to squeeze out the blood (Fig. 47.28). The pressure is maintained in the tourniquet during operation. If the operation continues for more than half an hour the surgeon may ask for the tourniquet to be released in order to flush the limb with blood and reduce the risk of paralysis. In the leg an Esmarch bandage is applied under considerable tension in over-lapping turns from the toes to the upper thigh. A second bandage is then applied tightly *over a pad* in the upper thigh after which the first one is unwound leaving the limb exsanguinated, or a pneumatic tourniquet is used inflated to 200 mm. If these bandages have been correctly applied the limb is completely bloodless and the operation can continue safely for at least an hour. There is a risk in applying the first bandage if the turn which is taken round the leg at the level of the head of the fibula is too tight (Fig. 47.28). The lateral popliteal (peroneal) nerve winds round the neck of the fibula and may be compressed at this point. Following operation, weakness of foot dorsiflexion is then found and there may be loss of sensation.

Oedema is common in the limb to which a tourniquet has been applied for any length of time, and this is an additional reason for elevation of the limb following operation.

Volkmann's ischaemic contracture. This condition arises in the arm following obstruction of the blood vessels in the region of the elbow. The obstruction may be produced by haematoma in the antecubital fossa or behind the knee, complicating a fracture or other injury. It has most commonly followed the application of a plaster for fractures in the region of the elbow. Insufficient padding has been used inside the plaster, which has been left unsplit: the greatly increased tension which has arisen from haematoma and oedema has compressed the nerves and blood vessels, leading to destruction of the muscles. Recovery is impossible and severe deformity of the hand or foot develops, with permanent disability. A similar condition arises in the calf muscles after injury involving the popliteal fossa. The dread of this condition is always present where there has been severe injury in the region of the knee or elbow and the utmost vigilance must be maintained for signs of nerve or vessel compression following injuries or operation.

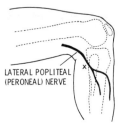

LATERAL POPLITEAL (PERONEAL) NERVE

Fig. 47.29   The outer side of the knee. The lateral popliteal nerve may be easily damaged by compression against the head of the fibula at the point 'x'. An Esmarch bandage, a tight plaster, faulty application of the Thomas splint, or allowing the leg to hang over the end of the operating table may produce foot-drop in this way.

48

Vascular Surgery

Enormous strides have been made in recent years towards solving some of the problems of cardiovascular disease by surgical means. In the hospitals of Great Britain surgery of the heart and great vessels in the thorax is undertaken by the thoracic surgeon, while the general surgeons deal with vascular disease of the extremities and abdominal aorta. With the tremendous increase of traumatic surgery, units dealing with large numbers of accident cases are bound to be involved in vascular surgery of the extremities.

Congenital vascular tumour

Overgrowth of blood vessel tissue in isolated areas of the body is quite common. A tumour of such tissue is an **angioma.** Not always visible at birth but enlarging later, the majority of these 'birth marks' are raised purple or red swellings which empty on pressure and refill when the pressure is released. They tend to fade during the first 4 years of life, but in certain areas whose blood supply is very rich the tumour may enlarge rapidly and require treatment by injection with sclerosing fluid, by radiation or by surgery (page 425).

Congenital arterio-venous fistula is a condition which occurs at several points in the circulation of a limb (Fig. 48.1). There is a direct shunt between some arteries and veins which allows great distension of the venous system; the limb becomes larger than the opposite one. Surgical measures may be necessary to block this communication.

Venous system

If the wall of a vein is damaged by injury or inflammation platelets become adherent to its lining and thrombosis may occur (page 58). Likewise if the rate of flow through a vein is considerably reduced by external pressure on the vein, thrombosis may result, without infection. In the portal system, obstruction to the main vein prevents a return of blood to the liver from the abdominal organs and result in portal hypertension and ascites (page 483).

Occasionally thrombosis occurs in the axillary vein with resultant oedema of the arm, or the vein may be occluded by enlargement of malignant glands in the axilla.

Thrombosis of an iliac or femoral vein is a complication of pregnancy.

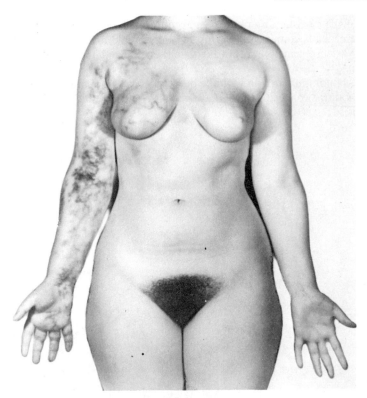

Fig. 48.1 Multiple arterio-venous fistulae affecting the right arm. The veins have been made clear by infra-red photography.

By far the most important lesions affecting veins are **varicosities** (Fig. 48.2). Such abnormal dilatations occur at the lower end of the oesophagus from obstruction to the portal venous return. Haemorrhoids may be produced similarly as a result of portal pressure or simply from chronic constipation and straining. The natural return of blood from the legs is dependent upon the presence of valves in the veins, and upon the upward movement of the stream of blood by the pumping action of the muscles. If these valves are defective, the veins become even more stretched and the valves are rendered completely useless. The weight of a full-length column of blood from the heart to the thigh or leg then exerts back pressure and produces a vicious circle of further dilatation. The incompetence of these veins is demonstrated by elevating the affected leg. This empties the veins completely. A tourniquet is then placed on the limb and the leg again lowered. The veins remain empty unless there is a patent communication with the deep venous system. The 'perforating' connections do not allow blood to flow 'outwards' unless they have been damaged. When the tourniquet is removed the veins will be seen to fill from above.

Stagnation in these dilated veins is apt to lead to thrombosis and a person who has varicose veins is subject to recurrent attacks of **superficial phlebitis**. These attacks, though painful, often result in the cure of the particular varicosity but they may be accompanied by infection of the surrounding tissue. On account of the impaired venous drainage, the skin of the lower leg becomes eczematous and may break down to form a varicose ulcer. Occasionally varicose veins burst, producing either external haemorrhage or haematoma under the skin.

The points of communication with the deep veins can be demonstrated by injection of radio-opaque Conray (page 264). Phlebography also helps to elucidate the presence of deep vein thrombosis.

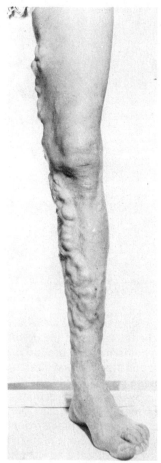

Fig. 48.2   Large varices of great saphenous veins. (From Kinmonth *et al.*, *Vascular Surgery.*)

Treatment

Many treatments are used to relieve the symptoms of varicose veins. Supportive elastic bandages or elastic stockings prevent overfilling of the varicosities and to some extent relieve pain and diminish swelling. The simplest surgical method is the injection of some irritant fluid (hypertonic saline, ethanolamine, sodium tetradecyl sulphate—Trombovar); this produces aseptic phlebitis and blocks the vein. Injection treatment to be effective requires multiple injections at weekly intervals with the application of sponge-foam pressure pads and elastic bandage to maintain pressure on the injected vein. This keeps it empty and ensures satisfactory thrombosis, while avoiding the formation of a large intravenous clot. After injection a large varicosity may, in fact, be tender for a long time and clot within it may liquefy (fibrinolysis) and need aspirating with a needle. Unfortunately, in many cases the channel is opened up again by the pressure of the column of blood in the vein above, so that recurrence is common.

In operative treatment, the main saphenous vein is tied in the groin, above and below the knee, and sometimes at the ankle to interrupt the stagnant column of fluid and produce thrombosis in the intervening segments. Injection is sometimes combined with this operation of ligature. A further method is to insert a long flexible wire from the groin to the lower end of the vein, or vice-versa, Fig. 48.3. The wire carries a small knob at one end.

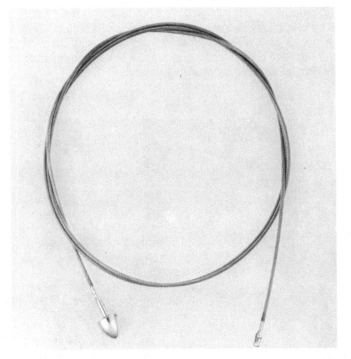

Fig. 48.3 Flexible vein stripper. The strippers have detachable heads enabling the stripper to be passed from above downwards if there is difficulty in the normal procedure. (Seward Surgical Instruments.)

The vein is tied to the knob and the wire pulled out at the other end of the leg, stripping the vein through the subcutaneous tissues. Recurrence is impossible as the affected vein has been extracted, though other channels may open up, particularly if deep perforating veins have not been isolated and tied.

Whatever method of treatment is used at operation, the precise nursing care will depend on the wishes of the surgeon. Usually, the patient is confined to bed for 3 or 4 days, pressure being maintained on the whole length of the limb by crepe bandages. Sometimes the lesser operation of ligature is performed in the out-patient department and the patient is allowed to go home.

There is rarely any severe disability following the treatment of varicose veins but sometimes pain is considerable, and very occasionally thrombosis occurs in the deep veins.

Chronic ulceration of the leg is in many cases due to the presence of varicose veins, but other 'gravitational' ulcers arise without any apparent cause. The treatment of these ulcers is essentially rest. Elevation of the limb in bed is almost always necessary, and the use of compression bandages. These may be of the 'Elastoplast' type or a gelatine paste with zinc oxide compound spread on cotton bandage (Unna's paste). The latter type sets as it dries, into a semi-rigid stocking, and commercially prepared bandages (Viscopaste) are clean and convenient to use, each one being wrapped in an airtight covering which retains the moisture; no soaking is required before application, and the bandage is left on for perhaps a month.

Long-standing ulcers may become malignant (Marjolin's ulcer) (Fig. 48.5). If there is doubt in any particular case, a biopsy is taken from the edge of the ulcer.

Skin grafts are used to aid the healing process when a chronic ulcer has been cleaned and its base has become covered by healthy granulation tissue.

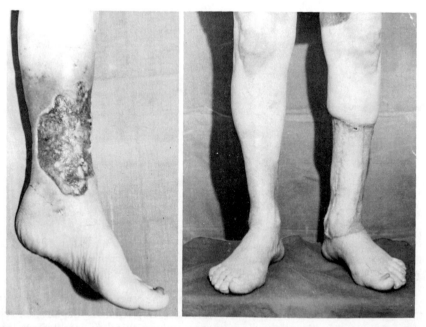

Fig. 48.4 Large varicose ulcer extending almost the whole way round the leg. This was treated by wide excision and the application of dermatome grafts. (From Kinmonth *et al.*, *Vascular Surgery*.)

Many patients tolerate their ulcers for 20 or 30 years as they are unable to afford the time to rest in bed. Even if healing occurs from intensive treatment, the ulcer is very likely to break down again.

Sometimes excision of the ulcer and overlying tissue is necessary. The area is covered by dermatome grafts.

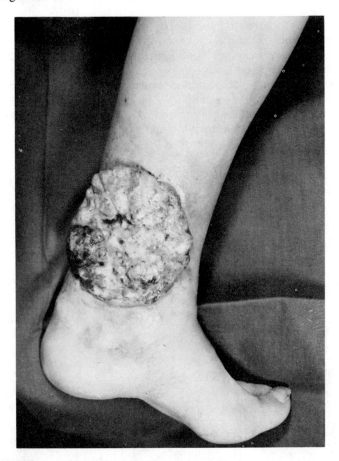

Fig. 48.5 Malignant (Marjolin's) ulcer of leg. This lady thought the ulcer was due to varicose veins and did not seek treatment: note the heaped-up edge of the ulcer.

Deep venous thrombosis arising after childbirth or operation is a factor which leads to chronic oedema of the legs and to the development of gravitational ulcer.

The skin around these ulcers is frequently the site of extensive varicose eczema and is liable to abrasion and infection. Various dressings are used, but the most important principle is to cover the ulcer with tulle gras or some non-adherent dressing through which serum can escape freely, and then to apply continuous pressure in order to prevent oedema. The pressure must of course not be sufficient to restrict the arterial supply.

Arterial disease

The whole of the normal arterial system is elastic. The muscular walls of the arteries are capable of expansion and contraction under nervous control in response to the oxygen requirements of the parts of the body which they supply. Each beat of the heart distends the entire arterial system and during cardiac diastole the flow of blood to the tissues is maintained by the elastic contraction ('tone') of the vessels. If this elasticity is impaired, the systolic blood pressure is automatically raised by an increased cardiac output in order to maintain an adequate blood flow. Consequently arterial hardening (**arteriosclerosis, atheroma**) inevitably leads to a high blood pressure and enlargement of the heart.

Injury to arteries may result from open wounds such as those inflicted by knives or gunshot, but the major arteries of the limbs are sometimes damaged when bones are broken. Figure 48.6 shows the effect of arterial injury. The small vessels, when divided, recoil and seal themselves off. Even one of the major arteries if cut across completely may retract and remain closed while the blood pressure is low and a state of shock persists. A puncture of a

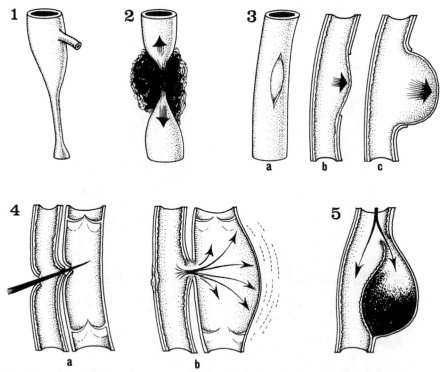

Fig. 48.6 Injury to arteries. **1.** Spasm—often occurs near a fracture. **2.** Complete division: haematoma: cut ends may be closed by spasm. **3.** Tear in outer coat, followed by aneurysm. **4.** Penetrating small wound through artery and accompanying vein (**a**) leading to arteriovenous aneurysm (fistula) (**b**). **5.** Dissecting aneurysm. The inner coat has broken and blood separates the layers of the wall causing obstruction to the lumen.

large vessel, however, does not allow the whole tube to retract and an enormous haematoma will occur if there is no open wound. The pressure from this haematoma on the surrounding tissue rapidly leads to complete occlusion of the blood vessel. Injury to the wall of the vessel without complete perforation weakens it and permits a bulge (**aneurysm**). Progressive enlargement of an aneurysm eventually leads to a rupture and in the case of the aorta this is immediately fatal. If, however, a diagnosis is made before rupture takes place the affected segment of the aorta can be removed and replaced by an artificial vessel.

Similarly, certain diseases of the arterial wall allow abnormal dilatation and the blood instead of being confined to the central channel escapes through a split in the inner layer of the artery and dissects it from the surrounding outer wall (**dissecting aneurysm**). This occurs particularly in the wall of the aorta. Usually the dissection starts in the arch of the aorta: if the stripping of the wall goes back to the aortic valve, a new valve may be put in and the separated wall of the aorta repaired or replaced with a graft. The dissection may track down to the abdominal aorta producing ischaemia of kidneys or viscera by blocking main branches of the aorta. The bulge in the wall of the vessel blocks the remaining lumen and cuts off the supply to the feet. Intense pain occurs and mimics serious abdominal disease such as perforation of an ulcer. Anuria, paralytic ileus, and cold pale feet indicate what has happened. An aortogram shows the extent of the block. Fig. 48.7 shows an aortic

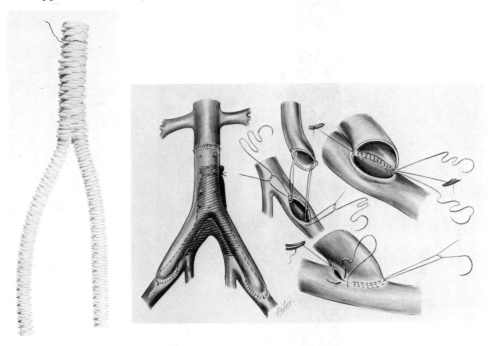

Fig. 48.7 Aortic prosthesis. Artificial aortic and iliac arteries made of synthetic woven fabric. The material is crimped to allow expansion and elasticity. It is tailored to fit each patient.

Fig. 48.8 A prosthesis has been used as a by-pass over the block at the bifurcation of the aorta. The diagram indicates the surgical technique involved. (From Kinmonth *et al.*, *Vascular Surgery*.)

prosthesis with two common iliac arteries. Such an operation takes many hours and the complications which may arise are those of any large abdominal operation together with all the hazards from ischaemia of the lower limbs.

A diseased artery may become obstructed slowly and if the block is confined to one particular length of the vessel a 'collateral circulation' develops between the branches arising behind and ahead of the site of obstruction. Sometimes, however, although there has been a gradually increased narrowing of the vessel, thrombosis occurs suddenly and the collateral circulation is insufficient to maintain the nutrition of the limb. Surgery to improve the blood flow may save the limb but amputation is frequently necessary.

Fortunately if the arterial supply to the legs is becoming insufficient the patient experiences symptoms in the form of cramps in the calf muscles after, exercise. The pain passes off if he stands still for a few minutes and returns when he goes on with his walk. This **intermittent claudication** calls attention to the danger and with care he may avoid any catastrophe. If the cramp is very severe or if there is evidence of impending gangrene in the toes, an operation is undertaken in suitable cases to increase the arterial blood flow.

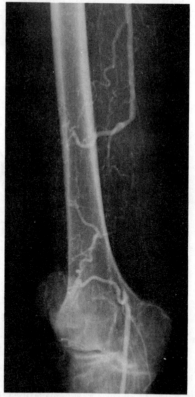

Fig. 48.9 Femoral arteriogram showing a gap opposite the lower third of the femur indicating a block of the upper part of the popliteal artery. This patient was 63 and suffered from claudication of the calf after walking 300 yards. While this did not interfere with his work, it prevented his weekend gardening. (From Kinmonth *et al.*, *Vascular Surgery*.)

Investigation

Radiological examination of the arterial system is performed by injecting Hypaque or meglamine into the artery through a needle or special plastic cannula. Occasionally the very act of penetrating the wall of the vessel with a needle dislodges part of the diseased lining which passes on down the artery forming an embolus. Figs. 48.9, 48.10 show examples of arterial obstruction demonstrated by x-rays.

Special tests are also undertaken to determine temperature changes of the limb, these giving an indication of the ability of the blood vessels to dilate.

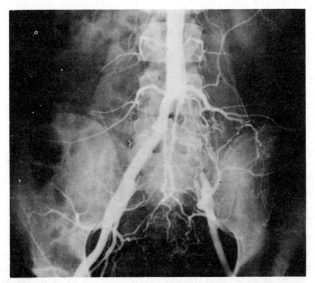

Fig. 48.10 A localised occlusion of the abdominal aorta with a good collateral circulation via the hypertrophied lumbar arteries. (From Kinmonth *et al.*, *Vascular Surgery*.)

An ultrasonic detector—Sonoscope—is used in the diagnosis of venous thrombosis (page 65) to scan the line of the blood vessels to detect pulsation that cannot be felt. By this 'probe' the level of block may be located. The instrument is used also in obstetrics to locate the placenta and in neurosurgery to locate tumours (page 864).

Treatment

Sympathectomy. Insufficient arterial supply to a limb may result in ischaemia of the tips of the digits only. In certain cases where the small vessels are involved and the blood supply to the muscles is not showing evidence of being defective, removal of the sympathetic nerves which control the diseased blood vessels is undertaken. This involves a cervical sympathectomy in the neck for an upper limb, or lumbar sympathectomy in the posterior abdominal wall for the lower limb. These operations have a very limited use and may in fact make matters worse by diverting blood away from the deep tissues and the muscles into the skin. Claudication will then become worse.

There are, however, other diseases of blood vessels such as Raynaud's disease in which the abnormal condition appears to be entirely one of nervous control of the small arteries (pages 946, 950).

Endarterectomy. When arterial obstruction is limited to a section of a main vessel as demonstrated by x-ray examination it is often possible to re-bore this vessel by removing the hard core and clot within it (Fig. 48.9). A good pulse may be restored immediately to the limb beyond the site of obstruction and the patient is saved from amputation. Clots may form post-operatively and the re-bored vessel will have to be cleared with a Fogarty catheter (page 67).

Carotid arteries are similarly affected with resultant minor and major strokes. If the lesion is found sufficiently early by carotid angiography, the obstruction may be removed from the carotid or a narrow portion widened by the use of a small patch-graft from a vein.

Hypertension is sometimes due to constriction of the renal artery: it too may be opened up again by vein patch-graft.

Post-operative nursing problems are related to the area which has been ischaemic. After carotid artery surgery, brain function may be affected; intensive care is often required. Renal artery surgery may result in temporary renal 'shut down'.

By-pass grafts. If the local obstruction in an artery cannot be treated by endarterectomy it can be by-passed by using a vein, an artery from a deep-freeze artery bank or by a prosthesis made from synthetic fibres such as crimped dacron or teflon. Common sites for a by-pass graft are ilio-femoral, and femoro-popliteal (Fig. 48.11). If the aorta is blocked above the renal arteries a by-pass can be inserted from the left subclavian artery to the femoral, thus feeding blood up the aorta to vital organs and the other leg.

Aneurysms. Reference has already been made to the abnormal dilatation of vessels which results from injury and to dissecting aneurysm of the aorta. Any aneurysm is dangerous in that it may burst. If the collateral circulation has been established and is adequate then the affected portion of the artery can be removed. Frequently, however, a by-pass graft has to be inserted and the aneurysm isolated by tying the artery above and below the bulge (Fig. 48.11).

Care of the ischaemic limb

Defective arterial blood supply renders the tissue especially liable to infection and to minor injury which in turn leads to non-healing. Tissues require less oxygen when they are cold and the limb in which incipient gangrene or actual gangrene occurs must be left exposed to the air. Any ulcer that is present can be protected by a light covering of gauze but it is essential that the gangrenous area should be kept cool and dry. On no account must radiant heat, hot-water bottles or coverings be used. If toenails require cutting the utmost care must be taken not to injure the nailbed since a very small injury may, as it were, set fire to the limb and result in amputation. From the nursing point of view the post-operative care of patients who have operations on arteries of the limb is essentially that of care of the ischaemic limb. One of the most important things to remember is that ischaemia also reduces skin sensation and as the leg is 'dead', pressure ulcers may develop very easily. Vigorous massage is extremely dangerous and even the friction of sliding a limb up and down on the sheet may cause abrasion of the skin.

Vascular surgery has been made possible by the introduction of anti-coagulant substances. Heparin is used frequently from the time of operation to prevent clotting within the graft or re-bored artery, and the patient may be given long-acting anti-coagulant substances. This means that he will be liable to haemorrhage and if the nurse should observe rectal bleeding or haematuria it must be reported at once.

Most arterial operations are carried out in specially organised units and the nursing routine will be very clearly laid down.

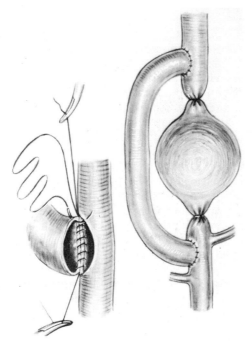

Fig. 48.11 A diagram illustrating the arterial ligature and by-pass operation for an aneurysm of a peripheral artery. Either an autogenous vein graft or a plastic prosthesis can be used as a by-pass. (From Kinmonth *et al.*, *Vascular Surgery*.)

In a community in which there is an increasing number of very old people the incidence of senile gangrene from advanced arterial disease leads to many social problems. Thickening of the nails of the toes, white patches, or little areas of gangrene may be observed by the nurse when she is blanket bathing an elderly person who is in hospital for some other condition. These little things must not be ignored as acute arterial obstruction can occur as a result of lowered blood pressure following an operation for some such condition as strangulated hernia.

In spite of the advances of modern surgery, amputation is still frequently required and an old person finds it very difficult by reason of frailty and dismay to adapt himself to the use of an artificial limb. The remaining tissues are also low in their resistance to infection and poor vitality in the amputation stump sometimes gives trouble which prevents the use of an artificial limb.

Arterial embolus (page 68)

Embolism occurs in arteries by detachment of atheromatous plaques on the wall of the aorta, or from clots in the heart. Sudden pain and pallor in a limb with loss of pulsation suggests embolism. Examination with the ultrasonic detector can locate the block, which can then be removed by Fogarty (page 67) catheter passed down the artery from above.

Cold injury

Conditions caused by exposure of tissues to cold are known as **cryopathies**. Literally this implies 'freezing' but it is usual to include conditions produced by a degree of cooling which has not in fact resulted in the tissues becoming frozen.

Frost-bite is not common in Great Britain, but in the severe winter of 1962, 5 patients were admitted to one London hospital suffering from a degree of frost-bite of the legs requiring amputation. Vagrants, often methylated spirit drinkers, who fall asleep in the open or live in disused buildings are liable to such injuries.

Similar injury arises from exposure to wet-cold following shipwreck or flooding (see Fig. 48.12). Frost-bite of the fingers and feet also occurs in high-altitude aviators.

Pernio or the development of chilblains is another reaction to exposure to cold.

The injuries that result from exposure with or without actual freezing of the tissues are in some ways similar to those of burns. The effect is not immediately apparent. Blistering is followed by necrosis and separation of the dead tissues takes a long time.

The nursing care of patients with these injuries is again that of the care of the injured limb but under no circumstances should artificial heat be applied as this will aggravate the damage. A cold limb must be protected from injury, preferably by being placed on a sheet of plastic foam, and it must be allowed to warm up at normal room temperature. The patient's general condition may need anti-shock treatment if the blood pressure is low. Pain is experienced as the tissues begin to recover their vitality; heavy sedation may be needed. Antibiotics are administered. Local toilet may be required to remove infected blistered skin, and if gangrene follows individual fingers or part of the limb may have to be amputated (Fig. 48.12).

Various degrees of exposure to cold produce spasm of the little blood vessels in the fingers, particularly in sensitive individuals. Relatively minor changes of temperature cause the fingers to blanch. This condition is known as Raynaud's disease and is a distinct entity due to over-sensitivity of the nerve supply of the blood vessels. Reference has already been made to its treatment with sympathectomy (page 943). Raynaud's 'phenomena' —spasm and blanching of the finger—occur as a secondary symptom in other diseases such as advanced cancer, lupus erythematosus and embolic disease. Angiography is used to show the condition of the digital vessels which are often permanently narrowed in secondary conditions.

Lymphatic vessels and lymphoedema

The lymphatic vessels are sometimes defective from birth and this may lead to enlargement of a limb. Lymphoedema may arise from pressure due to blockage of the lymph

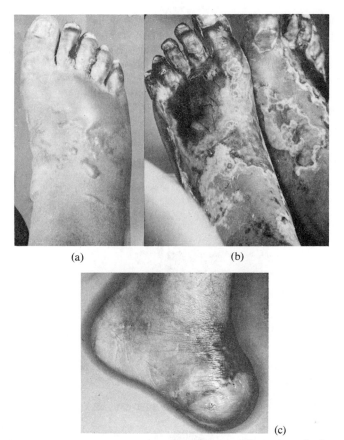

(a)   (b)

(c)

Fig. 48.12 Cold injury without frost-bite in a 26-year-old automobile washer who has worked with wet leaky boots in freezing weather. (a) The right foot on the day following exposure. (b) Both feet 10 days later. (c) The left foot 13 months later. (From Kinmonth *et al.*, *Vascular Surgery*.)

glands by malignant disease or parasitic infection (e.g. filaria, a microparasite occurring in tropical countries). It produces a chronic thickening of all the tissues. Perhaps the most common example of lymphoedema which a nurse will see is the swelling of an arm which occurs after radical mastectomy, or sometimes even without operation when carcinoma of the breast has invaded the lymphatic glands of the axilla.

Various operations undertaken for the relief of chronic lymphoedema have included the insertion of long strands of silk under the skin as 'wicks' to encourage the lymph to drain into other areas. Reversed skin flaps and extensive plastic procedures have been tried. Supportive elastic bandages help to control the swelling; prolonged elevation produces a temporary improvement.

Occasionally sarcoma develops in limbs with lymphoedema and this resembles the type of sarcoma endemic in certain countries, notably central Africa (Kaposi's sarcoma).

Lymphatic fistula. Removal of axillary glands in the treatment of breast carcinoma rarely leads to a leak of lymph as there are alternative pathways over the shoulder. When the groin glands are removed by 'block dissection' for a malignant condition such as melanoma in a leg, interruption of the main lymphatic pathway often results in a lymphatic fistula which is slow to heal and very liable to infection.

A continuous leak of clear fluid from an operation or accident wound at the root of the neck, especially on the left side, always suggests the presence of a fistula from the thoracic duct, the main lymph channel which returns lymph to the venous circulation.

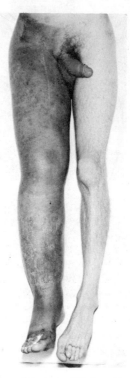

Fig. 48.13   Lymphoedema of sudden onset in a man of 23. Lymphangiography showed that his lymphatic system was congenitally defective. Sarcoma developed and the pigmentation shown in the photograph has arisen from perfusion of the limbs with anti-cancer drugs (page 434).

Lymphangiography is the study of lymphatic vessels by x-ray examination following injection of hypaque or some other radio-opaque material into one of the minute lymph vessels found in the hand or foot and sometimes the lymphatic pathways are traced visually by the injection of a dye such as Patent blue or Evans blue. By the injection of radio-opaque oily materials into the leg it is possible to demonstrate enlarged lymph glands in the abdomen, and to detect glands·involved with malignant disease.

Cystic hygroma. This is a congenital tumour of lymphatic vessels—a **lymphangioma**—which corresponds to the haemangioma or cavernous naevus. Unfortunately it is never confined to normal tissue planes and is extremely difficult to remove. It is most commonly found in the neck or axilla and is the site of repeated infection which may be very severe owing to the rapidity of spread (Fig. 48.14).

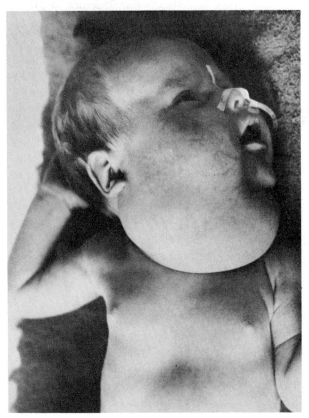

Fig. 48.14 Cystic hygroma involving the neck, tongue and floor of the mouth. Difficulty was experienced with swallowing and respiration (stridor). There were repeated attacks of infection but the main mass of the abnormal tissue in the neck and cheek was excised.

The autonomic nervous system

The sympathetic nervous system forms the unconscious control of organ function and the behaviour of the blood vessels. Its activity is mediated through release of chemicals at the nerve endings and various drugs can block this action in different areas. Generally speaking, overactivity of the sympathetic nerves produces excessive sweating and constriction of the blood vessels in the area affected—like the effect of adrenalin.

The two main areas of the system upon which operations are performed are at the root of the neck, supplying the upper arm, heart and head, and in the lumbar region behind the peritoneum, supplying the lower limbs.

Hyperhidrosis is a condition of excessive and embarrassing sweating, affecting hands, axillae or feet, and sympathectomy stops it.

Raynaud's disease in which there is excessive arterial spasm is treated by sympath-ectomy, and other conditions in which blood supply to the skin is poor may be helped by excision of the appropriate nerves. Four-limb sympathectomy deprives an individual of his normal temperature control but is sometimes needed.

Cervical sympathectomy may be performed at the root of the neck, but the more popular approach now is through the axilla, across the pleural space to the necks of the 1st and 2nd rib. The nursing problems are those of any thoracotomy: usually an under-water seal drain is not needed as the anaesthetist inflates the lung fully before the chest is closed.

Lumbar sympathectomy is carried out through a transverse loin incision. If both sides are done on the same occasion, post-operative distension and ileus is often trouble-some.

49

Plastic Surgery

The special surgical techniques included in plastic or reconstructive surgery are concerned mainly with the replacement of lost or damaged skin. There is considerable overlap between this specialty and general surgery, especially with the departments concerned with the surgery of the jaws and with orthopaedic surgery.

The uses of plastic surgery fall into four main groups:

(a) the surgery of congenital defects, such as the repair of cleft (hare) lip, cleft palate and hypospadias,

(b) the treatment of burns,

(c) the management of maxillo-facial injuries, the restoration of facial contours and the replacement of skin damaged or removed by other injury,

(d) the replacement of lost tissue, especially skin removed in the wide excision of malignant disease and ulceration,

(e) the removal of scar tissue which may have arisen from injury or previous operation. As well as being unsightly, scars interfere with free movement across joints or tendons such as those of the fingers, feet, or knees (Fig. 49.1).

Types of skin graft

The basis of grafting is that living skin is moved from one situation to another where it gains a fresh blood supply and becomes incorporated as living tissue. When small plants are moved from a seed bed, there is a critical period during which the life of the plant is in jeopardy until its roots are fixed firmly in the new soil from which they gain nutrition. Similarly, with tissue grafting, during this critical period the transplanted tissue is weak and susceptible to infections.

There are two main types of skin graft. A **free graft** is one in which a piece of skin is completely detached from the donor site and embedded on a prepared base of healthy granulation tissue elsewhere in the body. In order to obtain its new attachment, such a graft must be thin so that the nutrient serum and oxygen may reach the cells from the surrounding medium during this critical period of implantation. Free grafts are only suitable for situations where the new skin does not have to stand the wear and tear of weight bearing.

The second type of graft is the **pedicle graft** in which a larger piece of thicker skin is detached at one end and fixed to a new site. It gains a new blood supply through this transplanted end and in the interval draws on its own blood vessels coming through the base of the flap. When the graft has become firmly attached to the new site the original connection at the donor site is detached (Fig. 49.1).

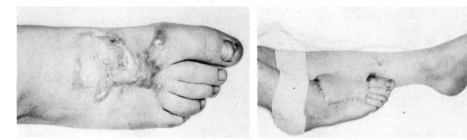

Fig. 49.1   Cross-leg pedicle flap. (*Left*) Adherent scar tissue on the foot limiting the movement of the underlying tendons. (*Right*) A pedicle flap has been cut from the opposite calf and applied to the area from which scar tissue has been excised. The legs are held together by Elastoplast. (By courtesy of Mr. P. H. Jayes.)

Table 62   Types of Skin Graft

Type of graft	Technique	Usual donor site	Thickness
Free			
SPLIT SKIN (Thiersch; Ollier)	Razor or Humby knife	Front of thigh or arm	Epidermis and part dermis
	Dermatome	Thigh, back, abdominal wall, etc.	
FULL THICKNESS (Wolfe; Krause)	Free excision	Back of pinna, mastoid area, abdominal wall	Epidermis, dermis
PINCH	Excision of disks, 1 cm	Upper thigh or arm	Epidermis at edges, with dermis and subcutaneous fat at centre
Pedicle			
FLAP	Multiple-stage operation	Calf for cross-leg flap: abdominal wall for hand or fore-arm	Epidermis, dermis, subcutaneous fat, and blood vessels
TUBE	Multiple-stage operation	Chest for arm or neck, forehead for face	Epidermis, dermis subcutaneous fat, and blood vessels
		Abdominal wall to forearm; thence to neck and forehead and finally to nose or face	

Pedicle grafts are used when a thick flap of skin is required as, for instance, to cover a bony prominence or to reconstruct part of a limb or to fashion a new nose.

Only a single operation is needed for a 'free' graft, while two or more operations are required to complete the transplant of a pedicle graft.

There are several methods of obtaining a free graft. Sometimes the full thickness of the skin is taken from an area of the body where the natural skin is already thin, such as the back of the pinna. A full-thickness graft of this type is sometimes used to fashion new eyelids. A strip of full-thickness hair-bearing skin is used from the mastoid area to make new eyebrows when the natural skin has been destroyed by burns. Full-thickness grafts are usually sutured in position in order to ensure satisfactory and continuous contact between the graft and surrounding tissue.

When a full-thickness graft is taken the donor area has to be closed by stitching the cut edges of the skin together. The split-skin graft, on the other hand, is taken by shaving off the surface layers of the skin leaving the basal layer from which new skin develops (Fig. 49.2). The deep portion of the normal skin has, protruding into it, dozens of tiny

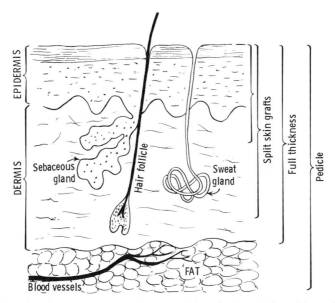

Fig. 49.2 Skin structure, showing varying graft thicknesses. The description of burns follows the same pattern—i.e. epidermal, epidermo-dermal (mixed) and full thickness.

papillae which contain blood vessels. When the split-skin graft is taken, the tops of these papillae are cut so that the surface bleeds, but heals completely without scarring. Consequently very extensive use can be made of this type of graft. When skin is required for covering a large non-weight-bearing area, split-skin grafts are used. The pieces removed can be utilised as a continuous sheet or cut up into 'postage stamp' grafts which are applied with small intervening gaps, to cover an even larger area than that from which the skin was taken. The grafted skin takes root in the bed of granulation tissue on which it is placed.

   The split-skin graft can be taken with a razor (**Thiersch graft**). Special knives are used, one of which, the Humby knife (Fig. 49.4), has a small roller attached to the blade so that the skin is flattened in advance of the cutting edge. These knives can only be used on surfaces of the body which can be flattened completely by pressure with a special board, the skin being sliced by to-and-fro movements of the blade similar to that used in carving a joint of meat. The **dermatome** is a mechanical contrivance for splitting the skin more accurately

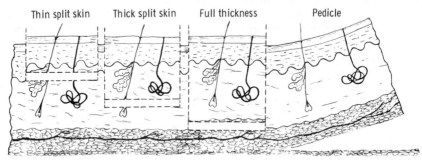

Thin split skin   Thick split skin   Full thickness   Pedicle

Fig. 49.3   Scheme of graft thicknesses. The line of separation between epidermis and dermis is irregular and even when a thick split-skin graft is taken healing of the donor area occurs by spreading of the remaining islands of epithelium from hair follicles and sebaceous cysts.

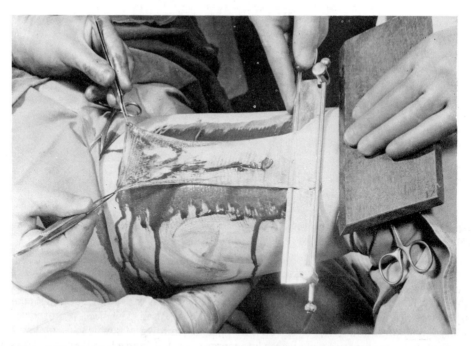

Fig. 49.4   Split-skin (Thiersch) graft being taken from the front of the thigh with a Humby knife. (By courtesy of Mr. P. H. Jayes.)

by means of a knife mounted on a drum. The surface of the drum is attached to the skin by a special rubber cement. The knife cuts the graft as the skin is lifted away from the body by its attachment to the drum. The advantage of the dermatome is that large grafts can be obtained from the abdominal wall, since the dermatome does not require a flat surface, if the skin is sufficiently movable to be picked up by the drum. The electric dermatome is now used extensively in special centres. The principle is similar, but rapid and smooth movements of the knife are carried out by an electric motor. Some patterns of mechanical dermatome are worked by compressed air.

Pinch grafts are occasionally used, particularly in areas where there is a risk of infection. The skin of the donor area is lifted with a needle, and a small disk of skin cut with a scalpel. This disk is thin at the edges and full thickness at the centre; and is less than a centimetre in diameter. Numbers of such pinch grafts are taken and applied to the raw area. They become incorporated in the granulation tissue and new epithelium grows from their edges so that the resultant scar is somewhat uneven but is more durable than that obtained from a thin split-skin graft. Each of the small areas from which skin has been taken by this method heals with scarring, so that an area normally concealed by clothing must be used as a donor site.

A pedicle graft may require several operations. Occasionally the graft is folded to make a tube, thus protecting its raw surface during the various stages of the grafting process. The tube pedicle is now rarely used. Fig. 49.1 shows a pedicle graft taken from the calf of one leg to replace thin scar tissue over the tendons of the opposite foot. When a particularly large graft is to be used, the first operation may consist only of cutting the sides of the flap and undermining it so that the graft may become accustomed to receiving a blood supply only from the ends. In the next operation one end is transplanted to the new site, the raw donor area being covered by a split-skin graft which is applied as a 'dressing'. In the third stage the pedicle is detached from its donor site, trimmed and finally sutured in place.

Cartilage and bone grafts are sometimes required in reconstructive surgery. Bone is taken from the crest of the ilium; cartilage is obtained from the front portion of the ribs.

Nursing principles

The main risk in any skin-grafting procedure is death of the graft. This will occur if the graft does not obtain sufficient blood supply from the receiving area. There are three factors which interfere with the blood supply, infection, haematoma, and movement.

It is important for those who have the post-operative care of plastic surgical cases, to attend in the operating theatre so that they may see exactly what has been done, the extent of the graft, and the way in which it has been immobilised.

Infection is prevented by adequate preparation of donor and recipient site. After burns, and in the treatment of chronic ulcers, the surface must be covered by healthy granulation tissue, which is flat and not too prolific. Sloughs may need surgical removal. Eusol dressing, applied over tulle gras, with a wool pad and crepe compression bandage, acts as a cleansing antiseptic and stimulates the formation of healthy granulation tissue. The pressure dressing keeps it flat. The area to be grafted may be freshly cut tissue (e.g. the bare area from which a pedicle graft has been lifted) and no special preparation is then necessary. Infection is controlled further by the use of antibiotics applied locally at the time of operation, and given by injection. Strict supervision is required for dressing skin grafts, and the surgeon may insist that dressings are changed only in the operating theatre.

Haemorrhage occurring beneath the skin graft lifts it up from its bed and prevents its invasion by healthy growing capillaries. The surgeon pays particular attention to this risk of bleeding at the time of operation, but the main factor in securing complete contact between the graft and its bed is by the use of compression bandaging. Special moulds of plastic material (Stent wax) may be made in the operating theatre. The split-skin graft is spread over the mould, which is held in place by bandaging. A mould of this type is used for skin grafting the orbit after the removal of an eye, and occasionally for the application of skin grafts in the separation of fingers fused together by a congenital defect (**syndactyly**, Fig. 49.5). In the majority of skin-graft cases, initial pressure bandaging is applied personally by the surgeon, but in cases of extensive burning where dressings may be changed frequently, the nurse is responsible for the re-application of this pressure, which must be firm and even.

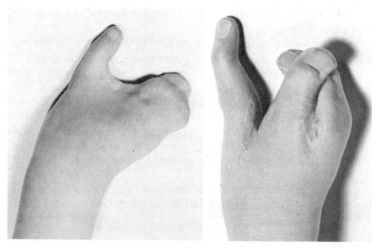

Fig. 49.5 'Lobster claw' deformity. The child was born with a fifth finger and a double thumb. (*Left*) The condition at 4 years old. (*Right*) At the age of 6. The little finger has been separated by extending the cleft, and the thumbs have been parted to provide more movement. A split-skin graft was inserted in the newly formed clefts.

Movement of the graft on its bed is avoided partly by secure bandaging and partly by the application of additional splints or plaster casts. The cross-leg flap is immobilised either by a plaster-of-Paris cast incorporating both legs, or as shown in Fig. 49.1 by encircling Elastoplast.

After the application of a split-skin or full-thickness graft, the dressing is usually left undisturbed for 7 to 10 days by which time the graft has become incorporated, though it may be easily detached by careless dressing.

A thick split-skin graft or a full-thickness graft frequently peels (like sunburn) as the outer layers of epithelium are shed. When the dressing is changed for the first or second time, this thin surface peel must not be mistaken for the graft itself.

Under no circumstances must heat in the form of poultice or hot bathing be applied to a recent skin graft. No strong antiseptic may be used and when the skin is being cleansed it must be dabbed and not rubbed.

Many patients who have plastic operations are in themselves quite fit and become restless during the period for which they have to remain in hospital until the graft is stable. In addition to this boredom is the further difficulty that cases of severe burns or extensive injury may require repeated admission to hospital for multi-stage operations.

After operations on the face, lips, or nose, particular care has to be paid to oral hygiene in a manner similar to that used in the treatment of fractures of the jaw (Chapter 42). Nostrils must be repeatedly cleansed and any nasal discharge wiped away very gently with a pledget of wool moistened by cetrimide. After cleft-lip operations this procedure should be repeated hourly, or more often if there is considerable nasal discharge.

In infancy, after the repair of a cleft-lip deformity which is frequently associated with cleft palate, a metal spring bow is frequently used. This is strapped to the cheek on either side of the upper lip to 'bunch up' the lip, thus taking the tension off the suture line during the period of healing. The baby's arms must be splinted with cardboard splints so that he is unable to move this bow or in any way disturb the lip except with his tongue. Feeding during this period must be carried out with a spoon or pipette. No bandages are applied but the suture line is dusted with penicillin powder or sometimes sealed with Whitehead's varnish (Fig. 49.6).

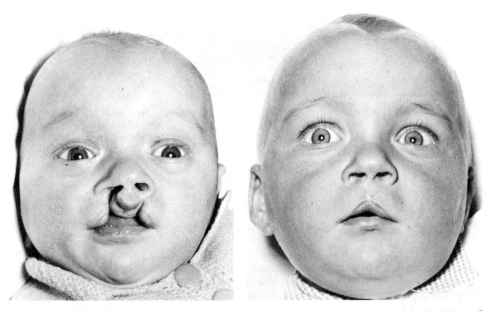

Fig. 49.6   Double cleft lip and palate showing deformity of the nose and the centre island of tissue. In the post-operative photograph the nose has been restored to normal contour.

Burns

Burns may be produced by dry heat. A flame or flash burn usually covers a wide area and involves those parts of the body not covered by clothing. Many burns are caused by contact with hot objects and these are usually deep and involve the full thickness of the skin over a smaller area. If the intensity of fire is sufficient, portions of the body may be roasted; that is, there is destruction of the skin, the fat, and deeper tissues. Burns caused by moist heat are usually described as **scalds** and are more superficial than contact burns, but if boiling water falls on clothing the prolonged contact may lead to deep burning.

For convenience in assessing the severity of burns, various grades are used to describe the depths of tissue involved.

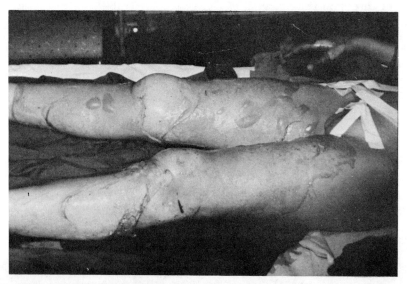

Fig. 49.7   Extensive flash burns of both legs due to kerosene explosion. The ignited vapour went up the boy's trouser legs and the trousers were scarcely damaged. Note the blistering and skin loss. A urethral catheter is strapped in place. Observation of urinary output is vital after severe burns. The damaged areas required over 200 patch (split skin) grafts.

Superficial burn (partial skin loss)

This is a simple **erythema** such as occurs with sunburn. It may extend over a wide area; it is intensely painful and produces marked shock with considerable general body reaction. Thus after exposure of the body to an abnormal amount of sunlight the patient may become feverish and feel ill for several days. There is oedema of the skin, and 'peeling' occurs during the 2nd week (compare effects of radiation in radiotherapy, page 443).

A slightly more severe burn leads to the formation of **blisters** (vesication). The skin is split and the gap between the layers is filled with serum. The skin covering a blister is dead and is usually removed by the surgeon. The base of the blister resembles the donor area after the taking of a split-skin graft. It heals in due course without scarring unless there has been deeper burning. Extensive blistering leads to the loss of large quantities of serum from the body (page 111), and it is this fluid loss which hastens the development of oligaemic shock. Fig. 49.8 shows extensive blistering on the hand of a child.

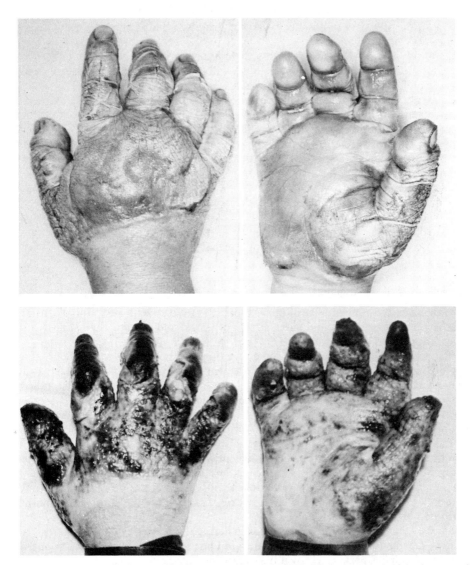

Fig. 49.8 Severe burn of the hand. (*Top*) Extensive deep blistering involving the whole of the fingers, palm and back of the hand. (*Below*) 20 days later. The dead skin has separated revealing destruction of underlying tissue with areas of gangrene in the finger pulp. Healthy granulation tissue covers much of the denuded area which is now ready for grafting. (By courtesy of Mr. P. H. Jayes.)

Deep burn (full thickness loss)

This term is used to indicate that the whole depth of skin has been destroyed by the burn, and will therefore be shed. Healing will be by granulation tissue with subsequent scarring. Before this is possible the dead tissue has to be separated as a slough and the devitalised tissue is very liable to infection. Severe toxaemia from the absorption of the decomposition products of the dead tissue, devitalises the patient and leads to severe anaemia.

In addition to full-thickness skin loss, subcutaneous fat and perhaps muscles may be involved in deeper burns. A very deep slough will form unless the dead tissue is removed surgically and replaced by healthy skin graft.

The treatment of burns depends upon the depth of the burning and the extent of the area involved, and frequently it is not possible to tell whether there is going to be full thickness loss or not, in any particular area. The majority of burns are therefore described as 'mixed'. There are areas in which there is blistering; in other areas there is clearly full thickness loss shown by the presence of white zones in the raw areas left after the shedding of a blistered skin.

Electric burns are of two types. First the electric flash or heat may produce a surface burn, in the same way as a flame. Second, there may be a very deep penetrating burn from the passage of the electric current through the tissues. Occasionally a whole finger may be coagulated by the passage of current. In such cases the dead tissue requires early removal, by operation. To await natural separation greatly prolongs the period of disability and runs the risk of severe infection.

Management of the burnt patient

At all stages in the treatment of burns there are two distinct aspects to be considered. First there is the prevention and management of shock, and second there is the treatment of the burnt areas.

First-aid treatment is directed to the prevention of shock and as far as the local treatment of burnt areas is concerned, there are two rules. **Exposed burnt areas should be covered** with clean, soft, non-fluffy material or even with clean paper, but **burnt areas to which clothing is adherent should be left undisturbed,** as the burnt clothing is a safe and sterilised dressing. Under no circumstances should any attempt be made to remove clothing from an individual who has been burnt. This must be deferred until admission to hospital.

Both neurogenic (vasodilatory) and oligaemic shock occur in cases of burns, the one passing fairly rapidly into the other where the burn is extensive. Certain areas of the body, especially those from which pain sensation is most intense, are more liable to produce severe shock than other areas, and it is the extent rather than the depth of the burn that determines the degree of shock.

Many schemes have been devised for calculating the percentage of the body's surface area involved in burns so that some estimate is obtained for the amount of plasma or plasma substitute which has to be given by infusion, to combat shock.

Fig. 49.9 shows the relative proportions of the body surface (Wallace's Rules of Nine). It is important to realise that a grave degree of shock may be produced by what may appear at first to be only a minor burn, involving perhaps both forearms and hands.

One of the nurse's primary duties is to keep a record of pulse rate and blood pressure in all cases, from the moment of admission, observations being made every half hour.

When the surgeon has made an initial assessment of the extent of burning and determined his plan for anti-shock treatment, intravenous infusion is commenced (except in minor cases which are treated as out-patients). It has been found that for every unit of 9 per cent surface burn, approximately 1200 ml of fluid is required by infusion. This is usually given as 1 unit of dextran and 1 unit of normal saline.

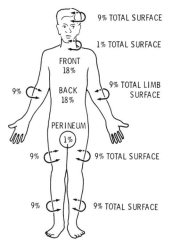

9% TOTAL SURFACE

1% TOTAL SURFACE

FRONT
18%

BACK
18%

9%

9% TOTAL LIMB
SURFACE

PERINEUM
1%

9%   9% TOTAL SURFACE

9%   9% TOTAL SURFACE

Fig. 49.9 'Rules of Nine' for assessing the area involved by burn.

Various methods of calculating infusion requirements have been devised, but these are based on bodyweight: very few severely burnt patients can be weighed but an approximate assessment is made, or a conscious patient usually knows his weight. This is in kilograms. By the 'Evans' formula' or 'Brook's formula' a total 24-hour requirement can be worked out.

By Evans' formula 1-ml normal saline or Hartmann's solution is given for every 'per cent' burn multiplied by the weight in kilograms. A '10-stone' adult (64 kilograms) with 20 per cent burn would need $64 \times 20 = 1280$ ml—and the same volume of plasma, blood or dextran, i.e. 2560 ml total minimum.

By Brook's formula 0·5 ml of saline or Hartmann's solution and 1·5 ml plasma, dextran or blood is given—the same total.

By simply using the Rule of Nine the total is almost the same, i.e. 20 per cent is approximately 2 'nines' thus giving $1200 \times 2 = 2400$.

Half the 24-hour requirement is given in the first 8 hours, the rest in the following 16 hours. The packed cell volume is then estimated and daily needs calculated.

Careful watch must be kept on urinary output and accurate records maintained. Not more than 7 litres of fluid should be given in 24 hours. Children require proportionately reduced quantities: for a child of 9 years, these quantities should be halved. In severe cases a catheter is left in place so that urinary output may be measured: output should be 20–40 ml per hour.

Treatment of the burnt areas

Attention is then turned to the treatment of the burns and the method employed varies in detail in different centres. The patient may need a general anaesthetic in order that the damaged areas may be cleaned and dead skin removed. Sometimes deeply burned tissue is excised at this initial cleansing operation and split-skin grafts applied to the raw area as a 'dressing' (see later).

In many cases, removal of clothing and the initial toilet of the burnt areas is carried out by an experienced nurse working under strictly aseptic conditions.

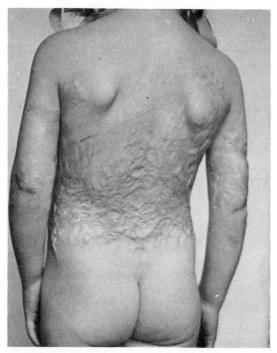

Fig. 49.10   Extensive keloid scarring on the back and arms, following severe burns. There has been full thickness loss over most of the area which was treated by patch grafts (split skin cut into small pieces). Many of the grafts can be seen as flat areas surrounded by keloid which has formed over the intervening granulation tissue. It is difficult to maintain adequate and even pressure over this area while the graft is 'taking'. The severity of this child's condition necessitated 6 litres of infusion: she was kept in an oxygen tent for 5 days.

There are widely divergent views about the subsequent treatment of burns. One of the main objectives is to prevent the loss of large quantities of serum from the skin and to this end various attempts have been made to coagulate the surface by the application of chemicals such as tannic acid or silver nitrate or mercurochrome. Tannic acid was given up as it can be absorbed and damage the kidneys. Silver nitrate is still used in some clinics and so is mercurochrome. However, the best natural dressing is a dry scab and the treatment used particularly in children, even with extensive superficial burns, is exposure in a warm room.

Very soon a dry crust forms which prevents the entry of infection and epithelialisation takes place underneath. If, however, there are deep areas of burn which the surgeon considers represent full thickness loss, although a crust may form over the surface, ultimately the dead tissue will separate as a slough and there is bound to be some infection. It is not possible initially to make accurate assessment of the depth of all burnt areas. Patches of white tissue suggest full thickness loss, but sometimes when vascular spasm passes off the blood supply returns to these areas. If facilities are available the ideal treatment is to excise the areas which are considered to be full thickness loss and apply an immediate split skin graft taken from elsewhere on the patient—an autograft. If the burns are extensive it may not be possible to obtain sufficient skin from the patient and a viable homograft may be taken from a parent for a child, or from another human being. Fresh skin can be stored after being frozen and is viable when thawed. Skin is also taken from a cadaver and treated by freezing in a special solution containing an antibiotic: this is 'lyophilised' skin and is stored in envelopes of Nylon film: it may be obtained commercially. Pig skin is similarly available. The application of 'foreign' skin whether human or porcine protects the dead area from infection and has been found to allow the formation of healthy granulation tissue before the body's reaction rejects the graft. By tissue typing between the human donor and the patient, a satisfactory tissue match may be obtained for a considerable period, perhaps 2 weeks. If this has not been possible the foreign graft is removed after 3 or 4 days and replaced by further grafts, and ultimately by an autograft of split skin.

With extensive burns lyophilised skin is used as a dressing on the *donor* areas from which autograft has been taken in order to diminish the fluid loss from the donor site and lessen discomfort. Thin split skin grafts will stay in place on a burnt area without a dressing being applied so that grafting can be combined with an exposure technique.

If it has not been possible to excise areas of full thickness loss and exposure treatment has been used (or, in difficult areas, non-adhesive dressings) the dead tissue begins to separate during the second week and a surgical toilet may be necessary to remove these sloughs to prepare a clean granulating area for subsequent grafting. In certain areas where a full thickness graft is required in order to provide mobile skin such as in the eyelids, split skin grafting is used initially and subsequently this may have to be excised and replaced by a thicker graft. If the eyebrows have been burnt, an inlay graft of hair-bearing skin from behind the ear is used. Severe facial burns involving the cartilage of the nose may produce such gross deformity that a nose reconstruction has to be undertaken at a later date.

Saline baths are used frequently in the treatment of burns of the limbs. In special centres, provision is made for lowering the whole patient into a bath. The cleansing effect of the irrigation with saline adds to the patient's comfort and diminishes the risk of infection, which thrives on dead tissue.

When the burning has been superficial only, the raw area at the base of the blister remains moist for approximately 10 days, depending upon the depth of skin involved; then, sometimes quite suddenly, it becomes dry and healing is complete.

Joint movement. The importance of maintaining function has already been described in the management of other limb injuries, and one of the most urgent considerations is the restoration of all joint movement. The bath method of treating burns has this additional advantage that the patient is able to move all his joints without the restriction of clothing. It is particularly important to prevent stiffening of the fingers. During World War II the Bunyan-Stannard transparent bag was introduced especially for the treatment of burns of the hand and arm. It was applied as a very large glove, the upper end being strapped with adhesive to the skin of the arm. Finger movements could take place freely within the bag which was irrigated from time to time with hypochlorite solution.

Diet. Patients who have been extensively burned, require a high-calorie diet to replace the protein loss from the exudate of serum. Infection is now uncommon, but when it occurs it produces anaemia which may be quite severe. A preparation of iron is therefore required during the convalescent period. The haemoglobin level should be estimated weekly and blood transfusion may be necessary. Additional vitamin supplies are given.

Sleep. It is known that adrenalin (which is produced by adrenal glands especially in conditions of stress) inhibits the normal division (mitosis) of skin cells, and severe or prolonged stress may have a profound effect upon the repair processes. More important is the knowledge that multiplication of skin cells is much faster during sleep than at other times. Lack of sleep may therefore actually *delay* wound healing. Convalescence is prolonged and depression is common. Sleep without heavy drugging is vital and is best achieved by mild sedatives with a tranquilliser action.

Other complications of burns. The respiratory tract may be burnt by a flame, by chemicals or by escaping steam. The treatment is essentially that of a patient who has been asphyxiated.

Burns involving the genitalia may lead to retention of urine.

The swallowing of hot fluids may cause ulceration of the oesophagus with subsequent contracture.

Victims of severe burning sometimes develop an acute duodenal ulcer (**Curling's ulcer**) which may bleed or perforate. If a patient during the recovery period (perhaps during the 2nd week) complains of severe indigestion this must be reported to the medical staff; severe stress and over-production of acid may be the cause.

Cover creams

After operation on the face, neck or arms, residual scars or areas of discoloration may be effectively disguised by the use of specially matched cover creams. When this procedure is necessary arrangements will be made for the patient to receive instructions in the use of the cosmetics.[1]

Wider applications of plastic surgery

The principles of plastic surgery outlined here are applied in many special departments. Split-skin graft procedures are commonplace in all surgical units. After excision of malignant tumours in certain positions reconstructive surgery is required for cosmetic or functional reasons. A knowledge of nursing management appropriate for skin graft cases is essential therefore in all surgical departments. The plastic surgeon is intimately involved with the dental surgeon in the management of facio-maxillary injuries.

Some plastic surgical units perform operations for hypospadias and other urethral abnormalities; such procedures are also undertaken in urological centres. Hare-lip and cleft-palate operations are in some centres within the realm of the paediatric surgeons. There is now such an overlap with other special surgical interests that a nurse may often be called upon to look after patients requiring this particular field of experience.

[1] Veil Cover Cream (Thomas Blake & Co.)

50

Accident Surgery

With the growth of the motorway system in Great Britain and the enormous general increase in road traffic, there has arisen a need to establish accident centres, fully staffed day and night and able to deal with patients suffering from multiple injuries. Accidents in the home account for many child deaths, and accidents in industry constitute an important economic problem quite apart from the suffering they cause. Modern methods of resuscitation, both in relation to the maintenance of artificial respiration and the institution of external cardiac massage have resulted in the immediate survival of many patients who would never have reached hospital before these techniques were evolved. It is clear that such patients are likely to have multiple injuries involving, for instance, brain damage and the rupture of abdominal viscera and several limb fractures.

Improvements in vascular surgery have made it possible to preserve limbs whose blood supply has been severely interfered with. The development of special techniques in hand surgery have made it possible to avoid the loss of even parts of fingers which in the past would have been amputated as a routine. Several important aspects of accident surgery have already been dealt with in the sections on resuscitation, care of the unconscious patient and asphyxia.

A nurse in charge of a casualty reception unit has one of the most exciting and rewarding duties in the profession. Even patients with relatively trivial injuries are apprehensive. They remember and recall to their friends their first impressions of hospital treatment. Here perhaps more than in any other department of surgery the nurse can be 'a pillar of strength' both to the patient and the surgical staff.

Accident prevention

There is a constant campaign of education throughout industry to prevent the occurrence of accidents. Legislation lays down standards of safety over the construction of buildings, the erection of scaffolding, the protection of machinery in factories, and safeguards against contamination with noxious chemicals in manufacturing processes. Much has been done in the design of motor vehicles to diminish the effect of accidents to passengers and the use of safety belts in motor cars has brought about a dramatic reduction in the severity of injuries. An increase of personal violence and assault with more frequent use of small arms has added to the accident load at hospitals.

Type of injury

A knowledge of the nature and mechanism of an accident is helpful to the surgeon who has to assess the injury in the first instance.

High-velocity impact injuries occurring in head-on collisions of road vehicles or in aircraft accidents often result in the head being thrown forward and the neck may be broken either by the forward thrust or the recoil of the head on the neck (whiplash injury). The face is literally pushed in by an impaction of the centre segment of the facial skeleton. The knees are often crushed against the dashboard of a car, resulting in fractures of the patella or the femur. Drivers whose movements are not restricted by an efficient safety belt are impaled on the steering wheel and sustain crush injuries of the chest. Safety-belt buckles, if not correctly placed to the side of the passenger, have been known to cause rupture of the liver and spleen.

'Run down' injuries to pedestrians invariably result in fractures of the legs and frequently in head injuries. Rupture of abdominal viscera is also common in this type of accident.

Personal assault injuries nearly always involve damage to the head or face, and frequently fracture of the mandible. Razor slash injuries may be extremely severe and the resultant blood loss may be fatal. Wounds resulting from gunshot will depend upon the type of weapon used. Revolver or rifle bullet injuries produce an entry wound and usually an exit wound with a trail of damage between the two small punctures. Such wounds necessitate complete exploration of the track of the bullet. Shotgun injuries, however, produce more widespread damage, particularly to muscle.

Crush injuries result from the collapse of buildings, or the fall of heavy packing cases on loaders and warehouse workers, and in motor accidents involving several vehicles. Tissue damage in such cases is often extreme and oligaemic shock severe.

Explosions unaccompanied by fire may produce head injury and rupture of the lungs or abdominal viscera, quite apart from the secondary injuries which occur if an individual is hurled some distance by the force of the explosion. Explosions accompanied by flash, followed immediately by fire, involve a double peril in that individuals may be rendered unconscious and therefore unable to escape from the fire.

Explosions occurring in a confined space such as a room invariably produce damage to the ear with rupture of the tympanic membrane: this injury is easily overlooked and nursing staff dealing with casualties should be on the lookout for deafness as a symptom.

Drowning may also be accompanied by limb or trunk injuries. In shipping and sailing accidents head injury may result in drowning and make resuscitation of the rescued patient much more difficult.

First aid and transport

Primary consideration in all injuries is to make sure that the patient has an unobstructed airway. If natural respiration has ceased, the immediate institution of artificial respiration is vital once the mouth has been cleared. If the patient has no palpable pulse in the wrist or in the neck, artificial respiration must be accompanied by cardiac massage. Bleeding is nearly always controllable by pressure at the site of injury and only on extremely rare occasions is the use of classical pressure points called for. Fractures must be immobilised to prevent further damage to other structures and to alleviate pain, and the provision of lightweight inflatable splints[1] which are easily applied has added very considerably to the efficiency of first-aid management. Accident ambulances are now equipped with positive-pressure artificial respiration apparatus and crews are fully drilled in resuscitation techniques.

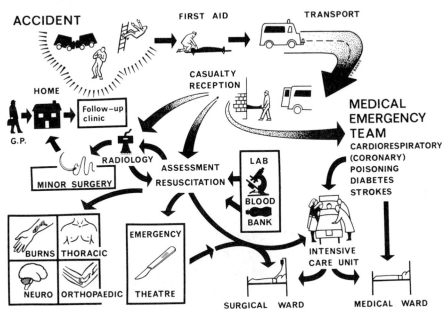

Fig. 50.1 Accident and medical emergency patients are 'processed' through the Casualty Department and adjacent ancillary services to a predetermined plan.

Casualty reception

At this stage the same primary considerations apply—the maintenance of an airway and of cardiac function, the control of haemorrhage and the avoidance of all unnecessary movement. If cardiac arrest has occurred, full resuscitation procedures are adopted with artificial respiration (ambu bag) and external cardiac massage. If there is shock or has been blood loss, blood is taken for cross-matching and an immediate intravenous infusion established, giving dextran (this must not be given before blood has been taken as it interferes with the grouping procedure). If drunkenness is suspected blood should be taken for alcohol estimation: not only is this important from the medicological view point, but intoxication may affect the management and recovery.

In patients with severe burns, blood is also examined spectroscopically for carbon monoxide. Poisoning with carbon monoxide is a common, often fatal, complication of those caught in fire in an enclosed area such as a house. They may not have suffered burns

---

[1] Inflatable splints which encase the limb may obstruct the blood flow if inflated to more than the recommended pressure for the particular make. Gangrene has resulted from such over-inflation.

or other injury, but this poisoning is often overlooked. The effective haemoglobin level is grossly reduced; transfusion and oxygen are required.

A specimen of urine should be obtained as soon as possible. If an unconscious patient is found to have a distended bladder, he should be catheterised under full aseptic conditions.

There then follows a general assessment of the patient's injuries by the casualty surgeon, who must be provided with all available evidence as to the nature of the accident and any changes in the patient's condition since he was first seen by the ambulance crew. The level of consciousness is estimated together with pulse rate and blood pressure so that there is a continuous minute-by-minute record from the moment of his arrival in hospital.

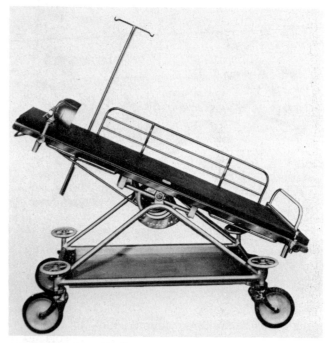

Fig. 50.2 Patient trolley designed specifically for accident reception work and resuscitation. This can be fully tilted in any direction and the base permits the positioning of x-rays so that the patient need not be moved for radiological examination. (Luton Trolley. A. L. Hawkins Ltd.)

Programme for treatment

If resuscitative measures are needed these have now been instituted, transfusion may have been started and initial assessment of injuries has been made. Usually at this stage x-ray examination is required and this may involve considerable discomfort for the patient, particularly if x-ray facilities are not readily available in the casualty department. If there is a delay in carrying out x-ray examinations the patient must remain under observation by a member of the nursing staff throughout and must never be left unattended even if he is fully conscious, for he will worry and wonder what is happening. All patients who have been unconscious and about whose state of consciousness there has been some doubt must be admitted to hospital and under no circumstances discharged simply because consciousness has been regained.

Patients with minor injuries will receive the appropriate treatment. This will include the suturing of wounds after adequate toilet, perhaps under local anaesthetic; reduction and plaster of minor fractures; and the injection of initial antibiotic dose. Necessary anti-tetanus measures will be taken (page 55). Arrangements must be made for transport for the return of a patient to his home or place of work, and this may involve calling the ambulance or hospital service. The nursing staff is responsible for the care of the patient during this waiting period and for ensuring that he has ample instructions about treatment and return to hospital if required.

Patients with major injuries may have to be prepared for the operating theatre while they are still in the casualty department. It is usual to leave the undressing and initial cleansing of patients with multiple injuries which need surgical treatment until the patient has been anaesthetised.

Types of wound

The management of accidental wounds depends on the method of injury, the extent of the wound in length and depth, the contamination with foreign matter, and the involvement of structures such as arteries, nerves or joints.

The effect on healing of tissue damage and other factors is described on page 31.

For descriptive purposes common terms are in use and these indicate to nurses and surgeons the type of treatment that is most likely. These terms are used in clinical notes and form a brief 'Casualty Department' description of a wound so that a surgeon can usually decide a programme without having to remove the initial dressings.

Incised wounds. These result from razor cuts, broken glass or sharp metal. The skin is cleanly divided with very little damage on either side of the cut and there is no contamination. The wounds are simply closed as with surgical incisions and very little scarring results. Extensive incised wounds of the face may, however, divide some of the muscles of expression and unless these are carefully repaired distortion persists afterwards.

Contused wounds. Here the tissue is bruised and the skin broken.

Blunt wounds. These are produced by blunt instruments such as a blow with a 'cosh', a fist or a boot, or a fall on the ground may crush the skin without in fact breaking its full thickness. As a result of the bruise the blood supply to the skin is jeopardised and quite large areas may die.

Burst wounds. These are also produced by blunt objects, usually with greater velocity inflicted on skin which is tight. The skin splits and is contused on either side of the tear. The edges and severely damaged tissue are excised so as to produce healthy straight margins for direct suture. If a large area of skin is contused it is excised and replaced by a graft, assuming there is no underlying damage.

Puncture wounds. These are produced by stabs with sharp instruments such as penknives, skewers and stilettos. The problem with puncture wounds is that without full exploration it is not possible to determine the depth. Internal organs may have been injured. Such wounds must be probed for the presence of foreign bodies and are usually explored unless it is obvious that they are very shallow.

Lacerated wounds. Severe jagged tears of the skin and underlying tissues are produced by sharp objects such as torn metal and are usually the result of major accidents or falls onto sharp objects. Full surgical toilet and excision of the wound edges is always needed.

Gunshot wounds may combine all the features of these types. Usually the entry wound made by a rifle bullet is a clean puncture and the exit wound is a burst with laceration around the centre. Bomb fragments, however, produce severe lacerated wounds and the pieces of metal become impacted in the underlying muscle, causing very extensive damage and a liability to gas gangrene.

Treatment of wounds

Minor wounds can be treated under local anaesthesia introduced by a needle inserted through the cut itself. Alternatively an area nerve block can be created 2 cm or so away from the edges of the cut. If, however, the wounds are grossly contaminated general anaesthetic is essential so that the depth of the wound can be explored and all other damaged tissue removed.

Whatever the involvement of other structures such as nerves and bones, soft tissues have to be dealt with by excision of all dead or badly bruised tissue and the conversion of the skin wound into a clean cut. Deep wounds are usually drained to prevent the accumulation of blood and the liability to greater infection. Sometimes the complete depth of the wound is left open for a few days until healing has commenced. When the risk of spreading infection has passed, the skin is then closed with stitches in the usual way. If there has been widespread damage and it is doubtful whether it is going to be safe to close the wound, or if there is already established infection in the wound, it is left open until it has become thoroughly clean. Subsequently the edges are freshened and the wound closed perhaps 2 or 3 weeks after the initial injury.

Initial closure of a wound is called **primary suture**. Closure a few days after the injury is called **delayed primary suture**, and a later closure is **secondary suture.**

Delayed rescue

Casualties who have been trapped by falling masonry or in a road or rail accident usually have severe crush injuries involving muscle damage. If, for instance, a thigh is caught under a girder the blood supply to the limb is impaired as if a tourniquet has been applied. When the limb is released, toxins from the damaged tissue are carried back by the returning circulation. Shock is increased rapidly: potassium from the damaged tissues causes a rise in serum potassium; the kidneys with a poor blood flow are unable to regulate the electrolytes and cardiac arrest can occur. Haemo- or peritoneal dialysis may be needed. This condition is described as 'crush syndrome'. Muscles that have been ischaemic either from direct pressure or from compression of a main artery undergo necrosis: the critical time of ischaemia is 6 hours and after that amputation may be urgent to save life.

Major accidents

Civil disasters such as railway accidents often result in the need to provide urgent treatment for far more patients than can possibly be handled by one casualty department.

In the British National Health Service there are area organisations in all regions to ensure that in the event of a major accident, casualties are distributed to suitable hospitals which are alerted by radio according to a predetermined plan. Mobile surgical teams are held at accident centres for immediate despatch to the scene of an accident for the rescue of patients who have been trapped and require surgical or medical assistance before they can be released.

Special references

	page		page
Artificial respiration	178	Head injuries	857
Blood transfusion	157	Jaw	787
Burns	958	Larynx	810
Cardiac arrest	193	Nose	797
Eyes	833	Shock	106
Gangrene	34	Tetanus and gas gangrene	55

51

Surgery of the Aged

Gerontology is the study of old age. The medical aspects of this subject are classed as **geriatrics.** In Great Britain this speciality is widely recognised as a distinct branch of medicine: special hospitals, self-contained units with full consultant and supporting services, have been organised. Nevertheless, while the care of old people presents its particular problems, in any general hospital all departments are involved in treating the aged, and the general practitioner especially has a continuing responsibility for these patients in their declining years.

Geriatric care, as distinct from specific surgical treatment, involves in particular the supportive services of physiotherapy, occupational therapy and welfare departments. Many old people have declining mental powers due to general ageing of the brain or perhaps from a more acute episode such as a stroke. If an old person is faced with an acute surgical emergency such as the sudden strangulation of a hernia which he has had for many years, the domestic problems may be very great—the aged wife unable to cope on her own, difficulties of hospital visiting, contact with responsible relatives and management of financial affairs.

In assessing the need for surgical intervention in less acute conditions such as uncomplicated hernia, diverticulitis, or arthritis of the hip, the patient's expected post-operative home environment has very great relevance. Arterial disease with its complications of claudication and gangrene, is very common, and yet such patients with poor circulation require the greatest degree of self-care with cleanliness, manicure and avoidance of minor injury. These old people may be least able to attend to their physical needs at home. Domiciliary care provided both from hospital geriatric centres and by the welfare services of the Local Authorities have to be mobilised to prevent complications of known disease and to maintain the greatest possible level of self-care and independence in the afflicted.

Cataract is essentially a problem of old age but operation to restore vision is fraught with danger. The patient may become confused and because of bad vision is apt to fall and sustain fractures. Defective hearing leads to misunderstanding of instructions given by doctor or nurse.

The background disorders which are most likely to affect elderly patients, each having a bearing on any necessary surgical programme, are:

1. Cardiac insufficiency shown by breathlessness, swelling of feet at the end of the day, engorged neck veins, frothy bloodstained sputum. The patient may already have had attacks of congestive failure and be having digitalis and diuretics.

2. Peripheral arterial disease shown by a history of claudication, blanching of the legs on elevation, irregular thickening of toe nails, loss of hair on the legs, and even areas of gangrene—all due to ischaemia. The patient may have learned to live with his disability, but sudden illness may cause rapid deterioration.

3. Arthritis affecting the big joints such as the hips and knees, preventing adequate mobility: this results in difficulty with toilet routine, bathing, position on the operating table and in obtaining a comfortable post-operative position in bed. Inability to change position frequently without help makes the development of bedsores more likely.

Rheumatoid (polyarticular) arthritis affecting mostly women, may prevent the use of hands in attending to hair, cutting nails or even feeding.

4. Urinary disorders. In men, frequency, dysuria and incontinence from prostatic obstruction may have been disregarded by the patient until the crisis of hospital admission from accident or other illness. Incontinence following prostatectomy or any nervous disorder can often be managed by the use of a penile clamp (Fig. 51.1) if the individual is not completely incapable. Alternatively a penile appliance (Fig. 51.2) may be used by day, with a night appliance draining into a bedside bag at night.

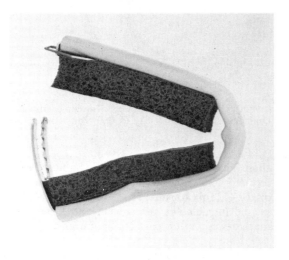

Fig. 51.1 Cunningham's penile clamp. This is available in several sizes and great care is needed if the skin of the penis or the urethra itself is anaesthetic as in paraplegia: the clamp may then be closed too tight and as no pain is produced necrosis occurs very quickly. This clamp's greatest value is for patients with normal sensation but incontinence such as sometimes follows prostatectomy or carcinoma of the prostate. (Seward Surgical Instruments.)

In women, incontinence especially on stress, is very common and in a minor degree is ignored by the patient, but in an acute illness the degree of urinary leak may become a major problem, and the use of a self-retaining indwelling catheter in the post-operative period is welcomed by the patient, relieving her of anxiety over incontinence.

5. Pulmonary disorders. Chronic bronchitis is accepted by old people as part of the 'ageing process', but when coughing results in the strangulation of a hernia it becomes the major disability and post-operative pneumonia is very likely to occur. Antibiotic therapy is started pre-operatively when possible in such patients.

6. Mental incapacity. Frank senile dementia is by no means uncommon, but even minor degrees of loss of reasoning power, or emotional control, in the patient or his spouse adds very considerably to the nursing problem. Deafness must be mentioned here as this often leads to lack of understanding between patient and nurse, particularly if the patient has not recognised, or does not admit, his deafness.

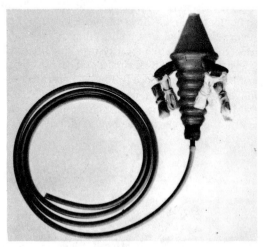

Fig. 51.2 Simplic male incontinence appliance for use in bed. The conical rubber top is cut to the appropriate size to fit the penis. Drainage is into a bedside bag. (J. G. Franklin & Sons Ltd.)

7. Chronic constipation. This arises from the patient habitually ignoring nervous impulses from a loaded rectum: in consequence the bowel becomes much less active and it is by no means uncommon for old folk to suffer from 'overflow incontinence' of the bowel. Huge faecal masses become impacted in the rectum and a manual evacuation of the bowel under general anaesthetic is often part of the initial programme of treatment in geriatric care.

8. Anaemia and malnutrition. Declining appetite and ready satisfaction with minimum but unsuitable diet leads frequently to shortage of vitamin intake in the elderly, and to anaemia. Low-income group patients often lack protein in the diet, and this affects the process of tissue repair. Lack of teeth may be a contributing factor, either because dentures have never been provided, or are several years out of date and no longer fit the ageing person's receding alveolar margins.

Thus it will be seen that when we apply the great principles of treatment (page 9) to the nursing of geriatric patients there is a very much greater emphasis on the rest, hygiene and diet aspects than with younger patients. Rarely is the condition for which an old person has been admitted to a surgical ward his or her sole medical problem, and the management of such a patient necessitates a full programme of treatment, including plans for resettlement at home or in an appropriate institution.

Ward routine

Meal times can be tedious and the elderly must be allowed to feed slowly. Rushing meals is unkind and dangerous.

Reference has already been made to the urological problems of old age: it is unreasonable and cruel to expect the aged—or for that matter any patient—to confine her toilet requirements to the times allotted in a fixed ward routine. Old people can be extremely troublesome, but their demands will be aggravated by lack of sympathy. *Some* discipline is necessary and in fact gives a sense of security to the aged as it does to children—it must never be aggressive or patronising.

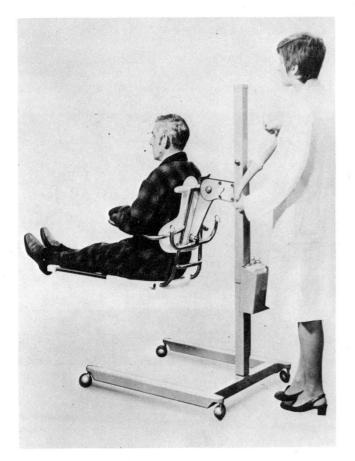

Fig. 51.3 Mecanaid Ambulift. Lifting and carrying device with which one person can transport a bed-fast patient for toilet and bath purposes. (Mecanaids Ltd.)

Osteoarthritis affects the joints between ribs and vertebrae and in consequence old people often have poor chest movement. Stimulus to activity is needed, but over zealous physiotherapy may result in fracture of the osteoporotic ribs. The patient with poor chest expansion is dependent almost entirely on the diaphragm movement for breathing. Abdominal distension, wound pain or tight abdominal bandaging further impedes respiration: sitting up further compresses the abdomen and raising the head end of the bed while allowing the patient still to be fairly flat is sometimes a great help.

Special toilet arrangements are required to provide access to lavatories by patients in wheelchairs. The provision of mechanical aids for lifting (Fig. 51.3) makes for efficiency, and when used intelligently these lifting devices remove much of the embarrassment which patients suffer when being 'manhandled'.

One of the latest devices is a plastic inlay tray which raises the inside level of the bath without requiring any plumbing or alterations (Fig. 51.4). These inlays are available in a variety of shapes and greatly lessen the strain of lifting elderly or heavy patients in and out of the bath.[1]

The Ladywell bath (Fig. 51.5), combined with a lifting device, takes much of the labour out of bathing routine and at the same time avoids the discomfort which has to be endured climbing into and out of the bath when a patient has severe arthritis.

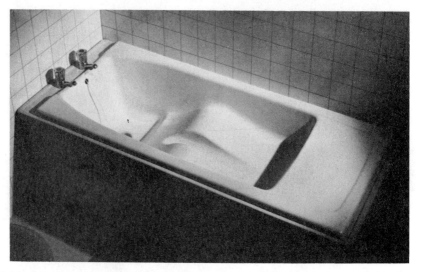

Fig. 51.4 Sunflower 'sit-in' type bath inlay. This is detachable and fits a standard bath. (F. Llewellyn & Co. Ltd.)

Comfort and furniture

Many elderly patients have a restricted range of movement and a nurse must pay particular attention to their position and physical comfort. The bed must not be too high, and the patient's feet must reach the ground while he is still sitting on the bed. Many

---

[1] The Sunflower bath was designed by St Bartholomew's Hospital, Research Unit for the Handicapped.

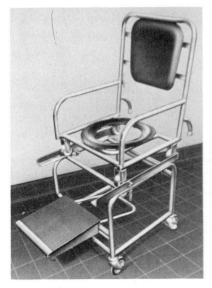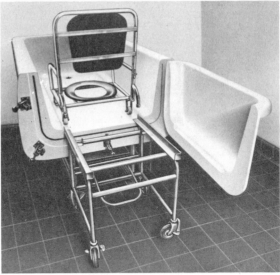

Fig. 51.5 Ladywell bath. Specially made 'Sani-chair' (*left*) in which the upper portion rolls forward into an open bath shown at right. (G. McLoughlin & Co. Ltd.)

old patients have a fixed kyphos (spinal flexion) and must therefore at all times have sufficient pillows to allow them to be comfortable without developing back strain. Bed-clothes must never be tucked in too tightly as this restricts patient's leg movements, with the resulting tendency to thrombosis and embolus.

Old patients must never be expected to sit in low armless 'fireside' type chairs from which it is difficult to rise. Spectacles, deaf aids and handkerchiefs must always be within reach.

Pressure sores

The skin in old age is thin, inelastic and easily damaged by any harsh surface. Sudden movement of a heel on a hard linen sheet may easily produce a blister. Polyether foam squares on which the patient can sit or lie are cheap, easily washed and disposable when worn or too soiled. The free use of foam without either a cloth or plastic cover does much to reduce maceration of the skin from sweat and pressure. Heel cups of foam protect sensitive feet. **Tubigrip**, an elastic cotton tube, is available with a thin foam lining. This is supplied in metre lengths which can be cut to provide pads for elbows, knees and ankles, or the ready-made product **Tubipad** can be used (Fig. 11.3).

If pressure ulcers have developed, the use of a ripple mattress or even a water bed is advisable (page 875). Once the ulcers have healed the likelihood of recurrence may be lessened by providing a 'Ripple Seat' cushion (Fig. 51.12).

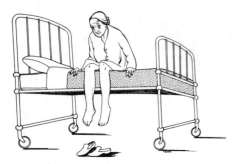

Fig. 51.6 Beds of varied height are useful. This old lady cannot reach the ground without slipping off the bed.

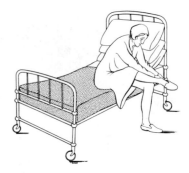

Fig. 51.7 A bed of correct height gives confidence and safety.

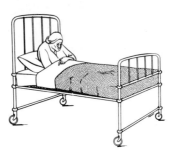

Fig. 51.8 This patient has no adequate back support; her movement is strictly limited by bedding which has been tucked in too tightly.

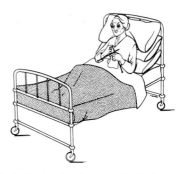

Fig. 51.9 In the absence of a back rest there must be sufficient pillows to support the neck. Where a cradle is not used over the legs the bedding must be loose to encourage leg movement.

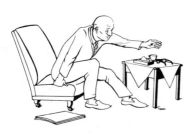

Fig. 51.10 Patients who are no longer confined to bed must have a chairside table. This man is having to rise from a chair which is much too low and reach a table which is too far away. This is an indication of thoughtless nursing.

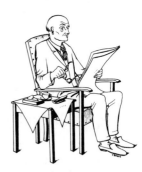

Fig. 51.11 Personal possessions must be within easy reach. A chair of this height produces less back strain and is easier to use.

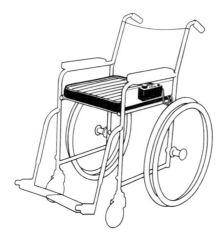

Fig. 51.12   Ripple cushion. This has a battery-powered inflation pump (cf. Ripple mattress, page 875). (Talley Surgical Instruments Ltd.)

Drugs

The elderly do not metabolise drugs rapidly and inadvertent overdosage is not uncommon. This arises because sometimes adult doses are prescribed without it being realised that some old people have lost a good deal of their body weight in declining years: the skeleton loses its density and the spine shortens and muscle activity is greatly reduced. It is vital that the patient's weight be recorded on admission and *if it is under 112 lb (8 stone; 50 kilos) the prescribing doctor's attention should be called to the fact.* Patients of greater weight are nevertheless still more susceptible to drugs on account of their advanced age. Heavy sedation may have alarming results by depressing respiration and lowering blood pressure. Cerebral thrombosis with a resultant stroke may ensue. Liability to venous thrombosis with subsequent embolism is undoubtedly increased.

These patients are often very susceptible to the quick-acting barbiturates such as pentobarbitone (Nembutal) and quinalbarbitone (Seconal). Amylobarbitone, given to those who are not used to the drug, can produce a state of confusion and delirium during which the patient may remove his drip, his catheter or his drainage tube. These have largely been discarded in favour of diazepam and dichloralphenazone (Welldorm) for sleeping.

Other drugs in common use—pethidine, ephedrine, Drinamyl (dextro-amphetamine) and amylobarbitone given for depression: propantheline and Nacton given for indigestion—particularly affect the bladder and may cause retention of urine. Stilboestrol given to control carcinoma of the prostate—a common condition in old men—may cause sodium and water retention in the body and precipitate heart failure. Biogastrone, a proprietary preparation used extensively as a palliative for duodenal ulcers, also may cause very severe water retention in the tissues with ascites and heart failure.

Many elderly patients who suffer from hypertension are on long-term treatment with hypotensive drugs and if a surgical problem arises very careful management of blood pressure level is needed.

After-care

Throughout treatment and on discharge from hospital it is important to maintain the patient's self-dependence and self-respect. It is very easy for us to fall into the trap of discharging a patient into the care of apparently devoted relatives without realising that the patient may now be dominated and subjected to the family's wish and convenience. Investigation by the local social welfare worker before discharge is arranged helps to determine the best course. The community nursing service must be brought into after-care.

The elderly, like children, require special 'protection' in hospital, but lack the resilience of children, and are far more sensitive; they are easily misunderstood, but the majority are only too ready to respond to kindness, courtesy and sympathy. It is a serious mistake to assume that because a patient is old and deaf no explanation of a nurse's intended action is needed and that the patient must simply comply!

The care of the aged when they are involved in surgical procedures is a challenge to good nursing and is most rewarding.

Sometimes the effect of surgery is disappointing and accelerates declining physical and mental powers of the individual, but on the other hand many elderly patients 'take on a new lease of life' after what proves for them to be a stimulating experience in hospital, quite apart from the relief of the particular disability for which they were admitted. Depression disappears as anxiety is relieved.

APPENDICES

Appendix I
Radiation Protection

Radioactivity is the emission of atomic particles. These 'rays' affect living tissues by producing chemical changes (**ionization**) in the cells: blood-forming organs and other tissues undergoing rapid cell division are most sensitive. Wherever radioactive materials are in use for scientific or industrial purposes, complicated and very thorough protective measures are required.

Sources of radioactivity used in medicine may be grouped into:

(**a**) **Fixed units**—x-ray diagnostic sets; x-ray, radium and cobalt 'bomb' therapy units; caesium and linear accelerator apparatus.

(**b**) **Mobile sources—sealed**, and therefore unspillable; radium needles, radon seeds and radioactive wire.

—**unsealed**, and spillable fluids (isotopes) such as radioactive iodine, gold, thorium paint, and other chemicals used as tracer substances in research and diagnostic work.

Safety measures must cover the protective screening of all persons working with these sources of energy. The danger of a particular isotope depends upon the length of its active life. For practical purposes the life of radioactive iodine is very short—several days—and the disposal of urine from patients given this substance is not dangerous. Nevertheless, every hospital where such substances are used has a 'code of practice' and rigid rules of nursing must always be observed. Radiographers, laboratory technicians and others whose routine duties involve exposure to radiation risks wear photographic film badges; these are developed regularly and give a record of exposure to radiation. There is an appointed radiological safety officer in each hospital.

The following general rules are suggested for nursing staff:

(*a*) Every nurse in a ward or department where radioactive substances are in use must read and sign a recommended code of practice drawn up by the hospital's radiological safety officer.

(*b*) Any loss of radioactive material, or accidental spillage, must be reported to the safety officer urgently: washing a contaminated area may spread the danger and any fluid spilled should be absorbed with blotting paper or cleansing tissue.

(*c*) The bed of any patient undergoing tests or treatment with radioactive substances must be clearly labelled: if the patient is undergoing treatment with radium or cobalt implants the bed must be at least 9 metres from any other patient, preferably in a separate room: this is *absolutely essential* if more than 50 mg of radium is being used. Nurses and visitors should spend the least time necessary for attention to the patient's comfort.

(*d*) After carrying out nursing procedures on a patient who has been given a radioactive isotope the nurse must wash thoroughly her hands and nails, *without* violent scrubbing (which may break the skin and allow penetration); in fact a 'barrier nursing' routine is in force.

(*e*) Radioactive materials must always be stored and conveyed in special containers.

(*f*) **Sterilisation of radioactive material.** Small sealed sources such as radium needles and gold grains require sterilisation before insertion in the body. The technique must ensure that the nursing staff is not exposed to radiation and that there can be no possible loss or damage to the radioactive source. When heat is used care must be taken that the temperature does not rise above 110 °C (which would happen if a steriliser boiled dry). Alternatively applicators can be immersed in antiseptic fluids (e.g. 0·5 per cent chlorhexidine, 1 per cent cetrimide in spirit).

Radioactive solutions that require sterilising will be prepared by, or under the direct supervision of, the radiological safety officer.

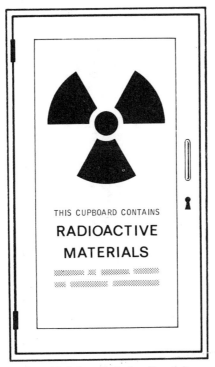

Three-bladed symbol of radioactivity

(*g*) **Contaminated laundry** must not be released with the general laundry until it has been monitored with a 'Geiger' counter and passed as safe. After contamination with short-life substances such as I^{131} (radioactive iodine) the articles are stored in a protective place or container until activity has fallen to a safe level. Washing in hot 3 per cent citric acid solution is recommended for assisting in the removal of radioactive isotopes from contaminated articles.

(*h*) **Radioactive waste**—contaminated dressings, soiled laundry, paper, etc., must not be placed in garbage bins, ordinary dressing incinerators, or in the case of fluids poured into sinks or drains. The method of disposal must be decided by the safety officer, and initially all such waste should be placed in polythene bags or containers.

The ultimate disposal of the waste depends on the degree of radioactivity, and when isotopes are rapidly decaying waste material becomes safe after short periods of storage. More permanent sources of radiation such as broken radium applicators have to be placed in lead containers and dealt with by a special disposal service.

(*i*) In areas where radioactive materials are being used an emergency decontamination pack should be available containing surgical gowns, masks, overshoes, polythene containers, forceps, blotting paper and other items as set out in *The Code of Practice for the Protection of Persons against Ionising Radiations arising from Medical and Dental Use*, H.M. Stationery Office, 1972. The accepted symbol indicating radioactivity is shown above.

Appendix II

TREATMENT OF SUDDEN CARDIAC AND RESPIRATORY EMERGENCIES

To be studied in conjunction with Chapter 10

Question		
IS THE AIRWAY OBSTRUCTED?	If the answer is—YES—Clear airway, extend head, lift chin forward, use gag, tongue-clip, etc. as necessary	
IS THE PATIENT MAKING RESPIRATORY EFFORT?	If the answer is—YES—Semi-prone coma position; keep airway clear. —NO —Positive pressure respiration, expired air (mouth-to-nose) or mechanical (e.g. Ambu bag)	
IS THERE A PULSE? (Carotid; or stethoscope over heart)	If the answer is—NO —CARDIAC ARREST HAS OCCURRED. THE BRAIN WILL BE IRRETRIEVABLY DAMAGED UNLESS EXTERNAL CARDIAC MASSAGE IS STARTED WITHIN THREE MINUTES	

TREATMENT OF CARDIAC ARREST (page 179)

IMMEDIATE TREATMENT BY EITHER MEDICAL OR NURSING STAFF

1. **Positive pressure ventilation**
   either by expired air (mouth-to-nose) or mechanical (Ambu bag or anaesthetic machine)
2. **External cardiac massage**
3. **Elevate legs**
4. **Send for:** anaesthetist, surgeon, transfusion apparatus, drugs, external defibrillator, and electrocardiograph

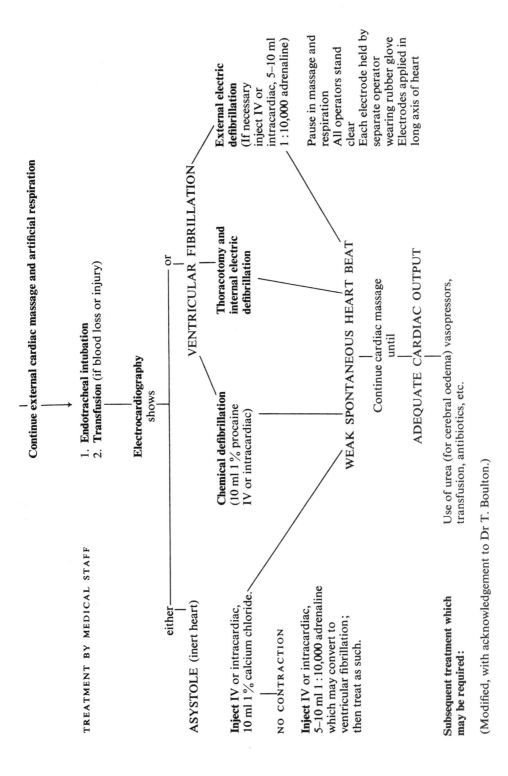

Continue external cardiac massage and artificial respiration

TREATMENT BY MEDICAL STAFF

1. **Endotracheal intubation**
2. **Transfusion** (if blood loss or injury)

Electrocardiography shows

either — or

ASYSTOLE (inert heart)

VENTRICULAR FIBRILLATION

Inject IV or intracardiac, 10 ml 1% calcium chloride.

NO CONTRACTION

Inject IV or intracardiac, 5–10 ml 1 : 10,000 adrenaline which may convert to ventricular fibrillation; then treat as such.

Chemical defibrillation (10 ml 1% procaine IV or intracardiac)

Thoracotomy and internal electric defibrillation

External electric defibrillation (If necessary inject IV or intracardiac, 5–10 ml 1 : 10,000 adrenaline)

Pause in massage and respiration
All operators stand clear
Each electrode held by separate operator wearing rubber glove
Electrodes applied in long axis of heart

WEAK SPONTANEOUS HEART BEAT

Continue cardiac massage until

ADEQUATE CARDIAC OUTPUT

Subsequent treatment which may be required:

Use of urea (for cerebral oedema) vasopressors, transfusion, antibiotics, etc.

(Modified, with acknowledgement to Dr T. Boulton.)

Index

Bold figures indicate main references to subjects.